Y0-BWY-921

THE JOURNALS OF CAPTAIN JAMES COOK ON HIS VOYAGES OF DISCOVERY

EDITED FROM THE ORIGINAL MANUSCRIPTS

FOUR VOLUMES AND A PORTFOLIO

II
THE VOYAGE OF THE *RESOLUTION* AND *ADVENTURE*
1772–1775

HAKLUYT SOCIETY
EXTRA SERIES No. XXXV

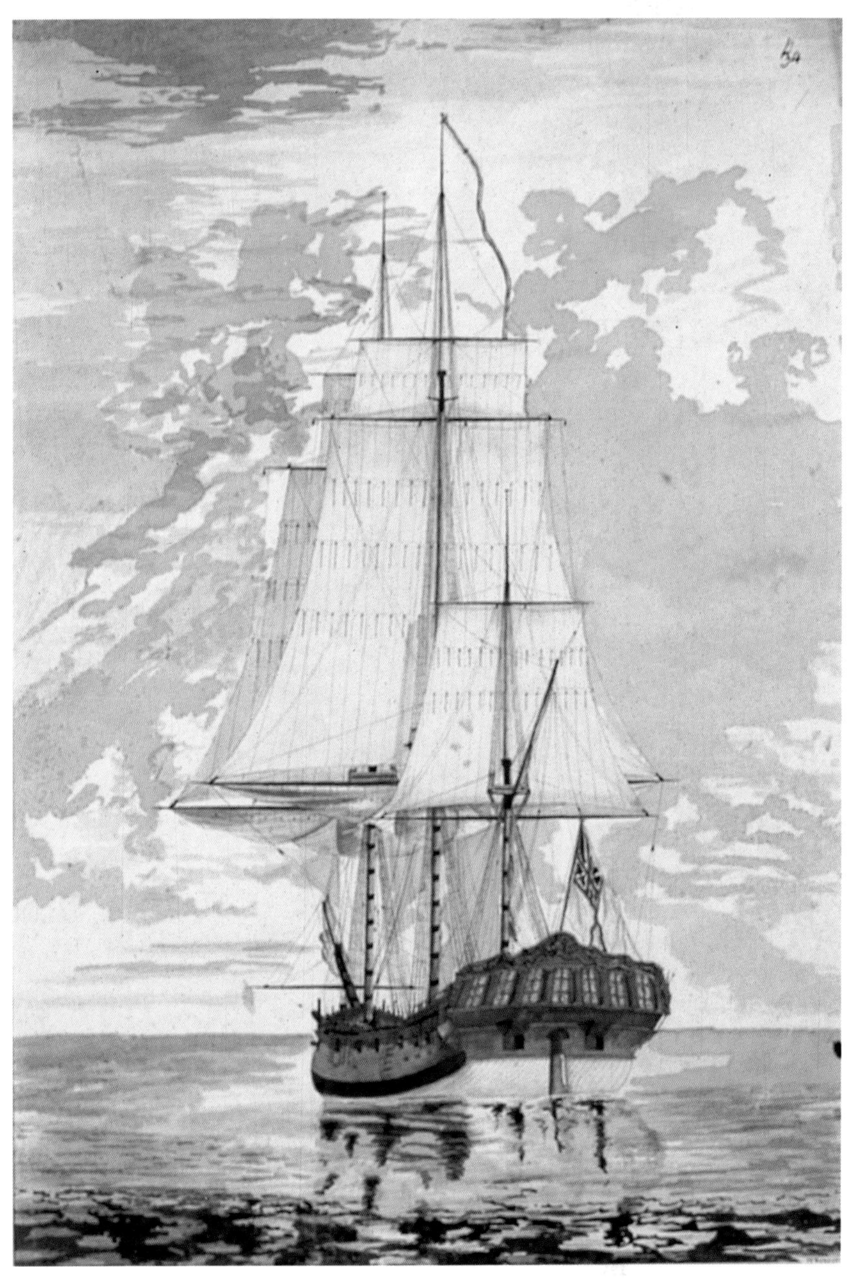

The *Resolution*

Water-colour drawing by Henry Roberts,
in the Mitchell Library, Sydney, D11, no. 14

THE JOURNALS OF CAPTAIN JAMES COOK
ON HIS VOYAGES OF DISCOVERY

*

THE VOYAGE OF THE *RESOLUTION* AND *ADVENTURE*

1772-1775

EDITED BY

J. C. BEAGLEHOLE

THE BOYDELL PRESS

in association with
HORDERN HOUSE, SYDNEY

Volume II first published 1961
Reprinted with addenda and corrigenda 1969

Reprinted 1999 by
The Boydell Press, Woodbridge
by arrangement with The Hakluyt Society

ISBN 0 85115 744 0 (set of four volumes and portfolio)

The Boydell Press is an imprint of Boydell & Brewer Ltd
PO Box 9, Woodbridge, Suffolk IP12 3DF, UK
and of Boydell & Brewer Inc.
PO Box 41026, Rochester, NY 14604-4126, USA
Web site: http://www.boydell.co.uk

A catalogue record for this book is available
from the British Library

Library of Congress Catalog Card Number: 99–18458

This publication is printed on acid-free paper

Printed in Great Britain by
St Edmundsbury Press, Bury St Edmunds, Suffolk

PREFACE

THIS volume is devoted to Cook's journal of his second voyage and to supplementary material which casts light from other sources on the history of the voyage. The plan of the volume follows very closely that of the first, allowing for the fact that certain preliminary matter in the first does not need to be repeated, or corresponding matter separately presented. Thus, what seems necessary to add to the Note on Polynesian History in Volume I is here included in the Introduction. Nor is documentation equally balanced: thus the amount of newspaper material on this voyage does not justify an appendix. But the relation of appendixes to text is the same, allowing, again, for greater or less bulk in individual appendixes.

It does not seem necessary to include a separate note on the printing of the text. The principles followed are virtually the same as those of the earlier volume—i.e. in the text, as far as possible to print what Cook wrote as he wrote it, with a minimum of silent correction for obvious slips, and a minimum of square brackets for omissions supplied editorially. In this volume, for example, the final 'ed' for a past participle, often omitted, has been only exceptionally added, when the sense has seemed to require it. If Cook's meaning is clear, there has been no attempt to make him a more careful or more 'correct' writer than he was. The reader will find inconsistencies, and if he cares to consult the holograph MSS will no doubt find more, which it may be best for an editor to admit in advance. The blank spaces Cook left for figures have been filled from the MSS as far as possible; some blanks still remain, which Cook himself did not think worth filling, or could not fill.

About the annotation it may be said in general that this second journal could be annotated for ever, and that one stops because one must stop somewhere. The voyage was not very much longer than the first, but for variety of experience it transcends most other voyages ever made, and the demands on an editor's industry are correspondingly great. In the end the editor is torn between anxiety over his reader's patience and shame over dealing inadequately with so many matters that call for an essay each. Nor can he be unappalled by the brute fact of expense.

Considerations of the same sort apply to the introductions. The voyage touched on so many things and people, on so many aspects of thought, even in the confined space of England—to go no further. Temptation lies everywhere, the filaments spread in every direction. Why not write more about the Banks episode, that strange person Forster and his unhappy son, the diverting story of Omai? How can one refrain from quoting at length Johnson and Boswell, how can one put Daines Barrington in a footnote, and say so little of Sandwich, and ignore Miss Ray, and Garrick, and virtually ignore the Royal Society? The answer can only be that this is an edition of Cook's journal, and neither a biography of Cook nor a history of the scientific-social life of England in the eighteenth century. Something will be found in the calendar of documents. Beyond that, one must simply say No; and surrounded by riches, like Clive stand astonished at one's own moderation.

The MSS I have printed or drawn on are preserved in the following collections: the British Museum Department of Manuscripts; the Public Record Office; the National Maritime Museum, Greenwich; the Royal Greenwich Observatory, Herstmonceux; the Royal Society; the Mitchell and Dixson Libraries, Sydney; the Alexander Turnbull Library and the General Assembly Library, Wellington; and by Viscount Hinchingbrooke, Lieutenant-Commander Palliser A. Hudson, and Mr J. A. Ferguson of Sydney. I am grateful to all these institutions and private owners for authority to print or otherwise use the documents in their possession.

Her Majesty the Queen has graciously permitted me to print five documents from the Georgian Papers in the Royal Archives, Windsor.

My list of acknowledgments otherwise is long. I have again taken advantage of the kindness of many of those mentioned in the Acknowledgments prefixed to Volume I; and rather than embarrass them by repeated thanks I merely add to the list there given. I cannot omit, however, to emphasize once more the continuous collaboration I have had from the Hon. Secretary of the Hakluyt Society, my friend Mr R. A. Skelton; and particularly his work on the 'graphic records' of the voyage and the illustrations to this volume. Nor can I fail to record the contribution again made to the scientific annotation by Dr A. M. Lysaght.

The editor of this volume was originally to have been Dr J. A. Williamson, and before it came to me he had done some preliminary work on the text. In England, also, Dr H. F. P. Herdman, of the National Institute of Oceanography, has been so very generous as to examine, and write for me a long discussion of, the antarctic portions of Cook's journal, and to give me the freest possible hand in making use of this. It will be found incorporated in the Introduction. Mr J. C. B. Redfearn has drawn the whole of the sketch-maps.

In Tonga, where I spent some time in June 1957, I became greatly indebted to H.R.H. Prince Tungi; the Hon. Havea Tu'iha'ateiho, then acting Prime Minister; H.B.M.'s Agent and Consul, Mr A. C. Reid, and Mrs Reid, the pleasantness of whose hospitality—to put it baldly—I shall not soon forget; Mr R. T. Sanders, Secretary to the Government; Mr E. Lawrence, Director of Agriculture; Ve'ehala, Keeper of the Palace Records; Lisiate Hingano, of the Department of Agriculture; and Netani Vete, of the Public Works Department. Thinking of Tonga, I think also of the whole launch-load of people at Eua, bound for Tongatapu, who, rather than incommode an utter stranger, cheerfully stayed an extra day and night at the island to give me the chance of seeing it. Friendly Islands indeed. To those islands I was taken in H.M.N.Z.S. *Lachlan*: my acknowledgments to Commander F. W. Hunt and his officers are very warm ones.

In Australia I am indebted to Mr G. D. Richardson, Deputy Principal Librarian of the Public Library of New South Wales; to Professor V. V. Hickman of the University of Tasmania; and to Mr M. Aurousseau, who has once again shouldered the labour of the Index. In New Caledonia, likewise, to Dr Jacques Barrau, of the South Pacific Commission; and Dr R. Catala, of the Station de Biologie Marine, Noumea.

In New Zealand, my new obligations are to Mr G. S. Parsonson, of the University of Otago, who has made a special study of the New Hebrides; Mr I. D. Thomsen, Director of the Carter Observatory, Wellington; Mr B. G. Hamlin, Dominion Museum botanist; Dr V. D. Zotov, of the Botanical Division of the Department of Scientific and Industrial Research; Mr V. F. Fisher of the Auckland Institute and Museum; my colleagues Professor H. D. Gordon and the late Mr N. V. Ryder; Mrs Falkner, of the Alexander Turnbull Library; Dr E. G. Jacoby, and Dr Ernest Philipp. Miss Rona Arbuckle, of my University, and Mrs Ilse Jacoby have done a vast mass of typing for me.

In Scotland (to spring back to the Northern Hemisphere) Messrs MacLehose have given to the printing of this volume the same infinite care, patience and generosity as they gave to the first.

To all these I record my grateful thanks.

J. C. B.

Victoria University of Wellington
January 1959

CONTENTS

ILLUSTRATIONS AND MAPS

The approximate linear reduction of original drawings is indicated by a fraction in brackets, e.g. (½). Reference to engravings is made only to those in the printed edition of the *Voyage* (1777). Sketch maps are indicated by an asterisk *.

ACKNOWLEDGMENTS

The reproductions have been made by courtesy of the Trustees of the Mitchell Library in the Public Library of New South Wales, Sydney (Frontispiece, Figs. 15–19, 23, 28*a*, 36, 39, 41, 46, 48, 50*a*, 59, 62*b*, 76), the Trustees of the National Maritime Museum, Greenwich (Figs. 3, 14, 25, 29, 30, 51, 61), the Trustees of the British Museum (Figs. 5, 7*b*, 11, 12, 37, 38, 47, 57, 60, 64, 67, 69, 71*a*, 77, 80), the Museum für Völkerkunde, Vienna (Fig. 9), the Trustees of the Dixson Collection, Sydney (Fig. [illegible]), the Astronomer Royal (Figs. 13, 56, 58, 65), the Trustees of the British Museum (Natural History) (Figs. 20, 21, 53, 71*b*, 75), the Lords Commissioners of the Admiralty (Figs. 14, 24–26, 29, 30, 40, 51, 61), the Committee of the Commonwealth National Library, Canberra (Figs. 27, 42, 50*b*, 52, 62*a*, 72, 73), the Dominion Archivist of Canada (Fig. 43), the Deputy Keeper of the Records (Figs. 74, 78), the Right Hon. the Earl of Birkenhead (Fig. 6), Sir Maurice Holmes, G.B.E., K.C.B. (Fig. 7*a*), H. O. Stafford Cooke Esq. (Fig. 8), Rex de C. Nan Kivell Esq. (Fig. 49).

The sketch maps (Figs. 1, 2, 10, 22, 31–35, 44, 45, 54, 55, 63, 66, 68, 70, 79, 81, 82) were drawn by Mr J. C. B. Redfearn, M.B.E.

PORTFOLIO

The original charts and views reproduced in the Portfolio (published in 1955) are here cited as Chart I, II, etc.

SELECT BIBLIOGRAPHICAL REFERENCES

(with abbreviations used in the Introduction and Notes)

I. *Logs and Journals by Cook*

The MS	Holograph MS journal in British Museum, Department of Manuscripts, Add. MS 27886. The text here printed.
B	Holograph MS journal in British Museum, Dept. of Manuscripts, Add. MS 27888. Text here partially printed.
Admiralty MS A	MS journal (transcript) in Public Record Office, London, Adm 55/108.
Greenwich MS G	MS journal (transcript) in National Maritime Museum, Greenwich. Formerly in Royal Library, Windsor.
Palliser Hudson MS H	MS journal (transcript) in the possession of Lieut.-Commander Palliser A. Hudson.
Add. MS 27889	Holograph papers in volume entitled *Cook's Second Voyage. Fragments* in British Museum, Dept. of Manuscripts, Add. MS 27889.
M	Holograph fragments in Mitchell Library, Sydney, Safe PH 17/12, 17/14.
D	Holograph fragment in volume entitled *Captain James Cook Relics and MSS* in Dixson Library, Sydney.
Log	Holograph log in British Museum, Dept. of Manuscripts, Add. MS 27956; and MS transcript, Add. MS 27887.
Voyage	*A Voyage towards the South Pole, and Round the World. Performed in His Majesty's Ships the Resolution ana Adventure . . . Written by James Cook, Commander of the Resolution* . . . 2 vols. London, 1777.

II. *Other MS Logs and Journals Kept in the* Resolution *and* Adventure, *or later MSS*

Bayly	Journal of William Bayly, astronomer *Adventure*, in Alexander Turnbull Library, Wellington.
Browne	Journal of Robert Browne, A.B. *Adventure*, in P.R.O., Adm 51/4521/9–10.
Burney log	Log of James Burney, 2nd lieutenant *Adventure*, in P.R.O., Adm 51/4523/1–2.

Burney, Ferguson MS	Journal-letter of James Burney, in Ferguson collection, Sydney.
Burr	Log of John Daval Burr, master's mate *Resolution* in P.R.O., Adm 55/106.
Clerke	Transcript of log of Charles Clerke, 2nd lieutenant *Resolution*, in P.R.O., Adm 55/103.
Clerke 8951 [–2, –3]	Clerke's log in British Museum, Dept. of Manuscripts, Add. MSS 8951–3.
Constable	Journal of Love Constable, midshipman *Adventure*, in P.R.O., Adm 51/4520/7–8.
Cooper	Journal of Robert Palliser Cooper, 1st lieutenant *Resolution*, in P.R.O., Adm 55/104, 109.
Elliott	Log of John Elliott, midshipman *Resolution*, in P.R.O., Adm 51/4556/208.
Elliott *Mem.*	*Memoirs of the early life of John Elliott . . . written by himself* . . . in British Museum, Dept. of Manuscripts, Add. MS 42714.
Furneaux	Log of Tobias Furneaux, captain *Adventure*, in P.R.O., Adm 55/1.
Furneaux Add. MS 27890	Account of the *Adventure*'s voyage written by Furneaux, in British Museum, Dept. of Manuscripts, Add. MS 27890.
Gilbert	Log of Joseph Gilbert, master *Resolution*, in P.R.O., Adm 55/107.
Harvey	Journal of William Harvey, midshipman *Resolution*, in P.R.O., Adm 51/4553/184–7.
Hawkey	Log of William Hawkey, master's mate *Adventure*, in P.R.O., Adm 55/4521/11.
Hergest	Journal of Richard Hergest, A.B. and midshipman *Adventure*, in P.R.O., Adm 51/4522/13.
Hood	Journal of Alexander Hood, A.B. *Resolution*, in P.R.O., Adm 51/4554/181–3.
Kempe	Log of Arthur Kempe, 1st lieutenant *Adventure*, in P.R.O., Adm 51/4520/1–3.
Lightfoot	Log of Henry Lightfoot, midshipman *Adventure*, in P.R.O., Adm 51/4523/5.
Mitchel	Log of Bowles Mitchel, midshipman *Resolution*, in P.R.O., Adm 51/4555/194–5.
Pickersgill	Log of Richard Pickersgill, 3rd lieutenant *Resolution*, in P.R.O., Adm 51/4553/205–6.
Pickersgill E	Journal of Richard Pickersgill, Enderby MS, in National Maritime Museum, Greenwich, MS 57/038.
Smith	Log of Isaac Smith, master's mate *Resolution*, in P.R.O., Adm 55/105.
Wales	Journal of William Wales, astronomer *Resolution*, in Mitchell Library, Sydney, Safe PH 18/4.

Wales log — Log of William Wales, in Royal Greenwich Observatory, Herstmonceux.

Wilby — Journal of John Wilby, A.B. *Adventure*, in P.R.O., Adm 51/4522/14.

Willis — Journal of Thomas Willis, midshipman *Resolution*, in P.R.O., Adm 51/4554/199–200; and log, Adm 51/4554/201–2.

III. *Printed Works*

[*Cook's Journals*,] I *The Journals of Captain James Cook on his Voyages of Discovery*, I. *The Voyage of the* Endeavour, *1768–1771*. Edited by J. C. Beaglehole. Cambridge, 1955.

Corney *The Quest and Occupation of Tahiti by Emissaries of Spain during the years 1772–1776*. Edited by Bolton Glanvill Corney. 3 vols. London, 1913–19.

Dalrymple, *Collection* *An Historical Collection of the several Voyages and Discoveries in the South Pacific Ocean*. By Alexander Dalrymple. 2 vols. London, 1770–1.

Forster *A Voyage round the World, in His Britannic Majesty's Sloop, Resolution, commanded by Capt. James Cook, during the Years 1772, 3, 4, and 5*. By George Forster, F.R.S. . . . 2 vols. London, 1777.

Forster, *Reply* *Reply to Mr Wales's Remarks*. By George Forster. London, 1778.

Forster, *Observations* *Observations made during a Voyage Round the World, on Physical Geography, Natural History, and Ethic Philosophy* . . . By John Reinold Forster, LL.D. F.R.S. and S.A. London, 1778.

Mariner *An Account of the Natives of the Tonga Islands, in the South Pacific Ocean . . . compiled and arranged from the extensive communications of Mr William Mariner, several years resident in those islands*. By John Martin, M.D. 2 vols. 3rd ed., Edinburgh, 1827.

Marra *Journal of the Resolution's Voyage . . . by which the Non-Existence of an undiscovered Continent, between the Equator and the 50th Degree of Southern Latitude, is demonstratively proved* . . . London, 1775.

Sparrman *A Voyage round the World with Captain James Cook in H.M.S. Resolution*. London, 1953.

Wales [and Bayly] *Astronomical Observations* *The Original Astronomical Observations, made in the course of A Voyage towards the South Pole, and Round the World* . . . By William Wales, F.R.S. . . . and Mr William Bayly . . . London, 1777.

Wales, *Remarks* *Remarks on Mr. Forster's Account of Captain Cook's last Voyage round the World, In the Years 1772, 1773, 1774, and 1775*. By William Wales, F.R.S. London, 1778.

INTRODUCTION

§ *The Plan*

A NUMBER of damaging charges have been made against the management of the British navy in the two decades after 1763; and certainly the characters of the Earl of Sandwich, as First Lord, and Sir Hugh Palliser, as Comptroller, do not—for whatever reason—radiate an effulgence altogether unsullied. They were not in this respect remarkable or alone. Though both were able and perceptive men, they were children of their time; and their time was not propitious to a too rigid pursuit of the administrative virtues. This at least can be said for them, however, in our present context, that they recognized a supreme virtue in a third man, that they perceived the strategic value of a plan of discovery as masterly as anything in the late repertory of war, and that they threw the resources of their department into the realizing of Cook's plan with all the concentration of a Pitt. Though the strategy was not theirs, they could have marred it. They left nothing undone to foster it, and with justice Cook placed their names upon his map. This was a map, the result of a voyage, such as had never been made before.

In the Postscript to his first journal Cook had put forward the tentative plan for a further Pacific voyage.[1] Experience and the history of his predecessors had made it plain to him that a discoverer in those seas could not rely for support merely on the casual supplies of almost accidental islands. He needed a base, known, reliable, which he could take into his calculations before ever he left home—a base as useful, indeed, and calculable, once he was on the full stretch of exploration, as Plymouth at home or the Cape on an East Indian voyage. Experience again, his own and others', had made plain the general pattern of the southern wind system—west to east in the higher latitudes,[2] east to west in the lower. He had also what one may call a lively seasonal sense. He had become interested in the question of the Southern Continent. He had in the voyage he had just completed considerably pushed back its possible northern limits. What was needed now was a summer passage in a higher latitude clean across the Pacific from west to east. Where could that passage start?

[1] I, p. 479.

[2] That is, in the higher latitudes as far as they had been sailed into.

Obviously from the New Zealand base he had already discovered, Queen Charlotte Sound. Leave Queen Charlotte Sound at the beginning of October at the latest, 'when you would have the whole summer before you and . . . might, with the prevailing Westerly winds, run to the Eastward in as high a Latitude as you please and, if you met with no lands, would have time enough to get round Cape Horne before the summer was too far spent'.[1] If there was no continent, 'and you had other Objects in View', then haul to the northward, pick up the east-west trade, visit some of the islands already discovered, search for those heard of but not yet seen, and 'thus the discoveries in the South Sea would be compleat'. The prescription was simple; the method it inculcated was admirable; the Admiralty, having Cook at disposal, was immediately convinced that it was both feasible and desirable; and the new voyage was decided on. But as a solution it was too simple; for it left out half the problem. The discoveries in the South Sea might be complete. But the Continent, if it existed, was much more than a fact of the South Sea. By hypothesis, it circled the world, it was Atlantic as well as Pacific. Cook, inevitably, realized the hiatus in his planning; and when the preparations for the new voyage were well under weigh, in February 1772, submitted to Sandwich a memorandum that was lucid and comprehensive.

'Upon due consideration of the discoveries that have been made in the Southern Ocean [Cook writes], and the tracks of the Ships which have made these discoveries; it appears that no Southern lands of great extent can extend to the Northward of 40° of Latitude, except about the Meridian of 140° West, every other part of the Southern Ocean have at different times been explored to the northward of the above parallel. Therefore to make new discoveries the Navigator must Traverse or Circumnavigate the Globe in a higher parallel than has hitherto been done, and this will be best accomplished by an Easterly Course on account of the prevailing westerly winds in all high Latitudes. The principle thing to be attended to is the proper Seasons of Year, for Winter is by no means favourable for discoveries in these Latitudes; for which reason it is humbly proposed that the Ships may not leave the Cape of Good Hope before the latter end of September or beginning of October, when having the whole summer before them may safely Steer to the Southward and make their way to New Zealand, between the parallels of 45° and 60° or in as high a Latitude as the weather and other circumstances will admit. If no land is discoveried in this rout the Ships will be obliged to touch at New Zealand to recrute their water.

[1] When Cook actually came to make that passage, towards the end of 1774, it took him just over six weeks from Ship Cove to his Tierra del Fuegan landfall; Furneaux, in December 1773–January 1774, was just over a month from New Zealand to the Horn.

'From New Zealand the same rout must be continued to Cape Horn, but before this can be accomplished they will be overtaken by Winter, and must seek Shelter in the more Hospitable Latitudes, for which purpose Otahieta will probably be found to be the most convenient, at, and in its Neighbourhood the Winter Months may be spent, after which they must steer to the Southward and continue their rout for Cape Horn in the Neighbourhood of which they may again recrute their water, and afterwards proceed for the Cape of Good Hope.'

Cook accompanied this memorandum with a map,[1] on which he had laid down the tracks of preceding navigators, Tasman, Wallis, Bougainville, and his own in the *Endeavour*, and those of the East Indiamen on their regular voyages, together with a broad yellow line round the Pole, weaving in and out of the sixtieth parallel. Of this he says,

'The Yellow line on the Map shews the track I would propose the Ships to make, Supposeing no land to intervene, for if land is discovered the track will be altered according to the directing of the land, but the general rout must be pursued otherwise some part of the Southern Ocean will remain unexplored.'[2]

This then was the matured plan; and with all its lucidity it was no easy one. With all Cook's reference to the proper seasons of year and safe steering to the southward he was speaking in the dark; for no one had yet made what could be properly called an antarctic voyage. Of the peculiar dangers of those seas Cook knew virtually nothing. He inferred coldness; to some extent, from Bouvet's experience, he inferred ice;[3] what picture otherwise he had formed in his mind we ourselves have no means of knowing. How far south he would have to go would be determined solely by the existence or non-existence of the continent. How far south he could go he perhaps never deliberated upon. Of two of his points of reference—if we may consider them as such—the meridian of 140° W runs down through the Marquesas group and the Tuamotus, and it may be doubted if he thought it very possible, after his previous voyage, that the continent would be found there, or east of it, north of 40° of latitude. That parallel runs between Australia and Tasmania, passes through New Zealand at the Taranaki Bight, and meets South America just south of Valdivia: along it the ocean is in fact as empty of land as it is

[1] Chart XXV; and in a simplified form, Fig. 2 in this volume.

[2] Mitchell Library MS, Safe PH 17/11. I have already printed this memorandum, or letter, to Sandwich in I, pp. cxiii–iv; but it seems necessary for clarity to give it again here.

[3] Among the supplies he asked for from the Navy Board were 'Ice Anchors and Hatchets'; see Calendar, p. 918 below.

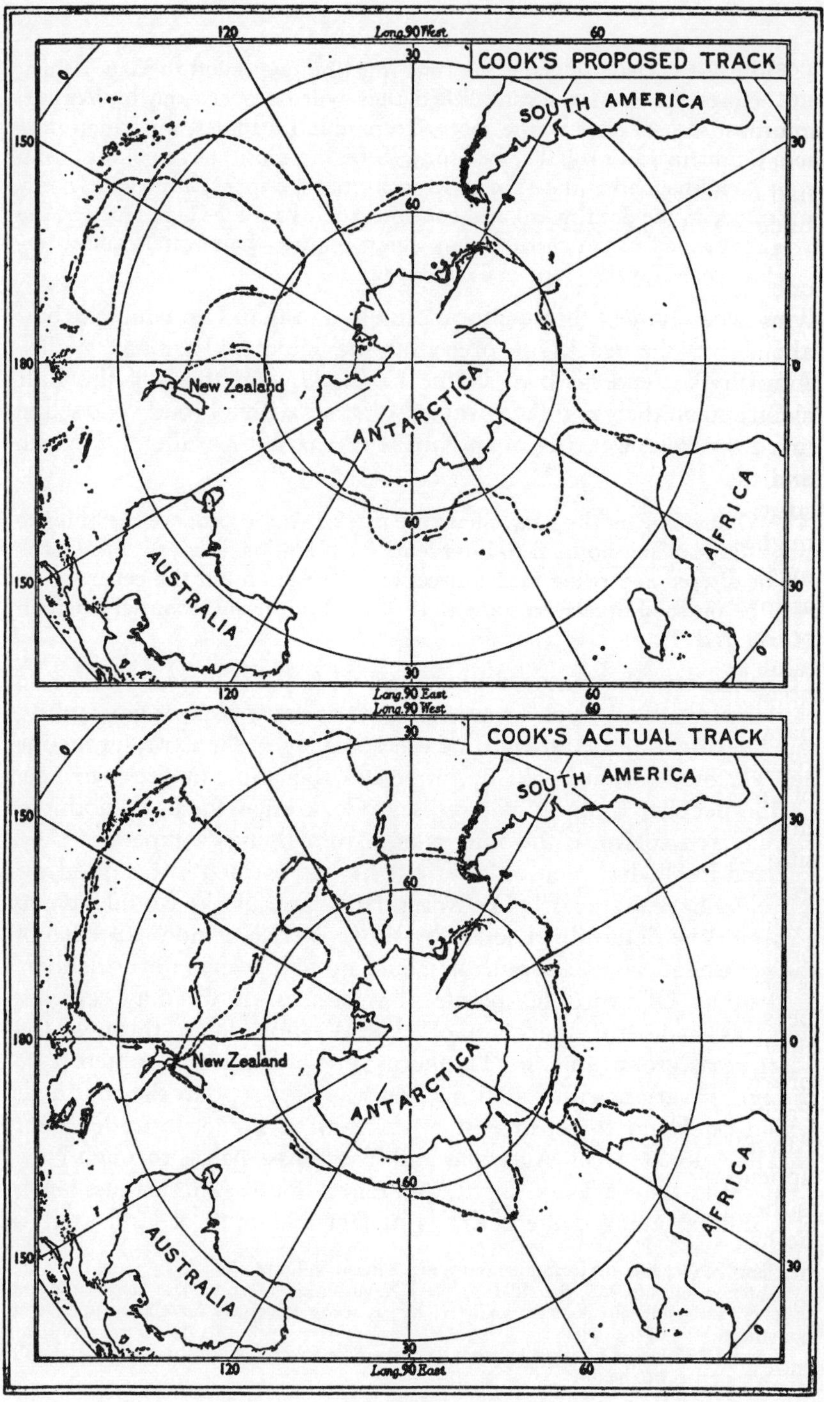
COOK'S PROPOSED TRACK
Long. 90 West
120
60
30
150
SOUTH AMERICA
60
180
0
New Zealand
ANTARCTICA
AFRICA
AUSTRALIA
150
30
120
Long. 90 East
60
COOK'S ACTUAL TRACK
Long. 90 West
SOUTH AMERICA
New Zealand
ANTARCTICA
AFRICA
AUSTRALIA
Long. 90 East

FIG. 2

possible for an ocean to be, while on each side of it the depths, though not as great as any of the fabulous 'deeps' or troughs, are sufficiently enormous. Yet there was a hiatus along the line, between long. 110°, where he had crossed it in February 1769, and long. 145°, where he had crossed it in September 1769, untraversed by any ship; the continental possibility, however remote, could not be lightly brushed aside.

There were two further points of reference. Neither was a Pacific one. The first was the Cape Circumcision sighted by Bouvet in 1739, lying about 54 degrees south and in longitude—so it was said—about 11° 20′ east of Greenwich—that is, well south of the familiar Atlantic—sighted, as it were, for a brief moment, and then lost in cloud and fog. This Cook had marked, with the fragment of coastline that Bouvet had reported, on the map he drew for Sandwich; and this received specific mention in his Secret Instructions, the instructions which one must regard as drawn up by himself. This cape might indeed project from a continent, though if it were a fair specimen of the land it belonged to the continent could hardly be an attractive one. Attractive or not, it must be diligently explored. The other point Cook also inserted in his map, with a mark of dubiety: 'Gulf of S[t] Sebastian Very Doub[t]full'—a huge gulf which opened fifteen degrees east of the Horn, and stretched far below the sixtieth parallel; inherited from the sixteenth-century cartographers, and recently, and recklessly, revived by Alexander Dalrymple on a chart of the South Atlantic Ocean that also gave Bouvet's track. This gulf, however, received no mention in the instructions, which may possibly be a measure of the faith felt in Dalrymple, as a general cartographer, by Cook as a circumnavigator. Between the gulf and South America land had been twice reported earlier by vessels driven east on homeward passages round the Horn—most recently in 1756: there is no doubt that Cook had these reports at the back of his mind, because in due course they came to its forefront. In the mean time, they were merely part of the Atlantic problem, and that had been provided for in his total plan. If one thinks of Cook primarily as a Pacific explorer—as one tends to do, not without justice—this Atlantic passage, when it does come, seems almost no more than an appendix to the main body of his voyage. But it is more than that: it is the foreseen and fore-planned closing of the gap in the circuit that he has already made; the circuit on his map realized in strict and necessary practice. If we seek for an appendix—or at least, to be more logical, for an extension of the plan—we can see it when the voyage is studied as a whole, in a second great incursion into warmer latitudes; for, although the essence of Cook's character is to make a plan and realize it in practice, we might almost add that the essence of the practice itself is elasticity. There is proof of that in the first voyage; there is ample proof of it in the second. He is like an artist: his solid design stands firm; within it he works out a detail that is not wholly preconceived, but develops as a development of thought, elaborate yet clear, subordinate yet continuously complementary to the main structure. There is this difference, that with the artist his technique is the servant of pure thought and feeling; the difficulties, given the technique, are within his own mind. With the navigator, whatever his accomplishment, the difficulties are outward as well as inward; he must be the master not merely of his own directed thought, but of the hundred shocks of brute and external circumstance.

§ *The Ships*

There seems no doubt that Cook's appointment to the *Scorpion* at the end of August 1771 was simply a 'holding' one, that he might be kept in full employment, and perhaps on full pay; for without a ship at all he would have been in the position of any other unemployed officer, and the half-pay of the unemployed was meagre. We do not know the precise moment when another voyage was resolved on—probably the resolution was taken as soon as Cook's journal had been read by the requisite persons—but in less than a month after the *Scorpion* appointment the Admiralty directed the Navy Board 'to purchase two proper vessels of about 400 tons for service in remote parts'.[1] Nor do we know precisely what arguments were advanced for the use of two vessels on the new voyage, rather than one, but the main argument is obvious enough—Cook was not a romantic, and had no wish for any repetition of the harrowing hours on the Great Barrier Reef, with no imaginable aid to look for. What extra safety lay in a consort he was very willing to embrace. He would have been quite glad to sail again in the *Endeavour*. She had proved her worth, but she had already been sent to the Falkland Islands as a store ship. There was no other ship like her in the navy, as there had been none before, and there seems to have been no doubt on the part of anyone that her build was the build required. Cook was accordingly instructed to go over the Pool of London and see what could be bought. He recommended three ships, of which the Navy Board early in November bought two—the *Marquis of Granby*, 462 tons (and so a

[1] Admiralty to Navy Board, 25 September 1771; National Maritime Museum, ADM/A/2647. I do not document every precise statement in this introduction, as that would be merely to repeat the Calendar of Documents, Appendix VIII below.

larger ship than the *Endeavour* by almost 100 tons) and the *Marquis of Rockingham*, 340 tons.[1] Their respective measurements were: length of lower deck 110′ 8″ and 97′ 3″, extreme breadth 35′ 5½″ and 28′ 4¼″, depth in hold 13′ 1½″ and 12′ 8¾″. They were both barks, and both built at Whitby by Fishburn, who built the *Endeavour*; the first fourteen months, the second eighteen months before. Their owner, or part-owner,[2] was Captain William Hammond of Hull, who may have been known to Cook already, but was certainly on friendly terms later. On the naval establishment they were classed as sloops (i.e. to be rigged as sloops-of-war), and on 28 November were commissioned under the names of *Drake* and *Raleigh*—honourable names, to be sure, for vessels of enterprise—the *Drake* to carry 110 men under the command of Cook, the *Raleigh* 80 under Tobias Furneaux. They were to be 'sheathed and filled' as was the *Endeavour*,[3] and fitted out, the one at Deptford, the other at Woolwich, in the very best manner possible. This fitting out proceeded apace, as it was agreed at first that the ships should sail as early as March 1772; and at the end of December, on the suggestion of Lord Rochford, the secretary of state, their names were changed. It had been in January 1771 that the difficult Falklands Islands question had been resolved without a Spanish war, and Rochford had no desire to provoke once more the susceptibilities of Spain. The Spanish court could be affronted if it liked by a new voyage into an ocean it regarded as its private property; nevertheless a voyage by ships with the chosen names might be needlessly wounding. The King agreed with Rochford. But what to substitute? *Aurora*? *Hesperus*?[4] We do not know, again, who thought of the two names that have taken on for us a sort of classic inevitability. The ships became *Resolution* and *Adventure*.

One has only to look through the correspondence recorded in the Calendar to realize what stature Cook had come to have at this time with the Admiralty and its subordinate departments. There was

[1] The prices paid were £4151 and £2103. Alterations to the *Marquis of Granby* (or *Resolution*), first and last, cost £6568—largely wasted money. Kitson, pp. 226–7.

[2] 'or part-owner': I say this on the authority of the *Memoirs* of John Elliott (see p. cxxxvi below), according to which Hammond was only a partner with Elliott's uncle John Wilkinson, a great ship-owner and broker and general merchant of the day; though it is hardly likely that Cook simply 'applied to my Uncle', as Elliott has it. Wilkinson 'furnish'd him with Two nearly new, of which he was the principal Owner, but he had a partner, in one or both, a Mr Hammond of Hull, and as my Uncle was becoming much connected with Ministers, he did not choose to have much to do about the Ships, He therefore introduced Mr Hammond at the Admiralty, and he transacted all the business respecting the Two Ships—and which, by the by, has been the making the fortunes of all the Hammonds since'.—Elliott, *Mem.*, ff. 7v–8. The last statement, like the first, may be open to question, but we know very little of the matter.

[3] I, p. cxxv.

[4] Rochford's letter to Sandwich, 20 December 1771, is printed on p. 908 below.

scarcely a request he made that was not immediately complied with; and even if there was delay because of the necessities of interdepartmental communication, compliance was the rule. The day the Navy Board reports to the Admiralty the purchase of ships, the Victualling Board seeks authority to supply Cook with the salted cabbage he has already asked for. Improved compasses, extra tools, ice anchors and hatchets, sugar instead of raisins, 'warping machines', patent medicines, extra anchors, stockfish, better quality seine-nets, different guns, deck-awnings, rob of oranges and lemons—the concession is almost automatic. Warping machines were not understood, but Cook got them. To only one demand did he receive a direct negative—he wanted brass instead of iron for the metal furnishings throughout his great cabin, and against that demand regulations stood adamant. On the Admiralty side, the voyage was regarded as an excellent opportunity for experiment, particularly in relation to antiscorbutic measures: hence the openness to suggestions from outside. The Baron Storsch, with his carrot marmalade, received a good hearing; so did Dr Priestley, with his device for sweetening water by the application to it of 'fixed air'; so did Mr Pelham, the secretary of the Victualling Office, with his recipe for experimental beer; Mr Irving's apparatus for distilling fresh water from the sea was installed in both ships; Mr Irving's improved fire-hearth was tried and rejected by Cook as unimproved while fitting-out was in progress. There was correspondence about the ships' companies—particularly that of the *Resolution*; if Cook wanted a particular man, he did not hesitate to ask for him. On the other side, the Admiralty had ideas. It found desirable a drummer who could play the violin, marines who could play the bagpipes—perhaps as an anticipated reply to the native musical endeavours of South Sea islanders. Cook himself, the papers make obvious, perfected a method of getting with speed what he wanted: he would go to an office—Navy Board, Victualling—and explain his need, and then write the necessary formal application on the spot; so many of his letters are headed and dated at the office itself.[1] And while all the quantities of official supplies, conventional and experimental, were being sent down for stowage, while odd combinations of qualities in seafaring men were being discussed, and commissions were being issued and altered, further supplies of a more extraordinary nature were building up, and a different sort of recruitment was going on: for we now have to reckon with Mr Joseph Banks.

Banks, there was no doubt of it, had made a great success of his

[1] Cf. I, p. 617, n.

voyage in the *Endeavour*. He had a taste for travel as yet unslaked. He was a friend of Lord Sandwich, and when the First Lord asked him, almost as soon as the new voyage was decided upon, whether he would like to go this time too, his response was immediate. He would; and so would Dr Solander. What followed in the next eight months, with its effects, in terms of personal relations, on the whole voyage, can be explained only on the assumption that young Mr Banks was not merely extremely sure of himself, but had an absurdly swollen head. Contemporary publicity was almost all in favour of Banks; the papers that have since been studied make what has been for nearly two hundred years a somewhat confused and cloudy story, alas! all too clear.[1] The *Resolution*, it must be remembered, was selected by Cook: to quote his own words, 'she was the ship of my choice and as I thought the fitest for the Service she was going upon of any I had ever seen'.[2] The service she was going upon was one of geographical discovery. She was not chosen as a passenger ship or a floating laboratory or an artist's studio, but precisely because she was what she was—a soundly-built collier, with adequate room for her crew and her stores. When Banks first saw her, he did not like her. Though she was larger than the *Endeavour*, he feared she was not large enough for him and his entourage; and he must already have begun to picture an entourage more complete than his earlier one. To him the idea of geographical discovery was quite secondary—he had a romantic view of standing upon the South Pole and turning full circle on his heel through 360 degrees of longitude,[3] but with that cheerful wish he was prepared to forget about it. What he could not forget was that the previous voyage had been 'Mr Banks's voyage', and that in consequence of it he had been—he still was—a great success in the learned as well as the social world; that the announcement of his intention to go on this one had created another sensation, and that applications were beginning to pour in on him from all parts of England, and even from some parts of Europe, from persons of a most unusual variety of types, couched in the most flattering language, to be taken with him. Nor, is it to be feared, could he forget—or rather, cease to take for granted—that as Mr Joseph Banks, a landed gentleman of a very considerable estate, he occupied a

[1] I have discussed this episode in Banks's life with some care in the introduction, 'The Young Banks', to *The* Endeavour *Journal of Joseph Banks* (Public Library of New South Wales), and need not go into undue detail here. The essential documents are printed in Appendix II.

[2] Add. MS 27888, f. 5. He says the same thing, at rather greater length, p. 7 below.

[3] Banks to the Comte de Lauraguais, December 1771, Mitchell Library MSS; and H. C. Cameron, *Sir Joseph Banks* (1952), pp. 319–20.

position in English life that made all other considerations trivial; and the First Lord was his friend. There is no need, on our part, to forget the disinterested side of Banks: he was willing, in the cause of science, to spend money, to undergo discomfort, to give—as he said—pledges to all Europe; but there is no doubt that he meant to astound all Europe. This voyage, too, was to be 'his' voyage; and though it is improbable that he said so at the beginning, he was to be the commander, and Cook was to be his servant, his executive officer, the ship's master rather than its captain.

He was even prepared to dogmatize on nautical matters; and he must have the vessel altered. Some adaptation was necessary, as a matter of course, and on some matters it was indispensable to consult Banks. He came to think that he should be consulted on all matters. From the beginning there was one firm obstacle in his way—Palliser. The Comptroller of the Navy was a good judge of ships, and he agreed entirely with Cook about the type of ship needed on this occasion; and beyond necessary details he did not want the ship altered at all. Banks removed that obstacle by going to Sandwich. The Navy Board—Palliser was not alone in his objection—was overruled. Cook's sentiments at the large reconstruction that followed can be established with a good deal of certainty. He disapproved, he was anxious to oblige Banks, he hoped for the best; he forced himself, against all reasonable expectation and in spite of all naval experience, to think it might do. In the end the vessel got a heightened waist and an additional upper deck, necessarily solidly built, and a raised poop or 'round-house' on top to accommodate the captain, who had relinquished his own quarters to Banks. The extra space otherwise provided, or its equivalent, was to be occupied by Banks's followers and the staggering amount of impedimenta, useful or useless, which for months he was accumulating. This programme made the *Resolution* the sight of the river, and she was visited not merely by those whose business it was, but, as Cook remarked, by 'many of all ranks... Ladies as well as gentlemen, for scarce a day past on which she was not crowded with Strangers who came on board for no other purpose but to see the Ship in which Mr Banks was to sail round the world'.[1] Whenever there was a hitch in the work, by which some little setback to Banks seemed possible, he brought out his sovereign argument—he threatened not to go.

It can at least be said for Banks that he could make himself useful, and that he had some interesting ideas on whom should be employed. It was he who ordered the brass medals struck by Matthew

[1] B.M. Add. MS 27888, f. 4–4v.

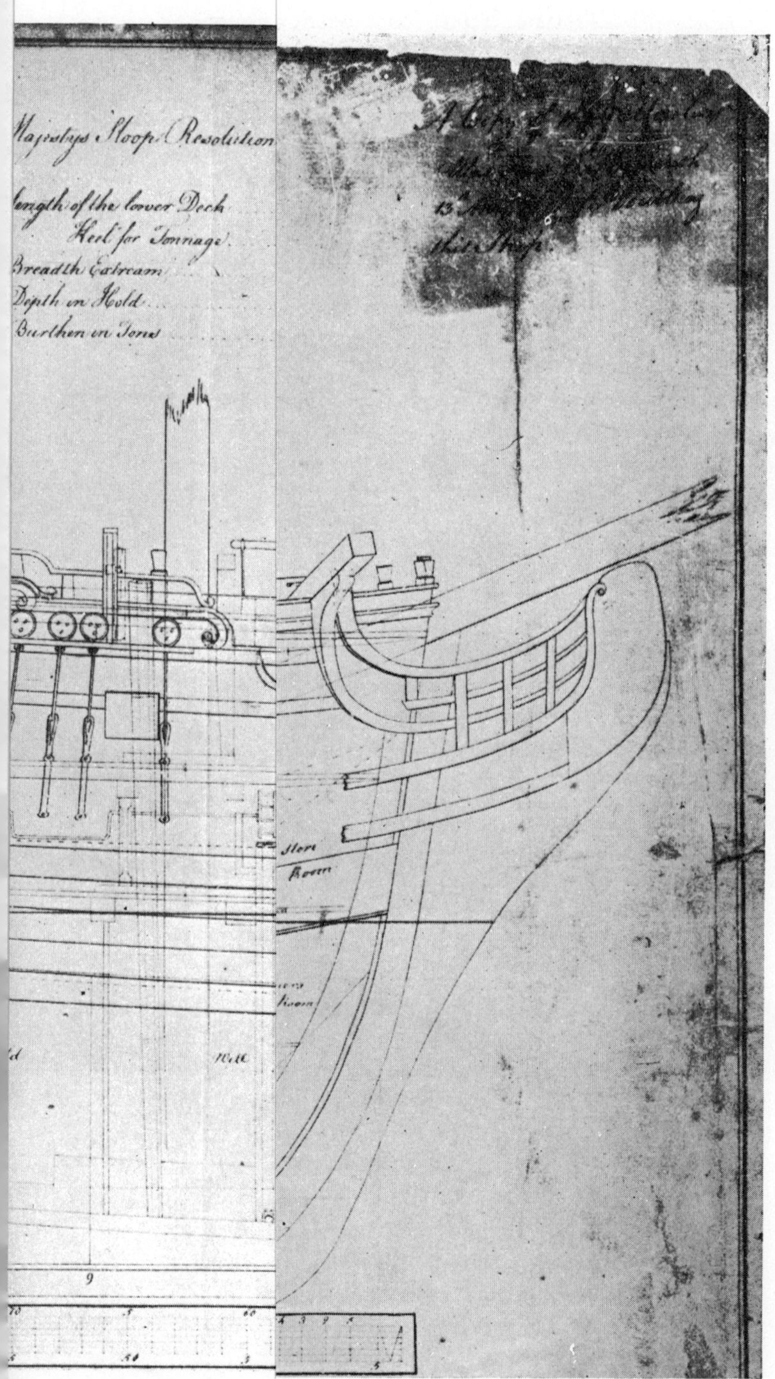

f the *Resolution*, March 1

Boulton, taken over by the Admiralty, and so freely distributed by Cook on the Pacific islands.[1] The Board of Longitude, or perhaps someone on it, having asked him and Solander for suggestions for the post of astronomer—as if Maskelyne, the Astronomer Royal, had not a strong enough will of his own—he proposed to Joseph Priestley that he should go (Priestley was not an astronomer), and then rebuffed him with the argument that his name, as that of a Unitarian, could not be put up before a Board on which sat Christian professors. He then turned to Dr James Lind, a young Edinburgh physician who had dabbled in astronomy as well as in other branches of science;[2] he did not know Lind, but Solander did, and Solander's letter[3] indicates the excitement pervading New Burlington Street. 'From not knowing how to properly equip ourselves we were not half so well provided last voyage as we now shall be. . . . Good God, we shall do wonders if you only will come and assist us.' Lind agreed to come, whatever the Board of Longitude's selection might be, and Cook was puzzled over his possible function. He would at least have been an agreeable companion. John Zoffany was engaged as principal artist; and as artist he had some qualities that might have made him very useful. The rest were simple draughtsmen, secretaries, servants (including two horn-players), thirteen in all: of these, two were to sail in the *Adventure*, the other eleven, with Banks himself, Solander and Lind in the *Resolution*. The most interesting idea of all did not come to light until the ships reached Madeira, at the end of July. Then it appeared that the thoughtful young philosopher had provided also for the companionship of a lady.[4]

In the end, none of them sailed. The reconstruction of the ship had put a March departure quite out of the question, but in the third week of April, she could be moved to Longreach to take in her

[1] See the Birmingham Assay Office pamphlet by Arthur Westwood, *Matthew Boulton's 'Otaheite' Medal* (1926). There are three letters from Boulton, or his firm, Boulton and Fothergill, to Banks, in the volume of MSS bearing on the voyage, called by him 'Voluntiers, Instructions, Provision for 2d. Voyage', now in the Mitchell Library, pp. 291–300. Banks ordered two gold and a number of silver medals, as well as the general supply. One regrets the profile head of George III. The pamphlet prints much of the Boulton and Fothergill side of the correspondence; Banks's letters seem to have disappeared.

[2] Banks finally had the effrontery to say: 'I had had influence enough to prevail on the board of Longitude to send with us Mes[s] Bailey & Wales as astronomers'.—MS Iceland Journal, McGill University Library, p. 4.

[3] pp. 901–3 below.

[4] Elliott's account (*Mem.*, f. 13–13v) would be almost incredible were it not directly borne out by Cook, p. 685 below. The British consul's story 'both surpriz'd, and amus'd Capt[n] Cook, very much', says Elliott. One does not of course know under what circumstances Banks issued his invitation to Mr, or Mrs, or Miss Burnett, but she was either a very great fool or a woman of spirit; 'unless this Lady had been *very prudent indeed*, she might have been the cause of much mischief', moralizes Elliott. Prudence, however, hardly seems to have been one of her characteristics.

ordnance stores. Here Cook found her already too deep in the water and took out twenty tons of ballast. Early in May she was ordered to the Downs, and sailed on the 10th. At the Nore, on the 14th, the pilot gave up. The ship was so top-heavy that she could hardly carry sail without capsizing. Cooper, the first lieutenant, temporarily in charge, gave Cook his private opinion that she was 'an exceeding dangerous and unsafe ship'; and the more ebullient Clerke gave his to Banks: 'By God, I'll go to sea in a grog-tub, if required, or in the Resolution as soon as you please, but must say I think her by far the most unsafe ship I ever saw or heard of'. Cook's error of judgment in hoping that all might be well was apparent to him, and he immediately told the Admiralty secretary that the upper works would have to be cut down again. A day of rapid communications between Admiralty and Navy Board settled the matter: the *Resolution* was to go to Sheerness, the round-house and new upper deck to be removed, the guns reduced in weight; and within a week it was decided to shorten the masts as well. Accommodation was to be made for the passengers such as would fit in the ship, not such as would fit the ship to the passengers. And Cook began to hear the most favourable reports of the ship as she was in the merchant service. The effect on Banks, when he saw what was happening, was instantaneous. A plan for the best accommodation that could be contrived (of which the Navy Board informed the Admiralty) was not good enough for him; and the Navy Board's letter was minuted, 'M[r] Banks does not go in her and that therefore only to make accommodation for Captain and Officers and astronomer'. To quote the memoirist Elliott, 'M[r] Banks came to Sheerness and when he saw the ship, and the Alterations that were made, He swore and stamp'd upon the Warfe, like a Mad Man; and instantly order'd his servants, and all his things out of the Ship'.[1] This time the Admiralty took him at his word.

[1] It is possible that Elliott has heightened the drama—if it needed any heightening—for he was very young at this time, and he wrote a good many years later. But he may quite well reflect the impression Banks made upon the less important members of the ship's company. He is worth quoting further: 'we were order'd into Sheerness, and the next morning at daylight, I believe two Hundred shipwrights were cutting, and tearing the ship to pieces, in all parts of her, so much, that it was dangerous to stir about . . . when this was done, M[r] Banks was requested to go to Sheerness, and take a View of the Accomodations, as they now stood, to try if he could go out in her, for in no other state could she go to sea, and go she must. . . . [Zoffany and Solander were] a loss to us, but upon the Whole, it has always been thought, that it was a most fortunate circumstance for the purposes of the Voyage, that M[r] Banks did not go with us; for a more proud, haught[y] man could not well be, and all his plans seemed directed to shew his own greatness; which would have accorded very Ill, with the discipline of a Man of War, and been the means of causing many quarrels in all parts of the Ship: We had on board in coming down the River, belonging to him, thirteen servants, in Scarlet and Silver; composing a full Band of Music; which was very delightful, as to the Music, but who I fear would some-

But Banks did not quite give up hope. He wrote a long letter of passionate self-justification to Sandwich. Why could he not have a West Indiaman or a man-of-war for his voyage? And a captain whose prudence and perseverance would be of more importance than any build of ship? (The side-blow at Cook can be explained only by the knowledge that this writer was beyond all reason and all gratitude.) Sandwich was no fool, and it is apparent that for the time being he had had enough of his friend. He complied with what Banks called scornfully 'the forms of office' by taking the opinions of the Navy Board and of Palliser in person on the young man's outburst, which there was some fear might be made public, and then he prepared a detailed reply. This must be taken as conclusive. It did not see the light, though it was submitted to the king; for Banks himself thought better of rushing into print. He had a party; there were questions in the Commons, adequately ignored; the anti-ministerial scribblers were all on his side, and other persons were supplied with information of a suitable cast.[1] Burke was involved, and Lord North was held off from reviving the question by Sandwich. Banks had some ill-justified hope of getting assistance from the East India Company; and when that faded, chartered a ship and took his whole company on a voyage to Iceland. He took with him also John Gore, who after three voyages round the world was no doubt in need of relaxation;[2] he would have perhaps liked Clerke as well, and anyhow professed concern for Clerke's future—but, said Clerke, '[I]

times have produc'd sounds not altogether harmonious: Nor has it been thought that Capt[n] Cook, and M[r] Banks would have agreed.'—Elliott *Mem.*, ff. 10–11. We cannot swallow all this, unless we are to assume that all Banks's people, including Zoffany, belonged to the private band.

[1] e.g. *Gentleman's Magazine* for June 1772 (XLII, p. 254): 'Mr Urban, As the expedition with a view to new discoveries, which Mr. Banks, Dr. Solander, and M. Zoffani, were to embark in, is now, after raising the expectation of the Literati throughout Europe to the highest pitch, abruptly laid aside; the following facts, that have been communicated to the public, deserve to be recorded in your useful Magazine as a memorable instance how little it is in the power of Majesty to perform, when the servants of the Crown are determined to oppose the Sovereign's will . . .'.—and so on. Cf. the *Gazetteer and New Daily Advertiser*, 11 June, letter from 'A Briton': 'From what I can see, Mr. Banks, Dr. Solander, Dr. Lind, and Mr. Zoffani, are likely to be excluded from a voyage which, from their sharing it, did honour to the nation; and in all probability, the noblest expedition ever fitted out will dwindle to nothing, and disgrace this country. I wish some one would point out to the public the dirty manoeuvre, which is now subverting the intentions of the King and Parliament of Great Britain, and of all the nation in general. I hope by laying this train of jobbing and meanness before the public, we may be led to see many other striking iniquities which are now going on . . .'. To this an anonymous person replied (16 June) that 'The whole of the matter is, Mr. B. did not chuse to go the voyage, unless he could ride the waves triumphantly, in all the pomp and splendour of an Eastern Monarch' There were further letters on 17 June ('An Englishman', anti-Banks) and 23 June ('Detector', 1½ columns pro-Banks). I have not studied the other newspapers; but it is unlikely that they would be sources of light.

[2] I am in error in saying, I, p. 595, that Gore 'Took Banks to Iceland'. Banks chartered a ship, captain and crew complete, and Gore went simply as a friend and guest.

have stood too far on this tack to think of putting about with any credit',[1] and was happy with Cook. From this Iceland voyage the young man gained some credit, though little compared to what would have come to him from the greater one. He must have had regrets; on the expedition's return he certainly felt embarrassment. His friendships suffered no irreparable harm; there was a temporary coolness with Cook, and a rift with Sandwich for a year or two. The man Banks could not forgive was the man whose judgment had been unwavering from the start: to the end of his life he maintained an unrelenting resentment against Palliser and the memory of Palliser.

The *Resolution* thus returned to her original condition, and men were indeed fitted into the ship—with no superfluity of room, it is true, but with room to do their work and to survive in health. There had been no need, and no attempt, to alter the *Adventure*, and about her no controversy ever centred. Banks's two men left her. She shared the virtues of her build; she served her purpose admirably. She was not quite the ship her consort was; she was harder to bring round into the wind, to which must be attributed the final parting of the ships, off the New Zealand coast in October 1773. As for the *Resolution*, that honest product of Mr Fishburn's yard at Whitby, she proved one of the great, one of the superb, ships of history; of all the ships of the past, could she by magic be recreated and made immortal, one would gaze on her with something like reverence.[2]

§ *The Men*

To make sure that the vessels should be adequately manned, the Admiralty forbade the carrying of officers' servants, promising the gentlemen thus deprived monetary compensation at the end of the voyage.[3] This may have made some difference, though the officers' servants on the *Endeavour* were mostly midshipmen-in-training, and the *Resolution*, at least, carried a large number of these 'young gentlemen', who fluctuated in *de facto* rank on the voyage between mid-

[1] 31 May 1772; p. 936 below.

[2] In the Dominion Museum, Wellington, is what purports to be the 'figure-head' of the *Resolution*, bought from the effects of Admiral Isaac Smith, after his death in 1831, by the 5th Viscount Galway, and presented to the Museum by his great-grandson, the 8th Viscount, Governor-General of New Zealand, in 1941. It is a carved wooden head, cut off at the neck, of a particularly savage animal (a wolf?), which may correspond with the forepart of the figure described as a sea-horse by W. Laird Clowes in his discussion of Holman's painting (Fig. 4 in this volume) in the *Geographical Journal*, LXIX (1927), p. 230. If this is authentic, then there is something at least still left of the great ship.

[3] Then how did Furneaux get both a servant, James Swilley, the negro, killed at Grass Cove, and compensation at the end of the voyage? Some of the lists, certainly, class Swilley as A.B.

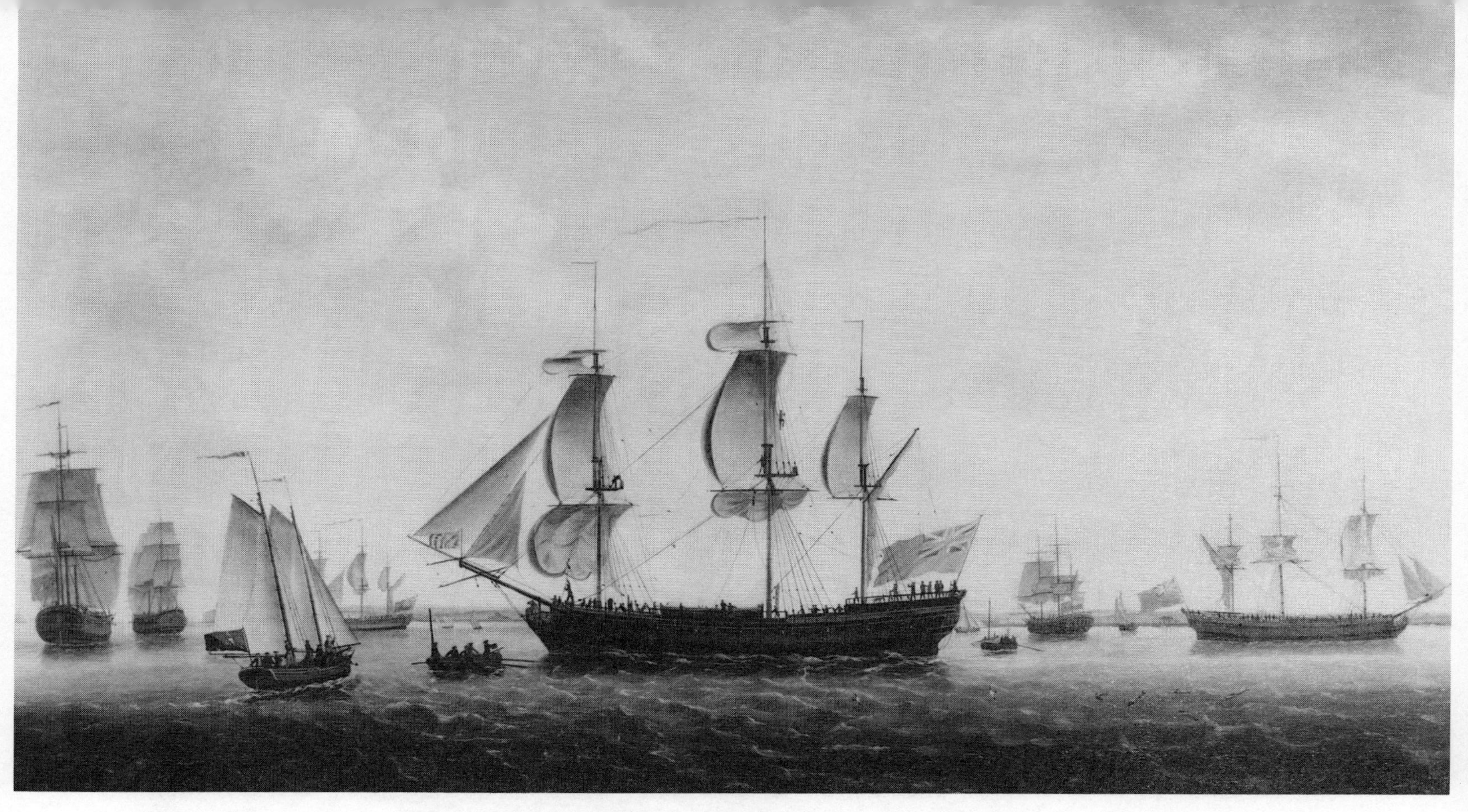

FIG. 4. The *Resolution* and *Adventure* in the Downs, 26–27 June 1772

Oil painting by Francis Holman, in the Dixson Collection, Sydney

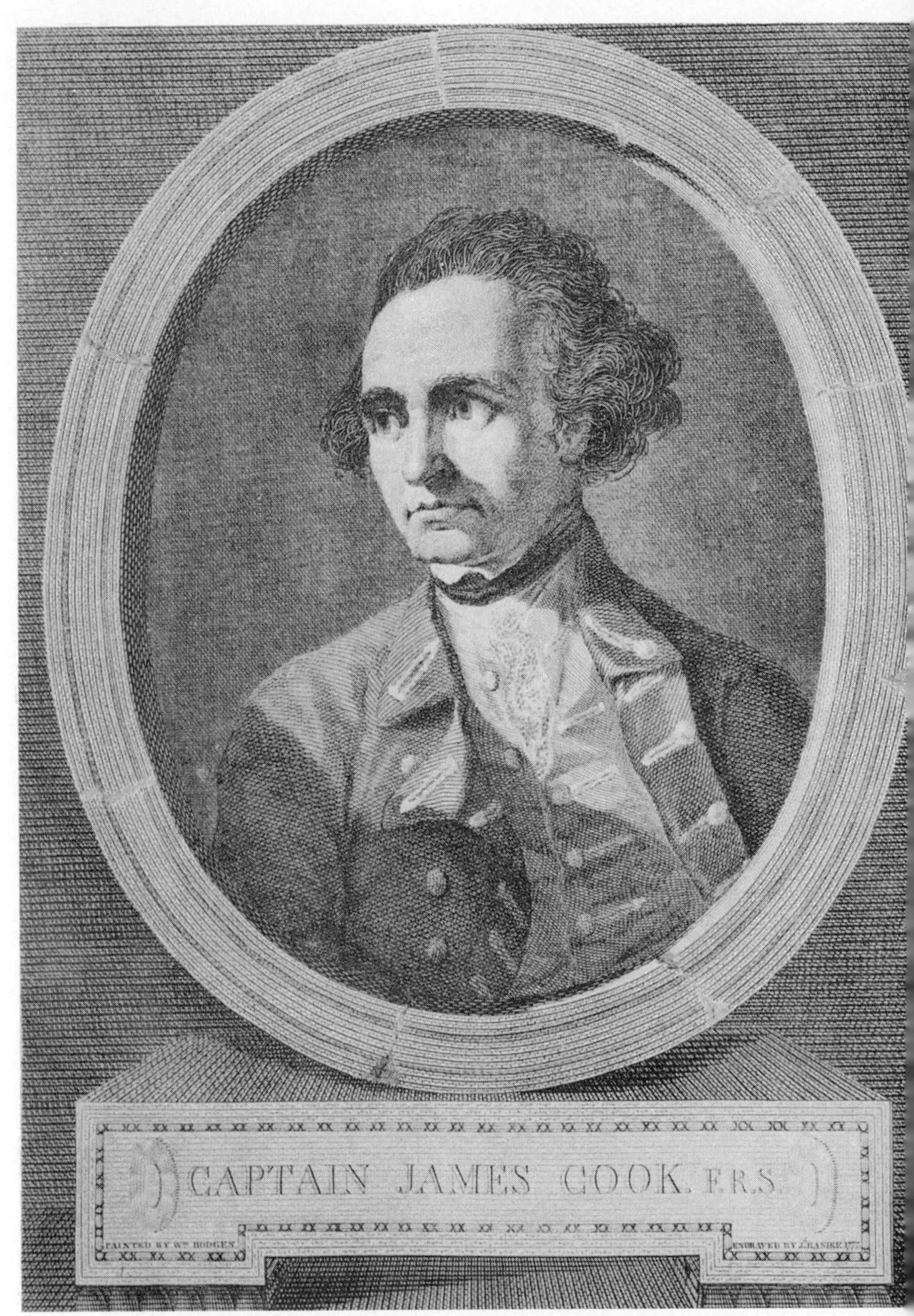

Fig. 5. Portrait of Captain Cook

Engraved by John Basire after William Hodges, 1777

shipman and A.B. The *Vestal* frigate was appointed to receive men until the ships were ready for them. Contrary to what has generally been said, the completion of the crews was not an entirely smooth process: the men, once their names had been put on the muster-rolls, had a habit of 'running'. There must have been a good deal of discussion of the chances of the voyage. To get the 90 seamen of the *Resolution*'s company, about 200 men were entered; to get the *Adventure*'s 69, about 122. Of these not many were discharged as superfluous, though Cook at one stage did get Admiralty permission to retain some men beyond the proper number, to allow him the chance of final selection. Nor were the old *Endeavour* men who volunteered for the new voyage as many as has sometimes been thought. Apart from the officers Clerke, Pickersgill and Edgcumbe, there were thirteen seamen and one marine. The marine, curiously enough, was Gibson, who had tried to desert at Tahiti, and was now promoted corporal. There were three midshipmen, Manley, Harvey and Isaac Smith. Six of the seamen received promotion, the others remained A.B's.[1] Yet these probably provided a stiffening, particularly the midshipmen and the other petty officers—with the exception of Marra, whose example could hardly be anything to anyone but unsettling. Whether a stiffening was needed we may doubt; for the men were the ordinary British sailors of the time, the majority in their twenties, not very civilized: the sort of men on whom an anthology of abuse could be culled from the pages of George Forster, so savage, brutal, drunken, insensitive, and blasphemous that one wonders that even a kindly Deity permitted the ship to put to sea; of whom Cook could say, with a charity that he extended to every savage race, 'they shewed themselves capable of surmounting every difficulty and danger which came in their way and never once looked upon either the one or the other to be a bit heightned by being seperated from our companion the Adventure'.[2] If that, said of the *Resolution*'s men, seems rather conventionally phrased, one has to remember that Cook, however he might write, never paid idle compliments; and if one wants a supporting statement, there is Elliott: 'I will here do them the justice to say that *No Men* could behave better, under every circumstance than they did, the same must be said of the officers; and I will add that I believe their never was a Ship, where for so long a period, under such circumstances, more happiness, order, and

[1] Dawson became captain's clerk; Peckover gunner's mate; Marra gunner's mate; Ramsay cook; Anderson (quartermaster) became gunner; Gray (quartermaster) became boatswain; Collett, Terrell, James Cook, Nathaniel Cook, remained A.B's.

[2] p. 647 below.

obedience was enjoy'd'.[1] There is no evidence that the *Adventure*'s men behaved less than well. One allows, of course, for the misdemeanours that earned floggings; for the individual crimes and failings that got more mention in other people's logs and journals than in Cook's. Forster, more than once, holds the marines and the sailors up in contrast, very much to the advantage of the former. It occurred to no one else to do so. Cook does not discriminate between them. They came from the same classes of society; they were punished and praised alike. If Cook had to make constant efforts, it was to keep them clean. If they had a clearly marked characteristic, it was their conservatism: although, when they came to an inhabited island they had, it is true, clearly marked objectives of enjoyment, it was not privation they detested, but innovation. They were, for that century, standard uneducated Englishmen.

Of their superiors in rank there is more to be said. The one who ranked highest after Cook was Tobias Furneaux, who had been round the world once before, with Wallis in the *Dolphin*[2]—when he impressed Robertson the master as a 'Gentele Agreeable well behaved Good man and very humain to all the Ships company'.[3] Entering the navy rather late, at the age of 20, in 1755, as a midshipman, he had rapidly been promoted to master's mate on the Jamaica station, and then to lieutenant for his gallantry in action. He served on the coast of Africa and again in the West Indies, and after the war in the Channel fleet, from which he was moved to the *Dolphin* as second lieutenant. During the considerable periods when Wallis and his first lieutenant were both sick men, he was virtually in command; while his conduct in charge of landing parties was moderate and wise. Experience and character alike, then, seemed to mark him out as an excellent second in command to Cook. But the face in his portrait, though it conveys vigour, with its rather large nose and full

[1] He goes on: 'And yet we had Two or three troublesome Characters on board. Old Mr Forster (tho clever) was very hot, and petulant in Argument, and once got knock'd down by Mr Burr, for giving him the lie, they were to have fought, but Mr F. fell soft in the End, and apoligized. And Captn Cook too, has been known to shew him out of his Cabbin. There was likewise a Mess, which Cook call'd his *black Sheep*, who were at times apt to get too much grog and Quarel in their Cups, those were sometimes in one Mess, and sometimes, two or three Messes. Those were Willis, Logie, Price, Cogland, Maxwell; & the Father of our own Mess, Mr Whitehouse, tho very sensible, was very Intriguing, hypocritical, and Mischievous. As to myself, I never had one angry word with any one the whole time, except once with my friend Grindal, whom I challeng'd at 16 years old, for giving me a blow, half in jest, half in anger, but which I conceiv'd an affront, and he Apoligiz'd'.—Elliott, *Mem.*, ff. 40v–1. It may be added that Elliott finished up the voyage with a bout of fisticuffs with Loggie.

[2] Furneaux was related to Wallis by the marriage of his aunt Anne Furneaux to Wallis's uncle, another Samuel Wallis.

[3] *The Discovery of Tahiti* (Hakluyt Society, 1948), p. 202.

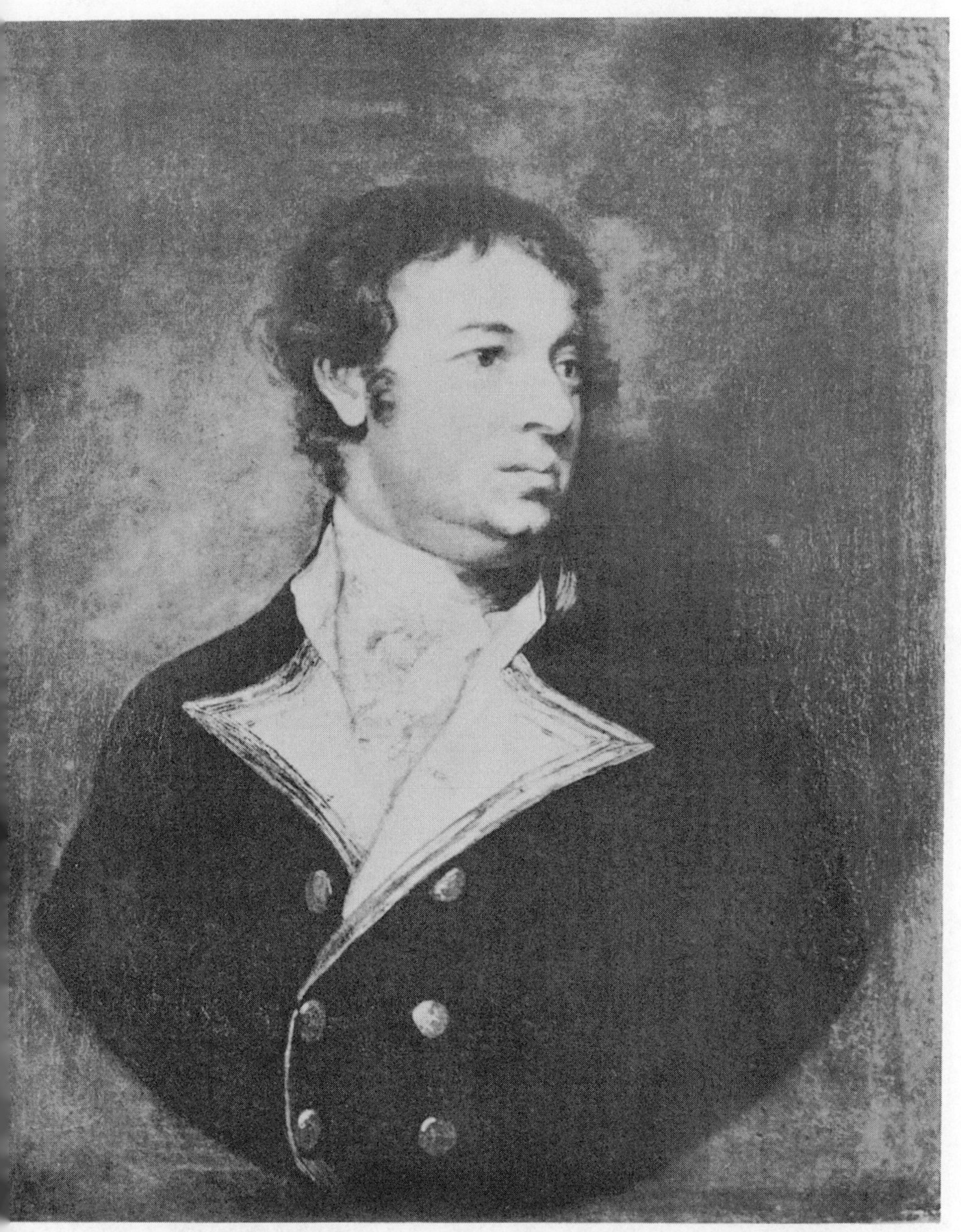

Fig. 6. Portrait of Captain Tobias Furneaux, by James Northcote, 1776

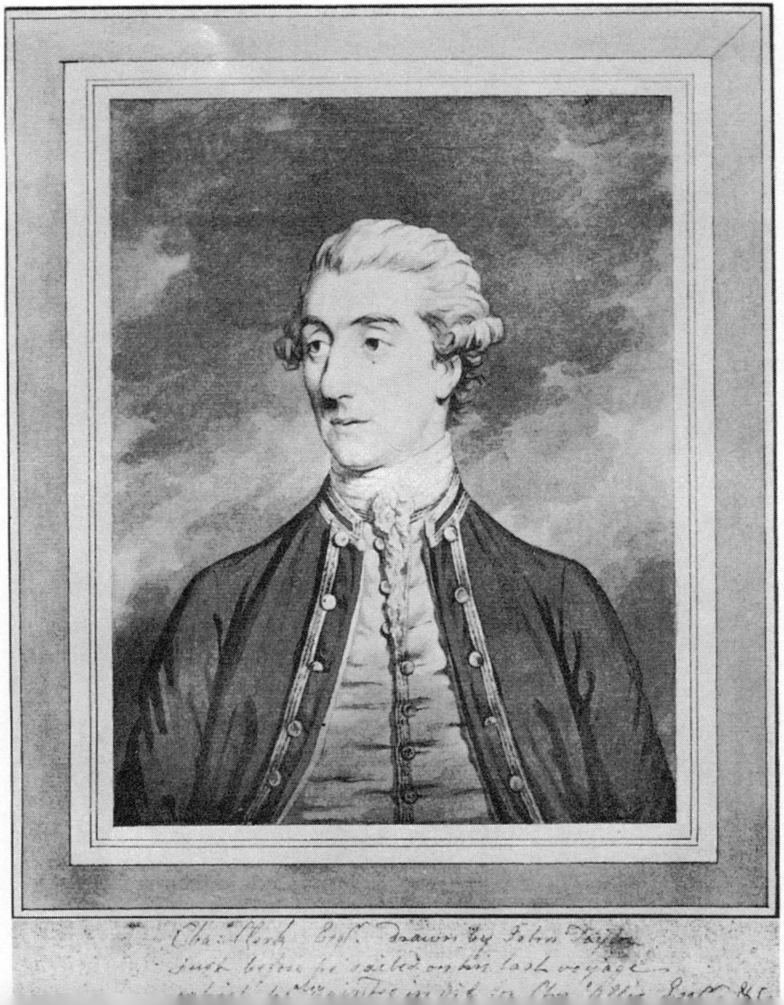

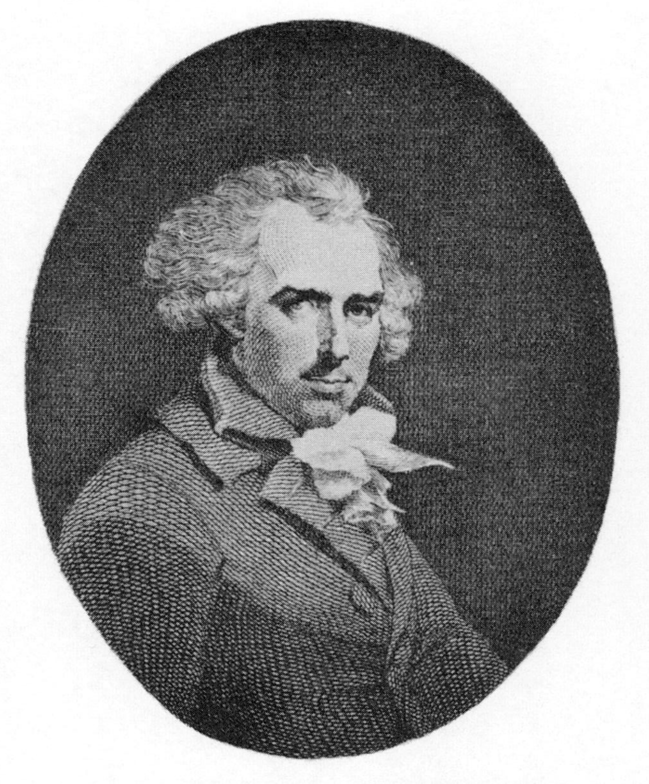

Fig. 7. (*left*) Portrait of Charles Clerke, by John Taylor, 1776

(*above*) Portrait of William Hodges, after Richard Westall, 1791

eyes and lips, does not give one a sense of thought; and Furneaux was indeed an executive rather than a ruminative officer. He was certainly an admirable seaman. As long as he was with Cook one finds no criticism that one would make. Separate them: and he was not, one immediately feels, really an explorer. There was an in-curiosity about Furneaux that made for strained relations more than once between him and Bayly the astronomer, whom he could certainly have helped more; there was a readiness to settle down into winter quarters, as a matter of routine, in April 1773 that must have received a shock when Cook turned up at Queen Charlotte Sound; Furneaux on his own would certainly have had deaths from scurvy. And a really curious man, one feels, would not finally have left the coast of Van Diemen's Land without making certain, from visual evidence, that it was or was not an island, especially knowing what his officers thought on the subject. At the critical moment he clings to assumption, rather than to enquiry; so that he hardly passes into the ranks of the original discoverers.

Returning to the *Resolution*, we find in Robert Palliser Cooper, the first lieutenant, another man whose mark is competence rather than originality. Cook speaks well of his conduct of the ship, and that must be his praise. He perhaps owed his place to his kinsman the Comptroller, like whom he became, in due course, a rear-admiral. Charles Clerke, second lieutenant, we have met on the first voyage, by reputation rather than otherwise. He now becomes three-dimensional, a positive personality of the most lively description, through both his journal and his letters to Banks;[1] and the journal in particular gives us an enlarged and matured personality as well as a lively one. He is a man capable of systematic observation and recording; able to generalize, also, and to think, and the light touch of his descriptions does not destroy their validity. It is Clerke, too, with whom we sometimes feel the tedium of the voyage, the irritation at, rather than the fear of, endless icebergs; it is Clerke whom, returned from the voyage, we should like to hear talk. Cook we should like to hear talk, of course, but Clerke would be more indiscreet, he would laugh more. Would Pickersgill laugh? Perhaps not. There was something desperately serious about Pickersgill, as about so many romantics; viewing his life as a whole, perhaps one sees also a little of the pathetic. There are the good intentions, never realized; there is the reach to something beyond his grasp, whether because of lack of training or lack of mental stamina one does not know. When

[1] Printed below in the Calendar.

he amuses us, it is not of set purpose. Yet as a writer, he has an idea of narrative. As a seaman and officer, he was fit for responsible work, he could be given a job to do, and Cook found him very useful. Some of his charts are good—notably that of Dusky Sound. He seems to have got on well with the island peoples, and to have earned their trust. He is certainly a less striking figure than Clerke, certainly a more complex one, less on good terms with the world, more likely to brood; and where Clerke writes down a jest, Pickersgill explains a grievance. Joseph Gilbert, the master, was the last of the senior officers, apart from the excellent Edgcumbe, of the marines. Gilbert was old as ages went on that ship, about 40; one of the growing list of men from Lincolnshire who had to do with the Pacific, and one whose career, like Cook's, had been marked by his part in the Newfoundland-Labrador survey. He was a sound officer, in principal charge, underneath Cook, of the surveying work of the voyage. Cook says the right things about him, in due form, but even more indicative is the reason given for certain action, that 'Mr Gilbert the Master, on whose judgement I had a good opinion',[1] was of a particular opinion himself. Gilbert was a good draughtsman, too: when it came to a 'view', a much better one than Cook, who had no pretensions in that line.

We know more about the midshipmen than usual, largely through the reminiscences of John Elliott, himself one of these 'young gentlemen'; and we know how Cook trained them. Some of them no doubt got their positions on their known merit, like the three who had been out in the *Endeavour*; some, like Elliott, through 'interest'; some perhaps through accident. It was thought, says Elliott, 'it would be quite a great feather, in a young man's Cap, to go with Captn Cook, and it requir'd much Intrest to get out with him; My Uncle therefore determin'd to send me out with him in the Resolution'—and took the boy to Palliser to secure his patronage, who passed him on to Cooper, who introduced him to Cook, 'who promis'd to take care of me,' and did. Elliott wrote brief characterizations of all the officers and civilians on his ship,[2] and he thought highly of most of his fellows. They were in general 'steady', some of them steady and clever as well. Roberts indeed was a 'very clever young man'. Burney was outside the usual run, and was 'Clever & Excentric'—though what his eccentricity led him to in the *Resolution* we never learn. Then

[1] See p. 546 below.

[2] I give all these in the appendix on the Ship's Company, but cannot resist giving here also his remarks on the three lieutenants: Cooper 'a sober, steady good officer'; Clerke 'a Brave and good officer, & a genal favorite'; Pickersgill 'a good officer and astronomer, but liking ye Grog'.—Add. MS 42714.

there was the small 'wild & drinking' set, one of them, Price, even 'unsteady' and drinking; and there was poor Loggie, with the trepanned head, drinking 'from misfortune', who was a trial to the captain, and once unjustly treated, thought Elliott, who liked him. There were two whom our memoirist disliked—the 'Hypocritical canting fellow' Maxwell, who got Loggie into trouble; and the 'Jesuitical' Whitehouse, 'sensible but an insinuating litigious mischief making fellow'; with whom we may contrast the one who was to rise to fame himself as an explorer, 'Mr Vancouver', aged 'about 13½' (in fact nearer 15), 'a Quiet inoffensive young man'. Inoffensive or offensive, steady or unsteady, they all had to knock down together, and Cook made the best of them he could. To quote Elliott again, 'In the Early part of the Voyage, Captn Cook made all us young gentlemen, do the duty aloft the same as the Sailors, learning to hand, and reef the sails, and Steer the Ship, E[x]ercise Small Arms &c thereby making us good Sailors, as well as good Officers'; later on they were put to observing, surveying, and drawing, 'And Myself, Roberts & Hood, form'd a very good set, for observing the Lunar Observations, as any in the Ship (and very correct)'.[1] There is something very pleasant about the glimpse of Cook in the further remark: 'I survey'd this Group [the New Hebrides, a formidable test] Myself, and settled them by my own Lunar Observations, and Captn Cook told me, they were nearly as correct as his own'.[2] The training the young gentlemen got was highly regarded in important circles; for when after the voyage Elliott was appointed to an East India Company ship, his preliminary examination before the Directors consisted in their 'saying that they suppos'd I had been with Cook, that having been a Pupil of his, I must be a good Sailor; asking me how my Uncle did, and telling me to withdraw'.[3] It is difficult, indeed, to imagine a better education for a young seaman than three years in the *Resolution*. Lastly, we must notice the surgeon and his mates, all three 'steady clever' men. Patten, there can be no doubt, was good professionally: so far as any surgeon could, he saved Cook's life; and there must have been something sterling about a man who earned good words not merely from Cook and a midshipman, but from the Forsters. Anderson, his first mate, was to become surgeon on the third voyage. He was an extremely intelligent man, with a wide-ranging as well as agreeable mind, interested in mankind, its peculiarities and languages, and in all the branches of natural history: the

[1] Elliott *Mem.*, f. 27v.
[2] ibid., f. 30.
[3] ibid., f. 49.

journals which we know he kept, from his later references to them, are the great loss from the records of this voyage. Drawwater, the junior mate, remains but a name.

The men of the *Adventure*, with few exceptions, are more shadowy. Shank, the first lieutenant, departs early, at the Cape. Kemp or Kempe, there promoted, seems to have been the parallel of Cooper, educated, competent, without frills; he followed Cooper later up the ladder of promotion, and longevity (it is to be presumed) made him at last an admiral. Burney, transferred at the Cape from the *Resolution*, is our personality on board the *Adventure*, and a man we know something about.[1] At sea from the age of 10, he owes his inclusion on the voyage to the musical connection between his father and Sandwich; and sails, at 21, still only an A.B., but one who has passed his lieutenant's examination, and owing to a hint from Sandwich to Cook, now sees promotion reasonably near. It comes, and it is clear by the end of his voyage that he has made the most of it. Burney, though he sailed very little with Cook himself, is one of the most interesting of Cook's officers; a thorough seaman, and certainly one of the mainstays of the *Adventure*'s company; in addition lively, observant, and articulate. He was to become the great scholar of Pacific exploration; some of his other activities might have been regarded by Mr Elliott as further proof of eccentricity. Fannin, like so many other masters, was a good professional man, skilled in chart-work, hardly visible as a person otherwise. Rowe, the master's mate who was slaughtered by the Maoris in Queen Charlotte Sound, stands out better, though perhaps not altogether to advantage—Jack Rowe, of the Furneaux-Wallis-Rowe connection, who evidently thought you should take a high hand with 'Indians', but when he really needed his muskets, was parted from them by the length of the beach. We have glimpses of the others in the journal of Bayly the astronomer, with their occasional horse-play or melancholy or quarrelling; evidently in one case, that of James Scott, the lieutenant of marines, with some quite real derangement of the mind, which made him a difficult person to live with.

And there were, with important parts to play, the civilians—the astronomers, the artist, the naturalists. The astronomers, indeed, renew our consideration of the plan of the voyage; for there was, inset as it were in the main theme, a supplementary one of some

[1] See the entry on p. 877 below. G. E. Manwaring's biography, *My Friend the Admiral* (1931), is useful, though it tends to be irrelevant, like much writing about the Burneys. See also Percy A. Scholes, *The Great Dr. Burney* (1948), and Joyce Hemlow's extremely interesting volume *The History of Fanny Burney* (1958).

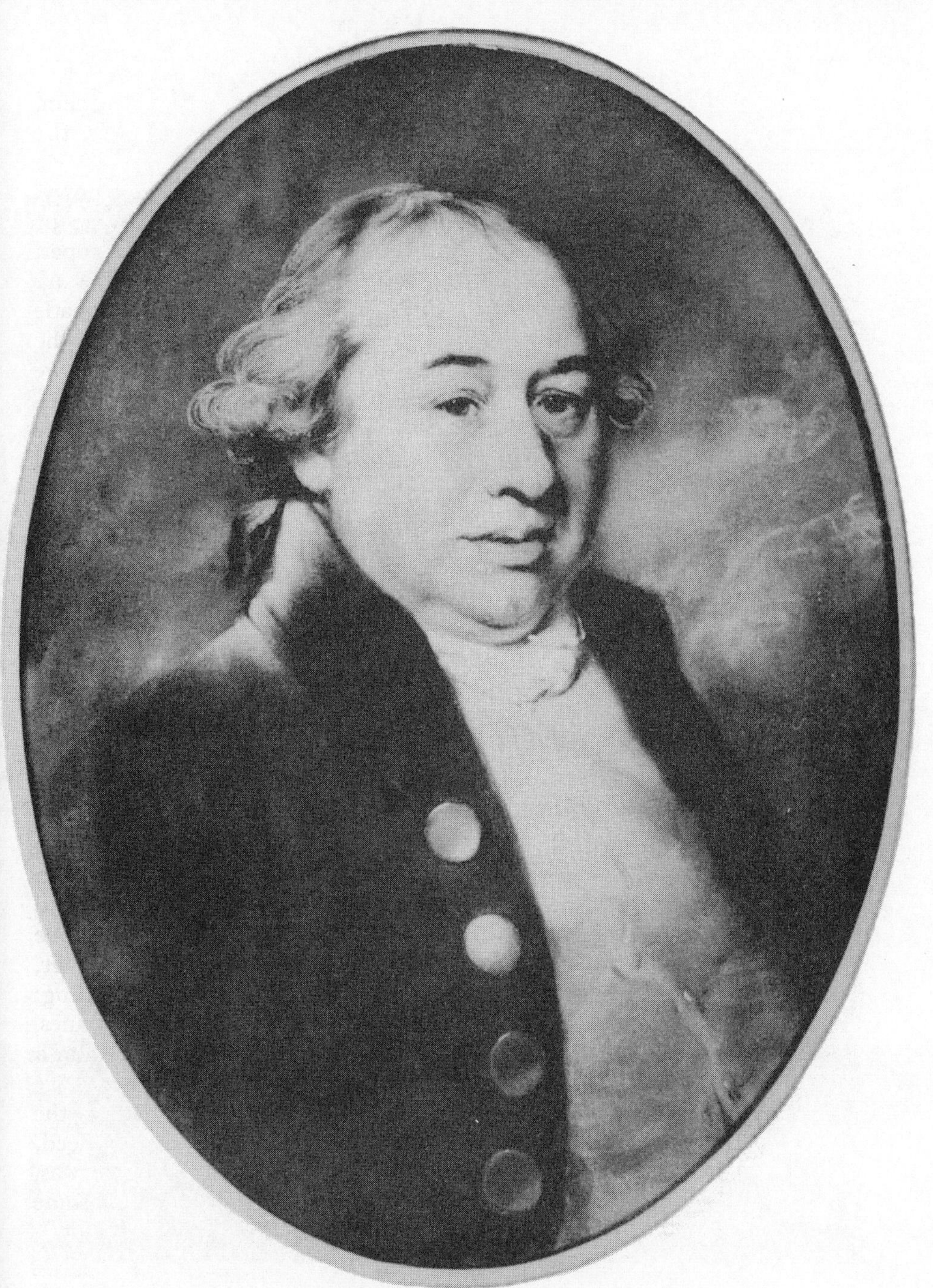

Fig. 8. Portrait of William Wales, by John Russell, 1794

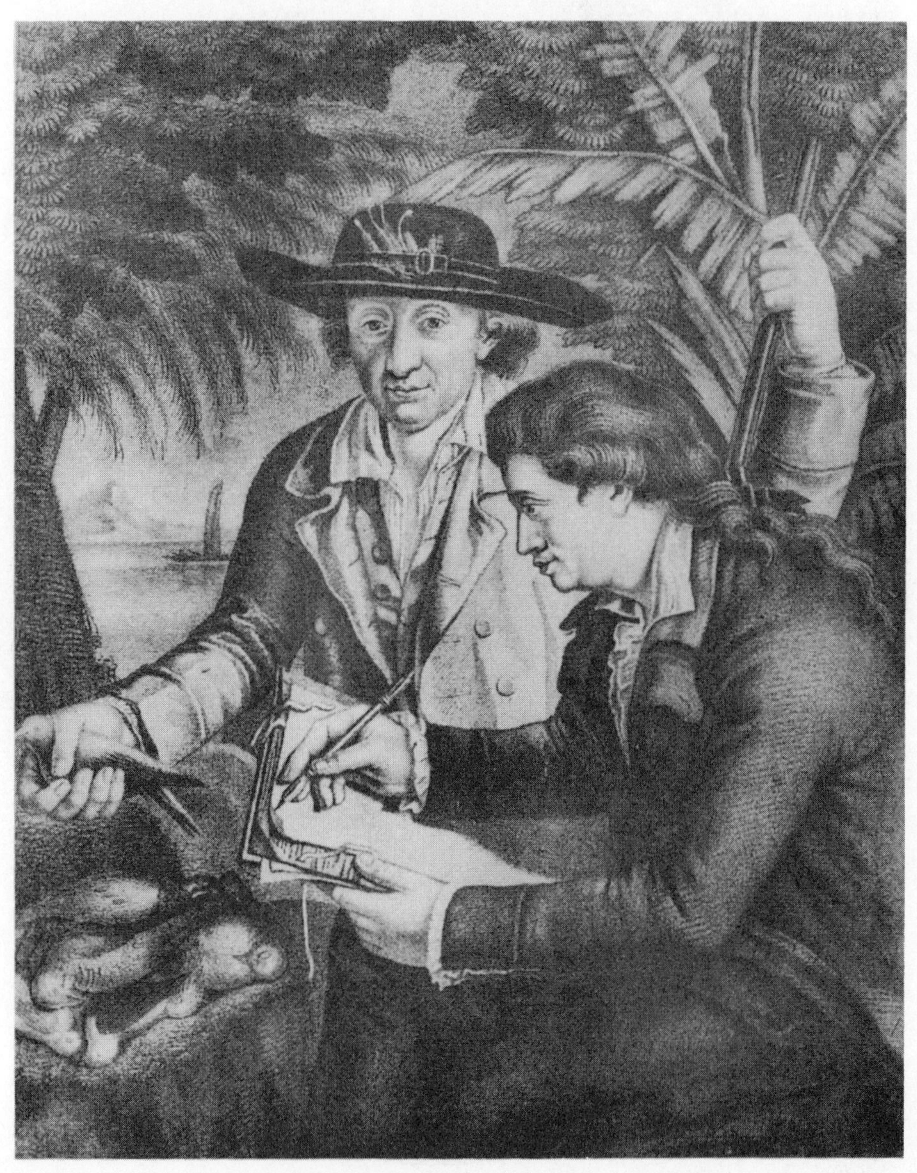

FIG. 9. Reinhold and George Forster at Tahiti

Engraved by D. Beyel after J. F. Rigaud

importance. This was the theme of finding longitude accurately at sea, in which Cook was interested as a surveyor as well as a sailor. The triumphs of the first voyage in the production of charts were due to lunar observation, and as observers Charles Green and Cook had shared the work. It was not intended that on this second voyage there should be less lunar observation: on that point the Board of Longitude, stepping forward in October 1771, was firm, but it also wanted something else—the exhaustive testing of the recently constructed chronometers, which could only be done against the check and control of constant astronomical work.[1] There were other matters, physical and hydrographical, on which the Board wanted regular observation and experiment, and there was a good deal of up-to-date apparatus supplied.[2] Scientific research, that is—whatever happened to natural history—was to be part of the voyage, sponsored this time not by the Royal Society but by Government itself. The Royal Society came into the plans only by giving its advice when invoked.[3] As Maskelyne, the Astronomer Royal, was a dominating member both of the Board of Longitude and of the Council of the Royal Society, there is no doubt that he got what he wanted, in advice, in observers, and in instructions to observers; and in spite of the feeling between himself, who had perfected the lunar system and distrusted machinery, and the clock-makers, who were out to win a prize of £20,000, there is no doubt that the voyage was the vindication of the chronometer, and of that great genius John Harrison.[4] Harrison, who was born in 1693, had given his life to the chronometer, but

[1] It may be scarcely necessary to say that the simplest method of finding the longitude of any place is to find the difference between its local time and the time at some fixed point of reference—e.g. Greenwich. To find this difference one needs a chronometer that will, anywhere it may be, at sea or on land, under any meteorological or marine conditions whatever, go at a uniform rate, and so show Greenwich time exactly. The man who could produce such an instrument, or something near enough to it, could claim the reward offered by the British government in 1714—for a 'generally practicable and useful method' of determining longitude at sea, at the end of a six weeks' voyage, within 60 geographical miles, £10,000; within 40 miles, £15,000; within 30 miles, £20,000. John Harrison was the first person who succeeded in the immensely difficult task of making the instrument needed—and in fact made one a great deal better than was asked for. The same act of Parliament that provided for these rewards set up the Board of Longitude, 'for the discovery of longitude at sea and for examining, trying and judging of all proposals, experiments and improvements relating to the same'. On the general question, see E. G. R. Taylor, *The Haven-Finding Art* (1956), Chap. XI.

[2] See Appendix III, pp. 721–2 below.

[3] See Calendar, pp. 900, 905 below. Weld rather gives a wrong impression of the Society as a moving force when he writes, 'This expedition . . . was strongly recommended to the Government by the Society, and in December, 1771, the Council were officially informed of the Admiralty's intention to send out an expedition, and requested to draw up such instructions and directions as they thought proper.'—*History of the Royal Society* (1848), II, pp. 54–5.

[4] The best brief account is by Lieut.-Commander R. T. Gould, *John Harrison and his Timekeepers* (National Maritime Museum, 1935).

made his way slowly with the Board of Longitude. The fourth chronometer he made, his 'Watch' or 'Watch-machine', had already been tried twice, on voyages to Jamaica, in 1762, and Barbados, in 1764, and had been proved a triumphantly successful piece of mechanism. The Board then settled down to make difficulties over paying the reward, but Harrison did, in 1765, get half of it, on condition of handing over all four models he had made.[1] Of the fourth, an exact duplicate was made by Larcum Kendall, and it was this that went on board the *Resolution* for further trial. Three other chronometers, all made by John Arnold, on principles of his own, were taken on the voyage experimentally, one in the *Resolution* and two in the *Adventure*. These were to go badly and finally all to break down, though Arnold was to do much better in the future. With the Harrison-Kendall instrument the story is different.

Whatever Banks's passion for the pleasing Dr Lind, Maskelyne was determined to have real astronomers in the ships, and he chose men he knew at first hand. William Wales had observed the transit of Venus at Hudson's Bay and helped on the *Nautical Almanac*. William Bayly had observed the transit of Venus at the North Cape and been an assistant at the Royal Observatory. There was no doubt about their capacities. Both were destined to have an important part in naval education; but Wales was the man who did the more varied work, had the more civilized, wide, and at the same time incisive, mind. It may have been a sort of luck that he taught at Christ's Hospital over the years when Charles Lamb and Leigh Hunt were there as pupils, so that he became enshrined in English literature, and we can remember, like Lamb, his Yorkshire accent, his 'constant glee', his severities that were without sting. The pastel portrait by John Russell,[2] one feels, gives us a too much softened Wales, a Wales rather blurred at the edges, fed fat on suburban sweets, who had never been severe or incisive, a Wales hard to reconcile with icebergs or poetry. Yet to read his journal is to be impressed by a personality quite austerely devoted to a fine sense of duty; to read his letters is to find him capable enough of severity in the presence of what he deems inadequate intellectual standards.[3] He noted, with

[1] He did not get the rest till 1773, after petitioning Parliament. He died in 1776, and one is glad that he lived long enough to learn of Cook's report on his work.

[2] Fig. 9 in this volume.

[3] e.g. Wales to Dr Douglas, 30 March 1784, after presenting compliments: 'Has returned the Log, which Capt King sent Last. W.W. has seen many bad reckonings but he thinks few so bad as it contains. He has however made out the track in the best Manner he could from it & Bayley's Book which is as bad as it'.—Eg. MS 2180, f. 187. And again: 'W. Wales presents Compliments to Dr Douglas & returns Forsters Characteres generum Plantarum; out of which he has not been able to extract any information whatever,

resignation, the rule of thumb conservatism of the sailors, and the meddling of midshipmen with his belongings; he registered his amusement at the large pretensions of the senior naturalist. He had a close eye for people and places alike. Yet he carried poetry in his mind—he knew his Thomson and Shakespeare and Milton—and he was humane. If, as one writer thinks, he may have given the young Coleridge the imagery of the *Ancient Mariner*,[1] we can concede that the poet was lucky. It was after the voyage that his severity flamed into the hottest of indignation, over the younger Forster's book, and there was no glee to take away the sting from that. With all this richness Bayly hardly compares; and it is obvious that in Furneaux he had a less sympathetic spirit to deal with than Wales had in Cook.[2]

One of the men Wales got on well with was Hodges, the ten years younger artist. If Zoffany had the qualities necessary for the 'official artist' of this voyage, then Hodges certainly had not; for his interests and capacities were quite different. His interest, as a pupil of Richard Wilson, was landscape, and, more and more as he developed his own individuality in foreign climates, light. He was not, apparently, first choice for the post. Another young man from Wilson's studio, Thomas Jones, told Hodges that he had been approached by 'Mr Stewart (the Athenian, as he was called) in the name of the Dilettanti Society, to go out with Captain Cook in his next voyage':[3] Jones's parents had refused their consent to his going to Italy, but on this proposal they rapidly changed their minds, and Lord Palmerston, also a luminary of culture, threw in his influence on behalf of Hodges. Banks, writing the introduction to the journal of his Iceland voyage, in which once more he relieves his bitterness at some length, remarks that the young man had hurried on board secretly to escape his creditors; but this may be no more than ill-natured gossip.[4] We,

except that they found, in the whole, 75 New Plants: but whether those are all, or any of them, different from such as had been discovered by Mr Banks he cannot learn.—If Dr Douglas has Mattys Book concerning the squabbles in the [Royal] Society, & has read it himself, would thank him for a sight of it. W.W. cannot prevail on himself to lay out half a Crown on it . . .'.—ibid., f. 190–190v.

[1] Bernard Smith, 'Coleridge's *Ancient Mariner* and Cook's Second Voyage', *Journal of Warburg and Courtauld Institutes*, XIX (1956), pp. 117–54.

[2] It may be pointed out, parenthetically, that the astronomers formed a sort of 'set'. Wales, Bayly, and Green, and Wales's 'servant' or assistant, George Gilpin, all worked at some time under Maskelyne at the Royal Observatory. The three first all observed the transit of Venus. Wales married Green's sister. Gilpin married Green's niece. Gilpin followed Wales as secretary to the Board of Longitude.

[3] *Memoirs of Thomas Jones*, Walpole Society, XXXII (1951), p. 37. I owe this reference to Dr Bernard Smith. It may strengthen the connection between Athenian Stuart and Cook suggested below, p. 609, n. 3.

[4] Banks certainly knew neither Hodges's name nor anything about him as an artist. Forster was appointed, he writes, '& soon after M^r^ a young man who had cheifly studied architecture was joind to him as lanscape & figure painter this young man

at a later day, are happily in his debt: on the voyage he worked hard. We should be still happier had he had a talent for the figure; for we greatly lack any rendering of eighteenth-century Pacific peoples unprejudiced by the artist's national idiom, and Hodges in his own sphere was an unprejudiced man. The series of head and shoulder portraits he did are no substitute: the only conviction that some of them carry, indeed, is the conviction that he could not draw, and nothing could be more really lamentable than some of the formal groups put together for him in London, in stale classical poses, for the engravings of the printed *Voyage*. But his landscapes, the rapid drawings in wash of the New Zealand coast outside Dusky Sound, or the extraordinary shapes of sea-worn ice, his small oil sketches, his careful panoramic renderings of island cliffs and shores, these are a different matter. They seemed to Cook, who was an unsophisticated critic of art, to be masterly; and having in mind their purpose, the fundamental literal one, we may be content to follow Cook, if at some distance. There was a poetic Hodges too, the Hodges of light-filled skies and romantic recollection, but that is a different matter again. Gifted, likeable, making the most of his chances, he seems a rather enviable person.

But who is going to envy John Reinhold Forster? We have come to one of the awkward beings of the age, the patently conspicuous phenomenon of the voyage. Let us admit at once, where we can, the virtues of Forster, his learning, the width of his interests, his perceptiveness in some things, the fact that, sunk deep beneath the surface, there was said to be some geniality. Let us admit that the surface itself must have been, at first sight, sometimes impressive—or how else could he have taken in, temporarily, so many excellent persons? Let us concede, as a mitigating factor, that for ocean voyaging no man was ever by physical or mental constitution less fitted. Yet there is nothing that can make him other than one of the Admiralty's vast mistakes. From first to last on the voyage, and afterwards, he was an incubus. One hesitates, in fact, to lay out his characteristics, lest the portrait should seem simply caricature. Dogmatic, humourless, suspicious, pretentious, contentious, censorious, demanding, rheumatic, he was a problem from any angle; to say, with Elliott, that he was 'a clever, but a litigious quarelsom fellow', is to stop far too short; Cook was forced to conclude one interview by turning him

was so much in debt that he was obliged to leave town without acquainting a single soul of where he intended to go, & no sooner was it known that he was at Plimouth than Baylifs were sent down to apprehend him whoom he escaped by keeping continualy on board the ship'.—MS Journal, McGill University Library, p. 5.

out of the cabin, Clerke threatened to put him under arrest, Burr the master's mate knocked him down—and indeed it was not tactful to call Burr a liar; the seas broke over him, men grew tired of listening to him, he was treated summarily; he said, too often, that he would complain to the king, the crew mimicked him. He exasperates us, but he cannot be ignored.

Forster was one of those unsettled men who so often, in the eighteenth century, came to England in search of prosperity; born in 1729 in Polish Prussia, of a family Scottish in origin, growing up a student of languages, history, archaeology, and what passed for philosophy, but with little thought of the natural sciences; diverted from medicine by his father, who thought he ought to be a lawyer, and compromising on theology, and a period of solid old-fashioned orthodoxy as a minister near Danzig. In 1754 he took a cousin for wife, who suffered in that capacity for forty-four years—'an exemplary domestic woman', to quote his biographer,[1] as she had to be; and in that year his son George was born.[2] It was George, a very intelligent boy interested in natural history, who turned his father's mind in the same direction, while, with a growing family, an inadequate living, and a total lack of economy, Reinhold used up his inheritances, and plunged into the debts that became his way of life. In 1765 he got a year's leave of absence from his church, and went with George to St Petersburg, whence he was sent by Count Orlov to make a survey of conditions in the colony of Saratov, on the lower Volga; went, reported, but was not taken into the central administration, waited month after month in vain for the pay that was due to him, refused to consider an academic post, overstayed his leave, and found himself deprived of his ministry. To maintain his family in Danzig, he sold his library, and determined to try his luck, with George, in England. Here he landed in 1766, and found that his Russian travels gave him some useful acquaintances. A position in the North American colonies was offered him: this he declined, to become, instead, Priestley's successor at the Dissenters' academy at Warrington in Lancashire, where he gathered his family again and in July 1767 began to teach French, German and natural history. Here too a pattern was established. His teaching was not appreciated, he had personal friction, and he left in 1768. He left for the

[1] Alfred Dove, in *Allgemeine Deutsche Biographie*, VII (1878).

[2] George is the name as given by Dove, and is presumably to be accepted, not the German form Georg. It was not at all unknown for German families who wanted to be a little 'different' to anglicize the name. In full the boy was called Johann George Adam. Johann Reinhold Forster played tricks with his own name: in England he called himself John Reinhold (which I have adopted), but also, for some reason, John Reinold.

church school in the same town, where he proposed also to give private lessons in—of all things—the science of war. This lasted till the autumn of 1770. Another man of large hopes, Alexander Dalrymple, then invited him to London, to take a post with the East India Company, which Dalrymple did not have to give away. He came—always with George—and Dalrymple was himself dismissed by the Company. For the next two years he drudged in poverty at minor literary work, George simultaneously translating hard (his rendering of Bougainville's voyage was done at this time): producing pamphlets on botany, zoology, mineralogy and geography, plentifully interlarded with quotations in Greek and the oriental languages, supplying George with notes, making natural history excursions, and somehow getting himself known in scientific circles and picking up patrons—picking up, even, an F.R.S.[1]

Then came his chance. Banks, Solander, Lind all left the expedition; and Parliament had voted £4000 for the support of a scientific man. Relinquished by Lind, where would the sum descend? At this moment Daines Barrington stepped in, that 'worthy and learned gentleman', lawyer, antiquary and naturalist, but more important perhaps, a man with one brother a highly thought of post captain in the navy, another a bishop, a third secretary at war: a friend of Banks, but not a blind friend, and a friend of Lord Sandwich.[2] Forster himself was an embarrassing friend, with his assorted learning, his self-confidence, his complaints, his persistence, and his improvidence; and Barrington made what might be considered a master-stroke—he got the £4000 for Forster.[3] It would provide for him, and inevitably, for George as his assistant; it would provide

[1] He was elected 27 February 1772. His certificate of candidature was signed by Banks, Solander, Daines Barrington, and eight others.

[2] The Hon. Daines Barrington (1727–1800), F.R.S., fourth son of the first Viscount Barrington. The quotation is from Boswell's *Johnson*, III, p. 314. At this time he was a county judge (Jeremy Bentham spoke highly of him, but not as a judge), with very wide interests and a large number of friends, from Gilbert White of Selborne to Bishop Percy and Dr Johnson. His *Observations on the Statutes* (1766) gave him some fame; his tracts on the possibility of reaching the North Pole gave him some importance in the history of exploration, and lay behind the northern voyage of Phipps in 1773. Forster, for the time, was all gratitude. He wrote to Thomas Pennant, 23 June 1772, 'Mr Barrington has done more in this affair, than a father could have done'.—*Banks Papers*, Mitchell Library, X3. And again, 19 November 1772, from the Cape, 'I am not a Man to hide knowledge from the learned world, but I will be repaid in the Friendship & esteem of my Friends, among whom You are next to Mr Barrington the First'.—ibid., Y1–2. He named the beautiful flowering tree *Barringtonia speciosa* (the Tahitian *hutu*) after his benefactor.

[3] A number of writers have made play with Cook's printed statement (*Voyage*, I, p. xxxiv) that Forster and his son were 'pitched upon' for employment as naturalists, finding something contemptuous in the phrase. But there was in the eighteenth century nothing contemptuous about it—it merely meant to choose. Johnson illustrates it with Tillotson's 'Pitch upon the best course of life, and custom will render it easy'. The sense of casual selection is quite modern.

amply for the exemplary woman and the family left behind for three years; and such a voyage, if Forster were the man he made himself out to be, must inevitably be the prelude to better things. Poor Barrington, like a good many other people at this time, was deceived. He did not sufficiently know his man. How Forster got through the thousands is a mystery, like most of his financial dealings; but the voyage was scarcely over before he proclaimed himself ill-paid as well as ill-used.[1] Even taking into account his needless engagement of Sparrman at the Cape as an assistant, the sum, though not as good as Hawkesworth's £6000, compared very favourably with Wales's £400 a year, and Cook's 6s a day. Having said so much about this abusive, and naturally much-abused man, it is only fair to let him speak for himself, even at some length; and if he speaks through his son, in print, it gives him the advantage of making a deliberate and measured statement, rather than such furiously extravagant remarks as form the substance of so many of his unpublished letters.[2]

'It will not be improper to acquaint the reader, that we were so situated on board the Resolution, as to meet with obstacles in all our researches, from those who might have been expected to give us all manner of assistance. It has always been the fate of science and philosophy to incur the contempt of ignorance, and this we might have suffered without repining; but as we could not purchase the good will of every petty tyrant with gold, we were studiously debarred the means of drawing the least advantage to science from the observations of others, who of themselves did not know how to make the proper use of a discovery when they had made it. Circumstances which were known to every person around us, remained impenetrable mysteries to us; and it was assuredly not owing to the good nature of our shipmates, if we have been fortunate enough to obtain even such trifling information, as has enabled me to give the true and exact situations of every place in this narrative, and in my chart. If it had been possible, they would have deceived even our eyes. It may seem extraordinary, that men of science, sent out in a ship belonging to the most enlightened nation in the world, should be cramped and deprived of the means of pursuing knowledge, in a manner which would only become a set of barbarians; but it is certain, that the traveller who visits the ruins of Egypt and Palestine, cannot experience greater mortification from the ignorant selfishness of Bedouins and other Arabs, than fell to our lot; since

[1] He began to lament, indeed, before the voyage. He wrote to Pennant, 23 June 1772, 'I get 4000£ for this Expedition, but 1500 go for the Equipment, which on acc[t] of its suddenness is very expensive'.—*Banks Papers*, Mitchell Library, X1. I frankly disbelieve this £1500 story. What equipment could he have possibly bought that made up that sum? Even Banks, after spending money lavishly for months, had bills amounting to less than £2200.

[2] Among, for example, the Sandwich Papers, Hinchingbrooke; or the Banks Papers in the Mitchell Library.

every discovery we attempted to make, was supposed to contain a treasure, which became the object of envy. The world will, however, derive one advantage from this proceeding; we shall have little to offer, but what we have seen with our own eyes, and for the truth and precision of which we can be answerable. If there had not been a few individuals of a more liberal way of thinking, whose disinterested love for the sciences comforted us from time to time, we should in all probability have fallen victims to that malevolence, which even the positive commands of captain Cook were sometimes insufficient to keep within bounds.'[1]

With these heavy charges Wales dealt in his *Remarks* on George's book, pertinently but not very respectfully. To traverse them now would do no good. It can only be said that Forster's demands on other people were very great, his ideas of his own rights extreme, his ability to compromise little; and his opinion of his own virtues permanent.[2] Knowing what Cook had suffered from the natural historians of this voyage, potential or actual, one need not refuse to believe a later story, even if it has passed through the hands of Forster. When Lieutenant King was appointed to the *Resolution* for the third voyage, he called on the captain to pay his respects, and he added his regret that there were no scientists going on the expedition. He was startled to hear Cook reply, 'Curse the scientists, and all science into the bargain!' 'This discourteous reply so shocked Mr King that he repeated it to me the next day,' writes Forster, 'and his respect for the man under whose command he was to sail was considerably diminished until I took the opportunity of setting things right by describing Cook's character and pointing out that it was in reality not so bad as it appeared, but that he was a cross-grained fellow who sometimes showed a mean disposition and was carried away by a hasty temper; and to this was added the overbearing attitude which was the result of having his head turned by Lord Sand-

[1] This is a note in George Forster's *Voyage*, II, p. 420. The passage which stimulates it is as follows (pp. 419–20): 'One of the surgeon's mates, who went on this excursion, collected a prodigious variety of new and curious shells upon the island of Ballabeea, and likewise met with many new species of plants, of which we did not see a single specimen in the districts we had visited; but the meanest and most unreasonable envy taught him to conceal these discoveries from us, though he was utterly incapable of making use of them for the benefit of science'. This monster of envy and ignorance could only have been William Anderson, whose version we should like to have.

[2] To strive visibly for justice once more, however, one may quote from one of Solander's letters to Banks: 'Mr Forster overwhelms me with civilities upon your account. He is of all men I know either the most open or the greatest fool. He certainly has made some clever remarks during the Voyage; but he talks rather too much of them. You cannot imagine how much the Man is mended since he came home: the Officers say they hardly know the Man. He came home thinking himself very great—now he, like Bruce, is reduced even in his own opinion'.—5 September 1775, *Banks Papers*, British Museum (Natural History), Botany Library, I, p. 98. Bruce was the Abyssinian traveller. The reduction in opinion could not have lasted very long.

wich. . . . On his first voyage Cook was accompanied by Banks and Solander, who were the representatives of science and art (*emollit mores nec finit esse feros*); and on the second voyage I and my son accompanied him and were his daily companions at table and elsewhere. He therefore of necessity acquired through our presence a greater respect and reverence for his own character and good name. Our mode of thought, our principles, and our habits had their effect upon him in the course of time through having them constantly before his notice . . .'.[1]

We have, unfortunately, in Cook no parallel statement of the civilizing influence thus brought to bear upon his life, unless we are to take his remark to King as an adequate summary. Of Forster as a maritime character enough has perhaps now been made. Nor is it really necessary here to go into the complications of his later years—even those immediately following the voyage—the debts, the dunning, the denunciations, the attacks on Sandwich and Cook, the long uneasy academic sequel at Halle; the long list of discarded friends, or friends forced to discard him—the good Barrington included. It requires a great deal of charity to feel that the story is melancholy, and not merely tedious.

Yet one might still scrape up some charity towards Forster if he had not ruined George. He exploited George, and that was shameful; but it did not matter so much, and it could be argued that George had a duty to help support his family. One must remember, too, that the father gave full scope to the son's early botanical leaning, and was in fact himself the one to be influenced. Nevertheless for half of George's too short life the heavy paternal figure weighed him down, determining his work and his words—or most of them—and his fate. Occasionally George could substitute a word. In 1787 he wrote from Vilna, that 'savage and dreary retreat', where he was a professor, to Thomas Pennant the naturalist. He was quite out of touch with his old friends and patrons.

'Perhaps even in this respect, as in many others, my fortunes have been influenced by the unsuccessful career of my father. In that case I have only the satisfaction of recollecting, that whilst I acted under his direction and by his positive order, the offence I might give, was involuntary, for which, if I now suffer, I stand acquitted in my own mind. Nay, I may add with some share of self-approbation, that by taking it upon me to plead

[1] This extract is from Forster's preface to the Berlin edition (1781) of Rickman's anonymous account of the third voyage (*Journal of Captain Cook's last Voyage to the Pacific Ocean, on Discovery*, London 1781), which was eagerly bought, and translated into German at once. I have quoted from the version by Miss U. Tewsley, appended to her translation of Zimmermann's *Reise um die Welt* (Wellington 1926), pp. 48–9.

my father's cause on several occasions, the poignancy of his invectives was in many instances mitigated by passing through my pen, though I could not prevent the admission of many severe expressions, which exasperated his adversaries, and hurt the justice of his plea in the eye of the unprejudiced.'[1]

To be the voice of John Reinhold Forster was a demoralizing training for any young man; and though in the end George broke from his father, he remained a divided personality, a man without a will. On shipboard men discriminated between them—Elliott remembered George as 'a clever, good young man'; and it may have been, partly, the remembrance of this goodness also that made it impossible for Wales to believe that George, with all his cleverness, wrote the Forster history of the voyage.

Before he went on the voyage George, as we have seen, had been his father's constant companion. He was a boy serious and intellectually alive, with a brilliant gift for languages as well as a taste for natural history observation, but physically never robust. His first ten years were his happiest: then, with little formal education but great capacity for assimilation, came the period of indigent following at his father's heels, a short unsuccessful too hard-worked apprenticeship to a London merchant, a short pupilage at the Dissenters' academy at Warrington; then language teaching (he was still only 14 or 15) to assist Reinhold, and the Grub Street years of translating travel books. To him, four months short of his eighteenth year, the voyage must have come as a release; and it certainly released and developed his mind. George's mind was that of a romantic, by some odd switch of endowment south German rather than Prussian in character. But his early lack of training left him with too many of the defects of the romantic: with great capacities, he remained superficial; his enthusiasms wilted; his attempts at stability foundered. Like his father, he tended to collect academic degrees and memberships of learned bodies as a substitute for real ambition. He wrote much, and influenced the development of German prose, but nevertheless remained a writer of the second rank.[2] He strongly influenced the work of one

[1] George Forster to Pennant, 5 March 1787; *Banks Papers*, Mitchell Library, Z 1–2, Another passage in this letter gives one aspect of the truth about J. R. Forster very well: 'You know him too well, you know his active mind, his fiery temper, his contempt for money and his perpetual want of it, the very consequence of his not setting a just value upon it, in short, you know that the situation can hardly be imagined, where he might be said to be perfectly at his ease and in the enjoyment of real happiness'.—'He still owes Sir Joseph Banks £250', George continues, and goes on (the typical Forster touch) to attack Banks for thinking the sum should be repaid.

[2] Thought worth reprinting, however, as recently as 1954; but in East Germany, and for his revolutionary sentiments rather than for his prose.—Gerhard Steiner and Manfred Häckel (eds.), *Forster: Ein Lesebuch für unsere Zeit* (Weimar, Thüringer Volksverlag). A

great man, Alexander von Humboldt. With less dissipation of his talents, he might have been a seminal force in the thought of his whole country. But real force, real independence he showed only for a few brief months as a leader of the Rhineland revolution in 1793; and his death in Paris, shortly after his thirty-ninth birthday, was that of a solitary and neglected man. It cannot be said, thinking of his precocious youth and his premature death, that George Forster did everything too early; because in the interim, when he might have risen to some real height, he tended to do nothing till he had to. We have, however, passed far beyond the *Resolution*, and we must continue to think of George as youthful, clever, good, hard-working, full of interest at the novel and astounding world, doing his best to smooth over the difficulties that arose daily between his shipmates and his uncomfortable parent, the amiable in attendance on unamiability.

That last phrase may characterize, too, Anders Sparrman, the young Swedish graduate from the university and the hands of Linnaeus, to whose presence Cook recurs only as the victim of misfortune; clever and steady, a little prim, a little upset by swearing, an ardent collector, interested in food and drink and in the habits of sailors, not at all a controversial figure. Nothing one knows about him tells against him; and for that very reason, perhaps, neutral among these natural historians he seems a point of rest.

§ *The Voyage*

The voyage is to be seen in terms of Cook's plan. But the plan is broad, and the journal is large, and one may best understand the happenings of those three years through a preliminary analysis. One may thus take the passage to the Cape and the time spent there, 13 July–22 November 1772, as a prologue; and the refitting at the Cape and the passage home, 22 March–29 July 1775, as an epilogue. From November 1772 to March 1775 the great achievement unrolls in five sections, as three 'ice-edge cruises' into the Antarctic, broken by two sweeps into the tropics, which are pinned on Queen Charlotte Sound in New Zealand as base, and, in the islands, on Tahiti-Huahine-Raiatea. Between the second tropical sweep and the last antarctic cruise is the sort of 'bridge-passage' across the South Pacific

monumental edition of his collected works, to be published at Leipzig, is also in preparation. Dove, op. cit., remarks that George's introduction to the German edition of Cook's third voyage (1787) was a particularly fine piece of writing: 'one of the soundest and at the same time most popular essays in the whole of our literature'.

from New Zealand to Tierra del Fuego and the Horn. We thus have, in broad terms chronologically:

(1) First ice-edge cruise (Atlantic-Indian Ocean sector), December 1772–March 1773
New Zealand (Dusky Sound and Queen Charlotte Sound), April–May 1773

(2) First tropical sweep (Tuamotus, Tahiti and Society Islands, Tonga), June–October 1773
Queen Charlotte Sound, November 1773

(3) Second ice-edge cruise (Pacific sector), November 1773–February 1774

(4) Second tropical sweep (Easter Island, Marquesas, Tuamotus, Tahiti and Society Islands, Niue, Tonga, New Hebrides, New Caledonia, Norfolk), February–October 1774
Queen Charlotte Sound, October–early November 1774
Passage to Tierra del Fuego, November–December 1774

(5) Third ice-edge cruise (Atlantic sector), January–February 1775.

Each of these five divisions has its own points of crisis or dramatic interest; of geographical interest almost always; in the islands, of extreme anthropological interest. The three southern cruises were a systematic attack on the main, the continental, problem; the two northern sweeps and the interludes at base give us so much that at times we forget that the voyage was an antarctic voyage at all. Indeed, between leaving the Cape in 1772 and arriving there again in 1775, considerably less than half the time was spent in latitudes south of New Zealand. But that is irrelevant, except purely as a note of time, as a bare fact of the voyage as a whole. The important thing is the nature of the experience. Yet one must not underrate the experience of the islands. The second northern sweep alone would have rendered a man memorable in the history of exploration, both as consolidation of earlier discovery and—by far the more important part—quite new discovery, across the boundary of Polynesia into the Melanesian area of the ocean. In following Tasman and Quiros, Cook clarifies, makes precise; in going beyond them, his charts are, for essential purposes, clarity itself.

These things were in the future. The immediate passage was the passage to the Cape, calling at Madeira and the Canaries. It might be regarded as routine, but is not without interest. Cook lost one man overboard, which was a fair hazard of the sea; and Furneaux two by sickness, which a proper hygiene would probably have prevented. Wales began to measure the temperature of the sea; the 'watch-machines' were carefully tended and observed, and though Cook was far from reposing the faith in one of them that he later did, already on 2 September, noting the effect of the currents on the ship's position, he could say that it was such as 'Mr Kendalls watch tought us to expect'. The experiments with diet began, in the brewing of beer from his 'inspissated juice of malt'. It was a shaking-down period for the crews, and we have an entry in Pickersgill's log that indicates that he at least was shaken. Cook had evidently put up a notice, because Pickersgill begins, 'Public Log Book Copy, "The Cask of Beer on Deck ordred to be Bung'd up so that no one must drink no more to night."—capts hand underneath'. And the first lieutenant had given the reason, 'because the Officer of the Watch Permited it to run about the Decks'.

'an Observation [our diarist proceeds] as Erronious as unjust I say for myself R-P-l. This Occaison'd a little dispute in the Ship therefore it will not be improper to speak of it. As an Officer I never saw it run about the Deck's nor ever heard that it did till this: as a Purser the Captn knew how to Prolong it which he endeavours to do till Past 12 in order to save the days allowance of wine by the Ships Company—this was seen thro by the People who drank it out as soon or nearly as soon as it was broch'd which Baulk'd the Affair—The Beer was Experimental beer sent out by Goverment to make trial of and not King's Allowance. Querry wheather they had not a right to wine and beer both; or wheather Goverm^t^ design'd it as a Perquesit to the Purser'.[1]

There is more to be got from this than an impression of righteous indignation (Pickersgill himself may have been the officer of the watch in question). Water would not keep fresh at sea; the water taken on at Porto Praya, we know from Clerke, was none of the best; and Cook thought it worth while to try the 'experimental beer' at once. He evidently put out a cask for the day in lieu of, or in addition to, the 'scuttle'—the cask of water on deck to which everyone had free access—and for one reason or another, it went too fast. To withhold beer from thirsty men, argued the sea-lawyers, was not fair; and this beer, being experimental, must of necessity be additional to the usual allowance.[2] Pursers were notoriously given to lining their own pockets at the seaman's expense; but it is odd to see the accusation levelled against Cook, in his capacity as purser, and odd to see it levelled by Pickersgill, who knew him. Cook knew his men, how-

[1] 17 September 1772, with the note, 'This Circumstance happend next day', so that indignation caused him to misplace his entry.
[2] Cf. Calendar, pp. 927, 928–9, 6 and 11 May.

ever: we have ample evidence that he knew how to humour them, and how to make a punishment fit a crime: he tried the beer, he kept the ship dry and aired and the ship's company clean, and when they reached the Cape more than one officer remarked on the fact that everybody was healthy and in good spirits. The contrast was seen in the Dutch ships that arrived from Europe shortly afterwards.

At the Cape Cook could once more consider what he was to look for. His instructions ran, 'You are, if possible, to leave the Cape of Good Hope by the end of October or beginning of November next, and proceeding to the southward, endeavour to fall in with Cape Circumcision . . .'. He could not leave the Cape of Good Hope at the stated time, but this was secondary. The position of Cape Circumcision was given as latitude ('nearly') 54° South, and longitude ('about') 11° 20′ East of Greenwich. It was something Cook could never find, and it may be remarked upon here. It existed, though as the point of a very small island and not of a continent, and the fact that Bouvet found it himself is one of the most remarkable chances in the history of discovery.[1] He was a French East India Company captain, who was anxious to give the Company what it much needed, a base for refreshment on the voyage to and from the East, which would not, like the Cape, be snatched away in time of war. His cogitations took him to the land which the French Sieur de Gonneville was said to have discovered in the South Atlantic in 1504, an agreeable land—possibly in hard fact the southern coast of Brazil, but placed in theory wherever the geographers wanted it; and in Bouvet's mind south, but not too far south, of the Cape, in a latitude which, going on the analogy of northern hemisphere latitudes, must be quite pleasant. The Company gave him two ships, the *Aigle* and *Marie*. He left Lorient in July 1738, and after touching at Santa Catharina, an island on the coast of Brazil, was far south, in the supposed neighbourhood of Gonneville's land, in November. That summer the ice was exceptionally far north—and the presence of ice, it was then held, with seaweed, seals and penguins, argued the nearness of land—and in conditions made dangerous by fog, as well as bergs and pack ice, Bouvet cruised for some weeks. On 1 January 1739, the day of the feast of the Circumcision, he sighted out of the fog his high snow-bound cape—rocky, desolate, rising sheer from the sea, flanked

[1] To quote Gould, 'Striking southward at a venture, he happened to fall in with a small, glaciated island, not five miles across, which is the most isolated spot in the whole world. It is possible to draw, round Bouvet island, a circle with a radius of 1000 miles—having an area equal to that of Europe—which contains no other land at all. It is the only spot on the earth's surface possessing this peculiarity'.—*Captain James Cook*, p. 111. See also Gould's notes on Bouvet Island, in *Oddities* (London 1944), pp. 136–40.

by glaciers and overhung by a massive ice-cap. He could not land; it could not be determined, even after ten days in the vicinity, whether the cape was part of a continent or an island (though his chief pilot was quite convinced it was only a very small island); and after sailing south to 57°, and 400 leagues eastward along the ice-edge in that latitude, Bouvet turned north-east as far as about 38°.[1] Thence, perforce, he steered homewards. Though the nature of Cape Circumcision might be dubious, he was convinced that beyond the great coast of ice must be the coast of the continent. This sub-antarctic voyage was a notable one, on the edge of the Antarctic if not in it; and Cook, who was to experience the same sort of conditions, though for much longer, came to have a great respect for Bouvet.

Bouvet gave the position of the Cape as latitude 54° 10′–15′, longitude between 27° and 28° east of Teneriffe (i.e. something like the Admiralty's 11° 20′) by dead reckoning from Santa Catharina. Under the conditions of his cruise, his dead reckoning cannot be called bad, but it suffered from the initial disadvantage that his longitude for Santa Catharina was 4° 20′ too far east. Correction for that error would have given him 5° 17′ east of Greenwich—which was still nearly two degrees from the truth.[2] The position of Bouvet Island—for it was an authentic island and neither a continent nor an iceberg—is latitude 54° 26′ S, 3° 24′ E. The Admiralty longitude was reckoned from Greenwich and not from Paris, and the difference of almost seven degrees between it and reality made a vast difference to Cook's chances of finding anything. The island, of which Cape Circumcision is the north-western extremity, extends only 5 miles from east to west, and 4¼ from north to south, an ice- and snow-covered speck which was not seen again for almost seventy years after Bouvet, and which scientific navigators still refused to believe in a hundred years after. But there the report was: credible, because Bouvet had not simply glimpsed something between the clouds and sailed instantly away; and if there was a cape, why then not a continent?

There were other accounts, rather garbled, of French voyages picked up by Cook at Cape Town; and one of these provided him with a new problem to be looked at on his own voyage. This was Kerguelen's foray (it can hardly be called much more) southwards from Mauritius; he, it was said, had found land in latitude 48°, and had rather basely left to perish a boat's crew lost in the fog. The latter

[1] i.e. 55° east of Teneriffe, to go on his own reckoning.

[2] It must be added that the figures one finds given for Bouvet in different places tend to plunge one into confusion. Burney, *Chronological History*, V (1817), p. 34, says the *Aigle*'s journal made the position lat. 54° S and long. 53° 45′ east from Santa Catharina, equal to 4° 30′ E of Greenwich—which argues very good dead reckoning indeed.

part of the story, put nakedly, may have been a libel, and Cook himself does not mention it in this form; but Kerguelen, through the strange extravagance of his enthusiasm at finding land at all, was none the less drawn into disgrace. He was a Breton nobleman who had built up for himself a visionary picture of Gonneville's country, and prevailed on the Crown to give him two ships, the *Fortune* and *Gros Ventre*, with which to rediscover it. Sailing from Mauritius on 16 January 1772, he did sight land—a small island on 12 February and next day something more extensive. The latitude was nearer 50° than 48°, the longitude about 70° E, fifteen degrees east of Mauritius.[1] The two ships were separated by a storm. Kerguelen himself could not get ashore, but his second in command, the Comte de St Allouarne, of the *Gros Ventre*, managed to land in 'Sea-Lion Bay' and annex 'la France Australe'. In spite of sea-lions and the dangers of tempest and fog, Kerguelen hastened back to France with a preposterously-coloured report of 'the central mass of the Antarctic continent', which must, he thought, produce all the crops of the corresponding latitude in the northern hemisphere (almost that of the Scillies), together with all the minerals and precious stones and men of the traditional Terra Australis. There was scepticism among his compatriots: nevertheless Kerguelen managed to get two more ships with which to return to the continent, establish a post, and consolidate his discovery by an eastward coasting voyage. He sailed in March 1773, and reached 'la France Australe' again in December of that year, when Cook was far to the east and south, only to find complete disillusion: cold, tempest, and sterility which made him change his name of Southern France to the Land of Desolation; and no continent but an island. It was impossible to leave men there, it was impossible with the sick and feeble men he commanded to explore further; there was nothing for Kerguelen to do but face the other misery of returning and confessing his ineptitude—which, to those at home, was not condoned by his endurance and his real, though limited, achievement. Cook, coming to the southern scene between these two voyages, found little to go upon—it was not until his homeward passage that he got explicit and reliable information: in the meanwhile there was this new continental rumour to be verified or disproved.

The other story Cook heard at the Cape was that of Marc Macé Marion du Fresne,[2] who had set out to take back to Tahiti the young

[1] Kerguelen's longitude, 61° 10′ E of Paris (63° 30′ E of Greenwich) was seriously out.

[2] I give here the correct names of this captain, on which I have erred, like practically everybody else, in the index to Volume I. I owe the correction to the researches of Mr

Ahutoru, the Tahitian brought to Paris by Bougainville. Ahutoru had died before Marion reached the Cape from Mauritius, his starting point; and probably Marion, during his stay at the Cape in December 1771, gave wrong information upon his route into the Pacific ('to proceed round Cape Horn after touching upon the Coast of Brazil'), because his instructions too were to visit the Southern Continent, and New Zealand, on the way. He was a good sailor, active, brave, with a marked lack of discretion, and he did not see Tahiti. For Cook he was a name that vanished on the ocean, to be caught up with, deceptively, at Tahiti, and to come into full view, at last, only at the Cape again in 1775, through his second in command, Crozet. In the meanwhile Marion had made his own discoveries in the southern ocean. Sailing from the Cape on 28 December 1771 and going south-east, on 13 January he discovered two small islands in the Prince Edward group (about 46° 50′ S, 37° 30′–38° E), the larger of which he called *Terre d'Espérance*—his hope being that the continent lay close by. He did not care to become entangled in the ice further south, so turned east, to find, on 23 January, the Crozet group, like the others high and snow-clad. These he called after his second in command; and then, with rather damaged ships, he made for Van Diemen's Land, passing north of the island that Kerguelen, a few days later, was in his turn to sight, and so strangely to rejoice in.

Cook was to validate and co-ordinate all these discoveries, though not on his present voyage—with one exception. The exception was the only one for which he had a position; precisely what else he had heard or read about Bouvet's voyage we do not know.[1] Meanwhile, having completed his stores, and reorganized his officers after the departure of poor Shank from the *Adventure*, on 23 November 1772 he sailed south, directing his course for Cape Circumcision.

(I) THE FIRST ICE-EDGE CRUISE[2]

Whatever Cook found in the Southern Ocean, he was sure to find ice: ice on the grand scale, awe-inspiring, whether the pack or the tabular iceberg, and the iceberg whether early in its drift or in its

J. D. Dunmore. The Marions in Brittany who had some connection with the seigneury of du Fresne have only recently been disentangled.

[1] Presumably he knew the brief account in Callander's *Terra Australis Cognita* (1768), III, pp. 641–4, a translation of the abstract given by de Brosses, II, pp. 255–9. Nothing fuller appeared in English until Dalrymple's *Collection of Voyages chiefly in the Southern Atlantic Ocean*, 1775. Dalrymple's account (a journal) came from D'Après de Mannevillette, the hydrographer to the French navy. He draws the track in his chart of the Southern Ocean of 1769: Cook had both this and the accompanying memoir.

[2] I repeat here my acknowledgments of the work of Dr H. F. P. Herdman on the antarctic portions of the journal, which I have incorporated in this introduction.

fantastic decay. He must certainly have met with sea ice before—very likely in the Baltic, no doubt on the Newfoundland and Nova Scotian coasts—although he says nothing about it: Wales in Hudson's Bay, and one or two of his men in the Greenland fishery, had had more experience. Some of his readers therefore have found it a little difficult to understand the apparent indifference with which he records his first encounters with both the antarctic bergs and pack ice. They come into the journals as quietly as if Cook had been among them all his life: he says little about the dimensions of the bergs, he says little about ice as a hazard; he is, as a rule, more descriptive about birds and animals. On the other hand, by the time one has arrived at the end of the journal one has no doubt that his mind was stirred, and while there are pages on which he almost ignores the presence of ice, the comments that, after due thought, he does make are extremely pertinent: comments for example both on its origin and on its movement. He built up his knowledge gradually, and to the modern student he gives some very interesting information. We are now aware of much concerning the distribution of the antarctic pack, especially in the summer months, while for most months of the year it has been possible to suggest a mean northern limit. On every occasion when Cook met pack ice, the northern edge lay within what might be called striking distance of the mean suggested by Mackintosh and Herdman in 1940.[1] That the actual northern limit varies from year to year is now an established fact: even in mid-winter, when it might not unreasonably be expected to remain fairly constant for some time, varying conditions of wind and temperature can alter the position of the ice-edge in one night. A temporary shift of a hundred miles or more has been recorded over a period of two and a half months.[2] The modern student, therefore, who through Cook can carry his observations back almost two hundred years, can also throw some light on phenomena that Cook found surprising, and sometimes distressing. In the higher latitudes, to give further examples, beyond 60° S, the prevailing wind is not westerly, but easterly; so that the grand strategy of the west to east voyage was not necessarily, in those latitudes, the best one. If Cook had known about the resultant currents set up by these winds, the West Wind Drift and the East Wind Drift, he could have answered more easily some of the questions that puzzled him. If he had known about the Antarctic Convergence—but there were so many things

[1] N. A. Mackintosh and H. F. P. Herdman, 'Distribution of the Pack Ice in the Southern Ocean', *Discovery Reports*, XIX (1940), pp. 285–96, pls. LXIX–XCV.

[2] H. F. P. Herdman, 'The Antarctic Pack Ice in Winter', *Journal of Glaciology*, 2, No. 13 (1953), pp. 184–93.

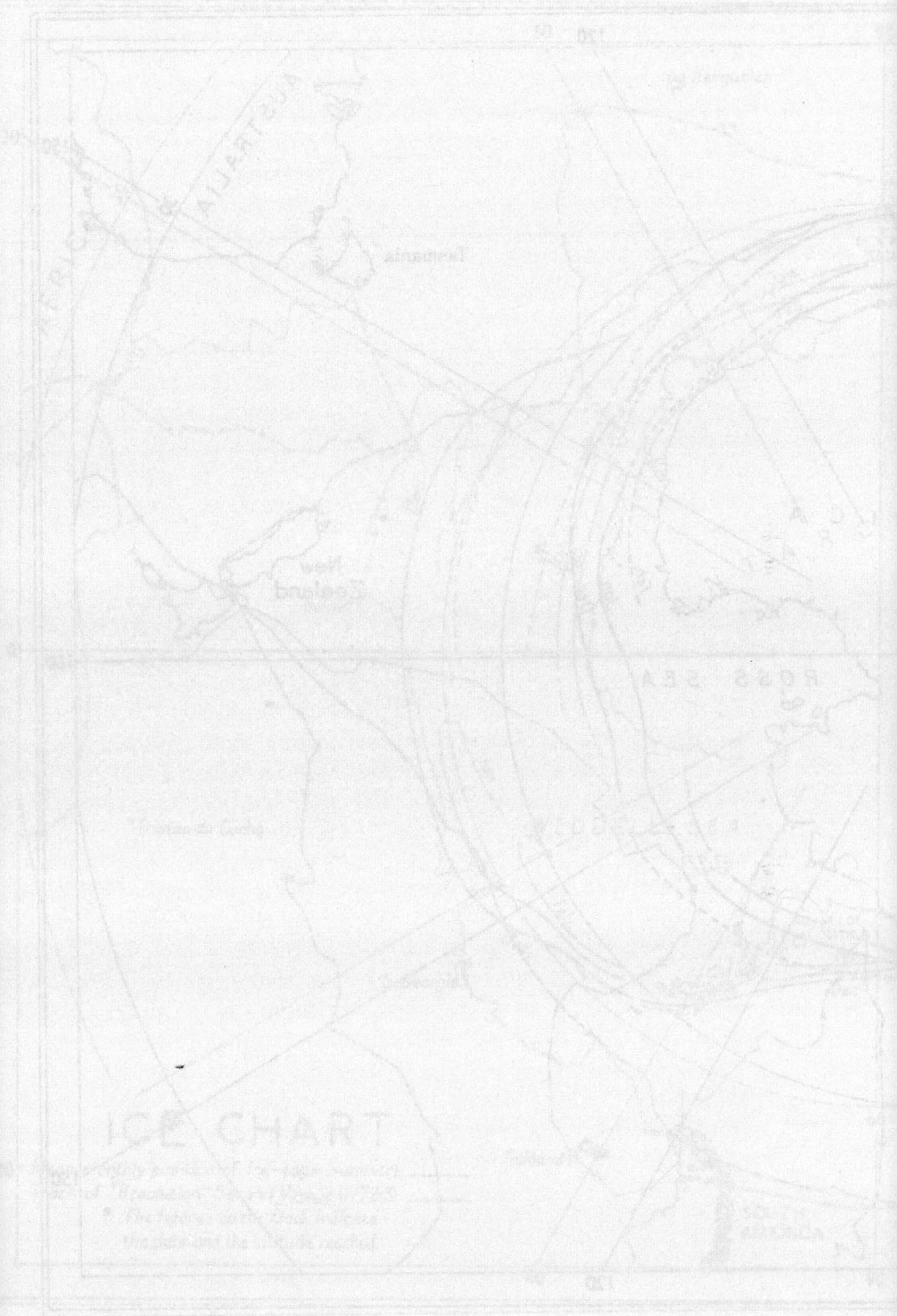

that he did not know, which he would have had no comfort in knowing, as he struggled through that icy, fog-stricken sea. There were some, certainly, that would have helped him.

The first 'ice island' recorded in the journal was on 10 December in lat. 50° 57′ S, long. 20° 45′ E, and it was a rather striking coincidence, and a fitting conclusion to the work in the Southern Ocean, that the last one seen, slightly over three years later, was in lat. 52° 52′ S, long. 26° 31′ E, not far away. Cook appears to have used the term 'Ice Island' to describe any type of iceberg, whether tabular in shape or not. It is a descriptive term, very applicable to the sometimes immense tabular bergs of antarctic waters (one has been recorded more than 100 miles long and 30 miles wide), but nowadays reserved for a rare form of iceberg found only in the Arctic.[1] The term 'tabular berg' is now used to describe any iceberg—no matter what its size—which has had its origin in shelf ice; and it is very likely, considering the date and the position, that the first berg sighted from the *Resolution* was a tabular one. Since the position lies well within the influence of the very cold surface water flowing away to the north and east from the Weddell Sea it is reasonably certain that the icebergs seen by Cook had their origin in the ice shelf of this sea. Pieces of shelf ice breaking away during the summer would not have reached water warm enough to melt them, before being imprisoned in the swift northerly advance of the pack ice in winter. Remaining thus inactive during the winter months, but moving generally in an easterly direction with the main body of pack, they would have had little chance to melt after the break-up of the pack in late November.

The two ships continued to the south despite bad weather conditions, strong westerly winds and poor visibility, due to snow and fog, which made it difficult at times to avoid the numerous bergs. Fog, in conjunction with strong winds, is very prevalent in these latitudes, especially in the vicinity of the Antarctic Convergence, which is the line of demarcation (by no means a straight one) between antarctic and sub-antarctic waters. Here it is that the cold antarctic water sinks below the warmer waters of the sub-antarctic zone, causing an abrupt change in the surface temperature. Nevertheless, on 14 December they fell in with the pack ice, in lat. 54° 55′ S, long. 22° 13′ E, some 120 miles north of the mean northern limit for the month but only 60 miles north of the position where it was found on 12 December in 1938. Here they were stopped 'by an

[1] Terence Armstrong and Brian Roberts, 'Illustrated Ice Glossary', *Polar Record*, 8, No. 52 (1956), pp. 4–12.

immence field of Ice to which we could see no end'. Influenced no doubt by the prevailing winds, and hoping to get round this field of ice, Cook proceeded along its edge south-easterly. The edge trended SSE, SE and SE by S during the remainder of the day, but on 15 December, after steering SE, the ships turned a point and hauled SSW, as there appeared to be clear water in that direction. It was not long, however, before they found themselves embayed and were forced away to the north and east before clearing the ice. A surface temperature taken while they were standing off for the night is recorded as 30° F. Little movement was possible the next day, on account of fog and snow, but on the 17th Cook was again steering south, until in a short time heavy pack ice once more stopped him. The pack was obviously breaking up fast, since many bergs and much loose ice were found to seaward of the main body, but there still remained an impenetrable body of ice to the south.

The ships thus continued on 18 December in an easterly direction along the edge, much hampered by an even greater number of icebergs and quantities of loose ice. Cook, that day, comments on the serenity of the weather as a rare event. He was right—by the next morning the normal ice-edge conditions of fog and strong winds once more prevailed. Seldom is the weather good near to seaward of pack ice—due, no doubt, to the difference in sea and air temperatures, especially when the winds are westerly and blowing off warmer water. Inside the pack, as many expeditionary ships have found, the weather is often fine and clear, but Cook—not without good reason—did not attempt to force a passage inside. On this same day he comments, for the first time since he met the antarctic pack ice, on the dangers of navigation in these waters. He preferred to navigate among icebergs—even in thick fog—to the danger, as he thought, of being frozen in, with almost certain damage to the ships. He also attempts to compare conditions with those of the Greenland ice—of which he himself had no experience. He was not to know, however, that the pack was then breaking up, and that from late December until early April the waters in which he was sailing are cleared of pack ice. But at this time the break-up had obviously only just begun. The ice-edge (as we have seen) lay well north of the mean position now tolerably well established in this region (and we have little reason to think that the mean has shifted significantly since Cook's day), and icebergs were not sighted in December 1772 until the *Resolution* was well south of the mean northern limit of bergs for this month. Many bergs, of course, are to be found throughout the summer months, because, with the rapid retreat of the ice edge to the south, they are constantly being freed and move east and north under the influence of the prevailing winds and currents. Cook had already remarked on 'High hills or rather Mountains' which he had seen 'within this Field Ice'.

Observations over the years since that time have shown that the incidence of icebergs in antarctic and sub-antarctic waters is probably greatest in the Atlantic and western Indian Ocean sectors, due to the diversion of the surface current system of the Weddell Sea by the long east coast of Graham Land and the southern section of a submarine ridge which, passing through the South Orkney and South Sandwich Islands, finally connects the volcanic mountains of Antarctica with the Andes in South America.[1] The very cold water from the Weddell Sea is thus forced north and, finally, north-east to join the current called the West Wind Drift, which persists around Antarctica, in all seasons, in the region of the prevailing westerly winds. The influence of this wide belt of very cold surface water can be shown to persist eastwards to the longitude of 30° E, and in winter it extends northwards, near the South Sandwich Islands, for about 1000 miles from the coasts of Antarctica; and it takes the icebergs with it.

By 18 December the ships had sailed some 90 miles eastwards along the edge of the ice, which lay nearly east and west, except for the bays. There was no sign of any opening by which they could get farther south, and Cook (like Bouvet under the same circumstances) thought it reasonable 'to suppose that this Ice either joins to or that there is land behind it and the appearence we had of land the day we fell in with it serves to increase the probability . . .'. He now intended, after getting a few miles farther north, 'to run 30 or 40 Leagues to the East before I haul again to the South, for here nothing can be done'. So he continued in an easterly direction, in poor weather, and with many bergs in sight, until 23 December. By this time he was in lat. 55° 26′ S, long. 31° 33′ E, and course was altered to the south, but it was not until lat. 57° 50′ S had been reached that he again met pack ice. This was on Christmas Day, when the weather—luckily, as will be seen—had improved. The ships then passed through several narrow fields of loose ice stretching SE and NW as far as they could see—varied by 'several Islands of the same composission'. On 26 December they were in 58° 31′ S, 27° 37′ E and were still moving through such fields of loose ice. The state of the ice was typical of break-up conditions, with rotten, honeycombed pieces

[1] See p. cii below.

in some fields,[1] and in others pieces four to eight inches thick, closely packed, broken into various sizes and 'heaped 3 or 4 one upon the other'.[2]

The following day the position was 58° 19′ S, 24° 39′ E, and they were then 240 miles almost due south of their position on the 19th. There can be little doubt that Cook had now worked his ships around the end of a wide tongue or belt of pack ice, and he continued to stand west. The ice cannot, however, have been very far away, as a Snow Petrel[3] was shot on the 30th, when the noon position is given as 59° 23′ S, 17° 1′ E. This same day Cook decided that having a clear sea ahead, and a favourable wind, he would continue west as far as the meridian of Cape Circumcision, provided he met with no impediment. Almost certainly he must have assumed that he was clear of pack ice, and it must therefore have been a surprise when, on the following day (the last of the year), to avoid loose ice ahead, the ships were hauled three points more to the north—only to find the ice so thick that they were obliged at 4 a.m. to stand back to the southward to clear it. When they were in 59° 20′, a vast ice field was seen to the north, 'extending NEBE & SWBW in a compact body farther than the eye could reach'.

Many years were to elapse before the modern pelagic whaling fleet was to establish the existence, in the early summer of most years, of this wide tongue of ice, stretching out in an unbroken mass far to the east from the Weddell Sea.[4] The whalers found that, in mid- or late December of most years, it was possible to push south through loose or scattered pack ice between the longitudes of 10° W and 30° E and reach clear water beyond, in latitude *c.* 60° S. In early January this area of clear water may stretch to within 100 miles of

[1] This type of ice is quite common in this sector. It almost certainly comprises ice several years old, i.e. ice which did not melt the previous year but remained in the cold Weddell current and was frozen-in again the next winter. Cook's description of it as exhibiting 'such a variety of figuers that there is not a animal on Earth that was not in some degree represented by it' is truly descriptive, and might well have been written today.

[2] A condition now described as 'rafted ice'. It is common in pack ice associated with the cold Weddell current, and on the western side of the Weddell Sea itself is caused by pressure of the mass of pack ice against the coasts of Graham Land. Here, where the pack ice is some feet thick, the 'rafting' of ice can crush a ship caught in the pack. In such way was the *Endurance* sunk in 1916.

[3] Observations in recent years have shown that seldom, if ever, does the Snow Petrel (*Pagodroma nivea*) range further than 100 miles from the edge of the pack ice. Other species of petrels have a wider distribution, but the Snow Petrel's range, quite definitely, is limited. Cook notes that Bouvet makes mention of these birds when he was off Cape Circumcision.

[4] It is seldom that this tongue of ice disappears completely. In most years the western part of it will persist throughout the summer and be incorporated in the new ice formed in the autumn (cf. Mackintosh and Herdman, loc. cit., pls. LXXX, LXXXIII, LXXXVI and LXXXIX).

the antarctic continent, and by mid-February only a small fringe of pack will remain around the coasts. If Cook had not been so anxious to look for Cape Circumcision he might well, at this time, have gone south and sighted, or perhaps even reached, the antarctic continent. As he did not find Cape Circumcision we may, by hypothesis, mourn the lost chance.

By 3 January 1773 the *Resolution* and *Adventure* were in lat. 59° 18′ S, long. 11° 09′ E, and so south and west of the position assigned to the cape in the instructions. Not knowing of the error in Bouvet's longitude, and because he assumed that it was a large area of land for which he was searching, Cook now came to the opinion that what Bouvet had taken for land was in fact 'nothing but Mountains of Ice surrounded by field Ice'. He admits that he himself and his officers were deceived by the 'Ice Hills' the day pack ice was first sighted. That the cape might have been merely an island, to be pin-pointed, does not at this time seem to have occurred to him. He was quite certain that no continent existed immediately in this area, and regretted the time spent in the search—time which would become the more valuable to him as the season advanced. His journal continues, summarizing alike geographical theory, his own experience, and his own plan. 'It is a general recieved opinion that Ice is formed near land, if so than there must be land in the Neighbourhood of this Ice, that is either to the Southward or Westward. I think it is most probable that it lies to the West and the Ice is brought from it by the prevailing Westerly Winds and Sea. I however have no inclination to go any farther West in search of it, having a greater desire to proceed to the East in Search of the land said to have been lately discovered by the French in the Latitude of 48½°South and in about the Longitude of 57° or 58°East'. He was right in thinking that the pack moves in an easterly direction, though it is driven by the current engendered by the wind—the West Wind Drift—rather than by the wind itself. Like the geographers, or the practical men to whom he had talked, he was wrong in assuming that the ice was invariably formed near land. In view of the short summer season, he was now obviously wasting his time in tacking against the westerlies, contrary to the west-east voyage he had designed, and the rumour of Kerguelen's discovery argued that there might be something to be found by reverting to this course.

On 4 January the ships were running to the east, some eighteen miles north of the position where there had been an impenetrable field of ice four days before. Cook infers correctly that such a large body of ice could not have melted in that time, and that it must have drifted northward. By 10 January they were in lat. 61° 58′ S, long. 36° 7′ E and on a course SE by S. Observations this day on the drift of loose ice led Cook to believe that there was a current setting NW, which was confirmed by the differences observed in the previous daily reckonings. Westward, the ship was ahead of the reckoning by 8 to 10 miles daily; eastward, astern by the same amount. The boundary between the West Wind Drift, moving in its easterly direction, and the west-moving current which, in general, surrounds the antarctic continent—the East Wind Drift—lies approximately in lat. 65° S. In the eastern part of the Atlantic sector (where Cook now was) the boundary is not so well defined; it probably lies between 60° and 65° S, and there is an intermediate area between the two currents where the movements of the surface water are irregular. Conditions, however, vary from year to year, quite possibly in relation to the extreme northern limit of the pack ice, and, bearing in mind the standard of accuracy demanded by Cook for all observations, the speed and direction of drift recorded was, no doubt, correct at that time. Further observations of the current were made on 13 January, when the ships were in lat. 64° 18′ S, long. 30° 48′ E: these showed that the surface current was setting NW, at $\frac{1}{3}$ knot, a very comparable speed to that of about 7 miles per day observed in the same area a few years ago. It was on this day also that Cook made the entry in his journal, 'Some curious and intresting experiments are wanting to know what effect cold has on Sea Water in some of the following instances: does it freeze or does it not, if it does, what degree of cold is necessary and what becomes of the Salt brine? for all the Ice we meet with yeilds Water perfectly sweet and fresh.'[1] It is the first of his recorded cogitations on the subject: he is obviously beginning to think out again the accepted physical and geographical principles. He was stimulated by the success achieved a few days before in watering the ship from floating ice—not, as was the arctic practice observed by Wales, at streams running from an iceberg—a triumph that caused some jubilation in the ships, even though its accomplishment entailed much discomfort.[2]

The Antarctic Circle was crossed, for the first time in history, on 17 January, shortly before noon, in long. 39° 35′ E. Icebergs had been scarce for some days and Cook was hoping that he had reached

[1] J. R. Forster discusses this problem at some length, quoting experimental work by Nairne and Higgins. The results seem a little indeterminate, but Forster himself (*Observations*, pp. 76–102), in a rather drawn-out dissertation on the subject, suggests that pack ice (I use the present-day term) is, in fact, formed *in situ*.

[2] e.g. Burney, Ferguson MS, 'we have more water than when we left the Cape of Good Hope'.

a clear sea. Many Antarctic and Snow Petrels were reported during the day and, as we now know, the presence of the latter in numbers is a sure sign of the close proximity of pack ice; indeed forty miles' more sailing brought the ships to the loose pack. Progress to the south was now possible only for a short distance and, in lat. 67° 15′ S, the ice became so heavy that they were forced to turn away. Although Cook was not, of course, aware of it he was then only some 75 miles from the antarctic continent, and his description of the ice which stopped the ships as comprising 'high Hills or Islands, smaller pieces packed close together and what Greenland men properly call field Ice', might well be a description of the types of ice often met with close packed around the coasts of Antarctica, especially in the deep bays and indentations—in fact, an accurate description of the ice conditions off this coast in mid-January of most years.

Taking into consideration the safety of his ships and the fact that the summer was half spent, Cook did not think it prudent to try to get round the ice field. He was wise. It probably reached south to the continent, and another month might have passed before it could show any signs of disposal. Standing away to the northward the ships made towards the position where Cook hoped to find the land lately reported by the French. Icebergs were seen every day except one[1] until they reached lat. 48° 36′ S, long. 57° 47′ E, on 2 February, when Cook began his search for the reported land. Not only was he unable to find it, he also, on 8 February, in thick weather—for the ships were again in the region of the Antarctic Convergence—lost contact with the *Adventure*. This was in lat. 49° 53′ S, long. 63° 39′ E, some five degrees west of Kerguelen's land. Cruising about the rendezvous, the position where she was last seen, for two out of the stipulated three days, without seeing any further sign of her, he at last concluded that she had been driven well to leeward (as he himself had been to some extent) and on 10 February stood to the east and south. Furneaux, on his side, cruised for three days, but driven to leeward, as Cook thought, could not regain position, and at the end of the time turned his mind to winter quarters and New Zealand—'distant fourteen hundred leagues, thro' a sea intirely unknown'.

On 13 February, in lat. 53° 54′ S, long. 72° 34′ E, many penguins were seen around the ship, which gave rise to the hope that they were near land—as indeed they were. Heard Island (lat. 53° 10′ S, long.

[1] On this day (30 January) Cook remarks on the absence of icebergs, but it is of interest to note that for several days previously no mention of them had been made in the journal. Presumably they had become so common as not to be worth mentioning.

73° 35′ E), still unknown, with large rookeries of four species of penguin, lay some 40 miles north-east, according to the noon position. As the ship's course was south-east they could not have passed any closer. On the other hand they must have passed uncomfortably close to an off-lying danger of Heard Island—two small rocky islets, now known as McDonald Islands—which lie about 28 miles to the westward. It is entertaining to note Cook's remarks in the journal '... and various were the oppinions among the officers of its [the land's] situation. Some said we should find it to East others to the North, but it was remarkable that not one gave it as his opinion that any was to be found to the South which served to convince me that they had no inclination to proceed any farther that way'. The comment is both perceptive and characteristic of a man who not merely knew what he wanted to do, but kept a keen eye on the feelings of his subordinates. He placed his own inclination before theirs, and kept south.

We have no mention of icebergs until 16 February, when the noon position was lat. 57° 8′ S, long. 80° 59′ E. Two were then seen. Cook also mentions the presence of a single penguin 'of the same sort as we usually saw near the Ice'; he continues, 'but it is now impossible for us to look upon Penguins to be certain signs of the vicinity of land or in short any other Aquatick birds which frequent high Latitudes'. Once again traditional dogma was going down before observation.[1] The Aurora Australis was seen on 16/17 February, to the general interest, and again the following night. Watering ship from pieces broken off icebergs was now routine in the *Resolution*, and on the 18th the ship was brought-to under an 'Island of Ice which was full half a mile in circuit and two hundred feet high'. While the boats were being hoisted out 'an immence quantity broke from the Island, a convincing proof that these Islands must decrease pretty fast while floating about in the Sea'. Cook also remarked that the loose pieces which had broken off drifted fast to the westward, i.e. 'it quited the Island in that direction'. He supposed this 'to be occasioned by a current, for the Wind which was at ESE could have little or no effect upon the Ice'. Cook's interpretation of the facts is here probably wrong. He knew that the greater part of an iceberg is submerged; and so it is amenable to the influence of the surface current, here the West Wind Drift moving east. It seems likely that the berg was accordingly moving east, but that the loose ice on the surface, which would be more affected by wind than by current, was stationary

[1] Clerke also was making a careful study of birds in relation to signs of land. See p. 753 below.

through the effect of wind against current—a difference of opinion from Cook which the following diagram will make plain. Numerous

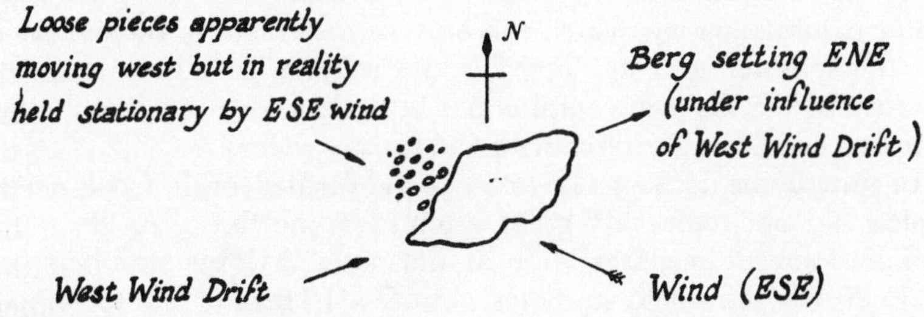

icebergs were seen in the course of the next few days, some of them 'of a considerable magnitude', and on 22 February, when in lat. 59° 35′ S, long. 93° 36′ E, they approached a berg estimated to be 'about half a mile in circuit and three or four hundred feet high'. As we now know, these dimensions indicate an extremely unstable berg, likely to overturn at any moment. This one did so, turning almost bottom up and, apparently, without breaking up further. Fortunately, the ship's boats, which were collecting pieces of ice in the vicinity, were not damaged.

It had been Cook's intention, before leaving antarctic waters to refit and refresh, to cross the Antarctic Circle once more. In this longitude and for some 50° eastwards of it he would have been hard put to it to do so; for seldom is the circle more than a few miles from the coast, while often it is inland. The ever-increasing number and size of the icebergs he was meeting, however, caused him worry. It was now late February, daylight hours were decreasing rapidly, and weather conditions—never very good here at this time of year—were poor. In these circumstances he decided, 24 February, when in lat. 61° 21′ S, long. 95° 15′ E, to turn away from the ice. The danger from bergs extended to the pieces which broke off from them in stormy weather. In his own words, 'the pieces which break from the large Islands are more dangerous then the Islands themselves, the latter are generally seen at a sufficient distance to give time to steer clear of them, whereas the others cannot be seen in the night or thick weather till they are under the Bows'.[1] He continues,

[1] There is not much to choose between this warning and that given in the current edition of the Admiralty's *Antarctic Pilot*. This latest warning reads, 'On a clear, dark night, a berg will not be seen with the unaided eye farther than one quarter of a mile, . . . On such a night when any sea is running, growlers are the most pressing danger; if they are sometimes visible on the wave crest and at other times awash or invisible in the trough,

'. . . great as these dangers are, they are now become so very familiar to us that the apprehensions they cause are never of long duration and are in some measure compencated by the very curious and romantick Views many of these Islands exhibit . . . in short, the whole exhibits a View which can only be discribed by the pencle of an able painter and at once fills the mind with admiration and horror'. Much the same opinion has been expressed by all who have followed Cook in these often wild and stormy waters.

In spite of his decision not to try to get further south, Cook nevertheless did not make any great attempt at northing. As he sailed almost due east icebergs were at first seen in large numbers; on 28 February, however, he notes, 'but few Islands of Ice to impede us, the late gale having probably destroyed great numbers of them'. It is unlikely that this was so—the surface temperature at this time of year precludes any melting, and if the bergs had been broken up by the gale, Cook should have seen vast quantities of 'pieces'. It is much more likely that with favourable winds (south to south-west) and a current setting to the north-east, the bergs had moved away quickly in the same direction. They are last reported on this easterly course on 8 March, in lat. 59° 44′ S, long. 121° 9′ E, and on 17 March the *Resolution* bore away north-east and then north—inclining to east—towards New Zealand. To complete four months in high latitudes in a small ship would in itself be an achievement; to navigate without accident in one of the stormiest oceans of the world, hampered by fog, and constantly among icebergs, was a very remarkable achievement of seamanship indeed. The whole voyage was great, but no one who has had much experience in antarctic waters will deny that those first four months were by far the worst part of it, and by implication the greatest in accomplishment. The dangers faced were quite unknown and the antarctic ice-edge is no place for the chicken-hearted. Even in summer the weather often is bad, as Cook found, and the dodging of icebergs in fog, sleet or snow, often with a gale thrown in for good measure, when one's only motive power was sail, must have been—to say the least of it—disquieting. Others did it after Cook, but with the benefit of his experience; none again was faced with the long-continued crisis of first experiment. His experience and experiment taught him when he had gone far enough, and if we have read his journal so far, we shall not be deceived by the apparently casual note at the end of his statement that 'the time was

speed should be reduced and great caution observed'. Words which—with the exception of those concerning speed—could well have been penned by Cook himself. Bouvet also had said something very like this.—Callander, *Terra Australis Cognita*, III, p. 642.

approaching when these Seas were not to be navigated without induring intense cold, which however by the by we were pretty well used to'. We shall rather be surprised that he seems to feel it necessary to indicate to the reader that he had some real reason, at this point, for breaking off the antarctic cruise: 'If the reader of this Journal desires to know my reasons for taking the resolution just mentioned I desire he will only consider that after crusing four months in these high Latitudes it must be natural for me to wish to injoy some short repose in a harbour where I can procure some refreshments for my people of which they begin to stand in need of, to this point too great attention could not be paid as the Voyage is but in its infancy'. One is unlikely to do anything but assent.

When Cook changed course for the north-east he had two visits in his mind—New Holland and New Zealand (by which one must understand Queen Charlotte Sound). New Holland interested him because of the possible or probable connection between Van Diemen's Land and New South Wales. Nevertheless he resolved to make his landfall, in the first place, at the southern end of New Zealand; and this he did on 25 March. At some time previously he had decided to call in at a southern port, instead of sailing directly up the west coast, as he had done in 1770, to the rendezvous in Queen Charlotte Sound,[1] and we can perhaps trace this decision back to the difference of opinion with Banks in that year, when he had felt himself forced to deny his friend the pleasure of stepping ashore at Dusky Sound.[2] Now there was no Banks to gratify, but certainly Cook had his own curiosity about this part of the country, and most certainly he felt that the sooner he could give his men 'repose' and large change of diet the better. To this decision we owe some interesting pages not only in Cook's own journal, but in the journals of others who wrote at length; we owe to it also an exceedingly brilliant piece of chartmaking; and, it must be said, a little later the brief and remorseless burst of activity from the New South Wales sealing-gangs that left scarcely an animal alive from one end of the coast to the other. Doubtless, however, that sort of onslaught on wild nature was bound to come, Cook or no Cook. We may be grateful for another glimpse of wild nature, in the Ngati Mamoe people who sparsely inhabited that watery country, and appear so infrequently in records of the

[1] Originally, it seems, he had envisaged coming in to New Zealand from the east, direct to Queen Charlotte Sound.—Fig. 2, and Chart XXV. But on such a point it is doubtful what evidential value this chart has: the main purpose was to stress the importance of New Zealand.

[2] I, pp. 265–6.

Maori. One thing we fail to get, any adequate impression of the sheer size of the fiordland cliffs and heights, all so much in just proportion that the eye is bound to underestimate, till some ridiculous piece of minute artificiality, like the *Resolution*, floats on the water at their feet. Romantic the poet Thomson may be, worthy to be quoted by William Wales, but he is a mild and chastened poet by these immensities.

The minds of men generally subsist on less elevated matters. The rain fell, the sandflies bit; the bagpipes, the fife and drum sounded to entertain the autochthonous friendly family; the boats surveyed daily, ducks were shot, seals knocked on the head, bellies crammed with fish—'The Happy taughtness of my Jacket excites in me a gratitude to do some justice to this good Dusky Bay, before I take my final departure from it', writes Clerke[1]—the tide was measured, the longitude ascertained, spruce beer brewed and found palatable; Cook, among others, was continually soaked, and suffered, it appears, from some acute form of rheumatism; Hodges busily painted waterfalls, the Forsters collected, Pickersgill's name was immortalized through the harbour he found; on 11 May the *Resolution* passed out through the northern entrance and Cook wrote some masterly sailing directions. The passage up the coast and into Queen Charlotte Sound had little of incident, apart from the spectacular and not very comfortable waterspouts off Stephens Island, and Cook's amendment of his previous view of the bay where Tasman anchored. On 18 May he was in the Sound, and there, to the general joy, was the *Adventure*.

Nothing could more clearly show the difference between Cook, the born explorer, and Furneaux the good seaman, than their respective journals during the time they had been parted. Furneaux wanted to cover the 4000 miles between him and a landfall as soon as possible, and get into harbour. But he knew that Cook had the Van Diemen's Land problem in his mind; and indeed Cook may have already discussed the probability of his calling there. Furneaux did another sensible thing: he had a fair idea what course Cook was intending to sail, and he knew what course Tasman had sailed across the southern Indian Ocean, and he therefore sailed roughly midway between them. In this way, though it would be possible to miss islands, the possibility of any large piece of land escaping notice would be reduced to a minimum. Furneaux, as we shall see, misinterpreted his Tasmanian landfall, and the southern coast (never very much visited) was a most unpromising one for men who wished

[1] Add. MS 8951, 11 May 1773.

to land; but he did find good anchorage, and water, in Adventure Bay. He was not the first voyager to come to the country since Tasman: he had been preceded, just over a year before, by Marion du Fresne. Marion had had bad luck. When coming to anchor off his *Terre d'Espérance* his ships had collided, the *Mascarin* lost her mizen mast and the *Marquis de Castries* her bowsprit, and he had accordingly made for Van Diemen's Land in the hope of both spars and water. He sighted the land a little north of Port Davey, on the west coast not far from Furneaux's landfall, on 3 March 1772, and similarly sailed round the south coast, to find anchorage, unlike Furneaux, near Tasman's Frederick Henry Bay. Close by, in Marion Bay, he remained six days: unlike Furneaux again, he made contact with the natives, who proved hostile; and able to get nothing he wanted, on 10 March he sailed for New Zealand and disaster. He does not appear to have been interested in the geography of the country. Furneaux was; but he cannot be thought to have made a very satisfactory attempt to clear up the main problem, whether it was insular or not. He was sailing up the east coast towards a solution when on 17 March Cook, far to the south, decided to make for New Holland or New Zealand; and on 25 March, when Cook sighted New Zealand, he was already six days out into the Tasman Sea, having left the problem as it was. Furneaux, with Bass Strait lying open before him, beat off into the south-easterly wind. His distaste for a lee shore may be understood; but how one wishes that, at the moment of decision, prudence had not so easily got the upper hand! Reading Cook on the subject, also, one would like a little further explanation of his reasons for accepting, apparently so easily, Furneaux's conclusion. There is perhaps here another instance of his principle, always patent though always unstated, of never criticizing his subordinates in a document going to his superiors.

In Queen Charlotte Sound the *Adventure*'s people had settled down for a pleasant few months. On them fell Cook with his determination not to 'Idle away the whole Winter in Port', and his theory that a winter voyage to the east was feasible. He had thought of making the investigation of Van Diemen's Land his winter task; 'but sence Captain Furneaux hath in a great degree cleared up this point I have given up all thoughts of going thither'. He summarizes his programme anew—a programme which would take him east, north, and then far south between New Zealand and the Horn. The first part of this is 'to proceed immidiately to the East between the Latitudes of 41° and 46° untill I arrived in the Longitude of 140° or 135° West and then, providing no land was discovered, to proceed to

Otaheite, from thence to return back to this place by the Shortest rout'. That is, he would cross a part of the ocean that he had not touched on his previous voyage, when he had come down from Tahiti to latitude 40° and turned west to New Zealand. He had not at this time considered land likely in this untouched part, because of the run of the sea, but it must now certainly be explored to remove all doubt. 'It may be thought by some an extraordinary step in me', he goes on, 'to proceed on discoveries as far South as 46° in the very depth of Winter for it must be own'd that this is a Season by no means favourable for discoveries. It nevertheless appear'd to me necessary that something must be done in it, in order to lessen the work I am upon least I should not be able to finish the discovery of the Southern part of the South Pacifick Ocean the insuing Summer, besides if I should discover any land in my rout to the East I shall be ready to begin with the Summer to explore it; setting aside all the[se] considerations I have little to fear, having two good Ships well provided and healthy crews'.

His own crew was certainly healthy; that of the *Adventure* at least appeared so. To the fish of Dusky Sound had been added the greens of Queen Charlotte Sound. Relations with the Maoris had been pleasant enough, vegetable gardens had been planted for their advantage, and that no doubt of the ships', pigs and goats had been left ashore. The carefully-tended ewe and ram ate a poisonous shrub and died; thus all Cook's 'fine hopes of stocking this country with a breed of Sheep were blasted in a moment'. The observations of Wales and Bayly seemed to prove that New Zealand had on the *Endeavour*'s voyage been charted a little too far to the east, a matter which nagged at Cook's mind for some time; and fresh observations of his own on the morals of the 'Indians' certainly proved that English visits had not tended to raise the local standards.[1] The birthday of King George III was celebrated 'in Festivity'. On 7 June the ships put out into the Strait, and next day were heading into the ocean itself, south and east.

(2) THE FIRST TROPICAL SWEEP

Cook sailed down to latitude 47° 7′ (not quite as far as that of the southernmost point of New Zealand), when he was in longitude

[1] Cook has a little bit of moralizing, part romantic and part historical: '. . . we debauch their Morals already too prone to vice and we interduce among them wants and perhaps diseases which they never before knew and which serves only to disturb that happy tranquillity they and their fore Fathers had injoy'd. If any one denies the truth of this

172° 49′ W, before he altered course north-east; and then more gradually and irregularly lessened his latitude over almost forty degrees of longitude till he crossed the fortieth parallel at about 133° 30′ W, and on 17 July turned almost directly north. That is, he had sailed over a more southerly course in this part of the ocean than had been before traversed, and coming up north, was bisecting the area between the course he had sailed north-west to Tahiti in early 1769, and that southward from Tahiti in August 1769. This ruled out still another area of possible continent—the last area possible, in fact, in a temperate zone. On this Cook comments in his entry for 2 August, by which time he had crossed Carteret's northward track of 1767. Obviously there was nothing to be discovered in this neighbourhood, except perhaps islands. 'As I have now in this and my former Voyage crossed this Ocean from 40° South and upwards it will hardly be denied but what I must have formed some judgement concerning the great object of my researches (viz) the Southern Continent. Circumstances seem to point out to us that there is none but this is too important a point to be left to conjector, facts must determine it and these can only be had by viseting the remaining unexplored parts of this Sea which will be the work of the remaining part of this voyage.' The seaweed he met with must have drifted from the New Zealand coast; the swell, from whatever direction it came, indicated the absence of any large land.[1] Meanwhile the men were beginning to find the passage tedious, the *Adventure* was badly afflicted with scurvy, and even in the *Resolution* there were symptoms. As Cook came into the islands he deemed it necessary once to send the cutter ahead at night with proper signals for use in case of danger, to avoid lying-to and thus delaying the arrival of the sick men at Tahiti. The precaution was perhaps the fruit of his experience within the Great Barrier Reef in 1770; and the four islands he saw before picking up those he recognized from his last voyage convinced him, if any convincing was necessary, of the justice of Bougainville's name, the Dangerous Archipelago. We may note that he had a copy of the English translation of Bougainville's book on board with him, as well as the translator—a book he scrutinized closely and with some exasperation. It is at this time that he makes the first of several criticisms of Bougainville[2] that were scrupulously excised from the text he prepared for publication.

assertion let him tell me what the Natives of the whole extent of America have gained by the commerce they have had with Europeans'.—p. 175 below. This was probably one of the things talked about in the great cabin.

[1] The argument, pp. 189–90 below, is a very characteristic bit of Cook writing.

[2] 12 August 1773, p. 195 below; see also pp. 234–5, 458, 526.

The weeks spent at Tahiti and the Society Islands do not call for prolonged analysis. Cook's narrative is clear, it is hoped that the annotation is sufficiently adequate, and Pickersgill[1] adds some lively detail for us. But the reader may be reminded that since Cook's departure from Tahiti in July 1769 there had been the period of warfare that had removed from the scene some of his friends of that year, and had for the time being radically altered the balance of power among the districts.[2] The death of Tuteha in March 1773 released the young Tu from his surveillance, and gave that timid yet cunning 'prince' a key position in the part of the island most visited by the English, while the death of the old Vehiatua brought to that title and dignity the young, charming, and short-lived man whose own death gave to his remote cousin Tu, through his brother, the first step towards his hegemony. Purea was no longer the commanding figure she had been four years earlier. There were chiefs, *arii*, powerful in 1769 who remained powerful in 1773; but necessarily, after the first meeting with the young Vehiatua, it was Tu who impressed Cook, and Tu with whom, at Matavai Bay and Pare, he had most dealings. There had been another incident in the island history, which might conceivably, under other circumstances, have been a complicating factor for Cook, but remained merely an incident. This was the first visit of the Spaniards to Tahiti, in 1772—a visit that denotes almost the last flicker of Spanish interest in the ocean that Spain had once claimed as its own.[3] The Spanish vessel was the frigate *Aguila*, her commander Don Domingo de Boenechea; she remained at the island from 8 November to 20 December, almost all that time anchored within the reef off the neighbourhood called Vaiurua, on the east coast of Taiarapu. Boenechea sent a boat round the island to explore and chart, whose company met the timorous Tu and a number of chiefs well known to Cook; all was amicability and charm; and when the Spaniards left they took four Tahitians with them, between 10 and 30 years of age, for the wider experience of Lima and instruction in Christian principles. For this visit, it was hoped, was one of reconnaissance only, to be followed by others which would ensure the benevolent sovereignty of Spain, and Boenechea conferred upon the island the name Amat, in honour of Don Manuel de Amat, the viceroy of Peru who had sent him to it. He did not return till November 1774, when he anchored in Vaitepiha Bay, Cook's anchorage of August the preceding year; by then Cook had

[1] Appendix IV.
[2] See the Note on Polynesian History, I, pp. clxxii ff., especially clxxxv.
[3] I, pp. cxvii–cxix.

been and gone from Tahiti twice since the Spaniards' first visit. Cook, who knew nothing about viceregal anxieties in Peru, but did know that a French expedition might be in the Pacific and had with him Bougainville's book, naturally enough thought at once of the French on hearing that others had been at the island.

Tahiti, or its reef, to begin with, was nearly fatal. As a place of refreshment, it was this time unrewarding. At Huahine, 2–7 September, and at Raiatea, 8–17 September, the ships did better, even lavishly, and the principal *arii*, 'Oree' and 'Oreo', were both welcoming and nobly generous. Oree was pleasanter than his Huahine people, the least generally pleasant of the islanders in that sea; it was they who waylaid and stripped poor Sparrman. It was from Huahine also that Furneaux took Omai, amiable and rather simple, whose later career in England was so suffused with glory. There was no lack of islanders who fancied travel, though Cook's Porio, from Tahiti, was enticed back to land by a young lady of Raiatea; but Raiatea supplied to the *Resolution* in exchange the charming young 'Odiddy'—Hiti-hiti or Mahine—who won hearts so universally that there was general lamentation when in the following June he was, in his own interests, returned to his island. Poor delightful Odiddy; it is he among the tempests and icebergs and New Zealand cannibals, not the pretentious Omai, who is the Polynesian hero of the voyage. According to the muster book he had a servant, Poetata; but that is the only mention Poetata gets on the voyage, he remains an accidentally-discovered shadow. They filled the place left by Isaac Taylor, the consumptive marine who died just after the arrival at Tahiti. The *Adventure*'s scurvy patients had rapidly regained health. Whatever the incidents and accidents of island life, indeed, no one of the ships' companies but was fit for another season in the south, and Cook left Raiatea very cheerfully, to return to Queen Charlotte Sound, by way of Tonga: 'I directed my Course to the West inclining to the South as well to avoid the tracks of former Navigators as to get into the Latitude of Amsterdam Island discovered by Tasman in 1643, my intention being to run as far west as that Island and even to touch there if I found it convenient before I proceeded to the South'. This was a change from his earlier design of 'the shortest route', and here we have the beginning of the programme of verification and co-ordination of earlier discoveries which was one of the great works of this voyage.

The Tongan islands are like a narrow net thrown irregularly over the ocean, reaching 175 miles from north to south. The net falls into a number of clusters or sub-groups—Tongatapu in the south,

Nomuka and Ha'apai as one moves north, Vava'u in the north; while beyond these limits, both north and south, are outliers that by settlement or nearest contiguity must be reckoned part of the same system. The majority of the more than hundred islands and islets, ranging from quite considerable pieces of land to specks almost awash, are coralline—Tongatapu itself is a raised atoll—and stretch up on the east; while to the west of a ship's track northward through the group is a shorter volcanic line, the units of which are very scattered. On the eastern side only Eua, Tongatapu, and Vava'u are of any height, but most bits of land are green with island vegetation, from the common beach hibiscus with its yellow blossom, one of the simplest and loveliest of flowers, up to the tall congregations of the coconuts. On the windward side of the islands the breakers curve and explode infinitely along the coast, in a continuous line from one end of a group to the other; and they have worn away and undercut the low ledges of coral, the *liku*, which mark the raised island—low, except the great cliffs of Eua, looking down to the thick leafy covering of the flats, and beyond them the vast surface of the sea, beneath which plunge the six miles of the Tonga Deep. The defect of the islands, as places to live on, is the scarcity of fresh water. Rain seeps away through the coral formation and the sea seeps in; ponds and wells are few and brackish, and it does no good to dig for water. There is a little stream among the hills of Eua, which makes that island enviable;[1] beyond that, fresh water must be stored in tanks, and in the days of Cook and Tasman wise men drank from the coconut. In one respect, therefore, these islands were not highly profitable places of call: in other respects they were, for they were well cultivated, fresh food abounded, and the people were friendly—as both Cook and Tasman found. Freshness of water, also, to seafarers was a relative matter.

Tasman, Cook's only predecessor in the main groups, had visited the islands in the last days of January 1643, and landed on two: Tongatapu, 'a low-lying island, much like Holland', which he called Amsterdam, 'because of the abundance of refreshments we got there'; and Nomuka, which he called Rotterdam, 'seeing that here we got our casks filled with water'. To the eastward of Tongatapu was Eua, which he called Middleburg; and it was here that Cook first came, to the general excitement of the populace, it was this that seemed to the English 'one intire Garden'. Besides refreshments, Tasman found on Tongatapu a 'king', and Cook looked for one. He did not find one on this voyage, though he did on his next; for Tonga, alone among

[1] In spite of which, it is today hardly settled, and the stream is the ornament of the government forestry estate.

Polynesian societies, did indeed have a king,[1] of a peculiar sort, at the head of a tight and complex social organization. Hence the grades of nobility by which Cook was perplexed on this first visit, when chief superseded chief, and the greatest seemed the stupidest. But even this was not the king. The king of Tonga—or at least the most exalted personage—was the *Tu'i Tonga*,[2] highly sacred as the descendant of the god Tangaloa and a woman of Tongatapu. In the fifteenth century the twenty-fourth of this line found the combined weight of sacred and secular functions too much for him, and made over the burden of temporal government to one of his brothers, the *Tu'i Ha'a Takalaua*. At the beginning of the sixteenth century this secular king also became wearied with office, and gave to his son the functions of ruling and collecting tribute, with a new title, that of *Tu'i Kanokupolu*, while he himself maintained the prestige and privileges of a higher formal rank. It was this last created dignitary who, therefore, became the effective king, while the Tu'i Tonga remained the sacred spiritual, and senior, leader of the community, and the Tu'i Ha'a Takalaua tended more and more to sink into the background. There was also a female Tu'i Tonga, the eldest daughter of the Tu'i Tonga by his principal wife: as time went on, it was first the eldest daughter of the Tu'i Ha'a Takalaua and then the eldest daughter of the Tu'i Kanokupolu who was chosen as principal wife; and the eldest daughter of this union, the *Tu'i Tonga fefine*,[3] was so sacred that no Tongan could marry her, and her traditional mate was the Fijian chief the Tu'i Lakeba. Their first born, male or female, was the *Tamaha* or sacred child—and if this was a daughter she was so sacred that neither the Tu'i Tonga nor the Tu'i Tonga *fefine* could eat in her presence, and had to carry out the *moemoe* or ceremony of obeisance, placing the head between her feet, before departing from her presence. Nobility in general, it may be added, descended through the female line, and daughters were superior in rank to sons. This discussion bears on some of the dignitaries whom Cook met on this voyage; for his 'Otago' was Ataongo, the son of the Tu'i Kanokupolu, and his 'Latoo-Nipooroo' or 'Latooliboula' was Latunipulu, a male Tamaha. As for his other chiefs, they were chiefs, but we are never quite certain of what order of importance, though all infinitely superior to the *tua* or peasants, who lived on the chiefs'

[1] Niue did also for a while, in the eighteenth century, under Tongan influence, but abandoned the institution.

[2] I give the formal spelling of this title, and of the other titles following. They are rendered in a variety of ways, frequently without capitals and each as one word—e.g. *tuitonga*.—*Tu'i*, a king or governor.

[3] *fefine*, woman; cf. Tahitian *vahine*, Maori *wahine*.

hereditary lands. All this was dark to Cook, though on his third voyage, on a longer visit, he began to get some enlightenment; and indeed, it took a good deal of enquiry to disentangle the system, even after the information gathered by William Mariner during his four years' captivity.[1]

What Cook could do to describe the appearance, habits, and 'material culture' of the people he did, and he observed a good deal. The *kava* plant grew much more freely in Tonga than in Tahiti, and Tonga was one of the places where the *kava* ceremonial reached its most complex development. The people were great weavers, the *tapa* mallets sounded from morning to night. Their carving and tattooing had developed different idioms from those of the Society group; they were skilful seamen and canoe-builders, though their best canoes came from the Lau islands of Fiji, where the timber was superior; their great men passed constantly between their own islands, and the voyage to Fiji was a sort of grand tour. They were excellent gardeners. The *faitoka*, the characteristic Tongan tomb-structure, was a thing Cook could not miss; but on this voyage he did not see any of the *langi*, the royal tombs, the huge stepped piles which were the Tongan contribution to the Polynesian art of accurate building in stone. He had difficulty with the language, harsher than Tahitian, with consonantal differences that can be seen in the words already here used; even Odiddy threw up his hands in despair. The people could not help stealing—which led to comic as well as serious situations, but it could not be denied that they had charm; and Cook was lucky in seeing them while their society was still stable.

He left Tongatapu on 8 October, and sighted New Zealand on the 21st. It was on the 22nd that the east coast chiefs came off to the *Resolution*, and received such lavish bounty of live-stock, seeds, and nails; it was on the 23rd that the long storm began that a week later finally parted the two ships; it was 3 November when Cook, having looked through the entrance to Port Nicholson and decided to take advantage of a southerly wind rather than to explore it, was at last anchored again in Ship Cove. Refreshment here and good relations with the Maoris were now a matter of course; and for the most part the incidents of this visit might be described as minor and normal. There was one exception that startled everybody. Cannibalism among the New Zealanders had been very strongly suspected, even regarded as a fact from the signs that had been seen of it: it was now

[1] John Martin, *An Account of the Natives of the Tonga Islands . . . compiled and arranged from the extensive communications of Mr William Mariner*. London, 1816; 3rd ed. Edinburgh, 1827. Mariner was a member of the crew of the *Port au Prince*, cut out by the Tongans at Lifuka in 1806, and remained in benevolent captivity till 1810.

seen in practice, and on board the *Resolution*. The severed head that caused all the excitement was bought for preservation by Pickersgill —how true to their characters our sailors are!—the alert and curious enquirer who acted as chef was Clerke. The incident led Cook to say all he could in favour of the New Zealanders—'few considers what a savage man is in his original state'; it led the Forsters to conclude that the English were to blame, because if they had not wanted to buy so many curios the New Zealanders would not have had to send out a war party to replenish their stocks, and if they had not done so no one would have been killed, and consequently no one would have been eaten.[1] Two days after this incident Cook sailed, 25 November. He had abandoned hope of seeing Furneaux again. He left a message in a bottle buried at the foot of a tree, with the words LOOK UNDERNEATH carved on it; fired guns along the eastern side of Cook Strait; then, seeing and hearing nothing, concluded that his consort had made for the Cape of Good Hope; and headed south. Four days later the *Adventure* at last got into Queen Charlotte Sound.

Furneaux had had his fill of bad weather. His ship was now light and crank. Driven up the coast at the beginning of November, he had put into Tolaga Bay for wood and water, sailed again and been driven back, repaired his rigging, and sailed once more on the 16th, to find gales off the mouth of the Strait that kept him beating backwards and forwards till the end of the month—a most infuriating experience. Only on 30 November did a favourable wind blow. At Ship Cove the bottle was soon discovered, and he set out to prepare for sea as quickly as possible. But then he found that his bread needed rebaking, a slow process; and when he was ready for sea, 17 December, came the tragedy. The cutter went to gather greens, and failed to return; and Burney, sent next day to investigate, made a report that struck the world as much as most other things in Cook's journals.[2] Ten men had been killed and their bodies gone into the Maori *hangi*, or cooking-pit. This was cannibalism indeed, by the side of which the spectacle on board the *Resolution* was almost an innocent joke.

Yet it is not altogether surprising that such a thing should happen. It was one of Cook's constant anxieties to see that no such thing did happen, whoever might be the sufferers, his own men or natives of the islands. The precautions he took to maintain good relations are written at large through his journals. If his justice erred, it was not in favour of his own men; but what he could do by tact and forethought to avoid the necessity of violent justice he was eager to do. He held his hand

[1] Cook, pp. 294–5 below; Forster, I, pp. 508, 512.
[2] See Appendix IV, pp. 749–52 below.

many times in Tahiti; he made demonstrations of force elsewhere with reluctance. He remembered—there is no doubt—his unhappy first attempts to make friends with the New Zealanders in 1769, and the slain men in the bay and by the river. He put his offering on the *faitoka* at Tongatapu; when he saw the images, 'I who had no intention to offend either them or their gods, did not so much as touch them'; he was properly respectful to those to whom respect seemed due; he was not negligent of others. He was not slow to recognize admirable qualities. He could not rearrange Polynesian—or later, Melanesian—mentality to suit his own convenience; and sometimes, as he frankly admitted, in the general contest of wits he came off worst, simply because he saw the consequences of too rigorous action. Theft was a constant problem—disinterested theft, so to speak, an exercise of the enlightened intelligence and a fine art—and was extremely difficult to deal with. Cook flogged his own men for theft from the islanders, as he did on the visit he had just concluded, and he gives his sentiments in general on the matter:

'It has ever been a maxim with me to punish the least crimes any of my people have commited against these uncivilized Nations, their robing us with impunity is by no means a sufficient reason why we should treat them in the same manner, a conduct we see they themselves cannot justify, they found themselves injured and sought for redress in a legal way. The best method in my opinion to preserve a good understanding with such people is first to shew them the use of fire arms and to convince them of the Superiority they give you over them and to be always upon your guard; when once they are sencible of these things, a regard for their own safety will deter them from disturbing you or being unanimous in forming any plan to attack you, and Strict honisty and gentle treatment on your part will make it their intrest not to do it.'[1]

There were two defects in this: the first was the assumption that savages, any more than civilized persons, always acted reasonably; the second was the assumption that fire-arms never missed fire, or that if they did, 'these uncivilized Nations' never noticed it. But they did notice it, and could take advantage of it, as Cook himself made clear.[2] He put considerable importance on native persuasion that their visitors were of a rather superior order—as we learn from Elliott, writing of Tonga 'one Anecdote, which occur'd while we stop'd here;

'And that was, that upon some occasion, one of our men gave one of the Natives a blow, which he return'd immediatly, and a battle ensued, in

[1] See p. 292 below.
[2] e.g. pp. 414, 417.

which the Islander had the advantage of the Britton, which surpriz'd us very much, and Captn [Cook] forbad such tryals of skill in future for it [would] be highly impolitic to let them suppose that they were equal to us in anything.'[1]

It was not possible to have seamen always under supervision, nor did those who should have acted responsibly always do so. Too many men were 'careless and imprudent'. Burney in his turn has a significant passage in one of his descriptions of the Society Islands, on what he calls the islanders' 'sending us to Coventry';

'they mentioned something of a woman being wounded, but how or which way we could not clearly make out—'tis likely they had too much reason for their Complaints Some of our young folks behaving in a very foolish, arrogant manner drawing their swords to fright them & pretending to be in a passion at trifles—this probably may be the occasion of others being ill used, as Mr Speerman was at Huaheine—it is not safe at any of the Islands, for a single person to wander too far from any houses, Speerman was not the only instance of people suffering by it—however in the houses, or amongst a Multitude you are safe from Robbers but not from pickpockets, of which there are always enough on the watch to take advantage of your Negligence.'[2]

Theft and blows, threats, cheating and blackguardism generally, whoever was the guilty party, these could be understood and appropriate measures taken whenever it seemed wise or possible to do so. But there was a further area of conduct which may sometimes have produced trouble, though we hear nothing of it as the cause of trouble because the seamen were naturally quite insensitive to it. They were average sensual Europeans set down in a society whose complexities were quite un-European, whose psychological filaments might be blundered into with the best intentions in the world, or without intention at all; the jolly sailor might commit the very blackest of blasphemies, shatter the most sacred conventions, and go equably on his way quite unwitting of the outrage of which he was guilty. How many breaches of *tapu* there were on these voyages no one will ever know. They should have been visited by divine, and condign, punishment. Europeans, it seems, were not governed by the ordinary laws the gods imposed upon mankind. But sometimes the Polynesian mind must have meditated the ordinary vengeance, and sometimes what seemed to Cook unmotivated mischief must have been very strictly motivated indeed. We know also that many Polynesians were inordinately proud, of fiery temper, taking insult with

[1] Elliott *Mem.*, f. 22.
[2] Burney, Ferguson MS.

quite sudden explosions of furious and unrestrained rage. We know, or can guess pretty well, what sort of discussions were held on board the ships about the people on shore: what sort of discussions the people on shore had are hidden from us. They kept no journals. We are to remember, finally, what it is too easy to forget, the difficulties of communication. Neither Cook nor any of his people properly understood or spoke a single Polynesian language. There were vocabularies; there were the bare elements on many sailors' lips; there was enough to carry on trade, make greetings, express friendship; but to go beyond the concrete, to discuss, that was a different matter. Even in quite elementary things, the pitfalls were many. A coast can be charted accurately, the sea sounded. To chart a savage society, to sound the savage mind, called for a new technique and for illimitable time. Over this branch of discovery hung an invisible mist of incomprehension. The ground on which men stood might seem firm; but it could fall away at a touch.

In this context we are, surely, to consider the massacre at Grass Cove. On his third voyage, in February 1777, Cook enquired into it, on the spot. The story he was told, through Omai, by a chief he felt he had every reason to trust, may be perfectly true, and we are anyhow not likely to get beyond it. Rowe, the master's mate, who commanded the boat's crew, and all his men except one, were sitting eating their dinner of bread and fish two hundred yards from the boat. They were surrounded by Maoris, in the usual way. They had, it appears, only three muskets with them; the rest were left in the boat, and one man was left in the boat to look after her. Some of the Maoris snatched at the food, and were beaten, a general quarrel flared up, two of the muskets were fired and two Maoris shot dead, the rest fell on the sailors before the third musket could be used and killed them all, including the man in the boat. It was exactly the sort of thing (to repeat) that Cook took every precaution to obviate.[1] It seems clear that these people had been making far too free with the

[1] Another story told to Cook, not irreconcilable with this one, has a Maori hit with a stick for stealing something from the boat, his cries bringing on the attack. A further, but later, story comes to us in George Clarke's *Early Life in New Zealand* (Hobart 1903) p. 27, according to which the sacredness of the chiefly head was involved. The massacre thus 'arose from unintentional violation of the tapu. I heard the story from a very old man when I was once on a visit to Blind Bay. He said that when the *Adventure's* boat landed in the cove, the men sat down to their meal, and one of them refused either to return or to pay for the stone hatchet of one of the Maoris; and that the latter snatched up a piece of bread and ran off. The white man ran after him with some kind of tin can in his hand, and coming back to a group of the natives sitting round the boat, he, sailor-like, put the tin, as if it were a hat, on the head of a chief. It had contained food, and it was to Maori feeling a very gross insult, and *that*, he said, was the direct cause of the massacre that followed'. Clarke (1823–1913) knew the Maoris and their language very well; but his old man's story may have been rationalization or adornment of the original facts.

Adventure's property, and that blood had already been shed; they may have come to hold Furneaux's men in low esteem; Rowe was certainly over-confident and careless in dealing with them;[1] and once the quarrel had started, on neither side was there anyone capable of beating it down. The vast excitement that followed may well have been an emotional release for most of the people in the Sound. There was nothing useful that Furneaux could do.

Cook's letter in the bottle was very indefinite about his future movements. He gave Furneaux no rendezvous and no orders. He was going south and then east. He might be at Easter Island about the end of March; he might go to Tahiti, but everything must depend on circumstances. He was in fact leaving Furneaux a free hand. Furneaux had his difficulties. His ship was not in good order, his sails and rigging were in bad order, though he had done what he could to refit in Ship Cove. The state of his provisions gave him no joy; and now he had lost ten of his best men. It does not seem, however, that he determined at once to make for home; he set out to sail over the south Pacific, and went as far south as 61°, when he was abreast of Cape Horn. He had met a good deal of ice, his men began to suffer from the cold, his provisions were damaged; and at this stage he decided that the prudent thing to do was to make for the Cape of Good Hope. He still conducted another search for Cape Circumcision, found nothing, and sighted the African coast on 17 March, the day Cook left Easter Island. He had at least sailed over some sea that Cook did not sail over; and it would be unwise to say that, after the great storm of October 1773, he did on his own less than was possible.

(3) THE SECOND ICE-EDGE CRUISE

Cook himself, on leaving New Zealand, registered possibilities in his journal even vaguer than those he had sketched in his letter to Furneaux. The exploring the southern parts of the Pacific Ocean was definite, 'in the doing of which I intend to employ the whole of the insuing season and if I do not find a Continent or isle between this and Cape Horn in which we can Winter perhaps I may spend the Winter within the Tropicks or else proceed round Cape Horn to Faulkland Islands, such were my thoughts at this time . . .'. The Falklands would give him a springboard for a South Atlantic cruise; but this is the only time he mentions them as coming into his calculations, before, later on, he dismisses them. He had already mentioned Easter Island and Tahiti to Furneaux, and it was undoubtedly

[1] See the extracts from Furneaux and Burney, and the annotation thereto, Appendix IV.

towards a further season among the Pacific islands that his mind was tending. He had probably not given the possibilities full scope; pushing south, he could see rather the weight of 'circumstances'. One circumstance did not yet worry him, that of his own health.

He left Cape Palliser on 27 November, making good progress roughly south-east, and on 12 December the ship was in lat. 60° 42′ S, long. 173° 4′ W. Icebergs are reported in 62° 10′ S the following day, and on 14 December, in lat. 64° 55′ S, long. 163° 20′ W, some 'loose ice'. The good progress south-eastwards continued—146 miles on 14 December and 116 miles on the 15th—through more icebergs and loose ice. In the latter part of the 15th an extensive field of loose ice was encountered, though with some leads and clear water beyond. Cook, however, thought it prudent to alter his course more to the east, especially as the weather was far from pleasant, with thick fog and a strong wind. In spite of the alteration in course the ship was embayed in loose ice, and was forced to return to the south-west before the wind veered to the westward and enabled her to stand northward. At this time the latitude was 66° 0′ S. The concentration of loose ice and icebergs is, as we have already noted, very typical of the break-up conditions and it is interesting to find that the edge of the loose ice (and presumably, the pack ice) lay only 20 to 30 miles north of the mean position suggested by Mackintosh and Herdman[1] for this month.

Cook was reluctant to navigate among so many icebergs, and, as he did not consider it probable that land would be found to the south of the ice, he sailed north-east to clear the pack, then setting his course eastwards. No doubt his decision to be cautious here was partly born of his experience in the Atlantic sector the previous summer. On the other hand, the remarks in his journal indicate that the ice conditions now found were quite different from any he had already met with. 'This feild or loose ice', he writes, 'is not such as is usually formed in Bays or Rivers, but like such as is broke off from large Islands, round ill-shaped pieces from the size of a small Ship's Hull downwards, whilest we were amongest it we frequently, notwithstanding all our care, ran against some of the large pieces, the shoks which the Ship received thereby was very considerable, such as no Ship could bear long unless properly prepared for the purpose'.[2] That the summer break-up of the pack ice was well established is shown by his remarks two days later, when the boats were collecting ice for watering ship. This ice 'was none of the best for our purpose,

[1] loc. cit.
[2] p. 305 below.

being composed chiefly of frozen Snow, was poras and had imbibed a good deal of Salt Water, this however dreaned of after it had lain some time, after which the ice yielded sweet water'.[1] Rotten ice of this type is common at this season on the ice edge, especially in the eastern part of the Pacific sector, where the advance and retreat of the pack is small.[2] Cook was, however, mistaken about its nature. There will, of course, be a certain amount of frozen snow associated with sea ice, but it is the snow that melts first. Unfortunately, little is known about the growth and dispersal of ice in the Pacific sector, other than that the range of these movements is small, and that the coasts of Antarctica are never clear. No one has yet penetrated to the continent by sea over the greater part of the sector.

Steering generally east but making southing whenever possible, Cook crossed the Antarctic Circle for the second time on 21 December, in about 143° W longitude. The weather was bad—thick fog accompanied by a strong gale, sleet and rain. It is not surprising that the ship 'came close aboard a large Island of ice' and that 'being at the same time a good deal embarrass'd with loose ice we with some difficulty wore and stood to the NW untill Noon . . .'. Most of the icebergs sighted this day were of the weathered type; Cook comments on their rugged appearance, with many peaks, and for the first time mentions that all those he had previously seen were 'quite flat at top' (i.e. tabular bergs). He remained south of the Antarctic Circle and, with northerly winds for the next three days, the ship did well on the eastward course: northerly winds, because she was by now well south of the region where the westerlies prevailed. On 24 December, in lat. 67° 19′ S, long. 138° 15′ W, they again met the pack, a large field of closely-packed floes stretching from south to east;[3] and again the weather was far from pleasant—a northerly gale 'attended with a thick fog Sleet and Snow which froze to the Rigging as it fell and decorated the whole with icicles'.[4] With such conditions, when sails became like boards and ropes like wire, it is not surprising that Cook was anxious to leave these waters. He had, apparently, made up his mind that land could not lie south of the ice and did not consider it prudent to go farther east, partly on account of the ice, but also because he was worried at leaving a space of 24 degrees of lati-

[1] p. 306 below.

[2] Herdman, *Journal of Glaciology*, I, No. 4, pp. 156–66, 172–3.

[3] Approximately 60 miles south of the mean northern limit for December, as suggested by Mackintosh and Herdman (loc. cit.). It should be noted, however, that, apart from Cook's own observations, there is only one other report of pack ice recorded for this month between the meridians of 160° and 80° W, and that was in 1841.

[4] One cannot better Cook's own descriptions of weather conditions which, if they are not the normal here for this time of the year, are certainly not rare.

tude unexplored to the north of him—the gap between his present position and his eastward track from New Zealand in July 1773.[1]

On Christmas Day, therefore, he turned away to the north-east, and then north. Very many icebergs were seen that day, but on the 26th during the morning 200 and upwards were sighted. The weather, fortunately, was clear, and although there was no wind early a breeze from the west-south-west later helped to free the ship from danger. As the journal says of the afternoon, a calm had been foreseen, and she was got 'into as clear a birth as we could where she drifted along with the ice islands and by takeing the advantage of every light air of wind was kept from falling foul of any one; we were fortunate in two things, continual day light and clear weather, had it been foggy nothing less than a miracle would have kept us clear of them . . .'—which dry statement conceals a world of vigilance and seamanship.[2] By 2 January 1774 she was in lat. 57° 58′ S, long. 136° 27′ W—some 560 miles north of the position on 24 December. Icebergs had been seen in great quantity during this passage north, but are not reported north of lat. 58° 39′ S. On 6 January course was altered to the north-east, and on the 11th Cook concluded that there was little probability of any large area of land lying between his present position and Tahiti. He therefore hauled round and stood back to the south-east, having decided some days earlier that the almost permanent westerly winds of these latitudes would prevent him from exploring to the west in that latitude (54° 55′ S). Cook's track on the chart makes visually quite clear his method as an oceanic explorer at this time. He had been 'down', 'up', and was now turning 'down' again, in a sort of giant irregular zigzag, and we can see how this last plunge south would complete his process. Sailing nearer to south than south-east the ship was, on 20 January, in lat. 62° 34′ S, long. 116° 24′ W—some 500 miles west of her northerly course at the end of December. Icebergs were sighted again that day, but no further mention is made of them until the 24th, in about lat. 62° 36′ S, long. 109° 32′ W. Cook crossed the Antarctic Circle for the third time, on 26 January, in long. 109° 31′ W. Icebergs were not seen the previous day, but nine—all small—are reported on this one. On the succeeding three days there was little or no wind but much fog, and on the 29th the *Resolution* was in lat. 70° 00′ S, long. 107° 27′ W and still making south in open water. Of this day Cook wrote 'Clear pleasent Weather, Air not cold'—rather

[1] See also his entries for 6 and 11 January 1774, pp. 314, 315.

[2] p. 310. It may be compared, as a matter of curiosity, with the passage quoted from Forster, p. cl below.

different conditions from those of 24 December when he turned north from the ice in 138° W. In January, it may be remarked, when south of the Antarctic Circle, the weather is often good; in fact it may be said that in this respect January is the best month of the year.

Later in the same day Cook reports the largest iceberg so far recorded in his journal—'not less than 3 miles in circuit'; it was, presumably, a tabular berg. Soon afterwards 'ice blink' was seen in the sky, denoting approach to closely-packed field ice, which stretched east and west as far as could be seen. To use Cook's own words, 'The outer or Nothern edge of this immence Ice field was composed of loose or broken ice so closely packed together that nothing could enter it; about a Mile in began the firm ice, in one compact solid boddy and seemed to increase in height as you traced it to the South; In this field we counted Ninety Seven Ice Hills or Mountains, many of them vastly large'. He contrasts it with the Greenland ice, which had no 'ice hills', and so was navigable to ships. The fact that the Greenland ships fished yearly among such ice kept him from asserting positively that the ice now seen 'extended in a solid body quite to the Pole', or that the 'ice islands' were formed in the pack, 'and afterwards broke off by gales of wind and other causes'; but he was obviously on the point of thinking so, and he was clear that the difference between navigating this icy sea and that of Greenland was made by 'these numberless and large Ice Hills' which 'must add such weight to the Ice feilds, to which they are fixed'.[1] It will be seen that he came to alter somewhat his hypothesis on the formation of icebergs; while his theory of 'weight' was certainly wide of the mark.

By noon next day, 30 January, Cook had managed to push still more to the south and east—in lat. 70° 48′ S, long. 106° 34′ W; and, finally, the following morning, to lat. 71° 10′ S, in long. 106° 54′ W. Then he was convinced he could get no farther. Nor has anyone else got here, by sea, since Cook's day. The R.R.S. *Discovery II*—a full-powered steamship, specially built for navigation in ice—penetrated to lat. 69° 49½′ S in long. 101° 25½′ W, on 6 January 1931, but was then forced to return.[2] Admittedly, this was nearly four weeks earlier than Cook, when the ice might reasonably, in any other sector, be expected to be farther north than at the end of the month. In the Pacific sector, especially in the eastern part, the belt of pack around the continent is relatively narrow; the seasonal movement has a

[1] pp. 321–2. There is an interesting revision of this in the following paragraph from Add. MS 27888, where Cook draws no inference at all from the Greenland fishery.

[2] Cf. Herdman, *Journal of Glaciology*, loc. cit., p. 173.

range of about 300 miles only, occurring between September and December. By January the northern edge of ice is relatively stable and there is little more retreat before the end of the summer. It seems fairly certain that, between the meridians of 70° and 140° there is, stretching out from the coasts of Antarctica, even in late summer, a permanent belt of pack ice some 60–100 miles wide.[1]

It is at this point in the voyage that Cook allows himself to make one of his few personal statements. On this day when he reached his farthest south he writes, 'I will not say it was impossible anywhere to get in among this Ice, but I will assert that the bare attempting of it would be a very dangerous enterprise and what I believe no man in my situation would have thought of. I whose ambition leads me not only farther than any other man has been before me, but as far as I think it possible for man to go, was not sorry at meeting this interruption, as it in some measure relieved us from the dangers and hardships, inseparable with the Navigation of the Southern Polar Regions. Sence therefore we could not proceed one Inch farther South, no other reason need be assigned for our Tacking and stretching back to the North . . .'.

It is possible, reading this passage quickly, to be struck primarily by the words in which he confesses his ambition, so different from the understatement habitually practised by this modest man; and they are proud and striking words. But they are not the most significant words. Those are the ones that follow: he 'was not sorry at meeting this interruption, as it in some measure relieved us from the dangers and hardships, inseparable with the Navigation of the Southern Polar Regions'. They may be compared with the passage, the other personal statement, he wrote on the first voyage after escaping from the Great Barrier Reef, on the pleasures and pains of discovery, and the attitude of 'the world'.[2] The situation was now rather different. Cook was not now the victim of the swell of the sea, he had not just been faced with inescapable doom, he and not the tide-race was the master of his ship. But he now had experience, full and superabundant, of the dangers and hardships which faced him and his small *Resolution*, among the icebergs and pack ice of the Antarctic; and he was turning back from them. The decision when to turn back is one which, at some time or other, faces every explorer. There is always the desire to go on still a little farther—a desire which may, and often does, lead to disaster. It requires courage to turn back in

[1] Cf. Herdman, *Journal of Glaciology*, loc. cit., pp. 156–66.
[2] See I, p. 380, and the discussion of this passage, p. clvii of that volume.

time, courage to face 'the world'—those who will perhaps say that you were prudent to save your own skin; for Cook, courage to contend with a phantom—his feeling that those who sent him out might hold that he had fallen short of his instructions. Yet the capacity to make this decision at the right time, judging individually, looking before and after, is the mark of the great explorer. Cook was right. His voyage was but part completed, there was still the western part of the Atlantic sector of the Southern Ocean to examine, the short summer season was ending. He had a duty to his crew and to his ship as well as to himself: he wisely decided that they had all had enough of the ice for a while.

Only a few icebergs were seen after leaving the edge of the pack, and the last was reported on 3 February, when the noon position is given as lat. 66° 25′ S, long. 101° 8′ W. Three days later, still in lat. 64°, Cook makes what almost seems to be a further apologia for his decision to turn north from the Pacific ice. It is in connection with his matured plan for the remainder of the voyage. He was this day, with all his reefs out and top-gallant sails set, steering north-east with a southerly wind behind him, having determined 'to proceed directly to the North'. His dubieties on leaving New Zealand at the end of November were now resolved: he had determined to spend the winter in the tropics. In the Pacific high latitudes he was convinced that there was no land. He thought none would be found on the other side of Cape Horn; but supposing he did now make straight for the coast laid down on Dalrymple's Atlantic chart, or for Bouvet's land, and found it to exist, the season would be too late to explore it, and have 'obliged us either to have wintered upon it, or retired to Falkland Isles or the Cape of Good Hope, which ever had been done, six or seven months must have been spent without being able in that time to make any discovery whatever, but if we had met with no land or other impediment we must have reached the last of these places [i.e. the Cape] by April at farthest'—and the quest for the southern continent would have been over. This would have been to decide much as Furneaux did; and if Cook had done so, and found nothing more, he would have been hard on Furneaux's heels; in any case it would have been the voyage he originally contemplated. But there was an alternative, which he had discussed with a not very enthusiastic Furneaux. Even if the Pacific continent had vanished, the ocean had 'room for very large Islands, and many of those formerly discover'd within the Southern Tropick are very imperfectly explored and there situations as imperfectly known'. As he had a good ship, a healthy crew, and 'no want' of stores and provisions—the result of very careful husbanding—the conclusion to him seemed obvious: 'I thought I cou'd not do better than to spend the insuing Winter within the Tropicks: I must own I have little expectation of makeing any valuable discovery, nevertheless it must be allowed that the Sciences will receive some improvement therefrom especially Navigation and Geography'. So he would first look for land said to have been discovered by Juan Fernandez in lat. 38° S, then for Easter Island, and then cross the ocean to the west 'on a rout differing from former Navigators, touching at, and settling the Situation of such Isles as we may meet with'; if he had time, he would go as far as Quiros's Austrialia del Espiritu Santo, Bougainville's Great Cyclades; and then he would make south again into latitude 50° or 60°, and steer east to the Horn—all this by November, so that he would have the best part of a summer in which to explore the southern Atlantic. 'This I must own is a great undertaking', says Cook, 'and perhaps more than I shall be able to perform'—for he did not dismiss the possibility of 'impediments'. As what has been called above an appendix to his voyage, and what may be better styled a parenthetical insertion, it was a quite astonishing undertaking—a summary and completion of almost everything done in the Pacific, as far west as the New Hebrides, up to his own first voyage. With anyone else the plan would have been preposterous. Cook carried it out precisely. He even added to it. On his time-table, when he arrived at Cape Horn at the end, he was one month overdue.

(4) THE SECOND TROPICAL SWEEP

The preceding words, it may be argued, go too far. But by 'completion' and 'precisely' it is not meant that Cook discovered or rediscovered every individual island in the area. He did not, for example, see the northern group of the Marquesas, or Mendaña's Santa Cruz. He was not a sort of Miltonic angel, standing on some superterrestrial vantage point and taking in the whole of the central and eastern Pacific at one view. 'Verification' might be a better word than 'completion': then how define his masterly survey of the whole of the New Hebrides? Verification, completion, precision—all these are words one must use; remembering, perhaps, that all words are relative. It may be noted that something like a third of his whole journal is devoted to this parenthetical portion of his voyage. So far, nevertheless, from the Miltonic angel is the navigator that to the attentive student of that journal he may possibly take on the faintest resemblance to a tourist—the first, the most eminent of Pacific tourists, a tourist with a guide-book. The guide-book is Alexander Dalrymple's *Historical Collection of Voyages to the South Seas*.[1] These two volumes of 1770–1 certainly went the voyage, and they could never have had a more devoted reader. As a compendium of documents in a field which Dalrymple, among geographical scholars, had taken peculiarly to himself, they were invaluable.[2] They presented the earlier discoveries as a series which could be checked, with enough detail to make identification possible—to make it possible, that is, if the discovery existed at all. For to Dalrymple any statement that declared, or could be made to declare, in favour of the continent, that sovereign subject, was as good as any other statement; and Cook, on his tour, his guide-book always in his hand, could never be merely the dutiful admirer of the given object: he was inevitably forced into the role of critic, examiner, appreciator beneath whose incorruptible gaze much might expand into a new clarity, but something might fade away. Luckily for Dalrymple he had collected a great deal that turned out to be fact, and the dissipation of Juan Fernandez' land is balanced by the solidifying of Quiros's Bay of St Philip and St James.

From latitude 64°, in the first week of February, Cook had for the most part favourable weather, though the westerlies forced him a little more to the east than he meant to go, and by the 22nd and 23rd of the month he was between lat. 37° and 36°, near enough to the longitude of the alleged Juan Fernandez discovery. There was nothing: 'circumstances gave us no hopes of finding what we were in search after, having continually a large swell from SW and West'. On the 26th therefore he bore away for Easter Island, north, and then west. Or was it Davis Land? Was the land sighted by the buccaneer in 1687, and described so lucidly by Lionel Wafer, copied so carefully by Dalrymple, the same as that visited by Roggeveen in 1722 and the Spanish in 1770?[3] This was a problem he never quite solved. The entries in the journal persuade us that he wanted to believe in the identity of the two, but the obstacles were large. In the

[1] As Cook tends to refer to it. Its correct title is *An Historical Collection of the several Voyages and Discoveries in the South Pacific Ocean*. The first volume was devoted to the Spanish voyages, the second to the Dutch. There was a good deal of Dalrymple deduction and argument in the work.

[2] After prolonged meditation, I withdraw the name of sciolist which I applied to Dalrymple in I, p. ci. But I confess I can think of none to substitute, and probably it would be ridiculous to try to find one. There was more than one side to Dalrymple—there was the disinterested hydrographer and the laborious student as well as the man of vanity, the projector and the rash controversialist. Unfortunately his scholarship, valuable as it was, could never be disinterested—he could not help being propagandist as well as historian, on his favourite subject he had no reserve of scepticism. He is a figure ripe for more extended study.

[3] Cook erroneously thought the Spanish visit was in 1769. See I, p. cxvii.

meanwhile, about the time he gave up the land of Juan Fernandez, he had himself posed a problem to Patten the surgeon. He had fallen sick of what he calls rather vaguely 'a Billious colick'—what was obviously a very painful intestinal complaint which, it seems, might quite well have been fatal. How long the crisis lasted and Patten's skill was extended we do not know,[1] but when Easter Island was sighted on 11 March Cook was still weak. He could potter about the beach with a watering party, engaging in minor trade, while an expedition marched along the southern shore and back over the hills, but that is all; so that his quite full observations on the island, the best we have from that century, are largely second hand. He did not think much of it: 'No Nation will ever contend for the honour of' its discovery, 'as there is hardly an Island in this sea which affords less refreshments and conveniences for Shiping than it does'; but his observations on the ethnic links of the people are acute, and it is obvious that even from the ship and on the beach he used his own eyes to good purpose.

To turn Easter Island into Davis Land there was needed a small sandy isle to go with it, and if the island had provided fresh water Cook would have looked for this (which would have been a waste of his time). We are brought back suddenly to one of the primary conditions of successful exploration, which, so often in reading Cook, we are liable to forget. Many of the crew were now beginning to show signs of scurvy; and a note found in one of the copies of the journal is very significant: 'It was afterwards found, that the few Roots &c[a] we got at this isle proved of infinate service to us and made us once more relish salt Beef and Pork, for which most of the Officers and some of the Crew had quite lost all appetite, nor is this to be wonder'd at, sence we had had no other flesh Meat for near four months'.[2] When the *Resolution* sailed, these few roots were uneaten, and seemed a small lot, and jaded palates might affect the voyage a good deal. But water was the main need. So Cook let the sandy isle go, 'as I . . . had a long run to make before I was assured of getting any and being at the same time in want of refreshments . . . as a small delay might have been attended with bad consequences'.[3] The long run was that to the Marquesas, about 29 degrees west of where he was, and 17 north. There, if Quiros spoke truth, he would certainly get fresh water, and he hoped all else he needed. A north-westerly course in continual fair weather, with easterly winds and the ship making good

[1] Marra's anonymous volume makes it from 23–28 February—for what that is worth as evidence.

[2] p. 349, n. 1.

[3] p. 349.

daily runs, brought him to latitude 9° 30′, where the Marquesas were supposed to lie, by 1 April; and turning west, he sighted them on the 7th. The visit was a little disappointing. High, precipitous, wildly romantic, these mountainous islands fall to the sea by ridges that end in steep volcanic cliffs; between them, down the valleys, sweep sudden gusts of wind perilous to ships; and Cook, turning into the 'port' that Mendaña in 1595 had called Madre de Dios, in the island of Santa Christina, was very nearly driven on to the rocks in his lee. The people were handsome above all other Polynesians, with an extra and special grace; and before a boat had even landed one who had snatched an iron stanchion was shot dead. Trade was nevertheless opened for fruit and pigs; and was ruined by some of the 'young gentlemen' who rashly abandoned the prescribed rules. It was difficult to get off wood and water, or to give the ship repairs. Cook therefore decided to depart for the known advantages of the Society Islands: his men were after all not so bad in health, though since last leaving New Zealand they had been nineteen weeks at sea, almost entirely on a salt diet. The anti-scorbutic articles on board had been well used; and the roots and bananas and sugar-cane of Easter Island had probably come in the nick of time. Possibly, if conditions had been more favourable, Cook would have heard of and explored the northern group of the islands; as it was, he did what he wished to do geographically, and settled accurately the position of Mendaña's group; he renamed the 'port', on the western side of Tahuata, Resolution Bay (it is now called Vaitahu); and on 12 April set his course south-west. This course brought him through the northern Tuamotus, where Byron and Roggeveen had been before him, and where the natives were not all friendly. On one only, Takaroa, was a landing made, fleetingly; and ten days after leaving the Marquesas the ship was once again anchored in Matavai Bay.

It was the last visit of the voyage to Tahiti, and the Society Islands. Cook did not think he would ever see them again, and over his journals hangs a rather valedictory air; more than once he confesses to some emotion. While very necessary repairs were going on, however, some exasperating incidents took place, and Tu was an exasperating person to deal with. There was the theft of the water-cask, the theft of the sleeping sentry's musket, and the public flogging of a Tahitian for the former (for the latter the sentry was punished equally). The marines were put through their exercise to impress the natives fully with the power of fire-arms, while, both to impress and oblige, the ship's guns were fired and an exhibition of fireworks presented. But what impressed the Tahitians most was a quantity of red parrot feathers that had been got at Tongatapu: and as the island had now recovered its wealth of hogs and other provisions, trade went on at a tremendous rate. What impressed Cook most in his turn was the 'Tahitian fleet'; and here again his misapprehension of the political structure of the island misled him. Great numbers of large canoes had certainly assembled, with all the appearances of preparation for war, and their destiny, it was made clear, was Aimeo, or Moorea. Cook concluded that the fleet was Tu's, that the commanders were Tu's admirals, and that Aimeo was in revolt against 'Tahiti'—i.e. Tu. Tu simultaneously complained to Cook that Towha (the principal 'admiral'), the chief of Faaa, and Potatau, the chief of Punaauia, who was also concerned with the fleet, were not his friends. The matter remains somewhat obscure. Certain Aimeo chiefs may have owed tribute to certain chiefs of Tahiti, but the one island was certainly not tributary or in any other way subject to the other. There was a struggle in progress on Aimeo, between Teri'itapunui, and his uncle Mahine. Teri'itapunui was Tu's wife's brother, but the last thing Tu wanted to do was to engage in war for his brother-in-law. Towha and Potatau did, on the other hand, and at this time they were bringing pressure on Tu to join them. He agreed, and then drew back. By the time Cook came to Tahiti again, on his third voyage, Tu had quarrelled with Towha; and when the *Bounty* arrived in 1788, he was under general attack, from Towha, Potatau, and their old enemy Mahine of Aimeo. Tu, however, had great capacity for survival, particularly with English support.[1] In the meantime Cook continued under his misapprehension of Tu's 'kingship', which Tu and his people were quite anxious to foster. No doubt there were times when he wished Tu were a more kingly person.

In one further way Cook was misled by the fleet—in calculating the population of the island.[2] It was a magnificent thing visually—Hodges sketched it, Cook had a measured drawing made of one large canoe, and bestowed some English equipment on a fine vessel then building. He would have liked to have seen manoeuvres at sea, but it was time for him to leave. He refused steadfastly to take anyone away with him from the island—much to the elder Forster's disgust; he saw no prospect of ever returning such an adventurer home, and he had not approved of Furneaux's enterprise. He very nearly lost a man himself, on 14 May, as the ship was under sail—Marra the gunner's mate, the rootless Irishman who wanted to stay at the island; and

[1] R. W. Williamson has co-ordinated the evidence, *Social and Political Systems of Central Polynesia*, I, pp. 197–200.

[2] p. 409; and I, clxxiv–clxxvii.

Cook's comments on the attempted desertion show how the situation, and his own feelings, had changed since the like attempt of 1769. He had some sympathy with Marra: 'I know not if he might not have obtained my consent if he had applied for it in proper time.' If Marra had ever thought of this way of going about it he might have been put off by the reminiscences of Corporal Gibson, to whom, in 1769, Cook's attitude had not been at all benevolent.

A week was spent at Huahine, where again the islanders showed their less amiable side. This time it was Forster's servant, that 'feeble man', who was set upon, while the officers more than once, when out shooting, had their belongings stolen. An expeditionary force to catch the robbers was quite abortive. As for the victims, thought Cook, it was partly their own fault: 'the careless and imprudent manner many of our people have rambled about in their country from a Vain opinion that fire Arms rendred them invincible hath incouraged some of these people to commit acts of Violence no man at Otaheite ever dar'd attempt'. He remained attached to 'Oree' the chief—the 'good old chief' who wept when Cook said he would come to Huahine no more, and replied 'Then let your sons come, we will treat them well'. At this stage trade goods were running short, and the smiths had to be set to work to hammer out nails and iron tools. There was a last ten days at Raiatea, where it was difficult, and hardly necessary, to add very greatly to the stock of provisions, and the principal attraction was the drama; for there were *arioi*, 'strolling players', on the island, and the chief's daughter was a leading lady very much in demand. Here poor Hiti-hiti, lost in tears, left the ship, to the general regret; he had on Forster's advice declined to stay at Tahiti, where he would have been a well looked-after hero, and returned home to Raiatea, where he was no hero at all. Orio, the chief, parted as affectionately from Cook as had his colleague of Huahine. Cook had thought of visiting Borabora; now, however, with his repairs done, and plentifully supplied with foodstuffs, he decided it would answer no end to go there, 'and directed my Course to the West and took our final leave of these happy isles and the good People in them'. This was on 4 June.

His intention was to visit 'Quiros's discoveries'—that is, the islands he was to call the New Hebrides, through which Bougainville had passed in 1768, identifying nothing Quiros had seen but bestowing some names of his own. Cook sailed rather south of west, so that he must have had it in mind to visit Tonga again on the way: a course that brought him on 16 June to the atoll he called Palmerston, and on the 21st to the upthrown coral cliffs of Niue, which for sufficient reason he called Savage Island. He landed here, and his description of the reception he got is as vivid as the present-day Niuean explanation of it is circumstantial. Fortunately no one was killed on either side, though more than one person had a fright; and Cook continued his course till he judged he was near Tasman's Rotterdam or 'Annamocka'—Nomuka, the largest of the south-central group of Tonga. Tasman had been there for the last week of January 1643, and got plenty of water that he regarded as fresh from a bay on the north coast called by him Justus Schoutens bay. On the morning of 25 June Cook was off the reefs and breakers of the subsidiary 'Otu Tolu group; next day he was able to work his way through, and in the evening of the 27th was anchored off Tasman's bay. He had already been asked for by name off the other end of the island—'a proof that these people have a communication with Amsterdam', and that the captain was a person worth talking about. Cook stayed here only three nights and the two days in between. The natives were by turns helpful and troublesome, and the water not good. There was outrageous thieving, the men were jostled, muskets had to be fired. Here also occurred the amusing episode of the presentation to Cook of a young lady, and the abuse to which he was subjected when he declined the gift; and here, for the only time on the voyage, Wales forgot to wind the chronometer. By the time the ship was ready to sail the people were 'very submissive and obligeing', and Cook, writing up his journal, did not hesitate to call their islands the Friendly Archipelago. With a good supply of fruit and roots as well as the dubious water he sailed on the 29th, making first for the near islands, the truncated active volcano Tofua and its extinct neighbour Kao of the beautiful cone; and then struck west, north-west, and again west for 'Quiros's discoveries', Bougainville's Great Cyclades.

A few days out from Tonga the islet Vatoa was sighted, a very small outlier of Fiji; but to encounter that large group, which would have provided an explorer with ample employment, Cook would have to have been sailing on a course much more north of west than he then was. He altered course when he was to the west of it, so that he came north between it and the New Hebrides, and turned west finally when he was in the latitude of the northern islands of this group—those, that is, that were sighted by Quiros and Bougainville; and on 17 July he picked up the east side of Bougainville's Aurora, or Maewo.[1] What he now did, between this date and the end of

[1] In giving the names of the New Hebridean islands accepted and used today I have followed the Admiralty *Pacific Islands Pilot,* II, 7th ed., 1943, and the Admiralty chart

August, may be contrasted with his proceedings at the Marquesas. There, for reasons already given, his stay was very brief, his investigations quite confined. Here he was well supplied with food, he found it possible to get more, he was not pressed for time; and, of course, the land of Quiros was one of his main objectives. The investigation and charting of the New Hebrides, therefore, however far they may rank below the antarctic cruises as a test of endurance, are one of the great triumphs of this voyage: we have a running survey comparable with that of New Zealand on the first voyage, though on a smaller scale, and one that, in general enquiry, was certainly made no less complicated by the attitude of the natives of the country. True, of the whole of the New Hebridean group there were some that Cook quite missed, the Banks and Torres islands, in the north, nearer to him when he was off Maewo or Espiritu Santo than were the islands to the south; but, as it happened, it was to the south that he turned initially, and when he came north again it was Quiros's Espiritu Santo that he regarded, naturally enough, as his point of departure.

What then, in short, did he do?—for to analyse at length the proceedings of those six weeks would be both to usurp the task of annotation and to obscure one's outline in detail. To the Miltonic angel, the New Hebrides would present the form of an immense Y, two oblique arms, as it were, and a single rather elongated leg.[1] Cook came into the group round the top of the eastern arm, sailed down inside, and out again through the northern part of the leg on to its eastern side. He then followed the leg almost, but not quite, to its southern extremity, turning between the two southernmost islands, to come up on its western side, and in at its top between the arms again; then, passing right round the western arm, first inside and then outside, he took his departure SSW. In terms of islands with their modern names, he sailed into the group round the northern point of Maewo (18 July), tacked his way between that island and Omba (or Aoba) and down the western sides of Raga and Ambrim.[2] He crossed over to land at Port Sandwich (22–23 July) just above the south-eastern point of Malekula, and then crossed back inside Epi, to tack out to the east again through the smaller islands between Epi and Efate, and south to the east of Eromanga and Tana. An attempt

3033. It should be noted that some of these names and spellings differ from those used generally in the islands; but I have tried, so far as possible, to give the variants as well. The Admiralty has followed the rulings of the Permanent Committee on Geographical Names; the local inhabitants are less amenable to discipline.

[1] On p. 472, n. 3, I have used the metaphor of a screen, but perhaps the reader will not object to some variety.

[2] See the sketch-map, Fig. 66.

to land at Eromanga (4 August) was abortive; at Tana he was successful, and remained there, in Port Resolution, for a fortnight, 6–20 August. Then, passing between Tana and Aneityum, he sailed north up the west side of Tana, Eromanga, Efate and Malekula, through Bougainville Strait at the north of Malekula and up the east side of Espiritu Santo, and (25 August) into the Bay of St Philip and St James which is the main feature of the northern coast of that island; then out of the bay and down the west side till he could see into Bougainville Strait again, and away on 1 September. This, with an enormous number of astronomical observations for fixing latitudes and longitudes, and the constant running survey, is the geographical achievement. On this last matter Cook discriminates. He must not be taken, he explains, as claiming too much: 'The word Survey, is not to be understood here, in its literal sence. Surveying a place, according to my Idea, is takeing a Geometrical Plan of it, in which every place is to have its true situation, which cannot be done in a work of this kind'.[1] His reader must be quite clear, that is, that he does not claim the same accuracy for his chart of these islands that he does for his charts of Newfoundland. He never, in explaining his own shortcomings, lost a faint touch of naïvety.

The reader who is not devoted to an intense geographical scrutiny may well prefer to consider the human situation, the problem of 'race-contacts', the nature of the people Cook was now among. There was, in the language heard at some of the islands, evidence of Tongan influence; but to all intents and purposes Cook had sailed clean out of Polynesia into a new world—the world of Melanesia, marked by a multiplicity of tongues, a multiplicity of clans, a social structure, a system of beliefs and observances of which he could in six weeks obviously form no notion at all. To this there is one exception: he did find it plain that all these people had no partiality for strangers, and another of his triumphs was that he and his men did manage to get a little beyond the beach at Tana. He could conceive that the stranger might quite naturally be their enemy, and he could sympathize with them:

'thus we found these people Civil and good Natured when not prompted by jealousy to a contrary conduct, a conduct one cannot blame them for when one considers the light in which they must look upon us in, its impossible for them to know our real design, we enter their Ports without their daring to make opposition, we attempt to land in a peaceable manner, if this succeeds its well, if not we land nevertheless and mentain the footing we thus got by the Superiority of our fire arms, in what other light can

[1] p. 509, n. 4. This he explains off the coast of Efate.

they than at first look upon us but as invaders of their Country; time and some acquaintance with us can only convince them of their mistake.'[1]

And again, 'there are few Nations who will willingly suffer you to make excursions far into their country'. But he could not conceive—he had no possible means of conceiving—that they lived so close to the supernatural, that the border between them and the unseen was so much non-existent, that a ship-load of white-coloured strangers could be immediately taken for ancestral ghosts. The Tana people must have revised their opinion on this point, or anyhow concluded that ghosts were not necessarily inimical. But native tradition combines with other indications and the known facts of Melanesian life to explain in this way much of Cook's difficulty in arriving at friendly terms with folk in comparison with whom, despite the pervasive power of *tapu*, Polynesians strike us as living in a clear light of rationalism. Cook's own feelings, in relation to a people 'civil and good-natured', explain his rage at the shooting on Tana, on the eve of the ship's departure, after so much painstaking care and consideration. Whatever the truth about this matter, it is one more illustration of the difficulties inherent in the meeting of different peoples. Before we leave the New Hebrides, we may perhaps observe that Cook's description of invaders landing in a country applies much more to his successors than to himself: if ever a man showed caution and goodwill there, though armed, he did.

Other incidents of the visit, though striking, curious, or entertaining enough, may be ignored.[2] Cook's intention, on leaving Espiritu Santo, was to call at Queen Charlotte Sound, to refresh further ere he crossed the South Pacific for the last time and made his final cruise in high latitudes. New Zealand had not come explicitly into his plan when he last stated it, before sailing north in search of the land of Juan Fernandez, and he had possibly thought he could finish his giant loop, or sweep, by sailing direct to the Horn or Tierra del Fuego. Forster makes some play with the inhumanity of this inten-

[1] p. 493.

[2] One should perhaps not ignore the complaint in Forster (II, p. 373), so reminiscent of Banks: 'Quiros had great reason to extol the beauty and fertility of this country; it is indeed to appearance, one of the finest in the world. Its riches in vegetable productions would doubtless have afforded the botanist an ample harvest of new plants, as next to New Zeeland it was the largest land we had hitherto seen, and had the advantage of having never been examined by other naturalists. But the study of nature was only made the secondary object in this voyage, which, contrary to its original intent, was so contrived in the execution, as to produce little more than a new track on the chart of the southern hemisphere. We were therefore obliged to look upon those moments, as peculiarly fortunate, when the urgent wants of the crew, and the interest of the sciences, happened to coincide'.—This is on departing from Espiritu Santo.

tion, the cruelty it entailed towards worn-out sailors,[1] and was forcefully rebutted by Wales: 'Captain Cook told me, on my complaining at Tanna, that I had but a very indifferent opportunity of ascertaining the rate which Mr. Kendall's time-keeper went at there, that it was of the less consequence, as I should soon have an opportunity of doing it, more completely, at New-Zealand'.[2] But it is quite possible that Cook brought up the idea again, perhaps not very seriously, and even discussed it with Patten, as Forster asserts;[3] which would do something to counter Forster's other charge that Cook never told anybody what he intended to do next, so that naturalists were always completely in the dark. At any rate, if he did consider it seriously, he wisely discarded it for a better plan—a plan that, on his passage to the south, almost inevitably brought him to New Caledonia (4 September); and this was a quite new discovery. The people here were easy to get on with; were, in fact, on their most excellent behaviour, and the stay in harbour for a week at Balade (till 13 September) was a pleasant interlude. If only, one thinks, Cook had had less confidence in the ability of his stomach to assimilate any food whatever! Possibly the opinion of Forster that the peculiar fish on this occasion was poisonous was enough to convince Cook that it was not poisonous; and possibly the fact that Forster was poisoned as well as Cook did not immediately improve the relations between them.

Leaving his harbour, Cook sailed first northwards for two days outside the reef, till he found that the shoals went farther than the land, and considered that possibly they filled the space of sea between this island and New South Wales (a theory that, unknown to him, had already been disproved by Surville on his passage south from the Solomons in 1769); and turned back to find himself in the afternoon of the 16th in a position that must have reminded him unhappily of his experience outside the Barrier on 16 August four years before—'At 3 PM it fell Calm and we were left to the Mercy of a great swell which set directly upon the reef which was hardly one league from us, we Sounded but could find no ground with a line of 200 fathoms'. And as before, he sent out the pinnace and cutter to tow, and they could do little. But a light breeze in the night this time saved the ship. On the passage to the south-east there was the long and (to the modern reader) amusing argument over whether certain natural phenomena were trees or pillars of basalt. We are not entitled to be too highly amused at John Reinhold Forster, how-

[1] Forster, II, p. 376.
[2] Wales, *Remarks*, p. 89.
[3] Forster, *Reply*, p. 35.

ever; basaltic pillars were all the fashion in the philosophical world, the Giants' Causeway in Ireland was causing both amazement and conjecture, and it was in 1772 that Banks added to his fame by his announcement of a like formation on the island of Staffa. Renewed danger to the ship came when, having rounded the Isle of Pines, she was caught on the night of 29 September within the reefs off the southern end of New Caledonia. A careful reading of Cook's entry for that afternoon does not convict him of undue rashness—after all, there were some risks he had to take, or he would not have been an explorer—but the night was certainly one in which only the most accomplished seamanship saved the *Resolution* and her company. The comment made by the captain is a true utterance of his mind, in its scrupulous and almost absurd moderation, combined with stubbornness. 'I was now almost tired of a Coast I could no longer explore but at the risk of loosing the ship and ruining the whole voyage, but I was determined not to leave it till I was satisfied what sort of trees those were which had been the subject of our speculation.' So next day he anchored and landed on an islet and took away specimens of *Araucaria columnaris* for spars. That having been done, and an examination of the whole vicinity made from the masthead, Cook determined to get clear of it; and next day was in a hard gale out of sight of land. He was driven to consider his time-table. It was now 1 October. The wind was in the wrong quarter for him to regain the land easily; the summer, which he needed for the high latitudes, was at hand; the ship again needed repair and stores; he could not afford to be kept in the Pacific by any accident for another year; in short he 'did not think it adviseable to loose time even in attempting to regain the Coast, and thus I was constrained as it were by necessity to leave it sooner than otherwise I should have done'.[1] He made an extremely good guess at the general direction of the south-west coast, the details of which were thus left to Bruni d'Entrecasteaux, who charted it in 1792—a not unworthy follower.

Cook sailed south to come into Queen Charlotte Sound from the west. On the way, 10 October, he made one more discovery, the small but agreeable Norfolk Island, the history of which was to be less than agreeable; and he landed there with more ease than those who later used it were to experience.[2] On the 19th he was moored in Ship Cove again, with a considerable amount to do in refitting the

[1] p. 562.

[2] The first ship to go there after Cook, the *Supply* from Sydney, in 1788, took a week to land her people; the second, the *Sirius*, also from Sydney, in 1790, was wrecked on the reef. As a convict settlement supplementary to Sydney, Norfolk had a very grim history indeed.

ship, and a considerable shortage of materials that a conventional shipbuilder would have deemed essential. With ingenuity, however, she was in three weeks made thoroughly ready for sea and another southern passage; and a diet of vegetable broth and fish made her company as ready. 'The market', says Clerke, 'was at the old stand'. It was obvious that the *Adventure* had been in the cove since Cook's last visit. He was somewhat disturbed by a garbled account of the wreck of a ship and the killing of its crew, though the natives, on being further questioned, took refuge in vagueness and denial; and after finding that the *Adventure* had certainly not been wrecked he put the unpleasant rumour out of his mind.[1] The discovery of another passage from the Sound into Cook Strait gave him some pleasure. Wales's further observations on the longitude of Ship Cove by this time had convinced him that he must accept with equanimity the fact that his chart of New Zealand was in error; but it is amusing to find him, with his own passion for accuracy, shrugging the matter off as one which would not 'much affect either Navigation or Geography'. On 10 November he stood out of the Sound, and next night was making south with all sails set, to cross the ocean in a mid-fifties latitude, 'so as to pass over those parts which were left unexplored last summer'. Half-way across, on 27 November, in lat. 55° 6′, long. 138° 56′ W, he concluded that no land could possibly be found; and decided, instead of going down to a higher latitude, to steer direct for the western entrance of Magellan Strait—not to pass through it, but to coast from it the southern side of Tierra del Fuego, a part not at all well known. The whole passage was uneventful. At midnight, 17–18 December, he sighted Cape Deseado.[2] The great work was almost over. 'I have now done with the Southern Pacific Ocean, and I hope those who honoured me with this employ will not think that I have left it unexplor'd, or that more could have been done in one voyage towards obtaining that end than has been done in this.'[3]

Cook was on this coast—if we may for convenience include Staten Island in it—until 3 January 1775. His observations were, considering its dangerous nature, detailed and good, and were not improved

[1] There was the language difficulty again; cf. p. 576, n. 5. One of the words these Maoris certainly must have used, *waka*, could have meant either a ship or a boat; and they demonstrated that, somehow or other, the *waka* was battered to pieces.

[2] Cook was right in thinking that his passage would be the first run that had been made across this ocean in a high southern latitude—unless the *Adventure* had preceded him, which it had. But those are wrong who say his voyage provided the first west to east circumnavigations. The French, more than once, were earlier: the first was the trading-vessel *Comtesse de Pontchartrain*, 250 tons, Captain Jean Baptiste Forgeais de Langerie, in 1714–16.—See E. W. Dahlgren, *Voyages français à destination de la Mer du Sud avant Bougainville, 1695–1749* (Paris, 1907).

[3] p. 587; and see the variants of this in n. 2 to that page.

on till the surveys of the *Adventure* and *Beagle* under King and Fitz-Roy in 1829–30. Of the whole period he spent a week in Christmas Sound, which runs into Waterman Island, part of Tierra del Fuego, and two days in New Year's Harbour on the north coast of Staten Island—both new discoveries. In the first, which was well surveyed, the ship's company feasted on geese and other birds; in the second, on penguins and seals; and though Cook was not really fond of boiled penguin, yet to him, and others, it was very tolerable after long-continued salt beef and pork. His account of birds and beasts is unusually full. He was cautious but acute about tides and currents. In Christmas Sound he had some contact with the natives, whose miserable state went to his heart; and here he lost another man, drunk, overboard and drowned in the darkness of the night—the last of the four to whom his voyage proved fatal. Of the region as a whole he did not think highly. Having refreshed his men, he did not need to stay, and on 3 January he sailed into the South Atlantic, on a cruise that took him no farther south than just beyond latitude 60°, but nevertheless revealed some interesting discoveries.

(5) THE THIRD ICE-EDGE CRUISE

Inevitably he found himself once again the adversary of Dalrymple: 'our course was SE with a view of discovering that extensive coast which Mr Dalrymple lies down in his [Atlantic] Chart in which is the Gulph of St Sebastian. I designed to make the Western point of that Gulph in order to have all the other parts before me. Indeed I had some doubts about the existence of such a Coast and this appeared to me to be the best rout to clear it up and to explore the Southern part of this ocean'. Dalrymple had been very rash. It was one thing to mark, on the other side of the ocean, a fragment of coastline for Bouvet; one thing to collate the perfectly genuine, if difficult to identify, discoveries of Antoine de la Roche of 1675 and the ship *León* of 1756; it was quite another to transfer to his chart this enormous gulf, with islands inside it, from a map published by Ortelius in 1587, supported by no evidence whatsoever; and it was the sort of thing that inevitably turned Cook into a sort of executioner—the executioner of misbegotten hypotheses. By 12 January this one had gone to join the rest. Two days later there was something solid—the island Cook called Georgia, and at first thought might be the continent. He spent eleven days in its neighbourhood, circumnavigating it, landing in Possession Bay on the north coast, and charting all the off-lying islets and rocks. He was surprised to find an island of this size, and in these latitudes, covered with snow and ice in mid-summer. But South Georgia, as we now know, is surrounded by very cold water throughout the year. The Andes of South America are connected with the Antarctic Continent by a submarine ridge, the Scotia Arc, through South Georgia, the South Sandwich Islands, the South Orkney Islands and Graham Land.[1] But between the Burdwood Bank and South Georgia there is a marked break in this ridge, which, it seems, normally causes a northward swing of the Antarctic Convergence and so allows the cold antarctic surface water to flow to the north and east of South Georgia. Whatever the reason, here was the snow and ice-covered island, and Cook, by analogy, no longer doubted the existence of Cape Circumcision, 'and did not doubt but that I should find more land than I should have time to explore'. Had he not seen more land, indeed, the previous day? He had, but it turned out to be only the collection of rocks to which he gave Clerke's name. He was right to reason in favour of Cape Circumcision, for the cape, or Bouvet Island, like South Georgia is surrounded by cold water: it lies south of the Antarctic Convergence by about 250 miles, and in winter is almost on the northern limit of the pack ice.

Cook learnt something else from South Georgia, and began to think again about the formation of ice and icebergs. The mountains here were cased with snow and ice, but the quantity which lay in the valleys was incredible, and 'before all of them the Coast was terminated by a wall of ice of considerable height. It can hardly be doubted but that a great deal of ice is formed here in the Winter which in the Spring is broke off and dispersed over the Sea: but this isle cannot produce the ten thousand part of what we have seen, either there must be more land or else ice is formed without it.'[2] In other words, he had seen glaciers and formed a theory of the glacier origin of bergs; and this was valid in general, though such bergs as calve from the South Georgian glaciers in particular are small and seldom get out of the bays and fiords before breaking up and melting. Again, he was thinking about the possible formation of sea-ice rather than land-ice. With these thoughts he parted from Georgia and its rocks (24 January) in storm and then fog; and steering south to latitude 60°, three days later decided he would go no farther unless he had

[1] J. R. Forster had some idea of this, when he conjectured the existence of 'submarine mountains' connecting Sandwich Land, Georgia, the Falklands, Staten Land and the broken lands belonging to Tierra del Fuego (*Observations*, p. 30). The general theory of submarine mountain chains, dividing the earth's surface into four basins, had been propounded by Philippe Buache in 1752.

[2] p. 625.

undoubted signs of meeting with land. A large tract of land near Cape Circumcision, he now thought, was at least as probable as land in the south; 'besides' (and he is honest) 'I was now tired of these high Southern Latitudes where nothing was to be found but ice and thick fogs'.

The first iceberg of the season was seen on 27 January, when the fog lifted slightly. A strong wind the next day brought fine, clear weather, the sea being 'strewed with large and small ice'. Later in the day the ship fell in 'all at once with a vast number of large Ice islands, and a Sea strewed with loose ice'. By this time weather conditions had deteriorated and it was again thick, with drizzling rain and sleet. Cook thereupon stood back to the west, not before he had observed that all the surrounding icebergs were flat-topped, and nearly all of equal height, some of them two or three miles in circuit. Much loose ice was around which he describes as 'what had broke from these isles'. His position was now lat. 60° 04′ S, long. 29° 23′ W, and it seems much more likely that the 'loose ice' was the northern edge of the pack. Its mean northern limit for this month lies very close to the position given, and the presence of so many new tabular bergs, carried in this direction in the ice which moves north-eastwards out of the Weddell Sea, is additional evidence in favour of its near neighbourhood. In the very cold water here in January (between 0° and −1° C)[1] there is little chance that any reasonable quantity of 'loose ice' could be formed by pieces broken off new tabular bergs. Little progress was made the following day, because of lack of wind, which made it difficult to avoid the numerous bergs. On the 30th the ship was still in much the same longitude, though some thirty miles north, having sailed through a good deal more loose ice. Later the same day Cook records the largest iceberg seen so far on the voyage, but without giving any reasonably accurate idea of its size.[2]

On 31 January, in hazy weather, land was sighted, a group of rocky islets, with what appeared to be a coast beyond them. The tallest of these islets Cook named Freezeland Peak, and the land beyond, Cape Bristol. Continuing south he saw more land, which he called Southern Thule; finding he could not weather this, he stood north again, passing Freezeland Peak, to sight on 1 February still

[1] N. A. Mackintosh, 'The Antarctic Convergence and the Distribution of Surface Temperature in Antarctic Waters', *Discovery Reports*, 23 (1946), pp. 177–212.

[2] In the course of the years many very large tabular icebergs have been recorded from these waters. Accurate measurements, unfortunately, are few, but one berg met by the R.R.S. *Discovery II* in 1930, between South Georgia and the South Sandwich Islands, measured *c.* 70 miles along one face.

more land, which received the name of Cape Montagu. Cook thought it probable that Cape Bristol was connected with Southern Thule (which is not surprising in view of the thick weather he experienced, the many icebergs and the loose ice in the vicinity). He also thought he saw land between Cape Bristol and Cape Montagu, but did not consider it wise to go nearer. What he saw was probably pack ice and bergs. In certain years the northern limit of pack ice in late January lies among the southern islands of the South Sandwich group, and although the sea may be clear of ice to its west, the ice often is found further north on the eastern side. To add to the confusion the weather was mostly foggy.

The northerly course brought the ship next day to more land still. She was unable to approach close but Cook was certain this was an island and continued north, having named it Saunders Island; and on 3 February the Candlemas Islands stood up out of the haze. He pronounced that there were two of them, with a small rock, perhaps more than one, between—a fact borne out in more recent times.[1] A heavy northerly swell led him to believe that there was no more land to the north of him—the remaining islands of the group were discovered by Bellingshausen in 1819—and he tried to return to the south to make a further examination of the supposed coast he had just left. Winds were contrary, however, and he was in long. 23° 34′ before he could make any real progress to the south. By noon on 5 February he was 3 degrees of longitude to the east of Saunders Island; and on the 6th, seeing neither land nor signs of land, concluded 'that what we had seen, which I named *Sandwich Land* was either a group of Islands or else a point of the Continent, for I firmly beleive that there is a tract of land near the Pole, which is the Source of most of the ice which is spread over this vast Southern Ocean'.[2]

At this point Cook enlarges on the possibility of a southern continent, reasoning very sensibly that if there was *not* a continent then the polar ice should lie approximately in the same latitude around the southern ocean—which neither he, nor other explorers of his time, found to be so. The greater part of the land must lie south of the Antarctic Circle, 'where the Sea is so pestered with ice, that the

[1] As usual, Cook was right. His original description was the most accurate of all given by those who visited the South Sandwich Islands between 1775 and 1930—when the group was surveyed by the R.R.S. *Discovery II*—S. W. Kemp and A. L. Nelson, *Discovery Reports*, III (1931), pp. 133–98. Since this survey of the Candlemas Islands so strikingly vindicated Cook's original description, the second island now bears the name of Vindication. Cf. p. 635, n. 1 below. It is a tribute to the remarkable accuracy of Cook's navigation that the running survey of the *Discovery II* confirmed, with minor differences in longitude, the positions assigned by him.

[2] pp. 636–7.

land is thereby inaccessible'. The risk of exploring a coast in these unknown waters was so great, he thought, that it was very unlikely that any man '. . . will ever venture farther than I have done and that the lands which may lie to the South will never be explored'. Then follows a forbidding account of the weather conditions one might expect to find in navigating towards such lands, and a description, which would certainly not attract the ordinary man, of 'the enexpressable horrid aspect of the Country'. It seems obvious that if Cook was not anxious to remain in the antarctic waters in the Pacific sector a year earlier, he was now even more determined to leave them. His reasoning is best put in his own words. 'After such an explanation as this the reader must not expect to find me much farther to the South. It is however not for want of inclination but other reasons. It would have been rashness in me to have risked all which had been done in the Voyage, in finding out and exploaring a Coast which when done would have answerd no end whatever, or been of the least use either to Navigation or Geography or indeed any other Science; Bouvets Discovery was yet before us, the existence of which was to be cleared up and lastly we were now not in a condition to undertake great things, nor indeed was there time had we been ever so well provided.' Surely the statement, 'we were not now in a condition to undertake great things', applies to the men as well as to the ship, to Cook himself as well as to his company. They had had enough; and their captain must have been very weary with the strain of navigating that small ship in that sea. Cook does not generally reiterate dangers and hardships.[1]

When it became obvious that to return to Sandwich Land would be difficult Cook turned east for Cape Circumcision. Icebergs were seen frequently but were not, apparently, numerous enough to cause worry. The meridian of Greenwich was reached a week after they had turned east and on the next day, 15 February, course was altered to north-east, to get into the latitude of Cape Circumcision. Again conditions were bad, with snow and sleet, and by the 18th a great swell from the south convinced Cook that what he was looking for could only be an island; nevertheless he did not think that, in lat. 54° 25′, he could miss seeing it. But once more he was misled by

[1] Cf. p. 647: '. . . our sails and rigging were so much worn that some thing was giving way every hour and we had nothing left either to repair or replace them. We had been a long time without refreshments, our Provisions were in a state of decay and little more nourishment remained in them than just to keep life and Soul together. My people were yet healthy and would cheerfully have gone wherever I had thought proper to lead them, but I dreaded the Scurvy laying hold of them at a time when we had nothing left to remove it. Besides it would have been cruel in me to have continued the Faitgues and hardships they were continually exposed to longer than absolutely necessary . . .'.

Bouvet's error in longitude; and when he altered course to look for it, in long. 4° 17′ E, he was already too far east. It was not an island he was ever to see. The search continued in approximately the correct latitude for 13 degrees of longitude, to 19° 18′ E. South Georgia had convinced Cook that Bouvet was right. Now something else convinced him, finally, that Bouvet was wrong. On 21 February he himself was not far from the position where he had seemed for a moment to have seen land over the ice, when south-bound in December 1772;[1] and here he was sailing in a clear sea. 'Ice hills' had deceived Cook and his officers: ice hills, he had no further doubt, had deceived Bouvet.[2] He set his course northwards, 'having no business farther South'.

The main purpose of the voyage was over, and Cook indulges in some conclusions. We have seen that he does not deny the possibility of a southern continent; on the contrary, he is of opinion that it does exist, for otherwise how could one account for the 'excessive cold, the many islands and vast floats of ice'? If it does exist, then, he suggests, the land will extend to the north in the Atlantic and Indian Ocean sectors, chiefly because of the colder temperatures found here in comparison wth the same latitudes in the Pacific sector. No doubt this was a very reasonable assumption to make in his day, when little was known of the oceanography of these regions. We are now aware that, as has been already mentioned, the presence of so much ice in the Atlantic sector is due to the cold water flowing away northeastwards from the Weddell Sea, and so influencing the surface temperatures as far as long. 30° E.

He goes on to formulate some generalizations on ice. What he says on the origin of 'Ice Islands' is, on the whole, very close to the facts now known. He does not agree that they have been formed 'by the freezing of the Water at the Mouths of large Rivers or great Cataracts and so accumulate till they are broke of by their own weight'; for none of the ice taken up contained any detritus.[3] He suggests rather that they have their origin in the valleys of the southern

[1] pp. 59, 63 below, 14 and 18 December.

[2] In 1808 the Enderby whalers *Swan*, Captain Lindsay, and *Otter*, Captain Hopper, acting on their owner's orders, searched for the cape on the 54th parallel eastwards from long. 10° W. They parted company but the *Swan* came upon it on 6 October and the *Otter* on 10 October. They found landing impossible. Sealers visited the island in 1822, and landed in 1825. In 1843 the *Erebus* and *Terror* could not find it: Ross was driven some miles to the northward shortly before reaching its meridian, and regained his course too late to sight it, though he passed it only eighteen miles away. Its position was finally settled in November 1898 by the German Deep Sea Exploration Expedition vessel *Valdivia*, Captain Krech; but even then a landing could not be made.

[3] Morainic icebergs are, on the other hand, occasionally found in antarctic and subantarctic waters. They are seldom large and are usually met with near the sub-antarctic islands.

lands, valleys which 'are covered many fathoms deep with everlasting snow and at the sea they terminate in Ice clifts of vast heights'. The remainder of his remarks so nearly agree with our present knowledge of the formation of tabular icebergs, that it is worth while quoting them in full.

'It is here where the Ice islands are formed, not from streames of Water, but from consolidated snow which is allmost continuallly falling or drifting down from the Mountains, especially in Winter when the frost must be intence. During that Season, these ice clifts must so accumulate as to fill up all the Bays be they ever so large, this is a fact which cannot be doubted as we have seen it so in summer; also during that season the Snow may fix and consolidate to ice to most of the other coasts and there also form Ice clifts. These clifts accumulate by continual falls of snow and what drifts from the Mountains till they are no longer able to support their own weight and then large pieces break off which we call Ice islands. Such as have a flat even Surface must be of the Ice formed in the bays and before the flat Vallies, the others which have a spired unequal surface must be formed on or under the side of a Coast, composed of spired Rocks and precepices, or some such uneven surface, for we cannot suppose that snow alone, as it falls, can form on a plain surface, such as the Sea, such a variety of high spired peaks and hills as we have seen on many of the Ice isles. It is certainly more reasonable to suppose that they are formed on a Coast whose Surface is something similar to theirs.'[1]

Commenting further on the shape of these spired 'Ice Islands' Cook observes that the 'perpendicular clift or side' so often seen is, to him, convincing proof that they must have broken off 'from a substance like themselves, that is from some large tract of ice'. This is on the whole a shrewd observation, and not very far from the truth; but more than half a century was to pass before Ross penetrated to Antarctica and discovered the ice barrier and the shelf ice which today bear his name. Today most of these ice islands would be described as tabular icebergs, and they derive mainly from the shelf ice in the Ross and Weddell Seas; though some, no doubt, have their origin in the smaller tongues of shelf ice (such as the Shackleton Ice Shelf located in, approximately, long. 100° E), which are found at a few points around the coasts of Antarctica. While Cook was so nearly right in his reasoning on the formation of tabular, or flat-topped, ice islands, he was quite wrong in thinking that the tall, irregular-shaped bergs were formed alongside a rugged coast. We are now in little doubt that all these large weathered icebergs have their origin in the tabular berg which, as it moves in a north-easterly direction into

[1] pp. 644–5.

warmer water, melts below the waterline and, when it has lost its stability, overturns.[1]

Cook concludes these remarks with the following paragraph, and again it is appropriate to quote him exactly: for here he goes close to working out a correct theory of the formation and movement of the pack.

'When I consider the vast quantity of Ice we have yearly seen and the vicinity of the places to the Pole where it is formed, where the degrees of Longitude are very small, I am lead to believe that these Ice Clifts extends in some parts a good way into the Sea, such parts especially as are sheltered from the Violence of the Winds; it may even be doubted if ever the Wind is violent in the very high Latitudes and that the Sea will freeze over, or the snow which falls upon it, which amounts to the same thing, we have instances in the Northern Hemisphere; the Baltick sea, the Gulf of S[t] Laurence, the Straits of Bell-isle and many other equally large Seas are frequently frozen over in Winter; nor is this attall extraordinary, for we have found the degree of cold at the surface of the sea, even in summer, to be two degrees below the freezing point, consequently nothing kept it from freezing but the Salts it contained and the agitation of its surface; when ever this last ceaseth in Winter, when the frost is set in and there comes a fall of Snow, it will freeze on the Surface as it falls and in a few days or perhaps in one night form such a sheet of ice as will not be easy broke up; thus a foundation will be laid for it to acumulate to any thickness by falls of snow, without it being attall necessary for the Sea Water to freeze. It may be by this means that these vast floats of low ice we find in the Spring of the Year are formed and after they break up are carried by the Currents to the North; for from all the observations I have been able to make, the Currents every where in the high Latitudes set to the North or the NE or NW but we have very seldom found them considerable.'[2]

It is—as he says—an imperfect account; but it is—as again he says—written wholly from his own observation. Winds are, in fact, violent in the high latitudes in winter, and in the very low air temperatures of autumn the sea itself does freeze. There are, however, quiet periods and, beginning with the freezing of the sea itself, the build-up of the winter pack ice of Antarctica proceeds much as surmised by Cook. Once this build-up is well under way the blizzards

[1] Small tabular bergs merely capsize when the underwater part melts away—the large ones often break up. In both instances the part now showing above water will bear a ragged and often fantastic shape (cf. Cook's entry for 24 February 1773, pp. 98–9). Some will resemble the towers and spires of a university city; others will seem as if they could exist only in the imagination of a disordered mind. In Hodges's drawings of 'Ice Islands' there is—even allowing for considerable artistic licence—more than merely an artist's conception of icebergs; they have a foundation in fact.

[2] pp. 645–6.

of winter can do little to break up the ice, since the weight of frozen snow on the water inhibits the formation of waves.

As he wrote the words last quoted he was already steering for the Cape. He had considered making a final search for 'the French discovery'—this time not Bouvet's but Kerguelen's. But he let it go. If the French had really made it, then there was no point in his doing their work over again:[1] it could only be an island, and an island not fertile; and the search would keep him two months longer at sea in a very unfit condition. Instead he thought he would look for the islands of Denia and Marseveen, closer to the Cape—which he did, in vain, because they did not exist. They were the islands which really were of ice, had been sighted, and had dissolved into the sea.[2] On 16 March, in the evening, the land of the Cape was seen, and next day ships; and Cook learnt from a Dutchman of the fate of the *Adventure*'s boat's crew. His immediate comment is interesting. The affair was melancholy. 'I must however observe in favour of the New Zealanders that I have allways found them of a Brave, Noble, Open and benevolent disposition, but they are a people that will never put up with an insult if they have an oppertunity to resent it.' There are instances we can find in his own journal of a lack of openness, even of a certain ignobility, in this admirable people; and one is led to wish that he had seen, from beginning to end, more of the best of them. But few explorers could have written precisely in this way, after this sort of disaster. On 21 March the *Resolution* was in Table Bay.

§

She remained here for five weeks, refreshing and refitting, and we need not wonder that only the standing rigging was good enough to be carried on. Cook, as in duty bound, at once sent off a copy of his journal and charts to the Admiralty by an English vessel homeward-bound. He discharged three men at their own request,[3] and took on four more for the passage home. He met a number of oblig-

[1] But what did he do on his third voyage, as soon as he left the Cape in 1776?—He made straight for Marion's and Kerguelen's discoveries as fast as he could.

[2] It is rather odd that Roberts, who was on this voyage, should in the 'General Chart' he drew to go with the account of the third voyage (Chart LVIII), have solemnly inserted these two suppositious islands. But Cook was not altogether satisfied (p. 651) that they did not exist, and he may have put them originally into Roberts's chart himself.—*Voyage to the Pacific Ocean* . . . (1784), I, p. lxxxii, n. 'Every other part of the chart not mentioned in this account, is as originally placed by Captain Cook'.

[3] Two of these were of the same name as himself, James Cook and Nathaniel Cook; perhaps they were brothers? By one of those oddities that turn up in the muster books, they both entered on 1 August 1773, just after the ship left New Zealand on her winter cruise. Both had been in the *Endeavour*, and Nathaniel at least returned to England in time to sail again in the *Resolution* on the third voyage.

ing people. The most interesting to him was Captain Crozet, of the French East Indiaman *Ajax*, for Crozet had been Marion's second in command, and knew all about the French discoveries. Cook now heard of Surville, and was given a chart showing the tracks of Marion and Kerguelen; he heard too of the Spanish voyage to Tahiti. The two captains were delighted with each other; and Cook was fired with the idea of making a chart which would show all the discoveries, 'both Ancient and Modern', and of providing 'an explanatory Memoir'. Was he, one wonders, a little inspired also by the idea of 'showing' Dalrymple, the author of so many charts and explanatory memoirs? Something else he met with at the Cape, a copy of Hawkesworth; and at this he was rather startled. He knew, when he sailed on 27 April, to the tune of a Danish band, that he would not meet icebergs or excessive cold; he did not know that his principal enemies on his homeward passage would be, not storms or calms, but the sprightly ladies of St Helena. Hawkesworth, speaking as Cook, had printed too much Banks, and Banks had been too uncomplimentary in his observations on that island. Cook managed to make his peace. Indeed he must have been human enough to have been hard to quarrel with on this last portion of the voyage; he must have had some pervading sense of satisfaction with what he had done. We can find traces in our records of a high-spirited geniality that may surprise us till we recollect that Cook was thought of as an affable conversationalist. He was now reposing great faith in the chronometer: he had left the Cape in company with the East Indiaman *Dutton*, to make a direct run to St Helena; and Elliott tells us, 'The day before we saw St Helena, the Dutton spoke us, and said they were afraid that we should miss the Island, but Captn Cook laughed at them, and told them that he would run their jibboom on the island if they choose, and on the 15th of May we made the Land'.[1] He had six days here, and three at Ascension at the end of the month, turtling; settled the position of Fernando de Noronha, without landing, on 9 June; called at Fayal to ascertain its longitude and to water; made the land about Plymouth on 29 July and next morning was anchored at Spithead.

His communications descended upon the Admiralty. The journal from the Cape had preceded him; but now came reports on inspissated juice of wort and sour krout and sugar and the keeping of bread and experimentally cured beef and health measures in general —enough to throw the Victualling Board and the Sick and Hurt Board into deep billows of thought for some time. Cook had returned,

[1] Elliott *Mem.*, f. 41v.

'Having been absent from England Three Years and Eighteen Days, in which time I lost but four men and one only of them by sickness'—and that not scurvy. It was safer to be with Cook in the Antarctic than it was to live in London. If only men had not fallen overboard or into the hold! A report he does not make, but might have made, was on his benevolent efforts to populate the Pacific with four-footed animals. Sheep and goats failed in New Zealand, pigs succeeded; pigs were presented and explained with great ceremony to the New Caledonian elders; dogs and bitches (Cook is particular) from New Zealand and the Society Islands were conferred upon almost every island where he landed for any time—Tongatapu, Nomuka, Tana, New Caledonia; and of those left on the last island he is careful to note the colours, 'because they may prove the Adam and Eve of their species in this country'.[1] Similarly he was generous, according to his means, and what he esteemed need, with cocks and hens and vegetable seeds—though few people came off so well as the East Coast Maori chief who on 22 October 1773 was presented with 'two Boars, two Sows, two Cocks and four Hens; the seeds and roots were such as are most usefull (viz) Wheat, French and Kidney Beans, Pease, Cabages, Turnips, Onions, Carrots, Parsnips, Yams &c[a] &c[a]'. The chief, it is true, was not so enraptured by all this as he was by a spike nail half the length of his arm; but we are to know that at least the cabbage did well.

There was another report written at large all over Cook's journal, over Wales's journal, over the careful records of daily observations which went to the Board of Longitude. That was the report on John Harrison's chronometer—or, to give it its ordinary name in the journal, 'Mr Kendall's watch'. The precious, the wonderful object we see last, in connection with this voyage, in the hands of Wales. 'On Monday [31 July] I brought the Watch up with me to London in a Post-Chaise and on Tuesday Carried it down to Greenwich in a Coach & delivered it to the Rev[d] M[r] Maskelyne.' It would be an error to say that this day Mr Maskelyne was presented with the end of his lunar system; for astronomers, and even seamen, continued to fix longitudes by astronomical observations for more than a hundred years. Nor had Harrison, or Kendall, solved the problem of longitude for every ship-master; for a cheaper instrument than this was necessary.[2] But the problem, as a problem, was solved beyond all

[1] No scholar seems to have gone systematically into the fate of these animals, though G. M. Thomson, *The Naturalisation of Animals and Plants in New Zealand* (Cambridge 1922), carefully examined the New Zealand case. On Tana, it is said, the noise the dogs made at night was unpleasing to the people, and they were slain.

[2] 'Mr Kendall's watch' cost £450, says Gould, *John Harrison . . .*, p. 14.

further cavilling, whatever other inventors and craftsmen might do. Arnold was to make good chronometers. Those of his that went on this voyage, however, were not good. Of the *Adventure*'s two, one stopped before ever it reached the Cape. The other stopped there, and was started again only to go with vast fluctuations of its rate—though this was not immediately apparent, for Cook remarks, 8 June 1773, that 'it hath hitherto been found to answer extremely well'. It was on this day that the *Resolution* one jammed when winding, beyond all remedy. But as early as 2 September 1772 Cook was writing about the Atlantic currents, as we have seen, 'Such is the effect [they] must have had on the Ship, and which Mr Kendalls Watch tought me to expect'. After more than two years, he pays his tribute to Wales's assiduity as an astronomer—'the situation of few parts of the world are better assertained than that of Queen Charlottes Sound'—and adds, 'Even the situation of such Islands as we past without touching at are by means of Mr Kendalls Watch determined with almost equal accuracy'.[1] He is not the only person to indicate satisfaction. Gilbert remarks of his chart of the Tierra del Fuegian coast, 'it is settled in Longitude from the mean of a number of observations of the ⊙ and ☽'s dist[ance] taken by Mr Clerk and my self and reduced to one point by Kendals watch which is most certainly the greatest piece of Mechanism the world have yet produced'.[2] The step is small to those almost affectionate phrases of Cook, when the piece of Mechanism had become part of the nautical family, 'our never-failing guide the Watch', 'our trusty friend the Watch'. There is really nothing more one can say in approval of Harrison's work, or that comments with a more pleasing turn on the measured phrases, the carefully composed instructions of the Commissioners for finding the Longitude at Sea.

If we are to judge by newspaper paragraphs, the general public interest in the completion of this second voyage was not as great as in that of the *Endeavour*, though there were some fantastic references[3] —certainly not as great as that surrounding the preparations for it and the exercises of Mr Banks. Among the more instructed, however, excitement ran high. The arrival of Omai just a year before and his impact on polite society had roused an agreeable emotion; so polite, so social, so genteel, was this modest young savage in the midst of civilization. But the return of Cook was something of a different order. 'Glorious voyage!' wrote Solander in London to Banks, lagging rather shame-facedly (one is driven to think) down Channel on

[1] p. 580 below. [2] Gilbert, after 3 January 1775.
[3] Kitson quotes a few, pp. 308–9.

a yachting holiday. The Lords of the Admiralty also were extremely pleased; and as information spread the learned and humane were alike delighted and amazed. Cook, summoned to St James's Palace on 9 August, presented his sovereign with a selection of maps and charts, and was presented in turn with his promotion to post-captain and his commission to H.M.S. *Kent.* He remained in command of that vessel a very short time. The Admiralty had a different plan for him, and three days later, his formal application having been made, he was appointed Fourth Captain of Greenwich Hospital, at a salary of £200 per annum, *plus* fire and light and 1s 2d per diem table money. It is doubtful whether Cook ever drew on that 1s 2d, or slept in a Greenwich bed; his correspondence over the next year is all dated from Mile End. Nor was he quite ready for dignified leisure, even had that been immediately possible. He writes rather ruefully to his old friend John Walker, 'I must . . . tell you that the Resolution was found to answer, on all occasions even beyond my expectation and is so little injured by the Voyage that she will soon be sent out again, but I shall not command her, my fate drives me from one extream to a nother[;] a few Months ago the whole Southern hemisphere was hardly big enough for me and now I am going to be confined within the limits of Greenwich Hospital, which are far too small for an active mind like mine, I must however confess it is a fine retreat and a pretty income, but whether I can bring my self to like ease and retirement, time will shew'.[1] He had, however, in applying for this ease and retirement, been very cautious; he 'would on no account be understood to withdraw from that line of service which their Lordships goodness has raised me to, knowing myself capable of ingaging in any duty which they may be pleased to commit to my charge'.[2] He was prepared, that is, to put himself on the shelf, if the Admiralty so wished it, provided he could slip off again at any moment.

[1] 19 August 1775; p. 960 below.
[2] 12 August 1775; p. 958 below.

TEXTUAL INTRODUCTION

THE textual problem with the second voyage is at first sight simple; but the more it is scrutinized the more complicated it becomes.[1] There are two holograph MSS, and where the first leaves off the story can be picked up and completed from the second. This is true; but it is only a minute part of the truth. Of Cook's journal of the first voyage there are copies, but they are all essentially copies of the same thing: the large differences are few, and can be comparatively easily accounted for: the variants in detail are many, but they can be noted as part of a single process of composition. One does not proceed very far in reading the copies of the second journal, however, before one realizes that they are all copies of different things, and that therefore a vast amount of manuscript must have disappeared; while, added to this, there are enough fragmentary remains in various stages of composition to convince one of the quite extraordinary amount of writing that Cook must have done on the voyage, as well as after it. The differences are innumerable, and great. True, there was plenty of time on the voyage for writing; but what made the man not merely revise, not merely fill out where detail was lacking, or compress where detail was too technical and too abundant, but fill out and compress in different ways in versions that thus became different re-writings of some text, the original of which we are hard put to discern? Why, when he was supplying blanks with the names of bays and headlands, did he supply those in his log and not in the journal? Why did he sometimes, even, add what one would call a 'journal entry' to the log and not to the journal? I confess that to some of the questions that arise I can find no answer at all.

Both holograph journals are in the Manuscript Department of the British Museum, Add. MSS 27886 and 27888. To the first of these, which I print as the main part of the text, I give no particular abbreviated name: it is referred to in the annotation, where necessary, as 'the text' or 'the MS'. The second I name B. There are three copies, mainly in the same hand, that of Cook's clerk William Dawson, though with the different variations of size and shape that would arise over a period of years. The first is in the Public Record

[1] The first sentence of the earlier Textual Introduction, I, p. cxciii, must therefore be somewhat modified.

Office, Adm 55/108: it is obviously the journal despatched by Cook to the Admiralty from the Cape in March 1775, and I name it A. The second is in the National Maritime Museum, Greenwich, and I name it G. The third is in the possession of Lieut.-Commander Palliser A. Hudson, and I name it H. Of the foregoing, Add. MS 27886 is a 'complete' journal up to Cook's last departure from Queen Charlotte Sound, 10 November 1774; B is 'complete' for the whole voyage ('complete' because in both cases modifications must be mentioned); A is complete up till the arrival at the Cape in March 1775; G is complete for the whole voyage; H is complete for the whole voyage. A, G and H, though all three containing a great deal that is identical, also vary, more or less, throughout. In addition to these versions, holographs or copy, there are also a number of holograph fragments: one in the British Museum, a portion of Add. MS 27889; two overlapping sections, clearly escaped from B, in the Mitchell Library; and twelve folio pages in the Dixson Library, another division of the Public Library of New South Wales—which are equally clearly part of the origin of H.

How, then, do all these MSS fit together, and what use can be made of them to give us a final text of the journal, as close to Cook as possible? The answer to the first of these questions must be still in some respects tentative; the answer to the second is a matter of practical solution.

(1) The basis of all Cook's journalizing is his log. We have a holograph log, Add. MS 27956. In this of course he entered navigational detail, on one side of a double open page, and on the other side the first notes on 'remarkable occurrences', whether on shipboard or on shore. The next step was the writing up of the, or a, journal, in which the navigational detail was compressed and generalized into winds, course sailed, distance run, latitude and longitude at noon, and sometimes other information of a standard sort—still on the left side of the double page; with the right side occupied by further generalization from the log, and by accounts, sometimes enormously expanded, of all that might pass as 'remarkable occurrences'—of which, indeed, there might be no trace in the log at all, because at a certain stage the log was virtually superseded. The journal of the first voyage was a journal of this type; and of this type too is Add. MS 27886. Here we are very close to the events, and here Cook is writing at fair length. But this, it appears, on the second voyage did not satisfy him; and he very soon began a second version. How soon we do not know, but in this second version he was content to generalize almost out of existence the history of the voyage up to his arrival at Madeira. The

[Nove]mber 28 1771 I received a Commission to comand his Majestys Sloop Drake at this time in the Dock at Deptford, Burdthen 462 Tons to be man'd with 110 Men including officers & to carry twelve Guns; at the same time Captain Tobias Furneaux was appointed to the Command of the Raleigh at Woolwich Burdthen 336 Tons, 80 Men & ten Guns. These two Sloops were both built at Whitby by Mr. Fishburn, the same as built the Endeavour Bark, the former about fourteen and the latter eighteen Months ago, and had just been purchased into the Navy from Capt. William Hammond of Hull in order to be sent on discoveries to the South Sea under my directions. The Admiralty gave orders that they should be fitted in the best manner possible, the Earl of Sandwich at this time first Lord interested himself very much in the Equipment and he was well seconded by Mr. Palliser and Sr. Jno. Williams the one Comptroller and the other Surveyor of the Navy, the Victualling Board was also very attentive in procuring the very best of every kind of Provisions in short every department seem'd to vie with each other in equiping these two Sloops; every standing Rule and order in the Navy was dispenced with, every alteration, every necessary and usefull article was granted as soon as ask'd for.

Two days after I received my Commission I hoisted the Pendant and took charge of the Sloop accordingly and began to enter Seamen the Vestal Frigate at this time in ordinary, was appoint to receive them untill the Sloop came out of Dock.

[De]cm: 25 The Admiralty changed the Sloops Names to Resolution and Adventure, and the Officers were order'd to take out new Comissions & Warrants accordingly

FIG. 11. The opening page of Cook's holograph journal

B.M., Add. MS 27886, fol. 5

The entries for 28 November–25 December 1772

145

Δ carved door post. Upon the whole ~~they~~ their houses are better
calculated for a Cold than a hot climate, & as there are no
partitions in their ~~houses~~ they can have little privacy —
Household Utensils are confined to very few articles, the larg[e]
Jarrs before mentioned is the only article worth noting, every
family has at least one of these, in which they bake their ro[ots]
and perhaps fish &c: The fire by which they Cook their victuals
is on the out side of the house in the open air: at each are
three or five pointed stones fixed in the ground, their point[ed]
ends being about six inches above the surface, in this form, Δ
those of three stones are only for one Jarr and those of five
for two: The Jarrs do not stand on their bottoms but ~~lay~~ lay inclined on
their bilge or side: the reason of these stones is obviously to k[eep]
the Jars from resting on the fire in order that it may burn
better: Their Chief subsistance must be in Roots and fish, Coco[a]
nuts, bread fruit, Plantains and Sugar cane are by no means plent[iful]
Bread fruit are very scarce and Cocoa nutt trees are small and
thinly planted and neither the one nor the other seem to yeild m[uch]
increase. To judge of the Inhabitants by the number ~~what~~ we saw ever[y]
day one must think them numerous but I believe it is no[t]
so, ~~but those~~ at this time they were Collected from all ~~that the greatest part came from distant~~ parts to
see us; Mr Pickersgill observed that down the Coast to the
West he had seen but few people and we knew they came dai[ly]
from the other side of the land over the mountains to see us. ~~I have~~
~~observed, that we met many the day we went to the hills, those~~
~~were not all, several companies were assembled on the hills, of~~
~~the other side of the land in order to see the Ship, as might be~~
~~supposed amongst these were several Women and even some~~
~~children. However~~ But although the ~~Inhabitants~~ may not be numero[us]
the Country upon the whole is not thinly peopled, especia[lly]
on the Sea Coast and in the plains and Valleys where it is
cultivatable. It seems not to be a Country able to suppor[t]

Δ The bark of a tree which I am told grows in the West Indies which they are almost continually chewing, it has a sweetish taste [illegible] by some of our people [illegible]

FIG. 12. A page from Cook's revised holograph journal

B.M., Add. MS 27888, fol. 280
Cook's description of New Caledonia, September 1774

separate left-hand page entries disappear altogether, and compression, expansion and re-wording are carried a considerable stage farther. We know that this must have happened; for otherwise how could the copy A have come into existence? A is a copy neither of Add. MS 27886 nor of B, though a large amount of it is identical with B; and it is hardly possible that that tidy clerk William Dawson composed a new version of Cook's journal, to be signed at the end by Cook, all by himself. The inference seems inescapable that there was at one time another Cook MS, complete from the end of July 1772 to March 1775—a considerable body of writing—which has now totally disappeared. But Cook was still not satisfied, and he started out to rewrite the story of the voyage as a whole, from its origins and planning in England. It is important not to overdo the amount of re-thinking and re-phrasing in all this, but re-thinking and re-phrasing there was, and the sheer physical labour in so much writing was enormous. This version is B; and the clerk's copy of it is G.

Cook was thus writing—it must have been more or less simultaneously—three different copies or versions of his journal: copies, for he did, a good deal, merely copy himself; versions, for there are enough divergencies to justify that word. If we concentrate on the two holographs, we can see the process quite clearly. The changes in B, even if small changes, are almost invariably changes of expansion; and the large changes are invariably so. Sometimes the recasting is not a matter of direct observation more fully set down; rather it is critical, ruminative, ratiocinative; or it is the result of discussion with other men or even of a sight of their journals. Or, finally, the differences are not differences of recasting at all, but are due to Cook's decision not to write some big pieces of description twice over, but to put them into B alone. Examples of small changes need not here be given. Of the first sort of recasting we may instance some of the passages on Bougainville. Of the second, we may take our example from the writing about Easter Island: in the original journal Cook quotes verbatim a report from Pickersgill; in B this report becomes part of an account in which there is a good deal more Wales than Pickersgill—because Cook (as he informs us) both discussed the matter with Wales and read his journal. Of the third sort of difference, we have the descriptions of the New Hebrides and of New Caledonia.

There is, then, some sort of logical connection, in development or straight transcription, between all the MSS so far discussed. Why Cook, with blanks to supply (e.g. with a name like 'Queen Charlotte's Foreland', excogitated after his initial writing) should prefer to add it to his log rather than his journal, is a point of composition it is hardly worth pursuing: perhaps he merely grasped the first book of record that came to his hand, left the matter for later attention elsewhere, and finally skipped some of the regular process. A more important question is, how do we account for the MS I have called H? To use a biological metaphor, it may almost be called a sport: it does not fit in to regular development at all. It is a copy, and it is a copy partly of Add. MS 27886, partly of B, partly of writing in neither of these MSS nor even in A; and it has small additions in Cook's hand found in no other source. A possible presumption is that Cook, feeling he needed another copy of the journal, put William Dawson to work, during the voyage, on whatever part of his own MS he had last completed, including redrafted material not in the other MSS and later rejected; and, because it was a fair copy, added figures and notes as he checked through it which are not in the other MSS—or are there, but in a different form. This would make H chronologically precede G, which indeed, everything indicates, was the last piece of copying done. And it was B, from which G was copied, that Cook worked on to produce the journal ultimately printed.

(2) The foregoing considerations make the production of a twentieth-century text far from simple. The stated objective is to print from Cook's manuscript. But there is in fact no complete manuscript that one can print. We are confronted with two: one of these, as we have seen, stops with the final departure from New Zealand; and B, as will be seen, is so chaotic and has lost so many of its pages that we are in no better case here. An easy way out, if we merely wanted a text, would be to print G, a highly legible, quite admirable copy, quite complete, of B before B began to be worked over in England. But G has the disadvantage that it is in William Dawson's hand, not Cook's; it is indeed too perfect. We miss the process of growth; and to annotate a copy from an original is not a process one cares to contemplate. Our text must therefore be a composite one. The plan has been adopted of printing Add. MS 27886 as far as it goes, and completing it from B, the latter part of which is fortunately almost unbroken. Where differences between the two versions are great, or where B contains large passages not in its predecessor, interpolations have been made, signified at the beginning and end by asterisks. Smaller differences, when they actually add to the history of the voyage, are included in the annotation. Where there is a break in B, such differences have been recorded from A and G; and when B becomes the text, significant differences have similarly been recorded from the copies. But no attempt has been made, as with the journal of the first voyage, to note merely verbal changes, unless they have

what might be termed a 'curiosity value' in relation to the working of Cook's mind; for though editorial work in collation has not been wanting, the conclusion has been reached that such recording would in this instance merely overweight the purely textual annotation, without serving any useful and compensating purpose.

The individual MSS may now be examined somewhat more in detail.

I. ADD. MS 27886

This is entitled, erroneously, 'Log-Book and Journal of Capt. Cook Nov. 1771–Nov. 1774', and on the fly-leaf of the volume as now bound is the note, 'Purchased of Mess[rs] Boone, 13 May 1868 (Sale at Puttick's 11 March. Lots 644, 645)'. We may therefore conclude that its history is closely linked with that of other MSS dispersed at the Puttick and Simpson sale—a history examined, so far as that seems possible, in I, pp. cxcvi–cc.

The journal was written in seven folio books, originally of 45 leaves each, bound in thick marbled paper; and it is possible that Cook broke off this version merely because he had come to the end of his store of this particular paper. The whole, except for the back marbled covers, has been taken to pieces and re-bound in a guard-book. There are a few interpolations in the bound volume, calculations, notes of observations and of expenditure of water, small fragments of draft, and so on, the notes mainly by Gilbert as master reporting to Cook: which presumably Cook simply placed between the pages to preserve them. There are 319 ff. in all, together with four slips pasted on to a separate page at the end, each numbered separately, 320–3, and then an unnumbered blank page. There are other blank pages here and there, no doubt left for later writing which was not done; and in writing Cook generally skipped the first and last leaf in each book. The first folio and its verso is headed 'Remarks in Long Island Sound', and looks like a clerk's writing——it is certainly not Cook's, nor Dawson's. The front marbled covers are numbered 1–7, and have the dates of their entries written on them, i.e. Book 1, 28 November 1771–2 January 1773; Book 2, 3 January–11 May 1773; Book 3, 12 May–17 September 1773; Book 4, 18 September 1773–6 February 1774; Book 5, 7 February–23 May 1774; Book 6, 23 May–17 August 1774 (breaking off at an incomplete entry); Book 7, 19 August–10 November 1774. Cook begins by writing his dates in the margin in red ink—a practice to which he is not very prone. After 6 April 1773 he gives this up; for which one may be grateful, as the red fades badly.

In Book 3, ff. 97–105, Furneaux's journal for 8 February–15 May 1773 is copied out in a clerk's hand, verbatim, with notes by Cook at the bottom of ff. 97, 98, 99. Cook's own writing has comparatively few deletions and alterations. Large sections of the MS indeed are in his best hand, small, neat and regular, like a very careful fair copy—though even in these sections he leaves blanks for names and other words. The thought presents itself that in such sections he was himself copying from his own now vanished MS, that from which William Dawson also copied A. Towards the end there are a great many blanks for figures of observations and measurements of various sorts which he did not carry in his mind; and which, for whatever reason, he did not later supply. This habit of hiatus, it may be parenthetically observed, is frequently a dismaying one for an editor. The journal is kept in ship time.

II. ADD. MS 27888: B

The MS has again on its fly-leaf the note, 'Purchased of Mess[rs] Boone 13 May 1868 (Sale at Puttick's 11 March)'. It is a small quarto, of 367 ff. Cook wrote in folded sheets of four pages, each four being at some early stage neatly numbered, though not by Cook. At a later date, presumably when the MS was bought by the Museum, there was consecutive numbering of each folio. In between these two systems of numbering Cook had carried out an extensive revision, giving his revised sections of 4 pp., naturally enough, the same numbers as those for which they were substituted; but as he preserved the original sections, and the whole was bound with no eye to order of composition, some initial confusion can be imagined. This confusion is added to by the fact that numerous sections have been lost altogether. For example, between ff. 20 and 21 (latest numbering) the original sections 12–18 are gone, i.e. 28 pages; and between ff. 30 and 31, the original 24–9 are gone, i.e. 24 pages. The original 32 and 33 are gone. There are two sections numbered 35, original and revised; 34 runs on to the second 35; the first 35 runs on to 36, but the second 35 to the last page of 36. The original 40 and 41 are missing; 42 is a misplaced section about Easter Island, followed by another 42 on Dusky Bay. Little good would be done to the reader of the present lines by asking him to follow a detailed analysis of the whole MS on this plan. The confusion is caused primarily by Cook's use of it as a draft for the text he was required, in the end, to produce for printing. He operated on the creature of his own mind, as any author should, quite mercilessly—deleting, adding, interlining, re-phrasing, incorporating footnotes in the text, transferring paragraphs from one place to another, writing sentences in the margin, drafting new sentences or paragraphs on scraps of paper marked A and B; all —in this most unliterary of men—the tricks of the writer in gestation. He is mindful of a public, and slips in a phrase like 'which I shall endeavour to convey to the reader'. Finally, when interlineations became confusing, or corrections were vital, he took to the thing with red ink—mainly in the second half of the text. It is hardly Cook's fault that his MS was arranged for binding by someone who had not read it, so that interpolations now came in the wrong place, and marginal additions end before they begin; but he certainly set his textual student a difficult problem. No doubt a textual student of his work would have been the last thing he could have envisaged.

What is the result of all this painstaking process of rewriting? Can we regard Add. MS 27888—B—in the end as a journal written on the voyage at all? It is kept in civil time; but so is A, which was certainly written on the voyage. It can be said that we have a very good guide to the answers to these questions in G, the Greenwich MS, an excellent copy, as has already been explained, of B—i.e. of B in its unrevised form, its 'first state', as it came from the voyage. B in this form is full of second thoughts, obviously, but not of thoughts that contradict earlier observation. Sometimes, indeed, the only difference between B at any stage and a passage of the earlier journal is a difference in the order of words—e.g. 'I also thought' becomes 'I thought also'. There is contraction and expansion, but the total effect is elucidation; and observation is supplemented by reflection. An excellent example of this is the treatment of the long excerpt from Furneaux's journal (pp. 143–61 below). Cook reduces Furneaux's severely technical entries to four of his own quarto pages, and at once clarifies and narrates, before he goes on with the discussion of Furneaux's experience that he has already written. We have this in the first state of B, and it is copied in G. But in the later state of B—B as it is now—we have his own observation supplemented, in many instances, by the observation of at least one other man, Wales the astronomer, between whom and Cook there grew up a high mutual regard. Cook, it seems possible, may first have discovered the worth of Wales's eye at Easter Island, when he himself was confined to the beach. It is in this part of the journal, at any rate, that he mentions his indebtedness to Wales. For what was beyond the beach he began by using Pickersgill's report direct (pp. 340–2 below). This must have gone into B, first state, as into Add. MS 27886 and into A, because G has it, with footnotes by Cook that go back as far as A. Then he had some conversation with Wales, and saw his journal, as a result of which he wrote the account of the island (B first state), copied in G, part of which is printed in the interpolation, pp. 354–9 below. Later on, he had the free use of Wales's journal, as a result of which he rewrote Pickersgill and filled him out from Wales, as in the interpolation pp. 343–8 below. I assume he did this last rewriting in London. The process is clear enough in B in its present state, ff. 174v–82v and 168v–72v. We have now left G behind, and as our latest version is to be printed, we have no need of William Dawson any more. But the debt to Wales is not a narrowly confined one—it goes far beyond Easter Island. Cook, it is clear, was a licensed plunderer, and there is no doubt that Wales gave the licence happily. It extends to phrases, to paragraphs, to thoughts on which Cook built. Knowing Cook's way of expression, one is sometimes staggered at his text till one has read Wales. On the first voyage, Cook had received an education from Banks and Solander: this time Wales was his master. Yet he was a discriminating borrower. His discussion of the morals of the women of Tahiti is enlightened, but it is Cook as well as Wales. He takes as much as he needs, his own thought is stimulated, but his own style is stimulated too. We find him on occasion balancing his sentences with some skill. He knows that, although he has been given a free hand, there are times when the wise man uses quotation marks; so that, though we may be rather startled to find him adverting to the jaws of all-devouring time, and wonder when he studied the Elizabethan sonnet, we find him comparing the heroes of Homer and the heroes of the New Hebrides in the character of Wales, quite explicitly, and not of Cook. It would be a pity to lose this side of Cook, the reflective man, making the best of his story, almost as much as it would be to lose the immediate day-by-day diarist. The combination of the two journals and of the extracts from Wales gives the reader at once a wholeness and a control; he knows where he is with Cook, and it is hoped that the textual footnotes will aid this knowledge.

One conclusion follows quite obviously: indeed it has already been stated more than once. B, not pure Cook, is not in its entirety a journal kept on the voyage. But it is, even in its last stage, a journal of the voyage. We are bound to deprive Cook of the credit of universal observation. But he ought to get some credit for knowing where and how to extend his report: where and how to build up the truth without either padding or, too often, speaking out of character. The last few pages of the text, with their two versions of the closing days of the voyage, will show him as the painful reviser quite independent of aid from other journals; and these pages have an interest of their own, quite apart from and alien to the interest of newly discovered reefs, or icebergs escaped from by inches, or anthropophagi.

III. HOLOGRAPH FRAGMENTS

(i) British Museum, Add. MS 27889. Entitled on the spine of the binding, 'Cook's Second Voyage. Fragments'. The fly-leaf has the note on purchase from Boone after Puttick's sale. The contents, ff. 138, are extremely varied, as if a bundle of every scrap of paper within reach had been tied up and sold together—including what appears to be an 8 pp. draft for Hawkesworth (neither in his hand nor in Cook's) and the long transcript printed as part of Monkhouse's journal in I, pp. 564–87. Some of the material has nothing whatever to do with Cook or the voyages. For the second voyage the material is as follows:

(*a*) ff. 1–10. Chapter-headings for the printed version of the journal.

(*b*) ff. 11–21v. A fair copy, with further deletions and alterations by Cook, of the printed introductory pages xxiii, para. 3, to xxxv, para. 1. Part of it is very directly drawn from Palliser's 'Thoughts', printed in Appendix II to the present volume; part, on antiscorbutic articles, is taken from the text of the present volume, pp. 13–15.

(*c*) ff. 22–4v appear to be drafts of the Explanation and Preface of the MS I have called A.

(*d*) f. 26–6v. Notes on the Azores (cf. pp. 674–82 below).

(*e*) ff. 35–62v. These are clearly some of the missing sections of B, originally numbered in sections of four pages, 8–21; but they are the last version we have of this B material, and were printed as Chapters I and II of the book, pp. 1–42, to l. 20—though with revisions and deletions. The final deletions may have been due to Cook, the revisions to his editor. In general the writing has been tightened up.

(*f*) ff. 63–6 are similar redrafted pages of B, ff. 350, 11v–13v, with turns of compliment to officials at the Cape and Madeira; and of the conclusion of the journal.

(*g*) ff. 68, 70, 72 are more scraps, notes of positions, a few isolated lines of draft at a time.

(*h*) f. 75–5v is part of a rewritten draft of the account of Dusky Sound.

(*i*) ff. 79–82v, 97–8 are miscellaneous notes, mainly of observations, with some pages blank.

(*j*) ff. 131–2v contain a discussion of the government of Tahiti and the nature of the *arii*, which appears to be a summary of the matter as it appeared to Cook, but not part of the journal.

From this volume a few footnotes have been extracted.

(ii) MITCHELL LIBRARY MSS. In this collection are two sets of 8 pp. each, and one isolated page, obviously strays from B. The two sets are numbered in fours, 72–5; but though they run consecutively, they overlap, and 74–5 seems to be later-written than 72–3. They comprise the description of Tonga, corresponding to the last ten lines of Chapter II and nearly the whole of Chapter III of Book II of the printed journal, I, pp. 210–24 (to l. 14). The first set, Safe PH 17/12, which is sumptuously bound, was acquired in 1935, after a long sojourn in America; the second is included in the volume of 'Cook Documents', Safe PH 17/4, transferred from the Australian Museum to the Mitchell Library in 1935—i.e. it is part of the papers sold by John Mackrell to the New South Wales Government in 1886 (I, p. cxciv). Annotations drawn from either section are signified by the letter M. The isolated page, numbered 76, is included in a volume entitled 'Papers in the autograph of Captain James Cook', Safe PH 17/2, acquired from the Sir Leicester Harmsworth collection in 1932.

(iii) DIXSON LIBRARY MSS. The Library has two items of great interest to the student of the journal.

(*a*) In a volume entitled *Captain James Cook Relics and MSS*, which contains some of Cook's scattered letters to the Victualling Board (see Calendar below) there are also 12 folio pages of journal, for 18–27 December 1774, when the *Resolution* was on the coast of Tierra del Fuego. The contents of the volume seem on the death of Mrs Cook to have gone to her servant Sarah Westlake (who married another of the servants, Charles Doswell) together with the furniture of a bedroom and some volumes of evangelical religion. From Sarah by way of her daughter the papers and some of the furniture came to her great-niece Ann Arbery, of Honiton, in Devon, who about 1900 sold or gave a number of articles to a Dr Shortridge—and then, persuaded of rather sharp practice on his part, refused to let him have more.[1] The volume in question has Shortridge's name written in it; and from him, or his estate, passed to Sir William Dixson. The portion of the journal is highly interesting: the twelve pages are an

[1] I take this information from a copy of an affidavit made by Ann Maria Sanford Arbery, in 1930, now in the National Maritime Museum.

almost immaculate fair copy by Cook—but of what? The text differs in numerous respects from B, A and G, and the differences are mainly differences of expansion. When or why Cook wrote it I cannot guess: and it does not help to discover that it is the original of the corresponding part of the Palliser Hudson MS, or H.[1] I refer to it in annotation as D.

(*b*) The second item is a 36-page draft of the General Introduction to the printed journal. That is, it is a copy by a clerk of Add. MS 27889, ff. 11–21v, with still further deletions and alterations, both by Cook and by his editor Douglas; but to these pages is prefixed an account of the earlier voyages of exploration in the Pacific, up to, and including, that of the *Endeavour*. This account does not seem to be the work of Cook; for it has not merely alterations by him, but his critical comments in the margins. The particular interest of the MS lies in the last five pages, which are almost entirely in Cook's hand, with their 'tributes' to Wales, Gilbert and Hodges (though the last has been drafted more than once before) and finally the conclusion in which he acknowledges 'the kind assistance of some worthy friends', and goes on to summarize, in famous words, his own unliterary career from prentice-boy to commander[2]—a passage also in the 'Explanations' prefixed to A. He was thinking latterly, no doubt, of Hawkesworth's polished pages; and though his own here referred to form no part of the journal as now printed, there is every excuse for printing his conclusion also in an introductory position,[3] unimproved by any kind assistance.

IV. THE ADMIRALTY MS: A

The MS, in the Public Record Office, Adm 55/108, is entitled *Journal of the Proceedings of His Majesty's Sloop Resolution In Exploring the South Atlantic, Indian & Pacific Oceans by James Cook Commander*. It is a clerk's fair copy, a large and closely-written folio of 302 pages. Of these, pp. 1–239 form the journal proper, from 13 July 1772 to 21 March 1775. Facing p. 1 is a page of 'Explanations', dated 22 March 1775 and signed by Cook, who also signs after the last entry, on p. 239. The text has a large number of footnotes, most of them in Dawson's hand, but a few in Cook's, which add references to 'views',

[1] I should certainly have supplied the gap in B, pp. 595–8 below, from this Dixson MS, in Cook's own hand, rather than from A, had I not come across it in Sydney only after the text had been set, with its footnotes. I have therefore used it, with some regret, for annotation only.

[2] In the printed *Voyage*, 'commander' has become 'post captain'.

[3] p. 2 below.

later observations, or register changes of mind on such things as currents or the formation and decay of icebergs. The extract from Furneaux's journal after the ships parted on 8 February 1773, which is given verbatim in Add. MS 27886, is here (as in B) compressed into a summary by Cook, indicating (among other indications) a later composition of this version of the journal. At the end are three blank pages: after which pp. 243–302 are occupied by vocabularies drawn up by William Anderson, the surgeon's mate, for Easter Island, the Marquesas, the Friendly Islands, Mallicollo, Tanna, New Caledonia, New Zealand, and Tahiti. Of these the largest is that for Tahiti, 28 pp., and this is the only one that was printed. The first two of these pages is on pronunciation, or rather the system adopted by Anderson to indicate pronunciation, so that this section of the volume deserves some attention from Pacific philologists. The journal originally included 14 charts: of these ten have been taken out and removed to the P.R.O. Map Room, leaving only those drawn on the pages—Easter Island (p. 326); the Marquesas (stuck down on p. 335); Georges Isle (p. 337); and Palliser's Isles (a charming little work, p. 338).

The contents of the pages of 'Explanations' are characteristic. 'I had begun this Journal', Cook explains, 'from the time the Voyage was first resolved upon and the Sloops put in Commission'—possibly a reference to Add. MS 27886; but when he considered that all the preliminaries were well known to the Admiralty, 'for whose information only I was to keep an account of my proceedings', he thought it would be sufficient to begin with the departure from Plymouth—and indeed, it takes him very few words to get to Madeira. Notes follow on the use of the 'Natural' and not the 'Nautical' day throughout the journal—i.e. the adoption of civil rather than ship time in the dates; the allowance for variation in courses and bearings; the adoption of Greenwich, for 'the first, or fixed Meridian' and reckonings east and west of it; praise of Gilbert's help with the charts and Hodges' masterly manner with the 'Views'; and the warning that some days were passed over unnoticed: 'on such days, no interesting circumstance accrued'. Finally, we get what must be the earliest form of his statement of the disadvantages of his career for literary composition. It differs from its later appearances, and one sighs in vain for Cook's first drafting of it. It is worth printing here, for the reader who wishes to compare it with the version given on p. 2.

'On reading over the Journal, I found I had omitted some things and others were not sufficiently explained; these defects are attempted to be made up by notes; In short, I have given the most candid and best account of things I was able; I have neither Natural, nor acquired abilities, for writing; I have been, I may say, constantly at Sea from my Youth and have draged myself (with the assistance of a few good friends) through all the Stations belonging to a Seaman, from a Prentice boy to a Commander:—After such a Candid confession, I shall hope to be excused for all the blunders that will appear in this Journal.'

This modest statement does much to explain the gratitude with which the Commander received permission to use the journal of an educated man like Wales, who was on such familiar terms with ancient and modern literature.

V. THE GREENWICH MS: G

This MS, like the Greenwich MS of the journal of the first voyage, was for many years in the Royal Library at Windsor, and was presented to the National Maritime Museum by His Majesty the King in 1937. It is a folio volume of 473 pp., signed at the end by Cook. The title-page reads, 'Cap^{tn} James Cook's Voyage from The Year 1772 to July 1775 Given me by Himself, Bristol'; at the head of p. 1 are the signatures 'Charles Paget 1797', and beneath this, 'Mulgrave'. Bristol was Cook's friend Augustus John Hervey, 3rd Earl of Bristol (see pp. 196, 241 below), who died in 1779; Mulgrave was the naval captain Constantine John Phipps (1744–92), 2nd Baron, a nephew of Bristol, who left him his naval library; he commanded the *Racehorse* and *Carcass* venture into northern seas in 1773. Paget was presumably Vice-admiral Sir Charles Paget (1778–1839), who acquired the first journal also in 1797. From the last named, one guesses, the volumes went into the royal possession: Paget commanded one of the royal yachts, 1817–19, was in attendance on the Prince Regent, and was appointed a groom of the bedchamber in 1822. The volume is all in the same hand—William Dawson's—which however becomes larger and larger as it moves on, so that the last pages have about twenty lines fewer than the first ones; and the charts from the printed *Voyage* are bound into it. It contains no original charts or views. It is, as has already been said, an excellent copy of B before Cook began to revise B for publication; and if there were nothing else to print as a full but unvarnished account of the voyage, one could be happy in printing this. It has no preliminary statements of any sort, but begins immediately with Monday 13 July 1772: 'At 6 o'clock in the morning sail'd from Plymouth Sound with the Adventure in Company . . .' and in a few lines is at 20 July.

VI. THE PALLISER HUDSON MS: H

This version has a title-page identical with A—i.e. *Journal of the Proceedings of His Majesty's Sloop Resolution In Exploring the South Atlantic Indian & Pacific Oceans by James Cook Commander*. It has 361 pp., numbered to p. 356 by Cook himself, and is signed at the end by him. The engraved portrait of Cook by Basire after Hodges is bound in at the beginning. There are signatures on the title-page of Graham Palliser and E. W. Palliser, and there seems to be no doubt that the volume was originally given by Cook to Sir Hugh Palliser, whence it has descended to its present owner.

The copy is carefully written throughout, but not entirely by Dawson. Perhaps Daniel Clark, a supplementary 'writer' (p. 881 below, no. 133) was also engaged. It begins differently from any of the other MSS, with the heading 'Equipment', and the words 'Soon after my return home in the Endeavour Bark it was resolved to equip two Ships . . .' and then goes on to an account of the fitting out which adds nothing to that in Add. MS 27886—indeed it lacks the list of officers and crew and stores there given. The account must be early; for Cook has not yet learned Hodges' Christian name, and supplies a blank with 'Jam^{s}', as the name is given in the MS last mentioned. These preliminaries having been noted, H runs much like this MS, up to the time of leaving Funchal, with minor differences such as the conversion of tenses—e.g. 'have' becomes 'had'; and the population figures given in A and B are missing. From 4 August 1772 we have the double-page form of journal, as in our printed text, till 30 October, when it goes over to B (or rather G, as here occurs one of the gaps in B). It reverts to Add. MS 27886 on 23 November and proceeds thus through the rest of 1772 and most of 1773, with slight incursions, as it were, into A and B, including some, but not all, of the footnotes in A and B—and when they occur, not invariably in the same form. The extract from Furneaux is verbatim. Sometimes we seem to have an even earlier form: e.g. for the text entry for 2 August 1773, 'Being in the Latitude of *Pitcair*[*n*]*s* Island discovered by Captain Carteret', we have '. . . latitude of   Island discover'd by [*him* altered in Cook's hand to] C. Carteret'. But when we come to 13 August 1773, and the naming of the coral islet Motu Tunga, we have an addition to the text, with the italicized words, '*Stephens Isle*, in honour of *Mr Stephens, Secretary to ye Admty*', inserted by Cook in blanks left for the purpose; while in B Cook drops Stephens (without mentioning him) for Sandwich and

Hervey (p. 196, n. 2 below). From 16 December 1773 we have B, but with the left-hand 'log-entries'; those for 2–6 February, and 22 February–11 March 1774 are omitted by the clerk and supplied by Cook. This combination goes on till the end of the last visit to the Society Islands; when, from 5 June 1774, we have B without the log-entries, with footnotes sometimes differing, and sometimes in Cook's hand. Then, on leaving New Zealand in November 1774, we have a reversion to the double-page journal again, from 11 November to 17 December, with Cook supplying the figures for the last date; and from then we may say we have a sort of B—perhaps B as a first draft. The MS fragment D, described above, has some bearing on this; some other differences from B will be found registered in the footnotes; and the large difference may here be noted that in the present MS is no account whatever of the visit to St Helena, except the bare mention of arrival, necessary repairs, fresh food and water, and departure. The MS is graced here and there with Cook's spelling corrections: 'seveliz'd' becomes 'civilized', 'exceptable' (a word he uses a good deal) becomes 'acceptable', and so on. One wonders who his teacher was. He never, one may add, became a brilliantly 'good speller', having more important things to do; indeed, in the holograph journal B, having managed 'petrel' successfully for upwards of three years, some unknown compulsion made him convert the name to 'peterel'. Such things are worth knowing only because anything about Cook is worth knowing.

At the end of the journal is bound in Sir John Pringle's *Discourse upon some late improvements of the Means for Preserving the Health of Mariners*.

SUBORDINATE MS SOURCES

(i) COOK'S LOG

As with the first voyage, there is no complete holograph log by Cook extant; but there is more for this voyage than for the first, in Add. MS 27956, which covers the period 16 October 1773 to 28 July 1775. This, like Add. MS 27955 (first voyage) bears the fly-leaf inscription 'Purchased of Mr C. J. Smith 12 Decr 1868', and its history must have been the same (I, pp. cxcix, ccxxvi). It is a large quarto of thick rough paper, originally it seems in two volumes, of ff. 86 and 74 respectively, each stabbed through the margin and sewn. The log occupies ff. 1–139. It is followed by two quite extraneous folio leaves, not in Cook's hand, headed 'Describtions of the Bearings and Harbours within Trinity Bay' (Newfoundland), numbered 140 and 141; ff. 142 and 143 are two separate scraps, stuck on f. 144, notes of figures made by Cook's men, the backs of which Cook himself has used for figures. The numbering then goes on to the end of the volume at f. 164; 164v has some odd calculations scribbled by Cook. The two volumes have been taken to pieces and the separate folios pasted into a guard book. The odd thing about the log, in relation to the journal, is, as already pointed out, Cook's habit of filling in blanks in the log and not in the journal; and, it may be added, of amending figures in the log and not in the journal. This makes the log a valuable source not merely for his first thoughts, but for his second thoughts also, and the use made of it will be frequently seen below in the text.

The Mitchell Library has two stray leaves of log, Safe PH 17/2, for 26–29 March 1773 and 12 November–4 December 1774.

There is a fair copy, Add. MS 27887, with the fly-leaf note of purchase from Boone after Puttick's sale, 'Lot 647'. This copy, folio, ff. 135, runs from 30 November 1771 to 28 December 1774, though the period up to 13 July 1772 is compressed into 1½ pp. of narrative abstract. There are a few additions and small corrections of figures in Cook's hand, showing some discrepancies with those given in Add. MS 27956. Most of them are too minute to be taken account of in the annotation. Early in the MS there are the following drawings: f. 4, two well-executed profiles of Porto Santo; f. 4v, a chart of 'Fonchall' Bay; f. 5, a chart of the island of Palma; f. 6v, profiles of St Iago and a chart of Porto Praya. Pasted in at the end, ff. 136–41, are a number of sheets giving daily ships' positions and meteorological observations on various passages during the voyage: all except the last are in a clerk's hand; the last, giving the route of the *Adventure* from New Zealand to the Cape of Good Hope, is written out by Cook. All are included in the 'Tables' at the end of the printed *Voyage*, II, pp. 295 ff. On the last page of the MS, otherwise blank, is stuck a fragment of memorandum, also in Cook's hand.

In the annotation 'Log' with a capital always refers to Cook's log. Up to the date when Add. MS 27956 begins the reference is necessarily to Add. MS 27887, thereafter it is to Add. MS 27956, unless otherwise specified; when it is necessary to discriminate between the two they are cited as Log 956 and Log 887.

(ii) OTHER LOGS AND JOURNALS

(a) *Resolution*

The general considerations that apply to the logs and journals of the ship's company on the first voyage apply also to those on the second. There is the usual copying or 'dog-eat-dog' process; but no general prototype, like the ship's log of the first voyage, appears to be extant. Some journals were concealed on the day of handing over: these could not have been many—we hear of four (pp. 961–2 below)—and it is most unlikely that they contained much of value. The majority of those extant are in the Public Record Office, their classification numbers in which are given in the list below. Only those elsewhere found have their whereabouts separately noted.

Cooper

Adm 55/104, 109; *Journal*. 'A Journal of the Proceedings of His Majesty's Sloop Resolution, on a Voyage upon Discovery, Towards the South Pole. Commencing from her first fitting out at Deptford, [i.e. 30 November 1771] to the 22 of April 1774 .... kept by Rob[t] P. Cooper'. Cooper did not hand over the document at the same time as the others, but retained it till the day after the ship left St Helena. It is carefully written, more of a log than a journal, detailed on the ship's management, with short journal entries when in port. These tell one little of the man, who appears competent, professional, without frills or brilliance.

Clerke

Adm 55/103; *Log*, fair copy, 28 November 1771–21 March 1775. Clerke calls it a log, but it happily crosses the indeterminate line between log and journal on very many occasions. We get a Clerke very much more mature in observation than on the previous voyage, and writing a racy style that is always a pleasure to read. This is not merely the merry, loquacious Clerke, though the man of humour is evident enough; it is a man capable of serious thought. The training he got from Green on the first voyage in astronomical work now bears fruit, while his observations of birds and of ice are as painstaking and regular. Clerke, who wrote so little on the first voyage, is now eminently worth quoting in conjunction with Cook; as a summarizer of island experience, and as a man who tried to generalize his observations into some sort of system, he is eminently worth giving, also, in Appendix IV below. It may be remarked that he never draws a chart or a view.

The MS just described is a fair copy by Clerke himself. He may have been allowed to retain his original, or to regain it from the Admiralty, for it is now in the British Museum, in three parts, quarto, Add. MSS 8951–3: (i) 23 November 1772–15 July 1773; (ii) 16 July 1773–23 August 1774; (iii) 24 August 1774–21 March 1775. The third part has two large draft folio sheets bound in. At the end (ff. 94–9v) is a careful table of co-ordinates for the daily ship's positions over the whole period from 8 September 1772 to 12 June 1775, together with a list of 'Phaenomena'—the state of the sea, birds, seals and whales seen, and so on: and this is followed by 20 ff. of French extracts, together with a chart and English translations, describing Bouvet's discovery. The Museum has also another fair copy of the log, in two parts, Add. MSS 8961–2: (i) 23 November 1772–28 December 1773; (ii) 29 December 1773–21 March 1775. Both the original and this copy have Banks's name-stamp in them, and the second has the spine-lettering, 'Mus. Brit. ex legato J. Banks Bart[t]'. Possibly Banks got the original not from Clerke himself but from the Admiralty, to have it copied, and failed to return it.

There are some variants between the original and Clerke's own P.R.O. copy. It is the latter that has been quoted generally in the footnotes: extracts from the original are distinguished as 'Clerke 8951 [2, 3]'.

Pickersgill

Adm 51/4553/205–6; *Log*, 28 November 1771–7 June 1773; 8 June 1773–4 June 1774. This is the sort of extraordinary production one would expect from Pickersgill. It begins with a page in praise of lunar observations and an explanation of his procedure (or proposed procedure) in keeping the log. This is followed by 2½ pp. of a table of latitudes and longitudes and notes on how different places were inhabited, of which the following are specimens:

'Drakes Island	English Soldgers
Cape Ortugal	Spaniards
Ohitapeah Bay	Freindly People
Herveys Isl[d]	I know not
Middleburg Isl[d]	Freinds to Strangers
Q. Charlottes Sound	Canibals
Savage Isle	Savages
Malicola	Negro Baboons
Cape Coronation	I belive so'

The odd thing about the log, apart from Pickersgill's own oddities, is the fact that it is kept in a number of different hands, and expressed in more than one style—as if sometimes someone had copied out the ship's log or something else for the lieutenant. For example, the Dusky Sound passages are quite different from anything Pickersgill ever wrote: they refer to 'an officer' when Pickersgill is obviously the officer, or to the 3rd lieutenant, and even the spelling is nicely regularized. Now and again we seem to be reading Cooper: and as Cooper kept the ship's log, it is possible that sometimes Pickersgill, now a man of status, got someone to copy out the ship's log for him; now and again we have a phrase of Clerke's. But there is enough Pickersgill direct to keep the book characteristic. It has a number of delicate outline or wash charts or 'plans': 'Prija Bay', Table Bay, the Marquesas, Easter Island, and—quite the best—a 'Plan of Dusky Sound in Tevipoenamoo New Zealand 1773 Lieut. R. Pickersgill Delin.'—which looks very much like the original of the engraved chart.

At the end of the second volume he writes, 'As this Book will contain no more, I shall keep on my further Account of this Voyage by Journal', with his signature. This presents a further problem; for there is no journal in the P.R.O. collection. The only journal we have is a fragmentary one, which breaks off on an unfinished page as early as 3 October 1773. This document, pure Pickersgill, somehow came into the possession of the great whaling family of Enderby: it has the bookplate of Samuel Enderby, underneath which is the inscription 'Given to William Enderby by George Enderby October 1849'. In 1957 it passed by purchase into the National Maritime Museum. It is a quarto of 143 pp. written, followed by a few blanks, and gives the impression that Pickersgill took his log and the missing journal and tried to write a narrative from them. It seems to have been worked up in England—it has an extended account of the discovery of Madeira, a story which evidently took Pickersgill's fancy, and even a quotation from Hakluyt—but when he gets down to the business of the voyage gives the impression that it cannot be very different from a journal kept currently. Some of it is certainly worth printing in Appendix IV; I refer to it as the Enderby MS, or, in footnotes, as Pickersgill E. Notes from the log are identified simply as Pickersgill.

Gilbert

Adm 55/107; *Log*, 3 January 1772–21 March 1775. 'A Log . . . Containing such Astronomical and Nautical Observations as may be usefull to Navigation. Have added Plans with Perspective views (in their proper places) of such Lands as have been Discovered during the voyage. New zealand, Otaheita and the Society Islands I refer to Captn Cooks Charts, Published in 1769 [*sic*][1] wherein the true situation of the Most projecting Points and Capes are well determined both in Latitude and Longitude the Reefs shoals &c are much better described than Many on the Coast of Great Britian.' This volume is pretty strictly a log; it has only a few concessions to journal writing, mainly brief summaries on places visited. Daily barometer and thermometer readings are given. Gilbert was a better draughtsman than handwriter, and his chief interest is in the many finely done charts and little water colour drawings or 'perspective views' which he gives. The best of these latter are Palliser's Islands, the volcano on Tana (Portfolio, Chart XXXVII*b*), Southern Thule, 'Christmas Bay', and New Year's Harbour (the last three Figs. 74*a*, *b* and 78 in this volume).

Isaac Smith

Adm 55/105; *Log*, 17 December 1771–11 March 1775. Again this is almost pure log, like Gilbert: it is a good log, but Isaac's 'Remarks' are formal and skimpy, and not highly literate. His attitude towards writing he perhaps sums up on 1 September 1774: 'As it will be impossible for me to describe the Situations of these Islands I have added a small map which I hop will Answer all Nautical Purposes, as farther Description I leave to Abler Hands'—and an excellent small map, of the 'Great Cyclades', it is. The log contains 15 charts and plans, and a wash drawing of icebergs; in most of the charts the ship's track is marked, and the work in general is precise—the master's mate had not been trained by Cook for nothing.

Burr

Adm 55/106; *Log*, 24 December 1771–15 March 1775. Burr is rather more literate than Smith, his fellow master's mate, and as a penman goes in for some rather superior flourishes; but, allowing for longer phraseology, his record is much the same—almost entirely confined to the nautical side of the voyage, good on observations; on the other hand, he has no charts.

Willis

Adm 51/4554/201–2; *Log*, 23 November 1772–18 October 1774; 19 October 1774–6 February 1775.—Adm 55/106 (a few pages stuck in

[1] From this it appears that, although Hawkesworth's volumes were not published till 1773, the charts for them must have been engraved before the *Resolution* left England in July 1772.

at the back); *Log*, 7 February–13 March 1775.—Adm 51/4554/199–200; *Journal*, 3 January 1772–23 December 1773; 24 December 1773–13 March 1775. There is nothing in all this beyond brief conventional entries; the log is quite good technically—better in fact than the journal.

Harvey

Adm 51/4553/184–7; *Journal*, 17 December 1771–7 March 1775. This is a log rather than a journal, in spite of the name which Harvey gives it. There are a few more extended entries in the islands, but nothing that shows original observation.

Loggie

Adm 51/4554/207; *Journal*, 18 January 1772–26 July 1773. At any rate, the writer denominates it 'Charles Loggie his Journal'; it is a very cursory production, probably all that one could expect from the unhappy Loggie.

Hood

Adm 51/4554/181–3; *Journal*, 5 March 1772–10 March 1775. This may be called a journal by courtesy—Hood does not give it a name at all. It is carefully written, without originality of phrase, which one could hardly expect from a boy who was only 14 when the voyage began.

Maxwell

Adm 51/4555/2–6; *Log*, 22 November 1772–13 March 1775. This is kept in several different hands on three different sizes of paper, sewn into a bit of old sail-cloth. It keeps to the general pattern, is strong on astronomical observations, and has nothing worth quoting.

Mitchel

Adm 51/4555/194–5; *Log*, 23 November 1772–14 March 1775. The spelling of the name with one 'l' is the writer's own, and he signs his name on the inside of the front and back covers of each of the large folio vellum-bound books. This is a very good and full log, with intelligent comment on islands, people, birds, etc., but rather lacking on the scientific side. The first two pages of the first volume give some interesting lists—an analysis of the crew in the watches when the ship sailed from the Cape, further broken down into officers, fo'c'sle men, waisters and afterguard; and a list which identifies the barber, the baker, and other functionaries who do not figure in the muster books as such.

Elliott

Adm 51/4556/208; *Log*, 23 November 1772–2 March 1775. Although Elliott was only 14 or 15 at the outset of the voyage (he says 14, the muster book 15) he was more capable of individual expression than the rest of the midshipmen, and appears a sensible and sensitive fellow, who keeps a neat log, illustrated with a few equally neat little wash drawings. He has a courteous turn of phrase most unusual in these documents: 'Since our Arrival [in Queen Charlotte's Sound], A friend of mine having been favor'd with the Track of the Adventure since our seperation was so good as to favor me with the Copy Which I Shall Insert in my Logg (Viz) . . .'. 'Houtahoyta' is an original rendering of Otaheite; and 'Snowyland' is his own name for South Georgia.

Elliott appears again, in the BRITISH MUSEUM, Add. MS 42714, 'Memoirs of the early life, of John Elliott, of Elliott House, Near Misson, Yorkshire, Esqr and, Lieut^t of the Royal Navy, written by himself, *at the request of his Wife* for the use, and Amusement of his Children only'. Fortunately these memoirs survived the children. Of an MS of 99 ff. +ii +3 plans of the Battle of Waterloo, ff. 7v–45v are devoted to the voyage. We do not know at what age Elliott wrote this; but he gives an extraordinarily vivid picture of his adventurous youth up to the Battle of the Saints, 12 April 1772, when an explosion of gunpowder put an end, so it seems, to his naval career. When he can be checked against the other records of the voyage, he is generally accurate, although it is quite possible that some minor detail may be inaccurate or confused: e.g. some of his guesses at the ages of his shipmates are rather rough ones. It is fairly safe to assume that the happenings of the voyage made such an impression on him, in his own impressionable adolescence, that a distorted account (where he cannot be checked) is hardly probable. There may be a little heightening at times, and no doubt we must allow for the personal view. But we can be thankful to Mrs Elliott for making her request. In the annotation log extracts are given as Elliott: those from the Memoirs as Elliott *Mem*.

Price

Adm 51/4556/190; *Log*, 1 September 1773–15 March 1775.—Adm 51/4556/188–9; *Journal*, 18 December 1772–15 March 1775. Price is described in the muster book as 20, Elliott thought he was about 15. The scribbling and experimenting with his signature, and the notes of working rules, on the fly-leaves of the log, would suggest that if 20, he was young for his age. The log is systematic but untidy, the handwriting awkward; the journal is no more than a slightly re-worked copy of the log, with half a dozen crude wash drawings of islands and coasts in the first volume.

Anon.

Adm 51/4555/218; *Log*, 22 November 1772–31 December 1773. The regular pattern, and quite commonplace.—Adm 51/4557/219; *Log*, 1 July 1773–9 March 1775. This contains notes of a great many lunar observations, and may possibly be a partial copy of the ship's log.

(b) *Adventure*

Furneaux

Adm 55/1; *Journal* and *Log*. The journal is headed 'Remarks onboard His Majesty's Sloop the Adventure (late called the Raleigh)' and runs from 28 November 1771–10 July 1774. It is a fair copy in two or three different hands. It is followed by 'The Logg of His Majesty's Sloop Adventure' in a different, smaller hand. Both are signed 'Tob^{s} Furneaux'. Furneaux was no journal keeper: the journal is simply a laconic abstract of the log, some of the entries in which are much fuller—such as a good description of Tonga, 3–8 October 1773. The journal however is fuller on the tragedy at Queen Charlotte Sound. It has not seemed worth while to print any of this material except in annotation of Cook. We are in different case however with B.M. Add. MS 27890—another of the Boone-Puttick purchases. This is in 20 ff. quarto, and is a fair copy by a clerk of an account written by Furneaux of the whole voyage, from 13 July 1772 to 3 March 1774, on which day he abandoned his independent search for Bouvet's land and hauled off northward for the Cape. From the appearance of the MS it was undoubtedly Furneaux's contribution to the printed volumes, suggested—one imagines—by Cook,[1] who has deleted everything on the periods when the two ships were together, as well as Furneaux's observations in Queen Charlotte Sound, and made a few corrections and minor alterations. What is left is printed in the *Voyage*, Book I, Chapter VII, and Book IV, Chapter VIII. Extracts—more than Cook gave—are now given in Appendix IV below.

[1] Perhaps to help Douglas when he was revising the journal for print. There is a letter extant from Cook to Douglas (dated only 'Sunday Morn'g') which reads in part, 'I am sorry Captain Furneaux's Journal has given you so much trouble, I am in some measure in fault for not looking over the Copy before it was put into your hands'.—Eg. MS 2180, f. 11. There could be no difficulty with the account in question.

In the ALEXANDER TURNBULL LIBRARY, *Holograph Letters and Documents of and relative to Captain James Cook*, is a fair copy of portion of the journal, 8 February–19 May 1773—i.e. the first period when the ships were parted; ff. 14 + 15 blanks. The individual entries are slightly shortened. It is in a hand rather like Furneaux's, but not, I think, his.

Kempe

dm 51/4520/1–3; *Log*, 13 July 1772–13 July 1774.—Adm 51/4520/4–5; *Journal*, 3 January 1772–13 July 1774. Kempe was evidently an educated man with a clear mind. The log is good and well-written, with some interesting detail; the journal, like Furneaux's, is a brief abstract of the log, with very little extra information.

Burney

Adm 51/4523/1–2; *Log*, 18 November 1772–23 January 1774.—Adm 51/4523/3–4; *Journal*, 19 November 1772–20 May 1774. Burney seems to have discarded from these records anything he wrote while in the *Resolution*. The log is a very good one technically, with a number of 'journal-entries'; and in it is pasted a copy of the report Burney made to Furneaux on his expedition to East Bay in search of the massacred boat's crew. The journal is, again, not as good or as full as the log, which it either repeats or abstracts. The log has so much of interest, however, what while Burney is one of our chief authorities for the *Adventure*, his observations extend also to the voyage in general. His chart of Van Diemen's Land is reproduced in the Portfolio, Chart XXVII. There is a copy, in Burney's hand, of his report on the massacre, and another of this chart, in the ALEXANDER TURNBULL LIBRARY, *Holograph Letters and Documents*. . . .

FERGUSON MS. There is an extremely interesting MS in the possession of Mr J. A. Ferguson, of Sydney, which gives us an unbuttoned Burney, and supplements his more formal records in a most valuable way. This, we remember when reading it, was one of the Burneys, Fanny's brother. It is a folio volume, of 35 ff., one or two of which are blank, and there are 9 ff. blank at the end. Some ff. in addition have been cut out, but this does not appear to affect the text. It runs from 22 June 1772 to 22 December 1773. Burney seems to have started it as a sort of long journal-communication to his family, and the account he gives is very frank, and now and again not uncritical of his shipmates. For the Tasmanian visit he copies his log, and draws the chart of Van Diemen's Land again, with an inset of Tasman's chart copied from Harris's *Voyages*. He has also a profile of

Cape Barren and charts of Adventure Bay and Vaitepiha Bay. Later on he puts down New Zealand and Tongan tunes in music notation. In the end the MS turns into rather disconnected notes, which nevertheless are always interesting. Burney, it is clear, could have produced a very good book on this voyage. This MS is cited as Burney, Ferguson MS.

Wilby

Adm 51/4522/14; *Journal*, 14 July 1772–13 July 1774. Wilby calls it a 'Journal of the Proceedings... on an Eastern expedition round the Globe'. It is the best of the midshipmen's journals, showing some direct observation and certainly more originality and personal feeling in the language than the rest. Why Wilby was allowed to retain it to the end of the voyage, instead of giving it up on 16 March 1774, we have no means of knowing: there are several other instances of this.

Constable

Adm 51/4520/7–8; *Journal*, 6 December 1771–14 March 1774. This is a fairly brief journal, clearly written, and spelt in a highly individual manner.

Lightfoot

Adm 51/4523/5; *Log*, 23 November 1772–14 May 1773. Unambiguously a log, with nothing much in it, and that much not always clearly expressed; it is hard to read because of its close writing and flourishes.

Hergest

Adm 51/4522/13; *Journal*, 13 July 1772–12 July 1774. Hergest also, curiously enough, managed to retain his journal till the end of the voyage. It is a tolerably good production, with some curious affinities to Browne the A.B. (see next entry); it is difficult to say who copied whom, but Hergest on the whole is fuller, writes more intelligibly, and spells better.

Browne

Adm 51/4521/9–10; *Journal*, 18 March 1772–16 March 1774. Brief, but not unintelligent, with one or two individual passages. Presumably he and Hergest were friends, and at times shared impressions.

Hawkey

Adm 51/4521/11; *Log*, 8 January 1772–14 March 1774. A neat full log, but hardly anything more. As Hawkey was master's mate for half the voyage, he probably drew largely on the ship's log.

Dyke

Adm 51/4521/12; *Log*, 4 June 1772–12 July 1774. Another puzzle in over-long retention of a log. It is neat, thin, and dull. Opposite the entries for the first half of November 1772 there are three pencil outlines of coastal profiles, one with a little shading.

Falconar

Adm 51/4524/1–2; *Log*, 23 November 1772–11 July 1774. 'Falconar' is the writer's own spelling of his name. He produces an excessively neat fair copy, presumably of the ship's log.

Anon.

Adm 51/4524/3–4 (labelled 17–18); *Log*, 23 November 1772–20 February 1774. An extraordinary production which just stops short of complete illegibility. So far as can be judged, it copies the ship's journal.

(iii) CIVILIANS' JOURNALS

Wales

MITCHELL LIBRARY MSS, Safe PH 18/4. *Journal*, 21 June 1772–17 October 1774. The MS is a large rather battered folio, very closely written, of 376 pp., most unfortunately incomplete. At the end is added a plan of an anchorage and fortified town, which we should willingly exchange for even one of the lost pages of the journal. Like everything else we have of Wales's, this serves to convince us of the breadth and play of his mind, his capacity for observation, his scientific exactitude, and his integrity as a man. It is both log and journal: that is, when at sea he does not write narrative or summaries, but seems to have used the ship's log pretty fully, and added his own observations. Thus he regularly notes two latitudes, by dead reckoning and by observation; four longitudes, by dead reckoning, by observation, by the watch at its Greenwich rate, and by the watch at its last observed rate of going; and the barometer and thermometer readings. He is most particular in his account of physical phenomena, and of his procedure in, e.g. tidal measurements. He appreciates natural scenery, and has a poet in his mind for his more ecstatic moments. Whenever he has a chance to observe mankind he writes at length and with talent. This journal is certainly the one that Cook read through so appreciatively. I have printed a good deal of it in Appendix V, omitting most of the detail of scientific observation, narrowly considered, which is now dead; not merely for its value in itself, but for its other value as—one might say—a source book for Cook. I have reduced cross-reference in the annotation to the barest minimum, and there is no need to print parallel passages in this place; but the reader can hardly fail to find Wales as excellent, in his way, as Cook, and comparison of the two journals highly interesting. This does not hold only for extended passages, such as occur in the description of Easter Island: a close student of Cook may occasionally wonder how he hit on an isolated and vivid phrase, such as the description of the man at the Marquesas, baling blood and water out of his canoe 'with a kind of hysteric laugh'. To find Wales's journal is to find the explanation of a great deal.

Royal Greenwich Observatory, Herstmonceux. Board of Longitude Papers, Vol. XLVI. *Log-Book of the Resolution.* This fortunately is intact, a fair copy, running from 21 July 1772 to 1 August 1775, and unfoliated. It is naturally enough, like the journal, kept in astronomical time—i.e. the day begins and ends at noon, but twenty-four hours later than ship time, so that the astronomer's 1st is the sailor's 2nd.[1] Wales's shorter entries in his journal tend to be virtually copied from this log, occasionally with some divergences, so that once or twice the log is more worth quoting than the journal. The great delight of the log is its twenty-two charts drawn by Wales, discovered too late for any inclusion in our volume of *Charts and Views*. Four are now reproduced. Wales may be quoted on this subject, for his characteristic mixture of professional pride and caution: 'As to Maps &c. which accompany this Volume, I can safely say they are my own both with respect to the Elements and execution: being done by my own hand, without either seeing or knowing any thing that was done on this head by other Persons. I was more particular in this, as I am convinced by much experience, that where

[1] Wales evidently had some difficulty over this with his shipmates: for at the end of the log he writes, 'I think, considering the connexion there is between them, it is much to be lamented that Seamen and Astronomers should not reckon their days alike, as this difference is very troublesome and causes much confusion, especially amongst younger hands in looking for, and taking things out of the Nautical Almanac. I have met with some whom I never could make fully comprehend it'.—Astronomical time was maintained till 1925.

Persons are continualy seeing what is done by others they are naturally lead to stretch their own Ideas & opinions towards those of their neighbours, and thereby loose all their own originallity, & become, in the End, little more than the notions and opinions of one Man, who happens to be more opinionated, or obstinate than the rest'. So Wales put down nothing that he did not see himself or have described to him by someone at the masthead—'I never went to the Mast Head myself'—and he drew attention to the possibility that what he put in as one island might be two or even more, and to other perils of the cartographer at sea. Altogether, we do not need to go to Charles Lamb or Leigh Hunt to find him an engaging figure.

Board of Longitude Papers, Vol. XLVII. *Observations.*[1] The astronomical observations made by Wales on the voyage are here entered in tabular form, with some notes on the instruments used, and calculations of longitude. The same volume contains (i) 'Journal of a voyage made by order of the Commissioners of Longitude on board of his Majesty's Sloop Resolution, 1772, 1773, 1774, 1775. W. Wales.' This appears to be the rough draft of the log. (ii) Record of the winding of the chronometers, signed by Cook, Wales, and one of the officers. (iii) Astronomical observations made at different places on shore; observations on the variation of the compass, rates of the clocks, tides, dip of the magnetic needle; lunar observations and observations of the solar eclipse.

Bayly

ALEXANDER TURNBULL LIBRARY. *Journal*, 23 June 1773–14 July 1774. A small folio volume of 135 pp. Bayly seems to have been a reasonably competent astronomer, but he had little of the education and none of the general abilities of Wales, and his rather short journal is by no means in the same class. Nevertheless, it contains a good deal of interest—on the *Adventure*'s experiences in New Zealand and in Tonga, on natural phenomena, on the peculiarities of the ship's officers. These last perhaps only the civilian would write about, and we are duly grateful to Bayly. His New Zealand pages have been printed by McNab in the *Historical Records of New Zealand*, II, pp. 201–18.

ROYAL GREENWICH OBSERVATORY, HERSTMONCEUX. Board of Longitude Papers, Vol. XLIV. *Log*,[2] 1 July 1772–13 July 1774.

[1] I have not seen this volume, and am indebted to Mr G. P. B. Naish for describing it to me.

[2] For notes on this and the volume of Observations next mentioned I am again indebted to Mr Naish.

This log has very few general remarks: the only descriptive passage of any length is on the Grass Cove massacre.

Board of Longitude Papers, Vol. XLV. *Observations.* This is devoted to the astronomical observations and calculations and to the daily record of the winding of the watches, signed by Furneaux, Bayly, and one of the lieutenants.

THE PRINTED SOURCES

COOK

A Voyage towards the South Pole, and Round the World. Performed in His Majesty's Ships the Resolution and Adventure, In the Years 1772, 1773, 1774, and 1775. Written by James Cook, Commander of the Resolution. In which is included, Captain Furneaux's Narrative of his Proceedings during the Separation of the Ships. 2 vols., 1777.

This is certainly Cook's book. There were to be no more Hawkesworths. 'The Journal of my late Voyage', writes Cook to his friend Commodore Wilson at Great Ayton, 'will be published in the course of next winter, and I am to have the sole advantage of the sale. It will want those flourishes which Dr. Hawkesworth gave the other, but it will be illustrated and ornamented with about sixty copper plates, which, I am of opinion, will exceed every thing that has been done in a work of this kind. . . . As to the Journal, it must speak for itself. I can only say that it is my own narrative, and as it was written during the voyage.'[1] This, though true enough, is not quite true; for we have already seen what pains he took to operate upon his journal, 'as it was written during the voyage', to make it fit for publication. And Cook had a collaborator, or editor, the well-known Dr John Douglas, Canon of Windsor, an expert and judicious practitioner in letters.[2] What Douglas did he estimated in two different ways at two different times. Writing to an unnamed correspondent in 1783 (when he was working on the third voyage), he protests against what he regards as contemptuous references to himself and to Cook in the

[1] 22 June 1776: quoted in George Young, *Life and Voyages of Captain James Cook* (1836), pp. 304–5.

[2] John Douglas (1721–1807), who appears frequently in Boswell's *Johnson*, 'the great detector of impostures', and in Goldsmith's *Retaliation*, as 'The scourge of impostors, the terror of quacks', was one of those 'respectable ecclesiastics' who did very well out of patronage in that century, the particular patron being the Marquis of Bath. Douglas became Canon of Windsor 1762, Canon of St Paul's 1776, Bishop of Carlisle 1787, Dean of Windsor 1788, Bishop of Salisbury 1791. He was a sociable man, wrote well, and was a good political and literary controversialist.

Morning Chronicle:[1] he asks this correspondent to find out from the editor 'who the Person is who told him I *digested* Capt Cook's former Voyage, which is absolutely false, as is also his other Assertion, that I am now *finishing* the last Voyage. The last as well as the former Voyage were prepared for the Press by the Captain himself, as may be seen by the M.S.S. in being; and even an Author by Profession, can never lay Claim to his own work, if the correction of a few Inaccuracies in Style, by a friend, can give the latter the least Share in the Merit or Demerit of the Composition'.[2] But in his autobiography he writes, 'In 1776 & 1777 I prepared Cap[t] Cooke's Voyage for the Press. I undertook this Task at y[e] earnest Intreaty of Lord Sandwich, & on Condition of Secrecy—His Majesty acquainted with it. I did a great deal to y[e] Cap[t]'s Journal to correct its Stile; to new point it; to divide it into Sentences, & Paragraphs, & Chapters & Books. Tho little appears to be done by me, the Journal if printed as the Captain put it into my Hands, would have been thought too incorrect, & have disgusted the Reader'.[3]

The first statement is obviously an understatement: 'the correction of a few Inaccuracies in Style' was in fact the correction of a multitudinous number, if by such corrections we understand the adjustment of spelling and matters of elementary grammar—the alteration of singular verbs to plural, the regularization of tenses, and so forth; or the substitution of one word for another to avoid too close repetition, or of 'which' or 'when' for Cook's phrases beginning with 'and'. Douglas is pretty consistent also in expanding the professional brevity of 'Thursday 24th. Winds from N.W. to N.E.' to the more

[1] 'It is unfortunate for this country, that she is never so happy in the choice of her Navigators as France. We force men into inches, without considering whether they will fit the space alotted or not. The navigators and explorers of France, have themselves always given the narrative of their voyages to the public, as well as the Spaniards and Portuguese; and recently we read with pleasure the excellent exotick accounts of Condamine, Belin, Bouganville, &c. But we were obliged to get Mr. Ben. Robbins to write Anson's Voyage for Walter, and Hawkesworth, to tarnish the Journals of Cook; and now Dr. Douglas, who digested and corrected Cook's Second Voyage, is finishing, grammatically, the last, which ended with the command of Capt. King: and surely these Marine Gentlemen's narratives must have been better told by themselves, than by those uninterested in their scenes of pleasure and distress. This observation is certainly verified in Parkinson's Narrative.'—*Morning Chronicle*, 18 January 1783, p. 2, col. 4. Parkinson's journal had of course been edited; see I, pp. ccliii–cclv.

[2] He goes on, 'I am sorry M[r] Woodfall [the editor] should have given his Sanction to such a heap of inconsistent Abuse.—It begins with insinuating that Cap[t] Cook was unfit for the service to w[ch] he was appointed. It soon after speaks of D[r] Hawkesworth as having *tarnished* his Journal, & then it proceeds to suppose him incapable of writing a Journal, by saying I had *digested* that of his former Voyage, & am now *finishing* that of the last'. He concludes by asking his correspondent to burn the letter.—19 January 1783; Eg. MS 2180, f. 68.

[3] Eg. MS 2181, f. 42v. Though styled an autobiography in the B.M. catalogue, the MS is really no more than a series of autobiographical notes, jotted down between 1776 and 1796.

polite 'On the 24th the wind blew from N.W. to N.E.'. Comparison of a few lines from Cook's MS with the printed page (M, 72 c, d; *Voyage*, I, p. 213) will show, as a fair average, what happened.

COOK. 'The Island of Amsterdam or Tongotabu is wholy laid out in Plantations, in which are planted some of the richest productions of nature, such as Bread fruit, Cocoanutts, Bananas, Shaddocks, yams, and some other roots Sugar Cane and a fruit like an nectarine called by them Feghega and at Otaheite Ahuya, inshort here are most of the Articles which the other islands produce besides some which they have not. M[r] Forster tells me that he has not only found the same Plants here as at Otaheite and the other isles, but several others which are not to be found there and I probably have added to their stock of Vegitables by leaving with them an assortment of garden Seeds Pulse &c[a]. Breadfruit here as well as at all the other isles, was not in Season nor was this the time for roots and Shaddocks, we got a few of these last at Middleburg; the produce and cultivation of this isle is the same as at Amsterdam with this difference that....'

DOUGLAS. 'The island of Amsterdam or Tongotabu is wholly laid out in plantations, in which are planted some of the richest productions of nature; such as bread-fruit, cocoa-nut trees, plantains, bananoes, shaddocks, yams, and some other roots, sugar-cane, and a fruit like a nectarine, called by them *Fighega*, and at Otaheite *Ahuya*: In short, here are most of the articles which the Society Islands produce, besides some which they have not. Mr. Forster tells me, that he not only found the same plants here, that are at Otaheite and the neighbouring isles, but several others which are not to be met with there. And I probably have added to their stock of vegetables, by leaving with them an assortment of garden seeds, pulse, &c. Bread-fruit here, as well as at all the other isles, was not in season; nor was this the time for roots and shaddocks. We got the latter only at Middleburg. [New paragraph] The produce and cultivation of this isle is the same as at Amsterdam; with this difference, that....'

This can not be regarded as drastic revision. Douglas certainly has taken pains to 'new point' the manuscript before him, and to new plan the sentences and paragraphs; and this, really, is what alters the feeling of the style. The quarter-deck rapidity has been slowed down; the gale, as it were, somewhat tempered; that elegantly professional punctuation has not turned the sailor into the canon of Windsor, but he has been brought home from the strand of Tongatapu to the Strand of London. As for the division into chapters and books, Douglas may have advised; but Cook did the work first, and the running analysis of the contents of the chapters was certainly his—we have his draft with all its alterations.[1] The draft gives us fifty-four

[1] Add. MS 27889, ff. 1–10, up to Chap. XLIV—i.e. Book IV, Chap. IV. Also we have his letter to Douglas, 26 April 1776: 'I have divided it into Books and Chap. takeing the

of the sixty-one chapters into which the book ultimately fell, with afterthoughts and insertions, and the directions which authors, that fearful race, sometimes give to printers—'Leave about 4 Inches between Book 1 & Chap. 1 for the Title'. Cook the writer is much like other writers.

We cannot say that Douglas claimed much too much for himself. Hard as Cook had worked, he remained 'incorrect'. Douglas was tactful, and Cook was appreciative. The gentlemen met, and corresponded. Advice was asked and given. We have a small sheaf of letters from Cook that are very revealing.

'I have recieved your letter of the 7th' [he writes on 10 January 1776] 'and also the Box with its contents. I have not had time to look over the corrections which you have made, but have not the least doubt but they were necessary, and that I shall be perfectly satisfied with them.

'The remarks you have made on Bits of loose paper, I find are very just. With respect to the Amours of my People at Otaheite & other places: I think it will not be necessary to mention them attall, unless it be by way of throwing a light on the Characters, or Customs of the People we are then among; and even then I would have it done in such a manner as might be unexceptionable to the nicest readers. In short my desire is that nothing indecent may appear in the whole book, and you cannot oblige me more than by pointing out whatever may appear to you as such.'[1]

On this last matter there was nothing much in the journal in its original state: indeed if the nice reader wishes to be affronted he must have recourse to the righteously pure pages of Forster. The correspondence continues. Cook thought he ought to write consistently in the present or the past tense—would Douglas give his opinion on which?[2] Captain Campbell and Sir Hugh Palliser were looking over the nautical part of the book.[3] The introduction was being sent by the stage.[4] He reports on the progress of negotiations between Sandwich and the elder Forster over the official publication of a volume by Forster, and over the progress of charts and other engravings.[5] He begs Douglas's acceptance of some Constantia wine,

former Voyages and Lord Ansons for my guidance, but submit the whole to your better judgement, with full hopes that you will make such alterations, as you may see necessary'. —Eg. MS 2180, f. 9–9v. And again, 'I should be glad to put of waiting upon you till next Saturday, when I will bring the whole Manuscript with me, to let you see how I have divided it into Books & Chapters. By that time I may have the Introduction ready for you to look over . . .'.—'Sunday Morn'g' [n.d.]—ibid., f. 11. It looks as if Douglas's memory transmuted his approval into original decision.

[1] Eg. MS 2180, f. 3.

[2] ibid., f. 7, 9 March 1776.

[3] ibid., f. 9, 26 April; f. 15v, 14 June; f. 17, 23 June.

[4] ibid., f. 15v, 14 June.

[5] ibid., f. 13–13v, 11 June; f. 15, 14 June; f. 17, 23 June.

and then of some Madeira which had made the voyage with the *Resolution*.[1] Finally there is the letter in which the captain, who had been hard at work preparing for a third voyage as well as in literary composition, bids farewell to his collaborator:

'It is now Settled that I am to Publish without Mr Forster, and I have taken my measures accordingly. When Captain Campbell has looked over the M.S. it will be put into the hands of Mr Strahan and Mr Stuart to be printed, and I shall hope for the Continuation of your assistance in correcting the proofs. I know not how to recompence you for the trouble you have had, and will have in the Work. I can only beg you will except of as many Copies, after it is published, as will serve your self and friends, and I have given directions for you to be furnished with them. When you have done with the Introduction, please to send it to Mr Strahan or bring it with you when you come to Town, for there needs be no hurry about it. Tomorrow Morning I set out to join my ship at the Nore, & with her proceed to Plymouth, where my stay will be but short. Permit me to assure you that I shall always have a due sence of the favors you have done. . . .'[2]

On this satisfactory note these two so dissimilar persons parted.

Besides the minor differences between the journal as written and the journal as published, for which Douglas was responsible, there were one or two major differences, which did not, however, affect the body of the account. All reference to Banks's intended part in the expedition was dropped, and the controversy over the *Resolution* was muted to a mention of 'various opinions . . . espoused by different people' over the sort of vessel most proper for the voyage; and to clinch the matter, Cook, as has been said already, took over into the text of his 'General Introduction' the paper written by Palliser for Sandwich on the subject. He incorporated in the introduction also both some of the early pages of the journal on the manning, fitting out and provisioning of the ships; and he prefixed a brief history of earlier exploration in the Pacific, up to and including the voyage of the *Endeavour*. In the text of the journal itself he inserted a paragraph or two he got from Sandwich on the career in England of Omai, and brought himself to take back some of his previously unfavourable opinion of that young person.[3] A number of appendixes were added: tables of the routes taken by the ships and various regular observations made, of which there has already been mention; Anderson's Tahitian vocabulary; a short comparative vocabulary of the islands from Easter Island to New Caledonia; a letter

[1] ibid., f. 5, 8 March; f. 9, 26 April.
[2] 23 June 1776, Eg. MS 2180, f. 17.
[3] *Voyage*, I, pp. 169–71; below, p. 428, n. 2.

from the secretary of the Board of Longitude to Sir John Pringle, requesting permission to print the presidential discourse on the delivery of the Copley medal into Mrs Cook's hands by the Royal Society on 30 November 1776; and that oration itself. The Board of Longitude made its request in March 1777—so long was the appearance of the book delayed by the engraving of the plates and the other incidentals of printing; and the great work was finally published early in May 1777. The public was not 'disgusted'; before the end of the year a second edition was needed, and in 1779 a third; a French translation appeared in 1778. The two quarto volumes would have given pleasure to any author; but Cook never saw them.

GEORGE FORSTER

A Voyage round the World, in His Britannic Majesty's Sloop, Resolution, commanded by Capt. James Cook, during the Years 1772, 3, 4, and 5. By George Forster, F.R.S. Member of the Royal Academy of Madrid, and of the Society for promoting Natural Knowledge at Berlin. 2 vols., 1777.

These volumes arose out of the quarrel between the Admiralty and the elder Forster over his contribution to the official account of the voyage—a quarrel into which Forster dragged everybody conceivable, to general distress and embarrassment. The documentation is formidable; the Forster claims fantastic; his accusations preposterous. The facts are simple, and may here be very briefly summarized. When Forster was appointed to the voyage he understood from Daines Barrington that on its completion he would be its official historian, and would in addition receive from the Admiralty provision for life. It is not in the least conceivable that Barrington would make any statement remotely resembling this, though he may possibly have expressed some hope that Forster might write the history of the voyage. After the voyage it seems to have been first thought that a joint book might be possible, with sections alternately by Cook and Forster. Naturally enough this hare-brained scheme was soon abandoned. But Sandwich, while quite clear that the main account must be Cook's, was willing to give Forster a hand in the publication on the general scientific side, in a separate volume, provided a specimen of his writing met with approval. An agreement was signed on 13 April 1776,[1] delimiting the ground to be covered by each man, allowing Forster to see proof-sheets of Cook's work as an aid to his own, and providing for the use by him of a certain

[1] Printed at the end of George Forster's *Letter to the Earl of Sandwich* (1778).

number of the copper-plates. The specimen provided by Forster was not at all satisfactory, but Sandwich was still prepared to accept the work if he would allow it to receive proper correction. This he refused under any circumstances, and regarded any advice to compromise as a gross betrayal of himself. There was nothing to do but break off negotiations, and forbid Forster to publish anything till after the official volumes had appeared. Thus propelled off the official stage, he remained as a fury denouncing vengeance from the wings. As a sort of vengeance, he set his son to work at once. George had no journal, but he had not been interdicted from publishing. George's father had kept a journal, and as a civilian he had not had to deliver it up to the Admiralty. George's task therefore was to produce a book from Reinhold's journal as fast as possible, and get it on to the market before Cook's.[1] As he was a quick worker, and did not have to wait while plates were engraved, he could have Dr Hornsby, the professor of astronomy at Oxford (a member of the Board of Longitude who may not have been acquainted with all the circumstances), look over his manuscript, rush it through the press, and publish in March 1777, six weeks before the official volumes.

Whatever may be thought of the Forsters, and their relations with their fellow human beings, it must be admitted that this is a remarkable performance for a young man of twenty-two. It is remarkable even though based largely on the record kept by his father; for J. R. Forster could not write like this. Nevertheless, only too clearly can we see that it was done with the father hanging over the desk. There are sentiments and turns of phrase that take us to the latter's *Observations*; there is the large footnote,[2] complaining of the obstacles put in the way of the Forster researches, which from its mingled bitterness and extravagance is unmistakeably from the father's mind; there is one large extract, on the expedition over Easter Island,[3] which professes to be a direct transcription from the elder man's journal. Yet no one can read J. R. Forster's English composition and not be con-

[1] 'The writing of a narrative of the voyage by the elder Forster having been forbidden by the Admiralty, George, to defeat the prohibition which had been imposed through jealousy, undertook to compile one out of Reinhold's journal. The hurriedly completed book appeared under his own name in 1777. It is unquestionably his work as regards the literary style; of the scientific matter however only a small portion can be ascribed to him. He admitted, in a confidential letter dated 19 September 1775, that during the voyage he took notes of only general interest, and that these were intended for his friends, and not for the public.'—Alfred Dove in *Allgemeine Deutsche Biographie*, VII, p. 173.—In the preface to the book (I, p. vii), George merely says, 'I had collected sufficient materials during the voyage . . . [the agreement] to which my father had signed, did not make him answerable for my actions, nor in the most distant manner preclude his giving me assistance. Therefore in every important circumstance, I had leave to consult his journals . . .'.

[2] II, p. 420; and printed pp. xlv–xlvi above.

[3] I, pp. 585–93.

vinced that he could not write this book. Of the two, George had the real gift for languages; it was George who did something to found a simple, rapid and attractive style in German; and there is more than one passage that, though no doubt not in the front rank of English satirical or descriptive writing, yet has a force and charm beyond the reach of a great number of English professional writers of the time. Consider his storm-scenes, or his description of morning at Vaitepiha Bay.[1] He has even humour, as in his note on the second anniversary of the departure from England, 12 July 1774, 'celebrated by the sailors with their usual mirth':

'One of them, of a fanatical turn, composed a hymn on the occasion, as he had done the first year; and after seriously exhorting his fellows to repentance, sat down and hugged the bottle heartily; but like all the rest, he proved unequal to the conflict, and sunk under the powerful influence of his adversary.'[2]

With which we may contrast another scene in which drunkenness, he alleges, played a considerable part, at Christmas time 1773:

'At six in the evening, we counted one hundred and five large masses of ice around us from the deck, the weather continuing very clear, fair, and perfectly calm. Towards noon the next day we were still in the same situation, with a very drunken crew, and from the mast-head observed one hundred and sixty-eight ice-islands, some of which were half a mile long, and none less than the hull of the ship. The whole scene looked like the wrecks of a shattered world, or as the poets describe some regions of hell; an idea which struck us the more forcibly, as execrations, oaths, and curses re-echoed about us on all sides'.[3]

There are times indeed when we feel that George is possibly writing for effect; and as usual, when a man is doing that, sometimes the effect comes off, and sometimes it does not.[4] His 'chilling horrors',

[1] e.g. I, pp. 486–9; and I, pp. 268–9.

[2] II, p. 196. I take it this is humour. Could the hymn-writer be Thomas Perry (cf. pp. 870–1 below)?

[3] I, pp. 537–8. Forster tends to harp on the bad language of the sailors: describing the gale off Cook Strait, 25 October 1773, he writes (I, p. 488), 'To complete this catalogue of horrors, we heard the voices of sailors from time to time louder than the blustering winds or the raging ocean itself, uttering horrible vollies of curses and oaths. Without any provocation to serve as an excuse, they execrated every limb in varied terms, piercing and complicated beyond the power of description'—and so on. On this Wales, insisting that the real writer is Reinhold, comments, 'had [the sailors] known the fright that he was in, or the uneasiness that their inconsiderate and unconcerned swearing gave him, they would, I am persuaded, have abated, at least in some measure, the variety of their imprecations; but the Doctor swears so dreadfully himself at times, that there was not a soul on board who ever dreamed that it gave him the least dissatisfaction'.—*Remarks*, p. 35.

[4] 'I talked to him of Forster's *Voyage to the South Seas*, which pleased me; but I found he did not like it. "Sir, (said he,) there is a great affectation of fine writing in it." '—Boswell's *Johnson* (ed. Birkbeck Hill), III, p. 180.

the fearful danger to which he subjects the ship at Plymouth (from which she was rescued only by the alertness of mind of J. R. Forster), the panic over a fire on board off Eromanga, would be more convincing if anybody else alluded to them. One reads with scepticism, one is continually discounting prejudices; the onslaughts on the British sailor are so continuous that in reaction one tends to forget that eighteenth-century sailors were not invariably patterns of all the manly virtues. It comes as a shock to light on the solitary balanced estimate: 'Though they are members of a civilized society, they are in some measure to be looked upon as a body of uncivilized men, rough, passionate, revengeful, but likewise brave, sincere, and true to one another'.[1]

Leaving on one side the Forster passions, the extraordinary hatred of Hawkesworth, the flattery of men with whom, presumably, Reinhold wished to stand well, leaving aside also the parade of learning which forces under our eyes half the Latin authors and a liberal selection of poets English, French, Italian and German, and dealing not too harshly with certain dogmatic assumptions, we may freely concede that George's book is valuable as well as long, and an indispensable supplement to Cook. It is valuable not so much because of its botany or zoology as because of its extended account of people; there is nothing in Cook, for example, as elaborate as the 175 pages which Forster devotes to the New Hebrides. The elder Forster was interested in such things as Tahitian religion. There is good use made of Burney's musical knowledge. We get acute observations on the Polynesian languages, and the subtle variations between them.[2] We get lively accounts of episodes in which George himself was implicated. We get some very good pictures of Cook. We get a certain amount of the romantic, but nothing as ridiculous as some of the pages of the elder man's *Observations*, which might have made even the hated Hawkesworth hesitate. All in all, the discriminating reader will not be sorry that George wrote the book, though as a moralist he may wish it had been written under other circumstances, and that the paternal figure that superintended the writing had shown less venom.

The Forster temper and the Forster recklessness being so prominently displayed in certain passages, it could hardly escape criticism. This was applied by Wales, 'our accurate and indefatigable astronomer', in an octavo pamphlet of 110 indignant pages, entitled *Remarks on Mr. Forster's Account of Captain Cook's last Voyage round the*

[1] This remark is the end of a long paragraph, some of it highly uncomplimentary.—I, pp. 535–6.

[2] 'Raiatea', rather than 'Ulietea', makes its first appearance in George's pages.

World (1778). Wales frankly disbelieved that George had written the book, its prejudices were so much and so transparently those of Reinhold—in which his acumen as a literary critic certainly failed him. But he made some damaging points. Not only did he spring to the defence of the 'poor seamen' but he took a series of specific statements that outraged him and rebutted them with a vigour and heat that are still alive, far removed from the genial fun he had poked in the private pages of his journal. 'On ne repousse point la verité sans bruit', he quoted from one of Forster's quotations. Apart from the controversy, he adds to our knowledge a little that is valuable in the annotation of Cook. George could not let this attack go unnoticed, and produced a quarto *Reply to Mr. Wales's Remarks* (1778), on the title-page of which he has now become 'George Forster, F.R.S. naturalist on the late voyage round the world, by the king's appointment'.[1] The attitude of calm dignity, quiet reason, detached and temperate irony, which he opposes to Wales's 'bruit' would be more appealing did we know less about its manufacture; and did it not all go down at times before a less attractive burst of vituperation. Thus the 'accurate and indefatigable astronomer' has now become something quite unpleasant, eaten up with envy over the Forsters' salary: 'what was hatched like a basilisk in the damp and noisome cabbins of the *Resolution*, might acquire its full growth, and produce a monstrous progeny in the dark cloisters of Christ's Hospital'.[2] No chance, however remote, is let go for an attack on Sandwich. Once or twice, it cannot be denied, George has the best of the argument; and to some readers he was persuasive, possibly on political grounds as much as on general controversial merit.

J. R. FORSTER

Observations made during a Voyage Round the World, on Physical Geography, Natural History, and Ethic Philosophy. Especially on 1. The Earth and its Strata, 2. Water and the Ocean, 3. The Atmosphere, 4. The Changes of the Globe, 5. Organic Bodies, and 6. The Human Species. By John Reinold Forster, LL.D. F.R.S. and S.A. And a Member of several Learned Academies in Europe. 1778.

This quarto volume of 650 pp. is solid not only with observations but with the characteristics of its author. Its extent is adequately described on its title-page; its nature is the nature of J. R. Forster, less

[1] He was elected F.R.S. on 9 January 1777, having been nominated by Banks, Solander and Maskelyne, among others. That at least is true.

[2] On his return, in 1775, Wales had been appointed master of the Mathematical School at Christ's Hospital.

the quarrelsomeness, which had gone into his son's book. It notes a number of facts which contribute to our knowledge of the voyage, but neither its merits nor its demerits as a philosophical disquisition need be gone into here. It is this which, according to George,[1] was intended as the Forster contribution to the official account, after the delimitation of fields between Cook and the philosopher. If so, it would have been a curious mate for Cook's volumes.[2]

WALES AND BAYLY

The Original Astronomical Observations, made in the course of A Voyage towards the South Pole, and Round the World.... By William Wales, F.R.S. Master of the Royal Mathematical School in Christ's Hospital; and Mr. William Bayly, Late Assistant at the Royal Observatory. 1777.

This, and not Forster, is the true appendix to Cook, though its serried ranks of figures are not likely to attract the modern reader. It was published at the order of the Board of Longitude, whose servants Wales and Bayly were. Bayly departed on the third voyage in the *Discovery* in 1776, and the volume was edited by Wales. He included in it certain remarks from his journal, and a most valuable introduction on the scientific equipment of the voyage. It also contains four plates: two scientific diagrams, a chart of Point Venus and the reef outside, and a seascape by Hodges—the last no doubt worked in because of the waterspouts.

[MARRA]

Journal of the Resolution's Voyage ... by which the Non-Existence of an undiscovered Continent, between the Equator and the 50th Degree of Southern Latitude, is demonstratively proved. Also a Journal of the Adventure's Voyage .... interspersed with Historical and Geographical Descriptions of the Islands and Countries discovered in the Course of their respective Voyages. 1775.

The origin of this small volume, on the face of it anonymous, is described in Appendix VIII, pp. 961–2 below. In spite of Admiralty precautions against publication of any surreptitious account of the

[1] *Reply*, p. 11.

[2] Although the Forster scientific works belong, strictly speaking, to the history of the voyage they need hardly be considered at length here. Botanically, they were the *Characteres Generum Plantarum* (London 1776), in which the descriptions were by Sparrman; and the following by George alone: *Florulae Insularum Australium Prodromus* (Göttingen 1786), of which, with the *Characteres*, the botanists speak despitefully; *De Plantis Esculentis Insularum Oceani Australis* (Halle 1786), a useful little handbook; *Fasciculus Plantarum Magellanicarum* and *Plantae Atlanticae* (both Göttingen 1787). J. R. Forster's *Descriptiones Animalium* (Berlin 1844), edited by Lichtenstein, dealt with the zoology.

voyage, the booksellers opened hungry mouths, and Marra the gunner's mate, whose career at sea was so checkered, was agile enough to thrust something like a journal into that of the enterprising Newbery. It may not have been to begin with very much of a journal; for, in spite of a great deal of editorial padding, and an account of the *Adventure*'s voyage which could have been picked up from some member of its company, the book is not a large one. Yet it does give a connected view of the voyage. The editor seems to have been David Henry, who ran the *Gentleman's Magazine*, which Newbery also published; he had already had experience in compiling voyages,[1] and would have had no difficulty in knocking together Marra's journal, or notes, and the other material. The illustrations are not very realistic, and the map is rather a rough and ready one. The book is by no means useless, however: strained through the meshes of our other accounts, it yields some grains of new information that have every appearance of authenticity; and though Marra himself was perhaps no great hand with a pen,[2] he had evidently a lively mind. He did not get into trouble through mere recalcitrance, and the scraps of his conversation reported to Cook by Anderson are further evidence. There may have been a good deal of talk, as well as the written word, for the editor to work on; and he may have seen other journals of sorts.

One gathers this from scattered remarks in a long abstract of the work which appeared in the *Gentleman's Magazine* from December 1775 to March 1776[3]—very likely the source of most public knowledge of the voyage before the appearance of Forster and Cook. If Henry edited the book, as he edited the magazine, then he displayed a laudable tolerance in letting pass the remark, 'As to the work before us, there cannot be the least doubt of its being written from the genuine journals [*sic*] of the voyage; but it appears to have been hastily written, and hastily printed'.[4] Generally, however, in referring to the basis of the book, the reviewer refers to 'our Journalist'—except in one other sentence,[5] which superimposes editorial comment

[1] *Gentleman's Magazine*, LXII, pt. 1 (1792), p. 579. This volume quotes or refers to Tasman, Campbell (the editor of the second edition of Harris), Hawkesworth, Dalrymple, Parkinson, Gonzalez (at Easter Island), Thevenot, Quiros, Byron, Sir William Temple—and the list is not complete.

[2] To judge from a letter he wrote to Banks: Smith, *Life of Sir Joseph Banks* (1911), pp. 45–6. This would not look half so silly, however, without the punctuation; and Smith might have known that every eighteenth-century full point is not equivalent to a twentieth-century full point.

[3] XLV (1775), pp. 587–91; XLVI (1776), pp. 15–20, 66–70, 118–22.

[4] XLV, p. 591. Or again, 'The writer has evidently paid greater attention to the choice of his matter, than to the refinement of his language'.—XLVI, p. 122.

[5] XLVI, p. 17.

in the midst of the 'review', on the question of language affinities between Tahiti and Tonga: 'but, say our Journalists, *their languages were totally different*, though this is denied by the Reviewer of this work, who appears to have been a party in the voyage he was employed to review and who, probably, may himself have some work of the like kind to present to the public'. This is piling up obscurity. Surely an editor knew whether or not his reviewer had been on the voyage? Or was he merely manufacturing an elaborate caution, to shield the gentleman from the possible consequences of divulging too much? He might not have fancied enquiries from the Admiralty. But then, how are we to account for the publication with his first instalment of a south polar chart, with the track of the *Resolution* marked on it—not at all a bad piece of work; and, with the last, of a chart of the 'Great Cyclades' and New Caledonia, with the track running down past Norfolk Island to New Zealand—which has the essential figures of the islands, though it makes the New Hebrides extend too far north and too far west, and New Caledonia a good deal too far west? And who supplied those to the *Gentleman's Magazine*? Obviously all the charts were not securely in the possession of the Admiralty.

Presumably the book itself sold reasonably well, though it did not go into a second London edition; for it was reprinted in Dublin in 1776, in which year also, at Leipzig, appeared a German edition. The Forsters denigrated it with zeal,[1] but whether that had any effect on German readers we do not know.

ANONYMOUS

A Second Voyage round the World. . . . By James Cook, Esq. Commander of His Majesty's Bark The Resolution. Undertaken by Order of the King, and encouraged by a Parliamentary Grant of Four Thousand Pounds. Drawn up from Authentic Papers. . . . 1776.

As this publication, 'Printed for the Editor', and sold by J. Almon in London, and Fletcher and Hodson in Cambridge, undoubtedly belongs to the bibliographical history of the voyage, it is mentioned here. But though it recounts a few incidents, not otherwise known, which do not seem out of key with the voyage as a whole, the rest is

[1] The late Mr J. B. Palmer, who did some useful investigation in these things, tracked down a letter from J. R. Forster in A. F. Büsching's *Wöchentliche Nachrichten*, 8 April 1776, which called the book an abortion, along with other strong words used. See also a prospectus, not then published, which George wrote for his own book, *Archiv für das Studium der neueren Sprachen*, 90 (1893), pp. 34–40.

so palpably fake, and in the most sensational terms, that it must be regarded as original invention—on the basis, perhaps, of a reading of Marra or conversation with a stray sailor. George Forster conjectured that the writer was a student of Cambridge; the new title-page of the reissue of 1781 boldly asserted that he was 'an Officer on Board'—which one feels as an affront to the intelligence even in the twentieth century. His obscure identity does not matter. The book got a bad press: the *Monthly Review* went as far as consulting Cook, and gave a list of fifteen alleged incidents pronounced, on his authority, to be false.[1] This was almost needless.

SPARRMAN

A Voyage round the World with Captain James Cook in H.M.S. Resolution. Translated by Huldine Beamish and Averil Mackenzie-Grieve; edited by Owen Rutter. 1944, 1953.

The bibliography of Sparrman is curious, and the easiest way for the English reader to consult him is in the translation noted above, first printed by the Golden Cockerel Press, and re-published in a less sumptuous form (London, Robert Hale) in 1953. As a witness Sparrman is embarrassing—though at times certainly valuable; for he left his testimony till 27 and 43 years after the event; and when he did publish, did not print a journal, but a narrative in which he drew not only on Cook and Forster, but Bougainville and later voyagers and historians like Vancouver, Turnbull, Crozet, La Pérouse or Labillardière. He did publish a book before then—the *Resa till Goda Hopps- Udden Södra, Pol-Kretsen och omkring Jordklotet, samt till Hottentot- och Caffer-Landen, åren 1772–6* (Stockholm 1783). This is one of the important works in South African literature, and its importance in travel literature was recognized at once. It went into a second Swedish edition, and was translated into German (1784); into English[2] (Dublin 1785, and a second edition corrected, of two volumes quarto, London 1786); and into French (1787). But it devoted only a single chapter, of 20 pages, to the author's years in the *Resolution*. Sparmann promised his readers a second volume on this theme. For various reasons[3] this suffered unconscionable postponement, and finally appeared in two parts, the first in 1802, the second not till 1818, with supplementary title-pages, *Resa omkring Jordklotet i Sällschap med Kapit. J. Cook och Hrr Forster, åren 1772, 1773, 1774 och*

[1] Vol. XXVIII (October 1776), pp. 270–3.

[2] *A Voyage to the Cape of Good Hope, towards the Antarctic Polar Circle and round the World, but chiefly into the Country of the Hottentots and Caffres, from the year 1772 to 1776.*

[3] *Voyage* (ed. Rutter), pp. xvi–xvii.

1775. The first part gave purchasers a sort of bonus in the shape of fragments of Tahitian and Tongan *tapa*. The volumes remained confined to the Swedish language, and became rare. From them, with certain modifications that do not appear to be important, the English edition of 1944 was produced.

Although Sparrman wrote a book, instead of publishing his journal, we can hardly blame him. But we should like the original document. There remains in the book, in spite of its elements of compilation, enough original observation to make him thoroughly worth consulting, and this rather sedate young man, with his dislike of swearing, his interest in food, his pleasure in being of help to Cook, his wonder at such barbaric English habits as boxing, and his rather pedestrian style, gives us a sense that when we have Sparrman himself—'But to return to my own Diary', he remarks at one point—we are on fairly safe ground. References in the notes are to the 1953 pagination.

THE GRAPHIC RECORDS[1]

ALTHOUGH Hodges was the 'official artist' on the voyage, and was prolific, he was not of course the only person to produce graphic records. There were the chart-makers; and there were the makers of natural history drawings. Charts were not infrequently adorned with 'views'; views, as well as charts, figured in some of the logs and journals, and there is no doubt that Hodges' technique in wash affected some of the seamen—for example, Gilbert and Roberts. We have indeed explicit testimony to this, in the memoirs of John Elliott: writing of the period at Tahiti, in April 1774, he says, 'Myself, Mr Roberts, and Mr Smith (Cooks Nephew) were when off Watch, Employ'd in Captn Cooks Cabbin either Copying Drawings for him, or Drawing for ourselves, under the Eye of Mr Hodges'.[2] The occurrence of charts and views in the logs and journals has already been noted; but the names of the draughtsmen may here be drawn together. Those who made charts were Cook, Pickersgill, Gilbert, Roberts, Isaac Smith, Vancouver, Wales, Burney, and Peter Fannin (master of the *Adventure*). Of these, Gilbert, Roberts, Smith and Fannin also did views, and Gilbert, Roberts and Fannin had some real aptitude in this department.

Hodges does not seem to have been concerned in the charts at all; and indeed it would have been quite out of character for him, as a professional 'artist', not a surveyor or hydrographer, to have had anything to do with them. He was above all a landscape painter, interested in atmosphere and light; rather to our misfortune, he was not given to the figure, and not very skilful at it, so that his portraits are confined to the head, or head and shoulders. He worked in water colour, for topographical subjects; oil, probably not direct from the subject, but from his water colour sketches (though certainly, often enough, while the subject was fresh in his mind, as at Dusky Sound); and red crayon, for his portrait drawings.

The chart-makers vary in skill. *Pickersgill's* work may be quite delicate, or quite rough. *Gilbert* was an experienced surveyor, with his style already formed, and a good topographical draughtsman;

[1] I have drawn this section up almost entirely on the basis of notes from Mr R. A. Skelton and Miss A. M. Lysaght.

[2] Elliott *Mem.*, f. 27v.

the rough charts in his journal are not at all the best he was capable of. *Roberts* was mature for his age (15 on joining), as his drawing of the *Resolution*, reproduced as our frontispiece, shows; but apparently picked up some of Cook's style in chart work, though he kept idiosyncrasies of his own. *Smith*, trained and overseen by Cook, drew charts exactly in Cook's manner; his single other drawing shows no talent whatever. *Vancouver*, with only two signed charts, in pen and ink, is extremely like Roberts. *Burney*, with his pen and wash, tends to be rough but is reliable. *Fannin* produces good controlled work both in charts and views and displays an agreeable taste in decorative ornament, fauna and flora predominating. *Wales's* work is beautiful, strictly impersonal in its pen and ink, with no touch of wash: throughout a severe scientific statement.

So much can be said of individuals, whose charts are either signed or clearly attributable because of their occurrence in logs and journals. There are, however, unsigned charts and views that appear separately, and though the charts display numerous differences in lay-out and minor variants in such details as nomenclature and soundings, together with distinctive differences, sometimes, in handwriting, there is almost a common style in many of them that stands in the way of clear attribution. Formal lettering approaches a sort of standard naval practice. We can associate roughs with signed fair copies, as we can associate unsigned sketches with Hodges' finished paintings; but what when drawings are repeated?[1] Unsigned topographical drawings, if not by Hodges, are more likely to be by Gilbert or Roberts than by others; unsigned charts by one of these two, or by Cook or Isaac Smith. The difficulty, having been indicated, can be relegated to the catalogue in Volume IV. There is no reason to attribute any of the unsigned portrait heads to any person other than Hodges.

An analysis may now be made of the material under the headings of (*a*) drawings and paintings, (*b*) charts and views, and (*c*) the more specialized natural history drawings.

[1] For instance, the three drawings of Sandwich Island and Resolution Harbour in the New Hebrides, and Freezland Peak in the South Sandwich Islands, occur as follows: (1) in Gilbert's log (P.R.O., Adm 55/107); (2) in B.M. Add. MS 15500. 13 and 17, unsigned; (3) as vignettes in the general chart, B.M. Add. MS 15500. 1, unsigned; (4) as vignettes in the general chart, Hydrographic Department but now in the National Maritime Museum, signed by Gilbert. We may conclude that all these were drawn by Gilbert—and this seems the most likely solution; or that the anonymous drawings were copied from Gilbert: or that they were all drawn by Hodges or copied from him (there is a Sandwich Island, Add. MS 15743. 6, drawn by him from the same viewpoint).

(a) *Drawings and paintings*

British Museum, Add. MS 15743. The collection was included in the Sir Joseph Banks bequest. It has 10 large unsigned drawings by Hodges, in pen and Indian ink wash, slightly tinted. They are perhaps sketches for oil paintings.

Print Room. Two drawings by Hodges.

Admiralty. 24 oil paintings by Hodges: some apparently painted on the voyage, and others after the return (when Hodges is said to have been employed by the Admiralty to work up his material). Cook refers to oil paintings made by Hodges on board (e.g. at Cape Town and Pare in Tahiti). The figures in the London paintings were perhaps from designs by other artists. A number of these pictures are on loan to, and hung in, the *National Maritime Museum*.

National Maritime Museum, Greenwich. Two oil paintings, attributed to Hodges (landings at 'Mallicolo' and Tanna, reproduced by Kitson when in the possession of Mr H. Arthurton).

Dominion Archives of Canada, Ottawa. 5 charcoal drawings of natives (head and shoulders). Unsigned; apparently Hodges' sketches for the red crayon drawings done for the Admiralty (now in the Commonwealth National Library, Canberra; see below).[1]

Mitchell Library, Sydney, D11. A volume of drawings, charts and profiles. It, or some of it, may once have belonged to Cook, but at any rate it has a very good descent: Admiral Isaac Smith, Canon Frederick Bennett, John Mackrell (?), Australian Museum. One drawing is signed by Hodges; four by Roberts. Canon Bennett's attributions are quite unreliable; nor are those by the Mitchell Library altogether to be accepted. We must probably not assume that every drawing not attributable to Hodges is by Roberts. Most (if not all) the second-voyage drawings are first or early sketches, direct from the subject; and criteria of style are here more valid than in more finished work. Besides the second-voyage material, the collection includes Newfoundland charts by Cook; two drawings from the first voyage (attributed by Canon Bennett to Isaac Smith: in fact copies of those in Add. MS 7085, and perhaps by Cook); and charts associated with Isaac Smith's service in the East Indies after this voyage.

[1] The Dominion Archives have also a water colour drawing of the 'Landing at Erramanga', signed by Cipriani, possibly made for Hodges to paint from: I am somewhat doubtful how far this sophisticated London production can be classed as a 'graphic record' of the voyage.

The Mitchell Library has also an oil painting of Polynesian natives, probably by Hodges.[1]

Commonwealth National Library, Canberra. 18 red crayon drawings (head and shoulders) of natives by Hodges; unsigned, formerly in Royal Naval Museum, Greenwich; presented by the Admiralty to the Australian Government in 1939. These are Hodges' final versions, worked up (perhaps in London?) from his sketches now in the Dominion Archives of Canada and the Mitchell Library (D11).

Petherick Collection. 4 pen drawings of Melanesian natives. Apparently these are preliminary sketches by Hodges.

Private collections. Mr R. de C. Nan Kivell, London, one water colour of Tonga. Dr H. J. Braunholtz, London, one oil of Tahiti. Mr William Fehr, Cape Town, one oil of Cape Town. All three pictures are by Hodges.

(b) *Charts and views*

Public Record Office. Adm 55/108 (larger charts removed to the Map Room, M.P.I. 86–95). The Admiralty MS of Cook's journal, with 'official' fair copies of charts; one view only. They are mostly pen and ink; some have a little wash. From the wording of Cook's 'Explanations' and from the style of drawing, I take these charts to be drawn by *Cook*.

Adm 55/107. *Gilbert's* log, with 21 charts (mostly accompanied by views) and a few separate views. Generally cursive but careful work. Mostly pen and wash; sparing of colour.

Adm 51/4553 205–6. *Pickersgill's* log. 6 charts, in pen and colour wash.

Adm 55/105. *Isaac Smith's* log, with 12 charts and a picture of icebergs: pen and colour wash.

Adm 51/4523/1. *Burney's* log, with 2 charts and a profile, all of Van Diemen's Land: pen and wash.

Adm 51/4556/208. *Price's* log, with a few rough coastal views: pen and wash.

British Museum. Add. MS 15500. This MS was formerly in the possession of the Duke of Sussex, illegitimate son of George III; it was purchased by the Museum from Thomas Rodd, bookseller, 5 April 1845.

[1] The Library has in addition a water colour of the 'Landing at Middleburgh', not signed, and possibly by Cipriani, which must be regarded with the same scepticism as the Cipriani drawing in the Canadian Archives, noted above.

It comprises 20 charts, most with views attached, and none signed. Closer comparison of style suggests that none of these is by Hodges. Some are related to corresponding ones in Add. MS 31360. One general chart (Add. MS 15500.2) has the *Adventure*'s track; the rest were drawn in the *Resolution*. A possible clue to the ownership of the volume is the two views of Trinidad and Martin Vaz, Atlantic islands never visited by Cook's ships.

Add. MS 27887 (fair copy of Cook's log). Three charts and two sets of profiles of Madeira and the Canary Islands.

Add. MS 31360. (See also Vol. I, pp. cxcvi–ix, cclxvi.) This includes 19 charts (accompanied by views) from this voyage, with some fragments. There are two charts signed by Roberts and two by Vancouver, both midshipmen: this volume almost certainly belonged to Cook, and it seems likely that he put into it the charts drawn for him by the 'young men'. Three charts were drawn in the *Adventure* (a general Mercator chart in 5 sheets, and two charts of Van Diemen's Land); the rest in the *Resolution*. The unsigned charts must be by Cook, Gilbert, Roberts, or Isaac Smith; some can be assigned on internal evidence.

Admiralty Library. Vz 11/55. Charts, views, and coastal profiles by Peter Fannin, master of the *Adventure*.

Royal Greenwich Observatory, Herstmonceux. MS journal by Wales (Board of Longitude Papers, Vol. XLVI), with 22 pen-and-ink charts. Preceded by an interesting note on methods of constructing them.

Alexander Turnbull Library, Wellington. A copy of Burney's chart of Van Diemen's Land, in his hand, in the volume *Holograph Letters and Documents of and relative to Captain James Cook*.

Ferguson Collection. The same, in the Burney MS in Mr J. H. Ferguson's possession.

(c) NATURAL HISTORY DRAWINGS

Botany

The botanical work of this voyage was practically all carried out by the Forsters. An account of the sets of plants distributed by them was published by Britten in 1885.[1] During the voyage George made 301 drawings of plants, which were bought with his other natural history drawings by Banks, and now comprise two volumes in the Botany Library, British Museum (Natural History). These contain

[1] 'The Forster Herbarium', *Journal of Botany*, xxiii (1885), pp. 360–8.

47 finished water-colour drawings, 41 outline drawings with some water-colour, 10 pen-and-ink drawings, and 203 pencil sketches. The artist signed only ten, but his name was written on a number of others by Dryander. A set of outline copper plates of the drawings was engraved, and 129 prints from them are bound with the originals. Their history is discussed by Britten: apparently only two sets of impressions were taken, one of which went eventually to Leningrad. In 1886 an annotated list of the Leningrad engravings was published by F. von Herder.[1] Herder gives references to the publications in which descriptions of the plants had appeared; most of the plates have never been published, but details from the drawings were the basis of the 75 illustrations in the *Characteres Generum Plantarum quas in itinere ad insulas Maris Australis, Collegerunt, Descripserunt, Delinearunt, Annis MDCCLXXII–MDCCLXXV, Joannes Reinoldus Forster . . . et Georgius Forster*, which was published in London in 1776, though the descriptions were by Sparrman.

Zoology

George Forster made a large number of careful studies of birds on the voyage, although his paintings and drawings of animals altogether amounted to only 272 sheets. (They are listed in the *Catalogue of the Library of the British Museum* (*Natural History*), 1922, Vol. VI, as 261 drawings, but several folios bear the same number and all the figures are not listed.) They comprise approximately 14 illustrations of invertebrates, 80 fishes, 140 birds and 35 mammals. Forster appears to have been more interested in birds than in the other animals, and some of his drawings of them have been painted against an elaborate background; these are for the most part signed. The less elaborate paintings and drawings are not generally signed, but nearly all have dates and notes on localities and sometimes on colour, with the vernacular name as well. They usually bear Forster's name in Dryander's hand. When Lichtenstein published J. R. Forster's MSS as the *Descriptiones Animalium quae in itinere ad maris australis terras per annos 1772 1773 et 1774 suscepto collegit observavit et delineavit Ioannes Reinoldus Forster . . .* (Berlin, 1844), he included Forster's notes on dates, and stated whether or not there was a painting by George (or another) of the animals described. Much of this information, together with the notes on the drawings themselves, has been recorded in a list of George Forster's bird paintings in A. M.

[1] 'Verzeichniss von G. Forsters Icones Plantarum in itinere ad insulas maris australis collectarum', *Acta Horti Petropolitana*, IX, fasc. 2 (1886), pp. 485–510.

Lysaght's catalogue of eighteenth-century ornithological paintings in the Banks collection.[1]

Another series of bird paintings was published by Sparrman in four fascicules of the *Museum Carlsonianum*, 1786–9. These paintings were not made by him, but after the voyage by J. C. Linnerhielm: some, perhaps all, were engraved by Fr. Akrel. They include fifteen species from the voyage, twelve of which Sparrman described; types of six of these are still preserved in Stockholm.[2]

There was another zoological artist on this voyage, but his work was poor in quality and not to be compared with George Forster's. He has not yet been identified, although three sets of bird paintings by him are known: one of 17 water-colour drawings in the Print Room, British Museum,[3] one of 38 in the Royal Scottish Museum, and one of 53 in the Mitchell Library, Sydney. They are discussed in detail in the catalogue of the eighteenth-century bird paintings mentioned above. The set in the British Museum belonged to Banks, who endorsed most of the paintings 'Captn Clarke, 1775' and noted the locality; these were not listed by Dryander, however, in his MS catalogue of the zoological paintings in Banks's library. The set now in the Royal Scottish Museum may well have been originally in William Anderson's possession, since he was surgeon's mate in the *Resolution*, and a copy of the general chart of her voyage, with place names in Anderson's hand, was with the drawings when they were presented to the Royal Scottish Museum by Professor Alexander Monro (secundus), one of Anderson's former teachers at Edinburgh University. The third set, now in the Mitchell Library, was originally in the possession of Admiral Isaac Smith; but though he too was on the voyage, his largely erroneous notes on the birds seem to have been written on the drawings long after. This set contains some fair copies of George Forster's drawings—fair copies which are much superior to some of the unknown artist's own work.

[1] A. M. Lysaght, 'Some eighteenth century bird paintings in the library of Sir Joseph Banks (1743–1820)', *Bull. Brit. Mus. (Nat. Hist.): Historical Series*, I, no. 6 (1959).

[2] Nils Gyldenstolpe, 'Types of birds in the Royal Natural History Museum in Stockholm', *Arkiv Zool. K. Vetensk. Akad.*, XIX A, no. 1 (1926).

[3] This is doubtless the set referred to by Solander in his letter to Banks, 14 August 1775 (below, p. 959): 'Mr Clerke shew'd me some drawings of Birds, made by a Midshipman, not bad, which I believe he intends for You.' This is the only clue to their authorship.

NOTE ON THE ANNOTATION

Where passages from Cook MSS (except from his log) additional to the text are given in the footnotes, the following practice has been adopted. (1) Quotation marks are not used. (2) Where such passages are fuller variants the initial and terminal words in the text, in italic, are followed by the variant in roman type. (3) Where they are simple additions to the text they begin with three full points [. . .]. (4) Where they are extracts from the MS called B, whence most of them come, they are normally unmarked. Other extracts are marked by the capital letters (A, D, G, H, M) signifying other MSS. (5) Folio numbers are given for each new folio quoted from B, but such folio or page numbers are not normally given for other MSS. (6) Parts of a note following such extracts are separated from Cook's words by a dash.

Where any of this practice has been varied or reversed (e.g. in the use of roman or italic type, or of quotation marks), it is hoped that the form employed is self-explanatory and unambiguous.

Extracts from other sources are enclosed in the usual way in quotation marks. Extracts from logs or journals kept in the *Adventure* are prefixed by the letters ADV. All others refer to the *Resolution*.

'Log', with a capital, always signifies Cook's log.

THE INSTRUCTIONS[1]

By the Commissioners for executing the Office of Lord High Admiral of Great Britain & Ireland &c[a]

Secret Instructions for Cap[t] Cook, Commander of His Majesty's Sloop Resolution.

Whereas several important Discoveries have been made in the Southern Hemisphere in the Voyages performed by the Dolphin under the command of Captain Byron, and afterwards under that of Cap[t] Wallis, by the Swallow Sloop under the Command of Cap[tain] Carteret, and by the Endeavour Bark commanded by Yourself; And whereas we have in pursuance of His Majestys Pleasure signified to us by the Earl of Sandwich, caused the Resolution & Adventure Sloops to be fitted out in all respects proper to proceed upon farther discoveries towards the South Pole, and from the experience we have of your abilities & good conduct in your late Voyage, have thought fit to appoint you to command the first mentioned Sloop, and to intrust you with the Conduct of the present intended Voyage, and have directed Capt. Furneaux, who commands the other Sloop, to follow your Orders for his further Proceedings; You are hereby requir'd & directed to proceed with the said two Sloops to the Island of Madeira, & there take on board such quantities of Wine as may be proper for their respective Companies.

Having so done, you are to make the best of your way to the Cape of Good Hope, where you are to refresh the Sloops companies & take on board such Provisions & Necessaries as you may stand in need of, & may be able to procure.

You are if possible to leave the Cape of Good Hope by the End of October or the beginning of November next, and proceeding to the Southward endeavour to fall in with Cape Circumcision, which is said by Mons[r] Bouvet, to lye nearly in the Latitude of 54°00′ South, and in about 11°20′ of Longitude East from Greenwich.

If you discover Cape Circumcision, you are to satisfy yourself whether it is a part of that Southern Continent which has so much

[1] Printed from the Canberra Letter Book, after collation with P.R.O. Adm 2/1332, pp. 196–203, as printed in Navy Records Society, *Naval Miscellany*, III (1928), pp. 351–6.

engaged the attention of Geographers & former Navigators, or Part of an Island. If it proves to be the former, You are to employ yourself diligently in exploring as great an Extent of it as you can; carefully observing the true situation thereof both in Latitude & Longitude, the Variation of the Needle, Bearings of Head Lands, Height, direction & Course of the Tydes & Currents, Depths & Soundings of the Sea, Shoals, Rocks, &c[a]; and also surveying & making Charts & taking views of such Bays, Harbours and different parts of the Coast, & making such Notations thereon, as may be useful either to Navigation or Commerce; you are also carefully to observe the nature of the soil & the produce thereof; the Animals & Fowls that inhabit or frequent it; the Fishes that are to be found in the Rivers or upon the Coast, & in what plenty; And in case there are any which are peculiar to that Country, you are to describe them as minutely, & to make as correct Drawings of them, as you can. If you find any Mines, Minerals, or valuable Stones, you are to bring home Specimens of each, as also of the Seeds of Trees, Shrubs, Plants, Fruits & Grains peculiar to the Country, as you may be able to collect, & to transmit them to our Secretary that we may cause proper Examination & Experiments to be made of them; You are likewise to observe the Genius, Temper, Disposition and Number of the Natives or Inhabitants, if there be any, & endeavour by all proper means to cultivate a Friendship and Alliance with them, making them Presents of such Trinquets as they may value, inviting them to Trafick, & shewing them every kind of Civility & Regard; but taking care nevertheless not to suffer yourself to be surprized by them, but to be always on your guard against any Accident. You are with the consent of the Natives to take possession of convenient Situations in the Country in the Name of the King of Great Britain, and to distribute among the Inhabitants some of the Medals with which you have been furnished to remain as Traces of your having been there. But if you find the Country uninhabited you are to take possession of it for His Majesty by setting up proper Marks & Inscriptions as first Discoverers & Possessors.

When you have performed this Service, if the State of your Provisions & the Condition of the Sloops will admit of it, you are to proceed upon farther Discoveries, either to the Eastward or Westward as your situation may then render most eligible, keeping in as high a Latitude as you can, & prosecuting your discoveries as near to the South Pole as possible; And you are to employ yourself in this manner so long as the condition of the Sloops, the health of their Crews, & the State of their Provisions will admit of it, having always great attention to the reserving as much of the latter as will enable you to reach some known Port where you may procure a sufficiency to carry you to England.

But if Cape Circumcision should prove to be part of an Island only; Or if you should not be able to find the said Cape from Monsr Bouvet's description of its situation; you are, in the first case, to make the necessary Surveys of the Island, & then stand on to the South ward so long as you judge there may be a likelyhood of falling in with the Continent, which you are also to do in the latter Case, and then proceed to the Eastward, in further Search of the said Continent, as well as to make discovery of such Islands as may be situated in that unexplored part of the Southern Hemisphere, keeping in as high Latitudes as you can & prosecuting your discoveries as before directed as near to the Pole as possible, until by circumnavigating the Globe you fall in again with Cape Circumcision, or the Spot where it is said to be situated; from whence you are to proceed to the Cape of Good Hope, & having there refreshed your People, & put the Sloops into condition to return to England, you are to repair with them to Spithead, where they are to remain til further Order.

In the prosecution of these Discoveries, whenever the Season of the Year may render it unsafe for you to continue in high Latitudes, you are to Retire to some known place to the Northward, to refresh your People & refit the Sloops, taking care to return to the Southward as soon as the Season will admit of it.

You are to observe with accuracy the situation of such Islands as you may discover in the course of your Voyage, which have not hitherto been discovered by any Europeans, & to make surveys & Draughts, & take Possession for His Majesty, of such of them as may appear to be of consequence, in the same manner as directed, with respect to the Continent.

But for as much as in an undertaking of this nature, several Emergencies may arise not to be foreseen, & therefore not particularly to be provided for by Instructions beforehand; You are, in all such Cases, to proceed as you shall judge most advantageous to the Service on which you are employed.

You are by all proper Conveyances, to Send to our Secretary, for our information, Accounts of your proceedings & Copies of the Surveys and Drawings you shall have made. And upon your arrival in England, you are immediately to repair to this Office in order to lay before us a full account of your Proceedings in the whole course of your Voyage; taking care before you leave the Sloop to Demand from the Officers & Petty Officers the Log Books & Journals they may have kept, & to seal them up for our inspection, and enjoining Them & the whole Crew, not to divulge where they have been, until they shall have permission so to do. And you are to direct Capt. Furneaux to do the same with respect to the Officers, Petty Officers & Crew of the Adventure.

If any Accident should happen to the Resolution in the Course of the Voyage so as to disable her from proceeding any farther, you are, in such case, to remove yourself & her Crew into the Adventure, & to prosecute your Voyage in her, her Commander being hereby strictly required to receive you on board & to obey your Orders the same in every respect as when you were actually on board the Resolution; And, in Case of your inability by sickness or otherwise to carry these Instructions into execution, you are to be careful to leave them with the next Officer in command, who is hereby required to execute them in the best manner he can.

Given &c the 25th of June 1772.

SANDWICH
LISBURNE
A. HERVEY
THOs BRADSHAW

By command of their Lordships
Php Stephens

JOURNAL ON BOARD
HIS MAJESTY'S BARK RESOLUTION

I shall conclude this preliminary discourse by publickly acknowlidging the kind Assistance of some worthy friends, in whose hands I left the Manuscript, when I embarked on a third expedition, who were so obliging as to superintend the printing and make such corrections as they found necessary, without altering the stile. For it was judged that it would be more exceptable to the Public, in the Authors words, than in any other persons, and that the Candid and faithfull manner in which it is written would counterbalance the want of stile and dullness of the subject. It is a work for information and not for amusement, written by a man, who has not the advantage of Education, acquired, nor Natural abilities for writing; but by one who has been constantly at sea from his youth, and who, with the Assistance of a few good friends gone through all the Stations belonging to a Seaman, from a prentice boy in the Coal Trade to a Commander in the Navy. After such a Candid confession he hopes the Public will not consider him as an author, but a man Zealously employed in the Service of his Country and obliged to give the best account he is able of his proceedings.

JOURNAL ON BOARD HIS MAJESTY'S BARK RESOLUTION

NOVEMBER 28*th* 1771. I received a Commission to comand His Majestys sloop Drake at this time in the Dock at Deptford, Burdthen 462 Tons to be man'd with 110 Men including officers & to carry twelve guns: at the same time Captain Tobias Furneaux[1] was appointed to the command of the Raleigh at Woolwich Burdthen 336 Tons 80 Men & ten guns. These two sloops were both built at Whitby by Mr Fis[h]burn the same as built the Endeavour Bark, the former about fourteen and the latter eightteen months ago, and had just been purchased into the Navy from Cap. William Hammond of Hull in order to be sent on discoveries to the South Sea under my directions. The Admiralty gave orders that they sould be fitted in the best manner possible, the Earl of Sandwich at this time first Lord intrested himself very much in the Equipment and he was well seconded by Mr Palliser and Sr Jno Williams the one Comptroller and the other Surveyor of the Navy, the Victualling Board was also very attentive in procuring the very best of every kind of Provisions in short every department seem'd to vie with each other in equiping these two Sloops: every standing Rule and order in the Navy was dispenced with, every alteration, every necessary and usefull article was granted as soon as ask'd for.[2]

Two days after I received my Commission I hoisted the Pendant and took charge of the Sloop accordingly and began to enter Seamen, the Vestal Frigate at this time in ordnary, was appoint[ed] to receive them untill the sloop came out of Dock.

Decemr 25*th*. The Admiralty changed the sloops Names to Resolution and Adventure and the officers were order'd to take out new Comisions & Warrants accordingly.[3]

[1] . . . who was Lieutenant with Captain Wallis in the South Sea and was promoted on this occasion.—f. 2.

[2] . . . under so many favourable circumstances it is reasonable to suppose that the equipment would meet with no interruption but so many people were concern'd in the expedition every one of which thought they had a right to advise and some even to direct, till in the end the old Proverb of more Cooks the worse broth, was never better verified, than in the equipment of the Drake as will be seen by and by.—f. 2v.

[3] It may be remarked that in the eighteenth century officers were commissioned to a particular ship, not simply as naval officers of a particular rank. Therefore—to take an example—Clerke, having been commissioned as second lieutenant of the *Drake* (and not as Lieutenant Clerke, R.N., appointed to the *Drake*) had to get a new commission as second lieutenant of the *Resolution*. Hence also Cooper's entry for 1 January 1772: 'Put up Bills

Mr Banks and Dr Solander who accompanied me in my last Voyage intended to embark with me in this in order to prosecute their discoveries in Natural History and Botany and other usefull knowlidge, for this purpose Mr Banks intend to take with him several Draughtsmen &c^a^. The Board of Longitude also came to a Resolution to send out an Astronomer in each sloop to make Astronomical Observations and also to make tryal of Mr Arnolds Watches and Mr Kendals Timepiece which were intended to be sent out with them. The Parliament voted Four thousand pounds towards carrying on Discoveries to the South Pole, this sum was intinded for Dr Lynd of Edinburgh as an incouragement for him to embark with us, but what the discoveries were, the Parliament meant he was to make, and for which they made so liberal a Vote, I know not.[1] Mr Zoffani the famous portrait painter was one of those who had engaged to accompany Mr Banks, all these gentlemen except one Astronomer were to embark in the Resolution and to have large and seperate apartments: three of these gentlemen were not thought of when the sloop was purchased (viz.) the Astronomer, Dr Lynd and Mr Zoffani. The addition of these three persons intirely altered the plan of accommodations and it was found difficult to find room for the whole and at the same time to leave room for her officers and crew and stowage for the necessary stores and provisions, for this end the Navy Board was prevailed upon, tho contrary to the opinion of some of the members particularly the Comptroller, to alter their former plan which was to leave her in her original state and to raise her upper Works about a a foot, to lay a spar deck upon her from the quarter deck to the forecastle (she having at this time a low waist) and to build a round house or couch for my accommodations so that the great Cabbin might be appropriated to the use of Mr Banks alone.[2] Things being thus resolved upon they were carried into execution with all possible dispatch and were about finished by the 6th of Feb^ry^ following on which day we hauld out of the dry into the Wet Dock, and began to taken in Ballast, stores and to Rigg the masts &c^a^ having by this time compleated our complement of men. On Wednesday 19th the Carpenters having nearly finish[ed] the different appartments of the Sloop,

for entering Seamen for the Resolution instead of the Drake, as did the Adventure instead of the Raleigh'.—For an interesting discussion of 'post and rank' see Michael Lewis, *England's Sea Officers* (1939), chap. V. Not until 1860 were 'ship commissions' formally superseded by 'general commissions'.

[1] *I know not:* will hardly ever come to the knowlidge of the publick much less to me as an individual.—f. 3.—But see p. 913 below, under 8 February, *Royal Society*.

[2] *so that . . . alone:* that the great Cabbin which was larger than that of a Sixty Gun Ship, might be appropriated to the use of Mr Banks alone a distinction which he claimed and which from a desire of obligeing him I very readily gave up . . .—f. 3v.

we hauld out of the Dock into the River and began to take in Provisions and the remainder of our stores &c^{a} which was not compleated untill the 9th of Ap^{r} when we saild from Deptford and the same evening stop'd a long side the sheer hulk at Woolwich where we were detain'd by contrary Winds untill the 22nd on which day with the Advantage of a Westerly wind we reached long reach and two days after were join'd by the Adventure.[1] On the 25th we got on board our guns Powder & other ordnance stores, our draught of Water at this time was 17 feet. Notwithstanding this great depth of water we had reson to think that she would prove Crank and that she was over built; but as all the Gentlemens appartments were full of heavy baggage and the sloop a good deal lumber'd a loft with heavy, and some useless articles, which we might soon get rid of, or get into the hold after we had consumed some of our Provisions I still entertain'd hopes that she would bear all her additional Works and suspended giving any other opinion untill a full tryal had been made of her foreseeing what would be the consequence in case she did not Answer in the manner she was now fitted.[2]

On the 29th we received on board our party of Marines consisting of Lieutenant Edgcumbe, one Serjeant two Corp^{ls} one Drum and fifteen Private. The Adventure also took on board her Marines consisting of a Lieutenant Serjeant Corperal, Drum and eight private. The Resolutions complement was now 112 men and the Adventures 81, their Lordships having, upon my application, added two Carpenters Mates to the former and one to the latter.

MAY *2nd.* Mr Banks gave an entertainment on board to the Earl of Sandwich, the French Embassador Cont de Guines and several other persons of distinction, the[y] were complimented at their coming on board and going a shore with all the honours due to their high ranks:[3] the Earl of Sandwich was so attentive to the equipment of these two sloops that he had honour'd us with his presence on board several times before in order to be an eye witness of their

[1] Cook ignores minor incidents: e.g., 'Sent Cutter up to Deptford for John Marra who was Confin'd on board the Grenville Brig for Security.'—Cooper, 14 April.—'Punish'd John Marra Gunners Mate one dozen for Mutiny & Desertion.'—Cooper, 22 April.

[2] *I still . . . fitted:* I still intertain'd hopes that after these things were properly stow'd away and once clear of the River that a Stop might be put to receiving any more on board, that she would Answer and bear all the additional Works that had been added to her and suspended giving any other opinion untill a full tryal had been made, foreseeing what would be the concequence in case any part of them were obliged to be taken away so as to lessen the gentlemens appartments and accommodations.—f. 4.

[3] 'Came on board the Right Honble The Earl of Sandwish with the French Ambassador and dined saluted them with three chears & 17 guns at their coming on board & going out of the ship.'—Gilbert, 2 May. And see Cook, p. xxviii above. The Comte (later Duc) de Guines was French ambassador in England 1770–76.

state and condition, a laudable tho rare thing in a first Lord of the Admiralty.[1]

In the night of the 7th Mr Sandford one of the Midshipmen fell out of the Launch, at this time laying along side of the Sheer hulk at Woolwich, and was unfortunatly drown'd, he was a young man of good parts and much esteem'd by the officers; some officious persons the next day inform'd Sr George Saville[2] that James Strong one of the Seamen[3] threw him overboard in concequence of which he was taken into custody, but upon examination this charge could not be proved and he thereupon was released, he however found means to escape from the officer who was sent to take him on board and we saw him no more.

Captain Furneaux having received orders to proceed to Plymouth she sail'd accordingly, at the same time the Resolution had orders to proceed to the Downs under the direction of the first Lieutenant, I having obtain'd leave to be absent untill she arrived at that place, accordingly on the 10th in the morning they got under sail with a light breeze at North where it did not continue long before it came to the Eastward and obliged her to work down the River in which she made so little progress that it was the 14th before she reached the Nore, in this short passage she was found so crank that it was thought unsafe to proceed any further with her. This being represented to me with all its circumstances by Mr Cooper the first Lieutenant I laid the same before the Admiralty and seeing that it was absolutely necessary that something should be done to remove the evil complain'd of I proposed to cut down her poop, shorten her masts and to change her guns from six to four pounders: the Navy Board who was immidiately consulted upon the matter, propos'd not only to cut down her poop, but to take of her spar deck, lower her waist and to reduce her as near to her original state as could conveniently be done. Orders were now sent down for her to put into Sheerness where she anchor'd on the 18th and the officers of that yard recieved orders to cut her down agreeable to a Plan sent them by the Navy Board and which was confirmable to their proposals. While these matters were under consideration of the Admiralty and Navy Board others of a contrary nature were in aggitation by Mr

[1] *a laudable . . . Admiralty:* and not out of Idle curiosity as many of all ranks did, Ladies as well as gentlemen, for scarce a day past on which she was not crowded with Strangers who came on board for no other purpose but to see the Ship in which Mr Banks was to sail round the world.—f. 4–4v.

[2] Sir George Savile (1726–84), F.R.S., M.P. for Yorkshire, an eminent Whig politician who never held office; he was ardent in political reform, and greatly looked up to for his integrity and unostentatious benevolence.

[3] This man did not go on the voyage.

Banks and his friends, as this gentlemen seem'd not to approve of the Ship at the first he now used all his influence to have her condem'd as totally unfit for the service she was going upon and to have a 40 gun Ship or an East Indiaman fitted out in her room, either of which would have been highly improper for makeing discoveries in remot parts. I shall not mention the arguments made use of by Mr Banks and his friends as many of them were highly absurd and advanced by people who were not judges of the subject one or two sea officers excepted who upon this occasion I beleive sacrificed their jud[ge]ment in support of their friendship, or some other montive be this as it may the clamour was so great that it was thought it would be brought before the house of commons. The Admiralty and Navy Boards however persevered in their resolution of clearing her of all her superfluous works and remain'd firm in their opinion that after this was done she would answer in every respect better then any ship they could get. I was accordingly ordered to join her immidiately, to inspect into and forward these works and to point out such others as might tend to remove the evil complain'd of a piece of service I went the more readily about as having not the least doubt with my self but that I must succeed indeed I had it much at heart as she was the Ship of my choice and as I then thought and still think the properest Ship for the Service she is intended for of any I ever saw. On the 20th I set out for Sheerness and arrived thier the same evening and found every thing in great forwardness, the Poop and Spar deck was already taken away and Mr Huntt the Builder only waited to consult me about some little alteration he proposed to make in the waist from the Navy Boards Plan which the Board afterwards approved of. The next day I proposed to the Navy Board by letter to shorten her lower Masts two feet which they approved of and it was done accordingly. On Sunday 24th Mr Banks and Dr Solander came down to take a view of the Sloop as she was now altered and return'd to town again the same even^g^ and soon after Mr Banks declared his resolution not to go the Voyage, aledging that the Sloop was neither roomy nor convenient enough for his purpose, nor noways proper for the Voyage, these were the principal reasons Mr Banks assign'd for giving up a Voyage the preparing for which had cost him about five Thousand pounds, he probably had others which he did not care to declare, at least whoever saw the Sloop and the appartments that were alloted to him and his people could not help but think so. Be this as it may, not only Mr Banks and his whole suite but Dr Lind gave up the Voyage and their Baggage &c^a^ were got out of the Sloop and sent to London, after which no more complaints were heard for want of room &c[a].[1]

On the 30th M[r] Palliser the Comptroller of the Navy paid us a Visit in order to inspect into the several alterations that had been & were still to make, for this gentleman had taken upon him in spite of all that had been alledged against her to make her compleatly fit not only for the sea but for the service she was intended for, indeed if his advice had not been over ruled at first a great deal of unnecessary trouble and expence would have been saved not only to the Crown but to M[r] Banks and every other person concerned.[2]

Every little plan of alteration being now fixed upon the whole was carried on with great allertness and for the sake of dispatch the Sloop lay all the time along side the Jetty head.[3]

On the 10th of June the Earl of Sandwich having imbarked on board the Augusta Yacht in order to Visit the several Dock yards and inspect into the state of the Navy, anchor'd at the Nore and soon after landed in the yard and came on board the Resolution. His Lordship inspected into and was pleased to approve of all the alterations that had been made, after a stay of about an hour he return'd on board the yacht and saild directly for the Downs. Every thing being now nearly upon the point of finishing and having some business to settle in London I set out for that place in the Even[g] and upon my arrival learnt that M[r] John Reinhold Forster and his Son M[r] George Forster were to imbark with me, gentlemen skill'd in Natural history and Botany but more especially the former, who from the first was desireous of going the Voyage and therefore no sooner heard that M[r] Banks had given it up then he applyed to go. The Earl of Sandwich favoured his proposals which were approved

[1] *after which . . . &c[a]:* after which several of the officers appartments were new model'd and finished without further interruption . . .—f. 6.—Banks's stores were not the only embarrassing ones. Cf. Pickersgill, 25 May: 'Empl[d] getting the Bread out of the Bread Room which was much damaged owing to the Rooms being lined with green furr the Juces of which the Bread had extracted and imbibed which had communicated a great way in but was luckily found out before we left England or its Consequence would have been very Bad.' The *Adventure* had the same trouble: Furneaux's 'Remarks . . . 31 October –23 November 1772' include mention of employment 'in getting up the Bread out of the Bread room, found a great quantity of it mouldy, & not fit to eat; had a Survey on it by order of Capt[n] Cook, & condemned 519[lb] it being in their Opinion milldew'd by the Green plank, which the Bread room was cas'd with'. Again, '. . . returnd several of the Officers Stoves there not being room sufficient to Carry them Receivd from London fresh Bread in Lieu of that return'd.'—Pickersgill, 29 May.

[2] '. . . at 1 PM fired 15 Guns being the Anniversary of King Charles's restoration'.—Furneaux. There was no disloyalty entailed in this Stuart celebration. King George got his own 21 guns on his birthday, 5 June.

[3] '. . . dry'd the ship betwixt decks with pots of charcoal fires & also the store rooms'. —Gilbert, 7 June.

of by His Majesty and a very handsome stipend allow'd him and his son; their Baggage and other necessarys being sent on board and I having finished my Business in Town I on Sunday morn the 21st tooke leave of my Family and set out, in company with Mr Wales the Astronomer for Sheerness where we arrived that evening and the next day saild out of the Harbour. Mr Hunt the Builder of the yard and some of the other officers attended us to the Nore where we try'd the Sloop upon a wind (having a fresh breeze at South) and found her to answer exceeding well:[1] her draught of Water at this time was 15 f^{t} 10 In. fore and abaft, a foot lighter than when she first went into Sheerness, one great point gain'd by cutting her down. At 6 o'Clock in the evening we anchord upon the Warp in 8 fathom where we were detaind untill the 25th when with the wind at sw we run over the Flatts and Anchored in Margate road and the next day got into the Downs where we lay but one night and than sail'd for Plymouth Sound where we arrived on Friday the 3rd of July and found our consort the Adventure Sloop waiting for us. The evening before we met between the Start and Plymouth Lord Sandwich in the Augusta Yatch, the Glory Frigate & Hazard Sloop. His Lordship was upon his return from vissiting Plym^{h} yard and where he had waited some days longer than he had occasion for my arrival, as soon as we join'd this little squadron we saluted his Lordship with 17 Guns, and soon after he and Mr Pallisser came on board. Their intintion for makeing us this Vissit was to be informed personaly from me of the true state and quallities of the Sloop and which I was now well able to give them and so much in her favour that I had not one fault to alledge againest her. So far from being crank I found her remarkably stiff and to work and sail better than could be expected from a ship of her burdthensome construction and at the same time deeply laden. Being able to give this information with so much Candor as could not be confuted they no doubt received great satisfaction therefrom. It is owing to the perseverance of these two persons that the expedition is in so much forwardness, had they given way to the general Clamour and not steadily adhered to their own better judgement the Voyage in all probabillity would have been laid aside. After a stay of something more than an hour they took their leave and we gave his Lordship three cheers at parting.

[1] 'at 2 cast off the Bridles & sail'd out of the Harbour to the Nore with several of the Officers of the Yard on board. A fine fresh Breeze—haul'd upon a wind on purpose to try what effect these alterations had made upon our Ship and soon found to our very great satisfaction that it had entirely remedied every ill quality she had—found her now a stiff Ship—work'd well—and readily got very good way through the Water.'—Clerke, 22 June. 'Bridles'—moorings.

On our Passage from the Downs to Plymouth I made tryal of Mr Irvings apparatus for distillation and found that our Coppers were not well addapted for that purpose.[1] Accordingly I applyed for others which were ordered to be got in readiness, indeed the Navy Board ever attentive to the fitting of these two Sloops had lodged orders at this place for them to be supplied with whatever I should think necessary to demand. However they were already so compleat that little was wanting, the design of their puting in here was to pay the Crews six Months pay and two Months Wages advance. I here received my Instruction the heads of which I had seen before I left London, indeed I was consulted at the time they were drawn up and nothing was inserted that I did not fully comprehend and approve of, a copy of these Instructions I gave to Captain Furneaux seald up and also some other necessary orders and Instructions relating to the Voyage.[2]

Having on board five men which were rather Invalides or at least such as I thought were not fit for the Voyage I applyed to Cap^tn^ Edwd Hughes, who at this time commanded His Majestys Ships at this port, to have them exchanged. He very obligeingly complied with my request and directing each Ship in the Harbour to furnish me with a good Seaman and such as was a Volunteer; this being done and having taken on board a fresh supply of Provisions and the Coppers being also nearly finished, on Friday the 10th the Officers & Crew of both Sloops were paid their Wages up to the 28th of May last and the Petty Officers and Seamen were also paid two months Advance.[3] The payment of Six Monthes Wages to the Offi-

[1] The apparatus depended on the fact that coppers on naval vessels were made double, so that while food was being cooked in one, salt water could be boiled for distillation in the other. There is a full description of it in an appendix to Phipps's *Voyage towards the North Pole* (1774), with a plate. The *Resolution*, not having been built as a naval vessel, presumably did not have coppers of the regulation design. Charles Irving (d. 1794) was an inventive surgeon in the Royal Navy, who petitioned the House of Commons in 1772 for public reward for this 'easy and practicable method of making sea water fresh and wholesome', having been granted £300 by the Admiralty in 1771. Both ships were also fitted with 'Lieutenant Osbridge's machine', which Cook refers to below (p. 508) as 'the Tin Machine . . . an excellent contrivance for sweetening Water at sea and is very will known in the Navy'. It is thus described by Sparrman, pp. 153–4: 'a machine employed in English warships; this is made of plated sheet-iron, with several flat-bottomed trays placed one above the other, with a space between. The bottom of each tray is pierced like a collender, so that, with the aid of a machine-driven pump, the water from the bottom of the usual drinking-casks on deck is raised six feet high to the topmost collender; it is then filtered through this in large drops, and falls from tray to tray in an increasingly finer rain, until it is down again in the cask, to be continually raised once more and dropped many times. It is plain that the breeze from windward takes away all the stench, and also cools the water.'

[2] . . . appointing the Island of Madeira the first place of Rendezvouze, Port Praya in the Island of St Iago the Second and the Cape of Good Hope the third.—f. 8.

[3] A The Ships Company where pay'd ye Six Months pay That They had do [due]

cers and crews of these two Sloops being nearly all they had due, was an indulgance never before granted to any of His Majestys Ships and was done with a view to enable them to purchase necessarys for so long a Voyage on which account people from the shore were allowed to come on board on this and the following day to sell them these necessarys. Every thing being at length compleated we on *Monday* the 13th at Six o'Clock in the morning left Plymouth Sound with the Adventure in Company[1] and stood to the SW with the wind at NW where I shall leave them and for the information of the curious give some account in what manner they are equiped and shall first begin with their established complement of Officers and Men, viz.

Resolution		
Officers	No.	Names
Captain	1	James Cook
Lieutenants	3	R. P. Cooper, Charls Clerk, Richd Pickersgill
Master	1	J. Gilbert
Masters Mates ..	3	
Midshipmen	6	
Boatswain	1	J. Gray
Boatswains Mates ..	3	
Gunner	1	Robt Anderson
Gunners Mates ..	2	
Surgeon	1	J. Patten
Surgeons Mates ..	2	
Carpenter	1	J. Wallice
Carpenters Mates ..	3	
Carpenters Crew ..	4	
Master at Arms ..	1	
Corporal	1	

& ye Two Months Advance besides, By Petioning to Lord Sandwich for it.'—Harvey, 10 July. Admiralty generosity evidently had to be instigated from below.

[1] It seems odd that a lieutenant of the *Adventure* should be at this date entirely vague about the purpose of the voyage, but Kemp writes, 'A few days since came in & join'd us, his Majestys sloop Resolution Capt Cook, being the sloop we are to accompany, as suppos'd on a Voyage round the Globe'. Pickersgill, who was no doubt more knowledgeable, provides the appropriate touch of sentiment, with the significant words 'Farewell Old England', written very large and surrounded by a scribbled border.

Sail maker	1	
Sail makers mate ..	1	
Armourer	1	
Armourers Mate ..	1	
Cook	1	
Cooks Mate	1	
Captains Clerk ..	1	
Quarter Masters ..	6	
Able Seamen includ[g] acting Midshipmen	45	
	92	
Marines		
Lieutenant	1	Jn[o] Edgcumb
Serjeant	1	
Corporals	2	
Drummer	1	
Privates	15	
Total Compli[t] ..	112	

Gentlemen & their Servants borne as Supernumeraries

M[r] W[m] Wales Astronomer with one Servant

M[r] Jn[o] Reinhold Forster & M[r] George Forster Botanists and Natural historians, with one Servant[1]

M[r] Jam[s] [2] Hodges, Landskip painter, this gentle[n] was sent on board by the Admiralty a few days after our arrival at Plymouth.

Total Number on board 118. As the Adventure's complement was about one third less than the Resolutions she had fewer officers in proportion, the whole number she had on board was 83 including M[r] Baily the Astronomer and his servant, which were all the supernumeraries she carried.

The manner in which they are victualed will best appear from the following account of Provisions which are now on board exclusive of what the officers have provided for themselves.

[1] Ernst or Ernest Scholient—a man, it may be assumed, in an unfortunate position. But we know very little about him.

[2] *sic;* for William. In H Cook carefully inserts the name: 'In order to make up for the want of M[r] Zoffany and some others who were to have gone out with M[r] Banks, the Admiralty engaged one M[r] Jam[s] Hodges to go out in the Resolution to make Drawings of such places and things as were curious, usefull, or worthy of note and he came onboard while we lay at Plymouth'.

Quallity	Resolution	Adventure
Biscuit ..	59531 pounds	39990 } Pounds
Flour	17437 D°	12767 }
Salt Beef ..	7637 four p^d pieces	4300 } pieces
D° Pork ..	14214 two p^d pieces	8820 }
Beer	19 Ton	30 Punch^s
Wine	642 Gall^ns	400 } Gallons
Spirit	1397 D°	300 }
Pease	358 Bushels	216 Bushels
Wheat ..	188 D°	820 } Gallons
Oatmeal ..	300 Gallons	460 }
Butter ..	1963 } Pounds	1000 } Pounds
Cheese ..	797 }	1200 }
Sugar ..	1959 }	1441 }
Oyle Olive ..	210 Gall^ns	237 } Gallons
Vinegar ..	259 D°	320 }
Suet	1900 } Pounds	1267 } Pounds
Raisins ..	3102 }	2776 }
Salt	101 Bush^s	51 } Bushels
*Malt	80 Bushels	60 }
		T. Cwt. Q. lb.
*Sour Krout ..	19337 } Pounds	5 5 0 4
*Salted Cabbage	4773 }	1 16 1 0
*Portable Broth	3000 }	2000 } Pounds
*Saloup ..	70 }	47 }
*Mustard ..	400 }	300 }
*Mermalade of Carrots ..	30 gallons	22 gallons
Water ..	45 Tons	40 Tons
Exper^l Beef ..	1384 pounds	298 peices 4 lb. each
Inspisated Juce of Beer ..	19 half Barrels	12 half Barrels

* The articles marked thus (*) are antiscorbuticks, and are to be issued occasionally

*Some readers that are unaquainted with the manner of Victualing the Navy may wish to know what is meant by whole allowance, which is a daly allowance of Provisinos allowed to each person without distinction. I will for brevity sake suppose four Men to mess or eat together which is very common, their daly allowance will be as followes, viz.

Each man is allowed every day one pound of Biscuit as much small Beer as he can drink or a pint of Wine, or half a pint of Brandy, Rum, or arrack, they will have besides on

Monday. Half a pound of Butter, about ten ounces of Cheshire Cheese and as much boild Oatmeal or Wheat as they can eat.

Tuesday. Two 4 pound pieces of Beef, or one four pound piece of Beef three pounds of Flour and one pound Raisins or half a pound of Suet.

Wednesday. Butter and cheese as on Monday and as much boild Pease as they can eat.

Thursday. Two 2 pound pieces of Pork with Pease.

Friday. The same as Wednesday.

Satrduay. The Same as Tuesday.

Sunday. The same as Thursday.

Sugar and Oyle are served in lieu of Butter and cheese a pound of the one or a pint of the other is equal to one lb of Butter or 21 ounces of Cheese.

If the above allowance is at any time through necessity shortened, the men are always paid for the Dificiency. But few of the anti-scorbutick articles before mentioned have been interduced into the Navy and those few only for the use of the Sick, indeed I do not recolect any thing but Portable Broth to have been put on board any Ship, excepting those latly sent on discoveries, or to other remote parts who have had some of these articles put on board partly for general use and partly for experiment. Some account of them may not be unexceptable to the curious.[1] Of Malt is made sweet wort and given to such persons as have contracted the Scurvey, and to such as from their habit of body are liable to contract it, at the discretion of the Surgeon.

Sour Krout, is Cabbage cut small, and cured by going through a state of fermentation (I am not acquainted with the proper method) it is afterward close pack'd in Casks with its own liquor, in which state it will keep any length of time, it is a very wholsome food and a very great antiscorbutick, a pound of it is served to each man each Beef day, it is much use[d] in several parts of Germony from whence it has its name which signifies Sour Cabbage, it having that taste to a high degree and may be eat either raw or boild.

[1] We had most of these articles on board the Endeavour Bark, but I have forgot if the use of them was explained in my Journal of that Voyage, and I have it not now with me. —Cook's note.

Salted Cabbage, is Cabbage cut to pieces well salted and close packed in Casks, it will keep good equally long with Sour Krout, but whether it be as great an Antiscorbutick or not the Faculty or experience must determine; it is served to the people in the same manner as Sour Krout, but must be freshened and boild before it can be eat.

Portable Broth is made from flesh meat, an Ounce of the former is said to contain the nourishing Juces of about three quarters of a Pound of the latter; the Commissioners of the Sick in their Instructions tells us that one ounce of Broth will be sufficient to make one Quart of liquid broth, so strong that it will Jelly when cold; but experience tells us that it will require double that quantity; it is dissolved in boiling Water and given to the Sick at the Discretion of the Surgeon; but to the well Men or Company in general, an Ounce to each Man is boiled in the Pease or Wheat on Banyan days, Days so call'd in the Navy, which are Mondays, Wednesday and Fridays because on these days they have no flesh meat.

Saloupe and Rob of Lemons and Oranges are intend[ed] for the Sick and Scorbutick only. Mustard is intended for all in general, it is allowed to be of an antiscorbutick quallity and its use is well known.

Marmalade of Carrets, is the Juice of Yallow Carrets Inspissated till it is of the thickness of flued honey or Treacle which last, it looks like and in some degree tastes like; it is recomended by Baron Storsch of Berlin, as a very great Antiscorbutick. He says 'a Spoonful of this Marmadlade, mix'd with Water, taken now and then will prevent the scurvey, it will even cure it if constantly taken'. It is much used by the poor people in Germany.

The Inspissated juce of Malt, which might be reckoned among the Antiscorbuticks, I shall speak of in another place. It will be unnecessary and tedious to enumerate the several articles of Naval Stores that are on board, nothing is wanting that was thought necessary, and the quantity Sufficient for so long a Voyage.*—ff. 9–11.

Besides the Provisions &c[a] mentioned above we have casks on board the two Sloops for the reception of about 4000[1] gall[ns] of Madeira Wine which we intend to take in at that Island, so that upon the whole includeing what the officers and gentlemen[2] have provided for themselves, we have full two years Provisions on board at whole allowance of most articles and of some much more and this exclusive

[1] Evidently a slip for 400, as elsewhere given. [2] *gentlemen:* Gentlemen Passengers.

of the antiscorbuticks before mentioned.[1] We were also provided with Mr Irvings apperatuses for distillation by which we can at any time get a small supply of fresh Water from the Sea, in case we should be short of that article. It will be both unnecessary and tedious to enumerate the Naval Stores that are on board, for besides their Furniture[2] of every kind which are all made of the very best materials, we have on board a variety of spare stores of every sort sufficient for so long a Voyage. We are also well provided with fishing Netts, Lines, Hooks, &ca &ca for catching of fish and in order to inable us to procure refreshments at such inhabitated parts of the World as we might touch at where Money is of no Value, the Admiralty caused to be put on board each of the Sloops several Articles of Merchantdize, as well to trade with the Natives for Provisions as to make them presents to gain their friendship, their Lordships also caus'd to be struck a number of Medals, on the one side the Kings head and on the other the two Sloops & the time they were at first intended to sail from England, these Medals are to be distributed to the Natives of, and left upon New Discoveried countries as testimonies of being the first discovereries. I have before mentioned that the Resolution carried Twelve carriage guns 4 pounds and the Adventure Ten, they have likewise an equal number of swivels with all other Arms and ammunition in proportion. On Board each of the Sloops is the frame, or all the parts compleat of a small Vesel of about twenty tons burdthen which can be put together in a little time whenever they may be wanting.

From this general View of the equipment the impartial reader who is a judge of Marine affairs will probably conclude with me that whatever may be the event of the expedition, the Ships are both well choosen and well provided.[3]

The Board of Longitude were not wanting on their part in providing the Astronomers with the very best of I[n]struments both for makeing Celestial and Nautical Observations but as the principal object these gentlemen are sent out upon is to assertain the going of Mr Kendall's Watch and three of Mr Arnolds, they employ'd themselves during our stay at Plymouth in makeing the necessary Observations on Drakes Island—& at 7 o'Clock in ye eveng on the Friday before we departed the Watches were put in motion in the presence

[1] . . . On board each of the Sloops is a Copper Oven for bakeing of Bread when ever the same is found convenient and necessary, but this can only be done a shore.—f. 9.

[2] 'Furniture' in the naval sense—i.e. apparatus in general for the working of the ship.

[3] *From this . . . provided:* H From this general view of the heads of the Equipment it must appear to every man conversant in marine Affairs, that no vessels could be better equiped or provided and I will take it upon me to say that none were more proper for the service they were going upon.

of my self Captain Furneaux, the first Lieutenant of each of the Sloops, the two astronomers and Mr Arnold and afterward put on board: Mr Kendals and one of Mr Arnolds on board the Resolution and the other two of Mr Arnolds on board the Adventure: the Commander, First Lieutenant and Astronomer on board each of the Sloops had each of them Keys of the Boxes which containd the Watches and were allways to be present at the winding them up and comparing the one with the other. Mr Kendalls Watch when put in motion was seven tenths of a second fast of mean time and its rate of going when try'd at Greenwich was five eights of a second per day slow of mean time. Mr Arnolds Watch when put in motion was Ten seconds and a half slow of mean time and its rate of going at Greenwich was fourteen Seconds & Sixty two hundreds part of a second Pr Day slow of mean time, from these datas the rate of their going will hereafter be determined.

By the observations made on Drakes Island its Lat. is 50°21′30″ N and Longitude 4°20′ West from Greenwich, hence by the help of a Survey of Plymouth Sound made by Mr Gilbert the Master I find Ram head from which I take my departure to lay in Latitude 50°19′ N and Longitude 4°23′ W. I shall now return to the Sloops which I left standing to the SW on the Monday ye 13th on the Noon of which day Ram head at the West entrance of Plymouth Sound bore NNE¾E distant Seven Leagues. Before I go on regularly with the Transaction of each day it will be necessary to premise that the day is supposed to begen and end at Noon, that is Tuesday will now begin on Monday Noon and end on Tuesday Noon, at which time Wednesday begins &ca, that all the bearings and Courses are the true bearings & Courses and not by Compass and that the proportion between the length of the Logg line and half minute glass by which the Sloops Way is measured, is as 50 feet is to 30 seconds of time,[1] the Longitude is reckoned west from the Meridian of Greenwh.[2]

TUESDAY 14*th*. The former part fresh breezes from the NW & Clowdy the remainder little wind and thick hazy weather with rain, at Noon we were in the Latd 49°10′ and Longitude 5°3′.

WEDNESDAY 15*th*. Foggy all this day with gentle Breezes from the NW with which we kept plying down Channell and at Noon we were

[1] Cook states the convention thus as a matter of habit, but in practical seamanship modifications were often made. Wales in fact remarks, at the end of his log, 'It should have been noted that whatever was the length of the half-minute glass, the Log-line had such proportion thereto as 49½ feet bears to 30 seconds'. It was generally considered prudent to divide the log-line at a smaller interval than 50 feet, so that the reckoning was ahead of the ship; Phipps indeed, after his experiments in 1773, recommended 45 feet.

[2] ... untill we are to the East of that Meridian when it will be reckoned East.—f. 11v.

in the Latitude of 48°51′ and Longitude 5°26′. Found by mustering the Sloops company that we have one Man More than our Complement owing to a mistake in the Clerk occasioned [by the hurry he was in in making out the advance Lists.][1]

THURSDAY 16*th*. Gentle gales from the NNE with which we stood to the SW with the Adventure in company and at Noon was in the Lat[d] of 47°29′ and Longitude 6°59′ W.

FRIDAY 17*th*. Winds from the NW to SWBW accompanied by a large swell from the NW. We stood to the SW untill 5 o'Clock am when we tacked and stood 4 hours to the NW and then again to the SW and were at Noon in the Latitude of 46°24′ and Longitude 7°24′ W. the NW swell still continues.

SATURDAY 18*th*. Fresh gales from the SW with squally, rainy unsettled weather which obliged us to reef our Topsails. At 6 in the pm we tacked and stood to the NW and at Noon had made 18 Miles upon a N 18° W Course since yesterday at Noon.[2]

SUNDAY 19*th*. Winds from the WNW a steady fresh breeze and clowdy weather. Stood closse upon a wind to the Southward all this day and at Noon we were in the Latitude of 45°20′ Long[de] 8°20′.

MONDAY 20*th*. In the pm had a fresh gale at West which in the am veer'd to SW increased and was attended with squals and rain which obliged the Adventure to take in her Topsails after which we did the same least we should run her out of sight. At 8 o'Clock in the am made Cape Ortegal on the Coast of [Spain] and which at Noon bore SSE distant 3 Leagues.

TUESDAY 21*st*. Winds variable and unsteady, attended with Foggs and rain in the pm but in the am it cleared up. At 2 o'Clock in the PM wore and stood to the NW Cape Ortegal bearing SSW distant 4 or 5 Miles. At Noon it bore ENE and the Groyn Light house SBE distant 3 Leagues.

WEDNESDAY 22*nd*. Had it calm from Noon until 9 o'Clock pm when a light breeze sprung up from the westward: took the opportunity of the Calm to send a Boat on board the Adventure with M[r] Wales in order to compare the Watches, at the same time I sent Captain Furneaux his orders how to proceed in case of seperation and not meet-

[1] The sentence is completed from H.

[2] At this point Forster (I, p. 5) is worth quoting for the recipe with which he concludes: 'Those who were not used to the sea, nay some of the oldest mariners, were affected by the sea-sickness, in various degrees of violence. It was of different duration with different persons, and after it had continued three days amongst us, we found the greatest relief from red port wine mulled, with spices and sugar'.

ing at the Cape of Good hope after a limeted time, also appointed Port Praya in the Island of St Jago to be the place of Rendezvouze in case of seperation between Madeira and the Cape de Verde Isl^{ds} and after waiting there [fourteen] days to proceed to the Cape of Good hope. As soon as the Boat returnd I sent her on Board of a sm^{l} French Vessel which we took for a fisher and as near as to be within hail, but upon the return of the Boat I learnt she was from Marceilles and bound to Ferrol, the Master inform'd that he had been brought too the day before by three Spanish Men of War under English Colours. After supplying him with some Water of which he stood in need of, having had none for several days we parted.[1] Here we found the variation by the mean of sever^{l} Az^{ths} to be 23°58′ West and in the morning 20°45′ West, our change of situation was by no means answerable to this difference. At Noon the Island of Cycearga[2] bore SEBS distant 4 or 5 Leagues.

THURSDAY *23rd.* A steady gentle gale from the Northward and clear weather. At 2 o'Clock in the PM pass'd by the Spainish Ships above mentioned the sternmost of which housed English colours and fired a gun to leeward and soon after hoisted his own proper Colours and spoke with the Adventure.[3] In the evening found the Variation by several Azth to be 24°50′ W and by the amplitude 24°39′ and in the morning by several Az^{ths} 19°22′. Every favourable circumstance attended the makeing of the observations of both yesterday and to day, they were all made by the same Compass and stood always

[1] 'We afterwards went on board a French Tartan bound from Marselles to Ferro with flower of whom we purchased 100 Bottles Frontenac Wine for 5£ Bottles included & about 60 Bottles of Syrup of Orgeat at 6^{d} ea., they informed us that 3 spanish Ships of war were crusing off Finistre.'—Wales. *Tartan[e]:* a small Mediterranean vessel, one-masted, carrying a large lateen sail and a foresail. *Syrup of Orgeat:* a syrup of barley or almonds and orange-flower water.

[2] The Sisargas islands, a short distance off the north-west corner of Spain.

[3] Cook's bare record of this incident may be enlarged—he being, evidently, not as quick to record offence as he had been at Rio de Janeiro in 1768. Clerke writes, 'Pass'd 3 Spanish Men of War, large 2 Deckers I beleive from 64 to 74 Guns, Commanded by an Admiral with red at ye F:T:G^{t} mast Head—the Admiral fir'd a shot at the Adventure, who taking no notice of it, the Spanish Admiral Tack'd and made ye Sig^{l} for his Squadron to follow him which they accordingly did—presently afterwards he fir'd another shot, upon which Capt Cook thought proper to bring too, as did the Adventure—the Spaniard hal'd him—wore and stood away for the Groyn [Corunna]. . . '. Elliott *Mem.* 11v–12, records that only 'Captn Foneraux' brought to, 'which displeas'd Captn Cook, as he consider'd it an Insult to the British Flag; the Spaniards ask'd what Ship that was ahead, and being told it was the Resolution, Captn Cook, He said Oh, Cook is it, and wish'd us all a good Voyage'. The Spaniards declined to give the name of their own ship, says Forster (I, p. 8), and 'We continued our course, after a scene so humiliating to the masters of the sea . . .'. So far from humiliation being intended, it seems obvious that the Spaniards, like the Viceroy at Rio in 1768, simply did not take the sloops for naval vessels. Cf. Bayly: '. . . when she found us belong to the King of England & was ships of war, they ask'd us whether we were bound, we answered them to Madiera, they wished us a good Voyage. . . .'

in the same place (viz) upon the Bitticle[1] and no one circumstance occured to render the observations the least dubious, the change of situation from the time of makeing one observation to the other, or even from one day to the other was too small to cause any material difference in the variation of the Compass, probably these differences might arrise from the vicinity of the land, be this as it may, they shew that these observations, however accurate they may be made, are not always to be depended upon. At Noon our Latitude was 42°18′ N and Longitude 11°0′. Thermometer 65.

FRIDAY 24*th*. A steady fresh gale at NNE and clear pleasent weather. At 7 in the pm found the Variation to be 22°45′ W. At Noon our Latitude was 40°2′ N and Longitude by Account 12°16′ and by observation 11°42′. Ther[r] 65.

SATURDAY 25*th*. Fresh gales at NNE with which we steer'd SSW and at Noon was in the Latitude of 37°41′ N and Longitude 13°22′. Ther[r] 70. At 7 o'Clock in the pm being than in the Latitude of 39°18′ and Longitude 12°0′ observed to be 21°35′ West.

SUNDAY 26*th*. A steady fresh gale at NNE and clear weather. Latitude at Noon 35°39′ N. Long[de] 14°39′. Ther[r] 72½.

MONDAY 27*th*. Wind and Weather as yesterday. At Noon Lat. 33°44′ N. Longitude 15°23′. Ther[r] 72.

TUESDAY 28*th*. In the PM being in the Latitude of 33°28′, Long[d] 15°50′ I took 9 observations of the Suns Azimuths immidiately one after another with M[r] Gregorys Compass. The Variation deduced therefrom was 20°35′ W. At the same time I took 9 others with D[r] Knights Compass which gave 21°19′ W—this last Compass is too well known to need any discription. M[r] Gregorys is made upon the same Principal but much larger and hath some improvements which I beleive in some measure lessen the too quick motion the D[rs] compass's are subject to, but more of this by and by. At Noon we were in the Latitude of 33°43′ and Longitude 15°23′ W.

WEDNESDAY 29*th*. Fresh breezes at NNE, North & NW, first part clear weather Remainder Hazey and Clowdy. At 7 o'Clock in the Evening saw the Island of Porto Santo bearing WSW. At 4 o'Clock in the AM it bore NWBW distant 4 Miles, and at Noon it bore NNE, the Brazen head on Madeira bore SWBW½W and the Deserters from South to SSW distant 3 or 4 Leagues.

[1] Binnacle; 'a wooden case or box, which contains the compasses, log-glasses, watch-glasses, and lights to show the compass at night'.—Falconer's *Dictionary of the Marine*, 1769.

Fresh gale at NE which by 4 in the pm carried us within 2 Miles of St Cruze where it left us and was succeeded by a Calm, and obliged us to hoist out our Pinnace to tow, with the help of which and a light air now and then we got into Funchal Road at half past 10 where we anchor'd in 25 fathom water as did the Adventure also. In the morning saluted the Garrison with 11 guns which was emmidiately return'd and soon after I went a shore accompaned by Captain Furneaux, Mr Forster and Mr Wales. At our landing we were received by a gentlemen from the Vice Consul Mr Sells, who conducted us to Mr Loughnans an English merchant resideing here and one of the contractors for supplying His Majestys Ships with Wine. To this gentleman and the Vice Consul who we found here I made known my wants at this Island and proposed to the latter to accompany me in the Visit I thought was due from me to the Governor

[1] but upon hearing that he was just going to set out for the country Mr Sells alone wint to know the truth who soon return'd with a message from the Governor, acquainting me that he could not now wait to receive the Visit I intended him but that he had given orders for every thing to be granted I had asked for, only desired that no Plans or drawings might be made of any of the Fortificasions, a very reasonable restriction and very readily promised on my part. Mr Loughnan in a very obligeing manner desired we would accommodate ourselves with him during our stay, Mr Forster and his son fixed themselves at his country house about two miles out of Town where they persued their Botanical discoveries; he also accommodated the Astronomers with an upper appartment in his house in Town very sutable for their purpose and into which they got their Instruments &ca to make the necessary observations: the very hansome manner this Gentleman obliged us with every thing we wanted deserve my personal acknowledgement.[2]

During our stay here the Sloops were supply'd with fresh Beef and Onions and a Thousand Bunches of the latter were distributed among the people for a Sea store, a Custom I observed last Voyage and had reason to think that they reçived great benifit therefrom. Having compleated our Water[3] and taken on board a large supply of Wine, fruit & other necessarys, we on Sunday the 2nd of Augt at 10 o'Clock in the pm weigh'd and put to sea with the Adventure in

[1] The blank space in the MS here Cook evidently left for the governor's name—which, however, he nowhere records.

[2] *the . . . acknowledgement:* indeed I am less indebted to this Gentleman for these favours than obliged by the very handsome manner, he procured me every thing I wanted.—f. 12v.

[3] . . . (which was put on board by Portuguese People and Boats at the [rate] of Shilling and pence per Ton).

company, and at Noon the same day the Town of Funchal bore NBW distant 11 or 12 Leagues.

The Town of Funchall which is the Capital of the Island is situated about the middle of the South side in the Bottom of the Bay of the same name in Latitude 32°33′[1] N Longitude 16°49′ West deduced from observations made on the spot by the late Dr [Heberden].[2] Mr Harrison in the year [1764] when he was sent to the West Indias[3] by the Board of Longitude in order to assertain the going of his watch or time piece, made the Longitude of Funchall by the said Watch[4] to be 17°10′ and Mr Kendalls Watch now on board and which is made after the very same manner as Mr Harrisons (parts like parts) 17°10′[5] from whence it should seem that its situation is more to the West than Dr [Heberden] makes it. Altho these two Watches point out the very same Longitude they may nevertheless have made some difference for Mr Harrison's was set agoing at Portsmouth, and Kendalls at Plymouth as has been before mention'd, concequently some difference may arrise from the difference of Longitude between these two places not being known to a presision sufficient to determine this point.[6] The Road of Funchall to which all Ships reasort that have any business at this Island, lies wholy exposed to Southerly Winds, with which winds it is very dangerous riding especially when they blow strong as they frequently do in the Winter; the best Anchoring is near the Loo Rock, at least it is there where the Portugueze Ships always lay who no doubt know the best ground, but the English and other Ships generally lay off the Town with the great Church bearing about North or NBE, in 30 or 25 fathom water, at the distance of ¾ or half a Mile from the Shore. The Deserters (3 small Islds laying off the East end of Madeira) are seen from the Road bearing SEBE.

For a more particular account of this Island I must refer to my last Voyage, to which I have only to add, that the Island is divided into two Captainships, *Funchal* and *Maxico*, the former containing twenty five parishes and the latter Seventeen: the following Table will exhibit at one view the number of Inhabitants that were in the

[1] ... 32°33′34″; and so A.
[2] AG Eberton.—In H the name is first written thus, and then altered by Cook, here and at its next occurrence, to the correct form. For Dr Thomas Heberden, see I, p. 8, n. 1.
[3] *to . . . Indias:* out to Barbadoes
[4] *his watch:* his famous watch
[5] ... 17°10′14″ West
[6] ... however it cannot be so great but what it must be allowed that the Watches have both gone well; so much cannot be said of the one of Mr Arnolds on board the Resolution, for the Longitude by it is only 14°26′, allowing it the same rate of going as at Greenwich which it has not once done, if we suppose Mr Kendals to have gone right, nor indeed has it kept any other equal rate from day to day.—f. 13.

Island in the year 1768, and also the number that were born and died, with a distinction of their Sexes, &c[a].[1]

Captain-ships	Grown men dead	Young men dead	Total	Grown Women dead	Young females dead	Total	Male children born	Female children born	Total
Funchal	735	657	1393	865	929	1495	712	704	1366
Maxico	699	421	1120	788	447	1235	402	400	802
Sum Total	1434	1078	2513	1653	1376	2730	1114	1104	2168

Captain-ships	Grown men Existing	Young Men Existing	Total	Grown Women existing	Young Women existing	Total	Total dead	Total living
Funchal	18055	3214	20995	19097	2904	22012	2888	42210
Maxico	8654	1648	10302	9083	1508	10591	2355	20883
Sum Total	26709	4862	31297	28170	4412	32603	5243	63093

[August 1772]

MONDAY *3rd. Winds NNE. Courses Sail'd SBW. Distce sail'd* 134 *miles. Latd at Noon* 29°44'. *Longd in at Noon West from Greenwich* 17°2'. A Steady fresh Trade and pleasent weather, cleaned and air'd betwixt decks with Charcoal fires.[2]

TUESDAY *4th. Winds NNE to East. Courses sail'd SSW½W. Distce sail'd* 84 *miles. Latd at Noon* 28°37'. *Longd in at Noon West from Greenwich* 18°13'. At 6 in the pm observed the Variation of the Compass

[1] Cook omits 'the following Table' from the MS: I take it from B, ff. 13v–14. It is also found in A (in a confused form) and G, but not H. What attracted Cook about the figures is hard to guess, as he did not normally collect statistics of known parts of the world. Perhaps he was simply presented with them by Forster, 'as a complete list extracted from the parish books was procured for us, from the governor's secretary' (Forster, I, p. 17). It will be seen that not all the figures given add up to the totals given; nor do the totals agree with Forster's. The whole thing was dropped from the printed *Voyage*.

[2] . . . We had no sooner got clear of the Island of Madeira than we got the settled NE Trade Wind, which carri'd us forward a pace; indeed this wind had blown ever sence we left Cape Finister, but it does not always happen that you meet with it there, on the contrary not till you approach the Canary isles.—f. 14v.—On this date the unfortunate Marra comes again into notice: '. . . punish'd John Marra with one dozen lashes for behaving Insolent to his Superior Officer'.—Log.

to be 15°49′ W and at half past a 11 saw the Island of Palma extending from SWBS to West distant 5 or 6 Miles, hauld to the NW in order to clear it, having at this time but little wind occasioned by being too near the Island. At Noon the body of it bore East half North distant 5 Leagues. The Island Palma is of a height sufficient to been seen 12 or 14 Leagues, and appears to be cover'd with Wood. Drawing N° 4 exhibets a view of this Island when it bears SEBE distant 4 Leagues. I judge the middle of it to lay in Latitude 28°38′ N and Longitude 17°52′ W.

WEDNESDAY 5*th. Winds Variable, ENE. Courses sail'd S* 23° *W. Distce sail'd* 46 *miles. Latd at Noon* 27°55′. *Longd in at Noon West from Greenwich* 18°33′. In the pm and most part of the night had little wind and at the same time very variable occasioned by being too near Palma for which reason ships passing to leeward of this Island ought to keep a good distance off. In the evening found the Variation to [be] 14°58′ West and in the morn saw the Island Ferro bearing SE ½S and soon after I brought too to wait for the Adventure she being far astern. At 11 we made sail and at Noon the Island Ferro bore SE Distant 14 Leagues.[1] I judge the middle of it lies in the Latitude of 27°42′ N and Longde 17°47′ W. It is of a great height and may be seen in clear weather 20 Leagues.

THURSDAY 6*th. Winds NE. Courses sail'd S½W. Distce sail'd* 11 *miles. Latd at Noon* 25°8′. *Longd in at Noon West from Greenwich* 18°45′ First part gentle breeze remainder a fresh gale & Clear weather. In the pm found the Variation to be 17°15′ West. At 6 o'Clock am I made the Adventures signal to make sail ahead with a view to try the two Sloops. Cap Furneaux accordingly set all the sail he could and was afterwards so far from geting ahead that he droped astern.[2]

FRIDAY 7*th. Therm.* 79. *Winds NE to East. Course S* 8° *W. Distce sail'd* 123 *miles. Latd in North* 24° 8′. *Longd in West pr. Reck.g & Obsern* 19°14′. *Variation of the Compass* 13°55′. A Steady fresh trade and pleasent Weather.

SATURDAY 8*th. Therm.* 78. *Wind East. Course S* 8° *W. Distce sail'd* 122 *miles. Latd in North* 27°7′. *Longd in West pr. Reck.g & Obsern* 19°33′; *Pr. Kendalls Watch* 20°3¼′. Hazey weather with gentle gales. Made 3 Puncheons of Beer of the Inspissated juce, the proportion being about ten of Water to one of Juce; I have mentioned in the account of

[1] . . . we saw it at Twenty from which a judgment may be formed of its height.

[2] 'Pump'd the Ship out, & put a foot of salt Water down the Pump, which has been done twice or three Times a Week & which will contribute greatly towards the health of the Ships Company, before this was observ'd the Stench of the Bulge water was exceedingly offencive'.—Cooper.

Provisions that we had 19 half Barrels of Inspissated Juce of Beer or Malt whereas only four were of Beer, the rest of Wort that was hopped before inspissated. Mr Pelham Secretary to the Commissioners of the Victualing having some years ago considered (and I think made tryal) that if the Juce of Malt, either made into Beer or Wort, was Inspissated by evaporation it would keep good a considerable length of time and by mixing it with Water a supply of Beer might at any time be had, several experiments were made last winter by Mr Pelham himself which so far promised success that the Commis^rs^ caused the quantity before mentioned to be prepared and put on board the Sloops for tryal, the inspissated Juce of Beer requires no other preparation to make to fit for use than to mix it with cold Water from one part in Eight to one part in twelve of Water or in such other proportion as might be liked and then stop it down and in a few days it will be brisk and drinkable but the other after being mixed in the same manner will require to be fermented with yeast in the usual way of makeing of Beer at least it was reasonable to think so, but experience teaches us that this will not always be necessary for what from the heat of the Weather and the agitation of the Ship both sorts are now in the highest state of fermentation and has hitherto evaded all our endeavours to stop it; could it once be prevented from fermenting in its Inspissated state it certainly would be a most valuable article at Sea. In the am Cleaned and smoaked the Sloop betwixt Decks.[1]

SUNDAY 9*th. Therm.* 79. *Winds NNE. Course S* 19°30′ *W. Distce sail'd* 128 *miles. Latd in North* 20°06′. *Longd in West Pr. Reck.g & Obsern* 20°19′. *Variation of the Compass West* 12°0′. A Steady fresh Trade & Clowdy.

MONDAY 10*th. Therm.* 79. *Winds NNE. Course S* 21°45′ *W. Distce sail'd* 150 *miles. Latd North* 17°47′. *Longd West Reck.g & Obsern.* 21°18′. Fresh Trade Wind and Clowdy.

TUESDAY 11*th. Therm.* 78. *Winds NEBN. Course S* 27°15′ *W. Distce sail'd* 109 *miles. Latd North* 16°10′. *Longd West Reck.g & Obsern.* 22°10′. *Vari^n^ of the Compass* 10°56′ *West.* D^o^ Weather: at 7 in the pm judgeing ourselves to be nearly the length of the Northermost of the Cape de verd Isles we shortend sail untill daylight when we made all sail and at 9 am made the Island of Bonavista bearing sw

[1] 'Brew'd some Beer with the essence of malt, which we have on board—it has several times fermented and blew the Bungs out—more then once the Head of the Cask out: by which accidents a considerable quantity of it has been lost which is rather unfortunate, as it makes a most agreeable and I believe a very salutary drink—proportion 6 Gall^ns^ to a Puncheon.'—Clerke.

distant about 5 Leagues, at Noon it extended from SSW to WBN, the middle or East point off which lay a Ledge of Rocks bore West by south distant 2 Leagues. Drawings N° 5 and 6 exhibets the appearance of this Island from the situations they were taken.

WEDNESDAY 12*th. Winds NNE. Course S* 29°40′ *W. Distce sail'd* 79 *miles. Latd North* 15°0′. *Longd West Reck.g & Obsern* 22°51′. Gentle gales and hazey with some showers of rain in the Morn. At 6 o'Clock in the pm the SW end of Bonavista bore NNW distant 4 Leagues. From this point to the Isle of Mayo, for which we now steer'd, the Course is dist. Leagues. At 6 o'Clock in the morning the NE end of this Island bore West distant 5 or 6 Miles. The Land in the Interior parts of this Island is high and mountainous but next the sea it is low and form'd of Rocks and Sand, near the NE end are two hills near to each other rather peaked and are remarkable by being intirely detatched from all the other hills; Drawing[s] N. 7 & 8 exhibet very accurate [the] appearence of this Island. We now steer'd SSW, SW and WSW for the Island St Jago, the South end of which at Noon bore SWBW distant 10 Miles, drawing N° 9 is the appearence of the Island in this situation where (A) is the East point of Port Praya Bay for which we now steer'd.

THURSDAY 13*th. Therm.* 84. *Latd North* 14°53½′. *Longd West Reck.g & Observn.* 23°1′; *Kendalls Watch* 23°2′. Fresh gales and hazey with some rain in the night. At 3 pm Anchored in the above Bay in 8 fathom water, the East point bearing East, the West SW½S and the Fort NW, the Adventure at the same time anchor'd without us. As soon as we Anchor'd I sent an officer ashore to wait on the Governor to acquaint him with the reason of my puting in here which was to procure a Supply of Water and such refreshments as were to be got, upon his return we saluted the Fort with 11 guns which was immediately returned.[1] [2] Governor of all the Cape de Verd Islands who happen'd to be here at this time promised[3] that I should be supply'd with every thing I wanted and on the morrow Bullocks and other things should be brought out of the Country for us. According in the Morn we set about filling our

[1] 'Saluted the Fort with 11 Guns they return'd 9 and made a thousand apologies for the other 2—the case was they really had no more in the Fort that would go off and to look at their Artillery I shou'd suppose the man possess'd of an eminent degree of Courage to fire so many.'—Clerke.

[2] Blank space left in the MS for the name of the 'Governor of all the . . . Islands'; which is supplied by Wales: 'and as I took a turn on shore to look round me for a few hours, I had the very singular honour of being introduced to Don Joachim Salarna Soldanha de Lobos, Governour-general of all his most faithfull Majesty's Dominions on the Coast of Africa, as one of his Britannic Majesty's learned Astronomers'.

[3] *promised:* he as well as the Governor or Commodant of the Fort, promised . . .

empty Water Casks at a dirty well at the head of the Bay under the foot of the fort,[1] I also set a person a shore to treat with the Companies Agent for Bullocks for the two Sloops and some people to buy refreshments &c[a].

FRIDAY 14*th*. In the PM had fresh gales from the NE attended with Squalls and showers of rain, the remaining part had Variable light airs and fair weather. This evening I received a message from the Governor acquainting me that there had not yet been time to collect the Bullocks &c[a] out of the Country, but if I would wait tomorrow I might depend on having them, as we had not fill'd all our empty water casks I readily acquiesced to this and sent him an invitation to dine with me and as many gentlemen as he choose to bring with him, he declined the invitation on account of his bad state of health, but Governor of Praya promised to favour me with his company. In the evening we received on board one Bullock which was kill'd the next Morning and weig'd 270 pounds, some Hoggs, Goats and fruits were brought on board at the same time, but in no great plenty. As our great dependance was on the next day accordingly in the morning I sent people from every mess to buy such necessarys as they wanted and the Clerk with money to purchas Bullocks, and at noon a Boat was sent to wait on the Governor to bring him and his company off to dinner.

SATURDAY 15*th*. After the Boat had waited some time she returnd with Lieutenant Pickersgill (who attended the duty ashore) with a message from the Governor excuseing himself from dining with me,[2] we therefore sit down to what was on the Table, piqued more at being kept so long from our dinners than the disapointment of his company. Mr. Pickersgill at the same time inform'd me that no Bullocks were come down or likely to come which in some measure may account for the rude beheavor of the governor who finding himself either unable or unwilling to perform his promise, probably did not care to come on board least I should upbraid him for a breach thereof. Trade however for other articles went on pretty briskly a shore, not a Boat return'd to the Sloop without Hoggs, Goats, Fowles or fruit of which she was pretty well stored by night at which time we had compleated our water and finding it was in vain to wait for Bullocks, we hoisted in our Boats, unmoor'd and at 9 o'Clock weigh'd and put to sea. As my puting into this Port was not confirmable to orders it may be expected I should give some

[1] 'and a damn'd bad watering place it is . . . what water we got was none of y[e] best; however 'twas tolerable'.—Clerke.

[2] *from . . . me:* with a lame excuse of the Comodants for not dining with me

reason why I deviated therefrom, the chief of which is that I found that I had not a sufficient quantity of Water on board even with the assistance of the Still to serve to the Cape of Good Hope without puting the People to a scanty allowance a thing I wished[1] to avoide. I also thought that if I could procure a Supply of fresh provisions it would be a means not only of saveing our sea store but many of our antiscorbutick articles untouched for some time longer; these were

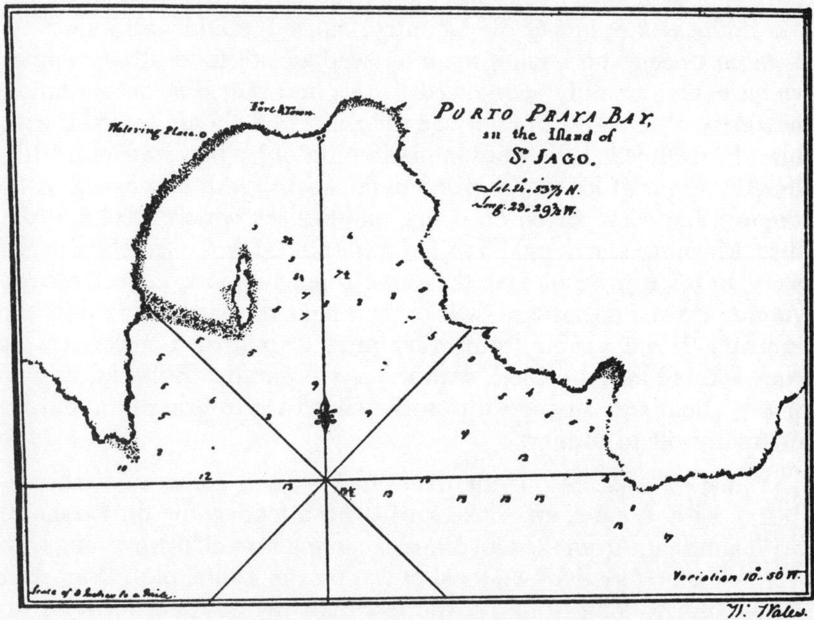

FIG. 13. William Wales, chart of Porto Praya

my montives for puting into Port Praya and altho' we have fallen short of my expectation in some articles, I how[ev]er make no doubt but what the People will recieve great benifit from the fruits and other refreshments they have got.

The Island of St Jago is one of the Southermost of the Cape de Verde Islands and by far the largest, it is of a very hilly and mountainous Surface and the Soil is said to be rich and firtile and to produce all the Tropical Fruits, besides grapes and some other European fruits, Indian Corn, Sugar and Cotton. Their domistick animals are Bullocks, Horses, Asses, Goats, Hogs, Sheep, Fowls and Turkeys and for any thing I know Geese and Ducks. The goats are of the Antilope kind and so extraordinary lean that hardly any thing can equal

[1] *wished:* wished much

them, indeed none of the other animals are overburden'd with fat. Bullocks & Hogs especially their Bullocks weigh from 200 to 300 lb. and must be purchased with money at the rate of Twelve Spanish Dollars a head. Other articles may be purchased with old cloaths &c[a] but buy them which way you will, you will find them to come dear enough.

Port Praya, which is only a small Bay, is situated about the middle of the South end of the Island in Latitude 14°53½′ N by observation, and in the Longitude 23°1′ W which I have reason to think is pretty near the truth altho' not ditermind by observation. Its situation may be known by the Southermost hill on the Island which is round and inclining to a peak at top and stand a little way inland in the direction of West from the Port. To sail in there is no danger but what shews itself (see the Plan). The two points which form the entrance are rather low and lay in the direction of WSW & ENE from each other distant 1½ Mile, it lies in NW 1¼ Mile and hath good Anchorage in every part of it from 14 to [4] fathom, the farther in the less water. Large ships ought not to anchor farther in then to bring the South end of y[e] Island, which lies under the West shore, to bear West where they will have eight fathom good ground. Your Water at a Well behind the Beach at the head of the Bay. I think the Water is tolerable good, it is however scarce for as the well is small it is soon emptyed and you must wait untill it recrutes again which may not happen that day if the Natives are in want of Water themselves in which case they generally carried it away as fast as it comes into the Well, so that the best time for strangers is early in a morning.[1]

*Its situation May be known, especiealy in coming from the East, by the Southermost hill on the Island which is round, inclining to a Peak at top, and stands a little way inland in the direction of West from the Port; therefore when the hill is upon that point of the Compass, the Port will be in the same direction, this Mark is the more necessary to be taken notice of, as there is a small Cove about a League to the Eastward of Praya with a sandy beach a Vally and Cocoa-nutt Trees behind, which strangers may take for Port Praya as we our selves did, tho' upon the whole I cannot say there is any great similarity between the two. The two points which form the

[1] From Wales, 13 August, we get a picture not only of ceaseless activity, but of Cook as assistant: 'Went on shore and measured the length of the small island mentioned above, which is very level. I measured it both ways, and differed only ten links of the Gunters' Chain. I set the line with the Azimuth Compass both ways, whilst Cap[t] Cook took the Angles subtended by the several points of the Bay from each station, with my Sextant from which Data the annexed Draught of the Bay is made'. A neat chart follows: see Fig. 13.

extremes of Port Praya are rather low, and lie in the direction WSW and ENE half a League from each other, close to the West point are some rocks on which the Sea Breaks pretty high; the Bay lies in NW near half a League and hath good anchoring ground in most parts of it from 14 to 4 fathom, the fa[r]ther in the less Water but large ships ought not to anchor in less than 8 fathom in which depth the south end of the Island which lies under the West shore, will bear west. The annexed Plan[1] will convey a better Idiea than any Words. You Water at a Well which is behind the beach at the head of the Bay, the Water is tolerable good but it is scarce and but bad geting it off, on account of the great surf which is upon the beach. Wood for fuel is scarce if attall to be got, it cannot be supposed that I can be particular in the Productions of a place on which I never set my foot, it is true some of the officers did and M[r] Forster made one Botanical excursion into the Island (where he collectd Ten or Twelve New Plants, I mean such as are unknown to Botanists) but two Days was too short a time to gain much knowledge of a place where they could hardly find a man they could attall converse with. It is however certain that the Island produceth all the Tropical Fruits, Grapes and some other European fruits, Indian Corn, Sugar and Cotton. Their domistick animals are Bullocks, Hoggs, Horses, Asses, Goats, Sheep, Fowles and Turkeys, Munkeys[2] and Guinea Hens which are Wild in the Island. The Goats are of the antilope kind and so extraordinary lean that hardly Any thing can equal them, and their Bullocks and Hoggs are not much better. Bullocks are to be purchased with Money only and the Price is Twelve Spanish Dollers a head, the one we had weighed 270 pounds. Other articles may be had in exchange for old cloaths &c[a] of the Natives themselves but the Sale of Bullocks is confined to a Company of Merchants, who have an agent residing upon the Spot.

The Island of S[t] Iago as well as all the other of the Cape de Verde Isles, belongs to the Portuguese, but the bulk of the Inhabitants are Blacks Migrated from Africa and I am told that many of the Military Officers, Cevil Magistrates and even the Clergy are of that complexion, we are however only to suppose that they fill the lowest

[1] 'The annexed Plan' has disappeared, but was presumably the original of the engraving in *Voyage*, I, pl. X. Wales has charts of Porto Praya Bay both in his journal and in his log, the fruit of the efforts in which he was aided by Cook, and there is one in Log 887, f. 6v.

[2] The sailors, as sailors will, bought many of these monkeys for pets, which was unfortunate for the monkeys, and caused Forster to moralize on the 'iron-hearted insensibility, and wanton barbarism' of the British seamen. The poor animals made the ship foul, and Cook had them thrown overboard.—Forster, I, p. 41. Wales sprang to the defence of the seamen; 'the Captain paid more attention to the health of his people, than to the lives of a few monkies'.—Wales, *Remarks*, p. 20.

of these Offices; this in my opinion is no bad policy in the Portuguese, especialy as these Island[s] are found not to agree with a European constitution but to agree very well with these people; was industry and cul[t]ivation of the Land properly incouraged, they might in time become very fine Islands: one very great disadva[n]tage will how[ev]er for ever attend them, the want of fresh Water, for from what I have been able to learn all or most of them are ill provided with that article. At Praya is a Fort wherein is a Governor, who is a Portuguese and I think has the rank of Captain, he however lives in no sort of state, nay, every thing about him has the appearence of poverty, he has a few black sold[i]ers who are kept here as a guard, who's Ludicrous appearence an Englishman cannot help laughing at, altho by such beheavour you offend them very much.

The Fort is wholy disigned for the Protection of the Bay and its situation seems not ill choosen for that purpose being upon elevated ground which runs directly from the Sea on the right, at the head of the Bay. I am told that it is in a manner quite in ruins and open on the Land side.*—ff. 17–18.

SATURDAY 15*th. Therm.* 80½. *Winds NNE. Course S* 32° *E. Distce sail'd* 77 *miles. Latd in North* 22°35′. *Longd in Wt. pr. Reck.g & Obn.* 22°19′. I have before mentioned that we put to Sea at 9 o'Clock in the evening, we had no sooner got clear of the land than we found a fresh gale at NNE with which we steer'd SEBS, in the morn the weather was squally attended with rain, at Noon the sun was nearly in our Zenith and being clowdy had no observation.

SUNDAY 16*th. Therm.* 81. *Winds NNE to SE. Course S* 12° *E. Distce sail'd* 91 *miles. Latd in North* 22°16′. *Longd in Wt. pr. Reck.g & Obn.* 22°0′. Fresh gales and squals with rain continued untill 8 pm, when it became fair but clowdy with Lightning, in the am had gentle breezes and clear serene weather.

MONDAY 17*th. Therm.* 80. *Winds Southerly. Course S* 60°15′ *E. Distce sail'd* 43 *miles. Latd in North* 11°58′. *Longd in Wt. pr. Reck.g & Obn.* 21°20′. Which continued all pm after which it became clowdy with fresh gales attended with showers of rain.

TUESDAY 18*th. Therm.* 82. *Winds SWesterly. Course S* 51°30′ *E. Distce sail'd* 56 *miles. Latd in North* 11°23′. *Longd in Wt. pr. Reck.g & Obn.* 20°35′; *Kendalls Watch* 21°25′. *Varn. of the Compass* 9°26′. First part fresh gales with flying showers of rain, the rem[r] little wind and fair. In the am got the Cables and every other thing up from betwixt decks in order to clear and air the Sloop.

WEDNESDAY 19*th. Therm.* 82. *Winds SW, W, & N. Course S* 27°15′ *E. Distce sail'd* 46 *miles. Latd in North* 10°42′. *Longd in Wt. pr. Reck.g & Obn.* 20°17′; *Kendalls Watch* 20°58′. Light airs and fair weather untill 10 o'Clock am when we had a very heavy shower of rain which lasted about an hour.

THURSDAY 20*th. Winds NW. Course SBE. Distce sail'd* 86 *miles. Latd in North* 9°17′. *Longd in Wt. pr. Reck.g & Obn.* 18°55′. Gentle breezes and Dark gloomy hot weather and fair untill 4 o'Clock in the am when we had squals attended with showers of rain. At Noon it rain'd excessive hard. In the pm we had the missfortune to loose Henry Smock one of the Carpenters Mates, he was at work over the side fitting in one of the Scuttles from whence we supposed he fell into the Sea for he was not seen untill the moment he sunk under the Stern when all assistance was too late.[1]

FRIDAY 21*st. Therm.* 79. *Winds Northerly, Calm, SW. Course S* 21° *E. Distce sail'd* 40 *miles. Latd in North* 8°40′. *Longd in Wt. pr. Reck.g & Obn.* 18°38′. During the hard rain which continued till about 3 o'Clock pm, we fill'd 7 Puncheons of rain water and might have fill'd as many more had we begun an hour sooner,[2] the havy rain brought on a Calm which continued untill Midnight after which a light breeze sprung up at sw which increased at times to squalls and continued all the time hazey with more or less rain.

SATURDAY 22*nd. Therm.* 80. *Winds SSW. Course SE* ¼° *E. Distce sail'd* 74 *miles. Latd in North* 7°50′. *Longd in Wt. pr. Reck.g & Obn.* 17°36′. Squally, Hazey rainy weather continued till near Noon, when it became fair and clear'd up and gave us an oppertunity to observe the Suns meridian Altitude which we have not had these 4 days past.[3]

SUNDAY 23*rd. Therm.* 79. *Winds SWBS. Course S* 48°15′ *E. Distce sail'd* 92 *miles. Latd in North* 6°49′. *Longd in Wt. pr. Reck.g & Obn.* 16°27′.

[1] He was, says Forster (I, p. 43) 'a rational fellow creature of a gentle and amiable disposition'; and displays the Forster amiability by remarking, with italics, 'His good-natured character, and a kind of serious turn of mind caused him to be regretted *even* among his shipmates. . . . Humanity stole a tear from each feeling traveller'. A few days later, feeling travellers were given in addition an appropriate touch of horror: they had 'had the misfortune to loose a man over board who was immediately siezed by the Shirks, & carried down', the *Adventure* was told.—Bayly, 26 August.

[2] . . . the rain powered down upon us not in drops but in streames, I never saw it rain harder in my life the Wind at the same time was variable inclining to blow in squalls and obliged the people to attend the deck so that few in the Ship escaped a good drenching, we however made the best use we could of it by filling most of our empty Water Casks. —f. 18v.

[3] ADV '. . . this day we saw great numbers of Boneta Fish some of which the men struck with the gig, we hawled in one of near 60^{lb} weight, they are very fine eating, rather more the tast of veal than Fish, I was taken very ill after dinner owing [to] eating some salt Beef & Pudding together, but got better of it in the Evening'.—Bayly.

Gentle gales and clowdy. A swallow disappear'd to day which has accompanied us for several days past, it was so tame that it came in & out our Cabbins.[1]

MONDAY 24*th. Therm.* 79. *Winds SSW & SBW. Course S* 69°30′ *E. Distce sail'd* 77 *miles. Latd in North* 6°28′. *Longd in Wt. pr. Reck.g. & Obn.* 15°16′. D° Weather. In the am set the Still to work.

TUESDAY 25*th. Therm.* 80. *Winds SSW. Course S* 62°15′ *E. Distce sail'd* 56 *miles. Latd in North* 5°53′. *Longd in Wt. pr. Reck.g & Obn.* 14°26′. A steady gentle breeze and hot clowdy weather. Got from the Still about 18 gallons of fresh Water in about 6 or 7 hours.[2]

WEDNESDAY 26*th. Therm.* 77. *Winds SW. Course S* 46° *E. Distce sail'd* 72 *miles. Latd in North* 5°3′. *Longd in Wt. pr. Reck.g & Obn.* 13°33′. Fore and middle parts D° Weather, the remainder fresh gales & hazey with rain.

THURSDAY 27*th. Therm.* 77. *Winds SWBS. Course SE. Distce sail'd* 85 *miles. Latd in North* 4°8′. *Longd in Wt. pr. Reck.g & Obsern* 12°36′. Fresh gales and Clowdy. Spoke with the Adventure and Captain Furneaux inform'd us that one of his young Gentlemen was dead.[3] At this time we have not one Sick on board.[4]

FRIDAY 28*th. Therm.* 77. *Winds Southerly. Course S* 70°30′ *E. Distce sail'd* 72 *miles. Latd in North* 3°44′. *Longd in Wt. pr. Reck.g & Obsern*

[1] *A swallow . . . Cabbins:* A little swallow has been our companion for several days, unable to fly about in the heavy rain it was taken up upon the deck and brought into the Cabbin, where it became so familiar that it went out and came in at the Windows at its pleasure; this familiarty continued for some days and then it disapeared.—ff. 18v–19.

[2] 'Employ'd working the Still its Produce being about three Gallons p[r] hour but is Productive of a great deal of Trouble and Expends a good deal of fewel.'—Pickersgill, 26 August.

[3] ADV '. . . at ½ past 7 PM Departed this life M[r] Jn[o] James Lambrecht Midshipman.'—Furneaux, 25 August.—'. . . of a Fever he caught at S[t] Iago by bathing and making too free with the water in the heat of the day'.—Add MS 27890. 'PM Sould by Oction the Affects of M[r] John Lambreath'.—Constable, 26 August. Wales reports that Furneaux's first diagnosis was 'a cold', so one suspects pneumonia, caused by carelessness and neglect of the precautions described in the next note; or could it have been typhoid? Independent advice was proffered in the case: 'I disired the Doctor to give him D[r] Norrises Drops, but he prefered D[r] Jam[s] Powders, we had many more ill but happily all recovered tho' another Midshipman (who was on shore with him) narrowly escaped.'—Bayly, 24 August. John Rayside, a stowaway in the *Adventure* from Madeira, was now entered in the ship's complement.—See p. 946 below.

[4] . . . altho' we had every thing of this kind to fear from the rains we have had, which is one of the greatest promoters of Sickness in these hot climates, to prevent which I took every necessary precaution by airing and drying the ship with fires made betwixt decks smoaking &c[a] and obliging the people to air their bedding, Wash and dry their cloaths whenever oppertunity offered: a neglect of these things causeth a disagreeable smell below, affects the air and seldom fails to bring on Sickness, but more especially in moist hot climates.—f. 19. Cf. Pickersgill, 'Made Charcoal fires below in the well and between decks which we found to be of great advantage in Expeling that damp moist Air Occaisoned by the Stagnated water's lying in her bottom altho We pour'd fresh into her every Day and Pump'd it out again.'

11°29′; *Kendalls Watch* 10°21¼′. *Varⁿ* 13°35′ *West.* Steady gales and Clowdy weather. Got by the Still 14 gallons of Fresh Water from one Copper the time the Pease was boiling (viz) from half past 7 o'Clock in the Morning till noon. Saw two Men of War Birds—and some Tropick Birds.[1]

SATURDAY 29*th. Therm.* 78. *Winds SWBS. Course S* 59° *E. Distce sail'd* 54 *miles. Latd in North* 3°11′. *Longd in Wt. pr. Reck.g & Obsern* 10°34′. *Varn* 14°12½′ *West.* Steady breezes and fair weather, Birds in sight as yesterday.[2]

SUNDAY 30*th. Therm.* 77. *Winds SSW. Course S* 62°15′ *E. Distce sail'd* 75 *miles. Latd in North* 2°36′. *Longd in Wt. pr. Reck.g & Obsern* 9°29′. *Varn* 14°54′ *West.* Gentle Breezes and clear weather.

MONDAY 31*st. Therm.* 77. *Winds Southerly. Courses East Southly. Distce sail'd* 51 *miles. Latd in North* 2°35′. *Longd in Wt. pr. Reck.g & Obsern* 8°37′. Gentle gales and Clowdy. In the pm bore down to and sent a Boat on board the Adventure with Mr Wales to compare the Watches. Tack'd at Noon to the sw.

[SEPTEMBER 1772]

TUESDAY 1*st. Therm.* 78. *Winds SSE. Course SW. Distce sail'd* 54 *miles. Latd in North* 1°57′. *Longd in Wt. pr. Reck.g & Obsern* 9°15′. *Varn* 15°35′ *West.* Little Wind and serene weather.[3]

[1] An entry of Bayly's of this date shows how easily ships could part company, whatever the justice of his remark about the watch of the *Resolution*. 'About 3 o'Clock this morning Mr Fanning (the Master) being Officer of the Watch, they lost the Resolution. Mr Fanning thought he saw her ahead on the Weather Bow, where she was some time before, two Midshipmen were sent to the main top who affirmed they saw her as aforesaid, & they all affirmed they saw her light; Mr Lanine [Lanyon] the Mate of the watch looked to Leeward & saw the Resolutions light in reality, near 4 Miles to leeward, the Master and Midshipmen still affirming they saw ships & lights & even thought they saw land & houses, so great is the strenght of Immagination, & of Course the Captain was acquainted, & before he came on deck (which was not long) two swivel Guns were fired, & when Capt Furneaux came on deck he saw the Resolutions light to leeward but could see no other nor any ship or any thing but water, notwithstanding the Master & Midshipmen still affirmed they saw every thing as aforesaid they then made two false fires but the Resolution took no notice of either Guns or false fires, from whence it is natural to conclude the Resolutions watch must be asleep, for otherwise must have seen the signals. The Ships were close to the wind, which rendered it impossible for us to go to windward of them in the time, therefore they must have let the Ship run away to leeward before the wind while we keept our right course.'

[2] The midshipmen were getting some practical training: '4 PM Unbent ye Main sail & Dipped a New one overboard & bent it, & Unbent ye Fore Topsail & Dipped a New one overboard which ye Gentlemen Bent'.—Harvey.—ADV '. . . this afternoon the Lieutenant of Marines, & Surgeon had som words &ca.'—Bayly. On the *Adventure* also Donald Stewart, marine, was punished 'with a dozen lashes for Fighting and Contempt to his Officers'.—Furneaux.

[3] 'Did not serve wine to the Ships Company to day, having experimental Beer'.—Cooper.

WEDNESDAY *2nd. Therm.* 76. *Winds Southerly. Courses S* 54° *W. Distce sail'd* 58 *miles. Latd in North* 1°23'. *Longd in Wt. pr. Reck.g* 10°2'. *Obsern* 6°39'. At half past 3 o'Clock in the pm I took nine distances of the Sun and Moon, the mean result of which gave 5°56' west. By the observations our Longitude at Noon is 6°39' which is 3°23' more east than that given by the Log. Such is the effect the Currants must have had on the Sloop, and which Mr Kendalls Watch tought us to expect.

THURSDAY *3rd. Therm.* 75. *Winds Southerly. Courses S* 71°45' *W. Distce sail'd* 83 *miles. Latd in North* 0°57'. *Longd in Wt. pr. Reck.g & Obsern* 7°58'. Fresh gales and Clowdy.

FRIDAY *4th. Therm.* 75. *Winds SBW. Course S* 84° *W. Distce sail'd* 67 *miles. Latd in North* 0°50'. *Longd in Wt. pr. Reck.g & Obsern* 9°14'. *Varn* 14°16' *West.* Gentle gales at times dark and Clowdy at other times clear.

SATURDAY *5th. Therm.* 76. *Winds Light Airs, Calms, &ca. Courses N* 78°15' *W. Distce sail'd* 10 *miles. Latd in North* 0°52'. *Longd in West pr. Reck.g & Obsern* 9°25'; *Kendals Watch* 9°16'. First part gentle breezes remainder Light airs and Calms, Weather dark and Clowdy; In the am hoisted out a Boat to try if there were any current,[1] found one seting North ⅓ of a Mile per hour; at the same time sounded but had no ground with 250 fathom of line. A Thermometer, which in the open air stood at 76½ in the surface of the sea 74 and when Immerged about 15' at the depth of 70 fathom it came up at 66. By this experiment it appears that the Sea Water was 8° colder at the depth of 70 fathom than it was at the Surface.[2]

[1] The traditional method of doing this is explained in Norie's *Epitome of Practical Navigation* (ed. 1900), p. 124: '... take a boat, in calm weather, a small distance from the ship, and, being provided with a half-minute glass, a log, a heavy weight, or kedge, and a small boat-compass: then let down the weight by a rope fastened to the boat's stem, to the depth of about 100 fathoms, by which the boat will remain nearly as steady as at anchor; then the log being hove, its bearing will be the setting of the current, and the number of knots run out in half-a-minute will be its drift per hour. This method is, however, very uncertain, owing to the effect of submarine currents.'

[2] 'The apparatus for trying the heat of the sea-water at different depths, consisted of a square wooden tube, of about 18 inches long, and three inches square externally. It was fitted with a valve at the bottom, which opened inward, and another at its top, that opened outward, and had a contrivance for suspending the Thermometer exactly in the middle of it. When it was used, it was fastened to the deep-sea line, just above the lead, so that all the way as it descended the water had a free passage through it, by means of the valves, which were then both open; but the instant it began to be thrown up, both the valves closed by the pressure of the water, and of course the Thermometer was brought up in a body of water, of the same temperature with that it was let down to.'—Wales in *Astronomical Observations*, p. liii. This apparatus, apparently invented by the Rev. Stephen Hales, F.R.S., had been used by Captain Henry Ellis in 1749 to make the earliest recorded measurements of deep-sea temperatures; 'with the bucket sea-gage' he drew water from a depth of 5346 feet.—*Phil. Trans.*, XLVII (1751), 211.

SUNDAY 6*th. Winds SW & SSW. Course S* 64° *E. Distce sail'd* 46 *miles. Latd in North* 0°32'. *Longd in West pr. Reck.g & Observn* 8°44'. First part light airs remainder gentle gales.[1] At Midnight pass'd a strong Ripling which we supposed to be occasioned by a Current.

MONDAY 7*th. Winds Southerly. Course S* 68°15' *E. Distce sail'd* 52 *miles. Latd in North* 0°19'. *Longd in West pr. Reck.g & Obsern* 7°56'. Gentle Breezes and clear the first part the remainder very clowdy and moist weather. At half past 7 in the am the Adventure made the Signal for seeing a sail which proved to be a Brig to Leeward standing to the westward.

TUESDAY 8*th. Winds SSE. Course S* 59° *W. Distce sail'd* 72 *miles. Latd in South* 0°18'. *Longd in West* 8°58'. *Reck.g & Observn* 9°50'. *Varian of the Compass* 14°12' *am West.* Steady breezes and Clowdy weather. In the PM I took several observations of the Sun and Moon, the mean result of which gave 9°00' which is 52' more than the Longitude by account carried on from the last observation.

WEDNESDAY 9*th. Therm.* 75. *Winds SEBS. Course SW*¼°*W. Distce sail'd* 60 *miles. Latd in North* 0°59'. *Longd in West pr. Reck.g & Observn* 10°35'. *Variation of the Compass* 12°59' *West.* Gentle gales and pleasent weather. In the PM after it was known that we were South of the Line or Equator, the ancient custom of Ducking &c[a] was observed and in the evening the People were made not a little merry with the liquor given them by the Gentle[n] on this occasion.[2] Took some observations of the ☽ and *s. The Longitude deduced therefrom was 9°58', nearly agreeing with yesterdays the mean of the two carried on to Noon as p[r] Column.

THURSDAY 10*th. Therm.* 75. *Winds SSE. Course S* 35° *W. Distce sail'd* 74 *miles. Latd in South* 2°0'. *Longd in West pr. Reck.g & Observn* 11°18'.

[1] ADV This day Bayly also was anxious to do some scientific investigation, and 'applied to the Cap[t] for a boat to be hoisted out in order to try the heat of the Sea water at different depths; but he refused one'.

[2] 'Brought too with M.T.S. to the mast Reeved a yard rope & ducked upwards of 50 people who had not before cross'd the Equator'.—Gilbert. No doubt the liquor given to the People by the Gentlemen was ransom: cf. I, p. 16. 'Those who had been obliged to undergo the briny submersion, changed their linen and clothes; and as this can never be done too often, especially in warm weather, the ducking proved a salutary operation to them. The quantity of strong liquors, arising from the forfeits of the rest, served to heighten the jovial humour, which is the predominant characteristic of sailors.'—Forster, I, p. 49. Evidence about the *Adventure* conflicts rather violently: 'Brought too with the Maintopsail to y[e] Mast. The Resolution emp[d] Ducking her People, a Custom we thought better broke than continued—therefore did not follow the example'.—Kemp.—'. . . Cap[t] Furneaux did not chose to let it be carried into execution on board the Adventure for fear of an Accident, though I confess I did not see any great danger in it.'—Bayly. But 'PM at 3 Bro[t] too with the Main Topsail to the mast and Duck'd Those that was not will[ing] to Pay the usual forfeit at the Line'.—Wilby. Young Mr Wilby must have been suffering from an illusion.

A Gentle Trade and clear weather. Exercized the People at Small Arms.

FRIDAY 11*th. Therm.* 76. *Winds SSE. Course S* 33° *W. Distce sail'd* 76 *miles. Latd in South* 3°5′. *Longd in West pr. Reck.g & Obsern* 11°50′; *Kendals Watch* 12°21′. *Varian of the Compass* 12°4½′ *West.* Gentle Gales & Clowdy weather.[1]

SATURDAY 12*th. Therm.* 76½. *Winds SEBE. Course SSW. Distce sail'd* 72 *miles. Latd in South* 4°11′. *Longd in West pr. Reck.g & Obsern* 12°18′. *Varian of the Compass* 10°24′ *West.* Pleasent weather. In the am Clean'd and smoaked betwixt decks.

SUNDAY 13*th. Therm.* 76. *Winds SEBE. Course S* 39°45′ *W. Distce sail'd* 78 *miles. Latd in South* 5°11′. *Longd in West pr. Reck.g & Obsern* 13°8′; *Kendals Watch* 14°20′. *Varian of the Compass* 9°52′ *West.* Weather as yesterday.[2]

MONDAY 14*th. Therm.* 75. *Winds SE. Course S* 30° *W. Distce sail'd* 94 *miles. Latd in South* 6°32′. *Longd in West pr. Reck.g & Obsern* 13° 55′; *Kendals Watch* 15°12′.[3] *Varian of the Compass* 9°20′. Captn Furneaux dine[d] with me to day, a nother of his Midshipmen is dead.[4] His crew are however healthy. At this time I have not one Sick on board.

TUESDAY 15*th. Therm.* 76. *Winds SE. Course S* 18°30′ *W. Latd in South* 8°17′. *Longd in West pr. Reck.g & Obsern* 14°31′. Fresh gales and Serene Weather the first part, remainder clowdy.

WEDNESDAY 16*th. Therm.* 75. *Winds SE. Course S* 26° *W. Distce sail'd* 81 *miles. Latd in South* 8°30′. *Varian of the Compass* 7°35′ *West.* AM Fresh gales and squally.[5]

[1] 'Punish'd Richard Lee, Seaman & Fras Taylor Marine, with 12 lashes Each for frequently insultg one of the petty Officers & behaving with Insolence to ye Officer of the Watch when repremanded for the same.'—Log.

[2] ADV 'Caught Plenty of Dolphin'.—Constable.

[3] 'Hitherto I have always deduced the Long, by last Observation, by allowing what the Log gave but as I find that Mr Kendall's Watch is infinitely more to be depended on, I shall in the future reduce it by allowing what is shown by that.'—Wales.

[4] He died on the 10th. 'Here we lost Mr Samuel Kempe (Midshipman) by the same unlucky means as Mr Lambrecht.'—Add. MS 27890. It appears that Dr Norris was no more successful than Dr James: 'at 11 oClock Mr Kemp, Midshipman departed this life of a Putrid fever which he contracted at St Jago, he recovered so far as to be able to walk about but for want of taking proper care of himself catched cold & had a relapse, the Doctor gave him Dr Norrises Antinomial drops regular according as pr Directions but they had not the desired Effect.'—Bayly.

[5] . . . The Wind now veering more and more to the East blowing a gentle Topgallant gale, which carried us in Eight days into the Latitude of 8°30′ South and Longitude 15° West, the Weather continuing clear and serene all the time; We daly saw of those Birds which are looked upon to be signs of the Vicinity of land, such as Boobies, Men of War Birds, Tropick Birds and Gannets, we supposed them to have come from the Islands of St Mathews and Ascension which Islands we pass'd at no great distance.—ff. 19v–20. For 'St Mathews' island see p. 668 below.

THURSDAY 17*th. Therm.* 73½. *Winds SE & SEBE. Latd in South* 11°17′. Fresh gales with squalls attended with light showers of rain.

FRIDAY 18*th. Therm.* 73½. *Winds SEBE. Course SSW½W. Distce sail'd* 84 *miles. Latd in South* 12°31′. *Longd in West,* 16°37′ *R.* 17°20′ *Obsern. Kendals Watch* 18°44′. Clowdy squally weather with showers, but 8 am it clear'd away long enought for us to take several observations of the Sun and Moon, the mean result of which carried up to Noon gave 17°20′ which is 43′ more to the West than the Longitude by Reckoning carried on from the last observations.[1]

SATURDAY 19*th. Therm.* 72½. *Winds ESE. Course S* 34°30′ *W. Distce sail'd* 116 *miles. Latd in South* 14°7′. *Longd in West pr. Reck.g & Obsern.* 18°26′. Fresh gales and squally with showers of Rain.

SUNDAY 20*th. Therm.* 72½. *Winds ESE. Course SSW½W. Distce sail'd* 103 *miles. Latd in South* 15°38′. *Longd in Wt. pr. Reck.g* 19°15′. *Obsern* 19°30′. *Variation of the Compass* 4°48′ *West.* First part fresh gales and squally, remainder moderate & Clear. The remains of the Inspissated juice of Malt, which has been on deck ever sence we arrived at Madeira, having left of fermenting was to day put into the hold (viz) 9 half Barrels, from the other 10 that were on board we have only made 11 Puncheons of Beer the rest of the juce having been lost by fermentation. The Beer made from this juce is of a very deep Colour, something of a burnt taste and without bitter and must be drinked soon after it has done firmenting otherways it turns hard and will Sour, in the Sloops Logg Book of this date it is said to be unpleasent to the taste, this however is only the opinion of some few and only happen'd to two Cask and was occasioned by their being made with the only Bad Cask of Water known to be in the Sloop.[2] In the am took several observations of the Sun and Moon the mean results gave 19°23′ at the time of Observation which carried on to Noon gives us as per Column.

MONDAY 21*st. Therm* 71. *Winds ESE. Course S* 24° *W. Distce sail'd*

[1] 'The Beer being all expended serv'd Wine to the People.'—Cooper. See also p. li above.—ADV '. . . this day Divided a 45 gallon Cask of Rum among the mess & it run something more than 6 Gallon each among 7 of us.'—Bayly.

[2] 'The Essence of Beer having left of fermenting put the remains which was 9 Casks down into the Hold after having brew'd 11 Puncheons, which prov'd a very salutary & I think pleasant drink. Many of our People dislik'd it vastly—prefer'd water to it—but I believe 'twas more caprice than any absolute distaste to it, I've seen many whims of this kind among Seamen—one on board the Dolphin I just now recollect & will relate. When we sail'd in the Dolphin & Tamer in 64 under Com: Biron the use of Portable Soup wch is now so universally esteem'd was quite in its infancy in the Navy. We gave it our Lads in their Pease, which brought on a complaint that there was so much damn'd nasty stuff put into their Pease that they cou'd not eat them.'—Clerke, 19 September.

107 *miles. Latd in South* 17°16′. *Longd in Wt. pr. Reck.g & Observn* 20°15′. Fresh gales and Clowdy with some Showers of rain.

TUESDAY 22*nd. Therm.* 72. *Winds ESE to EBS. Course SBW½W. Distce sail'd* 94 *miles. Latd in South* 18°46′. *Longd in Wt. pr. Reck.g* 20°44′; *Obsern* 21° 18′. *Varn of the Compass* 4°25′ *West.* Gentle gales and fair weather. In the pm took Number of Observations of the ☉ and ☽ which gave the Longitude at Noon as p[r] Column.

WEDNESDAY 23*rd. Therm.* 72. *Winds SE to East. Course SBW½W. Distce sail'd* 88 *miles. Latd in South* 20°12′. *Longd in West Reck.g & Obsern* 21°45′. *Varn of the Compass* 3° 14′ *West.* Gentle gales with some Squalls attended with Showers of Rain.

THURSDAY 24*th. Therm.* 72. *Winds EBS. Course SBW¼W. Distce sail'd* 86 *miles. Latd in South* 21°35′. *Longd in West Reck.g and Obsern* 22°6′. D[o] gales & Clowdy weather. At 8 AM made the signal for the Adventure to make more sail.

FRIDAY 25*th. Therm.* 71. *Winds ESE. Course S* 30°45′ *W. Distce sail'd* 92 *miles. Latd in South* 22°54′. *Longd in West Reck.g & Obsern* 22°57′. Moderate breezes, at times squally with rain. Sail-makers employ'd repairing Sails.

SATURDAY 26*th. Therm.* 73. *Winds ESE to ENE. Course S* 3°30′ *W. Distce sail'd* 83 *miles. Latd in South* 24°17′. *Longd in West Reck.g & Observn* 23°3′. *Varian of the Compass, G.* 2°2′ *West, R.* 2°45′ *West.* First part Moderate gales, remainder little wind & Clear.[1]

SUNDAY 27*th. Winds East. Course S½E. Distce sail'd* 30 *miles. Latd in South* 24°45′. *Longd in West Reck.g & Observn* 23°1′; *Kendals Watch* 23°57½′. *Varn of the Compass* 1°11½′ *West.* Light breezes and fair weather. In the am sent a Boat on board the Adventure to compare the Watches.[2]

MONDAY 28*th. Therm.* 72. *Winds E to NE. Course S* 15°30′ *E. Distce sail'd* 46 *miles. Latd in South* 25°29′. *Longd in West Reck.g and Observn* 22°54′; *Kendals Watch* 23°36′. *Varn of the Compass* 1°11′ *West.* Gentle breeze and Serene Weather. At 8 AM saw a Sail to the westward

[1] 'The Adventure run ahead of us which I think as times go is a very remarkable occurence and was oblig'd to shorten'd [*sic*] a good deal of sail and back her Mizen Tops[l] to get astern again. She is sharper about the Bows than the Resolution and in a heavy Head Sea she will sometimes wrong us a little this is the second time we observ'd it during the 10 weeks we've been out—every other of the 68 days out of the 70 our distance has been somewhat curtail'd and many of them very considerably by staying for Her.'—Clerke.

[2] ADV 'M[r] Wales came on board to compare the Watches . . . Cap[t] Fur[x] M[r] Falkener & my Self went on Board the Resolution to dinner & spent the afternoon on board, & Lieutena[n]t Char[ls] Clark dined on board the Adventure, returning on board our respective ships in the evenin after spending the afternoon very agreeable.'—Bayly.

standing after us, at 9 shortened Sail to speak her while the Adventure stood on.

TUESDAY 29*th. Therm.* 71. *Winds NNE. Course SEBE. Distce sail'd* 86 *miles. Latd in South* 26°17½'. *Longd in West Reck.g & Observn* 21°35'. *Varn of the Compass* 2°8' *West.* First part little Wind, latter fresh breeze and clear weather. At 1 pm finding that we could not speak the sail (which was a Snow) without being seperated too far from the Adventure we made sail and soon after she hoisted her Colours, which was either a Portuguese or St Georges Ensign, the distance being too great to distinguish the one from the other. At Daylight in the Morn she was seen out of the Main Top, bearing about NNW.

WEDNESDAY 30*th. Therm.* 71. *Winds Northly. Course S* 70°15' *E. Distce sail'd* 126 *miles. Latd in South* 26°59½'. *Longd in West Reck.g & Observn* 19°23'; *Kendals Watch* 20°12'. Fresh gales.

[OCTOBER 1772]

THURSDAY 1*st. Winds North, SSW. Course S* 75°15' *E. Distce sail'd* 118 *miles. Latd in South* 27°29'. *Longd in West Reck.g & Observn* 17°28'; *Kendals Watch* 18°11'. *Varn of the Compass* 3°45' *West.* First part D^o^ Wea^r^ latter light Wind and clowdy, inclinable to rain.

FRIDAY 2*nd. Winds Southerly. Course S* 75°30' *E. Distce sail'd* 40 *miles. Latd in South* 27°39'. *Longd in West Reck.g & Observn* 16°44'. *Varian of the Compass* 5°19' *West.* Gentle Breezes and some times Calm. Between 3 and 4 pm took several observations of y^e^ ☉ and ☽ the mean result of which gave 18°12' West Longitude which is 58' west of account carried on from the last observation, but nearly agrees with the Watch.

SATURDAY 3*rd. Therm.* 67. *Winds SW. Course S* 70° *E. Distce sail'd* 87 *miles. Latd in South* 28°9'. *Longd in West Reck.g & Observn* 15°11'. Gentle gales and pleasent Weather.

SUNDAY 4*th. Therm.* 62. *Winds SWBS. Course S* 67° *E. Distce sail'd* 135 *miles. Latd in South* 29°2'. *Longd in West Reck.g & Observn* 12°50'. Fresh gales and Clowdy. Saw an Albatross,[1] Pintado Bird[2] and several Sheer-waters.

MONDAY 5*th. Therm.* 61. *Winds Southrly. Course East. Distce sail'd* 83

[1] On this day Forster (I, p. 51) noted the appearance of the Wandering Albatross, *Diomedea exulans* Linn.

[2] The Cape Pigeon, *Daption capensis* (Linn.). Pintado is a Portuguese word meaning spotted or mottled, and is a term commonly used by sailors for this bird, which has a chequered appearance.

miles. Latd in South 29°2′. *Longd in West Reck.g & Observn* 11°16′. Fresh gales, latter part squally with rain; Birds as yesterday.

TUESDAY 6*th. Winds SE. Course S* 20°15′ *W. Distce sail'd* 50 *miles. Latd in South* 29°49′. *Longd in West pr Reck.g corr by Observn* 11°35′. Fresh gales and squally with Showers of rain.

WEDNESDAY 7*th. Winds ESE. Course S¾W. Distce sail'd* 92 *miles. Latd in South* 31°20′. *Longd in West pr Reck.g corr by Observn* 11°48′. D° Weather. In the evening took a reef in each Topsail.[1]

THURSDAY 8*th. Therm.* 62½. *Winds East. Course SBE¼E. Distce sail'd* 88 *miles. Latd in South* 32°45′. *Longd in West pr Reck.g corr by Observn* 11°23′. Weather continues the same, squalls a little stronger which obliged us to take the 2nd Reef in the Topsails.

FRIDAY 9*th. Therm.* 61. *Winds E to NE. Course S* 28° *E. Distce sail'd* 85 *miles. Latd in South* 34°0′. *Longd in West pr. Reck.g corr by Observn* 10°35′. First and latter parts, the Wind blowed fresh in Squalls. In the night it was Moderate, which occasioned the Reefs to be loosed out of the Topsls.

SATURDAY 10*th. Winds NE. Course ESE¼E. Distce sail'd* 85 *miles. Latd in South* 34°28′. *Longd in West pr. Reck.g corr by Observn* 8°58′. *Variation of the Compass* 8°53′ *West.* Fresh gales and squally with Showers of rain, at Noon gentle gales and clear weather. Fore Mentioned Birds about the Ship.[2]

SUNDAY 11*th. Therm* 63. *Winds NBE. Course S* 77° *E. Distce sail'd* 67 *miles. Latd in South* 34°45′. *Longd in West pr Reck.g corr by Observn* 7°39′, *pr. Mr Kendals Watch* 7°22½′. *Variation of the Compass* 8°30′ *West.* Gentle breezes and clear weather.

MONDAY 12*th. Therm.* 63. *Winds NBW. Course EBS. Distce sail'd* 36 *miles. Latd in South* 34°52′. *Longd in West pr. Reck.g* 6°56′, *Observn* 6°13′. *Variation of the Compass* 8°31′ *West.* Light breezes and clear weather. Many Birds about the Sloop especialy of the sort of Petrels, call'd Pintadoes, caught some with hook and line.[3] At 6h24′12″ by Mr Ken-

[1] ADV 'Saw Verias of Birds'.—Constable.

[2] ADV '. . . in the Evening The Surgeon & Lieutenant of Marines had some words & I belive some blows were given by the Surgeon.'—Bayly.

[3] ADV 'Caught three Pintarte Birds . . . AM Proformed Devine Service'.—Constable.—The birds may have been got by the rather unpleasant method described by Bayly, 3 October, for albatrosses; which, he writes, 'are easily catched, by the following method, take a piece of deal board about a foot square (mor or liss) fix a line to it so that the hook when baited with any sort of meat may lay on the board & be thereby floted, put the board on the water with the hook baited, laying on it, let the board fall a-starn by veering out your line perhaps 100 Yards the whiteness of the board attracts the bird so that he pitcheth on the water by it & swims along side of it, & seeing the bait greedily swallows it hook & all & is thereby catched'.

dals Watch the Moon rose about 4 Digits Eclipsed, the end of the Eclipse was observed as follows

	h	′	″	
By me at	6	53	51	with a Comon 4 f′ refractor
— Mr Forster Senr ..		55	23	— — 2 ft.
— — Wales		54	57	— — Quadt Telescope
— — Picke[r]sgill ..		55	30	— — 3 ft refractor
— — Gilbert		53	24	— — Naked Eye
— — Hervey		55	34	— — Quadt Telescope
Mean of all the observers	6	54	46½	
Watch slow of apparent time	0	3	59	
Apparent time at the end of the Eclipse ..	6	58	45½	
Do at Greenwich ..	7	25	0	
Diffce of Long at 4 pm when ye Altde for Corrg the Watch was taken	0	26	14½	Equal to 6°33½′

By the ☽ and α Aqula[1]	5°51′	Mean	6° 13′
By Do and Aldebn	6°35′		
By Mr Kendals Watch[2]			7° 9′

At 8 AM we brought too to wait for the Adventure and having but little Wind, we hoisted out a Boat and tryed the current, but found none, Mr Forster who was in the Boat shott an Albatross,[3] and some sheer waters, of the Petrels or Mother Caries tribe.[4]

TUESDAY 13*th. Therm.* 65. *Winds N to NE. Course S* 64° *E. Distce sail'd* 48 *miles. Latd in South* 35°13′. *Longd at West Reck.g Corr by Observn* 6°3′. Light gales and Clowdy.[5]

[1] G observed by Mr Wales

[2] N.B. we have lately found the Watch give a Longtiude more West than the Lunar observations.—A *adds* Soon after the Eclipse the Longitude observed by ☽ and Aquala. G *adds* Note, the Longitude resulting from the Eclipse of the Moon I beleive to be nearest the truth.

[3] The Grey-headed Albatross, *Diomedea chrysostoma* (Forster).

[4] Forster's records for this day do not include any storm petrels but he describes *Pterodroma macroptera* (Smith), the Long-winged Petrel, and it was figured by his son. They also took what appears to have been a Dusky Shearwater, *Puffinus assimilis elegans* Gigli and Salv., a bird that is very common in those waters.—ADV '. . . the Mackcannacks Variously Employ'd'.—Constable.

[5] 'at 3 PM The Adventure being up with us, sent ye Boat onboard of Her for some Paint ours being stowed away & Could not gett at it.'—Harvey.

WEDNESDAY 14*th*. *Winds NE. Course S* 77°30′ *E. Distce sail'd* 88 *miles. Latd in South* 35°32′. *Longd at West Reck.g Corr by Observn* 4°23′. First part gentle gales, remainder fresh gales and squally hazey weather.[1]

THURSDAY 15*th*. *Winds NE to N. Course S* 85°30′ *E. Distce sail'd* 87 *miles. Latd in South* 35°39′. *Longd at West Reck.g Corr by Observn* 2°36′. Fresh Breezes and clear weather. Saw some rock or Sea Weed, many Birds, Albatrosses, Pintadoes, Sheerwaters, &c^{a}.[2]

FRIDAY 16*th*. *Therm.* 61½°. *Winds NNW. Course N* 81°30′ *E. Distce sail'd* 134 *miles. Latd in South* 35°19′. *Longd at East Reck.g Corr by Observn* 0°7′ *E.* Fresh gales and fair. Hazey to wards noon.

SATURDAY 17*th*. *Winds Westerly. Course N* 79°30′ *E. Distce sail'd* 110 *miles. Latd in South* 35°0′. *Longd at East Reck.g Corr by Observn.* 2°16′. *Var^{n} of the Compass* 14°8′ *West.* Fresh gales and hazey with some rain. At 4 pm saw a Sail to the NW standing to the Eastward which hoisted Dutch Colours.

SUNDAY 18*th*. *Therm.* 60. *Winds SW. Course N* 79°45′ *E. Distce sail'd* 128 *miles. Latd in South* 34°37′. Moderate gales and Clowdy, a swell from SW.

MONDAY 19*th*. *Therm.* 57. *Winds SW, S & SE. Course N* 74° *E. Distce sail'd* 67 *miles. Latd in South* 34°20′. *Varn of the Compass* 15°12′ *West.* Little Winds and unsettled Weather, with some rain, the Dutch Ship yet in sight. At Noon Tacked and stood to the SE.[3]

TUESDAY 20*th*. *Therm.* 62. *Winds Easterly. Course S* 32° *E. Distce sail'd* 33 *miles. Latd in South* 34°48′. Little Wind and clear. Lost sight of the Dutch Ship having outsail'd her.[4]

WEDNESDAY 21*st*. *Therm.* 63. *Winds Easterly. Latd in South* 35°39′. *Longd at East Reck.g corr by Observn* 8°2′; *Kendals Watch* 7°20′. *Var^{n} of the Compass* 15°56′ *West.* Little Wind and clear weather. At 7^{h}30′20″ am the Longitude of the Ship deduced by the mean of five observed

[1] 'Brought too, and Muster'd the ships company, being Apprehensive there was a man Missing but found None.'—Pickersgill. Presumably there had been a signal from the *Adventure*: cf. Constable's entry for this date, '... at 5 PM Saw a Seal took it at first Sight for a man over board belonging to the Resolution'.

[2] A ... From this time [of the observations as above] to the 16th the wind was between the North and East, blowing a gentle gale, we were generally accompanied by Albatrosses, Pintadoes, Sheerwaters &c^{a} and a small grey bird less then Pigeons, they have whitish bellies and grey backs, with a black strake across from the tip of one wing to the tip of the other, these birds sometimes visets us in vast flights, they are as well as the Pintadoes, a southern bird, and are, I beleive, never seen within the Tropicks or north of the line.—They were Prions (*Pachyptila* sp.), but the species is not determinable.

[3] 'A Very Large Whale run some distance alongside of us'.—Cerke.

[4] ADV '... at 11 [AM] The Resolution's Boat came on Board: People in High Spirrets, and very Healthy'.—Wilby.

distances of the Sun and Moon was 8°4′30″ East. Mr Kendals Watch at the same time gave 7°22′.[1]

THURSDAY 22*nd. Winds Easterly. Latd in South* 36°52′. *Longd at East Reck.g Corr by Observn* 8°24′. First part moderate breezes and fair, remainder fresh breeze with some rain. Distilling fresh Water from Salt.

FRIDAY 23*rd. Winds NE & North. Course S* 63° *E. Distce sail'd* 44 *miles. Latd in South* 37°12′. *Longd at East Reck.g Corr by Observn* 9°13′. Little Wind with some Calms, in the am hoisted out a Boat and shott some Albatrosses and other Birds on which we feasted the next day.[2] Saw a Seal or as some thought a Sea Lyon.[3]

SATURDAY 24*th. Winds NW to SW. Course N* 70° *E. Distce sail'd* 96 *miles. Latd in South* 36°39′. *Longd at East Reck.g Corr by Observn* 11°6′. First part light breezes and clowdy, latter fresh gales and clear.

SUNDAY 25*th. Winds SW, S & SE. Course N* 65° *E. Distce sail'd* 140 *miles. Latd in South* 35°40′. Fresh gales and Clowdy.[4]

MONDAY 26*th. Therm.* 62. *Winds SE. Course N* 49°15′ *E. Distce sail'd* 92 *miles. Latd in South* 34°40′. Fresh gales and Clowdy.[5]

TUESDAY 27*th. Therm.* 60. *Winds SSE. Course N* 45° *E. Distce sail'd* 80 *miles. Latd in South* 33°44′. *Varn. of the Compass* 21°27′ *West.* D^o^ Weather. In the pm sounded without finding ground at 210 f^m^.

WEDNESDAY 28*th. Therm.* 67. *Winds SSW to NW. Latd in South* 33°43′. First part gentle gales remainder little wind. AM sounded no ground 210 f^m^.

FRIDAY 29*th. Therm.* 61. *Winds W to NNW. Latd in South* 33°53′. Gentle gales and Clowdy. pm Sounded no ground at 210 f^m^.

*The Wind Continued about two days at NW and SW then veered to the SE where it remain'd two days longer then fix'd at NW which carried us to our intended Port; as we approach'd the land the Sea

[1] A ... our Latitude [at this time] was 35°20′ S.—Midshipman Harvey gives us a more domestic detail: 'PM ... Muster'd ye Ships Company In order to stop there Wine who was Dirty'.

[2] A ... and found them exceeding good.—According to J. R. Forster (*Descriptiones Animalium*, p. 26), these included *Procellaria aequinoctialis* Linn., the Cape Hen, so called on account of its abundance at the Cape of Good Hope.

[3] AH ... which probably might be an inhabitant of one of the Isles of Tristian de Cunha, we being now nearly in their Latitude and about 15° East of them.

[4] 'Several Whales & some Thrashers about the Ship—Many Birds—Albotrosses, Pintada's, Peterels &c &c'.—Clerke. ADV 'Saw a Number of Parmmesita Wales'.—Constable.

[5] ADV 'The first Lieut^t^ taken with relapse of the Gout of which he has been confined to his cabbin this 3 Weeks past but had been able to walk a little for some days.'—Bayly, 25 October. This must be the sickness which put an end to Shank's participation in the voyage.

Fowl, which had accompanied us hitherto, began to leave us, at least they did not come in such numbers, nor did we see Gannets, or the black bird commonly call'd the Cape Hen, till we were nearly within sight of the Cape; nor did we strike soundings till Penguin Island bore NNE distant 2 or 3 leagues, where we had 50 fathom water; not but what Soundings may extend farther off, however I am well assured that they do not extend very far West from the Cape, for we could not find ground with a line of 210 fathoms 25 leagues West of Table Bay, the same at 35 Leagues and at 64 Leagues; I sounded these three times in order to find a Bank which I have been told lies to the West of the Cape but how far I never could learn. I was told before I left England by some gentlemen who were well enough acquainted with the Navigation between England and the Cape of Good Hope, that I sail'd at an improper season of the year and that I should meet with much Calm weather, near and under the line, this probably may be the case some years, it is however not general, on the contrary, we hardly met with any Calms, but a brisk SW Wind in those very latitudes, the Calms are expected, nor did we meet with any of those Tornadoes so much spoke of by former Navigators, a View of the Table of Winds &c^a[1] will explain these things better than many words, it is however true of what they have said of the Currants seting towards the Coast of Guinea, as you approach that shore; for from the time of our leaving St Jago to our arrival into the Latitude of 1½ North, which was eleven days, we were carried by the Currants 3½° of Longitude more East than our Reckoning, on the other hand after we had cross'd the line and got the SE trade Wind we always found by observations that the Ship out striped the Reckoning, which we judged to be owing to a Current seting between the South and West; upon the whole the Currents in this run seemed to ballance each other, for upon our arrival at the Cape the difference of Longitude by dead Reckoning kept from England without once being corrected was only three quarters of a degree less than that by observation.*—G, pp. 8–9.

SATURDAY 30*th*. *Therm.* 61. *Winds NNW. Latd in South* 33°53′. Fresh gales with rain in the night. At 2 pm Saw the land of the Cape of Good Hope, the Table Mountain which is over the Cape Town bore ESE Distant 12 or 13 Leagues.[2] At 7 AM Anchored in Table Bay (the

[1] This, I take it, refers to the daily 'log-entries' in the journal, given here in italics. A has a note in Cook's hand, 'This Table for want of Room is not inserted'.

[2] The passage from St Iago to the Cape, says Furneaux, took 77 days, 'which is reckoned long, but was overpaid by the continual fine weather we had, not meeting with a Calm exceeding Six hours, or more wind than we could wish for'.—Add. MS 27890, f. 2.

Adventure in Company) in 5 fathom Water Green Point or the West point of the Bay NWBW and the Church SWBS, Distant from Shore one Mile. Sent an officer to Notify our arrival to the Governor and on his return saluted the Garrison with Eleven Guns which was returned. Moored NE & SW a Cable each way, hoisted out the Longboat and began to prepare to heel and Water the Sloop &c^a^. At this time we have not one man on the Sick list, the People in general have injoy'd a good state of health ever since we left England.[1] Last night while we were off Penguin Island the Whole sea became all at once illuminated, or what the Seamen calls all on fire, some Water was taken up from along side in which were an immence number of small Globular Insects about the size of a Common Pins head and quite transparrant; this appearence of the Sea is very common in all parts I have been in, but the cause is not so generally known.[2]

As soon as I landed I waited upon the Governor Baron Plettenberg, who told me that he had received Instructions from Holland relating to these two Sloops and that I might be assured of every assistance the place could afford. My next care was to procure the necessary Provisions and stores wanting, to get the Sloops caulked and to prepare the Casks for the Brandy, Wine and other Provisions all which was set about without delay. But as the Bread we wanted was yet unbaked and all the Spirits to be brought out of the Country it was the 18 of the following Month before every thing was got on board and the 22nd before we could put to Sea. During this stay the Crews of both Sloops were served every Day with new baked Bread

[1] 'Our people all in perfect Health and spirits, owing I believe in a great measure to the strict attention of Captain Cook to their cleanliness and every other article that respects their Welfare'.—Clerke.—'Our people all in good health having been so from our sailing from plymouth sound from the great care & attention of our Capt.'—Gilbert. Cf. the following extracts from Clerke: 'Anchor'd here a Dutch East India Ship from Middleburg. She's been four Months upon her Passage—has buried 150 Men with the Scurvy and sent about 60 to the Hospital here, immediately upon her Arrival'.—2 November—'Anchor'd here a Dutch East India Ship from Zealand bound to Batavia, she has been out 23 Weeks and buried 41 Men'.—3 November. Cook takes due note of these fatalities in his Log, and in the extended version of his journal printed below.

[2] Cf. Wales: 'This Evening we amused ourselves with enquiring into the Cause of a very odd Phænomenon. The Sea all round the Ship, and as far as we could see was perfectly illuminated by the Number and brightness of those shining particles which are usually seen in a ship's Wake. We took up several Buckets full of the water & found it full of small Insects which when laid on a piece of paper were much like a bit of Jelly; but excepting these the Water was perfectly clear. When the Water was at rest in the Buckets, it ceased to be illuminated; but as soon as it was disturbed became as bright as that in the sea'. There are almost no insects at sea. A drawing by George Forster shows that these were *Noctiluca* sp., organisms which belong to the group Protozoa and are responsible for many of the astonishing displays of phosphorescence familiar to most voyagers. They had then been recognized as light-producing animals for about twenty years; the first accurate figure of them to be published was by Dicquemare in 1775.

fresh Beef or Mutton and as much greens as they could eat, they had also leave to go on shore 10 or 12 at a time to refresh themselves.

Messrs Wales and Baily the two Astronomers were on Shore all the time makeing the necessary astronomical observations in order to assertain the going of the Watches and other purposes. Mr Kendalls Watch thus far has been found to answer beyond all expecion, but this cannot be said of Mr Arnolds. The Longitude of the Cape Town pointed out by these watches is already mentioned in their proper Columns. By observa^ns^ made here Mr Kendals Watch is found to have altered its rate of going something more than one second p^r^ Day by gain^g^ $\frac{7}{8}$ of a Second p^r^ Day on mean time whereas at Greenwich it lost $\frac{5}{8}$ p^r^ day, this variation however is very inconsiderable. Mr Arnolds was found to loose on Mean time by the mean rate of its going for twelve days 1′31″, 0125 per day which is 1′17″, 63 more than at Greenwich and also varied in its rate sometimes more than half a minute p^r^ Day, however one of Mr Arnolds on board the Adventure kept time in such a manner as not to be complained on.[1] Mr Forster met with a Swedish Gentleman here, one Mr Sparman, who understood something of Botany and Natural History and who was willing to embarque with us, Mr Forster thinking that he would be of great assistance to him in the Course of the Voyage strongly importuned me to take him on board which I accordingly did.[2]

Mr Shank first Lieutenant of the Adventure having been in an ill state of health ever sence we left England and not recovering here, requested my leave to quit in order to return home for the reistablishment of his health, his requist appearing to be well founded I gave him leave accordingly[3] and appointed Mr Burney one of my

[1] The first casualty to the chronometers was suffered at the Cape. Wales (16 November) took down the instruments and the observatories which had been erected on shore, and 'in the evening the Captn sent boats to Carry them on board the ship, I sat in the stern sheets with one watch on each side me; both of which where going when we put off from the shore; In laying the boat alongside of the ship the person who steered it let it strike yet not so hard as to give me any Apprehensions at the time; however when I got on board the ship I found that Mr Arnolds watch had stoped for which I am not able to Assign any Reason if it was not caused by the Above mentioned stroke of the Boat against the ship's side.'

[2] This was done at Forster's expense: A 'The idea of gathering the treasures of nature in countries hitherto unknown to Europe, filled his mind so entirely, that he immediately engaged to accompany us on our circumnavigation; in the course of which, I am proud to say, we have found him an enthusiast in his science, well versed in medical knowledge, and endowed with a heart capable of the warmest feelings, and worthy of a philosopher.' —Forster, I, p. 68.

[3] 'I must beg leave to Assure their Lordships, that Mr Shank has quited the Sloop with the greatest reluctance and nothing but his bad State of Health would have oblig'd him to give up a Voyage on which he had Set his heart.'—Cook to Stephens, 18 November 1772, P.RO. Adm. 1/1610; below, p. 687.

Midshipmen second Lieutenant of the Adventure[1] in the room of M[r] Kemp whom I appointed first.

*FRIDAY 30*th* [October]. *Therm[r] 61. Winds NNW. Latt[d] in South* 33..53. Fresh Gales with rain in the night, at 2 PM saw the land of Cape of Good Hope; the Table Mountain, which is over the Cape Town bore ESE Distant 12 or 13 Leagues, at this time it was a good deal Obscured by clouds otherwise it might, from its height have been seen at a much greater distance, we now crow[d]ed all the sail we could thinking to get into the Bay before dark, but after we found this could not be accomplished we shortened sail & kept standing off & on behind Penguin Island (which lyes before the Bay) all night, which was none of the best being very squally with rain & dark withall, between 8 & 9 oClock the whole sea within the Compass of our sight became at once, as it were illumanated or what the Seamen calls all on fire, this appearance of the sea in some degree is very common, but the cause is not so generally known. M[r] Banks & D[r] Solander had satisfied me that it was occasioned by sea Insects. M[r] Forster however seemed not to favour this opinion, I therefore had some buckets of water drawn up from alongside the Ship, which we found full of an enumerable quantity of small globular Insects, about the size of a common Pins head and quite Transparrant, there was no doubt of their being living Animals, when in their o[w]n proper eliment tho' we could not perceive any life in them, M[r] Forster whose provence it is more minutely to describe things of this nature, was now well satisfied with the Cause of the sea's illumination.

At length Day light came & brought us fair weather and we stood into the Bay with the Adventure in Company, and anchored in 5 fathom water and afterwards moored NE & SW Green Point, on the West Point of the Bay, bore NWbW and the Church, in one with the Vally, between the Table Mountain and the Sugar Loaf, or Lyons head, bearing SWbS and distant from the landing Place, near the Fort, one Mile.

We had no sooner Anchor'd then we were Visited by the Captain of the Port or Master Attendant, some other Officers belonging to the Company and M[r] Brand, this last Gentleman brought us off such things as cannot fail of being exceptable to persons coming from sea, the purport of the Master Attendants Visit was according to

[1] Burney, though still only 22, had been at sea since the age of 10. He joined the *Resolution* as an A.B. in December 1771, but got his lieutenant's passing certificate in the following month. The boundary between A.B. and midshipman for 'young gentlemen' of his type was a very wavering one: indeed he hardly belonged any more to the category of 'young' gentlemen, and Cook had promised Sandwich to give him the first promotion that was available.

custom to take an account of the Ships, to enquire into the health of the crews, and in Particular if the Small Pox is onboard a thing they dread above all others at the Cape, and for these purposes, a Surgeon is allways one of the Visitants, my first Step after Anchoring was to send an Officer to the Governor to acquaint him with our arrival and the reasons that induced me to put in here, to which the officer received a very polite answer, and upon his return we Saluted the Governor With Eleven guns which complement was returned. Soon after I went on shore myself and waited upon him accompanied by Captain Furneaux & the two Mr Forsters; no proper Governor having arrived at the Cape since the death of Lieutenant Governor Baron Plettenberg acted as Governor in the room of who was daily expected,[1] this Gentleman received us with great politeness and Promis'd me every assistance this place could afford. From him I learnt that two French Ships from the Mauritius about 8 Months before had discoverd Land in the Latitude of 48° s and in the Meridian of that Island, along which they saild forty miles, till they came to a Bay into which they were about to enter, when they were drove off and seperated in a hard Gale of wind, after having lost some of their Boats and people, which they had sent to sound the Bay; one of the Ships (viz) the La Fortune soon after arrived at the Mauritius, the Captain of which was sent home to France with an account of the discovery, this captain reported, that the other Ship (Viz) the Grot Ventro [*sic*] was lost, this however was not the case, as will be seen by and by,[2] after having Visited the Governor and some other of the Principal persons of the place, we fix'd our selves at M[r] Brands, the usual residence of most Officers belonging to English ships, this Gentleman spares neither trouble nor expence to make his house agreable to those who favour him with their Company, & to accomodate them with every thing they want, with him I concerted measures for Supplying the Sloops with Provisions and all other necessaries they wanted and which he set out procuring without delay, while the Seamen onboard were employ[d] in overhauling the Rigging and the Carpenters in caulking the Sloops sides and Decks &c[a]. Mess[rs] Wales & Baily got all their Instruments on shore, in order to make astronomical observations, for assertaining the going of the watches and other purposes, the result of some of those observations shewed that M[r] Kendals Watch

[1] The great governor Ryk Tulbagh, whom Cook had met in 1771, had died in August of that year; no successor came immediately from elsewhere, and Joachim van Plettenberg remained as acting-governor till 1774, and then as governor till 1785.

[2] This was the report then current at the Cape of Kerguelen's expedition. See pp. liii–liv above.

had answerd beyond all expectations by pointing out the Longitude of this place to one minute of time to what it was observed by Mess[rs] Mason & Dixon in 176[1] they made the Longitude to be 18°23′ E of Greenwich and the Watch 18°8′, the Astronomers however found that it has altered its rate of going, something more than one second p[r] Day, by gaining here $\frac{7}{8}$ of a Second p[r] Day on Mean Time whereas at Greenwich it lost $\frac{5}{8}$ of a second: inconsiderable as this variation is, if it's rate of going had been allowed, agreeable to the mean of these it would have come still nearer the truth, little can be said in favour of the one of M[r] Arnolds on board of us, but one of those on board the Adventure promises fair to answer the purpose intended.

A Few days after our arrival a French ship arrived here from the Mauritius which brought us an account of the arrival of the Gros Ventre from Batavia two days before the other left the Island, in which time nothing about the discovery transpired, from all we could learn it appeared that discovery was not the principal object of these two ships and that they never set foot on the land they had seen, the one seems to have made the best of her way back to the Mauritius while the other went to Batavia and took in a Cargo of Arrack for the same Island and this was probably the chief intent of the Voyage, be this as it may, they are not the only Ships the french have fitted out from that Island, to go on either real or pretended discoveries, for in March last, two Ships, bound for the South Pacific Ocean touched here, on board one of them was Aotourou, the man M. Bougainville brought from *Otahieta* and who died of the small Pox before the ships sail'd from hence, one of them having that disorder on board, and for which the Dutch obliged her to lay at Penguin Island.[1] The death of Aotourou, who was upon his passage to his Native Isle, is the more unfortunate as this was the fate of Tupia and his Servant Tiato, the two we brought from the same Island, had any one of these three persons lived to Return, they must have prepossessed the Islanders with Ideas very much in favour of Europeans and been the means of their meeting with a good reception at Otahite or any of the neighbouring Isles; the contrary of which may in some degree be expected, especially to such as are unacquainted with their Language & customs; These two Ships were to proceed round Cape Horn after touching upon the Coast of Brazil, where probably they intended to spend the Winter and may be about leaving that coast now.

[1] The expedition of Marion du Fresne. But his ships were at the Cape in December 1771, not March 1772. See also pp. liv–lv, lxix above, pp. 656–7 below.

Three or four days after us, two Dutch Indiamen arrived here, the one from Middleburg, and the other from Zealand, after a passage of between four & five Months, in which one lost by the Scurvy & other putrid diseases 150 Men, and the other 41, and sent on their arrival great numbers to the Hospital, in very dreadfull circumstances; it is remarkable that one of these Ships which touched at Port Praya and left it a month before we arrived there and yet we got here three days before him. The Dutch at the Cape having found their Hospital too small for the reception of their Sick, are going to build a new one at the East part of the Town, the foundation of which was laid with great ceremony while we were there.

By the healthy condition of the Crews of both Sloops at our Arrival, I thought to have made my stay here very short, but as the Bread we wanted was unbaked and the Spirit, which I found scarce, to be collected from different parts out of the Country it was the 18th of November before we had got every thing onboard and the 22nd before we could put to Sea. During this time the Crews of both Sloops were served every day with fresh Beef, or Mutton new Baked Bread and as much greens as they could eat, the Sloops were caulk'd and Painted, and in every respect put into as good a condition as when they left England....

Mr Forster, whose whole time was taken up in the pursuits of Natural history and Botany, met with a Swedish Gentleman, one Mr Sparman who understood something of these Sciences having Stud[i]ed under [Dr Linnaeus][1] and being willing to embarque with us, Mr Forster strongly importuned me to take him onboard, thinking that he would be of great assistance to him in the course of the Voyage. I at last consented and he embarqued with us acordin[g]ly as an assistant to Mr Forster who bore his Expences onboard and allowed him a Yearly Stupend besides.

Mr Hodges employed himself here in Drawing a View of the Town and Port adjacent in Oyle Colours, which was properly packed up with some others and left with Mr Brand, in order to be forwarded to the Admiralty, by the first Ship that should [sail] for England.[2]

Mr Gilbert my Master, (by permission) Sounded the Bay and drawed a sketch thereof, which is here annex'd, and by which it will appear, that there is so little danger in sailing in and out of the Bay that any sailing direction I can give will be quite unnecessary.*—H, pp. 27–32.

[1] H has here a blank, which I supply from G. [2] Fig. 14.

MONDAY 23*rd. Winds NBW to NWBW. Course S.* 44° *W. Distce sail'd* 56 *miles. Latd in South* 34°36'. *Longd in East of Greenwich* 17°34'. *Longd made from the Cape of Good Hope* 0°49' *W.* First part moderate and Clowdy, remainder fresh gales and squally with rain. At 3 pm weighed and came to sail with the Adventure in Company. Saluted the Garrison with 15 guns which compliment was returned. Made several trips to get out of the Bay which we accomplished by 7 o'Clock at which time the Town bore SE Distant 4 Miles. Stood to the Westw^d all night to get an offing having the Wind at NNW and NW blowing in Squalls with rain which obliged us to reef our Topsails,[1] after having got clear of the land I directed my Course for Cape Circumcision.[2]

TUESDAY 24*th. Winds NW, SW to SE. Course S* 12° *E. Distce sail'd* 50 *miles. Latd in South* 35°25'. *Longd in East of Greenwch* 17°44'. *Longd made from the Cape of Good Hope* 0°39' *W.* Moderate gales and Clowdy Weather with a large swell from Southward. In the PM served to each Man[3] a Fearnought Jacket and a pair of Trowers which were allowed by the Admiralty. Many Albatroses about the Ship, some of which we caught with Hook and line and were not thought dispiseable food[4] even at a time when all hands were served fresh Mutton.

WEDNESDAY 25*th. Winds SE to ESE. Course S* 21° *W. Distce sail'd* 118 *miles. Latd in South* 37°15'. *Longd in East of Greenwch* 16°52'. *Longd made from the Cape of Good Hope* 1°31' *W.* Fresh gales and Clowdy weather.

THURSDAY 26*th. Winds E to NE. Course S* 10° *W. Distce sail'd* 111 *miles. Latd in South* 39°4'. *Longd in East of Greenwch* 16°27'. *Longd made from the Cape of Good Hope* 1°56'. Moderate gales and Clowdy, Swell from the Eastward.[5]

[1] A . . . the sea was again illuminated for some time in the same manner as it was the night before we arrived in Table Bay.

[2] 'This Day the Captain isued an Order out to be as sparing of ye Water as possible for we were going on a Passage we did not know how long, sett ye Still to work when ever ye Weather wou'd premitt, All ye Officers being allow'd a Quart of Water a Day for Tea'.—Harvey. Sparrman, p. 5, adds to this: 'There is seldom any extravagance with fresh water on sea voyages; but now particularly, with the uncertainty of the next landfall, every drop had to be carefully preserved. An armed sentry was placed on duty by the water-casks, and although he certainly allowed the people a thirst-quencher on the spot, he did not permit any water to be taken below deck. The Captain himself set an example by washing and shaving with seawater'. Irving's machine was kept working.

[3] *In the PM . . . Man:* A Judging that we should soon come into cold weather, I order'd Slops to be served to such as were in want, and gave to each man

[4] *were . . . food:* A were very well relish'd by many of the People

[5] Further provision for creature comfort in the *Adventure*: 'This day paid Capt Furneaux 23 Rix Dollers, as my share of the Extra Expences of the Miss: I likewis paid Mr Kemp 1st Lieu^t 14 Shilling as it being the Ballance of our joint expences of private Stock Viz—Capt Fur^nx Mr Kemp & my self bought of Mr Peter Fannin the Master 1 Hogshead of

FRIDAY 27*th. Therm.* 52½. *Winds W to SW. Course S* 24° *E. Distce sail'd* 66 *miles. Latd in South* 40°4′. *Longd in East of Greenwch* 17°2′. *Longd made from the Cape of Good Hope* 1°21′. Fresh gales with Squals. At 8 pm brought too untill day light in the Morn, then made sail.

SATURDAY 28*th. Winds SW to NW. Course S* 9° *E. Distce sail'd* 56 *miles. Latd in South* 40°59′. *Longd in East of Greenwch* 17°14′. *Longd made from the Cape of Good Hope* 1°9′. First and latter parts Fresh breezes, the Middle little wind or Calm.

SUNDAY 29*th. Winds WNW. Course South. Distce sail'd* 70 *miles. Latd in South* 42°9′. *Longd in East of Greenwch* 17°14′. *Longd made from the Cape of Good Hope* 1°9′. Strong gales with hard Squalls, rain & hail. At 7 pm brought too under the Fore Sail, and at 3 am Made sail under the Foresail, Mainsail and close reef'd Main Topsail, this last we were soon after obliged to take in and at 10 to hand the Main sail and lay-to under the Fore sail and to get down Topg[t] Yards. Adventure in Company.[1]

MONDAY 30*th. Winds WNW. Course S* 66° *E. Distce sail'd* 33 *miles. Latd in South* 42°24′. *Longd in East of Greenwch* 17°57′. *Longd made from the Cape of Good Hope* 0°26′. Very hard gales with rain and hail, lying-to under a Mizen Stay-sail most part of these 24 hours, the Sea running very high.[2] At 11 pm the Scuttle of the Boatswain Store-room (not being properly secured) Washed or broke loose and before

best Madeira Wine at 15 Pound Sterling Each having ⅓ Share which came to 5£ each. I being on Shore at the time M[r] Kemp paid my share then I bought of M[r] Brand [on] Mr Kemp[s] & my Joint acc[t] 28 Gallons of Arrack, & 20 Gallons of Best Cape wine, which together cost 36 Rix Dollers which is Equall to £8 8[s] Starling p[r] Bill & Rec[t]—M[r] Kemp[s] Share being £4 4[s] and 2[s] he had more therefore I was 14[s] in his Debt'.—Bayly, 25 November.

[1] Wales turned to a fresh scientific interest, having a meteorological as well as astronomical turn of mind: 'In the Midst of this heavy Gale, I tried D[r] Linds Wind Gage & found, that it was depressed by the force of the wind 0,45 of an Inch.' Dr James Lind's 'Portable Wind Gage' was described by him in a paper in the *Philosophical Transactions*, LXV (1775), pp. 355–65. It was what the physicist would now call a simple manometer: an apparatus consisting basically of a U-shaped tube half full of water, into one arm of which the wind was led to blow. The pressure of the wind was represented by the difference in levels of the water thus caused in the two arms; which, read off a scale between them, Lind claimed would give an accurate notation of any movement of the air from a gentle wind to the most violent hurricane. On shipboard there was the difficulty that the thing had to be held quite perpendicular. Wales's instrument was made by Nairne: he concluded that it 'would undoubtedly be very useful, if it could be made with a scale somewhat more extensive than that I made use of'.—*Astronomical Observations*, p. liii. Compare an entry in this volume, p. 337, for 25 July 1772: 'Tried Dr Lind's wind gage . . . but could not find that the wind had any sensible effect on it. At the time we had as much wind as we could well carry topgallant sails to'. Bayly also tried the gauge, but neither man seems to have made regular measurements with it—perhaps because of its uncertainty.

[2] '. . . the Adventure we find to be the most weatherly Ship in a Gale tho' this is as good a Sea Boat as can possibly swim.'—Clerke. The *Adventure*, that is, could sail closer to the wind without drifting to leeward.

it was discovered we had two feet and a half Water in the Sloop, however it was soon secured and the Water Pumped out without any other damage than weting some stores &c[a] betwixt Decks.[1]

[DECEMBER 1772]

TUESDAY 1*st. Winds WNW. Course S* 13° *E. Distce sail'd* 58 *miles. Latd in South* 43°21′. *Longd in East Greenwch* 18°10′. *Longd made from the Cape of Good Hope* 0°13′. Hard gales and fair Weather. At 2 pm made sail under the Fore sail and Staysails and at 4 set the Mainsail. At 8 bro[t] to under the Fore-sail untill daylight then set the Mainsail & M[n] Topsail which we could not carry Long, being so very squally with rain.[2] At 10 it was more moderate and we set the Main again.[3]

WEDNESDAY 2*nd. Therm.* 49½. *Winds Westerly. Course S* 40° *E. Distce sail'd* 40 *miles. Latd in South* 43°52′. *Longd in East of Greenwh* 18°45′. *Longd made C. Good Hope* 0°22′ *E.* First and latter parts fresh gales and Clowdy, the Middle little Wind. In the PM under our Courses and Staysails, in the night lay to under the Foresail, at 4 am made sail under the Courses and close reef'd Topsails. Sea running very high.

THURSDAY 3*rd. Therm.* 49. *Winds WNW. Course S Westerly. Distce sail'd* 36 *miles. Latd in South* 44°28′. *Longd in East of Greenwh* 18°43′. *Longd made C. Good Hope* 0°20′. Strong gales and Squally. At 8 pm brought to under the Fore sail and Mizen and could not make more sail untill 11 am when it was some thing moderater and we set the Mainsail and close Reef'd Topsails.[4]

FRIDAY 4*th. Therm.* 43. *Winds West to NW. Course S½W. Distce sail'd* 78 *miles. Latd in South* 45°46′. *Longd in East of Greenwh* 18°32′. *Longd made C. Good Hope* 0°9′ *Et.* Fresh gales and fair Weather, at

[1] 'About 12 oClock it was discovered that the ship was almost knee deep in Water between Decks; but on sounding the Well not more than about 20 Inches was there; and on examination it was found that the Inside scuttle of the Boatswain's store room had given way, which being on y[e] Lee side of the ship was almost constantly under water. Both hand Pumps were instantly set to work, & one of the quartermasters volontarily offered to go over the side and force in the out-side scuttle, which he effected after being three times washed up into y[e] fore chains.'—Wales. The chain-pumps had to be rigged to get the water out. Forster (I, pp. 89–90) makes a great deal more out of this incident than either Cook or Wales: 'every soul was filled with terror'; 'the officers encouraged the seamen with an alarming gentleness'; and so on.

[2] ADV 'This morning the Gale continued with hard rain which rendered it very uncomfortable the Sea breaking frequently with great violence over the Ship (but happy for us) she is an excellent Sea-boat & tho' she rowl much she does it with ease to herself.'—Bayly.

[3] One disease Cook could not obviate was the common cold. The conscientious Bowles Mitchel records its progress at this time: 27 November, 'Have ten Men sick & many complain of severe colds'.—28 November, 'People recovering.'—1 December, 'Have only 4 men slightly ill the rest recovered'.

[4] '[am] Put the Ships comp[y] to ⅞ allowance of bread'.—Mitchel.

8 pm took in the Topsails and stood on under our Courses untill the morning then set the Topsails with all the Reefs out. Got the spare Sails up to Dry, found them in the after Sail room very wet occasioned by the Deck over it being leaky and as it could not be come at to Caulk on account of the Fire Hearth I ordered it to be pull'd down and to be built in Midships betwixt the Fore and Main Hatchways.[1]

SATURDAY 5*th. Winds NW. Course S* 10° *W. Distce sail'd* 88 *miles. Latd in South* 47°10′. *Longd in East of Greenwh* 18°10′. *Longd made C. Good Hope* 0°13′ *Wt. Var. of the Compass* 15°55′ *West.* These 24 hours the Weather pretty moderate, the Sea however still continues high and the air begins to be pinching cold. At 8 p.m. Close reef'd the Topsails, at 4 am loosed two reefs out, got Topg[t] Yards across and set the Sails. Saw some Sea Weed.

SUNDAY 6*th. Therm.* 38. *Winds NNE, NW, SW. Course S¾E. Distce sail'd* 61 *miles. Latd in South* 48°11′. *Longd in East of Greenwh* 18°24′. *Longd made C. Good Hope* 0°1′ *E. Var. of the Compass* 18°11′ *West.* Fresh gales and hazey with drizling rain at times, the air so cold that every one complains.[2] At half past Eight pm bro[t] to under our Topsails untill the Morn, then made sail under the Courses and Double reef'd Topsails. A Large Sea from Westward. Many Birds about the Ship, Albatroses,[3] Sheerwaters, Pintadoes, Fulmers,[4] &c[a]

[1] 'This Afternoon the Carpenters set about making a new Sail Room between the Fore and Main Hatchways, the other being so Leaky in spight of all our Carpenters can do to the contrary that the Sails are continually wet.'—Clerke.—'This late gale, the ship has work'd the Ocham out of the Seams in general that there is scarce a dry Bed in the Ship & very weak in the Upper Works.'—Cooper. Of the fair weather of this day Wales writes, 'I remember to have read in some Author or other how that

"After a storm the sun more bright appears!"

And he adds

"That Joy is greatest which is rais'd from fears."

The latter part may be true for ought that I know to the contrary; but I am certain the former is so: for never did sun-shine & moderate Weather appear more delightfull than now to us, after near a week of the most turbulent weather that can be well imagined.'

[2] A ... The wind ... on the 29th [November] fixd at WNW and increas'd to a storm, which continued with some few intervals of moderate weather till the 6th of December, when being in the Latitude of 48°11′ South and Longitude 18°24′ East, which is nearly the same Meridian, as the Cape, the variation was 18°11′ West; this Gale which was attended with rain & hail, blew at times with such violence that we could carry no sail, by which means were drove far to the Eastw[d] of our intended Course, and left me no hopes of reaching *Cape Circumcision*, but the greatest misfortune that attended, was the loss of great part of our live stock we had brought from the Cape, which consisted of Sheep, Hogs and Geese, indeed this sudden transition from hot mild weather to extreme cold & Wet, made every man in the Ship feel its effects, for by this time the Mercury in the Thermometer was fallen to 38° whereas at the Cape it was generally at and upwards.

[3] Forster gives the names of three of these birds for this day: Wandering and Grey-headed Albatrosses and a Sooty Albatross, *Phoebetria* sp.

[4] The Silver-grey Petrel, *Fulmarus antarcticus* Stephens, the southern representative of the northern Fulmar Petrel.

and small grey Birds with a Black Strake a Cross the Back from the tip of one wing to the Tip of the other.[1]

MONDAY *7th. Therm.* 42½. *Winds SW, North, NW. Course S* 10° *E. Distce sail'd* 83 *miles. Latd in South* 49°32′. *Longd in East of Greenwh* 18°46′. *Longd made C. Good Hope* 0°23′ *E.* PM Fresh gales and fair Weather, the night clear and serene and the rising Sun gave us such flatering hopes of a fine day that we were induced to Loose all the reefs out of the Topsails and get Topg[t] Yards a Cross; before 8 o'Clock the Scene was changed, the Weather became hazey with rain and the gale increased so much as to oblige us to hand the Mainsail and close reefe the Topsails and to get down Topg[t] yards again. The Barometer at 28½ which is unusally low.

TUESDAY *8th. Therm.* 40. *Winds NW. Course S* 84° *E. Distce sail'd* 39 *miles. Latd in South* 49°36′. *Longd in East of Greenwh* 19°45′. *Longd made C. G. Hope* 1°22′ *East.* Very hard gales and Hazey with rain. At 1 PM took in the Topsails and Foresail Wore and brought to under the Mizen Staysail, Struck Topg[t] mast and got the Spritsail yard in fore and aft.[2] At 8 am Wore and lay too on the other Tack, the gale something moderater, but the Sea runs very high,[3] this together with the Weather which we think very cold, makes great distruction among our Hogs, Sheep and Poultry, not a night passes without some dying, with us, however, they are not wholy lost for we eat them notwithstanding.

WEDNESDAY *9th. Therm.* 36. *Winds NW to West. Course S* 68° *E. Distce sail'd* 27 *miles. Latd in South* 49°49′. *Longd in East of Greenwh* 20°24′. *Longd made C. G. Hope* 2°1′ *East. Var of the Compass* 16°34′. Hard gales and hazy weather. At 2 pm made the Signal for the Adventure to come under our Stern and Set the Fore Topmast Staysail, in the Even saw two Penguins and some Weed, Sounded without finding ground with 100 fathoms. At 8 Wore and lay to on

[1] Whale birds or prions, *Pachyptila* spp., or perhaps the Blue Petrel *Halobaena caerulea* (Gm.) (see pp. 65 and 68, n. 1).—Clerke's entry for this day ends, 'Serv'd Brandy to the People the Wine being out'.

[2] A . . . I thought proper to veer and lay the Sloops to under a mizen Stays[l] with their heads to the NE seing that they would bow the Sea, which ran prodigious high, better on this tack.

[3] 'A Very heavy Sea running these 24 hours—the Ship rowls very deep but exceedingly Easy—Very disagreeable Weather.'—Clerke 8951.—'Wore ship set the Maintopmast stay-sail to prevent her rowling. Thick weather so that was we Now to see land our Situat[n] must be better Immagined than discribed by them Who has ever been in a Gale of Wind at Sea.'—Pickersgill.—ADV 'Strong gales & Squally with a very heavy Sea from NW, Wore Ship up F Sail and lay too under M[n] & Miz[n] Staysails, Washed out of the M[n] Chains, 6 Oars the Decks being very Leaky, every Body below as wet as on Deck'.—Browne.—'Spliced the main brace being very wet and cold & people much fatigued'.—Furneaux.

the other Tack till 3 am, then wore again, Squaly with Showers of Snow. At 8 made the Signal for the Adventure to make sail and at 10 made sail our selves under the Courses and close reef'd Topsails, Weather more moderate and fair, but a very high Westerly Sea. Many birds in sight.

THURSDAY 10*th. Therm.* 36½. *Winds W to NW. Course SBE. Distce sail'd* 69 *miles. Latd in South* 50°57′. *Longd in East of Greenwh* 20°45′. *Longd made C. G. Hope* 2°22′. Fresh gales with a great Sea from the Westward, in the night Frost and in the am Showers of Snow and Sleet. At 6 pm took in the Topsails and at 8 the Mainsail and brot to under Foresail and Mizen. In the Morn made sail under Courses and Topsails and made the Signal for the Adventure to go a head. At 6 saw an Island of Ice to the Westward,[1] the Wind abating Loosed all the Reefs out of the Topsails, got Spritsail and Topsail Yards across and made the Signal for the Adventure to come under our Stern.

FRIDAY 11*th. Therm.* 34. *Winds N to Wt. Course S* 28° *E. Distce sail'd* 65 *miles. Latd in South* 51°37′. *Longd in East of Greenwh* 25°28′. *Longd in pr. Kendalls Watch* 25°28′. *Longd made C. G. Hope* 3°7′. Fresh gales Fogy and Hazy with Snow & Sleet. At 1 pm saw an Island of Ice right a head distant one Mile, which the Adventure took for land and made the Signal accordingly[2] and hauled her Wind till I made the Signal for her to come in under our Stern.[3] Reef'd the Topsails and sounded

[1] A . . . being then in the Latitude of 50°40′ South and Longitude 2°20′ East of the Cape of Good Hope.

[2] 'Passed very near to a large Island of Ice, which we mistook for land, at first, as did also the Adventure. This Island, I conceive, was at least twice as high above the Water as our Top Gallt Mast head, and appeared to be like those which I saw in Hudson's Straights in every respect, except that its top & sides were quite smooth & straight, & I never saw any there which were so.'—Wales. Burney, Ferguson MS, explains the mistake made now, as at other times when large 'ice islands' were sighted, until they became a commonplace: 'When the Sun shines and the Sky is clear they are of a fine light blue & transparent, in bad dirty weather they resemble Land coverd with snow the lower part appearing black'. On this day of fog, haze, snow and sleet no error, therefore, could have been more natural.

[3] *Fresh gales . . . our Stern:* A the weather coming hazy, I call'd the Adventure by signal under my stern, which was no sooner done than the weather became very hazy with snow and Sleet, in so much that we did not see an Island of Ice, which we were steering directly for, which we were less than a mile from, I judged it to be about 50 feet high, and half a mile in circuit, it was flat at top and its sides rose in a perpendicular direction, against which the sea broke exceeding high. Captain Furneaux at first took this Ice for land, and haul'd off from it untill call'd back by signal; as the weather was foggy, it was necessary to proceed with caution, . . . —Cf. Pickersgill: 'saw a Prodigious large Island of Ice, about a mile ahead which we took first for land so striking was the Appearence that the Adventure (who was astern of us) brot too & made ye Signal for Seeing Land, thus had we parted she would have reported us to be lost and with great reason for I never saw any greater resemblence of land in My life, nor could I have immagin'd that such a vast Body of Ice could have been form'd together, for it was at least 300 feet high above the water and Ice in general Swims ⅞ under water, its Length near half a Mile and in form a Pyramid. . . .' [AM] 'NB We being Now across M. Bouvets track to ye Eastwd of Cape Circumcision, expect to find land hourerly, tho' sailing here is render'd very Dangerous,

but had no ground at 150 f^{m} Spent the night makeing short trips under an easy Sail, the Wind blowing fresh in Squals with Sleet & Snow.[1] In the Morn stood to the Southward with the wind at West. A little before noon pass'd two Islands of Ice one on each side. Saw some Birds which were about the size of Land Pigions, shaped like Fulmers, Plumage White as Snow, with blackish Bills and feet. I believe them to be intirely new as I never saw any such Sea Birds before[2] and Mr Forster has no knowlidge of them.[3]

SATURDAY 12*th. Winds NW, North, & NW. Course S* 20½° *W. Distce sail'd* 71 *miles. Latd in South* 52°56′. *Longd in E. Greenwhich Reck.g* 20°50′. *Longd made C. G. Hope* 2°27′ *East.* Fresh gales and Hazy Foggy weather with sleet and snow. In the PM stood to the SW with the Wind at West & WNW which in the night veer'd to North at which time the Therm^{r} was one degree below the Freezing point, kept on a wind all night under an easy sail and in the Morn made all the Sail we could and Steer'd SW with the Wind at NW. Pass'd Six Islands of Ice this 24 hours, some of which were near two Miles in circuit and about 200 feet high,[4] on the Weather side of them the Sea broke very high, some Gentlemen on Deck saw some Penguins.[5]

Excessive Cold, thick snows, Islands of Ice very thick sometimes 40 in sight at once, the people Numb'd, ye Ropes all froze over with Ice & ye Rig^{g} & Sails all covered with Snow, such is the dispossion of ye Crew that every Man seems to try who shall be foremost in ye readest performance of his duty which calls for ye loudest acknowledgem^{ts} under such rigorous circumstances.'

[1] At ½ past 3 a.m., says Clerke, they carried away the fore topmast spring stay, 'which was so hard with Ice that we cou'd not at present splice it again'.

[2] A ... I beleive them to be of the Petrel tribe and Natives of these Icy sea's.

[3] The Snow-Petrel, *Pagodroma nivea* (Forst.)

[4] 'Pass'd by an Island of Ice—I believe as high as the Body of St Pauls Church.'—Clerke 8951.—'Pass'd by an Isl^{d} of Ice ½ a Mile in length, & I suppose 60 feet high, the Sea frequently breaking over it.'—Burr. The different estimates of height are interesting; cf. Wales: 'This afternoon passed pretty near to a large Island of Ice, and several small pieces. The Island was not very high; but I took the pains to measure its length, by taking the Angles subtended by it, & its bearings at two stations, & found it about half a mile. The sea broke frequently over it & yet was it not washed into gutters thereby but quite smooth and even—I therefore suppose it had not been long drove out to sea. We also saw a Pengwin.'

[5] A ... we was oblig'd to proceed with great caution on account of the Ice Islands, six of which we pass'd this day, some of them near two miles in circuit and 60 feet high and yet the sea broke quite over them, such was the force and height of the waves which broke against them and ex[h]ibits a view, which for a few moments is pleasing to the eye, but when one reflects on the danger this occasions the mind is fill'd with horror, for was a ship to get against the weather side of one of these Islands when the sea runs high she would be dashed to pieces in a moment; since we have got among the Ice Islands the Albatrosses have left us, that is, we see but one now and then nor do our other companions, Pintadoes, Sheerwaters, Small grey birds, Fulmars, &c^{a} appear in such numbers, on the other hand, Pinguins begins to make their appearance, two of these birds were seen to day ...—ADV '... we likewise saw 6 or 8 Penguins which seemed to have a Comb on the head like a Cock fesant, which is different from what I saw at the Cape in that part, other parts being to Appearance the Same.'—Bayly, 10 December. These penguins would be *Eudyptes*, but the species is hardly identifiable. The Cape penguin is the Jackass, *Spheniscus demersus* (Linn.).

SUNDAY 13*th*. *Therm.* 31½. *Winds North, NW to SW. Course S* 10° *E. Distce sail'd* 65 *miles. Latd in South* 54° 0′. *Longd in E. Greenwhich Reck.g* 21°9′. *Longd made C. G. Hope* 2°46′ *East.* Continued a SW Course With the Wind at NNW untill 8 pm then hauld close under our Topsails, the Wind soon after came to the west and in the Morn to SW and freshen'd, Hazey with Snow and Sleet all the 24 hours, the Thermometer generally below or at the freezing point so that our Sails and Rigging were chequered with Ice.[1] Pass'd 18 Islands of Ice, many loose pieces and saw more Penguins.[2]

MONDAY 14*th*. *Therm. In the Night* 29. *Winds Westerly. Course S* 34° *E. Distce sail'd* 66 *miles. Latd in South* 54°55′. *Longd in E. Greenwhich Reck.g* 22°13′, *Watch* 22°1′. *Longd made C. G. Hope* 3°50′. Fore and Middle parts fresh gales and hazy with showers of Snow. Stood to the SSE with the Wind at SW from Noon till 8 pm in which time twenty Islands of Ice[3] presented themselves to our View. We now sounded but found no ground with 150 fathoms of line. Tacked and stood to the northward under an easy sail untill Midnight then stood to the South and in the Morn set the Courses and staysails. At half past six we were stoped by an immence field of Ice[4] to which we could see no end,[5] over it to the SWBS we thought we saw high land, but can by no means assert it. We now bore away SSE, SE & SEBS as the Ice trended, keeping close by the edge of it, where we saw many Penguins and Whales and many of the Ice Birds, small grey Birds and Pintadoes. At 8 o'Clock bro^t to under a Point of the Ice and sent on board for Captain Furneaux, fixed on Rendizvouze in case of seperation, agreed on some other matters for the better keeping Company and after breakfast he return'd to his Sloop and we made sail along the Ice, but before we hoisted the boat in we took up several pieces which yeilded fresh Water, at Noon had a good

[1] A . . . they were all hung with Icikles.—'So very cold this last 24 hours that great part of ye Sheep bro^t from ye Cape died; Served fresh Mutton to ye People.'—Pickersgill.

[2] A . . . At Noon we were in the Latitude of 54°00′ South, which is the Latitude of Cape Circumcision discover'd by M. Bouvet in 1739, but we were ten degrees of Longitude East of it, which is near 118 Leagues in this Latitude.—Cook, in long. 21°9′, was working on the Admiralty definition of the longitude of Cape Circumcision, which was 11°20′ East.

[3] A . . . of various extent both for height and circuit.

[4] A . . . low Ice.

[5] A . . . either to the East, West or South; in different parts of this field were Islands or hills of ice like those we found floating in the Sea, and some on board thought they saw Land also over the Ice bearing SWBS. I even thought so myself, but changed my opinion upon more narrowly examining these Ice Hills and the various appearances they made when seen through the haze, for at this time it was both hazy and cloudy in the Horison, so that a distant Object could not be seen distinct.—The romantic Pickersgill was much struck with the 'Variety of shapes' among the 'very high Mountains of Ice . . . such as churches, Pillars, houses, forts & a Number of other things'.—This was unusually far north to meet the pack ice in December.

observation both for determining the Latitude and Longitude by the Watch.

TUESDAY 15*th. Winds NW, North, NE, NW. Course S* 47½ *E. Distce sail'd* 23 *miles. Latd in South* 55°10′. *Longd in Greenwich pr. Reck.g* 22°43′. *Longd in C. G. Hope* 4°20′. Gentle breezes and pretty clear weather in the PM, steer'd SE along the edge of the Ice till one o'Clock when we came to a point round which we hauled SSW there appearing a Clear sea in that direction, after running 4 Leagues upon this Course (always along the edge of the Ice) we found our selves in a manner surrounded by it which extended from the NNE round by the West and South to the East farther then the Eye could reach in one compact body, some few places excepted, where Water was to be seen like Ponds, in other places narrow creeks run in about a Mile or less, high hills or rather Mountains of Ice were seen within this Feild ice and many Islands of Ice without in the open Sea, Whales, Penguins and other Birds.[1] At 5 o'Clock we hauld away East with the Wind at North in order to get clear of the Ice, the extream East point of which at 8 o'Clock bore EBS, over which there appeared clear Water. We spent the night standing off and on under our Topsails as also the remainder of the Day being so Foggy at times that we could not see a Ships length.[2] Betwixt 12 at night and 7 in the Morn 4 Inches thick of Snow fell on the Decks the Thermometer most of the time five degrees below the Freezing point so that our Rigging and sails were all decorated with Icikles. We found a Current setting SE about ¾ of a Mile p^r hour,[3] at the same

[1] '... we have often been amused today with the Appearence of land but I beleave the whole to be a Deception.'—Log.

[2] A ... and we had much difficulty to avoide the many Islands of ice that surrounded us;

[3] '[9 AM] Bro't too, hoisted the Jolly Boat out to try the Current. [10] It came on a Thick Fog: fired a Swivel & Musquets for the Boat, & beat the Drum. At 11 Spoke the Adventure which our Boat had got on board of, She came on board, hoisted her in & found the Current to set SSE ½ a Mile an Hour'.—Cooper. Forster (I, pp. 99–100) makes a great deal of this little episode, with due acknowledgement of the care of Providence; Wales and the senior Forster were in the boat. Wales gives us less drama, less moralizing, and more science: 'Went with the Master in the boat to try the Current & heat of the sea.... Whilst we were doing this so thick a fog came on that we could not find the ship. About noon we fortunately found the Adventure and soon after saw ye Resolution & got on board. Thinking this a proper opportunity of trying ye state of the Air with respect to Electricity, I got my Apparatus over the Tafferel of the Ship....' This latter experiment was not successful —probably, he thought, because of the wind. Wales's 'Apparatus' was evidently a conducting rod, perhaps in sections, of the type described in Franklin's *Experiments and Observations on Electricity* (1751; 6th ed., 1774) and successfully used for the observation of atmospheric electricity in 1752 by John Canton in London and Charles Lemonnier in Paris. The apparatus was not among the equipment provided for Wales by the Board of Longitude, and it may have been supplied by or for Banks, whose bills relating to this voyage include one for 'rods' for this purpose; '2 rods to try the Electricity of ye foggs', for which he paid Edward Nairne 12s.—Mitchell Library, 'Voluntiers', p. 145. No record of Wales's observations was published.

time a Thermometer which in the open air was at 32°, in the Surface of the Sea 30° and after being Imerged 100 fathoms deep for 20 Minutes came up at 34° which is only 2° above freezing.[1]

WEDNESDAY 16*th. Winds NW. Course S* 30° *E. Distce sail'd* 2 *miles. Latd in South* 55°8′. *Longd in Greenwich pr· Reck.g* 22°45′. *Longd in C. G. Hope* 4°22′. Very thick Foggy weather with Snow, so that we could do nothing but make short boards first one way and then a nother. Thermometer generally at the freezing point and some times below it, Rigging and Sails hung with Icikles. Many Whales playing about the Ship.[2]

THURSDAY 17*th. Therm.* 33½. *Winds NW. Course S* 76° *E. Distce sail'd* 34 *miles. Latd in South* 55°16′. *Longd in Greenwh pr. Reck.g* 23°43′. *Watch* 23°28′. *Longd made C. G. Hope* 5°20′ *East. Varn of the Compass* 20°50′ *West.* At 2 pm the Weather clearing up a little we made sail to the Southward and 4 Saw the Main field of Ice extending from SSW to SE[3] and soon after to East, which obliged us to bear up to the East. At 10 o'Clock hauled upon a Wind to the Northward with an easy sail, Wind at WNW a gentle gale, Foggy and Hazy with Snow. At 4 am we stood to the South and after runing two Leagues was obliged to bear up again for the Ice along the edge of which we Steer'd betwix'd SSW and East, hauling into every opening without finding any inlet, snow showers continued but at times it was pretty clear so as to inable us to get observations for the Watch, Variation and Latitude. Many Islands and a great Deal of loose Ice without the Main feild, at Noon we saw a large dark brown Bird on the Water, which some thought was a land Bird and could not rise out of the Water, accordingly we stood towards it to take it up, but we were soon convinced that it was upon its proper element, it seem'd to be of the Albatross tribe, tho' some would have it to be a Goose or a Duck,[4] besides this Bird and the White one before mentioned, we

[1] A . . . This experiment proves, I think, to a demonstration, that these large bodies or Islands of Ice must accumulate while they remain in these high southern Latitudes. [Note appended] I have sence, had occasion to alter this opinion, and to be well assured that they are continually wasting.

[2] At 6 p.m. 'we cannot see the Length of the Quarter Deck'.—Clerke 8951.—'. . . at 11 the Weather clearing up a little, saw many Ice Islands about us—these 24 hours we've abounded rather too plentifully in Foggs & Ice Islands—either one or other we can very well cope with, but both together is rather too much.'—Clerke.

[3] 'About 3 oClock we began to discover a whitish hue in the horizon extending from about SE to SW which I ascribed to a field of Ice, having always found it so in the Northern seas, and was laugh'd at for my information; however at 4 oClock such a field was discovered from the Mast head extending without opening from SSW to SE.'—Wales. The 'whitish hue' was, of course, the phenomenon known as 'ice-blink', caused by the reflection of light from the ice. It is seen in a drawing by Hodges (Fig. 19).

[4] Probably the Giant Petrel, *Macronectes giganteus* (Gm.), known also as Nellie or Stinker

have seen a nother new bird sence we came among the Ice which is about the size of a Pin·adoe, its plumage is brown and white, I however never had good sight of it.[1] A Seal was also seen to day & many Whales.

FRIDAY 18*th. Therm.* 31. *Winds NW to NE. Course N* 20° *E. Distce sail'd* 18 *miles. Latd in South* 54°57′. *Longd in Greenwh pr. Reckg.* 24°6′ *Longd made C. G. Hope* 5°43′ *East.* From Noon till 8 pm kept steering along the Ice, SSW, SE,[2] East & NNE as we found it to trend, more broken Ice and small Islands without the Main Feild than usual, in so much that we had continualy some along side.[3] At 8 we sounded but had no ground with 250 fathoms of line, after this we hauled close upon a Wind to the northward the evening being clear and serene (a rare thing here) we could see the firm Ice extending from SSW to NE but this happened not to be the nothern point: for at 11 o'Clock we were obliged to Tack to avoide it, at 2 am we stood again to the northward thinking to clear it upon this Tack, but at 4 o'Clock we found this could not be done, it extending to our Weather bow in somuch that we were quite imbayed,[4] we therefore Tack'd and stood to the Westward under all the Sail we could set, having a fresh breeze and clear weather, but the serenity of the sky lasted not long, at 6 o'Clock the Weather became hazey and soon after a Thick Fog. The gale freshened and brought with it snow and sleet which freezed on our Rigging and Sails as it fell, the Wind however veer'd more & more to the NE which inabled us to clear the Field Ice, though at the same time it carred us among the Islands which we had enough to do to keep clear of, of two evils I thought this the least. Dangerous as it is sailing a mongest the floating Rocks in a thick Fog and unknown Sea, yet it is preferable to being intangled with Field Ice[5] under the same circumstances. The danger to be apprehended from this Ice is the geting fast in it where beside the damage a ship might receive might be detaind some time.[6] I have heard of a Greenland Ship lying nine Weeks fast in this kind of Ice and at present we have no

[1] The Antarctic Petrel, *Thalassoica antarctica* (Gm.). See Fig. 20*a*.

[2] [PM] 'Running along a field of Pack'd Ice, which at ½ past 1 we saw trend away to the SE—a very large field—we can't see over it from our Mast Heads—think theres very little doubt but these bodies of Ice reach to the Shore—but am much afraid this land is so environ'd with Ice that we shall never be able to make a compleat discovery of it.'—Clerke 8951.

[3] A ... we saild amongst it the most part of the day, and the high ice Islands without us were innumerable;

[4] A ... being then in Latitude 55°8′ South, Longitude 24°32′

[5] *Field Ice:* A these immence fields or floats of ice

[6] *where ... time:* A a circumstance that would be exceeding alarming....—But as a matter of fact the pack ice was then breaking up. Cook could not know this, and he might well be intimidated by the prospect of being frozen in.

more appearence of thaw than they can have in Greenland; on the Contrary Fahranheits Thermometer keeps generally below the freezing point and yet it may be said to be the middle of summer. We have now sail'd 30 Leagues a long the firm Ice, which has extended nearly East and West, the Several Bays formed by it excepted, every one of which we have looked into without finding one open[g] to the South. I think it reasonable to suppose that this Ice either joins to or that there is land behind it and the appearence we had of land the day we fell in with it serves to increase the probabillity, we however could see nothing like land either last night or this Morn, altho' the Weather was clearer than it has been for many days past. I now intend, after geting a few miles farther to the North, to run 30 or 40 Leagues to the East before I haul again to the South, for here nothing can be done.[1]

I have two Men onboard that have been in the Greenland trade, the one of them was in a Ship that lay nine Weeks and the other in one that lay Six Weeks fast in this kind of Ice, which they call Pack'd Ice, what they call field Ice, is thicker, and the whole field, be it ever so large, consists of one piece, whereas this, which I call field Ice, from its immence extent, consists of many pieces of various sizes both in thickness and Surface, from 30 or 40 feet square to 3 or 4, packed close together and in places heaped one upon another, and I am of opinion would be found too hard for a Ships side that is not properly armed against it; how long it may have or will lay here is a point not easily determined; such Ice is found in the Greenland Seas all the summer long and I think it cannot be colder there in the summer than it is here, be this as it may, we certainly have no thaw, on the contrary, Fahranheets Thermometer keeps generally below the freezing point altho' it is the middle of Summer. It is a general opinion that the Ice I have been speaking of is formed in Bays and Rivers, under this supposission we were led to beleive that Land was not far off and that it even laid to the southward behind the Ice, which alone hindered us from approaching it, and as we had now sail'd above 30 leagues along the edge of the Ice without finding a passage to the south, I determined to run 30 or 40 leagues to the East, afterwards endeavour to get to the southward and if I met with no land or other impediment to get behind the Ice and put the matter out of all manner of dispute.—G, pp. 15–16.

SATURDAY 19*th. Winds NE to NW. Course N* 42° *E. Dist. Saild* 54 *Miles. Lat. in South* 54°17′. *Longd. in East of Greenwich* 25°19′. *East of*

[1] 'Pass'd some Small Ice that appear'd to be River Ice'.—Cooper.

Cape G. Hope 6°56′. *Var. of the Compass* 22°26′. Foggy, Hazy weather with Sleet Snow and rain, stood to the North West from Noon till 6 pm with the Wind betwixt the NE and North, which afterwards veer'd to the NWward, we then Tack'd and stood to the NE untill 3 am when we bore away East with the Wind at NW and NWBW, meeting frequently with Islands of Ice of different Magnitude both for height and circuit and some loose pieces.[1]

SUNDAY 20*th. Thermr.* 34. *Winds NW to NE. Course N* 79°30′ *E. Dist Sail'd* 92 *Miles. Lat. in South* 54°0′. *Longde in East pr. Reck.g* 28°14′. *Long. made C.G.H.* 9°50′. In the PM had thick hazy Weather untill 6 o'Clock when it cleared up and continued so till 6 am when the gale freshen'd at NNE and brought with it hazey weather Sleet and Snow the Thermometer from 31° to 34. Ice Islands as usual of various extent both for height and circuit. Set all the Taylors to Work to lengthen the Sleves of the Seamens Jackets and to make Caps to shelter them from the Severity of the Weather, having order'd a quantity of Red Baize to be converted to that purpose.[2] Also began to make Wort from the Malt and give to such People as had symptoms of the Scurvy;[3] one of them indeed is highly Scorbutick altho he has been taking of the Rob for some time past without finding himself benifited therefrom, on the other hand the Adventure has had two men in a manner cured by it who came, even, from the Cape highly Scorbutick. Such another large brown bird or Albatross as we saw near the feild Ice I saw near the Ship last night:[4] the common sort of Albatross seem not to like an Icey sea for we have only seen one now and then sence we came a mong the Islands.

MONDAY 21*st. Thermr.* 31 *to* 33½. *Winds North to West. Course S* 76° *E. Dist. Sail'd* 42 *Miles. Lat. in South* 54°10′. *Longde. in East pr. Reck.g* 29°24′. *Watch* 29°23′. *Long. made C.G.H.* 11°1′. *Var. of the Compass* 21°47′. Fresh gales and hazy with Snow untill 8 AM the gale then

[1] 'From one to two o'Clock [p.m.] we passed by 4 Islands of Ice: the thickness of the weather hindered us from seeing one of the largest of them untill we had not time to wear ship; there was therefore but one way, and that very unlikely, to go clear of it—we however did weather it by a few fathoms. The Adventure had just time to wear and go to leeward of it.'—Wales.

[2] A ... weather very hazy with sleet and snow, and more sensibly colder then the Thermometer seem'd to point out, in so much that the whole Crew complain'd, and in order to inable them to support it the better, I caused the sleves of their Jackets (which were so short as to expose their arms) to be lengthen'd with baize and had a Cap for each man made of the same stuff, together with Canvas, which proved of great service to them. —Pickersgill, 28 December, gets his usual odd-looking version: 'Serv'd the People Bays Caps Covered with canvas to prevent there Ears being froze bit'.—Sparrman says the contractors had skimped the cloth on the jackets, which may very well have been true.

[3] 'Brewed Wort for some of the People who began to have symptoms of the Scurvy. I suppose I shall be believed when I say that I am unhappy in being one of them'.—Wales.

[4] The Giant Petrel.

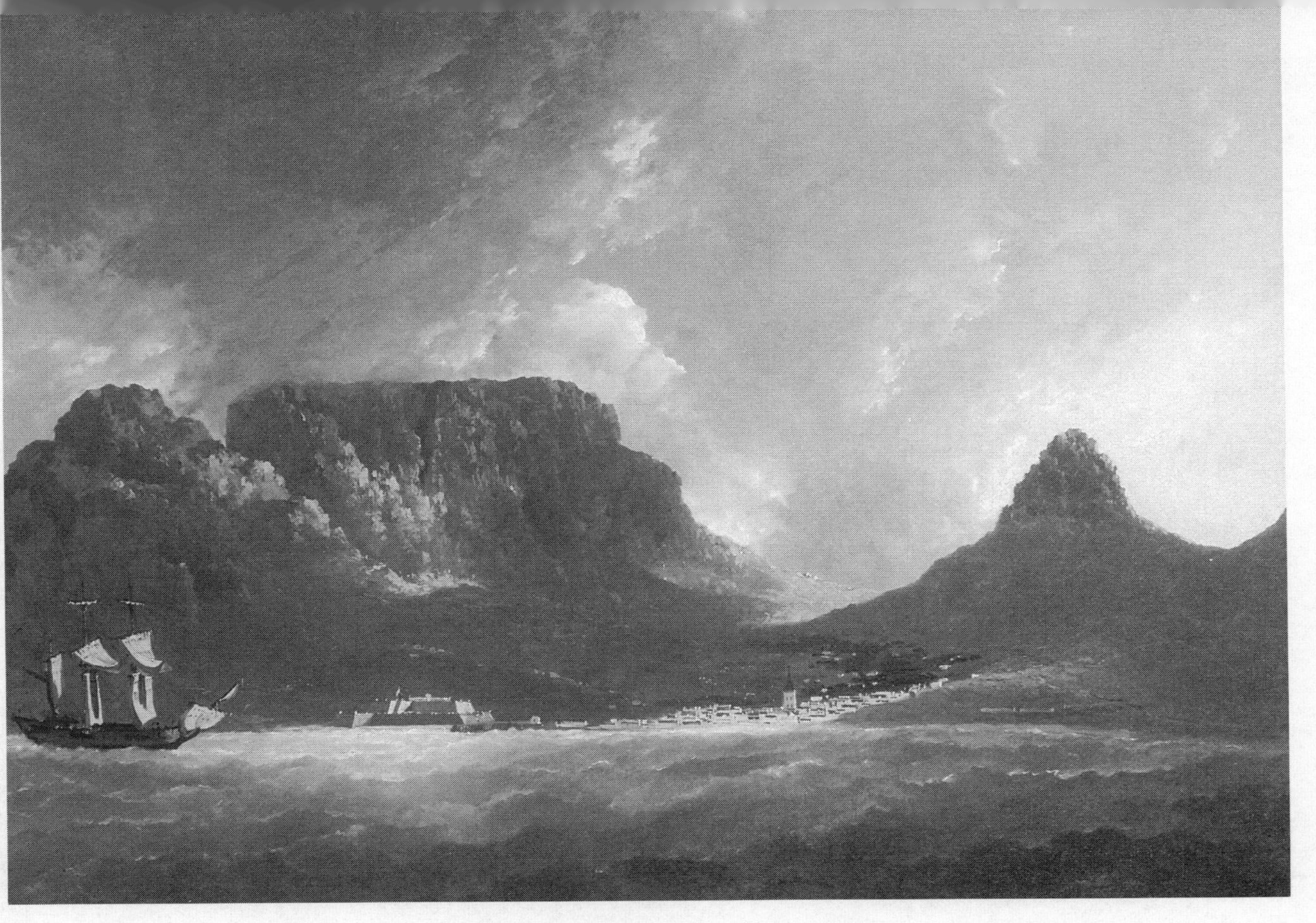

Fig. 14. Table Bay, November 1772

Oil painting by Hodges, in the National Maritime Museum

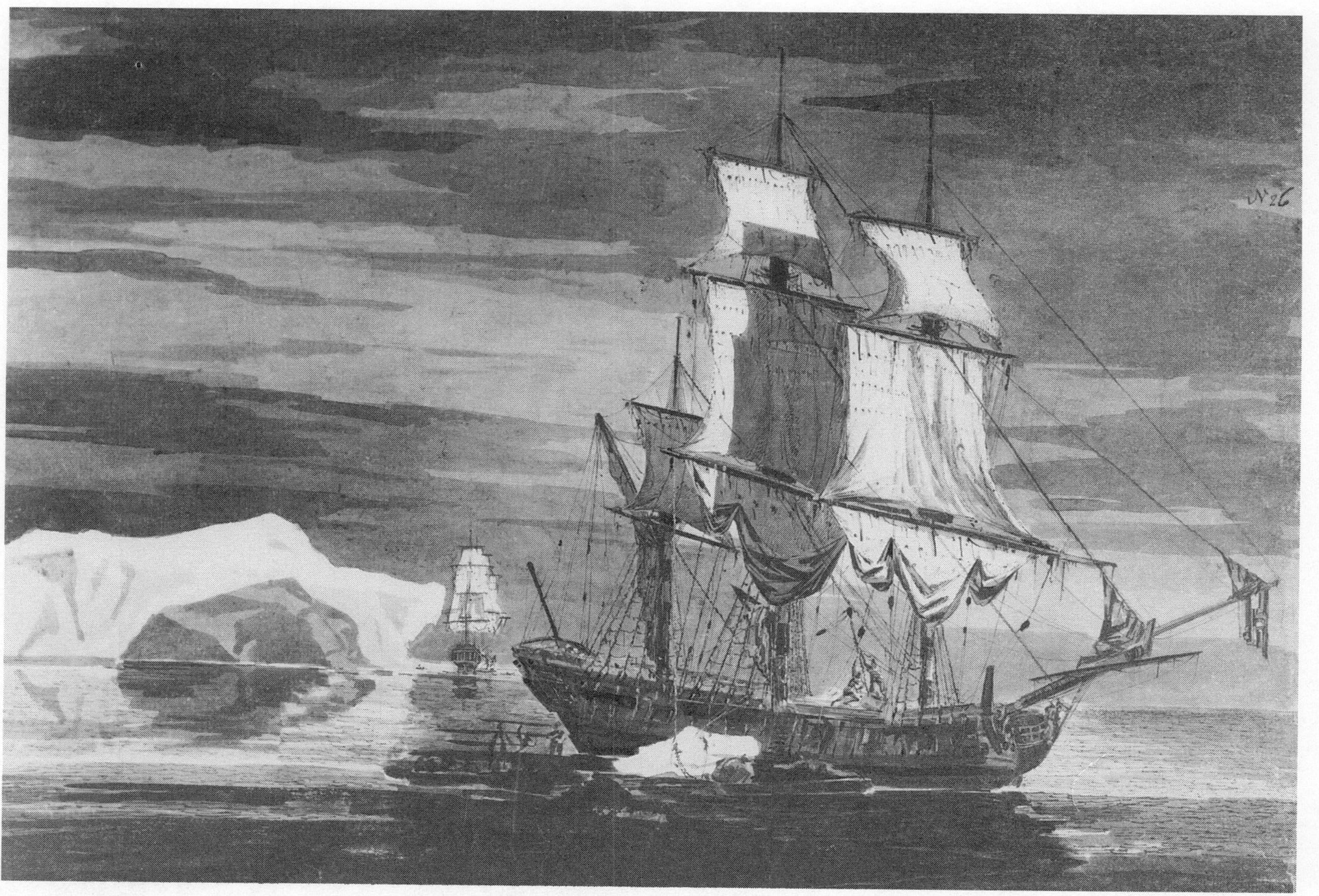

FIG. 15. The ships watering by taking in ice, in 61° S

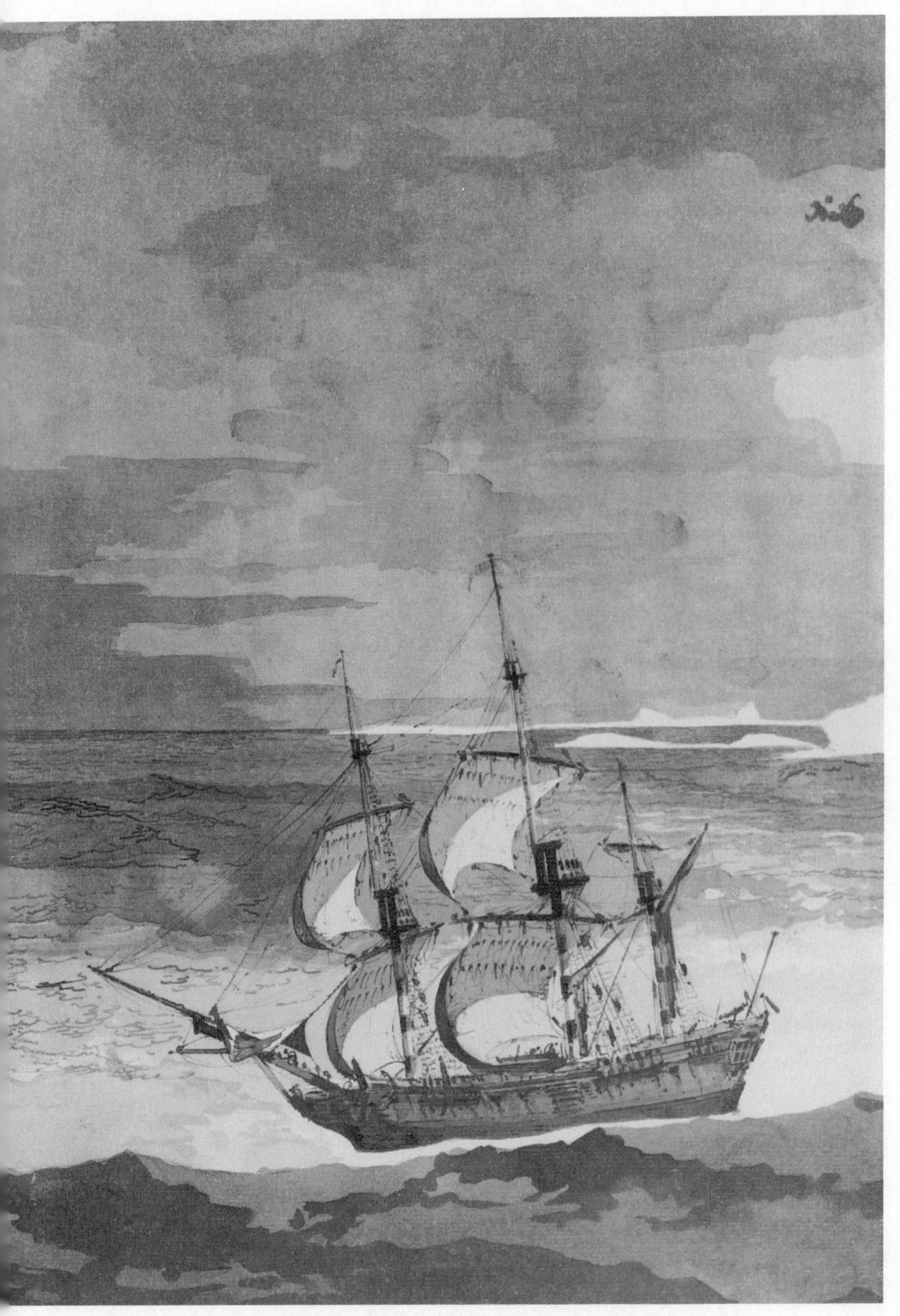

FIG. 16. The *Resolution* in a stream of pack-ice

Water-colour drawing by Hodges.—Mitchell Library, D11, no. 27a

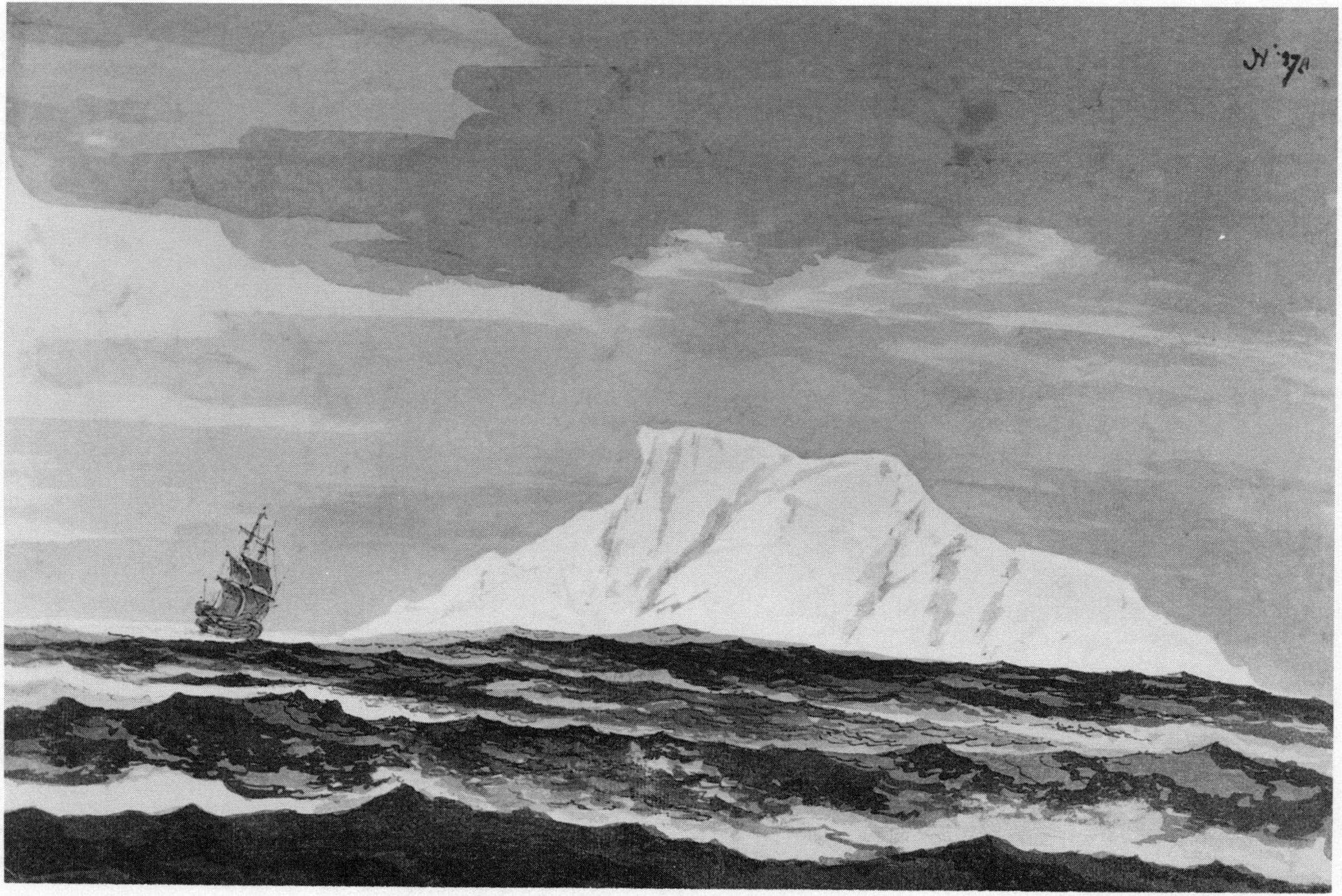

FIG. 17. The *Resolution* passing a tabular berg

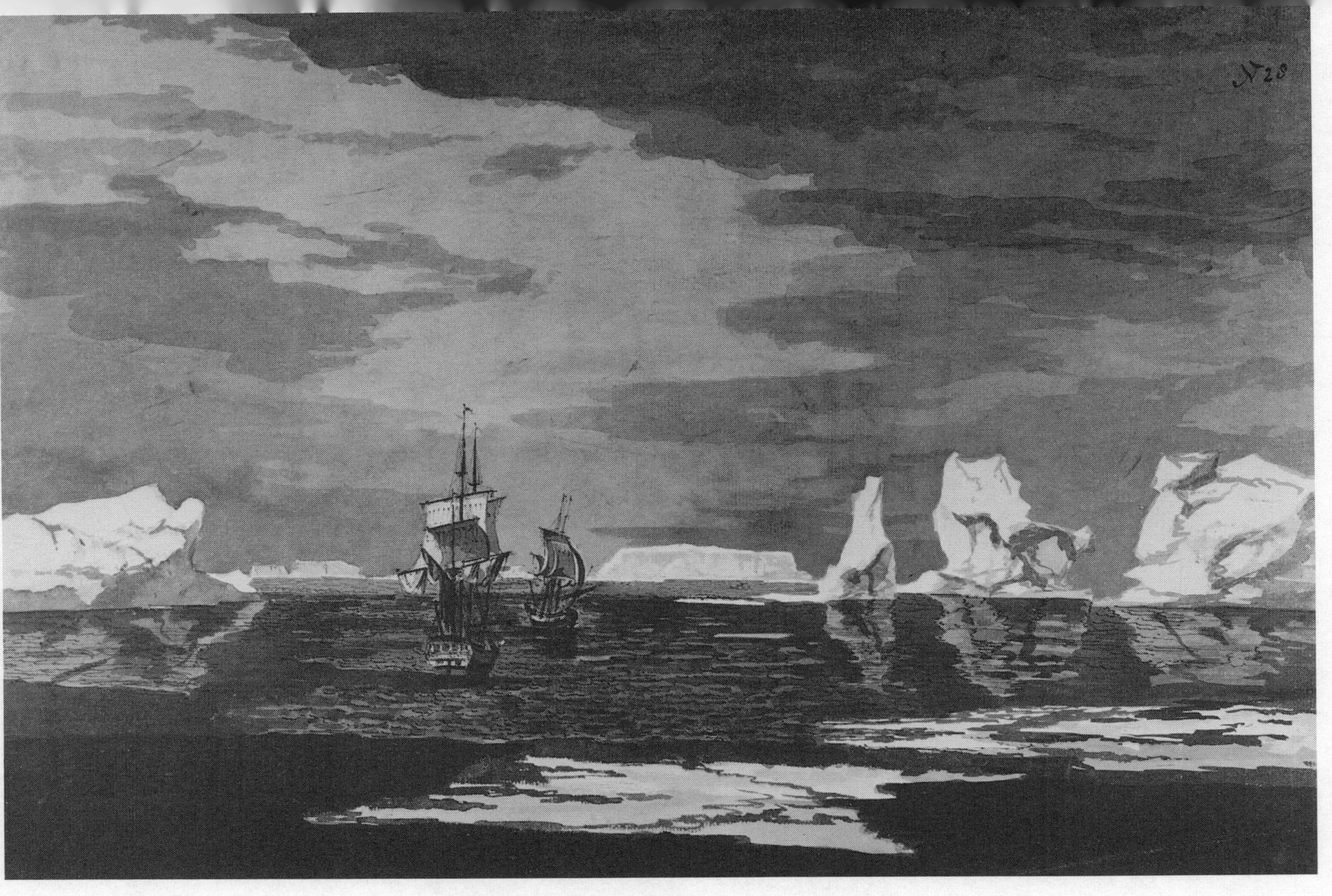

FIG. 18. The *Resolution* and *Adventure* among bergs

Water-colour drawing by Hodges.—Mitchell Library, D11, no. 28

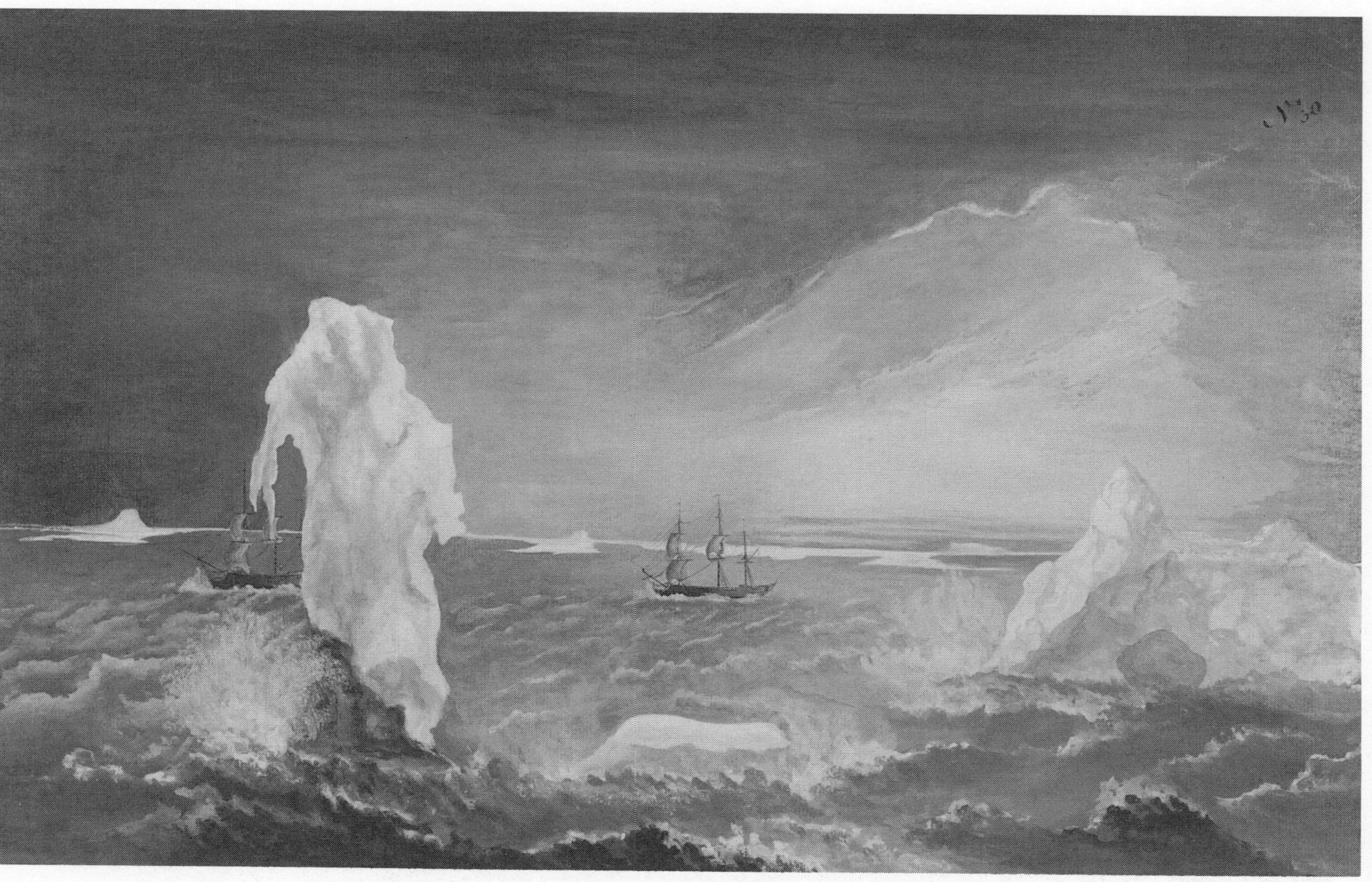

FIG. 10. The *Resolution* in the Antarctic

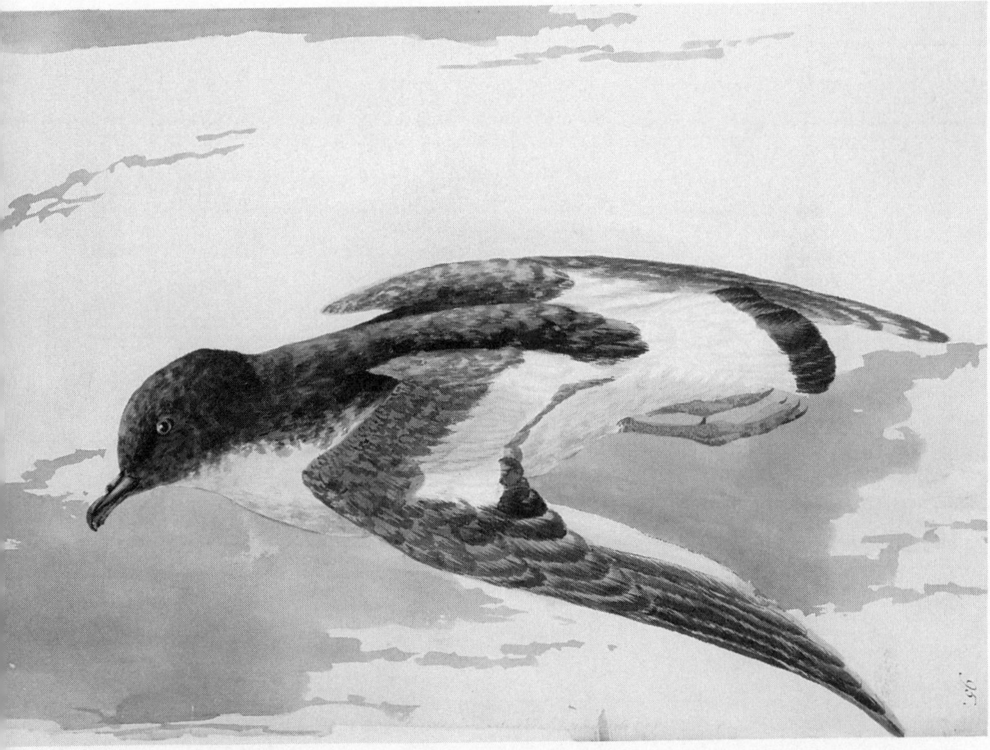

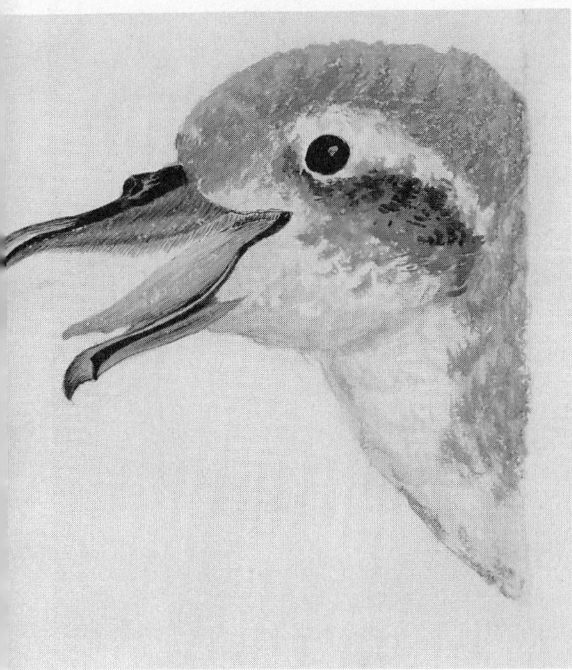

FIG. 20. Antarctic birds

(*above*) Antarctic Petrel; (*left*) head of Whale Bird. Drawings by George Forster in the British Museum (Nat. Hist.)—'Birds', pl. 95, 87

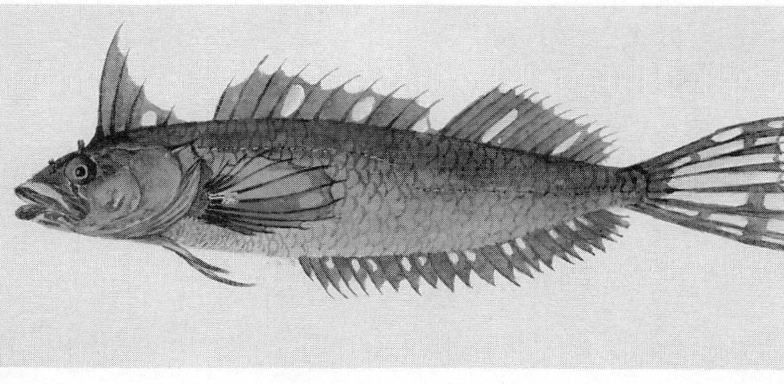

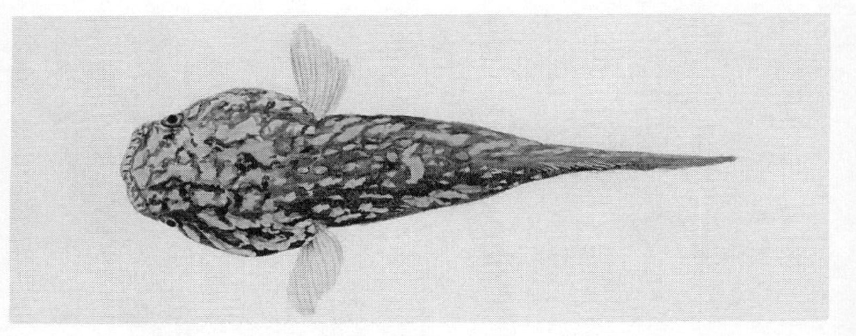

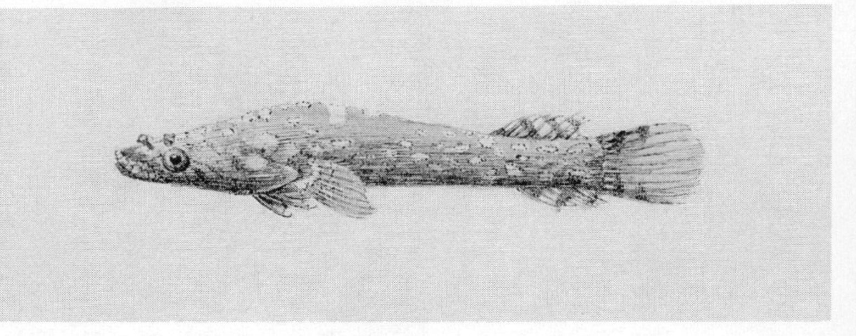

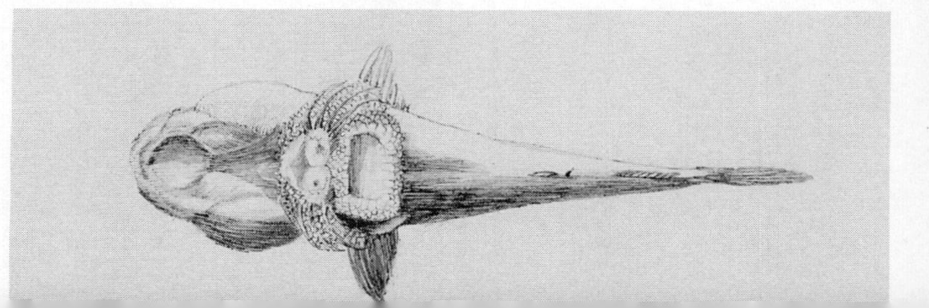

Fig. 21. New Zealand fishes

(above) *Blennius fenestratus*, Dusky Sound; (right) *Cyclopterus pinnulatus*, Queen Charlotte Sound. Drawings by George Forster in B.M. (N.H.)—'Fishes', II, pl. 186, 248

abating and the Weather clearing up, we hauld again to the Southward, the Course I now intend to Steer till I meet with Interruption. Ice Islands not so thick as usual nor quite so large. Had a Meridian observation to day which we have not had for some days past.

TUESDAY *22nd. Thermr.* 31½ *to* 33. *Winds NW to WSW. Course S* 32° *E. Dist. sail'd* 52 *mls. Lat. in South* 54°54'. *Longde. in East pr. Reck.g* 30°12'. *Long. made C.G.H.* 11°49'. Fresh gales, some times hazy with snow at other times tolerable clear. Stood South till 10 pm when seeing many Islands of Ice ahead we wore and stood under an easy Sail to the Northward till 3 am when we stood again to the Southward, but at 6 the thick Foggy weather made it prudent to stand again to the northward, at 8 the Wind came to West South West the weather cleared up, we Tacked and made all the Sail we could to the Southward, having seldom less than 10 or 12 Islands of Ice in sight.[1]

WEDNESDAY *23rd. Thermr.* 32 *to* 34. *Winds Westerly. Course S* 55° *E. Dist. Sail'd* 56 *Miles. Lat. in South* 55°26'. *Longd. in East of Greenwich pr. Reck.g* 31°33'. *Longd. from C.G.H.* 13°10'. *Var. of the Compass* 23°56'. Moderate gales and clowdy with some Showers of Snow and hail in the night. In the pm sounded but had no ground with 130 f^m^. In the am having but little Wind hoisted out a Boat to try the Current but found none, at the same time Mr Forster Shott some of the Small grey birds before mentioned which prov'd to be of the Petrel Tribe, they are rather smaller than our smallest Pigeons, the upper parts of their Boddys & Wings and their feet and Bills are of a blue grey colour, their billies and under parts of their wings are White a little tinged with blue, the uper Side of their quil feathers are dark blue tinged with black, this continues in a darkish blue strake along the upper part of the Wing and crosses the back a little above the tail and is very conspicuous when the Bird is on the Wing, the Bill is much broader than any other of the same tribe and the Tongue remarkably large. I shall for distinction sake call them Blue Peterls.[2] Having not much Wind and the day being such as would be called a tolerable good Winters day in England Cap Furneaux dined with us and returned on board in the evening.

THURSDAY *24th. Thermr.* 31 *to* 34. *Winds NW to NE. Course S* 7° *W.*

[1] 'People very hearty considering the damp sleety W^r^'.—Mitchel.

[2] A . . . these blue Petrels, as I shall call them, are seen no where but in the Southern Hemisphere from the Latitude of 28° and upwards.—The Broad-billed Prion or Whale Bird, *Pachyptila vittata* (Forster). The name Blue Petrel is nowadays given to *Halobaena caerulea* (Gm.), a bird very similar in shape and size to the prions and often to be found in company with them. See Fig. 20*b*.

Dist. Sail'd 65 *Miles. Lat. in South* 56°31'. *Longd. in East of Greenwich pr. Reck.g* 31°19' *Watch* 31°30'. *Longd. from C.G.H.* 12°56'. Gentle Breezes and clowdy, got up Topg[t] yards & Set the Sails, Isl[ds] of Ice as usual.

FRIDAY 25*th. Thermr.* 31 *to* 35½. *Winds East to South. Course S* 64½° *W. Dist. Sail'd* 88 *Miles. Lat. in South* 57°50'. *Longd. in East of Greenwich pr. Reck.g* 29°32'. *Longd. from C.G.H.* 11°9'. Gentle gales fair & Clowdy. Therm[r] from 31 to 35. At 2 pm being near an Island of Ice which was about 100 feet high and four cables in circuit I sent the Master in the Jolly Boat to see if any Fresh Water run from it, he soon returned with an account that their was not one Drop or the least appearence of thaw. From 8 to 12 am Sailed thro' several Floats or fields of loose Ice extending in length SE and NW as far as we could see and about ¼ of a Mile in breadth, at the same time we had several Islands of the same composission in sight. At Noon seeing that the People were inclinable to celebrate Christmas Day in their own way, I brought the Sloops under a very snug sail least I should be surprised with a gale [of] wind with a drunken crew,[1] this auction was however unnecessary for the Wind continued to blow in a gentle gale and the Weather such that had it not been for the length of the Day one might have supposed themselves keeping Christmas in the Latitude of 58° North for the air was exceeding sharp and cold.[2]

SATURDAY 26*th. Thermr.* 35 *to* 31. *Winds Southerly. Course S* 64½° *W. Dist. Sailed* 69 *Miles. Lat. in South* 58°31'. *Longde. East of Greenwich Reck.g* 27°37'. *Longd. made from C.G.H.* 8°34'. *Var. Compass* 19°25' *West.* Fresh gales fair & Clowdy till towards Noon when it cleared up and we had a very good observation; in the Course of this Days sail we

[1] 'Close reef'd y[e] Topsails & hauled y[e] mainsail expecting that y[e] people will be very soon not be [*sic*] in a Condition to take in sail should it be want[g] many Islands of Ice in sight.'—Log.

[2] A ... the weather was fair and cloudy, the air sharp and cold attended with a hard frost and altho this was the middle of summer with us, I much question if the day was colder in any part of England; at noon I brought the Sloops under a snug sail, seeing that the Crew were inclinable to celebrate the day in their own way, for which purpose they had been hording up liquor for some time past, I also made some addition to their allowance, had as many of the Officers and Petty Officers to dinner in the Cabbin as we [could] find room for, and the rest were entertain'd in the Gunroom, and mirth and good humor reigned throughout the whole Ship; the Crew of our consort seem'd to have kept Christmas day with the same festivity, for in the evening they rainged alongside of us and gave us three Cheers.—'Mirth and good humor' among the sailors, Forster translates as 'savage noise and drunkenness'.—I, p. 102. Besides getting boisterously drunk, adds Sparrman, the crew entertained themselves 'in fighting in the English fashion, which is called boxing'; and goes on for a number of pages to describe the passions and courtesies of this bloody sport.—pp. 12–16.

passed thro' Several Feilds of Broken loose Ice all of which lay[1] in the direction of NW and SE.[2] The Ice was so close in one that it would hardly admitt of a Passage thro, the pieces of this Ice was from 4 to 6 or 8 Inches thick, broke into various sized pieces and heaped 3 or 4 one upon the other, it appeared to have been constituted from clear water which occasioned some on board to think that it came from some River. The Ice in some other of the loose feilds appeared like Corral Rocks, honey combed and as it were rotten and exhibited such a variety of figuers that there is not a animal on Earth that was not in some degree represented by it.[3] We supposed these loose feilds to have broken from the large feild we had lately left and which I now determined to get behind, if possible, to satisfy my self whether it joined to any land or no.[4] To Day we saw some of the White Albatross with black tiped Wings,[5] some of the snow birds or White Peterls,[6] Blue Peterls &c and a nother kind of a Peterls, which are a good deal like the Pintadoes,[7] these as well as the White we have seen no where but a mong the Ice and but few at a time.

SUNDAY 27th. *Thermr.* 31 *to* 36. *Winds South to SW. Course N* 80° *W. Dist. Sailed* 72 *Miles. Lat. in South* 58°19′. *Longde. East of Greenwich Reck.g* 24°39′. *Longd. made from C.G.H.* 6°6′. Gentle gales and pretty clear weather. At 6 in the pm found the Variation by several Azm^ths^ to be 19°25′ West, our Longitude at the same time by Mr Kendalls Watch was 7°48½′ East of the Cape of Good Hope. Soon after Saw Several Penguins which occasioned us to Sound, as it is a received opinion that these birds seldom go out of Soundings, we however found no ground with 150 fathoms of line.[8] In the am we saw more loose Ice but not many Islands and those but small. The Day being

[1] *all . . . lay:* A they were in general narrow, but of a considerable length.

[2] ADV 'at 6 [PM] Passd through a Field of Broken Ice about 4 Leagues Long Stretching from North to South at 9 AM Passd through Another Field of Ice which Shook the Ship Verry Much . . .'—Hergest. Furneaux tells us that on board the *Adventure* the small pieces of broken ice were called 'plumpers from the frequent strokes they gave the ship's bows'.—Add. MS 27890, f. 3.

[3] *that . . . it:* A (as can hardly be conceived).—ADV Bayly, 20 December, exhibited more emotion: 'It is impossible to describe the Appearance of these larg masses of Ice, they strike terror & at the same time the fine hollow caverns or grottos made by the continual beating of the Sea, & the fine Arches mad[e] under them together with the most lively colours caused by the reflection of the Sea Water which (as the Poet says) is [a] noble Awfull Sean.'

[4] A . . . with this view, I kept on to the Westward with a gentle gale at South and SSW.

[5] Old male Wandering Albatrosses have white plumage with conspicuously black tips to the wings.

[6] The Snow Petrel.

[7] The Antarctic Petrel.

[8] 'A great Number of Penguins about ye ship where these penguins comes, causes Much consternation in the Ship, for it is well Known penguins retire to Land in order to bring forth their Young yet we have no other signs of land, nay every Indication (Except ye Ice) to ye Contrary.'—Pickersgill. Cf. p. 69, n. 2 below.

pleasent and the Sea Calm, we hoisted out a Boat from which Mr Forster shott a Penguin & some other Birds (Peterls).[1]

MONDAY 28*th. Thermr.* 35. *Winds East. Course S* 69° *W. Dist. Sailed* 70 *Miles. Lat. in South* 58°44′. *Longde. East of Greenwich* 21°55′. *Longd. made from C.G.H.* 3°32′. Had it Calm untill 6 PM when a breeze Sprung up at EBN which in the am Increased to a fresh gale: Whilest it was Calm we sounded but found no ground with 220 fathoms.[2] At 8 in the am I made the Signal for the Adventure to spread 4 Miles on our Larboard beam, the Wind and Weather favouring this Evolution.

TUESDAY 29*th. Thermr.* 31 *to* 36. *Winds East. Course S* 72° *W. Dist. Saild* 90 *Miles. Lat. in South* 59°12′. *Longd. E. of Greenwh pr. Reck.g* 19°1′. *Long. Cape Good Hope* 0°38′ *E.* First part a fresh breeze, the remainder a gentle Breeze and clowdy with Showers of Snow. At 4 pm called in the Adventure by Signal, the Weather being so hazy that we could but just see her, and at 6 took a reef in the Topsails, having at this time Several Islands of Ice in sight.[3] A[t] 4 am Saw Several Penguin. Loosed the Reefs out of the Topsails and Set Topgt Sails.[4] To Wards Noon I sent on Board for Captain Furneaux in order to communicate to him a resolution I had taken of runing as far West as the Meridian of Cape Circumcision, provided we met with no impediment, as the Distance is now not more than 80 Leagues the Wind favourable and the Sea pretty clear of Ice.

WEDNESDAY 30*th. Thermr.* 36. *Winds ENE. Course S* 80° *W. Dist. Saild* 60 *Miles. Lat. in South* 59°23′. *Longd. E. of Greenwh pr. Reck.g* 17°1′. *Long. Cape Good Hope* 1°22′ *W.* First part gentle Breezes and clowdy with Snow, at half past 1 pm hauled to the Northward for an Island of Ice, thinking if there were any loose peices about it to take some on board to convert into fresh Water: at 4 brought too close under the lee of the Isld where we did not find what we wanted, but saw upon it about 90[5] Penguins. We fired two 4 pound Shott at them,

[1] A ... some of the Petrels were of the blue sort, but differ'd from those before mention'd in not having a broad bill and the ends of their tail feathers were tiped white instead of dark blue, but whether or no these were only the destinctions between the Male and Female was a matter desputed by our Naturalists.— The difference was nothing to do with male or female. The 'blue sort' here described is the Blue Petrel proper, *Halobaena caerulea*; the others were *Pachyptila* sp. Cf. p. 56, n. 1 above.

[2] Scientific investigation was not confined to the *Resolution*. ADV '... at 7 [PM] tryd the Heat of the Water at 100 Fathom Deep & found it 2 Degrees warmer than ye Air'.—Hergest.

[3] *having ... sight:* A being surrounded on all sides with Islands of Ice.

[4] A ... at noon we were by observation in ... Longitude 19°1′ East, which is 3° more to the westward then we were, when we first fell in with the field ice, so that it is pretty clear that it joind to no land, as was conjectured.

[5] Mr Mitchel took credit for precision: 'Pass'd an ice island which had 86 Pengwins upon it (I counted them)'. A accepts this precise number.

the one struck the Ice near them and the other went over the Island, but they seemed quite undisturbed at both;[1] this piece of Ice was about half a mile in circuit, the West side on which the Penguins were ran sloping from the Sea like the roof of a house to the height of 100 feet and upwards for we lay for some Minutes with every sail becalmed under it.[2] In the night had little wind which did not increase till towards noon, some times clear and at other times hazey weather; at 9 am shott one of the White Birds upon which we put a Boat in the Water to take him up and by that means Shott a Penguin which weighed 11½ lb these Penguins differ only in some Minute particular[3] from those found in other parts of the World, their progression in the Water is however different to any I have seen, instead of swiming like other Birds, they leap or scip something like the Fish known to Seamen by the Name of scip Jacks.[4]

[1] 'Haul'd up for an Ice Island to try to get water which we are now in Much want of but found None. Saw on the Island a Number of those live things which we found to be Penguins, they set errect on their Leggs ranged in regular lines, which with their Breast's forms a very Whimsical appearence we fired two 4 Pounders at them but Mist them after which they wheeld off three deep and March down to y[e] water in a Rank (they Seemd to perform their Evolutions so well that they only wanted the use of Arms to cut a figure on Whimbleton Common)'.—Pickersgill—'. . . fir'd a shot at them some time afterwards they walk'd leisurely down the side of the Island into the sea.'—Gilbert. Wimbledon Common was a great centre for military exercises.

[2] A . . . it is a receiv'd opinion that Pinguins never go far from Land and that the sight of them is a sure indication of the vicinity of Land, this opinion may hold good where there are no Ice Islands, but where such are, these birds as well as many others, which usualy keep near the shores, finding a roosting place upon these Isl[ds] may be brought by them a vast distance from any land; it will however be said that they must go ashore to breed, probably the Females are there and these are only the Males which we saw; be this as it may, I shall continue to take notice of these birds when ever we see them, and leave every one to judge for themselves.—Clerke, as well as Pickersgill (p. 67, n. 8 above), thinks about the same subject: 'The meeting with Penguins has ever been suppos'd a sign of the vicinity of some Land but we've met with so many and are still at a loss for the least bit of Earth, that I begin very much to doubt that old (and I believe universally reciev'd) opinion as 'tis here evident they travel upon Islands of Ice which are Vehicles that may carry them an immense distance. . . . at 5 AM saw a Seal another suppos'd sign of Land.' In 8951 he adds, 'think 'tis by no means impossible nor improbable that they may bread on these Isles of Ice so that meeting them may give reason to suppose you may be near either an Isle of Earth or of Ice'. Wales throws in a sceptical note: '. . . It was thought by some that they might even breed here; but this seems however not probable, as the heat necessary to hatch the Eggs would melt the Ice where they lay and thereby defeat the very purpose it was intended to effect.' This reason against breeding, though a natural *a priori* one, was not valid. Wales did not know enough about penguins. Those that breed on ice hold their eggs on top of the feet, which thus insulate both the egg and the ice; the egg gets the necessary heat from the loose skin of the bird's lower abdomen, which forms a sort of enclosing purse over it. Nevertheless penguins do not breed on icebergs.

[3] A . . . distinguishable only to naturalists

[4] The penguin was the Antarctic Penguin, *Pygoscelis antarctica* (Forst.); Skipjack, *Katsuwonus pelamis* (Linn.), but see I, p. 166, n. 5. Cf. Wales, 26 December: 'This morning we saw prodigious numbers of Pengwins about the Ship. The progressive motion of these Birds in the water is odd enough; they do not swim like other Birds but leap forwards in the water by means of their Legs and Pinions, for they cannot be said to have wings. Their Note is not much unlike that of a Goose, which some of our People so happily imitated, that they could draw them almost close to the Ship's Side.' Cf. Fig. 75.

The White Bird is of the Petrel tribe, all its feathers are White; the Bill which is rather short is between Black & dark blue, and the Legs and feet blue.[1] Bouvet makes mention of these Birds when he was off Cape Circumcision.

THURSDAY 31*st. Thermr.* 31 *to* 36. *Winds East to SE. Course S* 60° *W. Dist. Sailed* 71 *Miles. Lat. in South* 59°58′. *Longd. in East of Greenwich pr. Reck.g* 16°19′. *Long. made from C.G.H.* 4°04′ *W.* PM Gentle gales and Clowdy, Steering WBS with some Ice Islands in Sight, at 8 o'Clock steer'd NW being nearly the direct course for Cape Circumcision. At Midnight seeing some loose Ice ahead we hauled three point more to the north in order to avoide it but the very reverse happened, for after standing an hour NBW the Ice was so thick about us that we were obliged to tack and Stand back to the Southward till half past 2 am, when we stood for it again thinking to take some up to serve as Water; but we soon found this impracticable, the Wind which had been at EBN now veered to SE and increased to a fresh gale and brought with [it] such a Sea as made it dangerous for the Sloops to lay among the Ice, this danger was much heightened by discovering at 4 o'Clock (being then in Lat 59°20′)[2] an immence field to the North of us, extending NEBE & SWBW in a compact body farther than the eye could reach, we were now near it[3] and already in the lose parts,[4] we immidiately wore, double reefed the Topsails, got our tacks on board and hauled to the Southward close upon a Wind, and it was not long before we got clear of the ice but not before we had receved several hard knocks for the pieces were of the largest sort.[5] Struck Topg^t yards, at Noon had strong gales and Clowdy hazy Weather and only one Ice Island in sight, indeed they are now become so familiar to us that they are generaly pass'd unnoticed. While we were in the ice a Seal was seen.

[JANUARY 1773]

FRIDAY 1*st. Thermr.* 31 *to* 31½. *Winds SE to SBW. Course S* 78° *W. Dist. Sailed* 66 *Miles. Lat. in South* 60°12′. *Longd. in East of Greenwich pr. Reck.g* 12°13′. *Long. made C.G.H.* 6°12′. PM Strong gales and Hazy, which obliged us to Close reefe our Topsails, and at 8 o'Clock to hand them, at which time we wore and stood to the East ward under our two Courses, having a hard gale blowing in Squals and

[1] The Snow Petrel.

[2] A . . . Longitude 15°30′ East.

[3] *now near it:* A not above two or three miles from the Main body.

[4] A . . . there was no time to deliberate.

[5] Cook had met the wide 'tongue' of ice that stretches out east from the Weddell Sea: p. lx above.

thick hazy weather with Snow and a very large Swell from the Eastward. At Midnight Wore and stood to the Westward, being in the Latitude 60°21′ s wind at South a strong gale which toward noon abate'd so that we could set our Topsails Close reefed, but the Weather still continued thick and hazy with Snow which ornamented[1] our Riging with Icikles.

SATURDAY *2nd. Thermr.* 31 *to* 32. *Winds S West. Course N* 48° *W. Dist. Sailed* 91 *Miles. Lat. in South* 59°12′. *Longd. in East of Greenwich pr. Reck.g* 9°45′ *Watch* 10°17′. *Long. made from C.G.H.* 8°38′. Fresh gales and hazy, with Showers of Sleet and Snow, till 9 am when it became fair and we loosed two Reefs out of the Topsails, the Wind had veered from South to West with which we stood to the Northward Pass'd 7 Ice Islands this 24 hours and saw some Penguins.

SUNDAY *3rd. Thermr.* 31 *to* 32. *Winds West, NW to NE. Course S* 82° *E. Dist. Sailed* 44 *Miles. Lat. in South* 59°18′. *Longde. in East of Greenwich pr. Reck.g* 11°9′. *Longd. made C.G. Hope* 7°14′. In the PM the Weather cleared up and we were favoured with a Sight of the Moon, which we had seen but once before sence we left the Cape,[2] we did not loose this oppertunity to observe the Distance betwixt her and the Sun, the Longitude deduced th[e]refrom was 9°34½′ East from Greenwich, being the mean of no less than 12 observations, Mr Kendals Watch at the same time gave 10°6′E and our Latitude was 58°53½′s. The Variation of the Compass by the mean of several Azimuths was 12°8′ West. We were now about 1½° or 2° of Longitude to the West of the Meridian of Cape Circumcision and at the going down of the sun 4°45′ of Latitude to the Southward of it,[3] the Weather was so clear, that Land even of a Moderate height might have been seen 15 Leagues, so that there could be no land betwixt us and the Latitude of 48°.[4] In short, I am of opinion[5] that what M. Bouvet took for Land and named Cape Circumcision was nothing but Mountains of Ice surrounded by field Ice. We our selves were undoubtedly deceived by the Ice Hills the Day we first fell in with the field Ice and many were of opinion that the Ice we run along join'd to land to the Southward, indeed this was a very probable supposission, the probabillity is however now very much lessened if not intirely set

[1] *which ornamented:* A which froze on the rigging as it fell and ornamented

[2] . . . by which a judgment may be formed of the kind of weather we have had since we have been at sea.

[3] . . . as it is laid down in Mr Dalrymple's chart

[4] Altered to 58°; and so also AH. In H the figure is inserted in Cook's hand.

[5] *15 Leagues . . . opinion:* G 14 or 15 leagues distance, which reduceth the extent of the land of Cape Circumcision to 70 or 80 leagues, which it cannot possibly exceed in the direction of North and South; it is however very probable . . .

a side for the Distance betwixt the Northern edge of that Ice and our Track to the West, South of it, hath no where exceeded 100 Leagues and in some places not Sixty, from this it is plain that if there is land it can have no great extent North and South, but I am so fully of opinion that there is none that I shall not go in search of it, being now determined to make the best of my way to the East in the Latitude of 60° or upwards, and am only sorry that in searching after those imaginary Lands, I have spent so much time, which will become the more valuable as the season advanceth.[1] It is a general recieved opinion that Ice is formed near land, if so than there must be land in the Neighbourhood of this Ice, that is either to the Southward or Westward. I think it most probable that it lies to the West and the Ice is brought from it by the prevailing Westerly Winds and Sea. I however have no inclination to go any farther West in search of it, having a greater desire to proceed to the East in Search of the land said to have been lately discovered by the French in the Latitude of 48½° South and in about the Longitude of 57° or 58° East.[2]

The Clear Weather continued no longer then 4 o'Clock in the AM, by that time the Wind had veered to NE and blowed a strong gale attended with a thick Fogg with snow and sleet which froze on the Rigging as it fell, the fine Even^{g} had tempted us to loose the Reefs out of the Topsails and get Topg^{t} yards across, but were now fain to get them down again & close reef the Topsails.

MONDAY 4*th. Winds NE to NNW. Course N* 82° *E. Dist. Sailed* 112 *Miles. Lat. in South* 58°55′. *Long. in East of Greenwich per Reck.g* 14°43′. *Long. Cape G. Hope* 3°40′. First and middle parts strong gales attended with a thick Fogg Sleet and Snow, all the Rigging covered with Ice and the air excessive cold,[3] the Crew however stand it tolerable well,

[1] ADV 'Standing now to the Eastward having given up our Searches after Cape Circumcision concluding if any such place, a small spot extending it self near East and West may be supposed from the Track we run down. The Feilds and Islands of Ice prevented our steering the Course we intended which detain'd us greatly, and now growing rather short of water with ye prospect too, of a long Passage, determin'd our departure'—Kemp, 5 January. Kemp was evidently a man who did some thinking for himself, and was reluctant to relinquish Cape Circumcision entirely; for he writes on the day after this: 'on the 14 of December last in the Morning, as we run down by a Feild of Ice, some had a notion they saw the Land, for my part I saw it not—neither do I beleive it was seen by any one—yet, I am of opinion that Land was not far distant from us by the quantity of Ice, both Feild's and Islands, which must have Drifted off from some Land & most likely from the Westward, being then nearly in the Latitude laid down of Cape Circumcision'.

[2] He refers to Kerguelen's discovery, which in fact lies 10½ to 12½ degrees farther east.

[3] . . . The Snow and Sleet continued till the Evening and as usual fixed on our Rigging as it fell, so that every Rope was covered with the finest transparent Ice I ever saw and afforded an agreeable sight enough to the Eye, but conve[ye]d to the mind an Idea of coldness much greater than it really was, and made the Sails and Rigging bad to handle. —f. 23.—Cf. Cooper: 'very hard Frost, the Rigging all glaz'd over with transparent Ice

each being cloathed with a fearnought Jacket, a pair of Trowsers of the same and a large Cap made of Canvas & Baize, these together with an additional glass of Brandy every Morning enables them to bear the Cold without Flinshing. At Noon we judged our selves to be in or near the same Longitude as we were when we fell in with the last Feild Ice and about Six Leagues farther to the North so that had it remained in the same place we ought to have been in the middle of it, or at least so many Leagues advanced within it; as it cannot be supposed that so large a body of Ice as that appeared to be could be wasted in so short a time as 4 Days, it must therefore have drifted to the northward and if so there can be no land to the north in this meridian, that is between the Latitude of 55° and 59° a part where we have not been and which I believe to be mostly covered with Ice, be this as it may, we have not only met with better weather, but much less Ice of every kind to the Southward of the above mentioned Latitudes, than we did to the northward. We had been steering ENE for some time with a view to make the Ice, but not seeing any thing of it we steer'd EBS½S in order to get to the Southward of our old Track.[1]

TUESDAY 5*th. Winds NW. Course EBS½S. Dist. Sailed* 159 *Miles. Lat. in South* 59°51′. *Long. in East of Greenwich per Reck.g* 19°40′. *Long. Cape G. Hope* 1°17′ *E.* Strong gales and Foggy with sleet and snow all the pm, in the am Moderate and fair with a large Sea from the NW which indicates no land near in that Quarter, in the Course of this days run we fell in with only 2 Islands of Ice.[2]

WEDNESDAY 6*th. Thermr.* 34½. *Winds NW. Course EBS. Distce. Sailed* 143 *Miles. Lat. in South* 60°18′. *Long. in East of Greenwich Reck.g* 24°21′. *Long. made C. G. Hope* 5°57′ *East.* Fresh gales am hazy attended with Snow Showers. We kept on to the East under all the sail we could carry having daylight the whole 24 hours round and the Weather realy milder than it was farther north, the gales more Moderate, and we are less incumbered with Ice having seen only four Islands this 24 hours.[3]

THURSDAY 7*th. Winds NW to West. Course S* 79°45′ *E. Distce. Sailed*

from the Mast head to the Deck & exceeding Cold'. Clerke: 'the frost is so severe and the Snow and Ice so thick and hard upon the Rigging that 'tis with great difficulty we render the Ropes through the Blocks—this has frequently been the case within this month past'.

[1] *be this . . . our old Track:* As we were now only going over a part of the Sea we had already made our selves acquainted with and for that reason wished to avoide it I directed the Course E by South half South, in order to get farther to the southward.—ff. 22v–23.

[2] 'the ice which fell from the Rigging measur'd 4 inches Thick.'—Mitchel.

[3] . . . indeed the Ice Islands were now so familiar to us that they were generally pass'd unnoticed.—f. 23.—'Mr Loggie Midshipman was Discharged from that Station for having had some Dispute with the Boatswain.'—Elliott.

126 *Miles. Lat. in South* 60°41′. *Long. in East of Greenwich Reck.g* 28°33′ *Watch* 28°8′. *Long. made C. G. Hope* 10°10′. Fresh gales and Hazy with frequent Showers of Snow, towards noon it cleared up and gave us an oppertunity to take some altitudes of the Sun to rectify our Longitude by the Watch and also to assertain the Latitude, Saw only three Islands of Ice and but few Birds.

FRIDAY 8*th. Thermr.* 35½. *Winds Westerly. Course S* 73° *E. Distce. Sailed* 135 *Miles. Lat. in South* 61°22′. *Long. in East of Greenwich Reck.g* 33°2′ *Watch* 32°33′. *Long. made C. G. Hope* 14°39′. *Var. of the Compass* 29°5′. Fresh gales and hazy with Showers of Snow. At 5 in the am being then in the Latitude of 61°12′, Long[d] 31°47′ E found the variation to be 29°5′ West.

SATURDAY 9*th. Thermr.* 35. *Winds NW. Lat. in South* 61°36′. *Var. of the Compass* 30°8′. Gentle gales and clowdy. In the PM passed Several Islands of Ice more than we have seen for some days past, and at 9 o'Clock came to one that had a quantity of loose Ice about it, upon which we hauled our Wind with a view to keep to windward in order to take some of it up in the Morn, at Midnight we tacked and stood for the Island, at this time the Wind shifted two or 3 Points to the Northward so that we could not fetch it, we therefore bore away for the next Island to Leeward which we reached by 8 o'Clock and finding loose pieces of Ice about it,[1] we hoisted out three Boats and took up as much as yeilded about 15 Tons of Fresh Water, the Adventure at the same time got about 8 or 9 and all this was done in 5 or 6 hours time; the pieces we took up and which had broke from the Main Island, were very hard and solid, and some of them too large to be handled so that we were obliged to break them with our Ice Axes[2] before they could be taken into the Boats, the Salt Water that adhered to the pieces was so trifleing as not to be tasted and after they had laid on Deck a little while intirely dreaned of, so that the Water which the Ice yeilded was perfectly well tasted, part of the Ice we packed in Casks and the rest we Milted in the Coppers and filled the Casks up with the Water; the Melting of the Ice is a little tideous and takes up some time, otherwise this is the most expeditious way of Watering I ever met with.[3]

SUNDAY 10*th. Winds NWBN to WNW. Course S* 54° *E. Dist. Saild* 37

[1] ... (part of which we our selves saw break from the Island) ...—f. 23.

[2] *Ice Axes:* Pic[k] Axes ...—f. 23. See the drawing by Hodges, Fig. 15.

[3] 'About 22[h] the Boats returned loaded with Ice, which were hauled into the Ship, and the Boats sent for another Cargo, of much more real value than Gold!'—Wales.—'We are now much distressd for want of Water & Keep a good lookout for a Convenient Opportunity to take on board some loose Ice in order to melt by which we hope to supply ourselves.'—Pickersgill, 8 January. [9 January, pm] 'Saw some loose Ice near an Ice

Miles. Lat. in South 61°58′. *Longd. in East pr. Reckg. Corrected* 36°7′ *Watch* 35°48′. *Long. made from C.G.H.* 17°44′. Gentle gales, first part fair and Clowdy, remainder hazy with showers of snow. In the PM hoisted in the Boats after having taken up all the loose Ice with which our Decks were full;[1] having got on board this seasonable supply of fresh Water,[2] I did not hesitate one moment whether or no I should steer farther to the South but directed my course South East by South, and as we had once broke the Ice I did not doubt of geting a supply of Water when ever I stood in need. We had not stood above one hour and a half upon the above Course before I found it necessary to keep away more East and before the Swell to prevent the Sloops from rowling occasioned in some measure by the great weight of Ice they had on their Decks which by 9 o'Clock in the Morning was a good deal reduced and the Swell gone down we resumed our former Course. By the drifting of the loose Ice I had reason to beleive that there was a Current Seting NW and the late difference between observations, the Watch and our reckoning confirms this, for while we were runing to the Westward the Ship outstriped the reckoning Eight or Ten Miles every Day, on the other hand in returning back to the East the reckoning was a head of the Ship and the error would have been nearly equal had we not made some allowance for it.

Island which was likely to Answer our purpose shortned sail & hauld our wind. Employ'd getting ready the boats [2 am] could not find the Island so bore away [6 am] Saw another stood for it, hauld close for it shortned sail & hoisted out all y[e] boats & took up y[e] decks-full of loose peices of Ice, which we found to yeild excellent water, as Every body was employed it afforded a very humorous sight, thus to see people buised some hacking away at a large peice of Ice, others drawing it up out of y[e] sea in basketts & I beleive is y[e] first Instance of drawing fresh water out of y[e] Ocean in hand basketts.'—Marra, pp. 7–8, describes the less humorous side of the work of picking up ice out of the water, 'whereby [the men's] arms in a very short space of time put on the appearance of icicles, and became so numbed as for the present to be totally incapable of use'. A number of the men got swollen jugular glands from drinking the ice water, says Sparrman, p. 23; also Forster, I, p. 107. Wales, going on his Hudson's Bay experience, laughed at this theory, *Remarks*, p. 22. The disease is obscure: possibly, my friend Dr Ernest Philipp suggests, lowered physical resistance in one or other of the crew, due to the cold and the diet, gave scope to some dormant organism which became virulent and spread as a throat infection, producing the glandular swellings in the neck. We can hardly blame the iceberg

[1] 'Put the people to watch & watch, employing them in breaking the ice very small, & filling the casks with it, the coppers melting it very slow—At noon had filled 13 butts'.—Mitchel. 'Employed as before. At noon had compleated; having filled 25 butts—the water of it proves exceedingly sweet & good'.—Mitchel, 11 January.

[2] . . . of which we stood in much need.—f. 23v.—'At ½ past 6 oClock hoisted in the Boats, and made Sail, with our *invaluable* cargo. It may possibly be usefull to remark that this method of watering, although rather more tedious on account of having the Ice to melt after it is on Board is notwithstanding greatly to be preferred to that of filling the Casks from the water which runs off the Islands, as is sometimes practised in Hudson's Straits, as this may be done with the greatest safety; whereas the other is attended with much danger to the Boats and people even there, and would be much more so here, in an open sea where the surf is almost continually breaking off large pieces from the sides of the Islands.'—Wales.

MONDAY 11*th. Thermr.* 35½. *Winds NNW to North. Course S.* 27¼° *E. Dist. Saild* 83 *Miles. Lat. in South* 63°12′. *Longd. in East pr. Reckg. Corrected* 37°29′. *Long. made from C.G.H.* 19°6′. *Variation of the Compass* 28°15′ *W.* Gentle gales and Clowdy with showers of Snow in the PM. In the Morn it was fair and so clear as to admit of our observing the Suns Azimuth by which we found the Variation of the Compass to be as p^r Column, being then in Latitude 62°44′, Long^d 37°0′ East. Islands of Ice continually in sight.

TUESDAY 12*th. Winds NE, East, & SE. Course S* 18½° *E. Dist. Saild* 63 *Miles. Lat. in South* 64°12′. *Longd. in East pr. Reckg. Corrected* 38°14′ *Watch* 37°47′. *Long. made from C.G.H.* 19°51′. *Variation of the Compass* 23°52½′. Gentle gales and Clowdy, at 4 in the AM it was clear and I took 12 observations of the Suns Azimuth with Mr Gregorys Compass which gave 23°39½′ West Variation. I also took a like number with two of Dr Knights Compass's, the one gave 23°15′ and the other 24°42′ West Variation, the Mean of all these Means is 23°52¼′; our Latitude and Longitude was the same as at Noon. At 6 o'Clock, having but little Wind, we brought to a mong some loose Ice, hoisted out the Boats and took up as much as filled all our empty Casks and compleated our Water to 40 Tons, the Adventure at the same time filled all her Empty Casks; while this was doing Mr Forster shott an Albatross whose plumage was of a Dark grey Colour, its head, uper sides of the Wings rather inclining to black with white Eye brows, we first saw of these Birds about the time of our first falling in with these Ice Islands and they have accompanied us ever sence.[1] Some of the Seamen call them Quaker Birds, from their grave Colour.[2] These and a black one with a yellow Bill[3] are our only Companions of the Albatross kind, all the other sorts have quite left us. Some Penguins were seen this morning.

WEDNESDAY 13*th. Winds Southerly—Calm. Course ESE. Dist. Sailed* 16 *Miles. Latitude in South* 64°18′. *Longd. in East Greenwich Reck.g Corrct.* 38°48′. *Longd. made Cape G. Hope* 20°25′. At 4 o'Clock in the PM hoisted in the Boats[4] and made sail to the SE with a gentle gale at SBW attended with Showers of Snow. At 2 am it fell calm, and at 9 hoisted out a Boat to try the Current which we found to set NW near

[1] . . . but we seldom see more than two at a time.—f. 24.

[2] The Light-mantled Sooty Albatross, *Phoebetria palpebrata* (Forster).

[3] A Giant Petrel.

[4] On this day, after the boats returned, Wales meditates on icebergs and land. Pieces were breaking off the ice islands continually, he remarked: 'as this circumstance happened several times during the few Hours we lay by it [the berg near which they watered], it must follow that these Islands (even the largest of them) cannot last long, &, of course cannot come very far'.

one third of a Mile an hour which is pretty confirmable to what I have before observed in regard to the Currants;[1] this is a point worth inquiring into, for was the direction of the Currants well assertained, we should be no longer at a loss to know from what quarter the Islands of Ice we daily meet with comes from.[2] At the time of trying the Currant Fahrenheits Thermometer was sent down 100 fathom and when it came up the mercury was at 32 which is the freezing point, some little time after, being exposed to the surface of the Sea, it rose to 33½ and in the open air to 36. Some curious and intresting experiments are wanting to know what effect cold has on Sea Water in some of the following instances: does it freeze or does it not?[3] if it does,[4] what degree of cold is necessary and what becomes of the Salt brine? for all the Ice we meet with yeilds Water perfectly sweet and fresh.

THURSDAY 14*th. Winds Calm, South to SE. Course N* 26° *E. Dist. Sailed* 23 *Miles. Latitude in South* 63°57′. *Longd. in East Greenwich Reck.g Corrct.* 39°38½′ *Watch* 38°36½′. *Longd. made Cape G. Hope* 21°15′. *Varn. of the Compass* 28°40′ *E.* The Calm continued untill 5 o'Clock pm when it was succeeded by a light breeze from the Southward which afterwards veered to SE,[5] the Day was fair and part of the morning clear and Serene, so as to enable us to observe several distances of the Sun and Moon, the mean result of them gave 39°30½′ East Longitude. Mr Kendals Watch at the same time gave 38°27¾′ East, 1°2′ West of the observations whereas on the 3rd Instant it was half a degree East of them—probably neither the one nor the other points out precisely the truth.

FRIDAY 15*th.*[6] *Winds South to S.E. Course N* 26° *E. Distce Sailed* 23 *Miles. Lat in South* 63°57′. *Longde in East of Greenwich Reck.g* 39°38½′ *Watch* 38°35½′. *Longt. East of C.G.H.* 21°15′. Very gentle breezes of Wind with tolerable Clear and Serene Weather. We have now had five tolerable good Days succeeding one another, which have been

[1] . . . The Currants however seem to be subject to variation, for while we were to the northward of the Feild Ice, we had great reason to believe that they set to the Westward . . .—f. 24v.

[2] A *note* Since this was written, I have had oppertunities enough to be well assured that what Current there is, in these Southern Seas, must, and does always set to the North, NW or NE by which the Ice is brought from the South; that there [are] neither Westerly nor Easterly Currents worth notice and that the error in reckoning must have been owing either to a following Sea or the Log or both.—H has a similar, but shorter, note in Cook's hand.

[3] A has here a footnote in Cook's hand 'See page 231'. This refers to the passage containing his mature thoughts on this subject, pp. 645–6 below.

[4] *if it does:* if it does freeze (of which I make no doubt) . . . —f. 24v.

[5] . . . with which we stood to the NE with all our Sails set . . .—f. 25.

[6] The MS has here Thursday 14th for a second time, instead of Friday 15th.

usefull to us more ways than one; having on board plenty of Fresh Water or Ice which is the same thing, the People have had an oppertunity to Wash and Dry their Linnen &ca a thing that was not a little wanting.[1] We also made the necessary Observns for finding the Ships place and the Variation of the Compass.

In the evening I found the Variation by the Mean of three Azimuths taken by Gregorys Compass to be	28°14′ w.
By the Mean of Six Azth taken by on[e] of Dr Knights Compass's	28°32′
and by a nother of Dr Knights	28°34′

The near agreement of the Variation by these three Compass's is a proff of the accuracy of the observations, the mean result of them is placed in the proper Column against yesterday noon as the Latitude and the Longitude was the same. In the Morning the Longitude was observed by the foll[ow]ing persons (viz.):

			° ′ ″
By my self being the Mean of Six Distces of the ☉ and ☽ to be			40 1 45
—	Do	Do	39 29 45
—	Mr Wales	Do	39 56 45
—	Lieutt Clerk	Do	39 38 0
—	Mr Gilbert	Do	39 48 45
—	Mr Smith, Masters Mate	.. .. ..	39 18 15
	Mean		39 42 12

Mr Kendalls Watch at the same time gave 38 41 30

nearly the same differences as yesterday, but Mr Wales and I took each of us Six Distances with the Telescopes fitted to our Quadts, which agreed nearly with the Watch, the results were as follows

Mr Wales .. .. 38°35′30″
Mine .. .. 38°36′45″ } It is impossible for me to say

whether those made with or without the Telescope are the nearest the truth, circumstances seem to be in favour of both: we certainly can observe with greater accuracy with the Telescope when the Ship is sufficiently steady which however very seldom happens so that most observations at sea are made without, but let them be made either the one way or the other, we are sure of finding a Ships place

[1] . . . the Wind in this time has blowen in gentle gales and the Weather has been apparently mild yet the Thermometer has never exceeded 36 and has often been as low as the freezing point.—f. 26.—Mitchel notes, 'People order'd to wash . . .'. Clerke (15th), 'put the People to ⅔ allowance of bread'; so evidently Cook was keeping a careful eye on the stores.

at sea to a Degree and a half and generally to less then half a Degree.[1] Such are the improvements Navigation has received from the Astronomers of this Age, by the Valuable Table they have communicated to the Publick under the direction of the Board of Longitude contained in the Astronomical Ephemeris and the Tables for correcting the Apparent Distance of the Moon and a Star from the effects of Refraction and Parallax, by these Tables the Calculations are rendred short beyond conception and easy to the meanest capacity and can never be enought recommended to the Attention of all Sea officers, who now have no excuse left for not making themselves acquainted with this usefull and necessary part of their Duty. Much Credet is also due to the Mathematical Instrument makers for the improvements and accuracy with which they make their Instruments, for without good Instruments the Tables would loose part of their use: we cannot have a greater proof of the accuracy of different Instruments than the near agreement of the above observations, taken with four different Sextants and which were made by three different persons, viz. Bird, Nairn & Ramsden.[2]

SATURDAY 16*th. Thermr.* 34 *to* 35. *Winds East & EBS. Course S* 2° *W. Dist. Sailed* 58 *Miles. Lat. in South* 64°31′. *Longde. in E. Greenwich Reck.g* 39°35′ *Watch* 38°32′. *Long^{de} made E. of C.G.H.* 21°12′. After Dinner having but little wind we brought to under an Island of Ice and sent a Boat to take up some loose pieces, while this was doing we shifted the two Topsails and Fore sail. At 5 o'Clock the Breeze freshened at East attended with snow and we made Sail to the

[1] . . . Should the Watch be found to keep its uniform rate of going it will point out to us the greatest error this method of observing the Longitude at Sea is liable to, which at the greatest does not exceed a degree and a half . . .—f. 25v.

[2] *made . . . Ramsden:* made by different workmen, mine by Mr Bird, Mr Wales's and Mr Clerkes by Ramsden and Mr Gilberts and Mr Smiths, who observed with the same Instrument, by Mr Nairn. [footnote] This was also made by Mr Ramsden.—f. 25v. But for 'Nairn' the published *Voyage*, curiously enough, reads 'Dollond'. Jesse Ramsden (1735–1800), F.R.S. 1786, Copley medallist 1795, was probably the greatest of eighteenth century makers of scientific instruments, renowned alike for the delicacy and scrupulous workmanship of his products, and for his unpunctuality in delivering them—'the artist's genius disdained time restrictions'. A Yorkshireman, he began life as a clothworker, but coming to London, apprenticed himself anew to a mathematical instrument maker in 1758, setting up on his own in 1762. He supplied a number of instruments to the Royal Society for use on Cook's first voyage. John Bird (1709–76) also was a clothworker, a weaver, early in life, and became famous all over Europe for his astronomical quadrants. See I, p. 87. Edward Nairne (1726–1806), F.R.S. 1776, another well-known 'optical, mathematical and philosophical instrument maker', carried out independent scientific studies, principally on electricity, and contributed papers to the *Philosophical Transactions* of the Royal Society. Peter Dollond (1730–1820), like his father John Dollond (1706–61), the inventor of the achromatic telescope, started in life as a silk-weaver, but opened a shop as an optician in 1750. He married a daughter of Jesse Ramsden. No mathematician, he yet had wonderful technical dexterity and judgment; in addition to other useful work, he continued the development of the refracting telescope.

Northward, but finding that we were only returning to the North on the same track we had advanced to the South we at 8 Tacked and stood to the Southward close upon a Wind, which was at EBS, having alternatly snow showers and fair Weather and during the whole am saw but one Island of Ice.

SUNDAY 17*th. Thermr.* 34. *Winds EBS. Course South. Dist. Sailed* 125 *Miles. Lat. in South* 66°36½′. *Longde. in E. Greenwich Reck.g* 39°35′. *Long*[de] *made E. of C.G.H.* 21°12′. In the PM had fresh gales and Clowdy weather. At 6 o'Clock, being then in the Latitude of 64°56′ S I found the Variation by Gregorys Compass to be 26°41′ West, at this time the Motion of the Ship was so great that I could not observe with D[r] Knights Compass. In the AM had hazy weather with Snow Showers and saw but one Island of Ice in the Course of these 24 hours so that we begin to think that we have got into a clear Sea.[1] At about a ¼ past 11 o'Clock we cross'd the Antarctic Circle for at Noon we were by observation four Miles and a half South of it and are undoubtedly the first and only Ship that ever cross'd that line. We now saw several Flocks of the Brown and White Pintadoes which we have named Antarctic Petrels because they seem to be natives of that Region;[2] the White Petrels also appear in greater numbers than of late and some few Dark Grey Albatrosses, our constant companions the Blue Petrels have not forsaken us but the Common Pintadoes have quite disapeared as well as many other sorts which are Common in lower Latitudes.

MONDAY 18*th. Winds EBS. Course North. Distce Sailed* 44 *Miles. Lat. in South* 65°52′. *Longde. in East Greenwich Reck.g* 39°35′. *Longde. East Cape G. Hope* 21°12′. In the PM had a Fresh gale and fair Weather. At 4 o'Clock we discoverd from the Mast head thirty eight Islands of Ice extending from the one Bow to the other, that is from the SE to West, and soon after we discovered Feild or Packed Ice in the same Direction and had so many loose pieces about the Ship that we were obliged to loof for one and bear up for another, the number increased so fast upon us that at ¾ past Six, being then in the Latitude of 67°15′ S, the Ice was so thick and close that we could proceed no

[1] . . . but these thoughts were of short duration . . .—f. 26v.

[2] . . . they are undoubtedly of the Petrel Tribe, are in every respect shaped like the Pintadoe, differing only from them in Colour, the head and fore part of the body of these are brown, and the hind part of the body, tail and ends of the wings are white.—f. 27. Cf. Clerke's description, 17 January,: 'We've seen this Morning many Flocks of Birds a good deal like the Pintado, or Cape Pidgeon, and about its size—we've met with many of them before in high Southern Latitudes, but this morning they flew about absolutely in Flocks—the upper Edge of the Wing along the Pinion from the body to the extreme end is brown the lower part all white—for distinctions sake I'll hereafter call them Antartick Peterels.'—The Antarctic Petrel, *Thalassoica antarctica* (Gm.) is here well-described.

further but were fain to Tack and stand from it. From the mast head I could see nothing to the Southward but Ice, in the Whole extent from East to WSW without the least appearence of any partition, this immence Feild was composed of different kinds of Ice, such as high Hills or Islands, smaller pieces packed close together and what Greenland men properly call field Ice, a piece of this kind, of such extend that I could see no end to it, lay to the SE of us, it was 16 or 18 feet high at least and appeared of a pretty equal height.[1] I did not think it was consistant with the safty of the Sloops or any ways prudent for me to persevere in going farther to the South as the summer was already half spent and it would have taken up some time to have got round this Ice, even supposing this to have been practicable, which however is doubtfull.[2] The Winds Continued at East and EBS and increased to a strong gale attended with a large Sea, hazy weather Sleet and Snow and obliged us to close reef our Topsails.[3]

TUESDAY 19*th. Winds ESE. Course N* 10°30′ *E. Distce. Sailed* 84 *Miles. Lat. in South* 64°29′. *Longd. East of Greenwich Reck.g* 40°12′ *Watch* 39°9′. *Longd. East of G.H.* 21°49′. Fresh gales and hazy weather with sleet and snow till towards Noon when the gale moderated so as to bear all the Reefs out, the Weather also became fair and Clowdy: only four Islands of Ice have been seen to Day.

WEDNESDAY 20*th. Winds EBS, ENE, EBS. Course N* 5¾° *E. Distce. Sailed* 30 *Miles. Lat. in South* 63°59′. *Longd. East of Greenwich Reck.g* 40°19′. *Longd. East of G.H.* 21°6′. PM gentle breeze and Clowdy. In the Evening[4] a Port Egmont Hen (Birds so call'd by us last Voyage on account of the great plenty of them at Port Egmont in Faulkland Isles) came hovering several times over the Ship and then left us in the direction of NE. They are about the size of a large Duck or Shag,[5] of a dark brown or Chocolate Colour with a White Strake in shape of a half moon under each Wing, it is said that these Birds never go far from land[6] and I believe it.[7] We saw of these Birds last

[1] ... Here we saw many Whales playing about the Ice ...

[2] ... I therefore came to a resolution to proceed directly in search of the land lately discovered by the French, and as the Winds still continued at EBS, I was obliged to return to the North over some part of the Sea I had already made my self acquainted with and for that reason wished to have avoided; but this was not to be done as our Course made good was little better than North.— f. 27v.—At this time the Antarctic continent was only about 75 miles away; but it is most improbable that Cook could have reached it.

[3] '... served a glass of brandy to the seamen as usual'.—Gilbert.

[4] ... being in the Latitude of 64°12′ S, Long^{de} 40°15′ E,

[5] *They ... Shag:* They are a short thick Bird about the size of a large Crow

[6] *it is said ... land:* I have been told that these Birds are found in great plenty at the Fero Isles North of Scotland and that they never go far from land.

[7] Probably the Brown Skua, *Catharacta skua lönnbergi* (Mathews), a southern form of the Great Skua; another form is abundant at the Falkland Islands. Cf. Clerke '... this Afternoon saw a Port Egmont (or Cape) Hen, which I think is a strong argument for supposing

voyage the day before we made the land of New Zealand being then between 30 and 40 Leagues off: but then we never saw less than two together whereas here is but one, which with the Islands of Ice may have come a great way from land, Mr Cooper says he has seen one of these Birds a Week ago which is very probable as our situation at that time was nearly the same as it is now. At Nine o'Clock the Wind coming to ENE we Tacked and stood to the SSE, but by 4 o'Clock in the AM the wind backed again to EBS with which we stood again to the Northward; as the Day advanced the gale increased attended with thick hazy weather and Snow, which at last obliged us to Close reef our Topsails and strike Topgt yards: this morning another Port Egmont Hen was seen or perhaps it might be the same as was seen last night.[1]

THURSDAY 21*st. Winds E to S. Course N* 23° *E. Distce. Sailed* 77 *Miles. Lat. in South* 62°48′. *Longd. East of Greenwich Reck.g* 41°25′. *Longd. East of G.H.* 23°2′. Dirty hazy weather with Snow: in the Evening the gale moderated so that we could carry whole Topsails and in the morning got Topgt Yards a Cross & Set the Sails. At this time the Wind was at South a gentle gale, but the high NE sea still kept up which is no sign of the Vicinity of land in that quarter and yet it is there we are to expect to find it. About 1 o'Clock in the pm Saw a White Albatross with black tiped wings,[2] I mention this because we had seen none to ye Srd of the Latitude we were then in.

FRIDAY 22*nd. Winds South to SW. Course N* 37¼° *E. Distce. Sailed* 93 *Miles. Lat. in South* 61°34′. *Longde. in East of Greenwich Reck.g* 43°25′ *Watch* 42°35′. *Long. E. of C.G. Hope* 28°9′. Fresh breeze and hazey, towards the Evening it clear'd away and we found the Variation to be 31°16′ E being then in Latitude 62°24′ S, Longde 4 ° ′ E. In the night had showers of snow and sleet, the air so cold that the Water in all our Water Vessels on Deck was froze.[3] In the AM had fair weather. Islands of Ice always in sight and the NE swell still keeps up.

SATURDAY 23*rd. Thermr* 36½, 32. *Winds SSE. Course N* 42° *E. Distce. Sailed* 122 *Miles. Lat. in South* 60°4′. *Longde. in East of Greenwich Reck.g*

some land near us; in any of my former Voyages I never saw, nor did I ever meet with any Voyager that asserted he ever did see this Bird above 40 or at most 50 Leagues from Land —'tis a brown Bird about the size of a Crow—hovers round about and over the Ship, as if curious to make observation—hardly ever flies low—there's a little white in the shape of a Horse Shoe under each wing but a little distant from the outer extremity of it.' The Cape Hen and Port Egmont Hen are not the same bird; the Cape Hen is the petrel *Procellaria aequinoctialis*.

[1] . . . as our situation was not much altered . . . f. 27v.

[2] . . . and a Pintado Bird . . .—f. 28.

[3] *was froze:* had been frozen for several preceding nights.

46°15′ *Watch* 45°31½′. *Long. E. of C.G. Hope* 28°22′. *Variation* 33°28½′. Fresh gales blowing in Squals attended with showers of Hail & snow till 5 o'Clock in the AM after which had fair Weather, the Sun appeared and we found by Several Azimuth the Variation to be 33°28½′ West our Latitude at this time was 60°27′ S.[1] At 9 o'Clock I spread the Sloops abreast of each other at 4 miles distant in order the better to discover any thing that might lay in our way.

SUNDAY 24*th. Thermr.* 34½. *Winds South to West. Course N* 39° *E. Distce. Sailed* 130 *Miles. Lat. in South* 58°24′. *Longde. in East of Greenwich Reck.g* 48°55′. *Long. E. of C.G. Hope* 30°32′. We continued sailing in this manner till 6 o'Clock in the pm when the Weather became hazey with showers of snow and made it necessary for us to join and at the same time to double reef the Fore and Mizen Topsails. At 11 o'Clock we hauled up our Courses, this occasioned the Adventure by some mistake to bring to, which obliged us to bring to also till two o'Clock in the am at which time we made sail again, having a fresh gale at West and fair Weather. We now began to see of those kind of Petrels which are so well known to Sailors by the name of black Sheer-waters.

MONDAY 25*th. Winds WNW, North to NEBE. Course N* 66° *E. Distce. Sailed* 62 *Miles. Lat. in South* 57°59′. *Longde. in East of Greenwich Reck.g* 50°42′. *Long. E. of C.G. Hope* 32°19′. Fresh gales and fair weather continued till 8 o'Clock in the am[2] when it became thick and hazey and the Wind having veered to NEBN we Tacked and stood to NW making but little way a gainest a very high Northerly Sea.

TUESDAY 26*th. Thermr.* 35. *Winds Easterly. Course N* 13° *W. Distce. Sailed* 44 *Miles. Lat. in South* 57°16′. *Longde. in East of Greenwich Reck.g* 50°24′. *Long. E. of C.G. Hope* 32°1′. In the PM the Wind veered to the Southward of East and by 8 o'Clock increased to a Storm attended with Sleet and Snow and very thick hazey weather, the Sea at the same time ran prodigious high and came from the NE, during night we went under the Fore sail and Main Topsail close reefed, at day light we added to them the Fore and Mizen Topsails. At 4 o'Clock

[1] Wales is again experimental: 'The Marine Watches being placed, one on each side of the great Cabbin, I judged it proper to put a Thermom[r] by each of them. Before a fire was kept in the Cabbin, I never saw these Thermom[rs] differ more than half a degree; but since there has been a fire, I have constantly found that Thermometer which was on the Weather side highest, and sometimes 3 Degrees. I have mentioned this Circumstance because it appeared to me curious; if it should be of no moment, nothing is lost but my labour in writing it down'.

[2] 'Shorten'd sail for the Night, as they begin now to be Dark for three or four hours.'—Wales.

it fell Calm, but the high Sea and a complication of the worst of weather, viz. Snow, Sleet and rain continued.[1]

WEDNESDAY 27*th. Thermr.* 35. *Winds Calm, SEBS, SBW. Course N* 14° *E. Dist. Sailed* 50 *Miles. Lat. in South* 56°28′. *Longde. in East of Greenwich Reck.g* 50°46′ *Watch* 50°32½′. *Long. made from C.G. Hope* 32°23′. *Varn. of the Compass* 31°23′ *West.* The Calm and thick hazey weather continued till 9 o'Clock in the PM at which time the Weather cleared up and a gentle breeze sprung up at SEBS, with which we steered NBE under our Fore sail and Topsails double reefd. At 8 o'Clock in the am the wind was at SBW a fresh breeze and clear weather. I now spread the Sloops four Miles from each other and steer'd NNE all sails set. Yesterday we saw a Grey Albatross[2] and last night a grey Sheerwater and a Port Egmont Hen.

THURSDAY 28*th. Winds South to West. Course N* 15° *E. Dist. Sailed* 124 *Miles. Lat. in South* 54°28′. *Longde. in East of Greenwich Reck.g* 51°46′ *Watch* 51°33½′. *Long. made from C.G. Hope* 33°23′. About 3 o'Clock in the pm the sun and moon appearing at intervals their Distance were observed by the following persons and the Longitude resulting therefrom was by

Mr Wales. Mean of two setts ..	50°59′
Lieutt Clerk	51°11′
Mr Gilbert	50°14′
Mr Smith	50°50′
Mr Kendalls Watch	50°50′

At 6 o'Clock being then in Latitude of 56°9′ the Variation was 31°23′ West. I now made Signal to the Adventure to come under my stern,[3] and at 8 o'Clock in the Morn spread them again having a fine fresh gale at West and pretty clear weather.[4]

FRIDAY 29*th. Thermr.* 38. *Winds WNW to NW. Course N* 29° *E. Dist. Sailed* 136 *Miles. Lat. in South* 52°29′. *Longde. in East of Greenwich Reck.g* 53°37′. *Long. made from C.G. Hope* 35°14′. At 2 o'Clock in the PM the sky became clowded, the weather hazey, the Wind increased to a fresh gale, blowed in squals attend[ed] with snow and drizling

[1] 'Many Birds about us—some remarkable large Albetrosses with white Bodies and Wings tip'd with black just at the extremety of each Wing—many of the common black and brown Albetrosses—these white Ones I don't recollect ever having met with before.' —Clerke: who is evidently describing old male Wandering Albatrosses, *Diomedea exulans* Linn.

[2] Unidentifiable.

[3] ADV '[10 pm] Saw a Number of Stars, which are the First we have seen for near six Weeks'.—Hawkey.

[4] 'Smoak'd the Ship between Decks with Gunpowder & Vinegar'.—Cooper.

rain, upon which I made signal to the Adventure to come under my stern and took a reef in each Topsail and at 8 handed the Main Sail till 3 in the Morn when we set it again. At noon it blowed a hard gale which obliged us to take the second reef in the Topsails, handed the Mizen Topsail and strike Topg[t] yards.[1]

SATURDAY 30*th. Thermr.* 39½. *Winds North W to North. Course N* 57° *E. Dist. Sailed* 101 *Miles. Lat. in South* 51°34′. *Longde. in East of Greenwich Reck.g* 55°55′. *Long. made from C.G. Hope* 37°32′. Very hard gale and thick hazey weather with drizling rain which obliged us to close reef our Topsails and at 8 o'Clock to hand the Main sail and Fore Topsail. We spent the night, which was dark and stormy, in making a trip to the SW, and in the morning made sail again to the NE under Courses and Double reefed Topsails, the Wind being some thing abated but it yet blew a fresh gale at NW and NNW attended with drizling rain and hazey thick weather. This is the first and only day we have seen no Ice sence we first discovered it.

SUNDAY 31*st. Winds North, NW, & West. Course N* 36°45′ *E. Diste. Sailed* 55 *Miles. Lat. in South* 50°50′. *Longde. in East Reck.g* 56°48′ *Watch* 56°49′. *Long. made from C.G.H.* 38°25′. Strong gales at North and hazey weather with rain, Stood to the Eastward till 8 o'Clock then Wore and stood to the Westward under the two Courses till 4 am, at which time the Wind had abated and backed to WBS and we again Stood North under double reefed Topsails, having a very high Sea from the NNW which gave us little hopes of meeting with Land in that direction. Some Islands of Ice seen to day.[2]

*. . . one of which we passed very near and found that it was breaking or falling to pieces by the cracking noise it made, which was equal to the report of a four pounder, there was a good deal of loose Ice about it and had the weather been favourable I should have brought to and taken some up, after passing this ice we saw no more

[1] 'We Yesterday saw two Cape Hens which is suppos'd a propitious Omen of being near Land—Wish with all my Heart we cou'd get hold of it. We've seen but 2 Ice Islands these 24 hours I believe we're getting to y[e] N[o]ward of them for what we have met with lately are dissolving fast'.—Clerke.

[2] Wales, 29–30 January, meditates on the marine barometer, which had begun to misbehave, going up for bad weather and down for good: [29] 'Quere, May not change of place, sometimes affect the Barometer? since bad weather is often local.' [30] 'It began to fall a few hours before the bad Weather began to abate, & continues falling'. His log adds to this, ''Tis an unfortunate circumstance for it, as it was just on the point of establishing its reputation with some of the greatest Sceptics in the Ship'.—Bad weather, as Wales says, is often local; and as the barometer indicates meteorological tendencies over a wider area, the sceptic could now and again scoff. It may be noted, on this occasion, and for the credit of science, that the weather was to deteriorate again.

till we returned again to the South.[1] We have however only missd seeing them one day sence we first fell in with them, by which it will appear what an immence extent of Sea these Islands of Ice are spread over, we have seen them from the Latitude of 50°45′ to 67°15′ and from Longitude 9½° to 56°48′ E and there can be no doubt of their extending a great way farther, not only to the South but to the East and West. Were the Islands of Ice which we only have seen, collected together they would from a moderate calculation, occupy a space of 208 Square Miles, when I consider the thick hazey weather and the many Foggy Days we have had, not above One hundred and tenth part of the Sea within the above mentioned limits, could com[e] within the Compass of our sight, and suppose-ing the parts unseen to be equally covered with Ice, which is certainly no unreasonable Supposision; the whole quantity of Ice collected together would occupy a space of 23002 Square miles, equal to about Six & half Square degrees, which is about a Thirty ninth part of the Sea within the limits above mentioned or more properly within the limits of our rout, for it is to this space my calculations are confind, in which I have not included the Feild-ice which for any thing I have seen to the contrary, may at one time of the year, extended over full as great a Space; nay I have even reason to believe that it occupies a much greater. I know it will be asked from whence this huge body of Ice comes, how and where it is formed and many such like questons, not one of which I am obliged to answer, at least I shall not do it now, but leave the further discussion of this subject, till some other oppertunity, as it can hardly be doubted but that I shall have occasion to resume it again, perhaps more than once in the course of the Voyage.*—ff. 29v–30.

[FEBRUARY 1773]

MONDAY 1*st. Thermr.* 41½. *Winds WNW. Course N* 18° *E. Diste. Sailed* 126 *Miles. Lat. in South* 48°51′. *Longde. in East Reck.g* 57°47′. *Long. made from C.G.H.* 39°24′. Fresh gales and Clowdy, at 2 pm passed two Isds of Ice. In the AM saw a small piece of rock weed.[2]

[1] after passing . . . South *altered from* these Islands have been so thin of late that it is not probable we shall meet with any more till we again turn to the South.

[2] 'PM at 3 pass'd by 2 Ice Islands. We run very near them; they made a continual noise a good deal resembling the firing of Musquets—they gave 2 or 3 Cracks I think full as loud as our 4 Pounders; an undoubted sign this, that they are dissolving fast. . . . at 11 pass'd some Seaweed which is in general deem'd a sign of being near some Land, but I think I've seen it a very great distance from any Land I'm sure I have from any thats been at all known'.—Clerke.—'[p.m.] Mr Coglan Midshipman was Disc[h]arged from that Station for haveing had a dispute with the Capts Servant; and was ordred to do his duty as a Foremastman.'—Elliott. Mr Coglan was one of the 'Wild & drinking' young gentlemen.

TUESDAY 2nd. *Winds NW to WNW. Course N 78° E. Diste. Sailed* 73 *Miles. Lat. in South* 48°36′. *Longde. in East* 59°35′ *Watch* 59°33′. *Long. made from C.G.H.* 41°12′. Hazey Clowdy weather and a fresh gale at NW with which we stood NEBN till 4 o'Clock in the PM when being in the Latitude of [48°39′] S and[1] nearly in the Meridian of the Isle of Mauritius, where we were to expect to find the Land said lately to have been discovered by the French, but seeing nothing of it[2] we bore away East and made the Signal to the Adventure to keep on our Starboard beam at 4 miles distance. In this manner we proceeded till half past Six o'Clock when the Adventure made the Signal to speak with me, we accordingly short[ed] sail, bro[t] to to wait for her to come up, when Captain Furneaux informed us that they just had seen a large Float of Sea or Rock Weed and several Birds (Divers)[3] about it. This was certainly a great sign of the vicinity of land but wheather it laid to the East or West was not possible for us to know. My intention was to have got into this Latitude four or five Degrees of Longitude to the West of the Meridian we are now in and then to have carried on my researches to the East but the West and NW Winds we have had the four preceeding Days prevented me (in spite of my endeavours) to put this in execution.[4] All I can say is that if this land lies to the West we are unlucky, I however have had no reason to believe that it does and therefore as the Wind will not permit going to the West shall search for it to the East. Accordingly we stood on till 8 o'Clock then brought to till 4 am when we re-asumed our Course to the East all Sails set four Miles North and South from each other the hazey weather not permiting to seperate farther. We passed two or three pieces of Weed[5] but saw no other sign of land. Swell from the West all this 24 hours. At noon we observed in Latitude 48°36′ S and not being able to see above 4 or 5

[1] 48°39′ [?] and Long[d] 58°07′ East

[2] 'We reciev'd intelligence at the Cape that a French Ship which had been upon discoveries, had confidently reported having met with Land due S[o] of the Mauritias in y[e] Lat[de] of 48° or 49°, we're now nearly in the Miridian of y[e] Mauritias and in the propos'd Lat[de] but cannot yet see Monsieurs Land'.—Clerke.

[3] '... some Divers (a bird with a black Back and white Belly about y[e] size of a Teal I believe hardly ever seen any great distance from Land) which gave them reason to apprehend being near some Land ...'—Clerke. The name was applied by Cook and other seamen to diving petrels, *Pelecanoides* spp., small birds rather widely distributed between latitudes 35° and 55° S.

[4] ... The continual high Sea we had lately had from the NE, North, NW and West left me no reason to beleive that land of any extent laid to the West, and therefore continued to steer to the E.—f. 30v.

[5] ... and saw two or three Birds know[n] by the name of Egg Birds, ...—f. 30v.—'at 11 saw an Egg Bird (or small white bird with a Swallow Tail) in general to be met with near land'.—Clerke. 'Egg Bird' was a name usually applied to the Sooty Tern or Wideawake, but was used by Cook and his men for terns in general.

miles farther I gave orders to Steer South half East and made the Signal to the Adventure to follow us.

WEDNESDAY 3*rd. Winds WBS, NW to North. Course S* 46° *W. Distce. Sailed* 33 *Miles. Lat. in South* 48°59′. *Longd. in East Reck.g* 60°11′. *Longd. East C.G.H.* 41°48′. Wind at West and NW, hazey weather till half past six pm when it cleared up so as to enable us to see four or five Leagues round us being now in the Latitude of 49°13′ S and seeing no signs of land I wore and stood to the Eastward and soon after spoke Captain Furneaux who told me that he thought the land laid to the NW of us as he had observed the Sea to be smooth when the Wind blowed from that quarter; altho this was just the very reverse to what had been taken notice of aboard us, who had been very attentive to this in particular, I resolved to steer to the NW, to clear up this point as soon as the Wind would permit for at present [it] blew directly from that Quarter, so that I thought it best to stand to the NE till 12 o'Clock when I brought it to till Daylight, when we made sail again to the ENE. At 8 o'Clock we were in Lat. 48°56′, Longde 60°47′ and 3°19′ East of the Meridian of the Mauritius, so that I almost despared of finding land to the East and as the Wind had now veered to North and NBW I tacked and stood to the Westward with a very fresh gale and which increased in such a manner as to oblige us to strike Topgt Yards and double reef the Topsails. Last evening I observed the Variation by several Azths to be 27°50′ W. At that time and likewise this morning we saw a Port Egmont Hen, probable it might be one and the same Bird which might have kept about the Sloops all night.[1]

THURSDAY 4*th. Winds NBW, West, & NWBW. Course S* 71°15′ *W. Distce. Sailed* 55 *Miles. Lat. in South* 49°16′. *Longd. in East Reck.g* 58°54′. *Long. East C.G.H.* 40°31′. *Varn. Compass* 27°50′ *West.* Strong gales with rain, which by 8 o'Clock in the evening increased to a Storm and obliged us to bring to under the Fore sail and Mizen Staysail. At Midnight the gale abated when we made sail under the Courses & Close reefed Topsails with the Wind at West and WNW, from which points we had a very high sea notwithstanding the strength of the gale blew from NBW & North. At 6 o'Clock in the am we saw a Port Egmont Hen, at the same time we loosed two reefs out of our Topsails, the Weather being fair and settled.[2]

FRIDAY 5*th. Thermr.* 41. *Winds NW, Calm, SW to WNW. Course N* 75°

[1] 'Mr Coglan was Ordred by the Capt to his former Duty as Midshipman'.—Elliott.

[2] ADV 'Served the Ship's Company an extraordinary allowance of Groag'.—Furneaux. He has similar entries from time to time at this period.

W. Dist. Sailed 31 *Miles. Lat. in South* 49°8′. *Longd. in East Reck.g* 58°8′. *Longd. East Cape* 39°45′. *Varn Compass* 30°26′. Fair Weather and a fresh gale at NW, with which we stood SW untill half past six o'Clock pm at which time we had run 31 Miles since Noon, we now Tacked and stood NE. Here we found the variation to be 27°50′ West. In the night had two hours Calm after which a breeze sprung up at SW, with which we stood NW all sails set but at noon could lay no better than North as the Wind kept veering round to the West & WNW. A Large Swell from the Westward.

SATURDAY 6*th. Thermr.* 43¾. *Winds West, North, NW, & WNW. Course N* 8° *E. Dist. Sailed* 68 *Miles. Lat. in South* 48°6′. *Longd. in East Reck.g* 58°22′ *Watch* 58°32′. *Longd. East Cape* 39°59′. In the pm had a fresh gale and fair weather, at 6 o'Clock the Variation was 30°26′ W. We continued our Course to the North and NE till 4 o'Clock am, by which time the Wind had veered to North, we Tacked and stood West with a fresh gale attended with rain. At 10 o'Clock the Wind veered back again to WNW, I now gave over all thoughts of beating any longer againest it and bore away East a little Southerly all sails set.[1] Indeed I had no sort of incouragement to proceed farther to the West as we have had continualy a long heavy Swell from that quarter which made it very improbable that any large land lay to the West.[2]

SUNDAY 7*th. Thermr.* 45. *Winds NW. Course S* 72° *E. Dist. Sailed* 146 *Miles. Lat. in South* 48°49′. *Longd. in East Reck.g* 61°48′ *Watch* 61°47′. *Longd. East Cape* 43°25′. Fresh gales, Hazey in the PM and Clowdy in

[1] . . . being satisfied that if there is any land hereabouts it can only be an is[l]e of no great extent, and it was just as probable I might have found it to the East as West. While we were plying about here, we took every oppertunity to observe the Variation of the Compass and found it to be from 27°50′ to 30°26′ West, probably the mean of the two extremes, viz. 29°4′ is the nearest the truth as it nearly agrees with the variation observed on board the Adventure. In making these observations we found that when the Sun was on the Starboard side of the Ship, the variation was the least and when on the Larboard side the greatest, this was not the first time we had made this observation, without being able to account for it.—ff. 35–5v. Cf. A 4 February: 'On the 4th being in the Latitude 49°37′ South, Longitude 58°12′ E, the variation was 27°50′ West, and the next day in Latitude 48°33′ South, Longitude 58°8′ East, it was 30°26′ West, as both the observations were equally well taken I can by no means account for this difference, I shall only observe that it hath frequently happen'd of late and that there must be some fault either in the Compasses, or observations or the variation does not follow that uniform law one might reasonably expect.'—See also p. 104 below.

[2] 'We've been for these 6 or 7 days past cruizing for the Land the Frenchman gave intelligence of at the Cape of Good Hope—if my friend Monsieur found any Land, he's been confoundedly out in the Latitude & Longitude of it, for we've search'd the spot he represented it in and its Environs too pretty narrowly and the devil an Inch of Land is there—this discovery being compleated run to the Eastward again.'—Clerke.—'. . . in this time we've made rather a disagreeable discovery—which is—that our friends the French were only amusing the good folks at the Cape with a little of the marvellous'.—Clerke 8951.

the night, Steer'd East Southerly till 8 o'Clock then took in the Studding sails and steer'd a point more to the South: before dark saw two Port Egmont Hens and in the Morning one more. At 4 o'Clock made the Signal for the Adventure to keep at the Distance of 4 miles on our Starboard beam. Having fair and clear weather, I had all the peoples Bedding &c[a] upon deck to air[1] a thing that was absolutely necessary.[2]

MONDAY 8*th. North, East to North. Course S* 54° *E. Distce. Saild* 103 *Miles. Lat. in South* 49°51′. *Longde. in East Reck.g* 63°57′. *Longde. East C.G.H.* 45°34′. At 6 o'Clock in the pm, made the Signal for the Adventure to come under our stern and at the same time took several Az[ths] which gave the var[n] 31°28′ but the observations were doubtfull on account of the rowling of the sloop occasioned by a very high Westerly swell. Fair weather continued till Midnight when it became Squally with rain and we took a reef in each Topsail. In the Morning saw several Penguins & Divers[3] and some were heard[4] at different times in the night, these signs of land continuing we at 8 o'Clock sounded but found no ground with 210 fathoms. We were now in the Latitude of 49°53′ s, Longitude 63°39′ East, Steering South by Compass close upon a Wind which was at ESE the Adventure was about a point or two upon our Larb[d] quarter, distant about one Mile and a half or as some thou[gh]t one Mile, about half an hour after a thick Fogg came on so that we could not see her. At 9 o'Clock we fired a gun and repeated it at 10 and at 11 and at Noon made the Signal to Tack and Tacked accordingly, but neither this last Signal or any of the former were answered by the Adventure which gave us too much reason to apprehend that a seperation would take[5] place. I have said that at 8 o'Clock we laid South by Compass with the wind at ESE but by 9 o'Clock or before the Wind veered to NNE so that we laid E½S, this must have brought the Adventure upon our weather beam or directly to Windward of us, provided she kept her Wind which she ought to have done as no signal was made to the contrary. In short we were intirely at a loss, even to guess by what means she got out of the hearing of the first gun we fired.

TUESDAY 9*th. Winds North, North, NBE & NNW. Course S* 66° *W.*

[1] . . . and the Ship cleaned and smoaked betwixt decks . . .—f. 35v.

[2] 'M[r] Loggie was ordred by the Capt[t] to his former Duty, as Midshipman.'—Elliott.

[3] *Divers:* Divers of two sorts, seemingly such as are usually seen on the Coast of England. Diving Petrels do not occur in the northern hemisphere but guillemots and razorbills dive for their food in the same way, and are common in the waters round the English coast.

[4] They were heard 'Croaking', says Cooper.

[5] *would take:* had taken . . .—f. 36.

Distce. Sailed 5 *Miles. Lat. in South* 49°53′. *Long*[d]. *in East Reck.g* 63°53′. *Longde. made C.G.H.* 45°30′. The thick Foggy Weather continuing and being apprehensive that the Adventure was still on the other Tack, we at 2 pm, after having run 2 Leagues to the West, made the Signal and Tacked, to which we heard no Answer, we now continued to fire a gun every half hour. At 3 o'Clock just after fireing our gun the officer of the Watch and others on Deck heard or thought they heard the report of a gun on the Weather bow, about the same space of time after fireing the next gun no one on deck doubted but what they heard the report of a nother gun on our beam, the different situations of these two sounds induced us to think that the Adventure was on the other Tack and standing to the Westward, and being to Windward of us I thought she might not hear our guns, but was only fireing half hour guns as well as us and that her fireing so soon after us was only chance. I therefore orderd a nother gun to be fire'd a quarter of an hour after to which we heard no answer, being now satisfied that she did not hear us both from her not answering and not bearing down, I prepared to Tack at 4 o'Clock but first ordered a Gun to be fired after which M[r] Forster alone thought he heard the report of a nother to Windward nearly in the same situation as the last, this occasioned my standing half an hour longer to the Westward in which time we fired two guns to which no answer was heard, we then Tack'd[1] and stood to the Westward after having stood some thing more than 8 Miles to the East. We still continued to fire half our guns and the Fogg dissipated at times so to admit us to see two or three Miles or more round us, we however could niether hear nor see any thing of her. Being now well assured that a Separation had taken place I had nothing to do but to repair to the place where we last saw her, Captain Furneaux being directed to do the same and there to cruze three days, accordingly I stood on to the Westward till 8 o'Clock, than made a trip to the East till Midnight and then again to the West till Day light and fired half hour guns and Bur[n]t false fires all night, the Weather continued Foggy and hazey and the Wind remained invariable at North and NBW, which, if the Adventure kept her Wind during the Fogg, was very favourable for her to return back to the apointed station. After day light at which time we could only see about 2 or 3 Miles round us, we tacked and stood to the East till 8 o'Clock, then again to the West and at Noon we were about 6 or 7 Miles East of the place were we last saw the Adven-

[1] A ... while we were in stays some of the people thought they heard four guns fired to leeward, this served only to perplex us, and made it doubtfull that any guns attall had been heard.

ture and would see about 3 or 4 Leagues round us: the Wind which was now at NNW had increased in such a manner as to oblige us to take in our Topsails and the Sea at the same time began to rise from the same point. We still continued to see Penguins and Divers[1] which made us conjector that land was not far off, it was for this reason I tacked yesterday at Noon which probably was the occasion of my loosing the Adventure for seeing such signs of the Vicinity of land, I thought it more prudent to make short boards during the Fogg, over that part of the Sea we had already made our selves accquainted with, than to continue standing to the Eastward at a time we could not see a quarter of a mile before us.

WEDNESDAY 10*th. Thermr.* 40½. *Winds NNW to WBN. Course S* 68°. *Distce. Sailed* 38 *Miles. Lat. in South* 50°7′. *Longde. in East Reck.g* 64°53′ *Watch* 64°49′. *Longd. C.G.H.* 46°30′. We stood to the Westward till half past 2 o'Clock pm having run 10 Miles sence Noon and neither hearing or seeing any thing of the Adventure, we wore and lay-too under the Mizen Staysail with our head to the Eastward, at 8 o'Clock the gale being somewhat abated we set the Foresail and this Sail we kept under all night; during the height of the gale the Weather was hazey with rain, but towards evening it cleared up so as to see 3 or 4 Leagues round us and in this state it continued all night, we however kept burning false fires at the mast head and fireing guns every hour, but neither the one nor the other had the desired effect for altho we laid too all the morning we could see nothing of the Adventure which if she had been with[in] 4 or 5 Leagues of us must have been seen from the mast head.[2] Having now spent two Days out of the three assign'd to look for each other, I thought it would be to little purpose to wait any longer[3] and still less to attempt to beat back to the appointed station will knowing that the Adventure must have been drove to leeward equally with our selves. I therefore made sail[4] to the SE with a very fresh gale at WBN accompanied with a high Sea, many dark grey Albatrosses, Blue Petrels and Sheerwaters about the Ship but only two or three divers were seen and not one Penguin.

THURSDAY 11*th. Thermr.* 40. *Winds WBN to NWBW. Course S* 54° *E. Distce. Sailed* 124 *Miles. Lat. in South* 51°25′. *Longde. in East Reck.g*

[1] 'Saw a Pengwin. This and those we saw yesterday are considerably different from those we saw amongst the Ice Islands to the Southward.'—Wales. Cf. p. 93, n. 2. Possibly these penguins and the 'divers' were from breeding grounds in the Crozet islands.

[2] 'Keep a good look out with a Man at each Mt Hd continually.'—Mitchel.

[3] A ... especially as we were now eight leagues to leeward of the appointed Rendezvouze

[4] *I therefore made sail:* I therefore gave over all hopes of joining her till we arrive at New Zealand which I had appointed to Winter at and made sail . . .—ff. 35, 37.

67°20′. *Longd. C.G.H.* 48°57′. Strong gale and fair Weather in the pm[1] at 7 Shortened Sail and at 11 brought to till 4 am when we steered again to the SE under all the Sail we could set, haveing hazey weather with some rain and a high sea from the West. Several Penguins were seen to day[2] and one Egg bird, which is also a sign of land as some think.

FRIDAY 12*th. Thermr.* 38. *Winds WBS. Course S* 55°30′ *E. Distce. Sailed* 148 *Miles. Lat. in South* 52°48′. *Longde. in East Reck.g* 70°20′ *Watch* 70°10′. *Longd. C.G.H.* 51°57′. *Varn.* 31°38′. Fresh gales, with Showers of hail and snow untill 6 o'Clock in the am when the Weather became fair and clear and we observed the Variation to be 31°38′ w. At the same time we found the Longitude by obser^{n} of the Sun and Moon nearly to agree with our Reckoning but the Latitude by observation was near half a degree to the north of that by account a circumstance neither owing to Winds nor Currents.

SATURDAY 13*th. Thermr.* 36. *Winds SW to WBS. Course S* 50°30′ *E. Distce. Sailed* 104 *Miles. Lat. in South* 53°54′. *Longde. in East Reck.g* 72°34′ *Watch* 72°24′. *Longd. C.G.H.* 54°11′. *Varn.* 33°8′. Gentle gales and pleasent Weather. In the Evening the Variation was 32°32′ w and in the morning 33°8′ w. We were now accompanied by a much greater number of Penguins than at any time before and of a different sort, being smaller, with Redish Bills and brown heads,[3] the meeting with so many of these Birds gave us still some hopes of meeting with land and various were the oppinions among the officers of its situation. Some said we should find it to East others to the North,[4] but it was remarkable that not one gave it as his opinion that any was to be found to the South which served to convince me that they had no inclination to proceed any farther that way. I however was resolved to get as far to the South as I conveniently could without looseing too much easting altho I must confess I had little hopes of meeting with land, for the high swell or Sea which we have had for some time from the West came now gradualy round to SSE so that it was not probable any land was near between these two points and it is less probable that land of any extent can lie to the North as

[1] 'People ordered from keeping the M^{t} H^{d} continually; but go as usual: which is every half hour.'—Mitchel.

[2] 'Saw several Pengwins, not like those which we have seen for several Days past; but those we saw formerly.'—Wales.

[3] Probably the Gentoo Penguin, *Pygoscelis papua* (Forster). In the eighteenth century English-speaking sealers commonly called this bird the Johnny Penguin. The Spanish translation of this was 'Juanito', which has degenerated into Gentoo.

[4] There was land near, and land where penguins bred—Heard Island, about 40 miles north-east, in lat. 53°10′ s, long. 73°35′ E.

we are not above Leagues South of Tasmans track[1] and this space I expect Captain Furneaux will explore, who I expect is to the North of me.[2]

SUNDAY 14*th. Thermr.* 35, 35½. *Winds WNW to SWBW. Course SE. Dist. Sailed* 120 *Miles. Lat. in South* 55°23′. *Longd. in East Reckg.* 74°48′. *Longd. East Cape G.H.* 56°25′. Fresh gales with Showers of snow and sleet in the night. Penguins accompanied us till the evening at which time we saw a Port Egmont Hen which flew away in the direction of NEBE. We also saw two or three Pintadoes, Birds which we have not seen for above this Week past. In the morning a Seal was seen but the Penguins had quite left us.

MONDAY 15*th. Thermr.* 36½. *Winds SWBS. Course SEBE. Dist. Sailed* 162 *Miles. Lat. in South* 56°52′. *Longd. in East Reckg.* 78°48′. *Longd. East Cape G.H.* 60°25′. Fresh gales, with now and then Showers of sleet and snow. In the evening the Variation was found to be 34°48′ West. The Wind now veered to SWBS or SSW and the Swell followed the same direction. About 6 in the AM a nother Seal was seen. Some petty thefts having lately been commited in the Ship, I made a thro' search to day for the stolen things and punished those in whose custody they were found.[3]

TUESDAY 16*th. Winds SWBS to South, Calm, NE. Course S* 77° *E. Dist. Sailed* 73 *Miles. Lat. in South* 57°8′. *Longd. in East Reckg.* 80°59′. *Longd. East Cape G.H.* 62°36′. First part fresh gales, remainder little Wind and calms. In the pm saw four Seals and observed the Variation to be 38° or 39°. At Day light in the Morn saw an Island of Ice bearing NBE which we steered for with a View to take some aboard, but at 6 o'Clock it fell calm and continued so till 10 when a breeze sprung up at North with which we stood to the East, not being able to reach the Ice, two Islands of which were now in sight and both to windward. A Single Penguin was about the Ship great part of the Morning, it was of the same sort as we usually saw near the Ice, but it is now im-

[1] *as we . . . track:* as we were only about 160 Leagues to the South of Tasmans track in 1642.—f. 38.

[2] Burney, Ferguson MS, 8 February (but clearly including a later decision under this date) writes that, as Cook intended running to the south as far as 55°, Furneaux thought it most advisable 'to Slant to the Southward to 52°30′ S & then haul again to the N°ward by degrees' till in the latitude of Van Diemen's Land: 'this was keeping nearly in the middle between Captn Cook and Tasman, & by sailing in 2 different routs we should be less liable to miss anything in our way'.

[3] 'Punish Wm Brisco & Francis Taylor with one dozen lashes each, Wm Atkinson, John Buttal & Phil. Brotherson with half a dozen each, all for Theft.'—Log. Atkinson was a seaman, Briscoe the tailor, Taylor and Buttal marines, and Brotherson the drummer. Cook followed up this disciplinary measure with another, we learn from Mitchel, who says, 'after which [i.e. the lashes] examin'd the peoples hands—those who had dirty where punish'd by stopping their daily allowance of Grog'.

possible for us to look upon Penguins to be certain signs of the vicinity of land or in short any other Aquatick birds which frequent high Latitudes.[1]

WEDNESDAY 17*th. Winds NBE to EBS. Course S* 36½° *E. Dist. Sailed* 57 *Miles. Lat. in South* 57°54′. *Longd. in East Reckg.* 82°4′. *Longd. East Cape G.H.* 63°41′. Gentle gales and dark clowdy weather with frequent Showers of Sleet and snow. At 9 o'Clock am Saw an Island of Ice to the westward distant 3 or 4 Leagues, which we bore down to with the same intention as we stood for the one yesterday. The Wind was now at East by South but the swell still continued to come from the West. Last night Lights were seen in the Heavens similar to those seen in the Northern Hemisphere commonly called the Northern lights, I do not remember of any Voyagers makeing mention of them being seen in the Southern before.[2]

THURSDAY 18*th. Thermr.* 30 *to* 33. *Winds SBW. Course S* 87° *E. Distce. Sailed* 48 *Miles. Lat. in South* 57°57′. *Longd. in East Reckg.* 83°44′ *Watch* 83°0′. *Longd. from the Cape G.H.* 65°21′. *Var.* 39°33′ *West.* A little past Noon we brought-to under the Island of Ice which was full half a mile in circuit and two hundred feet high. At this time there were but a few loose pieces about it but while we were hoisting out the Boats to take this up an immence quantity broke from the Island, a convincing proof that these Islands must decrease pretty fast while floating about in the Sea.[3] I observed the loose pieces to drift fast to

[1] This conclusion about penguins, at least, is certainly correct, though not about all 'Aquatick birds'. The distance penguins range from land in summer depends entirely on the whereabouts of food. Mitchel notes for this date that the needs of man at any rate were duly ministered to: 'People served their usual Grogg'.

[2] *commonly . . . before:* known by the name Aurora Borealis, or Northern Lights, but I never heard of the Aurora Australis being seen before; the officer of the Watch observed that it sometimes broke out in spiral rays and in a circular form, then its light was very strong and its appearence beautifull, he could not preceive it had any particular direction for it appeared at various times in different parts of the Heavens and difused its light throughout the whole atmosphere.—f. 39–9v. If it were not for Wales, one would say that Cook has somehow misdated the first appearance of this phenomenon: the other journal-keepers (including Clerke, 'the officer of the Watch', whose description he virtually quotes) all make it 18 February—except Pickersgill, who has it on the night of the 20th. But Pickersgill—who thought it 'superior to the Aurora Borealis, for the Colours are finer and the flashes more quick and beautifull'—told Wales about it on the morning of Wales's 16th—i.e. Cook's 17th. 'At leaving the Cape of Good Hope I had desired the Lieu[ts] & other Officers who kept Watch to be so obliging as to tell me if they saw extraordinary appearance[s] in the Heavens, and this Morning M[r] Pickersgill told me that he had seen something like the *Aurora Borealis*, but that he [had] not time to apprise me of it before the clouds returned and covered it'. Thereafter Wales gives pretty detailed descriptions of the phenomenon, as he had been instructed.

[3] *but while . . . Sea:* but while we were considering whether or no we should hoist our boats out to take some up, a great quantity broke from the island, upon which we hoisted out our boats and went to work to take some on board.'—f. 38v. Wales adds a touch of excitement: 'About Noon Came close under the Lee of the above mentioned Island of Ice,

the Westward, that is it quited the Island in that direction[1] and this I suppose to be occasioned by a current, for the Wind which was at ESE could have little or no effect upon the Ice.[2]

At 8 o'Clock we hoisted in the Boats and made sail to the Eastward with a gentle gale at South, having got on board as much Ice as yeilded nine or ten Tons of Water. In the morning the Variation was 39°33′ West. At Noon we had twelve Islands of Ice in sight besides an immence number of loose pieces which had broke off from the Island. The Southern lights were again seen last night. The Thermometer was 2° or 3° below the freezing point in consequence of which the Water in the Scuttle cask[3] was froze. Swell still continues to come from the West. The morning being clear Mr Wales and some of the officers took several Observations of the Sun and Moon which gave the Longitude reduc'd to Noon 83°44′ E one degree less then the Logg gives carried on from the last observations, which indicates that there is a current seting to the West.[4]

FRIDAY 19*th. Thermr.* 33 *to* 35. *Winds SBW to SBW.*[5] *Course S* 75°45′ *E. Distce. Sailed* 133 *Miles. Lat. in South* 58°30′. *Longd. in East Reckg.* 87°43′ *Watch* 86°59′. *Longd. from the Cape G.H.* 69°20′. *Var.* 37°8′ *West.* Fresh gales and Clowdy with frequent showers of hail and snow. In the Evening the Variation by several Azths was 37°8′ w. Shortened Sail during the night but in the Day set all the sail we could having continually a great number of Ice Islands in sight in every direction and many of them of a considerable magnitude.

SATURDAY 20*th. Winds SW to SBE. Course S* 82°15′ *E. Distce. Sailed* 124 *Miles. Lat. in South* 58°47′. *Longd. in East Reckg.* 91°44′ *Watch* 90°56′. *Longd. from the Cape G.H.* 75°41′. *Var.* 40°11′ *West.* Fresh gales with showers of snow in the pm, the remainder gentle gales and clear weather. Ice Islands as numerous as yesterday having never less than Ten or Twelve in sight. Swell still continues to come from the West.

SUNDAY 21*st. Thermr.* 36. *Winds South, SW to NWBW. Course S* 61° *E.*

and were by a kind of indraught or some means or other insensibly sucked so near that we had scarce any probab[ili]ty of escaping being drove against it which must have been inevitable destruction; and it was equally as unknown almost how we got off without, and we had scarce got to a Cable's length from it before several Pieces almost as large as the Ship broke off from that very part where we were'. Those pieces soon broke into lesser ones, and as soon as the ship was at a safe distance the boats were out watering.

[1] . . . and were in a few hours spread over a large space of Sea . . .—f. 39v.

[2] This circumstance greatly retarded our taking up ice . . .—f. 39v. For comment on Cook's theory of the absence of wind-effect on ice see pp. lxiv–lxv above.

[3] 'An open butt placed on the quarter-deck, and daily filled with fresh water out of the hold, for the use of the ship's company.'—Forster, I, p. 71.

[4] 'Served Wine to the Ships Company instead of Grog.'—Cooper.

[5] *SB W to SB W* looks like a slip. The Log gives the winds for this day as SW, W, WNW.

Dist. Sailed 27 *Miles. Lat. in South* 59°0′. *Longd. in East Reckg.* 92°30′. *Longd. E. of Cape G.H.* 76°27′. Gentle breeze and clowdy Weather. At 1 pm, thinking we saw land to the SW,[1] we Tacked and stood towards it, but at 3 o'Clock found it to be only clowds, which soon dissipated and we again resumed our Course to the SE. In the Evening the Horizon was unusally clear so as to see full 12 or 15 Leagues round.[2] The variation by several Az[ths] taken with D[r] Knights Compass was 40°8′ and by Gregorys 40°15′ West. Had but little wind all night which increased but very little with the Day and as the Sea was smooth and favourable for the Boats to take up Ice we steered for a large Island were we expected to meet with some and were not disapointed when we reached it. In the morning some Penguins were seen.

MONDAY 22*nd. Winds NBE to EBN. Course S* 44° *E. Dist. Sailed* 49 *Miles. Lat. in South* 59°35′. *Longd. in East Reckg.* 93°36′. *Longd. E. of Cape G.H.* 77°33′. *Varn. West* 40°51′. After Dinner hoisted out two Boats and set them to take up Ice while we stood to and from under the Island which was about half a mile in circuit and three or four hundred feet high, yet this huge body turned nearly bottom up while we were near it.[3] At 6 o'Clock having got aboard as much Ice as we could dispence with, we hoisted in the Boats and made sail to the SE with a gentle breeze at NBE having at this time Eight Ice Islands in sight and increased in such a manner as we run to the SE that in the morn[g] 23 were seen at one time and yet the Weather was generally hazey[4] with snow showers. Variation p[r] Az[ths] 40°51′ West.[5]

TUESDAY 23*rd. Thermr.* 35. *Winds ENE to East. Course S* 26° *E. Dist. Sailed* 95 *Miles. Lat. in South* 61°0′. *Longd. in East Reckg.* 95°2′. *Longd. E. of Cape G.H.* 76°39′. Gentle breeze and dark gloomy weather in the pm, in the am a fresh breeze with Snow. Passed this 24 hours 70 or 80 Islands of Ice many of them as large as any we have seen, at Noon observed in 61°0′ of Latitude.

[1] . . . the appearence was so strong that we doubted not but it was there in reality . . .—f. 40.

[2] *the Horizon . . . round:* we could see a considerable way round us, in which space nothing was to be seen but ice islands; in the night the Aurora Australis made a very brilliant and luminous appearence, it appeared first in the East a little above the Horizon and in a short time spread over the whole Heavens.—f. 40v.

[3] *while . . . it:* but its height was not apparently either increased or diminished by this.—ff. 36, 42.—If Cook had had a modern knowledge of icebergs he would have regarded the dimensions of this one as indicating extreme instability, and have kept well away from it.

[4] *hazey:* dark gloomy weather . . .—f. 42.

[5] 'All Hands very busily employ'd in bringing Onboard, melting in the Coppers & stowing away Ice—clear'd & clean'd the Launch & stow'd her full.'—Clerke.—'. . . at present have the Launch with other convenient places about the Deck filled with ice.'—Mitchel, 23 February.

WEDNESDAY *24th. Winds ESE. Course S 16° E. Dist. Sailed 22 Miles. Lat. in South* 61°21′. *Longd. in East Reckg.* 95°15′. *Longd. in C.G.H.* 79°12′. Fresh gales & hazey with Snow and sleet. Stood to the South till 8 pm at which time we were in the Latitude of 61°52′ s, the Ice Islands were now so numerous that we had passed upwards of Sixty or Seventy sence noon many of them a mile or a mile and a half in circuit,[1] increasing both in number and Magnitude as we advanced to the South, sufficient reasons for us to tack and spend the night making short boards, accordingly we stood to the north under Reefed Topsails and Fore sail till midnight when we tacked and stood South having very thick hazey weather with Sleet & snow together with a very strong gale and a high Sea from the East. Under these circumstances and surrounded on every side with huge pieces of Ice equally as dangerous as so many rocks, it was natural for us to wish for day-light which when it came was so far from lessening the danger that it served to increase our apprehensions thereof by exhibiting to our view those mountains of ice which in the night would have been passed unseen. These obstacles together with dark nights and the advanced season of the year, discouraged me from carrying into execution a resolution I had taken of crossing the Antarctick Circle once more, according at 4 o'Clock in the AM we Tacked and Stood to the North under our two Courses and double reefed Topsails, stormy Weather still continuing which together with a great Sea from the East, made great distruction among the Islands of Ice. This was so far from being of any advantage to us that it served only to increase the number of pieces we had to avoide, for the pieces which break from the large Islands are more dangerous then the Islands themselves, the latter are generally seen at a sufficient distance to give time to steer clear of them, whereas the others cannot be seen in the night or thick weather till they are under the Bows: great as these dangers are, they are now become so very familiar to us that the apprehensions they cause are never of long duration and are in some measure compencated by the very curious and romantick Views[2] many of these Islands exhibit and which are greatly heightned by the foaming and dashing of the waves against them and into the several holes and caverns which are formed in the most of them, in short the whole exhibits a View which can only be discribed by the pencle of an able painter and

[1] . . . in the morn of the 23rd twenty three were seen at one time and in the course of the day one hundred and upwards, many of them a mile or a mile and a half in circuit and from forty to three or four hundred feet high.—f. 42.

[2] *the . . . Views:* the seasonable supplies of fresh water these ice Islands afford us, without which we must have been greatly distressed, also by the very romantick views . . . f. 43.

at once fills the mind with admiration and horror, the first is occasioned by the beautifullniss of the Picture and the latter by the danger attending it, for was a ship to fall aboard one of these large pieces of ice she would be dashed to pieces in a moment.[1]

THURSDAY 25*th. Thermr.* 35 *&* 36½. *Winds East, Calm, West. Course North. Dist. Sailed* 32 *Miles. Lat. in South* 60°49′. *Longd. in East Reckg.* 95°15′ *Watch* 94°27′. *Longd. in C.G.H.* 76°52′. *Varn.* 43°6′ *West.* Fresh gale with snow and sleet till the evening when the gale abated, and in the night it fell calm after which a light breeze sprung up at West with which we steered East having fair weather. Pass'd this 24 hours a great number of Ice Islands, and in the morning saw a Port Egmont hen. We have seen but few Birds of late and these were Albatrosses, sheerwaters and blue petrels, it is remarkable that we have seen none of either the white or Antarctick Petrels sence we came last among the ice.

FRIDAY 26*th. Thermr.* 33 *&* 36½. *Winds NW to East. Course S* 76½° *E. Dist. Sailed* 80 *Miles. Lat. in South* 61°8′. *Longd. in East Reck.g* 97°52′ *Watch* 97°7′. *Longd. East C.G.H.* 79°29′. *Varn.* 42°18′ *West.* Fair and clear weather with a gentle breeze from NW, North to East from which last point came a very high swell so that no land could be near in that direction. In the evening the Variation was 43°6′ and in the morn 41°30′ W both found by several Az[ths]. At Sun set had 21 Ice Islands in sight, about the same time saw a Port Egmont hen and one more in the morning. At Noon could only see five Islands of Ice.

SATURDAY 27*th. Thermr.* 35. *Winds East to South. Course N* 61°15′ *E. Dist. Sailed* 83 *Miles Lat. in South* 60°28′. *Longde. in East Reck.g* 100°19′. *Long[d] East C.G.H.* 81°56′. Stood South till 3 o'Clock when being in the Latitude of 61°21′ S the Wind having veer'd to the South of East, we Tacked and Stood to the NE and East as the Wind veered round to the South. In the Evening it blew a very strong gale with squals attended with Snow and Sleet which brought us under the double reefed Topsails and obliged us to strike Topg[t] yards: in the night closed reefed the Topsails, the gail still increasing attended with very

[1] 'Ice Islands very large. As we were passing one this morning it fell all to peices—'twas about four times as big as the Ship.'—Clerke 8951.—'About 19[h] a very large Island of Ice burst in an Instant into three large, and many small pieces just as we came a breast of it: it made no report, or at least so little, that we could not hear it for the noise of the Sea & y[e] whistling of y[e] wind in the Rigging. About 22[h] we passed by one of the most curious Islands of Ice I ever saw: Its form was that of an old square Castle, one End of which had fallen into Ruins, and it had a Hole quite through it whose roof so exactly resembled the Gothic arch of an old Postern Gateway that I believe it would have puzzled an Architect to have built it truer.'—Wales. Cf. Fig. 19.

thick hazey weather, Snow, Sleet and rain and what made it still worse betwixt 8 o'Clock and noon we fell in with several large Islands of Ice from whence such vast quantities had broke of as covered the sea as far as we could see and so close as to make it difficult for us to get through it.[1]

SUNDAY 28*th*. *Thermr*. 36½. *Winds South to SW*. *Course N* 77°15′ *E*. *Dist*. *Sailed* 135 *Miles*. *Lat*. *in South* 59°58′. *Longd*. *in East Reck.g* 104°44′. *Long^d East C.G.H.* 86°21′. In the pm the gale abated and the Wind veered to SSW and SWBS. Hazey weather with sleet continued till 8 o'Clock in the am when it became fair and tolerable clear, at day light in the morn got Topg^t yards across and set all the sail we could, having a fine fresh gale and but few Islands of Ice to impede us, the late gale having probably distroyed great numbers of them. A large hollow sea hath continued to accompany the Wind that is from the East round by the South to SW, so that no land can be hoped for betwixt these two extreme points. We have a breeding sow on board which yesterday morning Farrowed nine Pigs every one of which were killed by the cold before 4 o'Clock in the afternoon notwithstanding all the care we could take of them, from the same cause several People on board[2] have their feet and hands chilblain'd, from the circumstances a judgement may be formed of the summer weather we injoy here.[3]

[MARCH 1773]

MONDAY 1*st*. *Thermr*. 35½. *Winds WSW*, *NW*, *& NEBE*. *Course S* 67°15′ *E*. *Dist^ce Sailed* 95 *Miles*. *Lat*. *in South* 60°35′. *Longd*. *in East Reck.g* 107°42′. *Longd*. *East C.G.H.* 89°19′. Fresh gales fair and Clowdy till 7 pm when it fell little wind and continued so about 2 hours and then a breeze sprung up at NNW which gradually veer'd to NEBE and increased to a very fresh gale attend with Snow sleet and rain, towards noon the Wind abated, but hazey weather with drizling rain still continued.

TUESDAY 2*nd*. *Thermr*. 38. *Winds Calm*. *Course S* 40° *E*. *Dist^ce Sailed* 13 *Miles*. *Lat*. *in South* 60°45′. *Longd*. *in East Reck.g* 107°58′. *Longd*. *East C.G.H.* 89°35′. At 4 o'Clock in the PM it fell calm[4] and con-

[1] *as covered . . . it:* as to cover the Sea all round us and rendered sailing rather dangerous, however by noon we were clear of it all.—f. 43v.

[2] . . . my self as well as several of my people . . . f. 44.

[3] 'A Number of Black & White porpoises about the ship.'—Log.

[4] Pickersgill for this night recounts a danger which might or might not have been met adequately by the means proposed. '[PM Calm] A large Ice Island SSW [4 am] Small Rain. Ship setting fast towards the Ice Island. Got the Warping Machines ready. A Heavy Swell setting to the S^oward Got the Ships Head round, by which we got clear of the Ice Island.'

tinued so untill noon with Foggy wet weather and a Prodigious swell from NW.[1]

WEDNESDAY *3rd. Thermr.* 38. *Winds SE to SW. Course NEBE¾E. Dist^ce Sailed* 66 *Miles. Lat. in South* 60°17′. *Longd. in East Reck.g* 109°59′ *Watch* 109°15′. *Longd. East C.G.H.* 91°36′. *Varn.* 39°4′ *West.*[2] Hazey Clowdy weather with a gentle breeze from SE to SW but a large Swell still continues to come from the NW, the air milder then usual, in the morning we loosed all the Reefs out of the Topsails, got Topg^t yards across & set all the small sails; a little before Noon some few Penguins were seen, but not above six or eight Islands of Ice have been seen these two days. About Noon saw the Sun which we have not done for these 3 days past.[3]

THURSDAY *4th. Thermr.* 36½. *Winds SW, NW to NE. Course S* 83° *E. Dist^ce Sailed* 106 *Miles. Lat. in South* 60°30′. *Longd. in East Reck.g* 112°50′. *Longd. East C.G.H.* 93°27′. PM gentle gales and Clowdy, at times the Sun appeared and inabled us in some degree to obtain the Variation and Longitude by the Watch. In the evening took in all the small sails, in the night the Wind veer'd by the NW North to NE and increased to a fresh gale attended with a thick haze, Sleet and drizling rain, we however feel the air warmer than usual. NW swell not yet gone down.

FRIDAY *5th. Thermr.* 37¼. *Winds NW, WSW, & East. Course S* 88° *E. Dist^ce Sailed* 112 *Miles. Lat. in South* 60°38′. *Longd. in East Reck.g* 116°50′ *Watch* 116°21′. *Longd. East C.G.H.* 98°27′. Rain continued till 4 pm when the Wind at once shifted to WSW and brought with it fair Weather.[4] At 9 am it fell little wind & shifted again to the East.[5] A Large swell still continues to come from NW and WNW. Passed only one Ice Island this 24 hours.

These were the 'machines' which Cook was at such pains to get out of the Navy Board when preparing for the voyage, after Captain Elliot's demonstration at sea in May 1771 (I, p. 470). Mitchel, writing of the same occasion as Pickersgill, refers to them as 'the Water (or towing) sails'. We shall see their attempted use in crisis later.

[1] . . . and at the same time a nother from the South or SSE, the dashing of the one Wave against the other made the Ship both roll and Pitch exceedingly, but at length the NW swell prevailed.

[2] . . . but the observations by which this was determined were none of the best; we are however obliged to make use of such as we can get at the very few & short intervals the Sun appears.

[3] Wales was trying the electricity of the air again, not with great success: 'Whether this was caused by the rolling motion of the ship, which hindered me from holding the things steady, or my want of skill in the operation I cannot say'.

[4] . . . in the night steer'd E½S, in order to have the Wind, which was at SSW, more upon ye beam, the better to inable us to stand back in case we fell in with any danger in the night, for we had not so much time to spare to allow us to lay-to.—f. 44v.

[5] . . . with which we Stood to the North.

SATURDAY 6*th. Thermr.* 37. *Winds EBS, SEBE, Calm, and WBN. Course N* 40° *E. Dist*ce *Sailed* 45 *miles. Lat. in South* 60°4′. *Longd. in East Reck.g* 117°59′ *Watch* 117°19′. *Longd. East C.G.H.* 99°36′.[1] *Varn.* 31°3′ *West.* Little Wind variable unsettled weather with drizling rain. In the even had three Islands of ice in sight, one of them larger than any we have yet seen, the side opposed to us seemed to be a mile in length if so it could not be less than three in circuit, however we saw it in the morning more plain when it did not appear quite so large. The sea for some distance from it was covered with large loose pieces of ice which probably had broke from it in the night as a cracking breaking noise was heard continualy,[2] this Island could not be less than one hundred feet high and yet such was the impetus force and height of the Waves which were broke against it[3] that the Water was thrown a considerable height above it.[4]

SUNDAY 7*th. Thermr.* 34½. *Winds SWBS, NW, NE to East. Course N* 84° *E. Dist*ce *Sailed* 58 *Miles. Lat. in South* 59°59′. *Longde in East Reck.g* 120°15′ *Watch* 119°36′. *Longd. East of C.G.H.* 101°51′. Gentle breeze and clowdy with some Showers of snow and sleet in the AM. In the PM found the Varn by several Azths to be 31°30′ West. Not one ice island seen this 24 hours.[5]

MONDAY 8*th. Thermr.* 40. *Winds East to SSW. Course N* 47° *E. Dist*ce *Sailed* 38 *Miles. Lat. in South* 59°44′. *Longde in East Reck.g* 121°9′ *Watch* 120°6′. *Longd. East of C.G.H.* 102°44′. *Varn.* 28°39½′ *West.* Little Wind between the South and East till 5 AM when it fell calm. Hazey weather with Sleet and Snow continued till the evening after which we had fair & clear Weather for the remainder of the day

[1] . . . the Latitude was determined by the meridian altitude of the Sun which appeared now & then for a few minutes till 3 in the afternoon indeed the Sky was in general so cloudy and the Weather so thick and hazey, that we had very little benefit of either the Sun or Moon, very seldom seeing the face of either the one or the other, and yet even under these circumstances the Weather for some days past could not be called very cold, it however had not the least pretention to be called Summer weather according to my Ideas of Summer in the Northern Hemisphere as far as 60° of Latitude which is nearly as far North as I have been.—ff. 44v–45.

[2] . . . and the Island itself did not appear so large as it had done the evening before.—f. 45.

[3] . . . by meeting with such a sudden resistance.

[4] 'Captain Cook having Observ'd many of the People in rather a ragged condition, this forenoon he gave them some Needles thread and Buttons, that they may have no excuse for their tatter'd [*sic*]—they also have every Saturday to themselves to wash &c—that they may likewise have no excuse for a dirty, or improper appearance'.—Clerke 8951.—'The Captain gave the People needles & thread, at the same time examined their hands—those who had dirty, suffered the usual punishment (the daily allowance of grog stopped)'.—Mitchel. This entry is followed by a very heavily deleted line and a half, as if Mr Mitchel had said something disrespectful, and then thought better of it.

[5] 'Served the people (stopped yesterday) their usual allowance'.—Mitchel.

even to a degree little known in this Sea,[1] it was however of short duration and proved to be the forerunner of a Storm. We nevertheless profited by it by observing some distances of the Moon and Stars[2] and geting some other necessary observations, only one Isle of Ice seen.[3]

TUESDAY 9*th. Thermr.* 37. *Winds ESE to SEBS. Course N* 49°45′ *E. Dist^ce Sailed* 76 *Miles. Lat. in South* 58°55′. *Longde. in East Reck.g* 123°1′. *Longd. East of C.G.H.* 104°38′. The Calm continued till 3 pm, when it was succeeded by a breeze from the SE which in the night veered more to the South and increased in such a manner as to oblige us to take in all our small sails close reef the Top-sails and strike Topg^t yards, the gale was attended with a prodigious Sea, Sleet and rain circumstances by no means favourable for sailing in an unknown sea, but as we had no prospect of meeting with land we carried a priss'd sail and by keeping[4] about two or three points from the Wind she went at a great rate and altho we went in the through of the Sea, which as I have just observed run very high, we ship'd no Water to speake of, nor indeed has she done it at any other time. Upon the whole she goes as dry over the Sea as any ship I ever met with.

WEDNESDAY 10*th. Thermr.* 33 *&* 34. *Winds South to SSW. Course N* 71° *E. Dist^ce Sailed* 155 *Miles. Lat. in South* 58°5′. *Longde in East Reck.g* 127°41′. *Longd. East of C.G.H.* 109°18′. Very hard gales with frequent Squalls attended with Showers of Snow and Sleet till the AM when it became some what more moderate so that we could bear two reefs out of our topsails especially as the Wind veered more aft, had a pretty smart frost in the night[5].

THURSDAY 11*th. Thermr.* 34 *to* 37. *Winds SWBS, West, NW, & NEBE. Course S* 88°45′ *E. Dist^ce Sailed* 85 *Miles. Lat. in South* 58°7′. *Longde in East Reck.g* 130°21′. *Longd. East of C.G.H.* 111°58′. *Varn.* 11°57′ *West.* In the PM the gale became so moderate that we could bear all the reefs out and studding sails set, during night had but

[1] *evening . . . Sea:* evening when the Weather became fair, the sky cleared up, and the night was remarkably pleasant as well as the Morning of the next day which for the brightness of the sky serenity and Mildness of the Weather gave place to none we had seen sence we left the Cape, and was such as is little known in this Sea.—f. 45v.

[2] which satisfied us with respect to our Longitude.

[3] 'Had the People's Bedding up to Air & Clean'd between Decks'.—Cooper.

[4] *by keeping:* having nothing to take care of but ourselves we kept

[5] 'About 10 this Fore Noon Fenton one of the Armourers Assistants fell from the Fore Cat-Harpens into the weather Fore Chains and wou'd have been overboard, but was caught with great presence of mind by Solomon Rarden one of the Boatswains Mates who happen'd to be walking the Fore Castle and saw him falling. He luckily reciev'd no material Hurt.'—Clerke.

little Wind attend with sharp frost,[1] in the AM the Wind veered to NE and blew a fresh gale with which we stood to the Southward. The Weather being tolerable clear I took several Az^{ths} when the sun was on the Larboard side of the Sloop which gave the variation 11°57′, also several when the Sun was on the Starb^{d} side which gave the Var^{n} 8°34′, however I believe the first to be nearest the truth, differences even greater than this under the same circumstances we have frequently found without being able to find out the cause.[2]

FRIDAY 12*th. Thermr.* 37 *to* 39½. *Winds ENE, EBN, E., EBS, WBN. Course S* 50° *E. Dist^{ce} Sailed* 54 *Miles. Lat. in South* 58°56′. *Longd. in East Reck.g* 131°41′. *Longd. East of Cape* 113°18′. Fresh gale in the PM attended with Showers of sleet, for the three preceed^{g} days we have had a long hollow swell from the SSE and SEBS, and the Wind which occasioned it has not only ceased for the two last days but has blowen from opposite points. I have just reason to conclude that there is no land near in that direction, however as the Wind remained at East I continued to stand to the South till 3 o'Clock in the AM when it fell calm and a few hours after was succeeded by a light breeze from West with which we steered East having both mild and tolerable clear weather. The SSE swell having gone down in the night was succeeded by one from NWBW.

[1] '[11 p.m.] A very heavy swell, the Ship rolling almost continually Gunnell-in.'—Wales.

[2] For earlier differences see p. 89, n. 1 above. Wales has an entry on this subject for his 11th (Cook's 12th) both in his log and in his journal, and as Clerke refers to the same subject on the 12th it is possible that Cook has erred in his entry—particularly as the weather was much more favourable on the 12th. 'Having frequently remarked very considerable irregularities in the Observed Variations of the Compass,' says the log, 'I sometime ago had occasion to examine into the circumstances under which they were made, and found that almost all those which gave the least Variation were made when the sun, in the morning, was on the Starboard side the Ship, and those which gave ye most on the Larboard. I mentioned this to some of the Officers and also to Capt Cook, who said *I was a Philosopher*. However this morning, the following were taken (I suppose) to confute me . . .'—the results, which Cook gives, beautifully bearing out the Philosopher. Cook does not mention his own preliminary gibe, to which of course he was equally open himself. Wales recurs to the subject later, 23 June 1773: the position of the sun would depend on whether the Ship's head was pointing north or south. Clerke's account runs as follows: 'AM We took several sets of Azimuths by Knight's and Gregory's Compasses. We've often observ'd 3° & sometimes 4° difference in the Angle of the Magnetic Azimuth by shifting the Tacks of the Ship, and taking the observations from the different sides—now this being a fine Morning, smooth Water, and just wind enough to veer her Head whichever way answers best our purpose; the following Observations were made with two different Compass's to attain this Difference which I'm totally at a loss to account for'. A table of observations follows. Pickersgill notes the same phenomenon, and its frequency, '& can by no means account for it'.—The position of the sun, of course, was merely incidental to the direction in which the ship's head was pointing. The immediate cause of the discrepancies was no doubt the position of the ironwork in the ship relative to the compass: when the head pointed in one direction, east of it, when in the other, west—with all necessary modifications as the ship veered. It was not until the work of Flinders, Bain and Barlow that the matter was thoroughly understood, and the problem of correcting the error solved by Barlow's invention of the neutralizing plate (1820).

SATURDAY 13*th. Thermr.* 35, 36¼. *Winds West, East to SSE. Course N* 74° *E. Dist*ce *Sailed* 51 *Miles. Lat. in South* 58°42′. *Longd. in East Reck.g* 133°15′. *Longd. East of Cape* 114°52′. *Varn.* 9°49′ *West.* Clowdy mild weather with a gentle breeze till the evening when it fell calm, the good Weather was of as short duration being succeeded by Snow, Sleet and rain; the Calm continued till 3 in the AM when a breeze sprung up at East which afterwards freshened and veered to SSE with which we stood to the Eastward under all the sail we could set.

SUNDAY 14*th. Thermr.* 36, 30 *to* 33. *Winds SBE to SSW, SE to SSE. Course N* 75°15′ *E. Dist*ce *Sailed* 86 *Miles. Lat. in South* 58°22′. *Longd. in East Reck.g* 135°54′ *Watch* 134°42′. *Longd. East of Cape* 117°31′. PM a fresh breeze from the Southward, Clowdy over head but so clear in the Horizon that we could see many Leagues round us. In the night had a few hours Calm, which was succeeded by a breeze from the SE attended with showers of snow and a very smart frost, as the day advanced the Wind increased and the Weather became clear and pleasent and afforded us an oppertunity to make several observations of the Sun and Moon, the result of those made by Mr Wales (for I did not observe my self) reduced to Noon gave the Longitude 136°32′ E which is 28′ more East than my reckoning, an error which in this Latitude is very inconsiderable. Mr Kendalls Watch at the same time gave 134°42′ and that of Mr Arnolds gave the same, this is the first and only time they have pointed out the same Longitude sence we left England, the greatest difference between them sence we left the Cape has not much exceeded 2 Degrees. The moderate and I might almost say pleasent weather we have had at times for these two or three days past made me wish I had been a few degrees of Latitude farther South and even tempted me to incline a little with our course that way, but we soon had Weather which convinced me that we were full far enough and that the time was approaching when these Seas were not to be navigated without induring intense cold, which however by the by we were pretty well used to.[1]

MONDAY 15*th. Thermr.* 32 *to* 34. *Winds South to West. Course S* 70°15′ *E. Dist*ce *Sailed* 125 *Miles. Lat. in South* 59°4′. *Longd. in East Reck.g* 139°40′. *Longd. East of C.G.H.* 121°17′. The Serenity of the sky was of Short duration, presently after noon it became Clowdy, the Wind increased to a fresh gale, blew in Squalls attended with very thick and heavy Showers of Snow and hail, in somuch that our decks and Rigging were continually covered with Snow and ice.

[1] 'Mustered the People and found them very clean.'—Mitchel.

TUESDAY 16*th. Thermr.* 32 *to* 35½. *Winds WBN, SE & SSW. Course N* 83° *E. Dist*[ce] *Sailed* 117 *Miles. Lat. in South* 58°52′. *Longd. in East Reck.g* 143°27′. *Longd. East of C.G.H.* 124°4′. *Varn.* 2°6′ *West.* The same Weather continued till the evening when it cleared up and became fair and the Wind veered back to SE,[1] we nevertheless had a long hollow swell from WSW, such as assured us that we had left no land behind us in that direction, in the night we had a very sharp frost and at times the whole Heavens were illuminated by the Southern lights:[2] fair weather continued all the am, a little clowdy over head, but very clear in the Horizon. At 10 o'Clock which was as soon as the Sun appeared, I found the Variation to be 2°6′ W being at that time in La[t] 58°31′ S, Long 143°10′ East. The WSW swell increaseth.

WEDNESDAY 17*th. Thermr.* 33 *to* 35½. *Winds South to SW. Course N* 86°40′. *Dist*[ce] *Sailed* 163 *Miles. Lat. in South* 58°40′. *Longd. in East Reck.g* 147°43′. *Longd. East of C.G.H.* 129°20′. *Varn.* 0°31′ *East.* Fresh gales, in the pm showers of Snow and hail, the remainder mostly fair but very dark and gloomy. In the evening being in the Latitude of 58°58′ S Longitude 144′27° E I found the variation by several Az[ths] to be 0°31′ East. I was not a little pleased with being able to determine with so much precision this point of the line in which the Compass hath no variation.[3] We continued to steer to the East inclining a little to the South till 5 o'Clock in the am at which time we were in the Latitude of 59°7′ S Long 146°53′ E. We then bore away NE and at Noon steer'd North inclining to the East[4] with a resolution of making the best of my way to *New Holland* or *New Zealand*, my sole montive for wishing to make the former is to inform my self[5] whether or no Van Diemens Land makes a part of that continent. If the reader of this Journal desires to know my reasons for taking the resolution just mentioned I desire he will only consider that after crusing four months in these high Latitudes it must be natural for me to wish to injoy some short repose in a harbour where I can procure some refreshments for my people of which they begin to stand in need of, to this point too great attention could not be paid as the Voyage is but in its infancy.

[1] *it cleared . . . SE:* the sky cleared up and the evening was so serene and clear, that we could see many Leagues round us, the Horizon being the only boundaries to our sight . . . f. 47.

[2] 'The Aurora Australes Displayed themselfs Exceeding Beautyfull to Night.'—Elliott.

[3] . . . for I look upon half a degree [as] next to nothing and that the intersection of the Latitude and Longitude just mention[ed] may be reckoned the point without any sencible error, at any rate the line can only pass a very small matter West of it.—f. 47v.

[4] . . . having the advantage of a very fresh gale at SW with dark gloomy weather.

[5] *my sole . . . my self:* first to the former had the Wind permitted just to satisfy myself.

THURSDAY 18*th*. *Thermr.* 41½. *Winds West to NW. Course N* 33° *E. Dist*[ce] *Sailed* 130 *Miles. Lat. in South* 56°52′. *Longd. in East Reck.g* 149°53′. *Longd. E. of Cape* 131°30′. Fresh gales and dark gloomy weather, in the night the Wind shifted to NW blew in Squalls which obliged us to reefe our Topsails, in the AM it blew a hard gale attended with thick hazey weather and rain. In the evening we saw a Port Egmont Hen and in the morn[g] a large piece of rock Weed.[1]

FRIDAY 19*th*. *Thermr.* 43. *Winds WSW to NW. Course N* 34° *E. Dist*[ce] *Sailed* 134 *Miles. Lat. in South* 55°1′. *Longd. in East Reck.g* 152°1′. *Longd. E of Cape* 133°38′. Thick hazey weather with rain till the evening when the sky clear'd up and we had fair Weather most part of the night and the Heavens beautifully illuminated with the Southern lights.[2] At 5 o'Clock in the pm the variation by several Az[ths] was 13°30′ E being then in the Latitude of 56°15′ Longitude 150°0′ E, soon after we hauld up with the Log a piece of Rock weed which was all covered with Barnacles. At 7 o'Clock in the Morning we saw a Seal and towards Noon some Penguins and more rock Weed, all these are what Navigators have hitherto looked upon as signs of the vicinity of land,[3] however at this time we know of none, nor is it probable that there is any nearer than New Holland or Van Diemens and from which we are distant [260] Leagues.[4]

SATURDAY 20*th*. *Thermr.* 46. *Winds WNW to NW. Course N* 45°20′ [*E*]. *Dist*[ce] *Sailed* 141 *Miles. Lat. in South* 53°22′. *Longd. in East Reck.g* 154°53′ *Watch* 153°13′. *Longd. E of Cape* 136°30′. *Varn.* 11°19′ *East.* Very fresh gales, Clowdy & sometimes thick hazey weather with a swell from the Westward. PM Variation p[r] Az[th] 11°19′ E. Either this or the Var[n] yesterday must be wrong as the variation is certainly increasing.[5]

SUNDAY 21*st*. *Thermr.* 46. *Winds West to NW. Course N* 34° *E. Distn. Sailed* 76 *Miles. Lat. in South* 51°14′. *Longd. in East Reck.g* 157°11′.

[1] *a large . . . Weed:* hauled up with the Logg a piece of Rock Weed, which was in a state of decay and covered with Barnacles.—f. 49.

[2] 'These Lights were once so bright that we could discern our shadows on the Deck'.—Wales.

[3] . . . I cannot however support the opinion.

[4] . . . We had at the same time several Porpuses playing about us one of which M[r] Cooper struck a Harpoon into, but as the Ship was runing seven knotts, it broke its hold, after towing the fish some Minutes before we could bring her to. As the Wind continued between the North and the West, would not permit me to touch at Van Diemens land I shaped my Course for New Zealand and being under no apprehensions of meeting with any danger I was not backward in carrying sail as well by night as day, having the advantage of a very strong gale . . .—f. 49v.—The nearest land at this time was much nearer than New Holland or Van Diemen's Land, and not very far to the east. It was Macquarie Island, lat. 54°37′S, long. 158°54′E.

[5] 'Set y[e] Topgallant sails in y[e] doing of which the maintopgallant blew all to pieces so as to be quite useless.'—Log.

Longd. E. of Cape 138°48′. Very fresh gales and Clowdy mild Weather. Seven or Eight degrees of Latitude has made a surprising difference in the Temperature of the air.[1] At 7 o'Clock in the AM Saw a Seal & some Rock or Sea Weed and at noon 2 Port Egmont Hens.[2]

MONDAY 22*nd. Thermr.* 47. *Winds NW, West & South. Course N* 48°15′ *E. Dist^ce Sailed* 117 *Miles. Lat. in South* 49°56′. *Longd. in East Reck.g* 159°28′ *Watch* 157°54′. *Longd. E of Cape* 141°5′. *Varn.* 13°59′ *East.* In the pm had strong gales and clowdy, in the night rain. AM fresh gales and fair Weather and a very large swell from WSW.[3] At 7 in the pm saw a Seal, took in reef in each Topsail and handed the small sails for the night as usual, at day light in the morn, loosed the reefs out again & set the Topg^t sails and studding sails, by so doing we lost a studding sail boom, yard and Fore top-gall^t sail the latter being an old worn sail blew all to peices, the Main topgall^t sail which was in the same condition went the same way two days ago.

TUESDAY 23*rd. Thermr.* 49. *Winds South to SEBS. Course N* 34°45′ *E. Dist^ce Sailed* 158 *Miles. Lat. in South* 47°46′. *Longd. in East Reck.g* 161°47′ *Watch* 160°8′. *Longd. E. of Cape* 143°24′. Fresh gales and for the most part fair Weather with a very large swell from the South. In the AM saw a Seal & some Port Egmont Hens.

WEDNESDAY 24*th. Winds SE. Course N* 50°45′ *E. Distn. Sailed* 114 *Miles. Lat. in South* 46°33′. *Long. in East* 164°18′. *Longd. E. of Cape* 145°55′. Fresh gales in thc pm fair Weather, in the am hazey with drizling rain. Saw several Port Egmont Hens at different times this 24 hours.

THURSDAY 25*th. Thermr.* 54. *Winds SE to WBS. Course N* 77°45′ *E. Dist^ce Sailed* 80 *Miles. Lat. in South* 46°16′. *Long. in East Reck.g* 166°11′. *Longd. E. of Cape* 147°48′. Foggy wet weather continued till the evening when the Wind abated and the Weather cleared up, about 2 o'Clock we passed a peice of Wood & a quantity of Weed. In the morning the Wind shifted to South and SW when we made all sail, saw more Weed, Egg Birds, Port Egmont Hens &c^a. These signs of

[1] . . . which we felt with an agreeable satisfaction.—f. 49v.

[2] 'Many Peterels, some Albetrosses and 3 Port Egmont Hens about the Ship—these Egmont Hens attack and beat the Albetrosses—we've seen several instances of it today; the Albetrosses to avoid them get into the water. Here are likewise a brown Peterel about the size of a Pidgeon with a white Tail which I dont remember to have seen before.'—Clerke. This last bird could have been a northern stray of the Antarctic Petrel, which, by a sort of optical illusion, appears when on the wing to be brown with a white tail; but of course Clerke had met with Antarctic Petrels before.

[3] A . . . on the morning of the 22nd the wind shifted to South, and brought with it fair weather, . . . for these three days past the Mercury in the Thermometer rose to 46°, and we feel the weather quite mild, seven or eight degrees of Latitude has made a surprizing difference in the temperature of the air, which we feel with an agreable satisfaction.

the vicinity of land we were to expect for at 10 o'Clock the land of New Zealand was seen from the Masthead and at Noon from the Deck extending from NEBE to East distant 10 Leag[s]. For two days past we have had a very large swell from the SW.

[FRIDAY 26*th.*] Intending to put into *Dusky Bay* or any other Port I could find on the Southern part of *Newzealand*,[1] we steered in for the land under all the Sail I could set, haveing the advantage of a fresh gale and tolerable clear weather till half past 4 in the pm when the Weather became very thick and hazey, at this time we were within 3 or 4 Miles of the land and before the Mouth of a Bay which I had mistook for Dusky Bay,[2] being deceived by some Islands which lie before it.[3] Fearing to run into a place in thick weather we were utter strangers to, I tacked in 25 f[m] water and stood out to sea. This Bay lies on the SE side of West Cape and may be known by a White clift which is on one of the Islands which lies about the middle of the Mouth of the Bay;[4] this part of the Coast I did not see[5] in my last voyage, indeed we have seen so little of it now and under so many disadvantages, that all I have said of it must be very doubtfull.[6] We stood off to the South under Close reefed Topsails & Courses till 11 o'Clock when we wore and stood to the Northward,[7] at 5 o'Clock in the am the gale abated and we bore up for the land under all the sail we could set, at 8 the West Cape bore EBN½N, for which we steered and entred Dusky Bay about Noon in the mouth of which we found 44 fathom water, a Sandy Bottom, the West cape bearing SSE and the[8] North point of the Bay North, here we found a vast swell roll in from the SW, the Water Shoalden'd to 40 f[m], after which we had no ground with 60, we were however too far advanc[d] to return and therefore pushed on not doubting but what we should find anchorage, for in this Bay we were all strangers, in my last Voyage I did no more than discover it.[9]

SATURDAY 27*th.* After runing about two Leagues up the Bay without find'g Anchorage and having pass'd some of the Islands which

[1] AH Tavai-poenammoo

[2] '... this Bay we mistooke for Duskey Bay which lies on y[e] North side of y[e] Cape, that is where we now fell in with, we did not see in my former voyage, it seems to form a large Bay in which appears to be many Islands and some sunken rocks, but y[e] thick foggy Weather prevented us from seeing anything distinct.'—Log.

[3] A ... and seeing some breakers and broken ground ahead,

[4] Cook seems from his description to have been off Chalky Inlet.

[5] A ... but at a great distance

[6] *all ... doubtfull:* A the less I say about it the fewer mistakes I shall make.

[7] A ... having a very high and irregular sea

[8] *and the:* A and Point Five-fingers or the

[9] *discover it:* A discover and name it.

lie in it, I brought to, hoisted out two Boats and sent one of them with an officer round a point on the Larboard hand and upon her makeing the Signal for anchorage we followed with the Ship and came to an Anchor in 50 f^{m} water so near the shore[1] as to reach it with a hawser after having been 117 Days at Sea in which time we have Sailed [3660] Leagues without once having sight of land.[2] I

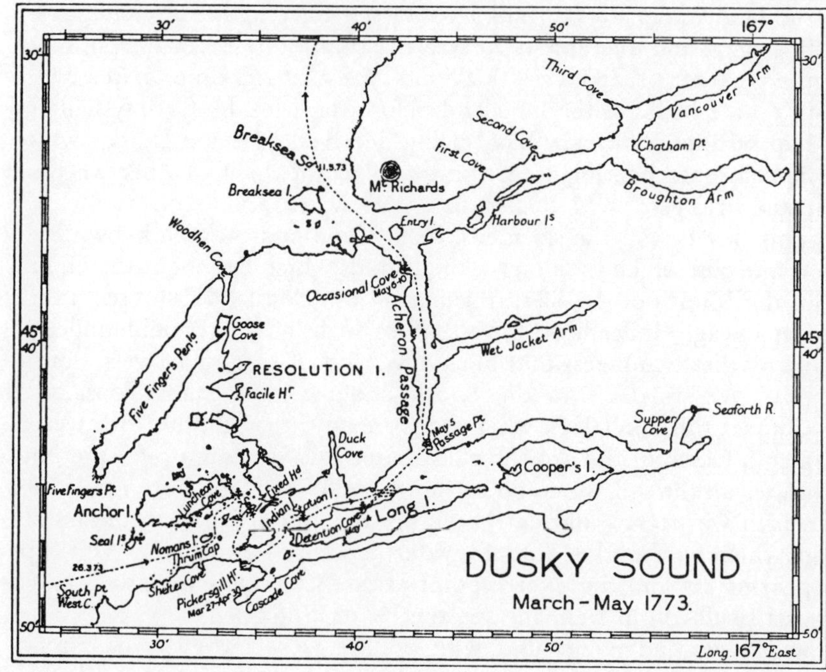

FIG. 22

cannot however help thinking but that there is some near the Meridian of the Mauritius and about the Latitude of 49° or 50° which I have been unfortunate enough not to find, at least the many Penguins and Divers we saw there seemed to indicate as much, but I shall refer makeing my remarks on this subject till I join the Adventure which cannot be far off if not already in *Queen Charlottes Sound* provided she hath met with nothing to retard her. It may be asked why I did not proceed directly for that place as being the Rendesvouze, the Discovery of a good Port in the Southern part of this Country and to find out its produce were objects more intresting, it

[1] Anchor Point, at the east end of Anchor Island.

[2] A gives the precise time of anchoring, 'at 3 in the afternoon'. The figure 3660 is from A and H (where it is inserted in Cook's hand).

is quite immeterial whether the Adventure joins us now or a Month or two hence. Mention has already been made of sweet wort being given to the Scorbutick People; the Marmalade of Carrots alone was also given to one man and we found that both had the desired effect in so much that we have only one man on board that can be called ill of this disease and two or three more on the Sick list of slight complaints.[1]

My first care after the Ship was moored was to send a Boat & People afishing,[2] in the mean time some of the Gentle[n] went in a Boat to a rock a small distance from the ship on which were many Seals,[3] one of which they killed which afforded us a fresh Meal. As I did not like the place we had anchored in I sent Lieut[t] Pickersgill over to the SE side of the Bay to look for a more convenient Harbour while I went my self to the other side for the same purpose, I found an exceeding snugg Harbour, but met with nothing else worthy to be noted. Soon after my return to the Ship M[r] Pickersgill returned also and reported that he had also succeeded in find[ing] a good harbour with every other conveniency. As I liked the situation of this harbour better than the one I had found I determined to go to it in the morning, the fishing Boat was equally as successful by returning with as much fish as all hands could eat for supper and in a few hours in the morning supplyed us with a Dinner. This gave us certain hopes of being Plentifully supplyed with fish.

We had rain in the night and untill 9 o'Clock in the Morning when we got under sail and with a small breeze at SW worked over to the NW side of the Bay where we anchored in M[r] Pickersgills Harbour which I found full as safe and convenient as he had reported.[4]

[1] *It may be asked . . . complaints:* A after such a long continuence at Sea in a high Southern Latitude it is but reasonable to think that many of my people would be ill of the Scurvy, the contrary however happen'd; mention hath already been made of Sweet Wort, and Marmalade of Carrots being given to such as were of a scorbutick habit of body, these had so far the desir'd effect, especially the former, that we had only one man onboard that could be call'd very ill of this disease, occasion'd chiefly by a bad habit of body, and a complication of other disorders; we are not to attribute the general good state of health in the Crew, wholy to the sweet Wort & Marmalade, this last was only given to one Man, we must allow Portable Broth and Sour Krout to have had some share in it, this last article can never be enough recommended.—Cf. Clerke, 28 March: 'We've now arriv'd at a Port with a Ships Crew in the best Order that I believe ever was heard of after such a long Passage at Sea—particularly if we come to consult Climates; this happy state of Health was certainly owing to the Extraordinary indulgencies of Govern[t] of Crowt, Wheat, Malt &c &c together with the strickt attention paid by Cap[t] Cook to the Peoples Clenliness.'

[2] 'and some hands to cut wood an Article that we were much in want of . . .'—Log.

[3] The New Zealand Fur Seal or Kekeno, *Arctocephalus forsteri* (Lesson).

[4] See the inset to Chart XXIX. It is rather difficult, looking at the chart, and also on the spot, to see why Cook brought the ship in through the narrow passage between the mainland and the high abrupt little Crayfish Island instead of round the other end of the island, but presumably that is the way Pickersgill went, and the boats were out to help. In any case, Cook generally knew what he was doing.

SUNDAY 28*th*. In the PM hauled the Sloop into a small creek and moored her head and stern to the Trees and so near the Shore as to reach it with a Brow or stage[1] which nature had in a manner prepared for us by a large tree which growed in a horizontal direction over the Water so long that the Top of it reached our gunwale. Wood for fuel was here so convenient that our yards were locked in the branches of the trees, about one hundred yards from our stern was a fine stream of fresh Water and every place abounded with excellent fish and the shores and Woods we found not distitute of wild fowl, so that we expected to injoy with ease what in our situation might be call'd the luxuries of life.[2] The few sheep and goats we had left were not likely to fair quite so well here being neither pasture nor grass to eat but what is course and harsh, nevertheless we were supprised to find that they would not eat it as they had not tasted either grass or hay for these many Weeks past,[3] nor did they seem over fond of the leaves of more tender plants and shrubs, upon examination we found their teeth loose and that many of them had every symptom of an inveterate Sea Scurvy; out of four Ewes and Two Rams I brought from the Cape with an intent to put a shore in this Country or any other I might have found, I have only been able to preserve one of each and even they are in so bad a state that it is doubtfull if they may recover.[4]

In the AM some of the officers went up the Bay in a small Boat on a shooting party, but returned again before noon and reported that they had seen Inhabitants in an Arm of the Bay[5] and as the Day was rainy and wet they did not think proper to land, but return to the Sloop and acquaint me therewith,[6] they had but just got on board when the Natives appeared in two or three Canoes off a point about a Mile from us and soon after retired behind the point out of sight probably owing to a heavy shower of rain which then fell.

MONDAY 29*th*. After the rain was over one small double Canoe in

[1] 'Brow', from Scandinavian *bru*, a bridge, a name for a ship's gangway still used in H.M. dockyards. 'Stage' in this sense seems to belong to the late eighteenth century. Fig. 24.

[2] A ... this determin'd me to spend some time in this Bay, in order to examine it thoroughly, as no one had ever landed before on any of the Southern parts of this Country, for in my last Voyage I had other and more greater objects in view, viz. the discovery of the whole Eastern Coast of New Holland.

[3] *nevertheless ... past:* A it was however not so bad, but that we expected they would devour it with great greediness, and were the more surpris'd to find that they would not taste it,

[4] A ... notwithstanding all the care possible had been taken of them.

[5] A ... for hitherto we had not seen the least vestigias of any.—This arm of the bay was Cascade Cove: see the entry for 12 April below.

[6] The Log version is that 'they discovered Inhabitants upon which they thought proper to return least they should be attack'd by the natives at a time when their fire arms would have been useless by reason of the rain which then fell ...'

which were Eight of the natives appeared again and came within musquet shott of the Ship where they [were] looking at us for about half an hour or more and then retired, all the signs of freindship we could make notwithstanding. After dinner I tooke two Boats and went in search of them in the Cove where they were first seen, accompaned by several of the officers and gentlemen, we found the Canoe[1] hauled upon the Shore, near two small mean hutts where there were several fire places, some fishing netts, a few fish lying on the beach and some in the Canoe; we however saw no people, they probably had retired into the Woods. After a short stay and leaving in the Canoe some medals, Looking glasses, Beeds &c[a] I embarked and rowed to the head of the Cove where we found nothing remarkable; in returning down the Cove we put a shore where we landed before but so still no people, they however could not be far off for we could smell the smoke of fire nor had any thing[2] I had put into the Canoe been touched to which I now added a hatchet[3] and then return with the night aboard.

In the AM no person went from the Ship, all hands were Employed clearing the Woods, making the Brow &c[a].

TUESDAY 30*th*. Showery Weather. In the PM a party of the officers made an excursion up the Bay and M[r] Forster with his party were out Botanizing, both partys returned in the evening without meeting with any thing remarkable. In the AM cleared places in the Woods near the Brook and set up Tents for the Water[er]s, Coopers, Sailmakers &c[a].

WEDNESDAY 31*st*. PM fair weather, Some hands assisting M[r] Wales to clear a place for his observatory. In the AM very stormy rainy Weather in so much that no Work could go forward.

[APRIL 1773]

THURSDAY 1*st*. Little Wind and tolerable fair. Began to cut down Wood for fuel, got our empty casks ashore to fill with Water and to repair such as were in want of repair, set up the Forge to repair our Iron Work[4] and put the Sail-makers to Work upon the Sails all of which were absolutly necessary occupations. Also began to Brew

[1] *Canoe:* A . . . Canoe, at least a Canoe,

[2] *fire . . . any thing:* A fire, but saw none, nor did I care to search farther or to force an interview they seem'd to avoid, well knowing that the way to obtain this was to leave the time and place to themselves; it did not appear that any thing . . .

[3] '. . . also a small hatchet sticking in a Tree & to Shew them the use of the latter we Bark'd a part of it.'—Cooper.

[4] A . . . we began to clear places in the Woods to set up the Astronomers observatory; . . . Tents for the Sailmakers and Cooper to repair the sails and Casks in . . .

Beer with the leaves & branches of a tree which resembles the Americo black Spruce Inspissated Juce of Wort and Melasses;[1] now I have mentioned the Inspissated Juce of Wort it may not be a miss to inform the reader that I have made several trials of it sence we left the Cape of Good Hope and find it to answer in a cold climate beyond all expectation: The Juce deluted in warm Water in the proportion of Twelve parts Water to one part Juce made a very good well tasted small Beer, some Juce I had from Mr Pelham himself[2] would bear Sixteen Waters to one of Juce, by making use of warm Water (which ought always to be done) and keeping of it in a Warm place if the Weather be cold, there will be no difficulty in fermenting it, a little grounds of either Small or Strong Beer will answer as well as yeast.[3] In the afternoon I went to the place where the Natives were first seen to see if any of the articles I had left there were taken away, but I found every thing just as I had left nor did it appear that any body had been there sence. We shott several curious Birds among which was a Duck of Blue grey Plumage with the end of its Bill as soft as the lips of any other animal, as it is altogether unknown I shall endeavour to preserve the Whole in spirits.[4] With the night I returned on board.

FRIDAY 2*nd*. A very pleasent Morning, Lieut^ts^ Clerk and Edgcomb and the two Mr Forsters went in a small Boat to the Indian Cove[5] to search for the productions of Nature while myself with Lieut^t^ Pickersgill & Mr Hodges went in the Pinnace to view the North West part of the Bay, in our Way we touched at the Seal rock where we killed three Seals one of which afforded us much sport. After passing several Isles we at length came to the most northern & Western

[1] A ... from the knowledge I had of, and the similarity this tree bore to the Spruce, I judged that with the addition of the other articles it would make a very wholsom Beer and make up for the want of Vegetables which this place did not afford and the event proved that I was not misstaken.—Cf. Cooper: '... began to make Beer from a Tree of a Rosinish quality intermixt with the Tea Plant.'—The tree was the Rimu, *Dacrydium cupressinum*; the Tea Plant the Manuka, *Leptospermum scoparium*.

[2] *from ... himself:* A of Mr Pelham's own preparing

[3] Clerke, 5 April, has a note on the beer: '... got Beer on board for the People and stopt their Spirits—this Beer I think is a very palatable pleasant drink; the Major part of the People I believe are of the same Opinion, for they seem to drink pretty plentifully of it....' Sparrman also has a note (p. 26): 'After a small amount of rum or arrack has been added, with some brown sugar, and stirred into this really pleasant, refreshing, and healthy drink, it bubbled and tasted rather like champagne; it was called *kallebogas*, after a similar mixture in North America'. Banks, in his early Newfoundland journal, describes the North American refinements: spruce beer with rum or brandy or gin added made Callibogus; with egg and sugar made Egg Calli; with spirits, drunk hot, made Kings Calli. But hot champagne sounds rather daunting.

[4] The Blue Duck or Whio, *Hymenolaimus malacorhyncos* (Gm.).

[5] Cascade Cove, not the Indian Cove, so named on the engraved chart, at the east end of Indian Isle.

Arm of the Bay the same as is formed by the Land of Point five fingers, in the Bottom of this Arm[1] we found many Ducks, Water Hens[2] and other Wild fowl. Some we killed and returned on board at 10 o'Clock in the evening when I learnt that the other party had had but indiffer[t] sport, they took with them a black Dog which we got at the Cape, at the first Musquet they fired he ran into the Woods from whence he could not be prevaled upon to return.[3]

SATURDAY *3rd.* Showery in the afternoon. Only the fishing Boat from the Ship to day. A four footed animal has been several times seen in the Woods near the Ship, but as we have not been fortunate enough to catch it, it is not easy to say what sort of an Animal it is, for although it has been seen by several no two have agree'd in their description of it, all however agree that it is of a   Colour and about the size of a large Catt and those who seem to have had the best view of it say that it is the most like a Jackal of any animal known.[4] To day we had an excellent dinner on fish, Seal and wild fowl.

SUNDAY *4th,* MONDAY *5th.* Wind Westerly with very rainy dirty Weather so that little or no work could be done. In the after noon of the latter being tolerable fair I imployed my self in surveying where I also met with good sport among the Curlews or Black Birds.[5]

TUESDAY *6th.* Early in the Morn a Shooting party made up wholy of the officers went in a small Boat to the place where I was on Friday last and my self accompanied by the two M[r] Forsters and M[r] Hodges set out in the Pinnace upon the Survey of the Bay, my attention was directed to the North side where and about half way up the Bay I discovered a very safe and capacious Cove in the bottom of

[1] Goose Cove.

[2] *Gallirallus australis* Sparrman, a flightless rail known as Weka by the Maoris.

[3] This misguided animal, after a fortnight's burst of freedom, came back to his masters, to be slain for a roast in mid-Pacific, on 9 June following.

[4] This other 'four-footed animal' was illusory, unless the report was founded on indistinct glimpses of a Maori dog, or possibly the wandering ship's dog. In a later passage of B (f. 61) Cook adds to the description, that it had short legs and a bushy tail and was of a mouse colour. The Maori dog had short legs and a thick tail, but was generally black or white in colour. Forster, *Observations*, p. 190, says the mysterious animal was seen at dawn, and must have been a mistake. Edward Bell, the clerk of the *Chatham* with Vancouver, who visited Dusky Sound in November 1791, wrote in his journal, 'We saw no animals here, nor the slightest marks of any, tho' Captn. Cook says there are animals here, and that one of his people saw one, but a Sailor when he goes ashore at a strange place is sure to see more than anyone else can. One of our Carpenters said he saw a Bear at the Wooding place, but on being question'd what it was like said it was White, like a Greenland Bear, which is so very improbable that he found few that wou'd credit his story'.—*Hist. Rec. N.Z.*, II, p. 500.

[5] The black phase of the New Zealand Oyster-catcher, the Maori Toreapango, *Haematopus ostralegus unicolor* Forst. Cook met them on the first voyage at Mercury Bay.

which is a fresh Water River and on the Western shore several beautiful small Cascades, and the Shores are so steep that a ship may lie near enough to convey ye Water into her with a hose. In this Cove we shott fourteen Ducks which occasioned my naming it Duck Cove: on our return in the evening[1] we had a short interview with three of the Natives, one man and two Women, they first discovered themselves on the NE point of Indian Island, named so on this occasion.

WEDNESDAY *7th.* The man called to us as we passed by from the point of a Rock on which he stood with his staff of destruction in his hand,[2] the two Women stood behind him at the skirts of the Woods with each a Spear in her hand, the man seemed rather afraid[3] when we approached the Rock with our Boat, he however stood firm. I threw him a shore two handkerchiefs but he did not desend the Rock to take them up. At length I landed went up and imbraced him and presented him with such articles as I had about me which disapated his fears[4] and presently after we were joined by the two Women, the Gentlemen that were with me and some of the Seamen and we spent about half an hour in chitchat which was little understood on either side in which the youngest of the two Women bore by far the greatest share.[5] We presented them with fish and Wild fowl which we had in our boat, which the young Woman afterwards took up one by one and threw them into the Boat again giving us to understand that such things they wanted not. Night approaching obliged us to take leave of them, when the young Woman gave us a

[1] i.e. the evening of the 7th, ship time. In the course of his narrative Cook has slightly misplaced this date.

[2] *The man . . . hand:* A we should have pass'd without seeing them had not the man holloa'd to us, he stood with his club in his hand upon the point of a rock.—But what exactly did the man have in his hand? A 'staff of destruction' would, one might at first think, be the 'spear' called *taiaha*; a 'club' might be some sort of *patu*; see I, p. 200. In Hodges' drawing of the 'Family in Dusky Bay, New Zealand' (*Voyage*, I, pl. LXIII) the man is leaning on a large *pouwhenua*, with one end rather paddle-shaped, equivalent to a long club; and this might also be regarded as a 'staff of destruction'. His *patu* hangs at his waist. One of the women is holding the long spear called *huata*, which ascends out of the picture. See also Fig. 26.

[3] *seemed rather afraid:* A could not help discovering great signs of fear

[4] George Forster, who is so often, for whatever reason, censorious of his shipmates, cannot refrain at times from implicit admiration of Cook, as here: 'Captain Cook went to the head of the boat, called to him in a friendly manner, and threw him his own and some other handkerchiefs, which he would not pick up. The captain then taking some sheets of white paper in his hand, landed on the rock unarmed, and held the paper out to the native. The man now trembled very visibly, and having exhibited strong marks of fear in his countenance, took the paper: upon which captain Cook coming up to him, took hold of his hand, and embraced him, touching the man's nose with his own, which is their mode of salutation'.—Forster, I, pp. 137–8; and for a like instance, p. 169. Cf. Elliott, p. 124, n. 3 below.

[5] AH . . . which occasion'd one of the Seamen to say, that weomen did not want tongue in no part of the world . . .

Dance but the man view'd[1] us with great attention. At midnight the sportsmen returned having had but indifferent success. In the morning I went again to the Indians[2] and carried with me various articles which I presented them with, most of which they received with a great deal of indifferency, except hatchets and spike nails, these they seemed to value very much. The interview was at the same place as last night and where we saw the whole Family which consisted of the Man, his two wives,[3] the young Woman before mentioned his daughter,[4] a Boy about 14 or 15 years of age and three small Children the youngest of which was at the breast, they were all well looking people except one Woman, Mother to the young Woman, who had a large Wan on her upper lip which made her look disagreeable enough and seemed[5] to be intirely neglected by the man. They conducted us to their habitation which was but a little within the skirts of the Woods and were two low wretched huts made of the bark of trees. Their Canoe was made fast in a creek near to them, a small double one just capable to transport the whole family from place to place. During our stay with them Mr Hodges made drawens of them which occasioned them to give him the name of Toetoe.[6] When we took leave of them the Chief presented me with a piece of Cloth and some other trifles and immediately after expressed a desire for one of our Boat Cloaks,[7] I took the hint and ordered one to be made for him of red Baize as soon as I came on board.

THURSDAY *8th.* Rainy Weather most part of this 24 hours. In the [morning?] hauled the Seine for the first time but caught only four fish. Hooks and lines make up for these difficiency.[8]

[1] *when . . . viewed:* when the youngest of the two Women whose Volubility of Tongue exceeding every thing I ever met with, gave us a dance but the man stood and viewed . . . —f. 52.

[2] *went . . . Indians:* made the Natives another Visit accompanied by Mr Forster and Mr Hodges

[3] . . . (as we supposed).—But in the Log Cook refers to 'a Man his Wife a Middle aged Woman sister to either ye man or wife . . .' Monogamy was the ordinary Maori custom, but polygamy was not unknown, mainly among the *rangatira* or chiefly class.

[4] 'one jolly Wench of a Daughter'.—Clerke, 11 April.

[5] . . . on that account

[6] *Toetoe:* Toe-toe, which word we supposed signifies marking or painting.—*Tuhituhi,* to paint, draw.

[7] 'Boat-cloaks are commonly of prodigious dimensions and great width, so that the whole body may be wrapped into them several times'.—Forster, I, p. 115. A boat-cloak, which is supposed to have belonged to Nelson's Hardy, preserved in the National Maritime Museum, is of blue or green baize; the body is a vast semicircle of material, of five feet radius, attached to the shoulder piece with a uniform 'anchor' button to fasten the neck; there is a hood, like that of a duffle coat.

[8] 'We abound every day in Excellent Fish: which one Boat supplies in 3 or 4 hours fishing'.—Clerke.

FRIDAY 9*th*. In the PM I viseted the Natives, we made known our approach by hollowing but they did not meet us at the shore as usual, they were perhaps better employed for when we came to their habitation they were all dressed, Man Women and Children, in their best Cloathing with their hair comb'd oyled and tyed upon the crowns of their heads and oramented with white feathers.[1] I presented the chief with the Cloak with which he seemed well pleased and took his Patta-pattou from his girdle and gave it me, after a short Stay we took leave and rowed over to the North side of the Bay in order to continue the Survey and on this service I spent the day.

SATURDAY 10*th*. Very heavy rain all the night which did not cease at Noon.[2]

SUNDAY 11*th*. Rain continued all the PM but the Morning was clear and Serene which afforded an oppertunity for us to dry our linnen a thing very much wanting, not having had fair weather enough for that purpose sence we put into this Bay. Mr Forster and his party profited by the day in Botanizing. About 10 o'Clock the family of the Natives paid us a visit, seeing that they approachd the Ship with great caution I met them in my Boat which I quited and went into their canoe, nevertheless I could not prevail upon them to put along side the Ship and was at last obliged to leave them to follow their own inclinations; at length they put a shore in a little creek hard by us and afterwards came and set down on the shore abreast of the Ship near enough to speak to us. I caused the Bagpipes and fife to be played and the Drum to be beat, this last they admired most, nothing however would induce them to come a board but they entered with great familiarity into conversation[3] with such of the officers & Seamen as went to them and paid a much greater regard to some more than others and these we had reason to believe they took to be Women,[4] to one man in particular the Girl shewed an

[1] *oramented . . . feathers:* stuck with white feathers, some wore a *fillet* of feathers round their heads and all of them had bunches of white feathers stuck in their ears, thus dress'd and all standing they received us with great courtesy.—f. 52v.—It looks as if this family had exploited the albatross. Bunches of albatross or gannet down, known as *pohoi*, were much favoured as ear ornaments among the Maori people.

[2] . . . no work was done.

[3] . . . (little understood).—But cf. Clerke, 12 April: 'their language seems much more harsh than the Language of the Northern Inhabitants of this Island but a great many of their words I find are perfectly alike and I believe this difference which we observe is principally the difference of the Dialect rather than the Language'.

[4] Possibly, as Sparrman says, because of a rather delicate, feminine appearance; partly perhaps because of the frocks worn by these seamen: it is difficult to think of any other explanation, if Cook's belief was justified. See also Wales, p. 780 below.

extraordinary fondness untill she discovered his sex and then she would not suffer him to come near her, whether it was because that she before realy took him for a Women or that the Man[1] had taken some liberties with her which she thus resented I know not.

MONDAY 12*th*. Being a fine afternoon I took Mr Hodges to a large Cascade which falls down a high mountain on the South side of the Bay about a League higher up than the Cove where we are anchrd. He took a drawing of it on Paper and afterwards painted it in oyle Colours[2] which exhibits at one view a better discription of it than I can give, huge heaps of stones lies at the foot of this Cascade which have been brought by the force of the Stream from adjacent mountains, the stones were of different sorts, none however appeared to contain[3] either Minerals or Mitals, nevertheless I brought away specimens[4] of every sort as the whole country, that is the rocky part of it, seems to be made up of these sort of stones and no other. This Cascade is at the East point of a Cove which lies in SW about [2 Miles] which I named Cascade Cove, in it is good anchorage and all other necessaries,[5] at the entrence is an Island with a good Passage on each side, that on the east side is by much the widest, near midd channell and a little above the Isle are two Rocks which are covered at high-water, it was in this cove we first saw the Natives. When I returnd aboard in the evening, I found that the natives had taken up their quarters not more than one hundred yards from our watering place which was a great mark of the intire confidence they placed in us. After dinner a shooting party made up of the officers went over to the North side of the Bay having the small Cutter to convey them from place to place. In the Morning I went in the Pinnace, accompanied by Mr Forster, to Survey the Isles and Rocks which lie in the mouth of the Bay, I found some of them to shelter a very Snug Cove, on the SE side of Anchor Isle, from all Winds, which we call'd Lunchen Cove because here we dined on Craw fish[6] on the side of a pleasent brook under the shade of the trees.

[1] . . . in order to discover himself.

[2] 'Some of these cascades with their neighbouring scenery, require the pencil and genius of a Salvator Rosa to do them justice: however the ingenious artist, who went with us on this expedition has great merit, in having executed some of these romantic landscapes in a masterly manner.'—Forster, *Observations*, pp. 51–2.—The painting mentioned by Cook must be one of those that now hang in Admiralty House, London. See Fig. 25.

[3] *appeared to contain:* according to Mr Forsters opinion, who I believe to be a judge, contains . . .—f. 53.

[4] The word in the MS is indeterminate, but reads most like 'spicumas'. As all the other MSS read 'specimens', I print it intelligibly thus.

[5] Cook's sober estimate falls far short, it must be admitted, of the eloquence devoted by George Forster to the description of this romantic spot, I, pp. 146–9.

[6] Probably *Jasus lalandi* (Lamarck), a large sea crawfish.

TUESDAY 13*th*. After dinner we proceed by rowing out to the outermost Isles where we saw many Seals, fourteen we killed and brought away with us, we might have got many more could we have landed with safty on the other Isles.[1] I returned aboard about 8 o'Clock in the evening and the next morning set out again to continue the Survey. I intend to have landed again on the Seal Isles but there run such a surf that I could not come near them, with some difficulty I rowed out to Sea and round the SW end of Anchor Isle, it happened very lucky that I took this round[2] in which we found the Sportsmen Boat adrift with no one in her, we lay hold of her the very moment she was going to be dashed against the Rocks. I was not at a loss to guess how she came adrift nor was I under any apprehensions for the safty of the People[3] who had been in her; after securing[4] the Boat in a little creek I proceeded to the place where we supposed the Gentlemen to be & which we reached between 7 & 8 o'Clock in the evening and found them upon a small Isle in Goose Cove, where as the tide was out we could not come with the Boat but was obliged to wait till the return of the flood and as this would not happen till 3 o'Clock in the morning we land upon a naked beach, not knowing where to find a better place, and after some time got a fire and broiled some fish on which we made a hearty supper without any other sauce than a good appetite. After this we laid down to sleep having a stoney beach of a bed and the canopy of Heaven four a covering. At length the Tide permited us to take of the sportsmen and with them we imbarqued & proceed for the place where we had left their boat which we soon reached having a breeze of wind in our favour attended with rain. When we came to the Creek which was on the NW side of Anchor Isle we found their an immence number of Blue Peterls, some on the Wing, others in the Woods, in holes in the ground, under the roots of trees and in the creveses of rocks where they had desposited their young;[5] as not one was to be seen in the day time they must be then out at sea seaking for food which they bring to their young in the evening, the noise they made was like the croaking of Frogs.[6] After restoring the sportsmen to their boat

[1] *could . . . Isles:* would the Surf have permitted us to land with safety on all the rocks . . . —f. 53v.

[2] MS rount: he may have intended 'route'.

[3] *People:* gentlemen

[4] *after securing:* after refreshing our selves with such as we had to eat and drink and securing . . .—Wednesday 14th is to be understood as coming in somewhere about this position in the narrative, as Cook is still writing in terms of ship time.

[5] *where . . . young:* where there was no getting at them and where we supposed their young ones where [*sic*] . . .—f. 54.

[6] . . . they are I beleive of the broad bill'd kind which sort are not so commonly seen at sea as the others, here however they are in great numbers and fly much about in the

we all proceeded for the Ship which we reached at 7 o'Clock not a little fatigued with our nights expedition.

Last night the natives returned to their habitations probably foreseeing that rainy weather was at hand.

THURSDAY 15*th*. Rain continued all the PM and most part of the night, in the morning it cleared up and became fair, when I set out with two Boats to continue the Survey of the NW side of the Bay accompanied by the two Mr Forsters and several of the officers which I detatched in one boat to Goose Cove, where we intended to lodge the night, while I proceeded in the other examining the harbours and Isles which laid in my way.

FRIDAY 16*th*. While I was rowing about the shores I picked up about a score Wild fowl and caught fish sufficient to serve us the night[1] and reached the place of rendezvouze a little after dark and found the Gentlemin all out Duck Shooting, they however soon returnd having had but indifferent sport,[2] by that time I had got a hutt built and Dinner & supper, for we joined them in one, was near ready,[3] after a hearty repast on what the day had produced we laid down to rest, but took care to rise before day in the Morning in order to have a little sport[4] among the Ducks before we left the Cove. Accordingly at Day light we prepared for the attack, those who had reconnoitred the place before choose their stations accordingly whilest I and one of the Petty officers remained in the Boat and rowed to the head of the Cove in order to Start the game which we did so effectually that out of some scores of Ducks we only detained one to our selves, sending all the rest down to those stationed below: after this I landed and walked aCross the narrow Isthmus which disjoins this Cove from the Sea or rather from a nother Cove which ru[n]s in from Sea about one Mile, it lies open to the [north winds] it however had all the appearence of a good Harbour and safe Anchorage, at the head is a fine sandy beach where I found a vast number of Water or Wood Hens[5] a score of them I shott which recompenced me for the trouble of crossing the Isthmus through the wet Woods up to the back side in Water and also made up for the loss of the Ducks. About 9 o'Clock we all got collected to-

night, some of our gentlemen at first took them for batts.—f. 54. Probably this was the Broad-billed Whale Bird, which breeds here.

[1] *us the night:* the whole party

[2] *having . . . sport:* not over loaded with game

[3] *by that . . . ready:* by this time the Cooks had done their parts, in which little art was required

[4] *a little sport:* the other bout

[5] Hence the name on the engraved chart, Wood Hen Cove. Again the Weka.

gether when the success of every one was known which was by no means great,[1] indeed the weather was unfavourable for shooting being rainy all the morning. After breakfast we set out to return aboard continuing the Survey in my way and picking up what game we met with.

SATURDAY 17*th*. We got on board in the evening with about seven dozen of wild fowls and two Seals, the most of them shott while I was rowing about exploreing the Coves and Harbours I met with, every place affording something especially to us to whom nothing came a miss. Rain all the AM which confind every body to the Ship.

SUNDAY 18*th*. In the AM fair and clear weather which we employed in drying our sails &c[a].

MONDAY 19*th*. In the PM the family of the natives before mentioned made us a nother Viset and in the morning the Chief and his Daughter[2] were induced to come on board while the rest of the family went out in the Canoe afishing, before they came on board I shew'd them the Sheep and Goats which they viewed for a moment with a kind of stupid insensibility, after this I conducted them to the brow, but before the chief set his foot upon it to come into the Ship he took a small branch in his hand with which he struck the Ship side two or three times repeating at the same time a speach or Prayer, which when done he threw the branch into the main chains and came on board[3] followed by the girl. I then took them down into the Cabbin and we set down to breakfast, they sat at table with us but would not tast any of our Victuals, the Chief wanted to know where I slept and to pry into every part of the Cabbin every part of which he viewed with some surprise but it was not possible to fix his attention to any one thing a single moment.[4] What seemed to strike them the most was the number and strength of the Decks and other parts of the Ship: the Chief (before I gave him any thing)[5] presented me with a piece of Cloth and a green talk hatchet,[6] he also

[1] *great:* answerable to our expectation

[2] A *note:* We learnt afterwards that this young Woman was not his Daughter

[3] . . . this custom and manner of makeing peace as it were is practised by all the nations in the South Seas I have seen; . . .—f. 55.

[4] . . . the works of art appeared to him in the same light as those of nature and were as far remov'd beyond his comprehension.—f. 55.—According to Marra (p. 29) the old man was much taken with the process of sawing plank on board, and took the pitman's place himself, but soon gave out; the sawyers and carpenters at work were his favourite sight. If this was so, it is curious that no one else mentions it.

[5] *before . . . anything:* before he came aboard

[6] i.e. a greenstone or nephrite adze, *toki pounamu.*

gave a piece of cloth to Mr Forster and the girl presented Mr Hodges with a nother piece,[1] this custom is common among the Natives of the South Sea Isles, but I never saw it practised in New Zealand before. Of all the various articles which I gave him, hatchets and Nails were the most valuable in his eyes, these he never would suffer to go out of his hands after he had on[c]e got them whereas many other articles he would lay down and even leave behind him, as soon as I could get quet of them they were conducted down into the Gun-room where I left them[2] and set out with two Boats to examine the head of the Bay[3] my self in one accompanied by the two Mr Forsters and Mr Hodges and Lieut^t^ Cooper in the other.

TUESDAY 20*th*. Without meeting with any thing remarkable we reached the head of the Bay by sunset where we took up our quarters for the night.[4] At day light in the Morn I took two men in one of the Boats and with Mr Forster went to take a view of the flat land at the head of the Bay,[5] we land on one side and ordered the Boat to meet us at the other, we had not been long landed before we saw some ducks which by creeping through the bushes we got a shott at and killed one, the moment we had fired the natives, which we had not discovered before, set up a most hideous and clamorous noise in two or three places close by us, we hollowed in our turn and at the same time retired to our boat which was full half a mile off, the natives kept up their clamoring noise but did not follow us, indeed we found afterwards that they could not because of a branch of the River between us and them.[6] As soon as we got to our boat and found

[1] Cloth—i.e. woven flax material. Mitchel says the Maoris ventured on board 'bringing with them, some new outside apparel, stuffed with feathers—(agreeable to the Climate) & made it a present to the Captain &c'. This looks like a description of a valuable *kahu*, or feather cloak—the feathers being very ingeniously incorporated on the outside of the woven surface. If Mitchel is accurate, then Cook hardly lays enough stress on the nature of the gift.

[2] The gunroom was aft, on the deck below the great cabin and steerage, and was where the lieutenants messed. Clerke has a characteristic account: 'the Old Gentleman and the Young Lady his Daughter ventur'd to pay us a Visit onboard the Ship—they seem'd a good deal delighted with viewing the various parts of the Vessel and were very desirous of Hatchets, Nails and Fish Hooks with which Articles I believe they got themselves very well pay'd for their complaisance in favouring us with this Visit. The Gallantry of our People in general made them very anxious to pay some Compliment to the Young Lady, as 'twas the first Female we had seen for many Months, but the Young Gypsey did not seem at all inclin'd to repay them in the Kind Indian Women in general trade in and indeed the Kind that's most esteem'd I believe by all men after so long an absence from the Sex'.

[3] That is, the head of the most southerly part of the Sound; they passed to the south of Long Island and Cooper's Island.

[4] . . . at the first place we could land upon for the flatts hindered us from geting quite to the head.

[5] . . . near to where we spent the night.

[6] . . . nor did we find their numbers answerable to the noise they made

that their was a river[1] I rowed into it and was soon after joined by Mr Cooper in the other boat, with this reinforcement I proceed up the River shooting wild Ducks, of which there were plenty, as we went along, now and then hearing the natives in the Woods, at length two appeared on the banks of the River a man and a woman, the latter waving some thing white in her hand as a sign of freindship. Mr Cooper being near them I calld to him to land as I wanted to take the advantage of the tide to get as high up as I could which did not much exceed half a mile before I was stoped by the rapidity of the Stream and great stones which laid in the bed of the River, upon my return I found that as Mr Cooper did not land when the natives expected him they had retired into the Woods, but two others appeared on the opposite shore whom I endeavoured to have an interview with, but this I could not effect[2] and as the tide was now falling I retired out of the River to the place where we laid the night and where we breakfasted, which done we imbarqued in order to return on board, but just as we were going we saw two men on the opposite side of the Bay hollowing to us, this induced me to row over to them and as the flatts would not permit the Boats to come near the Shore I waded out to them with two men more all unarmed, the two natives standing about one hundred yards from the Water side with each a spear in his hand, as we advanced they retired but waited when I advanced alone and beckoned with their hands for the others to keep back as they had seen me do.[3] At length one of them laid down his spear,[4] pulled up a grass plant and came to me with it in his hand giving me hold of one end while he held the other, standing in this manner he made a speach not one word of which I understood, in it were some long pauses waiting as I thought for me to make answer, for when I spoke he proceeded; as soon as

[1] . . . that would admit the boats.—This river is called on Pickersgill's chart of Dusky Sound (P.R.O. Adm 51/4553) the Alarm River; it is the Seaforth, which debouches into Supper Cove; there is deep soft mud at its mouth, the configuration of which has altered somewhat since Cook's day.

[2] . . . for as I approached the shore they always retired farther into the woods which was so thick as to cover them from our sight.

[3] Probably this is the episode referred to by Elliott *Mem.* ff. 16v–17, as one typical of Cook's character: 'Upon another occasion Captn Cook found more Natives, at a distance up the Sound, and took much pains to gain an intercourse with them, but they never came near the Ship; And certainly no man could be better calculated to gain the confidence of Savages than Captn Cook. He was Brave, uncommonly Cool, Humane, and Patient. He would land alone unarm'd—or lay aside his Arms, and sit down, when they threaten'd with theirs, throwing them Beads, Knives, and other little presents then by degrees advancing nearer, till by Patience, and forbearance, he gain'd their friendship, and an intercourse with them; which to people in our situation, was of the utmost consequence'.

[4] *At length . . . spear:* it was some little time before I could prevail upon them to lay down their spears which at last one of them did, . . .—f. 55v.

this ceremony was over, which was but short we saluted each other, he then took his hahou[1] or coat from off his back and put it upon mine after which peace seemed firmly established, more of our people joining us did not in the least allarm them,[2] we could see more people in the skirts of the Woods, none of them however joined us, probably these were their women and children. I gave to each of these men a hatchet and a knife having nothing else about me; perhaps these were the most valuable things I could give them. They wanted us much to go to their habitations telling us they would give us some thing to eat;[3] they took particular notice of such of us as had beards and those that had none but whether they took those without beards to be of the other sex or no I know not. When we took leave they followed us to our boat, seeing the musquets laying aCross the stern they made signs for them to be taken away which when done they came along side and even assisted us to launch her. At this time it was necessary for us to look well after them for they wanted to take away every thing they could lay their hands up[on] except the musquets which they took care not to touch, the Slaughter they had seen us make among the Wild Ducks had taught them to looke up[on] these as instruments of death. We saw no Canoes or other Boats with them, two or three logs of wood tied together serves the same purpose,[4] fish and wild fowl are in such plenty in the River [near] their habitations that they have but little occasion to go far for food and they have few neighbours to disturb them, I believe their whole number does not exceed three families.

WEDNESDAY 21*st*. It was noon when we tooke leave of these two men and proceeded down the Bay, the NW side of which I survey'd in my way and the Isles which lay in the middle,[5] night however at last overtook us and obliged me to leave one arm unlooked into.[6] At 8 o'Clock at night we got on board, when I learnt that the man and his Daughter stayed on board yesterday untill noon and that having learnt from our people of the things I had left in the place[7] where

[1] *Kahu*, a fine cloak: Cook uses the Tahitian form for a cloak in general, *ahu*. Very possibly the Maori was wearing something much more everyday—a plain *parakiri* or even a rough *pake* or rain cape.

[2] . . . on the contrary they saluted every one as he came up

[3] . . . and I was sorry that the Tide and other circumstances would not permit me to accept of thier invitation; . . .—f. 56.

[4] . . . and were indeed sufficient for the Navigation of the River on the Banks of which they lived and where

[5] Cooper's Island, Long Island, and a number of islets close by; Indian Isle and the others to the west must have been already surveyed.

[6] He means the passage running north, of which Resolution Island forms the western side; but there were more arms than one still to look into, as he later found. See Fig. 30.

[7] *in the place:* in Cascade Cove, the place

they were first seen, he sent and took them away, he had also learnt from our people to fire a musquet which he did two or three times.[1]

THURSDAY 22*nd*. In the PM I went with a party a Seal hunting, the surf was so high that we could only land in one place where we killed Ten, these animals serve us for three purposes, the skins we use for our rigging, the fatt makes oyle for our lamps and the flesh we eat, their harslets are equal to that of a hog and the flesh of some of them eats little inferior to beef steakes, nay I beleive we should think it superior could we get the better of prejudice.

FRIDAY 23*rd* & SATURDAY 24*th*. In the morning Lieut[t] Pickersgill and the Master[2] went to the Cascade Cove in order to clime one of the Mountains, the Sumit of which they reached between two and three o'Clock in the after-noon as we could see by the smoak of fire which they made; at the same time I went to the same Cove on a fishing party where we had but indifferent success and night brought us on board as well as those who had been in the Country, they reported that inland nothing was to be seen but barren mountains with huge craggy precipices frightfull to behold and on the SE side of *Cape West* four miles out at Sea is a Ledge of rocks on which the Sea broke very high, I believe these rocks to lie where we first fell in with the land for there we saw breake[r]s about that distance from shore.

Having five Geese left of those we brought from the *Cape of Good Hope* I went with them this morning to Goose Cove (named so on this account) where I left them. I choose this place for leaving them at for two reasons, first here being no inhabitants to disturb them, and secondly here appeared to be the most food, I make no doubt but what they will breed and may in time spread over the whole Country, which will answer the intent of the founder.

SUNDAY 25*th*. We spent the day shooting in and about the Cove and returned on board about 10 o'Clock at night. Lieut[t] Pickersgill who was one of the party shott a White Hern[3] which answers exactly with

[1] *he had . . . times:* he remain'd with his family by us till to day when they all went away and we saw them no more, which was the more extraordinary as he never went away empty handed, from one or a nother he did not get less than nine or ten hatchets, three or four times that number of large spike Nails besides many other articles, so far as these things may be counted riches among them he exceeds every man in New Zealand, at this time he is possessed of more Hatchets and axes than are the whole Country besides.—ff. 56–6v.

[2] . . . and two others . . .—Sparrman was one of these two.

[3] The White Heron was the Maori Kotuku, *Egretta alba modesta* (Gray). Supremely beautiful and striking in flight, it was comparatively rare even in Maori days, and correspondingly celebrated in legend and oratory. Pickersgill set an unfortunate precedent. The bird maintains itself still at about stable numbers in a single colony on the West Coast of the South Island. The European form is *E. alba alba* Linn.

Mr Pennants discription[1] of the White Herns that either now are or were formerly in England. For the Eight days past we have not had one single Shower of rain, a circumstance that I believe is very uncommon here especially at this time of the year. These few fair days has given us time to compleat our Wood and Water, Overhaul the rigging, caulk the Ship and put her in a condition for Sea.

MONDAY 26*th.* Continual rain till near noon when it became tolerable fair and we cast off the shorefasts,[2] hove the Ship out to her anchor and steadied her with a hawser to the shore.

TUESDAY 27*th.* Hazey Weather with showers of rain. In the Morning I set out in the Pinnace, accompanied by the two Mr Forsters and Mr Pickersgill, to examine the arm or Inlet I left unexplored when I was at the head of the Bay.[3]

WEDNESDAY 28*th.* After rowing about two Leagues up the arm, or more properly down it, for I found it to communicate with the Sea and to offer a better outlet for Ships bound to the northward than the one we came in by: after making this discovery and refreshing our selves on broiled fish and wild fowl, we at 7 o'Clock in the evening set out for the Ship which we reachd at 11, leaving two inlets which have their begining from this and runs in to the Eastward, unexplored. In proceeding up this arm we shott 39 Curlews or oyster catchers, three Ducks a Shagg and a Penguin[4] without going one foot out of the way or causing any great delay.[5] In the Morning we got the Tents and every other article from the Shore and only waited for a wind to carry us out of the Cove.

THURSDAY 29*th.* Mostly Calm with showers of rain, in the evening I set fire to the top wood &c^a that was on a part of the ground we had occupied in order to dry it, and in the morning dug it up and sowed in it several sorts of seeds, the ground was such as did not promise success to the planter and[6] yet it was the best I could find.

[1] . . . in his British Zoology . . .—Thomas Pennant (1726–98) of Downing, Flintshire, a great traveller in England and Scotland, a naturalist of considerable fame, and a man of enormous literary industry; F.R.S. 1767. His works on natural history were highly thought of, as repositories of the knowledge of his day, and his correspondence with Banks shows the range of his interest. His *British Zoology* first appeared in folio in 1766; the four volumes of the 8vo edition (London and Chester, 1768–70) are books likely to have been taken on the voyage by Forster, and perhaps by Anderson.

[2] A shore-fast was a hawser carried out to secure a vessel to a quay or to some object on shore—e.g. a buried anchor or a tree.

[3] '. . . the Armourers employ'd making Irons to guard the Carv'd work on the Quarters'. —Cooper.

[4] This was probably the Little Blue Penguin or Korora, *Eudyptula minor* (Forster), a specimen of which had been taken here and painted by George Forster on 31 March.

[5] *any great delay*: any other delay than picking them up.—f. 57.

[6] MS as.

FRIDAY 30*th*. At 2 o'Clock in the PM wieghed and with a light breeze at SW stood up the Bay for the new passage, soon after we had got through between the East end of Indian Island and the West end of Long Island, it fell Calm and obleged us to anchor in 43 fathom water under the north side and a little above the West end of the latter Island.[1] At 9 the next morning we wieghed again with a light breeze at West, which together with the assistance of all the Boats ahead towing was hardly sufficient to stem the current.

[MAY 1773]

SATURDAY 1*st*. After strugling till 6 in the evening, in which time we did not get above [five] mile from our last anchoring place we anchored close to the north side of the last mentioned Island[2] and made a hawser fast to the shore. At day light in the morning we got again under sail and attempted to work to windward haveing a light breeze down the Bay. At first we gain'd ground, but the breeze dying away we soon lost more than we had got and at last was obliged to bear up for a Cove on the north side of long isle[3] where we anchored in 19 fathom water. In this Cove we found two hutts not long sence inhabited.[4]

SUNDAY 2*nd*. Calm with Showers of Rain.

MONDAY 3*rd*. The Calm continued till near noon when a light breeze sprung up at SW tempted us to get under sail, which was no sooner done then it fell again Calm and obliged us to anchor in our old place.

TUESDAY 4*th*. The Calm continued all this Day, attended with continual rain.

WEDNESDAY 5*th*. At 1 o'Clock in the PM the Weather became fair and a small breeze sprung up at SW which with the help of our boats carried us to the entrence of the Passage leading to Sea when the Calm again returned and forced us to anchor in 30 fathom water before a Sandy beach at the East entrance of the passage, which anchoring place is only to be used in cases of necessity.[5] In the night

[1] About a third of a mile east from the tiny islet Cook called Station Isle; the anchorage is marked on the engraved chart.

[2] . . . not more than one hundred yards from the shore.—f. 57v.

[3] Long Island. Cook called the anchorage Detention Cove.

[4] . . . and near them two very large fire places or ovens such as they have in the Isles.

[5] . . . this anchoring place hath nothing to recommend it like the one we came from which hath every thing in its favour.—f. 57v.—It was a little cove just within Passage Point (Cook's name), only about three miles in a direct line from the previous anchorage. The 'Passage leading to sea' was to receive the name Acheron Passage, after the ship that made the later survey of the region, in 1851.

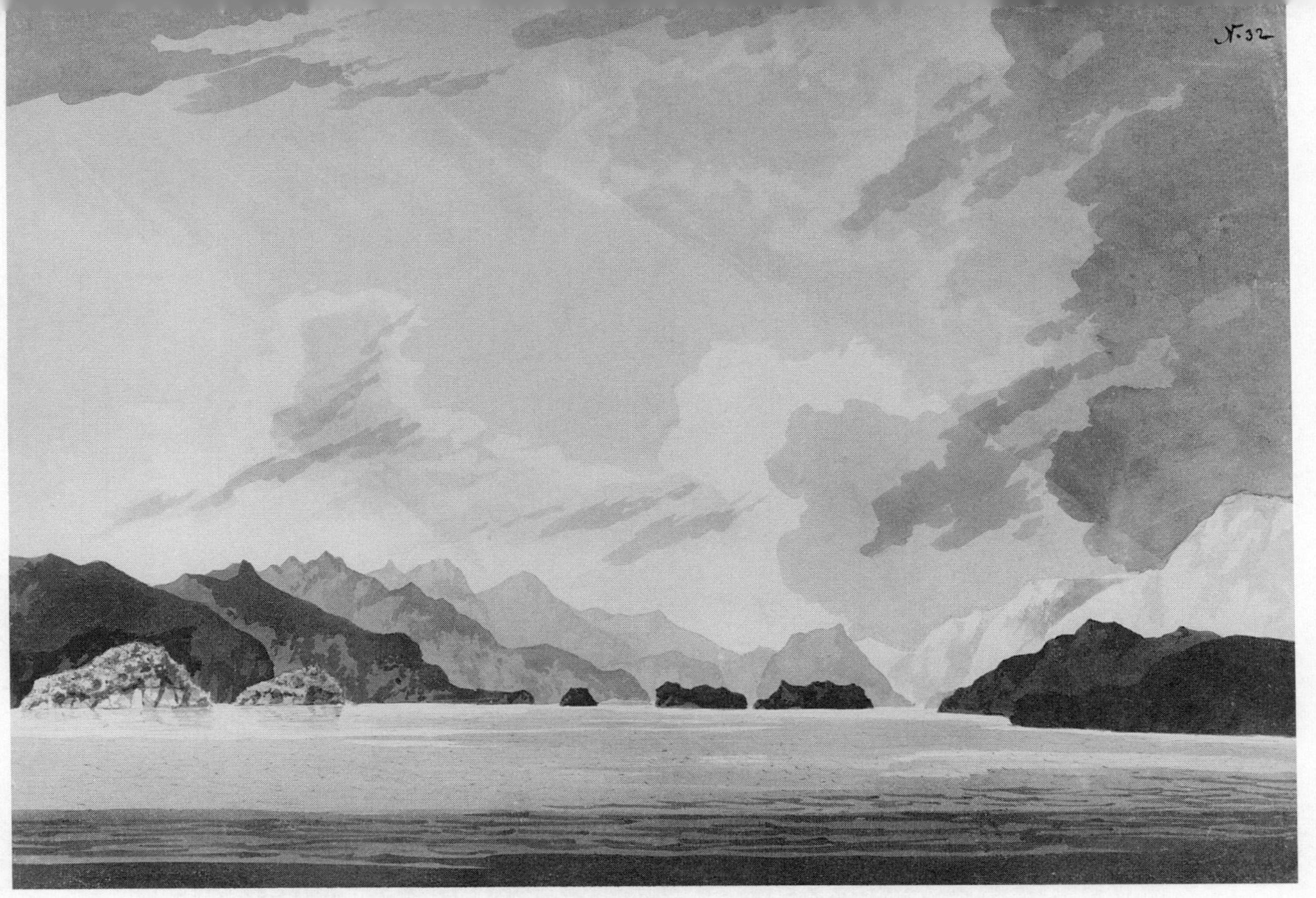

Fig. 23. View of Dusky Sound from the sea

Water-colour drawing by Hodges.—Mitchell Library, D11, no. 32

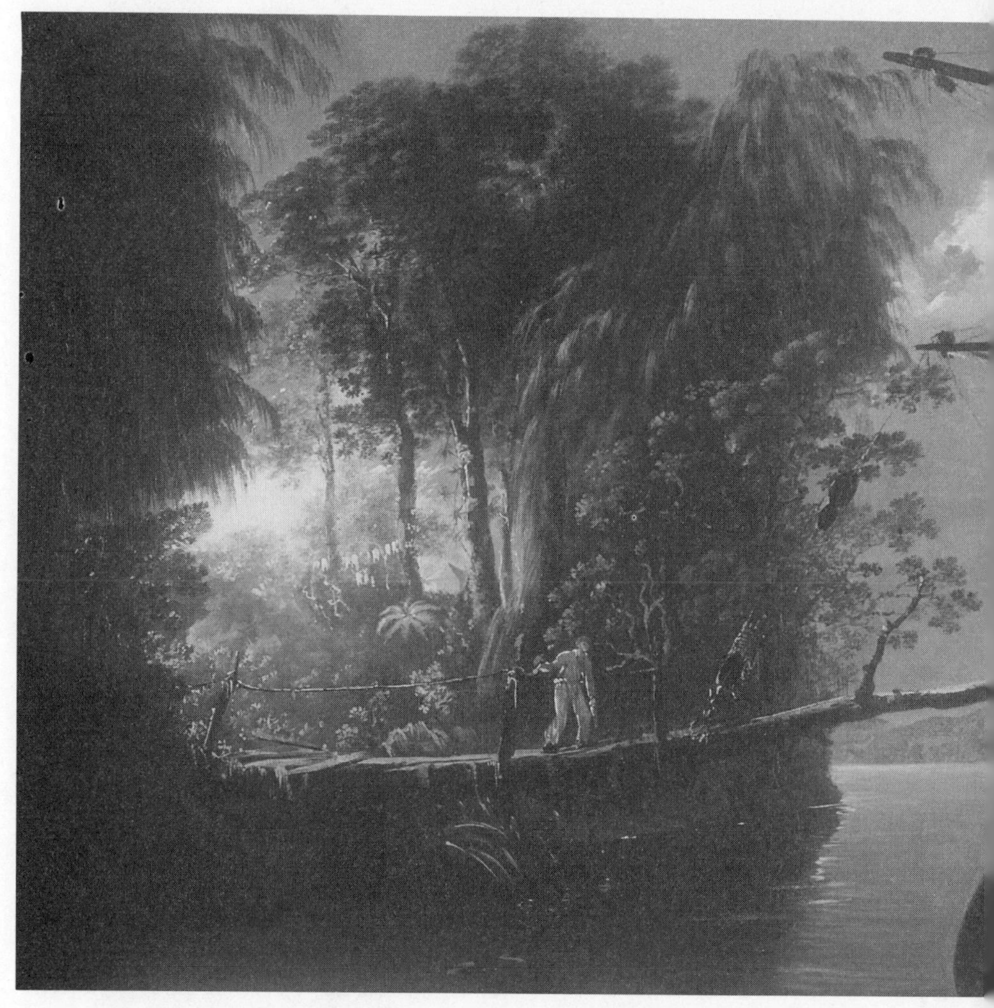

FIG. 24. The *Resolution* in Pickersgill Harbour, Dusky Sound

Oil painting by Hodges, in Admiralty House

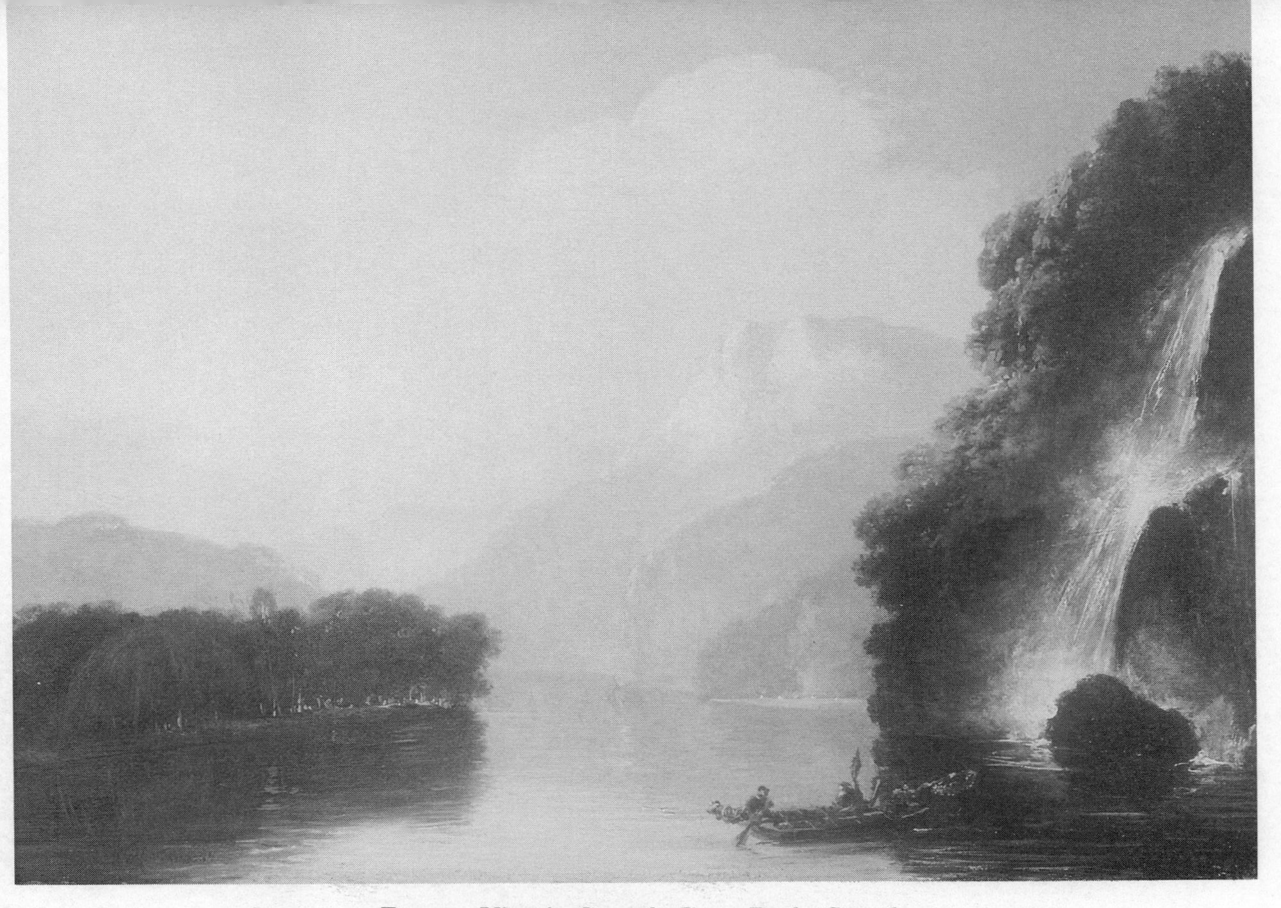

Fig. 25. View in Cascade Cove, Dusky Sound

Oil painting by Hodges, in the National Maritime Museum

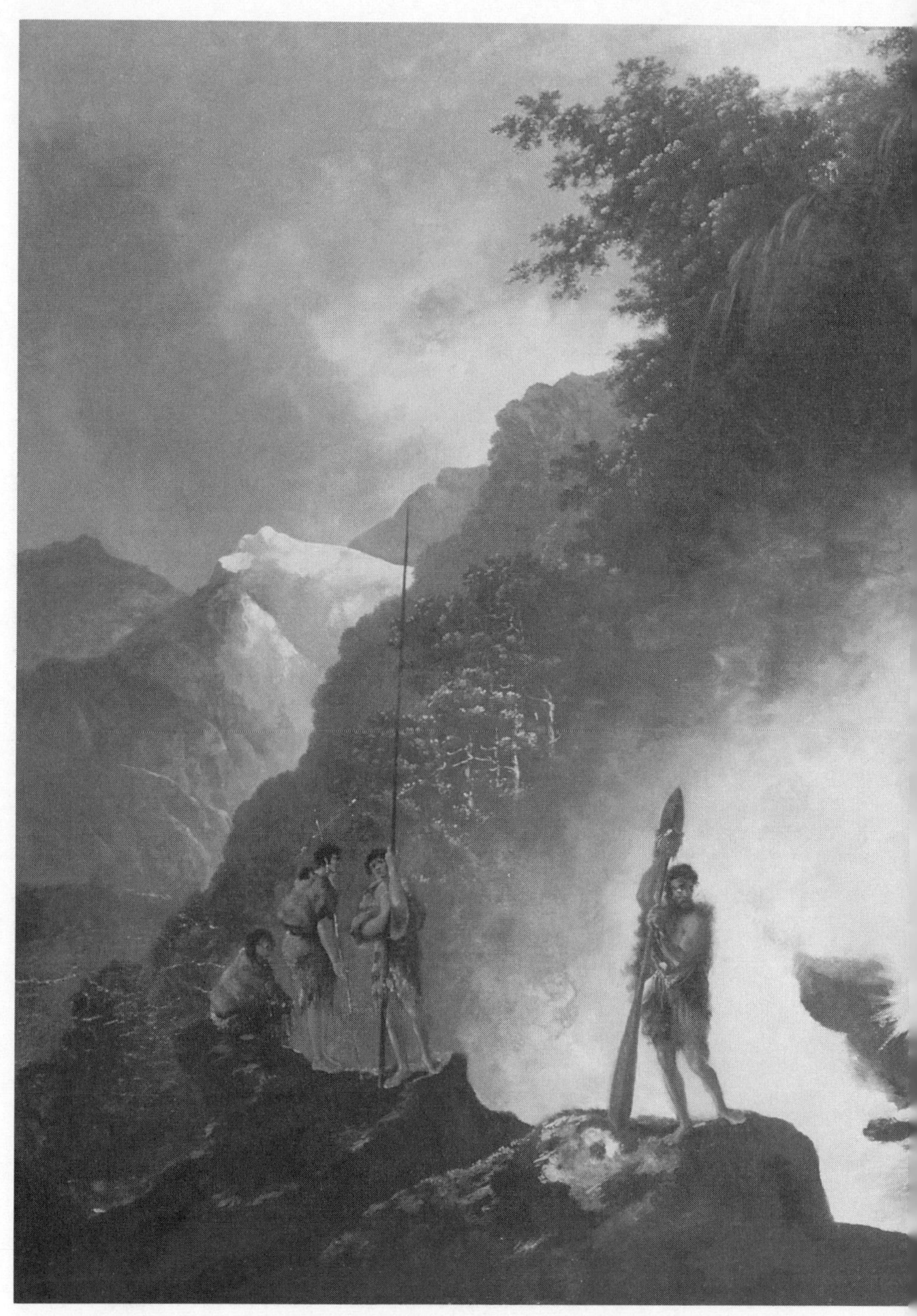

FIG. 26. Maori family at Cascade Cove

Detail of oil painting by Hodges, in Admiralty House

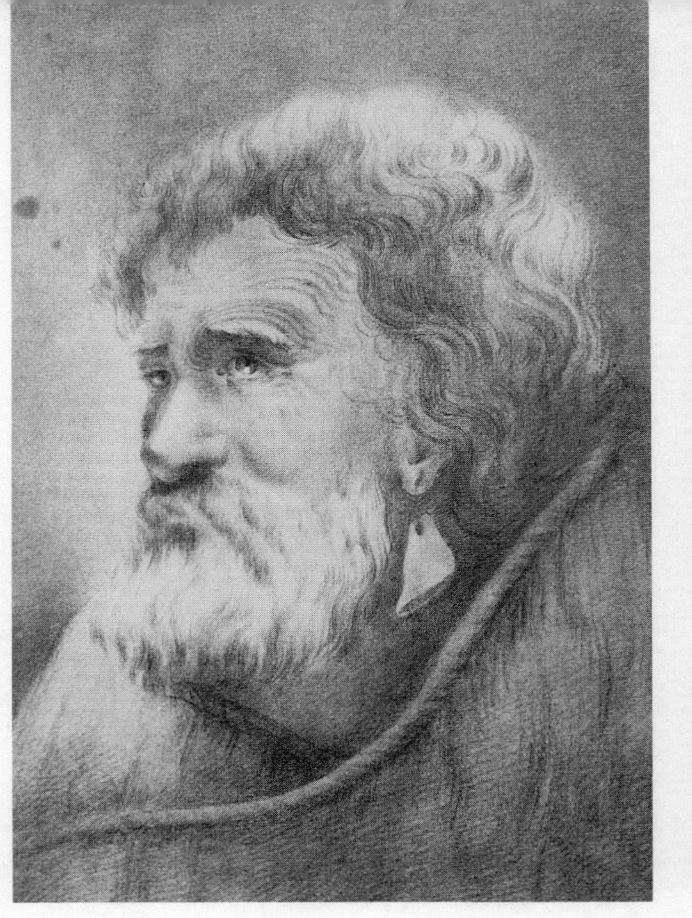

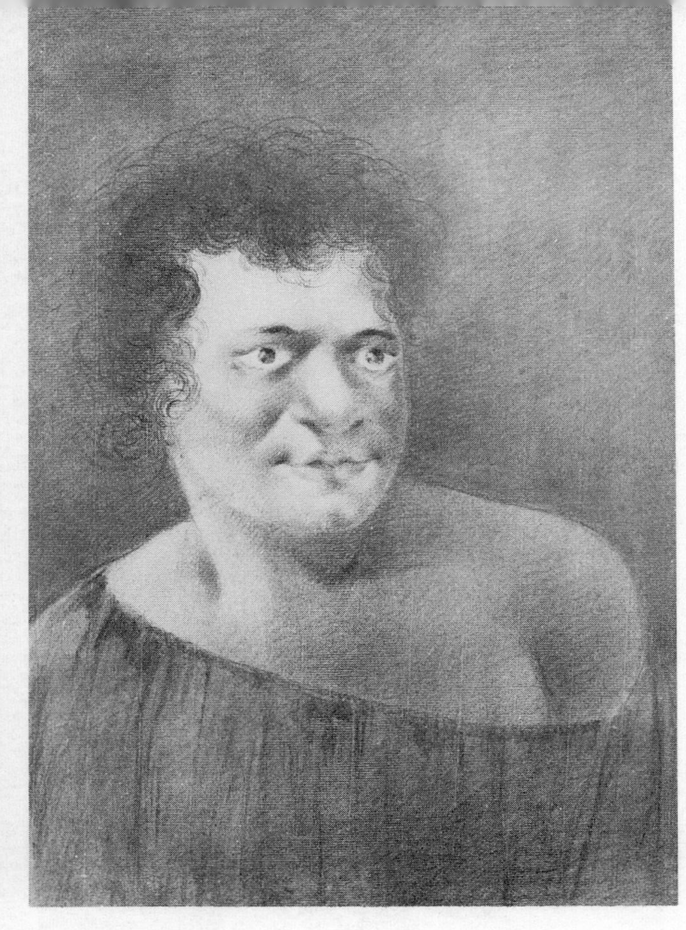

FIG. 27. Portrait heads of Maoris

(*left*) Old man; (*right*) Woman. Crayon drawings by Hodges.—Commonwealth National Library

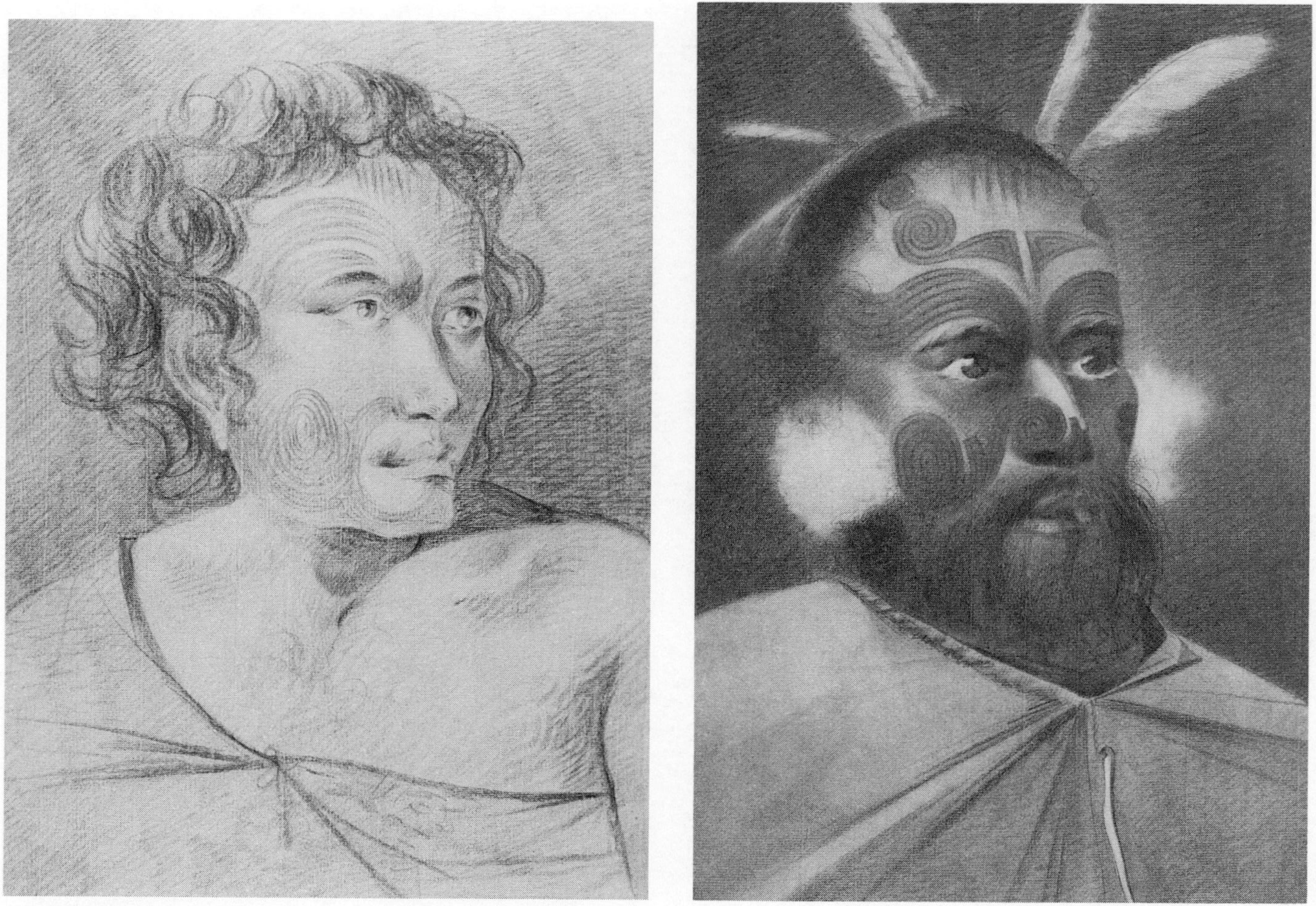

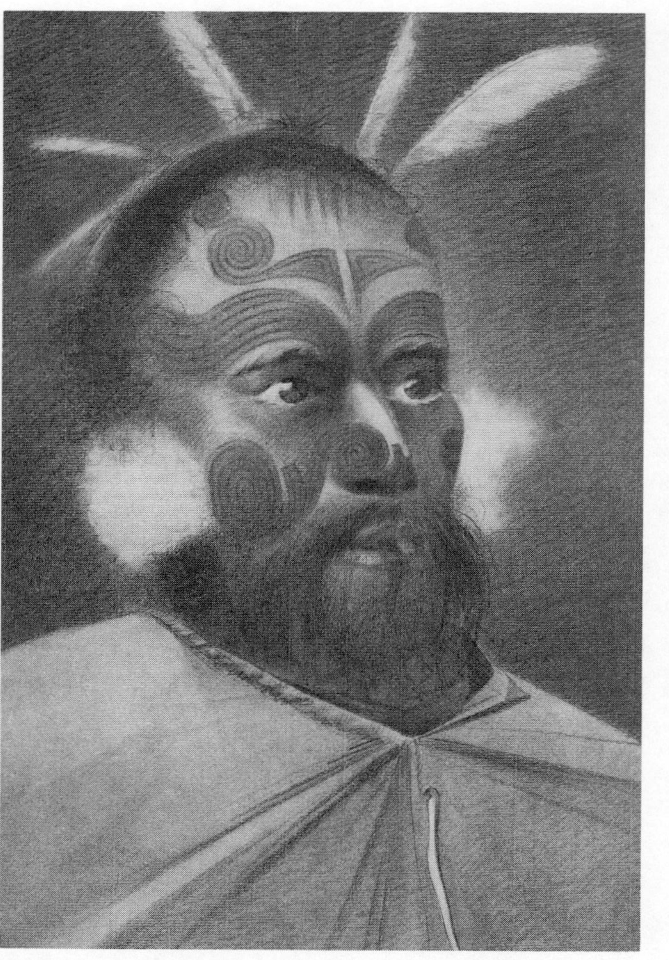

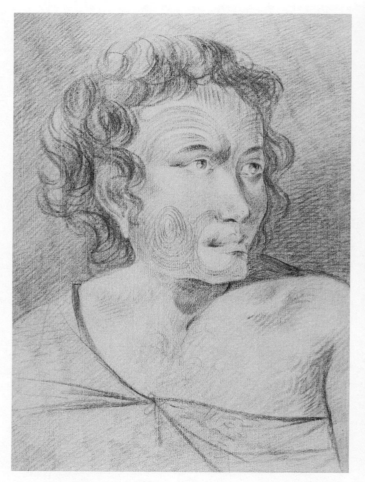

Fig. 28. Portrait heads of Maoris, tattooed

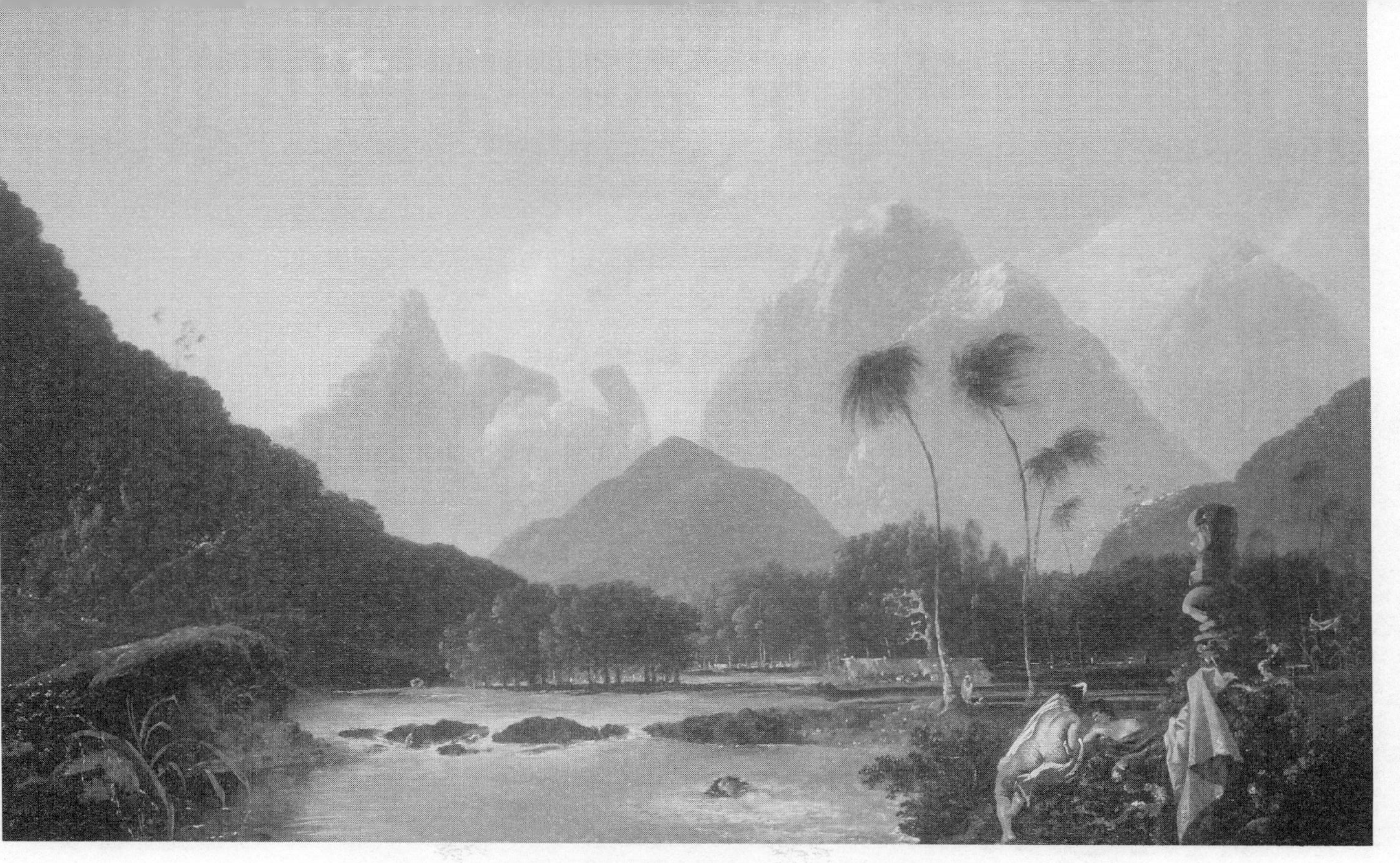

Fig. 29. View in Vaitepiha Bay, Tahiti

Oil painting by Hodges, in the National Maritime Museum

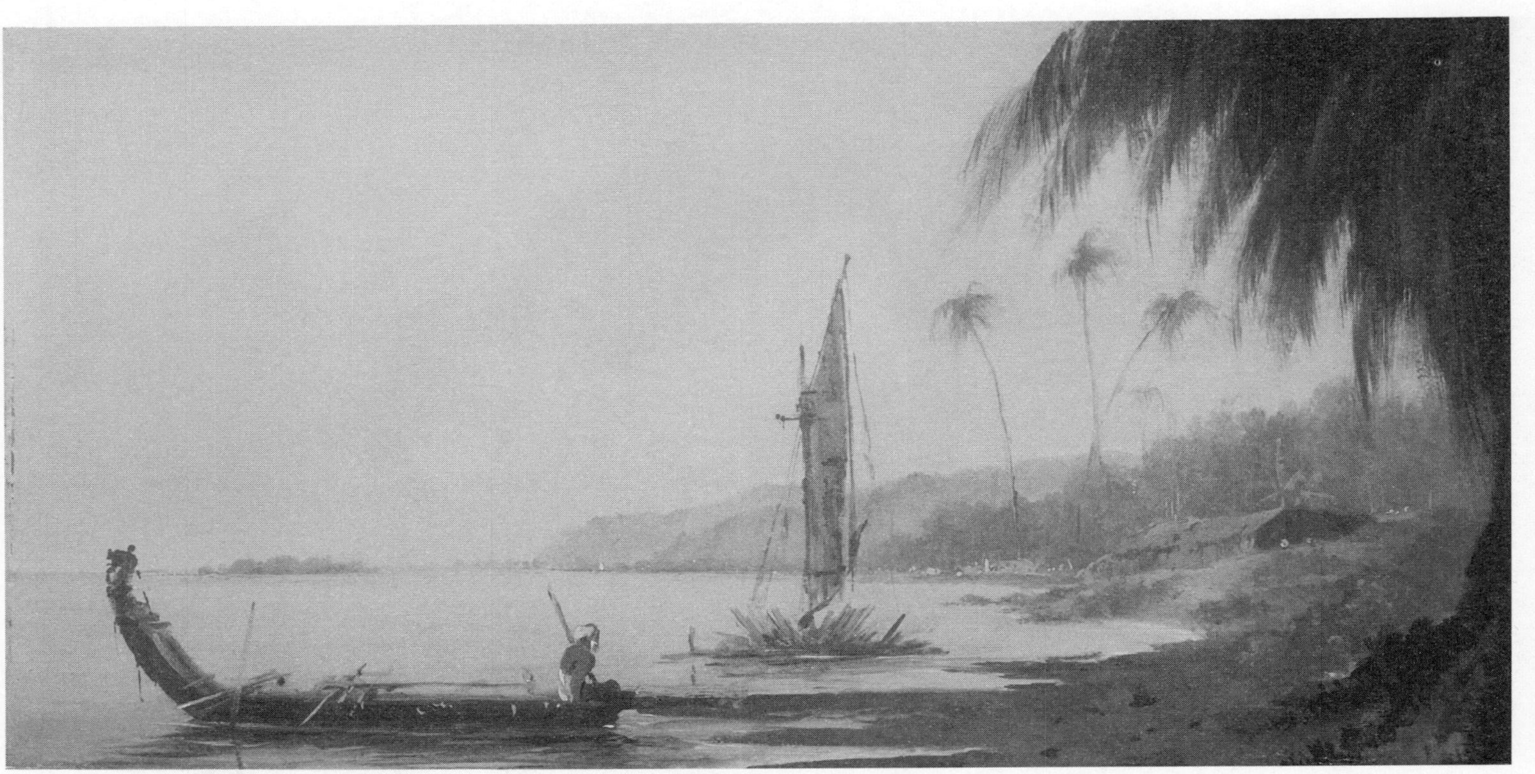

Fig. 30. View from Point Venus, Tahiti, looking east

Oil painting by Hodges, in the National Maritime Museum

had some very heavy squalls of Wind, attended with rain, hail & Snow and some thunder. Day-light exhibited to our view all the hills and mountains covered with Snow.[1]

THURSDAY *6th.* At 2 o'Clock in the PM we got under sail with a light breeze at SSW which with the help of our Boats carried us down the Passage to our intended anchoring place where we anchored at 8 o'Clock in 16 fathom water and moored with a hawser to the Shore, under the first point on the Starboard shore as you come in from Sea, which point covered us from the Sea and is within the Island which lies in the middle of the Passage.[2] In the AM being fair weather got the Cables and every other thing up from betwixt decks, cleaned the Deck and aired it with fires.[3] At the same time I sent Lieut[t] Pickersgill with the Pinnace accompanied by the two M[r] Forsters to explore the Second Arm or Inlet which turns in to the Eastward my self being confined on board by a Cold.[4]

FRIDAY *7th.* Fair Weather continued till 6 o'Clock in the AM when it was succeeded by a storm from NW which blew in hard squalls attended with rain, and obliged us to strike Topg[t] yards lower our lower yards and carry out a nother hawser to the Shore.

SATURDAY *8th.* The bad Weather continued till day light in the morn when it fell calm and the sky in some degree cleared up, at this time M[r] Pickersgill returned, after having spent a very disagreeable night,[5] he was at the head of the Arm which he judged to extend in about [8] Miles, in it are good anchoring places Wood Water Wild fowl and fish.[6] At 9 o'Clock I set out to explore the first inlet

[1] '... from 11 pm to 8 am the wea[r] exceedingly tempestious attended with hard squalls of hail & rain with much thunder and lightning, at daylight the Mountians covered with snow the wea[r] cold and every apperence of approaching winter great falls of water from the mountains'.—Gilbert.

[2] In Occasional Cove (Cook's name). The island Cook called Entry Island. In Roberts's chart, Add. MS 31360.55, it is called Parrot Island, but this name was still-born.

[3] ... a thing that ought never to be long neglected in wet moist Weather.

[4] This is Cook's version of a *malaise* otherwise described by Forster, I, p. 181: 'The captain was taken ill of a fever and violent pain in the groin, which terminated in a rheumatic swelling of the right foot, contracted probably by wading too frequently in the water, and sitting too long in the boat after it, without changing his cloaths'. No doubt this is correct anyhow in its definition of the cause.

[5] *at this time ... night:* At 7 in the morning M[r] Pickersgill return'd together with his companions in no very good plight, ...—f. 58.

[6] This was Wetjacket Arm, so called from the experience of the party there. Forster devotes three pages to the storm: 'in a word, it seemed as if all nature was hastening to a general catastrophe ... and our hearts sunk with apprehension lest the ship might be destroyed by the tempest or its concomitant aetherial fires, and ourselves left to perish in an unfrequented part of the world'.—p. 185. Pickersgill E is less dramatic: 'On the 7th I went with the Pinnace to explore a Sound, expecting to get back on the same Night but was disapointed for it came on a very voilent storm of Snow Hail and Thunder with a meer Hurrican of wind which confind us in a little Cove, and what was worse we had

which also runs in to the Eastward,[1] or that next the Sea and ordered Mr Gilbert to go out and examine the Passage out to Sea, while the People on board where employed hoisting in the Launch filling up our Water &c^a^.

SUNDAY 9*th*. I proceeded up the Inlet till about 5 o'Clock in the pm when I was overtaken by bad Weather and obliged to Return before I had seen the end of it, as this inlet lies partly Parallel with the Sea Coast I was of opinion that it might communicate with Doubtfull Harbour or some other inlet to the northward, appearences was however rather against this opinion and the bad weather hindred me from determin^g^ the point. I was about [10] miles up it[2] and found on the Northwest side three Coves wherein is good anchorage, also on the SE side between the Main and the Isles which lies [about 4] Miles up the Inlet is good Anchorage, Wood, fresh Water and all other necessarys such as fish and Wild fowl, of the latter we killed in this excursion three Dozen, after a very hard row against both wind and rain we reached the Ship at 9 o'Clock at night with not a dry thread on our backs. The bad Weather continued till the next Morn when it fill Calm, the weather cleared up and became fair and as we had not wind to put to Sea I went again to the Inlet to explore some Coves which I had not time to do in the PM and also to Shoot some Wild fowl for a Sea Stock, the two Mr Forsters and Mr Hodges[3] with me, the officers also formed a party and went to the Coves & Isles Mr Gilbert explored in the PM and where he found many wild fowl.

MONDAY 10*th*. Fair Weather continued all the PM and the evening brought my self and party and all the other sportsmen on board, I and party met with good sport, but the other party found little. In the AM had a strong gale from the Westward which blew in such flurries over the high lands as prevented us from geting under sail, it was also attended with heavy Showers of rain.

TUESDAY 11*th*. In the PM it moderated and my self, Mr Cooper and some of the gentlemen went out in two Boats to the rocks which lie out at Sea at the entrance of the Bay, in order to kill Seals, the Weather was rather unfavourable for this sport and the Sea run high

nothing to eat but a few Mussels which we gatherd at low water from the Rocks and nothing to drink but spring water; in this situation we were keept for 36 hours, quite wet and the woods so wet we could not get a bit of fire to burn and being intirely exposed to the inclemency of the weather'.

[1] This was Breaksea Sound.

[2] . . . and thought I saw the end of it.

[3] The name is conjectural: something has been badly written over something else badly written.

so as to make landing difficult, we however killed 10 but could wait only to take in five and with them we returned on board. In the morning I sent a Boat out for the other five, and at 9 o'Clock we got under sail with a light breeze at SE and stood out to Sea takeing up the Boat by the way with 13 Seals. It was noon before we had got well clear of the entrence at which time we observed in 45°30½′, the Entrance of the Bay bore SEBE Break Sea Isle which is the outermost on the South point of the entrance of the Bay bore SSE,[1] Point Five fingers or the Southermost land bore S 42° West and the no[r]thermost land NNE, in this situation we had a prodigious swell from SW which broke with great voilence on all the Shores which were exposed to it.

As there is no Port in New Zealand I have been in that affords the necessary refreshments in such plenty as Dusky Bay, and altho' it lies far remote from the tradeing parts of the World, nevertheless a short account of the adjacent Country and a discription of the Bay may not only be acceptable to the curious reader but may be of use to some future Navigators for we can by no means till what use future ages may make of the discoveries made in the present. The south[2] entrance of this Bay is situated on the North side of *Cape West* in the Latitude of 45°[3] South, it is formed by the Cape to the South and Point five fingers to the North, this point is remarkable by several peaked rocks lying off it,[4] the land of this point is still more remarkable by the little Similarity it bears to the lands adjacent being a narrow Peninsula lying north and South, of a moderate height and covered with Wood. To sail into this Bay[5] is by no means difficult as I know of no danger but what shows it self. The worst that attends it is the depth of Water which is too great to admit of anchorage except in the Coves or Harbours and near the shores and even in many places this last is not to be done, the anchoring places are however numerous enough and equally safe and commodious.

Pickersgills Harbour where we laid is[6] situated on the South shore abreast of the West end of Indian Island which Island may be known by its proximity to that shore, there is a Passage into this Harbour on both sides of the small Isle which lies before it, but the most room is on the upper or east side haveing regard to a sunken

[1] . . . distant 3 Miles.

[2] MS north, which is clearly a slip.

[3] 45°48′

[4] *peaked . . . it:* pointed rocks lying off it which when View'd from some situations has some resemblence to the five fingers of a mans hand from whence it takes its name . . .—f. 58v.

[5] . . . by this entrance

[6] *laid is:* laid is not inferior to any in the Bay for two or three Ships: it is

rock which lies between this end of the Isle and the main nearest to the latter;[1] the next Cove above on this side is Cascade Cove where there is room for a fleet of ships and may also be entered on either side of the Island which lies in the entrance takeing care to avoide a sunken Rock which lies towards the SE shore a little above the Island, this Rock as well as the one in Pickersgills Harbour appears at half Ebb. It would be needless to enumerate all the Anchoring places in this Capacious Bay, it is sufficient to point out one or two on each side.[2] Those who would anchor on the North side (which I must recommend to those who are bound to the South) will find no better place than Facile Harbour, to sail into it you need only consult the Chart which[3] will be a sufficient guide not only for this but all the other anchoring places as well as to sail quite through

[1] . . . Keep the isle close aboard and you will not only avoide the rock but keep in anchoring ground . . .—f. 59.

[2] . . . those who want to be acquainted with more need only consult the chart which they may depend upon, is without any material error.—f. 59.—Considering the duration of Cook's stay in Dusky Sound, this chart is indeed a brilliant piece of work, for which a good deal of credit must go to Gilbert, the master, and to Pickersgill, as well as to Cook himself. Archibald Menzies, the surgeon and botanist of Vancouver's *Discovery*, in 1791 was not slow in his praise of Cook: 'After kindling a fire & refreshing ourselves on whatever game & fish the day afforded, we drank a cheerful glass to the memory of Capt. Cook, whose steps we were now pursuing, & as far as we had opportunity to trace them, we could not help reflecting with peculiar pleasure & admiration on the justness of his observations & the accuracy of his delineations throughout every part of the complicated survey of this extensive Sound, where he had left so little for us to finish'. (*Hist. Rec. N.Z.*, II, p. 490.) All there was to finish was in fact the inlet that Cook, impeded by bad weather, explored on 8–9 May—Breaksea Sound. This did not, as he thought it might, 'communicate with Doubtfull Harbour or some other inlet to the northward', but divided into two at Chatham Point, the Vancouver Arm (the more northerly one) and the Broughton Arm. In spite of Vancouver's survey Cook's guess died hard, and on later maps (e.g. Wyld 1841) a fabulous 'Mac's Passage' runs north to Doubtful Sound, cutting off from the mainland an equally fabulous 'Paterson Island'. What wandering Scots were thus commemorated we do not know. On the engraved chart Cook has, opposite his Third Cove, a conjectural 'Apparent Island', with another behind it, both in front of a conjectural cove lettered 'No body knows what'. 'Apparent Island' is no doubt the steeply rising peninsula which divides the Vancouver from the Broughton Arm; the second 'island' one of the higher hills whose slopes fall to the southern shore of the Broughton Arm. Vancouver, having completed his survey, had the happiness of substituting for 'No body knows what' the legend 'Somebody knows what'. Cook conferred a good many names, most of which are self-explanatory, where he has not explained them: but one would like to know precisely why Station Isle, Prove Isle, Stop Isle, Fixt Head (a name moved on Stokes's *Acheron* chart to the end of the island off Cook's Fixt Head). They may have been points used in the survey. Presumably his Thrum Cap, being heavily bushed, was so named for the same reason as his Thrum Cap in the Tuamotus—I, p. 70, n. 2; and another islet of the same name in Halifax harbour. See *Voyage*, I, pl. XIII.

[3] *to sail . . . which:* To sail into this Harbour keep the inside of the land of five fingers point aboard untill you are the length of the Isles which lie abreast the middle of that land, haul round the north point of these Isles and you will have the Harbour before you bearing East, but the chart . . .—f. 59.—Facile Harbour was not so facile after all; Robert Murry, an officer of the 800 ton vessel *Endeavour*, which was abandoned there in a rotten condition in 1795, thought it was one of the worst havens in the Sound: 'The great height of the land about Facile Harbour and the immense depth of the valleys, or rather chasms between the hills cause the wind to come down in heavy gusts. . . . In no other part of Duskey Bay have I felt the gusts of so much violence as in Facile Harbour'; in addition

from the South to the north entrance; this last lies[1] in the Latitude of 45°35′ s and 5 Leagues to the Northward of Point Five fingers. To make this entrance plane it will be necessary to approach the Shore within a few miles as the land about it is of a considerable height, its situation may however be known at a greater distance as it lies under the first Craggy Mountains which rise to the northward of the land of Point five fingers, the most southermost of these Mountains is remarkable by having at the top or summit two small hillocks,[2] when this mountain bears SBE[3] you will be before the entrance on the south side of which lie several Islands, the Westermost or outermost is the most considerable both in height and circuit, in sailing in you leave this Isle[4] as well as the others to the South, the best Anchorage is in the first[5] Arm which is on the larboard hand going in, either in one of its Coves or with[in] the Isles which lie under the SE shore.[6] Mr Hodges has drawn a very accurate view both of the North and South entrance as well as several other parts of the Bay and in them hath deliniated the face of the Country with such judgement as will at once convey a better Idea of it than can be express'd by words nevertheless as it is somewhat singular I shall not pass it over in silence, the Country is exceeding Mountainous, not only about Dusky Bay but all the Southern part of this eastern Coast[7] and exhibits to our view nothing[8] but woods and barren cragy precipice's, no meadows or Launs are to be seen nor plains or flatt land of any extent;[9] the land near the Sea, shores of the Bay and all the Islands

there were straggling rocks and the ground tended to be foul. A more recent seaman, RNZNVR, whose admiration of Dusky Sound in general verges on the ecstatic, has made the remark, 'I never saw such a god-forsaken hellish place in my life'.

[1] *entrance . . . lies:* G entrance, but least any Navigator should come here possess'd of this Journal and not of the Chart, I shall give some directions for this Navigation. In coming in at the South entrance keep the South shore aboard untill you approach the West end of Indian Island which you will know not only by its apparent but real nearness to the Shore, from this Situation it will appear as a point dividing the bay into two arms, leave this Isle on your starboard side & continue your Course up the Bay which is EBN½N without turning either to the right or left, when you are abreast or above the East end of this Isle you will find the bay of a considerable breadth and higher up to be contracted by two projecting points, three miles above the one on the North side and abreast of two small Isles is the Passage out to Sea or to the North entrance and lies nearly in the direction of NBW & SBE, the North entrance lies . . .

[2] Mount Richards, about 3500 feet.

[3] SSE.

[4] . . . and which I have call'd breaksea Isle because it effectually covers the entrance from the violence of the SW swell which the other is so much exposed to.—f. 59v.—Roberts's charts, Add. MSS 31360.55 and 15500.4, have a variant of this name, Breakers; another chart, Add. MS 15500.3, calls it Breaksee.

[5] . . . or North

[6] The Harbour Isles on the engraved chart.

[7] . . . of Tavai-poenammoo . . .—f. 60.

[8] *nothing:* little else

[9] cf. Add. MS 27889, f. 75: 'The very Islands, which lay in the Bay and on the Sea

are thickly covered with Wood of various sorts fit for the Ship-wright joiner and other uses, excepting the River Thames I have not seen finer timber in all New Zealand, the most considerable here as well as in that River is the spruce tree as we call'd it from the similarity of its leaves to the America black spruce, but the wood is much more ponderous and of a redish colour, many of these trees run from Six to ten or twelve feet in girt[1] and from 80 to 90[2] or a hundred feet in length and are large enough to make a Main-mast for a 40 or 50 Gun Ship,[3] the wood land is however of no great extent and extends but a little way inland. From what we could see of the interior parts of the Country, it consists intirely of barren rocky mountains which are so crow[d]ed together as to leave room for no vallies of extent nor did we see a single acre of ground fit for a Plantation of any kind. The Inhabitants of this Bay are of the same race as those in the other parts of this Country, speak the same language and observe nearly the same customs; these indeed whether from custom or a more generous dispossision make you presents before they receive any, in this they come nearer to the Otaheiteans than the rest of their Country men. What could induce three or four families[4] to seperate themselves so far from the Society of the rest of their fellow creatures is not easy to guess, by our meeting with Inhabitants in this place makes it probable that there are Inhabitants in most of the Bays and harbours in the Southern parts of this Island,[5] the many vestigias we saw of People in different parts of this Bay[6] indicates that they live a wandering life never remaining long in one spott, and if one can judge from appearences & circumstances few as they are they live not in perfect amity one family with another, for if they do why do not they form themselves into some society a thing not only natural to Man, but is even observed by the brute creation.

If the Inhabitants of Dusky Bay feel at any time the effects of cold they never can that of hunger,[7] as every corner of the Bay abounds

Coast may each of them be called a mountain, and the whole Country a heap of steep, barren Mountains rising one above another till their lofty and craggy Summits are lost in the Clouds: and several of them were continually covered with snow'. This was greatly revised again for the printed version, *Voyage*, I, p. 95.

[1] *ten . . . girt:* eight and ten feet in girt (I have been told of some much more)

[2] 60 to 80 or 100

[3] 'it also makes good plank or boards . . .'—Log.

[4] . . . for I beleive there are not more

[5] *Inhabitants . . . Island:* people scater'd over all this Southern Isle

[6] . . . compair'd with the number of people themselves

[7] Sparrman, who was interested in food, thought that perhaps the ship was conferring a benefit upon the New Zealanders in giving them rats. In Pickersgill Harbour, the vermin

with fish, the Coal fish (as we call it)[1] is here in vast plenty, is larger and better flavoured than I have any where tasted,[2] nor are there any want of Craw and other shell fish,[3] Seals are also here in Plenty, they chiefly inhabit the Rocks & small Isles which lie near the Sea,[4] the flesh of many of them we found excellent eating, not a bit inferior to the finest Beef Stakes and the Harslets of them all are little inferior to a Hogs.[5] The Wild fowl are Ducks, Shaggs, Cormorrants, Oyster Catchers or Sea pies, Water or wood Hens, which are something like our English Rails, these inhabet the Skirts of the Woods and feed upon the Sea beach they are very like a Common Hen[6] and eat very well in a Pye or Fricasee, they are so scarce in other parts of New Zealand that I never saw one but at this place,[7] Albatroses, Gannets,[8] Gulls,[9] Penguins and other aquatick birds; the Land fowl

could walk ashore over the bridge. He incidentally casts some light on his shipmates and ship's diet. 'It may be that the less delicate among the savages will develop an appetite for their flesh, and thus the noxious animals may prove a lesser evil for them. Such [an] idea seems not unlikely for savages, but two Englishmen in the *Resolution*, one a midshipman inclined to drunkenness, the other an aged and staid quartermaster, developed this surprising taste. The former had a favourite cat who never failed to catch and carry rats to her master: he divided the prey so that the cat had the fore part, and the back part was cleaned, roasted, and peppered for himself. Both rat-eaters declared that their dish was good and tasty. Thus they often enjoyed fresh food while many of their shipmates were complaining of the monotonous daily ration of hard salt beef.'—p. 42. The Maori did not take to the rats, but the rats, in due course (like a ship's cat mentioned by Forster, I, p. 128) took to the New Zealand small birds.

[1] *Parapercis colias* (Bloch and Schn.), the New Zealand Blue Cod, Rawaru of the Maoris, one of the most delicious food fishes, which is at its best in deep waters round the southern coast of New Zealand. J. R. Forster (*Descr. An.*, pp. 122–4) gives a detailed description of it.

[2] *the Coal fish . . . tasted:* one boat with hooks and lines was always sufficient to supply the whole crew with this article.—f. 60v.

[3] . . . all excellent in their kind

[4] 'these seals differ from those we have in Europe in some particulars, especially in their skins, which is much finer, resembling much the skin of an Otter.'—Log. The publication of Cook's second *Voyage* and the foundation of British settlement at Sydney meant the virtual extinction of the New Zealand seal. The first sealing gang was left at Luncheon Cove, Anchor Island, in Dusky Sound, in 1792; by 1830 the seals were gone, not merely from Dusky Sound, but from the rest of the coast and the southern islands.

[5] Sparrman, p. 29, calls them 'sea-bears', and writes, 'The blubber from these animals is most useful for lamps, ropes, and other ship's requirements; their livers and hearts also provided good dishes, but as all kinds of liver disagree with me, at my suggestion they tried braising the flesh with cherry sauce, and this, after the oil had been removed, was more palatable to me, and later came into general use.' Whether cherry sauce had its origin with a benevolent Victualling Board, or the barrel of dried cherries that Banks had got specially from Copenhagen for Solander had failed to be unloaded, we do not know. The article does not come into the official correspondence. But the experiment is interesting.

[6] . . . and most of them of a dirty black colour

[7] . . . the reason may be, that as they cannot fly, are very tame, inhabit the skirts of the Woods and feed on the Sea beach, the Natives may have in a manner wholy distroyed them.—f. 60v.—The weka's well-known curiosity also betrayed him, all too frequently, into the Maori trap, as later the European bushman's.

[8] *Sula bassana serrator* Gray.

[9] The Silver Gull or Tarapunga, *Larus novae-hollandiae scopulinus* Forster, was taken here.

are Hawks,[1] Parrots,[2] Pigeons[3] and such other birds as are common to this country.

The Ducks are of five sorts, the largest are as big as a Muscovy Duck with a very beautifull variegated plumage, both male and feemale have a large white spot on each wing, the head and neck of the latter is white, but all the other feathers as well as those on the head and neck of the Drake are of a dark variegated colour;[4] the second sort have a brown plumage with bright green feathers in their wings and are about the size of an English tame duck;[5] the third sort is the blue grey Duck before mentioned or the whistling Duck as some called them from the whistling noise they made, what is most remarkable in these is the end of their beaks which are soft and of a skinny or more properly cartilaginous substance;[6] the fourth sort is something bigger than teal and all black except the Drake which has some white feathers in his wings,[7] there are but few of this sort, we saw of them no where but in the river at the head of the Bay; the last sort is a small brown Duck, very common, as I am told in England.[8]—f. 60v.

The flax plant is as common here as in any other part of New Zealand[9] and the natives apply it to the same use, in general the produce of the land is much the same with this difference that there is not so great a variety. Mention hath already be[en] made of our having seen a quadrupede, it is to be wished we could have given some better account of it as it is more than probable that it is of a new species: we are however now certain that this Country is not so clear of these sort of animals as was once thought. The most mischievous animal here is the small black sandfly which are exceeding numerous and are so troublesome that they exceed every thing of the kind I ever met with, wherever they light they cause a swelling and such an intolerable itching that it is not possible to refrain from

[1] A Bush Hawk or Karearea, *Falco novaeseelandiae* Gm., was taken on 4 April. Sparrman thought the hawks 'were really delicious roasted'.

[2] A Red-fronted Parrakeet or Kakariki, *Cyanoramphus novaezelandiae* (Sparrm.) was taken on 5 April.

[3] A New Zealand Pigeon or Kereru, *Hemiphaga novaeseelandiae* (Gm.), was taken on 3 April; generally thought to have been discovered by Crozet at the Bay of Islands in 1772, this species was noted by Sydney Parkinson on the first voyage, though he made no drawing of it.

[4] The Paradise Duck, *Tadorna variegata* (Gm.).

[5] The Grey Duck, *Anas superciliosa* Gm.

[6] The Blue Duck, *Hymenolaimus malacorhynchos*. It is sometimes called the Whistling Duck, and the Maori name, Whio, is also derived from its call.

[7] The New Zealand Scaup or Black Teal, *Aythya novaeseelandiae* (Gm.).

[8] The Brown Teal, *Anas castanea chlorotis* Gray.

[9] Forster gave it its name, *Phormium tenax*—unless he appropriated this, like other things, from Solander's papers.

scratching and at last ends in ulcers like the small Pox.[1] The almost continual rain may be reckoned a nother ilconveniency attending this Bay but perhaps this may only happen at some seasons of the year, yet the situation of the Country, vast height and nearness of the Mountains seems to subject it to much rain at all times. Notwithstanding our people were continually exposed to the rain yet they felt no ill effects from it, on the contrary such as were sick or ailing when we arrived recovered strength daily and the whole crew became strong and vigorous.[2]

I have already made mention of our brewing Beer which we at first made with a decoction of the leaves of the spruce tree mixed with Inspissated juce of Wort and Mellasses but finding that the decoction of Spruce alone made the Beer to astringent we mixed with it an equal quantity of the Tea plant which partly distroyed the Astringentcy of the other and made the Beer exceeding Palatable and esteemed by every one on board. This Beer we brewed in the same manner as spruce Beer, that is we first made a strong decoction of the leaves or small branches of the Spruce tree & Tea shrub by boiling them three or four hours, or untill the bark will strip with ease from the branches, then take the leaves or branches out of the Copper and mix with the liquor the proper quantity of Melasses and Inspissated Juce, one Gallon of the former and three of the latter is sufficient to make a Puncheon or 80 gallons of Beer,[3] let this mixture just boil and then put it into the Cask and to it add an equal quantity of Cold Water more or less according to your taste and the strength of the decoction, when the whole is but milk warm put in a little grounds of Beer or yeast, if you have any, or any thing else that will cause fermentation and in a few days the Beer will be fit to drink, after the casks have been brewed in two or three times the Beer will generally ferment of it self.[4] It is not attall necessary to have Inspissated juce of Wort for the making of this Beer. Melasses alone will do full as well of which Ten gallons will be sufficient to make a Tun of Beer: sugar will also answer the same purpose, I made use of the Inspissated juce of Malt because I had it, and could not apply it to a better use and to save sugar and Melasses, for of the

[1] Cook, it must be allowed, speaks with great moderation of this pest, writing as he was in pre-dimethylphthalate days. It was *Austrosimulium* sp., whose larvae breed in running water; the adults are not uncommon throughout New Zealand, but abound multitudinously in the Sounds district.

[2] . . . which can only be attributed to the healthiness of the place and the fresh provisions it afforded: the Beer certainly contributed not a little . . .—f. 61.

[3] *and Inspissated . . . Beer:* ten gallons of which is sufficient to make a Tun or 240 Gallon . . .—f. 61v.

[4] . . . especially if the weather is warm.

latter I had but one small cask and of the former little to spare for this use, had I known how well this beer would have succeeded and the great use it was of to the people I should have come better prepared, indeed I was partly discouraged by an experiment I made last Voyage which did not succeed, owing as I now believe to some missmanagement. The Spruce tree may be known from the other trees by the discription I have given of it even to such as are unacquaint[d] with spruce pine, the leaves have a resinous tast and smell. The Tea Plant is a shruby tree which grows on dry soil near the shores, it bears a small leafe of which this (   ) is the natural size, small white flowers and small [cones][1] which contain the seeds,[2] this Plant is not only usefull in making Beer but is a substitute for Tea, this we found out last voyage and used it as such then as well as now. In order still better to know these two usefull Plants I have added a Drawing of each, the account I have given of them and their use will hardly be thought foreign to this Journal.[3] It is the business of Voyagers to pass over nothing that may be usefull to posterity and it cannot be denied that these would if ever this Country is settled by a Sevelized people or frequented by shipping.

I shall conclude this account of Dusky Bay with inserting some Nautical Observations made at Pickersgills Harbour where the Variation of the Compass was 13° [30′] East, the Tides were observed to rise and fall on the days of the full Moon Eight feet and at the Change but five feet seven[4] inches, this difference in the tides between the New and full Moon is a little extraordinary and probably was occasioned at this time by some accidental cause such as Winds &c[a]. The Latitude of the observatory was 45°4′ s.

		° ′ ″
Longitude[5] by the Mean of all M[r] Wales's observations		166 2 46½ E
—	by M[r] Kendals Watch supposing it to have gone mean time from England	164 29 12¾
—	Supposing it to have gone mean time from the Cape	164 29 49½
—	Supposing it to have gone at its Cape rate	165 12 36¾

[1] BG coins; H cones [alteration by Cook].

[2] . . . this is the best description I who am no botanist can give of it

[3] Plates LI and XXII in *Voyage*, I; the originals have disappeared. In due course Cook's recipe found due praise: Edward Bell of the *Chatham* wrote in 1791, 'Our Spruce Beer, which was made after the directions given by Captn. Cook, prov'd excellent, and was served out to the Ship's Company in lieu of Spirits'.—*Hist. Rec. N.Z.*, II, p. 498.

[4] *seven:* 4

[5] *Longitude:* The Longitude of the observatory in Pickersgills Harbour . . .—f. 62.

—	Supposing it to have gone at its Greenwich rate	163 47 9
By M[r] Arnolds Watch supposing it to have gone at its	Cape rate	165 38 35½

To the above account I shall add by way of remark that the Longitude by observations is deduced from observed distances of the Sun and Moon and Moon and Stars, the almost continual clowded sky not permiting of any other, and even but few of these; the Longitude thus found is less than it is in my Chart of the Island constructed in my former Voyage by near three quarters of a degree; that in reckoning our Longitude by M[r] Kendalls Watch from England to the Cape of Good Hope we allowed it to go as at Greenwich and from the Cape to this place mean time from supposision that it would return back to its Greenwich rate but in this we were misstaken for it was found to gain here 6″,46 per day on mean time;[1] this uncertainty of obtaining the true rate of going of Watches and what is still worse their varying their rate will always render the Long[d] deduced from them a little uncertain especially in long runs. From the foregoing results it will appear that M[r] Arnolds watch goes the best of the two, but we know for certain that it varies from its self in its rate of going more than the other and that its coming nearer the true Longitude is owing more to chance than to any superior quallities it has over the other; we are to consider that if we had made no stay at the Cape of Good Hope[2] but have been obliged to abide by the rates given us by the Astronomer Royal, in this case M[r] Kendalls would only have been two degrees and a quarter out whereas the error in M[r] Arnolds would have been inconceviably great, more owing to its rate of going not being well settled than to any bad quallities in the Watch.

WEDNESDAY 12*th*. Having quited Dusky Bay as has been already mentioned I directed my Course along shore for Queen Charlottes Sound[3] having a gentle breeze at SE and South with fair weather.

At 4 in the PM Doubtfull Harbour bore ESE dist[t] three or 4 Leagues & the North entrance of Dusky Bay SSE distant 5 Leagues. In the night had little Wind with showers of rain, in the morning it was fair

[1] ... and M[r] Arnolds to lose upon a mean Seconds p[r] day, at the Cape this last was found to lose 1′31″012 Seconds p[r] day on mean time whereas the rate given us by the Astronomer Royal was 14,62 Seconds, this uncertainty of obtaining the true rate of the going of Watches and what is still worse thier varying thier rate will for ever render the Longitude deduced from them in all long runs a little uncertain.

[2] ... so that the going of the Watches could not have been rectified ...

[3] ... where I expected to find the Adventure

but the Weather was dark & gloomy and the Wind veered to NW. At Noon we were distant from the Shore 5 Leagues.

THURSDAY 13*th*. Wind at NW to West a fresh gale, first part rain latter fair. Course made good this 24 hours NEBN dist^{e} 120 miles.

FRIDAY 14*th*. Winds from West to South, first part fresh gales & Cloudy, Middle a gentle gale with Showers of rain, latter little wind and variable. At Noon we were by Observation in the Lat of 41°53′ and about 7 or 8 Leagues from the land.

SATURDAY 15*th*. Little [wind] and Variable between the South and East and East & North with fair Weather. At Noon observed in Lat 41°12′ Rocks Point ENE.

SUNDAY 16*th*. Wind at NNE and NEBN a fresh gale and Clowdy hazey weather. Plying to Windward, at Noon Rocks point bore NNE distant about 4 Leagues and being about 3 miles from the nearest shore which was a low sandy beach, in this situation had 25 fathom water.

MONDAY 17*th*. At 5 pm the Wind veer'd to West and afterwards to SSW and blew a Strong gale, at Middnight judgeing our selves the length of Cape Farewell, we brought to till 4 am when we made sail, at 8 the above Cape bore west half South distant six Leg^{s}. At Noon Stephens's Isle bore E½S dist 5 Legues.

TUESDAY 18*th*. At 4 o'Clock in the PM the sky became suddenly obscured and seemed to indicate much Wind which occasioned us to clew up all our sails, presently after Six Water Spouts were seen, four rose and spent themselves between us and the land,[1] the fifth was at some distance without us and the Sixth pass'd under our Stern at about fifty yards from us,[2] the diameter of the base of this spout I judged to be about fifty or sixty feet, during the time these Spouts lasted which was near a hour we had light puffs of wind from all points of the Compass.[3] Water Spouts are caused by whirl

[1] . . that is to the SW of us

[2] 'One, I was told, came within 30 or 40 yards of the Ship; but I was then below; when I got on deck it was about 100 fathoms from her. I am perswaded that if it had gone over her it would have torn away her sails & yards; perhaps her Masts and standing Rigging also'.—Wales.

[3] 'PM from 4 to 5 Ship's Head and Wind all round the Compass. Very dark Cloudy Weather a Number of Waterspouts forming around us, one of which came so near the Ship as to give us some disagreeable apprehensions, as the Wind wou'd not in the least assist us in getting from it . . . the whole Atmosphere seemed in a state of Strange purterbation: Puffs of wind from every point of the Compass, and whichever way we got the Ship's Head in a few seconds we were all back again, so we made the best preparation we cou'd for its reception by clewing up the Sails, throwing Tarpaulings over the Hatchways &c: &c: &c: there was the most violent motion of the water by far that I ever saw, or indeed cou'd

winds which carries the Water in a stream upwards, the Sea below them is much agitated and all in a foam[1] from which a tube or round boddy is formed by which the water is conveyed[2] up to the Clowds, some of our people said they saw a bird in the one near us which was whirled round in the same manner as the fly of a Jack while it was carried upwards;[3] we had thick hazey weather for some hours after with varible Winds, but by middnight the Weather was clear at which time we pass'd Stephens's Isle at the distance of one mile.

*After leaving Dusky Bay as hath been already mentioned I directed my course a long shore for Queen Charlottes Sound where I expected to find the Adventure. In this passage we met with nothing remarkable or worthy of note till Monday the 17th at 4 oClock in the afternoon being then about 3 Leagues to the Westward of Cape Stephens, having a gentle gale at West by South and clear weather. The Wind at once flattned to a Calm and the Sky became sudanly obscured by dark dense clouds which occasioned us to clew up all our sails and presently after Six Water Spouts were seen; four rose and spent themselves between us and the land, that is to the SW of us the fifth was without us, the sixth first appeared in the SW at the distance of two or three miles at least from us, its progressive motion was to the NE not in a straight but crooked line and pass'd within fifty yards of our stern without our feeling any of its effects. The diameter of the Base of this spout I judged to be about fifty or Sixty feet, that is the Sea within this space was much agitated and foamed up to a great height from which a tube or round boddy was formed by which the Water or air or both was carried in a spiral stream up to the Clouds, some of our people said they saw a Bird in the one near us which was whirl'd round like the fly of a Jack as it was carried upwards. During the time these spouts lasted we had now and then light puffs of wind from all points of the compass and some few slight showers of rain which generally fell in large drops and the Weather continued thick and hazy for some hours after with variable light breezes of Wind: at length the wind fixed in its old point and the sky reassumed its former serenity; some of these Spouts appear'd at times to be stationary and at other times to have a quick but very unequal progressive motion and always in a crooked line, some times one way and some times another so that once or twice we observed them to

form any idea of; the Spout drove at a great rate along the surface of the water, came directly for us to within about 40 or 50 Yards, then alter'd its direction run abreast and so ahead of us'.—Clerke.

[1] *all in a foam:* foamed up to a great height

[2] *is conveyed:* or air or both was carried in a spiral stream

[3] A *note,* On farther enquiry I did not find this well attested.

cross one a nother, from the assending motion of the bird and several other circumstances it was very plane to us that these spouts were caused by whirl-w[i]nds and that the Water in them was violantly hurried upwards and did not descend from the Clouds as I have heard some assert. The first appeerence of them is by the violent agitation and rising up of the Water and presently after you see a round column or tube forming from the clouds above, which apparently desends till it joins the agitated Water below. I say apparently because I believe it not to be so in reallity, but that the tube is already formed and that first from the agitated water below and assends, but that at first it is either too small or too thin to be seen, after the Tube is form'd or become visible, its apparent diameter increaseth untill it becomes pretty large, after that it decreaseth and at last it breaks or becomes invisible towards the lower part, soon after the Sea below reasumes its natural state and the tube is drawn by little and little up to the Clouds where it is dissipated; the same tube would some times have a vertical direction and at others crooked or inclined. The most rationale account I have read of Water spouts is in Mr Falconer's Marine Dictionary[1] which is chiefly collected from the Philosophical Writings of the ingenious Dr Franklin; I have been told that the firing of a gun will dissipate them and I am now sorry I did not try the experiment as we were near enough and had a gun ready for the purpose, but as soon as the danger was past I thought no more about it, being too attentive in viewing these extraordinary meteor's.[2]*—f. 63–3v.

About Six leagues to the Eastward of Cape Farewell there seems to be a spacious Bay covered from the Sea by a low point of land and is I beleive the same as Tasman first anchored in.[3] Blind Bay, which is to the SE of this seems to extend a long way in to the South, the sight in this direction was not bounded by any land, I think it not improbable but that it may communicate with Queen Charlottes Sound.[4] At Daylight in the Morn we were the length of Point Jack-

[1] William Falconer, *A New and Universal Dictionary of the Marine*... (1769).

[2] '... accordingly a four-pounder was ordered to be got ready, but our people being, as usual, very dilatory about it, the danger was passed before we could try this experiment.' —Forster, I, p. 192.—As a visual appendix to all this, one may mention Hodges's large canvas 'View of Cape Stephens' now in the National Maritime Museum—a view taken from the shore, with the *Resolution* and waterspout in the middle distance; a monument of stormy and romantic art which, in the different medium, out-Byrons Byron. There is an engraving of another picture by Hodges, from the sea this time, and also romantic, 'Painted from Nature', in Wales and Bayly, *Astronomical Observations* (1777), pl. IV.

[3] This persuasion was correct. It was Golden Bay—the Murderers' Bay of Tasman—covered by Farewell Spit.

[4] Cook seems now to have got the two great bays separated in his mind—on his first voyage (I, p. 273), sailing direct from Cape Farewell to Cape Stephens he had noticed only one huge bottomless—i.e. 'blind'—opening. It was left to d'Urville, in January 1827,

son at the entrance of Queen Charlottes Sound and soon after we discovered the Adventure in Ship Cove by the Signals she made,[1] what little wind we had was out of the Sound so that we had to work in, in the doing of which we discovered a rock which we did not see in my last voyage, it lies SBE¼E from the outermost of the two Brothers and in a line with the white Rocks on with the middle of Long Island, the top of it is even or rather above the Surface of the Sea and there is deep water all round it.[2] At Noon the Adventure's Boat came on board with Lieut[t] Kemp and brought us a dish of fish and some Salleting.

Little Wind and clear pleasent Weather. With the assistance of our boats and the tide which was in our favour we got to an Anchor in Ship Cove at Six o'Clock in the evening and the next morning we moved farther in and moor'd with a hawser to the Shore. A little while before we anchored Captain Furneaux came on board and informed me that he arrived here on the 7th of Apr[l] having first touched at Van Diemens Land but his transactions from the time we parted will best appear by the following Journal which is a transcription of his proceedings from that time to this day.

The Natives of this place gave him on his first arrival a friendly reception and hath at sundry times supplyed him with fish for Nails and other trifles, but as they have quite deserted the places they lived in when I was here before and remove'd higher up the Sound he only hath had Visits from them now and then.

[FURNEAUX'S JOURNAL]

[FEBRUARY 1773]

MONDAY 8*th.*[3] *Winds NNE, NEBN, East, EBS, NEBE, NE. Course S* 51°30′ *E. Dist.* 116 *Miles. Lat. in* 50°03′ *S. Long. made* 45°30′ *E.* First part, moderate and fair weather; middle fresh gales & hazey; latter thick fog, at 7 PM Join'd the Resolution p[r] Signal, hauld down the Studding Sails, at 12 took one Reef in the Foretopsail. At 8 AM the

to mark and name the division between the two, Separation Point. Cook's guess that Blind, or Tasman, Bay communicated with Queen Charlotte Sound was not a good one.

[1] . . . a circumstance which gave pleasure to every one aboard and I believe was no less exceptable to them.—f. 65.—Cf. pp. 160, n. 3; 161, n. 1 below. Wales (17 May) says they saw the flashes of the *Adventure's* guns when they were abreast of Cape Jackson.

[2] Cook Rock, as a line from the middle of Long Island through White Rocks makes amply clear: but the outermost of the Brothers lies SBE¼E from Cook Rock—not the other way round, as Cook states it. He will be found making this sort of slip more than once below. Why so careful a man should do this it is hard to fathom.

[3] The following copy of Furneaux's journal is in a clerk's hand. In B ff. 65–8v Cook summarises it, and this summary is copied in A and G. H copies the original. For a more readable account by Furneaux himself see pp. 731–41 below.

Resolution about three Miles dist^t from us.[1] At 9 fired a Gun in Answer to one from her, the report bore distant from what we expected; (Viz^t East) soon After we fired another Gun but heard no answer, Repeated it every half hour, at noon thick foggy wea^r, can see nothing of the Resolution.

TUESDAY 9*th. Winds NE, NBE, NNE, NEBN, NNE, NBE. Course S* 51°00′ *E. Dist.* 21 *Miles. Lat. in* 50°16′. *Long. made* 45°55′ *E.* First & Middle parts Fresh breezes & thick foggy Weather; latter part more clear, fired a Gun every half hour, but heard no answer from the Resolution, at 7 PM haul'd the wind, and judged she must have done the same when it first Shifted.[2] AM saw many Penguins & Dip chicks.[3]

WEDNESDAY 10*th. Winds NBE, NBW, NEBN, NWBW, WNW, NWBW, NW. Course N* 37° *E. Dist.* 30 *Miles. Lat. in* 49°52′ *S. Long. made* 46°30′ *E.* First & Middle parts Strong gales & Squally wea^r, latter part fresh gales and cloudy, at 2 PM handed the Topsails, at ½ past 4 handed the Mainsail and brought too under the Foresail & Mizen Staysail, at 8 got in the Jibb boom. At 5 AM more moderate, Wore Ship & made sail. Set the two Topsails. At ½ past 11 Wore. Saw a seal, at noon fair wea^r, can see nothing of the Resolution.[4]

THURSDAY 11*th. Winds NWBW, NBW, N°, NWBN, Course S* 21° *E. Dist.* 28 *Miles. Lat. in* 50°18′ *S. Long. made* 46°55′ *E.* Fresh gales and Squally weather, at 1 PM split the Main topm^st Staysail, at 7 Wore Ship, at 4 AM Wore ship, at noon can see nothing of the Resolution, bore away for the Rendezvouz in New Zealand.[5]

FRIDAY 12*th. Winds NWterly. Course S* 79° *E. Dist.* 119 *Miles. Lat. in* 50°40′. *Long. made* 49°50′ *E.* Moderate wea^r, at 2 PM out 2nd reefs, got the Main top Gall^t yard across & set Studding sails, saw many

[1] 'very thick fog'.—Furneaux.

[2] 'PM Fired a Gun every ½ hour till 4 Oclock as Sig^ls But had no Ans^r at which Time it Cleard up and I thought I see her ahead: we made Sail and at 5 have^g a Clear Horizon we Found it only the Strengh of Immagination.'—Wilby.

[3] Note by Cook: 'Dip chicks are the same as I call Divers. C.'

[4] At this point disaster struck Mr Bayly: 'This morning I found that my cask of Porter (which was stowed in the fore Hold) was entirely drank out by some of the Ships crew unknown, as likewis a quarter cask of Madiera wine belonging to Mr Shank our late First Lieu^t who stayed at the Cape on acc^t of his ill State of Health'.

[5] '[1 pm] Bore up to the Eastward having given up all hopes of joi[n]ing the Resolution after trying our utmost to Turn to windward to join Company, instead of which we lost ground—'twas then thought most prudent to waste no more time in searching for her, the Winter season advanceing so fast upon us.'—Kemp, 12 February.—'. . . this morning saw some Penguins with rose combs on their heads which is very different from any we have seen before & great numbers of Sea fowls of various kinds'.—Bayly. Penguins do not have 'rose combs'. The position was not far from Kerguelen Island, and the local penguin nearest to Bayly's description is the Macaroni, *Eudyptes chrysolophus* (Brandt).

Penguins,[1] at 8 haul'd down Studding Sails & took 2 reefs in the Fore & Main Topsails. At 4 AM got the Fore Top gallant yard across and Set Studding sails. Variatn pr Amplitude 29°43′ w.

SATURDAY 13*th. Winds WNW, SW, WSW. Course S* 78° *E. Dist.* 121 *Miles. Lat. in* 51°5′ *S. Long. made* 53°0′ *E.* Moderate & Cloudy wear. at 8 PM haul'd down Studding sails & took one reef in the Topsails, At 3 AM let out the reefs & Set Studding sails. Variation pr Azimuth 32°30′ West.

SUNDAY 14*th. Winds NW, WNW, West. Course S* 75°00′ *E. Dist.* 136 *Miles. Lat. in* 51°40′ *S. Long. made* 56°29′ *E.* Fresh breezes & Cloudy, with Sleet in the first part. At 8 PM haul'd down the Studding sails and took one reef in the Topsails. At 4 AM made sail. Saw many birds & Seals.[2]

MONDAY 15*th. Winds NWBW, West, SWBW. Course S* 77°00′ *E. Dist.* 140 *Miles. Lat. in* 52°12′ *S. Long. made* 60°13′ *E.* Fresh Gales & Cloudy wear. PM Variation pr azmths 34°14′ w. At 8 shorten'd sail, at 3 AM made sail, Variation pr Azimth 35°7′ w. Bent the small Bower Cable.

TUESDAY 16*th. Winds West, WNW, NNE. Course S* 79° *E. Dist.* 78 *Miles. Lat. in* 52°27′ *S. Long. made* 62°22′. Moderate & Cloudy wear with rain at times. At 7 PM haul'd down studding Sails & Shortend sail. At 4 AM made sail.[3]

WEDNESDAY 17*th. Winds NEBE, NW, West, WNW. Course S* 79°00′ *E. Dist.* 143 *Miles. Lat. in* 52°54′ *S. Long. made* 66°30′ *E.* Fresh gales & hazy with rain and Sleet at times, at 6 PM shorten'd sail, At 4 am made sail.

THURSDAY 18*th. Winds NW, W, WNW. Course East. Dist.* 144 *Miles. Lat. in* 52°54′ *S. Long. made* 70°34′ *E.* Fresh breezes & Cloudy wear. PM saw some Sea weed, at 7 shorten'd sail, AM made sail.

FRIDAY 19*th. Winds NWBW, SW, WSW, SWBW, SW. Course N* 84°30′ *E. Dist.* 148 *Miles. Lat. in* 52°40′ *S. Long. made* 74°41′ *E.* First

[1] Note by Cook: 'Under this meridian and 1° to ye South we also saw Penguins. C.'

[2] Note by Cook: 'Nearly under this Meridian & 2° to the South we saw many Penguins. C.'—'This morning I saw 2 Seals & one large whale, & such a great Number of sea fowl of various kinds but mostly Petrals (if not all) that the horizon seemed in motion with their flying to & fro.'—Bayly. These fowl were probably whale birds or prions.

[3] 'This Afternoon Mr Scott (the Lieut of Marines,) turned out of our Mess, he behaved in an Insolent manner to the Capt so that the Capt took him by the Shoulder & put him out of the great cabbin & shut the door after him, he was of an unhappy temper allway[s] quarreling with the Capt & officers, he being a great stikler for *Honour*, that if you spoke the least word in a Joke his scotch Blood would be up.'—Bayly.

& latter parts fresh breezes & Cloudy wea^r with small rain, Middle part hard Gales with violent Squalls. At 3 PM set the Larboard Fore Studding Sail, at 8 took two reefs in the Topsails and handed the Mainsail. At 4 PM let out the two reefs in the Topsails & set the Mainsail. At 5 set the Main Topsail. Variation p^r Azimuth 29°45′ W. At 9 handed the Mainsail & got down Top Gall^t Yards.

SATURDAY 20*th. Winds SWBS, SW, WNW. Course N* 83°00′ *E. Dist.* 146 *Miles. Lat. in* 52°22′ *S. Long. made* 78°45′ *E.* Fresh Gales & Squally wea^r. at 4 PM saw some sea Weed. at 8 close Reef'd the Topsails, at 4 AM thick Snow. Let out the 2nd reefs, at 7 split the Starboard lower Studding sail, at Noon thick Snow & hail.

SUNDAY 21*st. Winds SW, SWBS, SW, WNW. Course N* 89°00′ *E. Dist.* 108 *Miles. Lat. in* 52°20′ *S. Long. made* 81°47′ *E.* Moderate & Cloudy wea^r. PM Variation p^r Azimuth 28°30′ West. at 8 close reef'd the Topsails, at 3 AM Set ye Mizen Topsail, and got up Top Gall^t Yards, at 7 let out the 1st reefs, at 9 set Studding sails, at 11 saw a large Island of Ice. At Noon little wind & fair.[1]

MONDAY 22*nd. Winds NW, N, NEBE, ENE, East. Course S* 74°00′ *E. Dist.* 75 *Miles. Lat. in* 52°40′ s. *Long. made* 8°00′ *E.* First & Middle parts, moderate & fair, Latter part fresh & Gales hazy wea^r at 3 pm hoisted out the Boats & Sent them towards the Ice.[2] Variation p^r Azimuth 29°09′ West. at 7 the boats return'd but could get no Ice; hoisted them in & took one reef in the Topsails, at 11 in 2nd reef of the Main topsail, AM saw a seal.

TUESDAY 23*rd. Winds EBN, N, NNW, NWBN. Course N* 74°30′ *E. Dist.* 83 *Miles. Lat. in* 52°18′ *S. Long. Made* 86°10′ *E.* Fresh Gales & hazy with rain, at 4 pm Wore ship, at 5 shorten'd sail & sounded, found no ground with 140 fa^ms. AM made sail.

WEDNESDAY 24*th. Winds N, NNE, NW. Course N* 85° *E. Dist.* 89 *Miles. Lat. in* 52°10′ *S. Long. Made* 88°45′ *E.* First part fresh Gales, with Squalls & showers of rain, Middle & latter moderate with rain at times, at 7 PM in 2nd reefs, at 3 AM let out the Reefs, and got Top Gall^t Yards a cross, at 6 Set Studding sails, Exercis'd Great Guns & small arms. Saw some sea weed.

THURSDAY 25*th. Winds NW, WNW, West. Course N* 79°00′ *E. Dist.* 128 *Miles. Lat. in* 51°46′ *S. Long. made* 92°14′ *E.* Fresh Gales &

[1] 'Tho' lucky in a fair wind, yet this is the finest day we have known for some time, which we truly relish.'—Kemp.

[2] Note by Cook: 'This is the only Island of Ice they met with. C.'

cloudy wea^{r}. at 8 PM took two Reefs in the Topsails and handed the Mainsail, at 5 am let out 2nd Reefs & handed ye Mizen Topsail. saw some sea weed.

FRIDAY 26*th. Winds WNW, N. Course N* 80°00′ *E. Dist.* 143 *Miles Lat. in* 51°22′ *S. Long. made* 96°09′ *E.* Fresh Gales & fair wea^{r}. at ½ past 7 PM handed ye Mainsail and took two Reefs in ye Tops^{ls}. at 10 saw a Meteor in the NNW which directed its course to the SW.[1] at 3 AM let out 2nd reefs and set the Mizen Topsail, Mainsail & Studding sails, saw a number of Porpoises, spotted black & white,[2] at noon took one Reef in the Topsails.

SATURDAY 27*th. Winds NBE, N, NNW, NW. Course N* 75°15′ *E. Dist.* 145 *Miles. Lat. in* 50°54′ *S. Long. made* 99°58′ *E.* Fresh Gales & Squally wea^{r}, at 4 PM in 2 reef of the Maintops^{l} and got down Top Gall^{t} Yards, at 7 close Reef'd the Tops^{ls} and handed ye Mainsail & Miz Topsail, at 10 Shipt a Sea, which washed overboard the Larboard waistcloth. at noon more mod^{t}. let out ye 2nd reef of ye Topsails.

SUNDAY 28*th. Winds NNW, NW, WNW. Course N* 76°00′ *E. Dist* 145 *Miles. Lat. in* 50°20′ *S. Long. made* 103°26′ *E.* Fresh Gales & Squally wea^{r}. pm Variation p^{r} azimuth 18° West, at 7 in 2nd Reefs Tops^{ls} & handed the Mainsail, at 4 am out 2nd reefs and set the mainsail, at 8 sett the Studding Sails, at 12 Squally, haul'd them down.

[MARCH 1773]

MONDAY 1*st. Winds West, WNW, WBS, NWBW, NW. Course N* 57°00′ *E. Dist.* 140 *Miles. Lat. in* 49°04′ *S. Long. made* 106°37′ *E.* First & middle parts, fresh gales with very hard squalls & Snow. PM split the Jib, at 8 close reef'd the maintopsail and handed the Foretopsail and mainsail, at 12 set the Fore & Mizen Topsails. AM Variation p^{r} Azimuth 10°00′ W. at ½ past 7 thought we saw land on the Larboard Bow, haul'd down the Studding sails, took in the 2nd reefs of the Topsails & haul'd the wind towards it. AM out 2nd reefs & bore away, being mistaken in the sight of the Land.[3]

[1] '. . . this evening was remarkeably serene & clear, we saw the Aurora Astralis or southern lights very light, so that I could read common good print very distinct they appeared in white streaks terminating in a point at some distance from the Zenith, & in all respects resembled the Aurora Borealis or Northern lights: this was the first [time] we have seen it during the Voyage'.—Bayly.

[2] Possibly Hector's Dolphin, *Cephalorhynchus hectori* (Van Beneden).

[3] 'On the first of March we were alarmed with the cry of Land by the men at the Mast head on the Larboard beam which gave us great joy; we immediately hauled our wind and stood for it, but to our mortification were disappointed in a few hours, for what we took to be land prove'd no more than Clouds which disappeared as we sailed towards them . . .'—Add. MS 27890, f. 5–5v.

TUESDAY *2nd. Winds NWBN, NWBW, NW. Course N* 50°00′ *E. Dist.* 139 *Miles. Lat. in* 47°35′ *S. Long. Made* 109°26′ *E.* Fresh Gales & cloudy with a NW Swell, at 1 PM Got down the main Top Gall[t] Yard, at 7 handed the mainsail, at 2 AM Set it & made sail. Much Rock Weed has gone past us these 24 hours.

WEDNESDAY *3rd. Winds NW, NNW, NWBN. Course N* 52°00′ *E. Dist.* 121 *Miles. Lat. in* 46°22′ *S. Long. made* 111°38′ *E.* Fresh Gales & hazy rainy Squally weather, at 4 PM a piece of drift wood went past, at 7 close Reef'd the Topsails and handed the Mainsail, sounded but found no ground, at 3 AM made sail, much Rock weed gone past us.

THURSDAY *4th. Winds NWBN, WNW, WSW, SW. Course NE½N Dist.* 120 *Miles. Lat. in* 44°50′ *S. Long. made* 113°57′ *E.* First & Middle parts moderate breezes with Showers of rain, latter part, fresh gales with frequent Squalls & Rain. PM Variation p[r] Azimuth 6°00′ West, at 7 sounded but had no ground with 130 fa[ms] at 9 Shorten'd sail, at 2 am made sail, at 5 carried away a Topmast Studding sail Yard, saw many pieces of Sea Weed. Variation 3°09′ West.[1]

FRIDAY *5th. Winds SW, West. Course N* 67°00′ *E. Dist.* 126 *Miles. Lat. in* 44°01′ *S. Long. made* 116°52′ *E.* First part fresh Gales, & cloudy weather, Middle & latter, fresh breezes & fair. PM unbent the Maintopsail & bent a New One, Variation 3°03′ West, at 7 Shorten'd sail. AM made sail.

SATURDAY *6th. Winds West, WNW, WBN, WSW. Course N* 88°00′ *E. Dist.* 142 *Miles. Lat. in* 43°56′ *S. Long. made* 120°19′ *E.* First & latter parts, fresh Gales & cloudy, Middle Strong gales with hard Squalls. PM Variation 1°30′ w. at 6 Shortend sail, at 4 am made sail,[2] Variation 1°30′ E.[3]

SUNDAY *7th. Winds WSW, WBS, WSW. Course N* 85°00′ *E. Dist.* 100 *Miles. Lat. in* 43°47′ *S. Long. made* 122°42′ *E.* Fresh Gales & fair weather, PM Variation p[r] Azimuth 1°30′ East. At 6 short[d] sail & haûl'd the wind to y[e] Northward, At 1 AM Wore, at 2 bore away & made sail, Variation p[r] Azimuth 1°30′ East.

[1] '... at about 11½[h] evening an odd afair hapned, Viz M[r] Mory (a Midshipman) was on his watch on the Forecastle by himself, there happened not to be any one nearer than the quarter Deck to him. He run aft in violent Agitation crying out he should never see his father again & after he was a little pacified, he said that as he was walking to & fro his Father came & walked by him dressed the same as when he saw him last in England, this terified him so that he was ready to sink, & made him conclude his father was dead. This M[r] Mory is a very sober young man & not in the least given to d[r]ink.'—Bayly.

[2] '... this Morning Servd Fishing Lines &c to the Ships Company'.—Burney log.

[3] Note by Cook: 'Here it appears that the line of no Variation pasith through the Lat. of 43°58′ and Longitude 118°50′ East of the Cape of Good Hope. C.'

MONDAY 8*th. Winds WBS, WBN, WBS. Course N* 87°00′ *E. Dist.* 110 *Miles. Lat. in* 43°42′ *S. Long. made* 125°28′ *E.* Moderate & fair weather, at 7 PM bro[t] too & Sounded but had no ground with 150 fa[ms]. Shorten'd sail, am made sail, saw a piece of drift wood.

TUESDAY 9*th. Winds West. WSW, WNW, NW. Course S* 88°30′ *E. Dist.* 81 *Miles. Lat. in* 43°44′ *S. Long. made* 127°30′ *E.* Mod[t] brezes and Cloudy wea[r], at 7 PM Shorten'd sail, at 8 Sounded but found no ground, at 5 AM made sail, at 9 saw the Land bearing NNE.[1] haul'd the wind, at ½ past the most Southern part NEBE and a Rock about 5 miles without it, ENE; unstowed the Anchor & bent the Sheet Cable, at Noon the Northermost land in Sight bore NBW. Stand[g] in NNE½E for a bluff point of Land,[2] seeing sev[l] Isl[ds] [3] & broken land to y[e] SE.

WEDNESDAY 10*th. Winds Variable. Course N* 70°00′ *E. Dist.* 30 *Miles. Lat. in* 43°38′ *S. Long. made* 126°12′ *E.* First & Middle parts, moderate breezes and hazy wea[r], latter part Strong gale & Squally with rain, at 1 PM hoisted out the Cutter & sent her in shore, at ½ past 1 fired a Gun as a signal for her to return, at 2 she returned, Sounded 47 fa[ms] Coral ground, at 4 sounded 48 fa[ms] brown sand with small stones & broken shells. Standing in between the Mew Stone (a rock which resembles the Mew stone at Plymouth) & the main Land, at 8 the Eastermost Land EBN½N & the Southermost WNW 9 or 10 miles, at 10 Sounded but found no ground with 75 fa[ms], at 3 AM Sounded 72 fa[ms] fine dark brown Sand with small stones and Shells, at 5 Tacked, the Mewstone W½S & the SE Cape NE½E. at 9 hoisted out the Boat & Sent her on shore, with the 2nd Lieutenant to Sound & look for Water, at 11 it blowing very Strong, made the Boat Sign[l] to Return & Repeated it Often,[4] at noon the SE point ENE 4 Leagues.

[1] This was the land about the South West Cape of Tasmania. From this point the reader would be well-advised to add to these bare bones the flesh of Add. MS 27890, pp. 732–6 below; and see Fig. 31, p. 162.

[2] Cox bluff.

[3] The Maatsuyker group, so called by Tasman, of which the most southerly is the Mewstone (Furneaux's name—see next entry). Chart XXVII, by Burney, calls the islands generally 'Pedra blancs', a mis-spelling of Tasman's 'Pedra Brancka'; and here the mis-application of Tasman's names begins. His islands were further south-east, 14 miles SSE of South East Cape; they are called on the engraved chart (*Voyage*, I, pl. VIII) Swilly Isles, perhaps after Furneaux's birthplace Swilly, near Plymouth, and are the two large rocks now known as Pedra Blanca (not white, but named by Tasman after a rock he knew off the China coast) and Eddystone. Cook gave this latter name on his third voyage. The two lie on the same reef.

[4] 'but they did not see nor hear any thing of it, the ship then three or four leagues off, that we could not see any thing of the Boat, which gave us great uneasiness, as there was a very great Sea.'—Add. MS 27890, f. 6.

THURSDAY 11*th. Winds West, WSW. Course N* 54°00′ *E. Dist.* 30 *Miles. Lat. in* 43°20′ *S. Long. made* 126°48′ *E.* First part fresh gales and hazy, latter moderate, at ½ past noon our boat return'd,[1] hoisted her in & bore away. At 4 the Eastmost land NE½E, 4 or 5 miles, At 5 Marias Island (the most S.ern part)[2] N½E, at 7 came too with the small Bower, under a high bluff in 24 fa[ms] fine sand & mud, distant off shore ⅔[rds] of a mile, at 4 AM hoisted out the Boats & Sent them inshore to sound, at 8 they return'd having found a good anchoring place, convenient for wooding & watering, at 10 weighed, employd working into the Bay, which I called Adventure Bay.[3]

FRIDAY 12*th. Winds N.* First & latter parts little wind & Cloudy, Middle calm, at 6 PM came to with the small Bower, in 11 fathoms, fine sandy ground, moored a Cable Each way, the small Bower to the SSE, the Northermost part of the Bay (when moored) bore NNE¼E, the watering Place W½N, am Sent our empty Casks ashore, and a guang of hands to cut wood.

SATURDAY 13*th. Winds NNW.* Moderate breezes & cloudy with rain at times, Employ'd wooding & watering.[4]

[1] We have an account of this first experiment in landing: it was in a bay between two islets, Louisa Bay: 'AM . . . at 9 it fell Calm. Hoisted out the Large Cutter and sent her in Shore in search of fresh water, with our 2nd Lieu[t] a Mate and Midshipman, with 7 hands arm'd. We Row'd in Shore to the E[t]ward of the Bay just Mention'd [Cox Bight] where we Observ'd the Land to part, we conjectured a fresh water River was there, But being too far from the Ship, we row'd into a Small Bay to the E[t]ward where we attemp'd to Land on a Sandy Beach but could not for the Surf. However we Land a Little to right of it, under the Lee of some Rocks that Projectured out, We Climb'd up these Rocks inadvertantly without our Arm's, But on Reccolection by the Sight of Wood Ashes, we procured our Implem[ts] and proceed'd in our Attempt. We Observ'd a Path Leading in the Wood which had we followd, would in all Probability Led us to the Natives, but the Weath[r] growing Hazy and Likely to Blow, we took the Prudentest Method, of Return[g] on Board; Have[g] tak[g] [*sic*] a convince[g] proof of their Being natives near [at] hand. at the Larb[d] Hand come[g] out their is a fine Run of Water from the Rocks, but not safe, too near it in a Boat: ½ past 12 got Safe on Board to the great Joy of our Shipmates: They have[g] Fired Serv[l] Guns as Sig[ls] for us, which we heard nothing Off. The Ship was under Close Reef Tops[ls] and the Weath[r] Grew very dirty—Its very Bold in Shore, have[g] many Bays; and the Land coverd with Trees, mak[g] every[where] an Entire Wood.'—Wilby.—The boat, says Constable, 'Brought of Several Green Boughs which was a pleasent Sight to us'. See also pp. 732–3, 746 below.

[2] i.e. the southern end of the Tasman Peninsula, which was taken for a group of islands (Chart XXVII). Furneaux got his identifications wrong, through beginning to make them too far west.

[3] 'We first took this bay to be that by Tasman called Frederick Henry Bay, but find his laid down five leagues to the Northward of this.'—Add. MS 27890, f. 6v. That is, they had mistaken Bruni Island for the Tasman Peninsula, and a bay on the east side of the one for a bay on the east side of the other. Adventure Bay was in fact Tasman's Storm Bay. Though Furneaux is so briefly uninformative here, he describes the bay fairly fully in Add. MS 27890, ff. 6v–8; see pp. 734–5 below; and see Chart XXVIII.

[4] 'the People Discovered several Hutts, or Wigwams, on Shore, wth several Baggs made out of Grass; in which they Carry their Shell Fish, which I Believe is their Chief Food, for in all their Hutts, we found great Quantity of them and no Signs of any other food; they

SUNDAY 14*th. Winds Variable.* D° weather, employed wooding & watering.

MONDAY 15*th. Winds WNW, NNW.* D° weather. PM compleated our water & wood^{g}.[1] AM hoisted in the Launch, unmoor'd & hove Short, at ½ past 9 weighed & made sail out of the Bay, at 11 hoisted in the Boats, at noon the Eastermost land ENE¼E. Tasmans head SSW. distant from the Bottom of the Bay 5 or 6 miles.

TUESDAY 16*th. Winds SSE, WSW, SW, SWBS, West. Course N* 67°00' *E. Dist.* 41 *Miles. Lat. in* 43°06'. *Long. made* 0°52' *E.* Moderate breezes with Squalls, and showers of rain at times, at ½ past 6 the westermost land WSW½W & the Eastermost land NE½E. At 4 AM Out 1st reef of the Topsails, at ½ past 5, the Northermost point of Marias Island NWBN, at 8 the westermost land WBN and a small Island NWBN, dist^{t} off shore 4 or 5 Leagues. At noon the S.most part of Marias Isl^{d} SWBW½W & the N.most land NNW dist^{ce} off shore 5 Leagues.[2]

WEDNESDAY 17*th. Winds Variable. Course N* 60°00' *W. Dist.* 83 *Miles Lat. in* 41°44' *S.* Moderate breezes & fair wea^{r}, at 5 the South end of Marias Island SWBS 9 Leagues and the Northermost Island NWBW½W. 6 Leagues, Sounded no ground at 80 fathoms, at 8 AM the Southermost land SW½S 3 Leagues, saw many smokes along

makes Large fire[s] of the Woods so that most of the Trees, are Burnt near the Ground; and their's Scarce any but what the Bark, is Strip'd off, either to Build their Wigwams or Burn for we saw no Signs of their having any Canoes, nor any Kind of Istrument among them; for the Furm Branches, with which their Hutts are made are split & Torn; they are I Believe a Very Ignorant & Miserable set of People'.—Browne/Hergest. For this day Bayly has a little complaint of his own. He watched the tides ashore and found irregularity: 'but the cause of this Irregularity I had not an opportunity of trying our stay being so short, & not the Assistance of a Boat for if ever I wanted one the Capt was always furnished with an Evasive refusal'.

[1] 'This day we Found out Sev^{l} Huts or Wigwams with some Bags in them, made of weed But not the Least Appearance of any People. They have nothing to Live on but Shellfish, that we can Observe, for the Birds, what Few there are, is so shy, that its difficult to get a Shot at them. To the SW of the First Water^{g} Place there is a Large Lagoon which I believe has Plenty of Fish in it for one of our Gentlemen caught upwards of 2 Dozen Trout, and Shot a Possum, which was the only Animal we saw. Their are a great many Gum Trees and of a vast Thickness and Hight, one of Which Measured in Circumference 26 feet & ye Height under the Branches was 20 feet. The Tree seems most of 'em to have been Burnt down, for their was not the Least Appearance of any Ingenuitty. We see their Fires in a Sandy Bay to the Nward of us, but no way Inclineable to near us But seem'd rather to Fly From us.'—Wilby.—'We found plenty of the dung of some Animal that seemed of the dear kind, the dung being in hard buttons, we shot one animal that had a false belly, this in England is what is a Possom. . .'—Bayly. The animal of the 'dear kind' was no doubt a kangaroo.

[2] 'On the 16th passed the Island called Marias, so named by Tasman, they appear to be the same as the main land.'—Add. MS 27890, f. 8. Furneaux's constant reference to 'Marias Island', in the singular, has no significance, although there is only one Maria Island. In the foregoing sentence he refers to it as 'they', and in spite of the appearance he noted the charts show four main islands, apart from inconsiderable islets lying off them.

shore, at Noon the No.most land NBW. St Patricks head[1] WNW 4 Leagues. and the Northermost of Schouten's Island[2] S½E.

THURSDAY 18*th. Winds SSW, S°, SBW, S°, SBW, Course North. Dist.* 84 *Miles. Lat. in* 40°20′ *S.* First & latter parts fresh gales & cloudy weat^{r}. Middle part, Strong Gales & Squally wea^{r}. running along shore, at 4 PM St Helen's Point[3] NW½W 7 or 8 miles, at 6 in 3rd reef of the Topsails, handed the Mi^{z} Topsail & got down T.G. Yards, the N^{o}.most land NBW½W 6 or 7 miles, at midnight saw many large fires along shore,[4] at 1 PM handed the Foretopsail, at 2, our Maintopsail Staysail split all in rags and blew overboard, at 5 more moderate, sett the topsails, at 6 saw the Land and three small Islands laying off of it, the N^{o}most bearing WSW¼S and three other Islands to ye NW of them: the Westmost bearing NNW & the Northmost NWBN.[5] at 8 out 3rd Reef of the Foretopsail & 3rd and 2nd of the main topsail.[6]

[1] '... at Noon gave name to a Bluff Point Call'd it St Patrick's Head in Honour to the Day, have a great number of his Country on Board.'—Wilby.

[2] i.e. part of the Freycinet Peninsula, mistaken by Furneaux, like Tasman, for a group of islands. Schouten's Island lies off the southern point of the peninsula.

[3] Furneaux is most exasperating in his omission of the reasons for names; and here no one else supplements him. Perhaps after St. Helen's Point on the Isle of Wight?

[4] See, on Chart XXVII, the inscription 'Bay of Fires'; and within the coast-line, 'Low Level Land seemingly a fine country and Populous'. No doubt the fires provided the evidence for the population.

[5] These lines about 'three small islands ... and three other islands', taken in conjunction with the chart (either Chart XXVII or the modern chart), the ship's track, and the times and bearings given, are extremely confusing, and I do not know what precisely Furneaux saw. Presumably 'small islands' are islands lying off the main islands of the Furneaux group. They can hardly have been the Furneaux islands themselves, because that would make nonsense of the bearings given, and of most of the following entry. The northernmost group Furneaux could see may have been Babel, Cat, and Storehouse islets, off Sellar Point, where Flinders Island turns north-west. It might indeed be necessary to sail his course to find out what he meant.

[6] The *Adventure* was now off Cape Barren Island, the second in size of the Furneaux group, 'Barren Uninhabited Islands', according to Chart XXVII; Cape Barren was named. The chart shows the opening of the division between Cape Barren and Flinders islands, Franklin Sound, the entrance to which is spread with islets and sandbanks.—At this point it is necessary to advert to another sentence in Add. MS 27890, f. 8: 'In the Latitude of 40°50′ South the Land trenches away to the westward, which I believe forms a deep bay, as we saw several smokes rising aback of the Island from the deck when we could not see the least sign of Land from the Masthead'. A number of the journal-keepers on the ship could by no means accept this deep-bay assumption: indeed on the chart Burney writes without hesitation, 'Suposed Streights or Passage'. Cf. Hergest, 18 March: 'at 6 AM Saw the Land about 5 Leagues to the Northward of the Eddystone Point [the northern point of the Bay of Fires] it seemd to stretch to the Westward and at the same time saw More Land Bearing WSW¼S Stretching to the Northward which Appeard like Several Large Islands [Cape Barren Island and Clarke Island?] So that we Judge here is a Streights[.] at noon of a Cape which we namd Cape Barren Distant about 6 Mile it Appeard to be an Island and Formed the North head of the Supposd Streight in the Lat^{d} of 40..14 South'.—19 March: 'All the Land which we have Passd this Afternoon Appeard to be a Number of Islands if so they are a Strong Confirmation of the Supposd Streights & are in the Mouth of it between Van deiman Land and New Holland.' Kemp, 21 March, is more cautious: 'N.B. The opening which we discover'd on the 19th [?18th] Inst^{t} I take to be the Streights leading between New Holland and Van Diemen's Land, but this is

FRIDAY 19*th*. *Winds SSE, SSW, SWBS, SBE, S°. Course NNE. Dist.* 63 *Miles. Lat. in* 39°20′ *S.* Fresh breezes & cloudy weather, at 1 PM saw a number of breakers about 1 mile from us,[1] Sounded 8 fathoms, sandy ground; haul'd off & deepen'd the water, to 15 fathoms, at 4 a Small Island[2] bore WBS 4 Leagues, at 6 the N°most land WBN, 7 or 8 miles. Sounded 18 fa^ms^ fine white sand with small Shells, at 7 the N°most land W¼S, and an Island[3] without it, WBN½W. Close Reefed the Topsails & stood of to the Eastward, at 8 Sounded 22 fa^ms^ fine sand, set the mizen Topsail, at ½ p^t^ 11 Sounded 26 fa^ms^ bro^t^ too & at 12 Sounded 46 fa^ms^. at 1, 50 f^ms^, at 2, 53 f^ms^. at 3 am wore & made sail, at 6 the N°most land WBS½S distant 10 or 12 Leagues. Out 3rd Reef of the foretopsail, at 7 Sounded 26 fa^ms^, at 8, 22 f^ms^ sand & Shells, haul'd up for New Zealand.[4]

mere conjecture, as we were not nigh enough to be certain, whether there is a streight leading thro or not.' See also the notes from Bayly and Burney that follow. There was indeed a strait here between New Holland and Van Diemen's Land, though the Furneaux Islands intervened—Banks Strait, which leads right into the greater Bass Strait.

[1] Hence the name on the chart, 'Bay of Shoals'. Bayly finds here another reason for a strait: '. . . off these islands the water is very shole, having only 7 or 8 fathom water 5 or 6 Miles of shore, we immediately halled off to the Eastward to keep clear of the sand banks that run out to a great distance from shore, owing (probably) to the current setting out of the opening, & it seems very evident this is the mouth of a straight which Seperates new Holland from Van Diemans Land. . . . Another circumstance that convinceth me there is a passage thro, is that there was a very strong draft of Water directly in shore all the Time we were passing by these broken Islands, which was not the case on any other part of the Coast.' It seems that he was not writing of Banks Strait, but of the passage between Cape Barren Island and Flinders Island; which of course would equally have taken the ship into Bass Strait. On the other hand, Kemp on the 19th mentions 'A great Current, setting to ye Northward'—i.e. not directly 'out of the opening' as Bayly has it.

[2] Babel island.

[3] East Sister island.

[4] 'As we stood on to the Northward we made Land again in about 39° [? the Kent islands in Bass Strait, but see Burney and Wilby in this note, and p. 164, n. 6 below] and did not stand further to the Northward as we found the ground very uneaven and shoal water some distance off. I think it a very dangerous coast to fall in with. The Coast from Adventure bay to the place where we stood away for Zealand is S½W and N½E about 75 Leagues, and it is my opinion that there is no Streights between New Holland and Van Dieman's Land, but a very deep bay. I should have stood further to the Northward, but the wind blowing strong at SSE and looking likely to haul round to the Eastward, which would have blown right on the land, I therefore thought it more prudent to leave the Coast and steer for New Zealand.'—Add. MS 27890, f. 8v. It will be noticed that none of Furneaux's officers appeared to suspect the existence of a strait where they now were—which is curious: they all thought in terms of one farther south. Burney's journal for this date runs, '. . . at 6 Saw the Land we Set Last Night bearing wbs¾s 10 or 11 Leagues. All the Land we have coasted Since Yesterday noon from Cape Barren are a parcel of uninhabited Islands—Coast Dangerous—we now Steerd NW. at 8 finding we Shoald our water very fast as we stood in this direction & no Land being in Sight we hauld off & Stood for New Zealand—at 9 Saw Land from the Mast head bearing NNW 12 or 14 Leagues—this I take to be the South part of New Holland—for it appears very likely to me, that there is a passage between that & Vandiemen's Land at the Back of Cape Barren.'—Wilby strikes a different note: 'From the Mast head we Saw Land bear^g^ about NNW But our Soundings greatly Decrease'd and thick Foggy W^r^ come^g^ on and in all Probability should have it Blow^g^ We were Induce'd to Bear away for our Rendevous at New Zeal^d^ Every one being of Hopes to meet with our Concort, and Spending a Few Months in Ease & Quiteness, After Beat^g^ the Seas For 4 Months without Intermission.' Evidently the ship's company were all looking forward to a pleasant time doing nothing in winter quarters.

SATURDAY 20*th. Winds S E^t erly. Course S* 87°00′ *E. Dist.* 79 *Miles. Lat. in* 39°24′ *S.* Fresh gales, & cloudy wea^r with a SE swell, at 2 pm out 2nd Reef of the Maintopsail, at 6 close reef'd the Topsails, at 5 am out 3rd reefs, at ½ past 6 out 2 reefs.

SUNDAY 21*st. Winds S, SBE, SE. Course N* 87°00′ *E. Dist.* 72 *Miles. Lat. in* 39°20′ *S.* Moderate gales & fair with a great Swell from the SE. PM Variation p^r Azimuth 7°50′ E. at 7 took in the two Reefs in the Topsails, am let them Out.

MONDAY 22*nd. Winds SBE, SBW, South. Course S* 79°00′ *E. Dist.* 62 *Miles. Lat. in* 39°32′ *S.* First & Middle parts moderate breezes & cloudy, with a swell from the SE. latter p^t hard Gales, with rain & severe squalls, at 6 PM in 1st reef of the topsails, Variation p^r Amp^d 7°30′ E. AM Variation 6°00′ E. at 11 handed the fore & Mizen Topsails, got down Top Gall^t Yards & close reef'd the Maintopsails.

TUESDAY 23*rd. Winds S, SBW, SBE. Course N* 73°00′ *E. Dist.* 72 *Miles. Lat. in* 39°11′ *S.* First & Middle parts, strong gales & squally with rain, thunder & lightening; at 2 set the maintopsail & foretopsail, at 8 handed them.[1]

WEDNESDAY 24*th. Winds South, SBE, South. Course N* 79°00′ *E. Dist.* 62 *Miles. Lat. in* 39°00′ *S.* First & Middle parts Strong gales and squally wea^r with a heavy sea from the S.ward, latter part more moderate, at 1 PM shipt a Sea which stove the large Cutter and washed the Small Cutter out of her to the waist, at 5 double Reef'd the Mainsail and set it. AM swayed ye Main Yards up and let out the Reefs, at noon set the Topsails.

THURSDAY 25*th. Winds S, SBE, SBW. Course S* 75°00′ *E. Dist.* 93 *Miles. Lat. in* 39°24′ *S.* First & Middle part fresh gales & Cloudy with a Swell from the SE, latter part fresh breezes & Cloudy, AM Variation 10°10′ E.

FRIDAY 26*th. Winds SSW, S, SSW. Course S* 67°00′ *E. Dist.* 107 *Miles. Lat. in* 40°06′ *S.* Moderate breezes & fair wea^r. PM Variation p^r azimuth 10°56′ E, AM variation p^r Azimuth 11°04′ E.

SATURDAY 27*th. Winds SSW, SBE, SW. Course S* 80°00′ *E. Dist.* 66

[1] 'The morning was remarkably serene & fine, but about 10 AM it began to blow at South with thick rain & we soon had a Mountaneous sea—which lasted all day, & in the evening the Gale increased accompanied with Thunder, Lightning & Rain which lasted most part of the night & the violent agitation of the Sea made the water look like flashes of liquid fire, so that it is almost impossible for the Immagination to paint such an Awfull tremendous Sean.'—Bayly.

Miles. Lat. in 40°17′ *S.* Moderate breezes & fair weather; Set the Rigging up.

SUNDAY 28*th. Winds SW, Calm. Course S* 85°00′ *E. Dist.* 21 *Miles. Lat. in* 40°19′ *S.* Light breezes & fair: PM variation p^r^ Azimuth 10°30′ E.[1] AM hoisted out the Cutter & tryed the Current, found a Small drift to ye SW. Variation 11°45′ E. hoisted in the cutter.

MONDAY 29*th. Winds N.erly. Course S* 70°00′ *E. Dist.* 62 *Miles. Lat. in* 40°40′ *S.* Light breezes & fair wea^r^. AM variation p. Azimuth 12°40′ E.

TUESDAY 30*th. Winds N.Et.erly. Course S* 72°00′ *E. Dist.* 102 *Miles. Lat. in* 41°11′ *S.* Fresh breezes & fair wea^r^. PM variation p^r^ Az^th^ 11°56′ E and AM 11°20′ E.

WEDNESDAY 31*st. Winds Nerly. Course S* 75°00′ *E. Dist.* 91 *Miles. Lat. in* 41°36′ *S.* Fresh breezes & Cloudy weather.

[APRIL 1773]

THURSDAY 1*st. Winds N, NNW, NWBN. Course N* 86°30′ *E. Dist.* 80 *Miles. Lat. in* 41°30′ *S.* First & Middle part, fresh breezes & Cloudy wea^r^, latter part squally wth hard rain.

FRIDAY 2*nd. Winds NNW, NBW. Course N* 79°00′ *E. Dist.* 77 *Miles. Lat. in* 41°12′ *S.* Fresh Gales & Squally with hard rain in the latter part.

SATURDAY 3*rd. Winds N, ENE, SSE. Course N* 62°00′ *E. Dist.* 68 *Miles. Lat. in* 40°40′ *S.* First & latter parts, fresh breezes with rain, Middle part squally with hard rain, at ½ past 4 PM shorten'd sail, a very heavy swell from the N.ward, at 6 saw the Land bearing EBN dist. about 5 Leagues, made sail a longshore. At 8 the Eastermost land NEBE½E. at noon Cape Farewell EBN½N and Rocks point, SBE½E 5 Leagues, Offshore 3 or 4 leagues.

[1] For this night, Bayly, who seems always to have been at the centre of melodrama, reports another adventure that at its face value casts a lurid light on the senior officers of the ship. 'After I was in bed, Mr Kempe the 1st Lieu^t^, & Mr Burney 2^d^ Lieu^t^, Mr Andrews the Surgeon, & Mr Hawkey Midshipman, these All came to my door & Asked me to give them Brandy which I refused to do, thinking they already had enough, it being between 12 & 1 OClock at Night, I therefore beged them to go to bed, but they procured a hammer & chissel & began ripping the Hinges of my door. I then put my clothes on & went out of my Cabbin, the first I met was Mr Burney whome I took by the coller & put down on the Arm-chest. They all came on me & I was forced out of the steerage where this happened & felt several blows on my Head, & the Surgeon thretened to strike me with the Hammer which he had in his hand, but the Capt coming put an end to the scuffle.' One imagines that there was a good deal of concealed laughter about all this, whatever the gentlemen's consumption of brandy had been.

SUNDAY 4*th. Winds SSW, SW, SBW. Lat. in* 40°14′ *S.* First & latter parts, moderate & fair weather, middle part fresh Gales & fair. PM standing along Shore, at 8 PM entered the Streights, at $\frac{1}{2}$ past 11 bro^{t} too Sounded 48 fa^{m} with sand, mud, & broken Shells, at 4 AM made sail, at 5 out all reefes, at $\frac{1}{2}$ p^{t} 5, Mount Egmont bore NNE and point Stephen SE$\frac{1}{2}$E 6 or 7 Leagues, at 8 Mount Egmont bore NBE$\frac{1}{2}$E 10 or 11 Leag^{s} and the West part of Blind bay SBW$\frac{1}{4}$W about 5 Leagues distance, at noon Stephen's Island SE 5 Leagues and Mount Egmont NBE 12 Leagues.

MONDAY 5*th. Winds WNW, NW, Et.erly.* Moderate breezes & fair wea^{r}. at 4 PM Stephens's Island SE$\frac{1}{2}$S. Mount Egmont NBE and the west end of Blind bay SSW$\frac{1}{2}$W. at 12 Stephens's Island SBE$\frac{1}{2}$E. at 3 AM bro^{t} too & sounded but found no ground at 75 fa^{ms}, Stephens's Island then bearing SWBW about 4 Leagues distant, at 5 wore Ship and made sail, at $\frac{1}{2}$ past 7 taken aback, filled the other way, at noon Point Jackson ESE$\frac{1}{2}$S 3 Leagues & Stephens's Island NW$\frac{1}{2}$N, off shore 4 or 5 miles, had from 32 to 40 fathoms and then to 32 again, when we Tacked & stood off.[1]

TUESDAY 6*th. Winds East, SSE, SW.* Light breeze and fair wea^{r}, at 1 pm Tack'd, at $\frac{1}{2}$ past 2 found the tide set strong to the Westward, anchored in 39 fathoms, muddy ground, Point Jackson bore SE$\frac{1}{2}$E 3 Leagues, the East part of an Inlet SWBW$\frac{1}{2}$W about 4 Leagues to the Westward of Jacksons Point, at 8 found the tide slack: weighed and made sail, at 10 Sounded, no ground at 60 fa^{ms} at 12 no ground at 70 fa^{ms}. Point Jackson SSE distant 2 Leagues, at 8 am Cape *Koamaroo* SEBS & point Jackson WNW$\frac{1}{4}$W at $\frac{1}{2}$ past 10 found the Tide set strong on Some Rocks, about $\frac{1}{3}$ over the Sound from the East side, we then came too in 38 f^{ms} nigh them, Point Jackson then bearing NE$\frac{1}{2}$N the Northermost of the two brothers EBS & the middle of entry Island NE.

WEDNESDAY 7*th. Winds Variable.* First & latter part, fresh breezes and fair, middle Calm. at 2 pm weighed and stood in for Queen Charlottes Sound,[2] at 5 anchor'd in Ship Cove, with the Best Bower

[1] '. . . the land hereabouts is full of deep Bays & Openings—it is not unlikely that all the Land hereabouts are seperate Islands and that there is a Communication at the Back, between them & the main Land from Blind Bay all the Way to Charlotte Sound.'—Burney log.

[2] 'In coming in to Charlotte sound we saild over a Barr on which is at least 7 & 8 fms water and 18 fms both without and within the Barr we had regular sounding's afterward's all the way into the Anchoring place. We came the South Passage in, But the North is Equally good and safe, not less than 7 & 8 fms all the way through, tho' Capt Cook d[o]es not mention a word of the North Passage, neither did he sail in or out that way.'—Kemp. By the North Passage he no doubt means the passage on the north-western side of Motuara.

in 10 fa[ms]. AM hoisted out the Launch and moored ship the best bower to the Northward.[1]

THURSDAY 8*th*. *Winds NNW, SBE.* Little wind & fair, PM unbent the Sails, sent the launch for a turn of water. AM employ'd on an Island a shore in Clearing a place for our Tents.[2]

FRIDAY 9*th*. *Winds N, NNW, SSE.* Little wind and fair. PM Erected the Tent, AM got down the Top Gall[t] masts and lowered down the lower Yards. Sent on shore some empty Water Casks, several canoes came alongside and traded with us.[3]

SATURDAY 10*th*. *Winds SBE, NW, NNW.* PM Sent on Shore to the Tent our 2nd Lieutenant, a Midshipman and seven men & some

[1] 'Serv'd the Ships Company an Extra ½ Allowance of Brandy'.—Furneaux log.—'... found several very convenient Watering places with Excellent Water, & one where we judge Capt[n] Cook water'd in the Endeavour—the Names of several of his People being cut on the Trees—but no Signs of the Resolution'.—Burney log.

[2] 'On the top of the Island was a post erected by the Endeavour's people with her name and time of Departure on it.'—Add. MS 27890, f. 9v. See I, pp. 242–3. It appears that Furneaux carried out all his shore activities from this time to 27 April on Motuara, and not at Ship Cove. Bayly was settled with his instruments on the islet joined to Motuara at low water, which had been known on the first voyage as Hippa island, from the Maori pa built on it, and was now called merely 'the Hippa'; and the old Maori houses proved very comfortable to live in, when the floor was sunk an extra foot.—Add. MS 27890, f. 12. Bayly, 17 April, described the place in his journal: 'I went on Shore on a small Island called the Hippa by the Natives which I named Observatory Island, it is a rock whose sides are perpendicular in many places, & indeed the whole was well fortified by nature there being only one landing place, & the passage up from it exceeding difficult, but by hard labour I made steps in the rocks so that its ascent was much easier than before—on the top of this small Island was a Town consisting of 33 houses, the most elevated part was tolerably level for about 100 Yards long & 8 or 10 Yards wide; this was fortified with strong posts or sticks drove into the ground, & those interwoven with long sticks in a horizontal direction, & then filled with small brush wood with one place two feet square where was a wooden dore, so that only one man could get in at a time & that on his hands & knees & of course easy destroy'd if at war'.—p. 66.

[3] 'At 11, Came alongside two Canoes wth 16 Indians in them & gave us a great quantity of fish for nails & whatever we offered them; In one of the Canoes found the Head & neck of an Indian, which we suppose they had lately murdered, as they took great pains to conceal it from us, for, on our discovering it, the man in whose possession it was, appeared greatly terrified & trembled from Head to foot, but on our taking no further notice of it, they parted from us seemingly well pleased with the things we had given them; they frequently mention'd the name of Tobia, which we suppos'd was enquiring after him, but co[d] not make them sensible of his Death'.—Furneaux log. Cf. Burney log, which says the canoes, a single and a double one, ventured alongside after making a long speech, and goes on, 'they were much pleasd with the presents we made them, till by chance one of our gentlemen saw a human Head in the canoe, on our discovering this they all got out of the Ship & although we tried to get a second Sight of it, we could not without using force which we did not chuse to do. however they were so offended with our having seen it that they immediately went away'. Another version is Constable, who misplaces the date to 12 April: 'Came a Longside Several Canoes & Trade with us [we found?] the Inhabbitance to be Poor Creators by Ingeeness Discover'd one of the People to have a mans head Veery fresh, we attempted to take it from [him] but thought it would Make a confusion and Disturbance a mong them.'

Marines, Employ'd variously on board, several Canoes came alongside & traded with us.[1]

SUNDAY 11*th. Winds SBW to NW.* First & middle parts, light breezes and fair, latter fresh gales and cloudy. PM employ'd in clearing the Fish Room. AM received a launch load of water.

MONDAY 12*th. Winds SBE, West, NNW.* First part fresh gales and cloudy. Middle and latter, light airs and fair wea^{r}. AM Employed about the Hold, several canoes with about 120 of the Indians came a long side and trucked with us.

TUESDAY 13*th. Winds NNW to South.* Ditto weather. Employed about the hold, the Indians came alongside as usual.

WEDNESDAY 14*th. Winds Variable.* Ditto weather, Employed about the Hold and Rigging.

THURSDAY 15*th. Winds So.erly.* First part, moderate & cloudy, Middle & latter fresh breezes, employed as yesterday. Punished David Lewis for Theft.

FRIDAY 16*th. Winds So.erly.* Fresh breezes and cloudy, AM cleared Hawser.

SATURDAY 17*th. Winds SSE.* Fresh Gales and squally wea^{r}. Employ'd occasionally.

SUNDAY 18*th. Winds SSE.* First part fresh breezes and cloudy, Middle & latter Strong Gales and Squally, employed variously.

MONDAY 19*th. Winds S, SSW.* Fresh Gales and cloudy. Carpenters employ'd in Shifting a Plank on the Larboard side, and caulking between decks.

TUESDAY 20*th. Winds SSW.* Ditto weather, Carpenters employ'd as yesterday.

WEDNESDAY 21*st. Winds SWBS.* Moderate & fair, employed occasionally. Caulkers in caulking, sent the Cutter up the Sound.

THURSDAY 22*nd. Winds So.erly.* First part moderate & cloudy, middle & latter small rain, came alongside 3 Canoes, & Trucked with us for Fish, Our Cutter Returned, she had been 9 leagues up

[1] Five canoes and about fifty Indians, says Kemp: 'They Traded with us as Yesterday (but like Georges Island People) they Esteem Nails of more Value than anything else we cou'd offer them. A Looking Glass which I gave them yesterday they shew'd me was broke and wanted me to give them a large Nail in exchange for the Frame which remain'd perfect except the Glass that being entirely gone'.

the Sound, found very deep water all the way, the River[1] running to the WSW.

FRIDAY 23rd. *Winds South.* Strong gales and squally with rain, Caulkers employed between Decks.

SATURDAY 24th. *Winds SBW.* First part fresh Gales & cloudy. Middle & latter, moderate & fair. Caulkers employ'd as yesterday.

SUNDAY 25th. *Winds SBW to SSE.* Light air & fair, AM weighed our Anchor, and warped further in the Cove. Three Canoes came to our tent and truck't with the people.

MONDAY 26th. *Winds So.erly.* Ditto weather, employed in warping the Ship, at 4 anchored with y[e] best bower in 11 fathoms, and moored with a Cable and a half to the Southward the Small bower to the Northward, and Coasting Anchor towards the watering Place.

TUESDAY 27th. *Winds NW to SSE.* First & middle parts light airs & fair, Latter fresh gales, PM employed in clearing a place for our Tent near the watering place and in transporting the empty Casks from the Island.

WEDNESDAY 28th. *Winds SSW, West, NNW.* Light airs and fair, PM sent on Shore all our Spars, Sloops masts, Yards, &c[a]. AM bro[t] over the Tent from the Island to the watering place, one Canoe came alongside and truck'd with fish.

THURSDAY 29th. *Winds Variable.* First & latter parts light breezes and fair, middle fresh gales with Showers, Caulkers employed between Decks.

FRIDAY 30th. *Winds So.erly.* First & Middle parts light airs & fair, latter fresh Gales and cloudy, three Canoes came alongside & trucked with us.

[MAY 1773]

SATURDAY 1st. *Winds S, W, NW.* First part fresh gales and cloudy, Middle & latter light airs & fair, PM rec'd a turn of water, three Canoes came alongside.

SUNDAY 2nd. *Winds Variable.* Moderate & fair, Cleared hawser, employ'd caulking between Decks.

MONDAY 3rd. *Winds Variable.* First & middle parts D[o] wea[r], latter light airs with small rain.

[1] There is no river. This may be a slip on Furneaux's part, or he may have assumed that a river entered the bottom of the sound.

TUESDAY 4*th. Winds No.erly.* Fresh breezes and fair. Employ'd occasionally.

WEDNESDAY 5*th. Winds Variable.* Moderate & Cloudy with showers of rain. Employ'd in the Hold.

THURSDAY 6*th. Winds So.erly.* Fresh breezes and fair. Employ'd as yesterday.

FRIDAY 7*th. Winds Variable.* Fresh breezes and fair.

SATURDAY 8*th. Winds Wt.erly.* Moderate & fair, the Carpenters employed repairing the Boats.

SUNDAY 9*th. Winds NW.* D^o^ wea^r^. Employed in the Hold.

MONDAY 10*th. Winds SE.erly.* D^o^ wea^r^. Employed in the Hold. Carpenters on the Boats.

TUESDAY 11*th. Winds Wt.erly, So.erly.* First part cloudy with showers of rain, middle & latter fair. PM at ¼ past 5 Our people on shore felt the Shock of an Earthquake.[1]

WEDNESDAY 12*th. Winds Variable.* Moderate & fair, Employ'd overhauling the rigging.

THURSDAY 13*th. Winds Wt.erly.* Ditto weather. Employ'd occasionally, Came alongside two Canoes.

FRIDAY 14*th. Winds Variable.* Little wind and fair weather.

SATURDAY 15*th. Winds No.erly.* Moderate breezes and cloudy. PM Employ'd scrubbing between wind and water.[2]

SUNDAY 16*th. Winds NW.* First part moderate, middle & latter Squally with hard rain.

MONDAY 17*th. Winds NW, Et.erly, So.erly.* First part Squally, middle and latter moderate weather with showers of rain.

TUESDAY 18*th. Winds So.erly.* Light breezes and fair wea^r^. AM saw a sail in the offing. Sent our boat out.[3]

[1] 'PM ab^t^ 5, the people at the Tent felt two severe shocks of an Earthquake'.—Furneaux log.

[2] 'We now begin to dispair of seeing the Resolution which we expected before this time to have join'd us here'.—Kemp.

[3] '. . . this morning about Sunrise we were alarmed by 2 musquetoons being fired at the Astronomers Tent on the Hippa which we soon found to the great joy & satisfaction of every body was meant as a Signal for the Resolution—at ½ past 10 Mr Kemp went out to her with fish and Sallad from the Garden in the Small Cutter. Every thing we Set in the garden is in a fair way—nothing has faild.'—Burney log.

WEDNESDAY 19*th. Winds Variable.* Ditto wea^r^. PM got on board a Launch load of water. AM came in & anchor'd here His Majesty's Sloop Resolution.[1]

Now I have had the perusal of Captain Furneaux's Journal it is necessary to mention before I proceed with our transactions in this place, such general remarks as hath occur'd to me and not before taken notice of. My reason for quiting the high Latitudes in the latter end of January and Steering to the North was to search for the land said to have been lately descovered by the French; what am I now to think of that land? I cannot suppose as some doth that the whole is a fiction, no, if I had had no such information the several Signs of land we met with in that neighbourhood would have induced me to believe that there is land, the small divers which we saw there, which Captain Furnea[u]x calls Dip Chicks, we have no where else met with but on the Coast of New Zealand, these therefore must be looked upon as signs of the Vicinity of land without paying any regard to Penguins and Seals which are every where to be found, it is nevertheless certain that it can only be an Island and one of very small extent unless it lies to the West of the Longitude of 57°; there indeed is room for a pretty large land as will more fully appear by the Chart. If the French have realy made the descovery they will no doubt make it Publick and then this point will be cleared up, it was not my business to spend[2] much time in search of an Island I was not sure existed, the discovery of a Southern Continent is the object I have in view, besides at that time it was just as probable that I should meet with it to the East or South as any other way; I shall now drop this subject and follow Captain Furneaux to Van Diemens Land in which rout he seems to have met with nothing remarkable, one remark however hath occur'd to me which I shall not omit to mention as it appears intresting to Seamen. In this rout he seems to have had a constant sucession of Strong Westerly Winds, varying a few points to the North or South nor does it appear that he had one hours Calm in this whole run the greatest part of which was made between the Parallels of 51° & 53°, whereas 8 or 10° degrees farther South we not only had frequent Calms for many hours together but much easterly and variable Winds, seldom remaining in the same quarter twenty four hours together; in general I have observed that to the Southward of 58° or 60° the Easterly Winds prevail, at least they blow as often as any

[1] 'PM Saluted the Resolution with a 11 Guns which She Returnd whose Meet^s^ gave a general Joy to the whole Ships Comp^y^'.—Wilby.

[2] *it was . . . spend:* it would not have been prudent in me to have spent . . .—f. 67v.

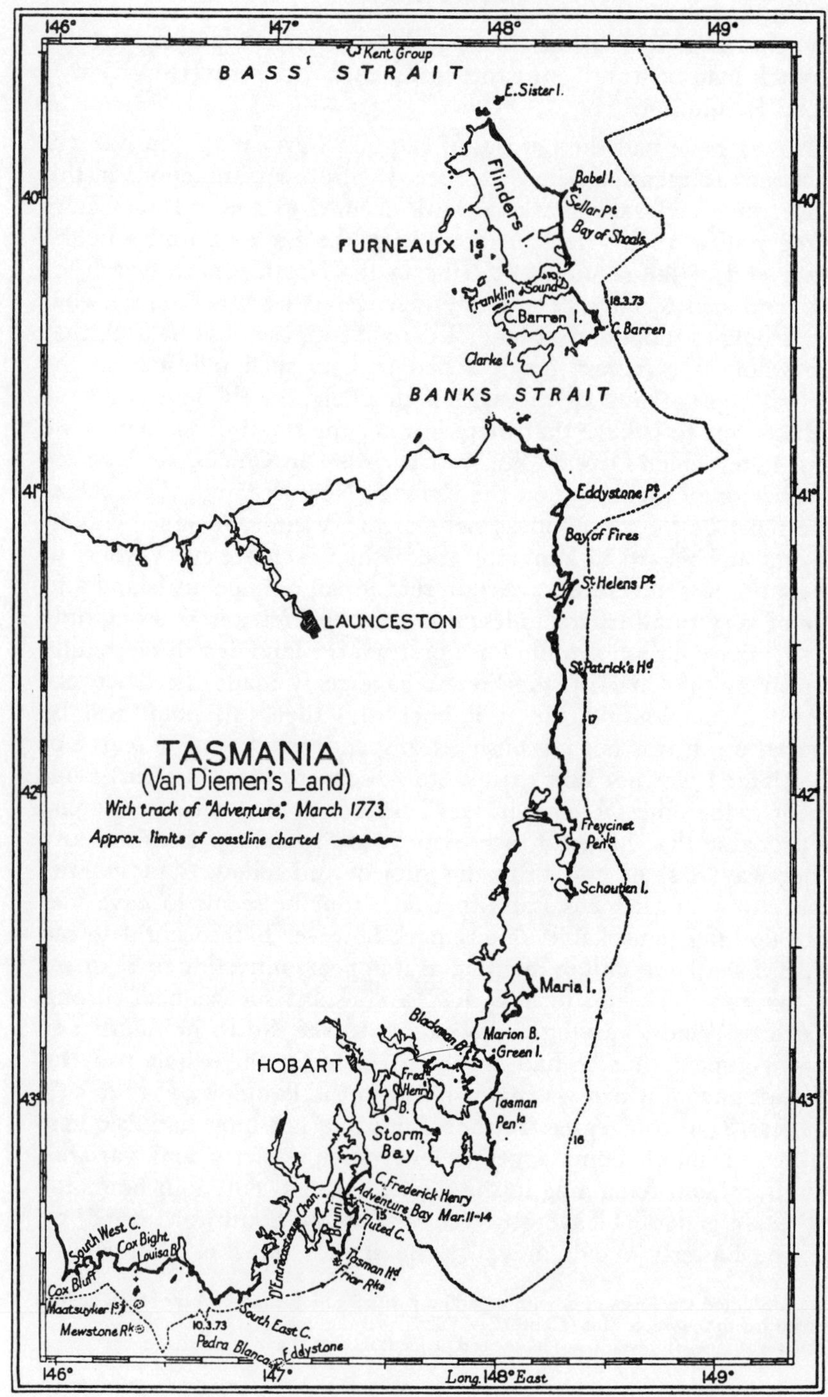

146°
147°
148°
149°
Kent Group
BASS STRAIT
E. Sister I.
Flinders I.
Babel I.
Sellar Pt.
Bay of Shoals
FURNEAUX Is.
Franklin Sound
18.3.73
C. Barren I.
C. Barren
Clarke I.
BANKS STRAIT
40°
41°
42°
43°
Eddystone Pt.
Bay of Fires
St. Helens Pt.
LAUNCESTON
St. Patrick's Hd.
17
TASMANIA
(Van Diemen's Land)
With track of "Adventure," March 1773.
Approx. limits of coastline charted
Freycinet Pen.
Schouten I.
Maria I.
Blackman B.
Marion B.
Green I.
HOBART
Fred. Henry B.
Tasman Pen.
Storm Bay
16
C. Frederick Henry
Adventure Bay Mar. 11-14
15
Fluted C.
Bruni
D'Entrecasteaux Chan.
South West C.
Cox Bight
Louisa B.
Cox Bluff
Tasman Hd.
Friar Rks.
Maatsuyker Is.
Mewstone Rk.
10.3.73
South East C.
Pedra Blanca
Eddystone
146°
147°
Long. 148° East
149°

FIG. 31

other, whereas to the North of 58° down to 40°, 35° or 30° the Westerly winds prevail, this is to be understood of the great Ocean for where Lands intervene this may not hold good. I shall conclude these remarks with a few observations on Van Diemans land founded on the account Captain Furneaux has given me of it and the map he hath made of the Coast[1] by which it appears that the most Southern point of that land call'd by him S W Cape lies in the Latitude of 43°38′ S, Longitude 145°56′ E[2] of Greenwich, the country about it is barren and of a moderate and unequal height, this point appears to be the same as Tasmans named South Cape for on the one side the coast trends NW and on the other East a little Southerly to the Longitude of 147°00′ E or to the S E Cape; between these two Capes lie several small Islands, the Southermost of which is call'd the Mewstone from its similarity to the Rock or Islet of the same name in Plymouth Sound, it lies in the Latitude of 43°44′ S and five Leagues & a half to the East of the S W or South Cape: this Island together [with] Swilly Island, which is much larger, and lies SEBS ten Leagues from the S E Cape, appears to me to be sufficient guide to distinguish these two Capes the one from the other. From the S E Cape the Coast turns more to the north to Tasmans head or the Fryars[3] which are Rocks lying off it, in the Latitude of 43°30′, Longitude 147°27′, on the West side of this head lies an Island pretty near the Shore which between the Cape and the head forms a Bay call'd Storm Bay. The land is here covered with Wood. FromTasmans Head the Coast trends NNE and North to Adventure Bay which lies in the Latitude of 43°20′.[4] This Bay is sheltered from most Winds and affords good anchorage in [11] fathom water, fresh Water

[1] *I shall . . . Coast:* In order to convey a better Idea of the Coast of Van Diemens Land than I could collect from Captain Furneaux's Journal, I have added the following observations of my own, founded on the Chart he hath drawn of the Coast. . . .

[2] 43°38′ S, Longitude 145°56′ E: 43°48′ S, Longitude 145°55′ E. Furneaux was a good deal out in his latitude; his longitude is much better. The position is lat. 43°05′, long. 146°03′.

[3] Called the Friars, it seems, because they were black.

[4] B leaves a space, unfilled, for the longitude. Furneaux, Add. MS 27890, f. 6v, gives it as 147°34′ E, from 'a good observation of the Star Antares and the Moon' on a fine clear evening.—At this point it is worth while to comment on Cook's comments on Furneaux, with whose information no doubt he did the best he could; and on Furneaux's interpretation of Tasman. Cook seems to have persuaded Furneaux that his South West Cape was Tasman's South Cape—'a point much like the Ram head off Plymouth, which I take to be the same Tasman calls South Cape' (Add. MS 27890, f. 5v); but they kept the name S.W. Cape on their charts. It was however Furneaux's South East Cape that was Tasman's South Cape. Swilly island (Tasman's Pedra Brancka) is drawn but not named on Chart XXVII, named Swilly Isles on pl. VIII in the *Voyage*, I. There is no island on the west side of Tasman's Head; what was taken for an island is a peninsula projected from Bruni Island, of which Tasman's Head is the southernmost point. The opening between S.E. Cape and Tasman's Head was, as we have seen, wrongly identified by Furneaux as Tasman's Storm Bay, and Cook adopted this. But it is in reality the wide entrance to D'Entrecasteaux Channel, between Bruni Island and the main. With this wrong, other

& Wood for fual. To the Northward of Adventure Bay in about the Latitude of 43°10′ is the Bay of Fredrick Henry where Tasman Anchored, before this Bay in the Longitude of 148° lies Maria's Isles,[1] extending nearly North and South from the Latitude of 43°16′ to 42°39′, North of these lies Schoutens Isles[2] which are 4 in Number extending from 42°23′ to 42°4′: as Captain Furneaux's Track after leaving Adventure Bay was without or to the Eastward of all these Islands he saw hardly any part of the Main untill he came to the Latitude of 42°, or to the Nothermost of Schoutens Isles which lies near the Main, from this place the direction of the coast is nearly North down to 40°50′, here the night and stormy weather obliged him to haul off the land which he got in with again the next day in the Latitude of 40°30′ and coasted along Shore to the Latitude of 39°46′ and the next day being [the 19th] of March he queted the Coast and hauld up for New Zealand; this last land he rainged along are[3] four Islands (Furneaux Islands)[4] and he supposes that there is a Strait or Passage behind them, this supposision implies a doubt of this land being Islands.[5] When they haul'd up for New Zealand they were in the Latitude of 39°20′ at that time they saw land from the mast head bearing NNW distant by estimation 12 Leagues[6] and is

errors follow, logically enough. Adventure Bay, still known by that name, was Tasman's Storm Bay. In due course the name Storm Bay was taken from where Furneaux wrongly put it, but applied, equally wrongly, to the large bay between Bruni Island and the Tasman Peninsula, at one head of which lies the capital city of Hobart—i.e. the bay of which Adventure Bay, close to its opening on the west, forms a part.

[1] Further error. Tasman's Frederick Henry Bay does not lie north of Adventure Bay, but north-east; and 'Maria's Isles' do not lie 'before' but 'behind' it. That is, it is *outside* the Tasman peninsula. Tasman was blown out of the present Storm Bay, and making again for the land, anchored off Green Island, in front of Marion Bay, and four miles south-east of the present Blackman's Bay, where his men landed. This latter was his Frederick Henry Bay. The engraved chart, pl. VIII, goes, quite illegitimately, much farther than Chart XXVII, in actually drawing, with a line as firm as anywhere else, the 'B. of Frederick Henry' and the coast north of it, where Burney leaves a blank.

[2] i.e. the Freycinet Peninsula with Schouten Island off it.

[3] *are:* Captain Furneaux has laid down in his Chart as . . .—f. 68v.

[4] Chart XXVII shows what may be three islands (apart from offshore islets), with the legend 'Barren & Uninhabited Islands', rather different from the elaborate shapes of the four 'Furneaux's Isles' of the engraved chart. This, with other details of the latter, raises considerable doubts of Burney's chart being its original.

[5] I do not follow this reasoning, or feel precisely certain what Cook means. Furneaux does not suppose anywhere on paper that there is a strait or passage behind these islands, but it would be a natural thing to suppose, whether on paper or in conversation. Cook goes on to the argument (so far as I can see) that it is therefore doubtful whether 'this land' (Van Diemen's Land) is islands—i.e. the Furneaux Islands must lie off a mainland. But as Van Diemen's Land might nevertheless be a single island, we are not much farther on our principal quest.

[6] I have suggested above (p. 153, n. 4) that Furneaux saw the Kent islands, but Cook now says (what Furneaux does not) that this land bore NNW—which would make it part of the Australian coast, probably the mountainous Gippsland country. We must assume then that the land to which Furneaux refers was not *in* lat. 39°, but sighted *from* lat. 39°—and thus reconcile Furneaux with Burney, Wilby and Cook.

distant from Point Hicks, the most Southern part of my discovery, 17 or 18 Leagues and about the same distance or some thing more from the nothern point of Furneaux's Islands; it is therefore highly probable that the whole is one continued land and that Van Diemens land is a part of New Holland, the Similarity of the Countrys, Soil Produce Inhabitents &c[a] all serve to increase the probabillity.[1] The direction of the Coast from the Southermost of Maria's Islands down to the Northermost land is nearly North[2] and lies under the Meridian of 148°06′ East. Captain Furneaux had no intercourse with the Natives, nor did he I beleive see any, but he saw many of their fires and some of their hutts, the same Custom of burning the Country prevails here as in *New South Wales*, upon the whole, by what I can learn, the account I have given of the Southern parts of this last Country in my former Voyage will convey a very good Idea of Van Diemens land, which I have now done with and shall return to our transactions in Queen Charlottes Sound.

WEDNESDAY 19*th*. I have some were in this Journal mentioned a desire I had of Viseting Vandeimens land in order to inform my self whether or no it made a part of New Holland, but sence Captain Furneaux hath in a great degree cleared up this point I have given up all thoughts of going thither, but that I might not Idle away the whole Winter in Port I proposed to Captain Furneaux to spend that time in exploring the unknown parts of the Sea to the East and North, acquainting him at the same time with the rout I intended to take and the time I meant to spend in this cruze. To this propossition he readily agreed; and in concequence thereof I disired him to get his Sloop ready for sea as soon as possible[3] for at this time she was striped.[4] Knowing that sellery and Scurvey grass and other vegetables were to be found in this Sound and that when boiled with Wheat or Pease and Portable Soupe makes a very nourishing and wholesom Diet which is extreemly beneficial both in cureing and preventing the Scurvey, I went my self at day light in the Morn in search of some and returned by breakfast with a boat load and having satisfied my self that enough was to be [got] I gave orders that it should be

[1] Here again it is rather difficult to follow Cook's reasoning, apart from the passage on 'Similarity': the geographical inference does not at all seem a necessary one. No doubt he was a good deal influenced by Furneaux's opinion.

[2] *North:* North and South as will appear by the annexed Chart

[3] *I had given . . . possible:* I could have no business there and therefore came to a resolution to continue our researches to the East between the Latitudes of 41° and 46° and acquainted Captain Furneaux therewith and ordered him to get his Sloop in readiness to put to Sea as soon as possible.—f. 69.

[4] . . . from a supposision that I should remain here the Winter.

boild with Wheat or Oatmeal and Portable Soup for the Crew of both Sloops every morning for breakfast and also with Pease[1] every day for dinner and I took care that this order was punctualy complied with at least in my sloop.

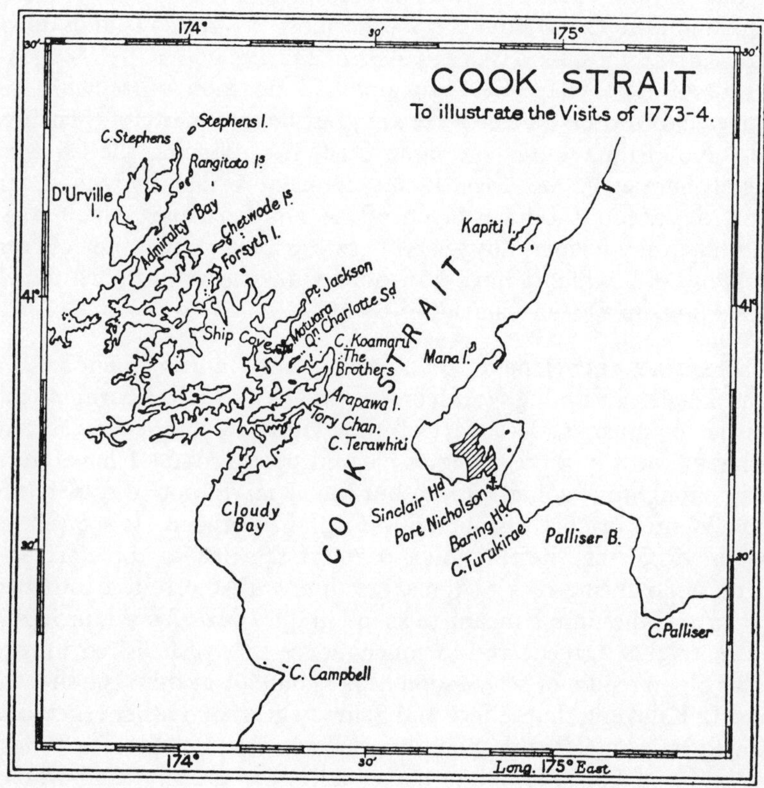

FIG. 32

THURSDAY 20*th*. This morning I put ashore at the Watering place near the Adventure 's Tent, a Ewe and a Ram (the only two remaining of those I brought from the Cape of Good Hope) untill I found a proper place to put them a shore for good for my intention was to leave them in this Country, at the same time I visited the different Gardens Captain Furnea[u]x and his officers had planted with garden seeds roots &c[a] all of which were in flourishing condi-

[1] ... and broth

tion and if improved or taken care of by the natives might prove of great use to them.[1]

FRIDAY 21*st.* My self with a party of men employed digging up ground on Long Island, which we planted with several sorts of garden seeds and return'd on board in the evening with a quantity of selery and scurvy grass.[2] Some hands a shore cuting Wood & filling Water.

SATURDAY 22*nd.* Some hands employed Wooding and Watering,[3] Lieut[t] Pickersgill with the Cutter collecting Selery and Scurvy grass, M[r] Forster and his party Botanizing, and my self accomp[d] by Captain Furneaux out in the Pinnace a Shooting.

SUNDAY 23*rd.* Last Night the Ewe and Ram I had with so much care and trouble brought to this place, died, we did suppose that they were poisoned by eating of some poisonous plant,[4] thus all my fine hopes of stocking this Country with a breed of Sheep were blasted in a moment. Towards noon we were visited for the first time by some of the Natives, they stayed and dined with us and it was not a little they devoured, they were dismiss'd in the evening Loaded with presents.

MONDAY 24*th.* Being a pleasent morning I sent M[r] Gilbert the Master out to Sea in the Cutter to sound about the Rock we discover'd in coming in, my self accompanied by Captain Furneaux & M[r] Forster went in the Pinnace to the West Bay on a Shooting party, in our way we met a large Canoe in which were fourteen or fifteen people, one of the first questions they asked was for Tupia the Otaheitean and they seem'd to express some concern when we told them he was dead. They all of them enquired after this man of Captain Furneaux when he first arrived: the people in this canoe seem'd as if they were going to the Ships but when we parted with them they

[1] 'AM sent what empty casks we had a shore and some hands to cut wood and wash linnen, also sent ye Launch with an Officer to look for grass for our sheep and to collect sallery & scurvy grass to boil with Wheat and pòrtable soup for the people's breakfast and in their pease for Dinner, set up the Forge to finish the repairs of our Iron Work two boats out afishing with hooks and one hauling the saine all of them return'd with success.'—Log.—'. . . at 5 the Pinnace returned with a great Quantity of Wild Selery and Scurvey grass; Its admired by every body as very wholesom Vegetables and is Exceeding Pleasent to the Palate.'—Elliott.

[2] . . . and Sow Thistles . . .—This plant was the Maori Puwha, *Sonchus oleraceus*.

[3] . . . and other necessary duties of the Ship

[4] Very likely this was the shrub Tupakihi or Tutu (*Coriaria arborea*), the New Zealand farmer's 'Tute', so often a bane to wandering cattle. It flourishes on the outskirts of the bush, and its deadly young green shoots would have been extremely attractive to Cook's unfortunate animals.

went another way. In the West Bay we had pretty good sport among the Sea Pies[1] and Shaggs and in the evening return'd a board when I lear[n]t that a Canoe from the northward or some place out of the Sound had been alongside, the people in her, who appear'd to be strangers, also enquired after Tupia,[2] Lieutenant Pickersgill away in the Launch collecting selery and Scurvy grass.

TUESDAY 25*th*. Wind at NW very stormy with rain, struck Topg[t] yards.

WEDNESDAY 26*th*. The same weather continued till the afternoon when the Wind abated & the Sky cleared up.

THURSDAY 27*th*. Employed geting on board Wood and Water, collicting Vegetables &c[a]. Drying and repairing Sails.

FRIDAY 28*th*. Employed as yesterday, Launch assisting the Adventure.[3]

SATURDAY 29*th*. This Morning several of the Natives came along side and brought with them some fish which they exchanged for Nails &c[a]. After Breakfast I took one of them over to Motuara and shew'd him the Potatoes planted there by M[r] Fannen the Master of the Adventure which he had brought from the Cape of Good Hope, there seems to be no doubt of their succeeding as they were in a very thriving state, the man was so pleased with them that he immidiately began to hough the earth about the plants, I call'd them Coumalla a root common[4] in many parts of *Eahei nomauwe* and is as I could find from this man not unknown to the Inhabitents of *Tavai-poenammoo*. I next carried him to the other of Captain Furneaux's gardens (this gentleman being with me) I explaned to him as well as I could the nature of the Turnips, Carrots & Parsnips roots together with Potatoes that will be of more use to them than all the other vegetables. I gave him a tolerable Idea of the Carrots and Parsnips by calling them Tara[5] a root to which they bear some likeness and is known to the Natives.

[1] According to Newton's *Dictionary of Birds* this is an old name for oyster catchers. 'Sea pie' was generally used in literature until in 1731 Catesby published the name of Oyster catcher for the birds common on the Carolina oyster beds exposed at low tides. But this name seems to have been an early popular term in Europe, since there are various non-English equivalents such as the Frisian *Oestervisscher* and the German *Austermann*.

[2] . . . Late in the evening M[r] Gilbert returned, having sounded all round the rock which he found to be very small and steep to . . .—f. 70.

[3] 'The Sailmakers employ'd repairing the spare Sails being a good deal damag'd by the Rats'.—Cooper.

[4] *I call'd . . . common:* I gave him a good idea of this root by calling them Coumalla a root in taste like a Potatoe and is common . . .—'Coumalla', i.e. Kumara, *Ipomoea batatas*.

[5] Taro, *Colocasia antiquorum*.

SUNDAY 30*th*. We were Viseted again by the Natives this morning who brought with them some fish to market, Two or three families having taken up their aboad near us.[1]

MONDAY 31*st*. This Day I employ'd in clearing and diging up ground on Motuara and planting it with Wheat, Pease and other Pulse Carrots Parsnips and Straw berries.

[JUNE 1773]

WEDNESDAY 2*nd*.[2] This Morning I went over to the East side of the Sound accompanied by Captain Furneaux and Mr Forster, there I put a Shore two Goats male and female, the latter was old but had two fine Kids, some time before we arrived in *Dusky Bay*, which were both kill'd by the cold as I have already mentioned, the male was something more than twelve months old: Captain Furneaux hath put a Shore in Canibals Cove a Boar and a Breeding Sow[3] so that we have reason to hope that in process of time this Country will be stocked with Goats and Hoggs; there is no great danger that the Natives will destroy them as they are exceedingly afraid of both,[4] besides as they have not the least knowlidge of them being left, they will grow so Wild before they are discovered as not to suffer any one to come near them. The Goats will undoubtedly take to the Mountains and the Hoggs to the Woods where there is plenty of food for both. In this excursion I saw the largest Seal I ever met with, it was Swiming on the Surface of the Water and suffer'd us to come near enough to fire at it but without effect for after a chase of near an hour we were obliged to give it up. By the size of this animal it is probable that it was a Sea-Lioness, it certainly very much resembled the one drawn by Lord Anson, our seeing a Sea Lion when we entred this Sound in my former Voyage increaseth the probabillity.[5] After Loading two Boats with Vegetables and Shooting some Pigeons & other Birds we return'd on board in the evening.

[1] *Two . . . us:* Two or Three families of these people now took up there aboad near us, employed themselves daily in fishing and supplyed us with the fruits of their labour the good effects of which we soon felt, for we were by no means such expert fishers as them, nor were any of our methods of fishing equal to theirs.—f. 70.

[2] Although Cook writes 'Tues. 1' in his margin, the MS has no entry for that day. BH read 'Nothing remarkable'. G passes straight from 29 May to 2 June.

[3] *a Breeding Sow:* 2 Breeding Sows

[4] A It afterwards appear'd that they soon found them and caught them too, as much as they seem'd to fear them.

[5] . . . and I am of opinion that they have their aboad on some of the Rocks which lie in the Straits or on those which lie off Admiralty Bay.—f. 70v.—It was probably *Neophoca cinerea* Péron and Lesueur, the New Zealand Sea Lion. The Anson reference is to Walter's *Voyage round the World . . . by George Anson Esq.*, popularly known as *Anson's Voyage*; London 1748 and often reprinted. Cf. I, p. 234, n. 3.

THURSDAY *3rd.* Sent the Carpenter over to the East side of the Sound to Cut spars, the Boat was chased by some of the natives in a large Canoe but with what intent is not known. Early in the morning our friends the Natives brought us off some[1] fish and we had there company at breakfast. One of them agree'd to go away with me, but he afterwards[2] was of a nother mind as were some others that offer'd to go away in the Adventure, it was even said that some of them offered their Children to sale but this certainly had no foundation in truth, the report took rise on board the Adventure where they were utter strangers to their Language and Customs: It was not uncommon for them to bring their children with them aboard and present them to us in expectation of our making them presents, this happened to me yesterday morning a Man brought his Son a boy about 10 years of age and presented him to me and as the report was then currant I thought he wanted to sell him, but at last I found out that he wanted me to give him a Shirt[3] which I accordingly did the Boy was so fond of his new dress that he went all over the Ship presenting him self to every boddy that came in his way, this liberty of the Boy offended old Will the Ram Goat who up with his head and knock'd the boy backwards on the Deck, Will would have repeated his blow had not some of the people got to the boys assistance, this missfortune however seem'd to him irrepairable, the Shirt was dirted and he was afraid to appear in the Cabbin before his father untill brought in by Mr Forster, when he told a very lamentable story against Goure[4] the great Dog, for so they call all the quadrepeds we have aboard, nor could he be pacified till his shirt was wash'd and dry'd.[5] While these people were on board a large double Canoe in which were twenty or thirty people appear'd in sight, our friends on board seem'd much alarmed telling us that the others were enimies, two of them, the one with a Spear and the other with a Stone hatchet in his hand, got upon the Arm Chists which were on the Poop and there in a kind of bravado set those enimies at difiance while the others took to their Canoes and padled ashore probably to secure the Women & Children and effects. All I could do I could not prevail on these men to call the Canoe alongside on the Contrary they seem'd displeased at my doing it,[6] at length after

[1] *some:* a large supply of

[2] . . . that is when it came to the point

[3] *a Shirt:* a white Shirt

[4] *kuri*, a dog.

[5] This story [i.e. not of 'old Will', but of Cook's mistake over the 'sale' of the boy], though extreamly trifling in its self, will show how liable we are to misstake these peoples meaning and to ascribe to them customs they never knew even in thought.—f. 71.

[6] . . . and wanted me to fire upon them; the people in the Canoe seem'd to pay very little regard to those aboard, but kept advancing slowly towards the Ship and after performing the usual ceremony put along side.

some ceremony perform'd by the people in her they put along side after which the chief was easily prevail'd upon to come aboard followed by many others and Peace was immidiately istablished on all sides indeed it did not appear to me that the people in this Canoe had any intention of making war upon their Brethren at least if they did they were sensible enough to know that this was neither time nor place for them to commit hostillities. One of the first questions these Strangers ask'd was for *Tupia*, and when I told them he was dead, one or two of them express'd their sorrow by a kind of lamentation which appear'd to me to be merely formal. A trade soon Commenced between our people and these, it was not possible to hinder the former from giving the clothes from of their backs for the merest trifles, things that were neither usefull nor curious, such was the prevailing passion for curiosities and caused me to dismiss these strangers sooner than I would have done. When they departed they went over to Moutara[1] where, by the help of our Glasses we discover'd four or five more Canoes and a number of people on the Shore, this induced me to go over in my boat accompanied by Mr Forster and one of the Officers, we were well received by the Chief and the whole tribe which consisted of between 90 & 100 people Men Women and Children, having with them Six Canoes and all their utensils which made it probable that they were come to reside in this Sound, but this is only conjector for it is very common for them when they even go but a little way to carry their whole property with them, every place being equally alike to them if it affords the necessary subsistance so that it can hardly be said that they are ever from home, thus we may easily account for the migration of those few small families we found in *Dusky Bay*. Living thus dispers'd in small parties knowing no head but the chief of the family or tribe whose authority may be very little, subjects them to many inconveniences a well regulated society united under one head or any other form of government are not subject to, these form Laws and regulations for their general security, are not alarm'd at the appearence of every stranger and if attack'd or invaded by a publick enimy have strong holds to retire to where they can with advantage defend themselves, their property & their Country, this seems to be the state of most of the Inhabitents of *Eahei-nomauwe*, whereas those of *Tavai-poenammoo*, by living a wandering life in small parties are distitute of most of these advantages which subjects them to perpetual alarms, and we generally find them upon their guard traveling and

[1] Motuara.

working as it were with their Arms in their hands even the Women are not exempted from carrying Arms as appear'd at the first interview I had with the family in *Dusky Bay* when each of the two Women were Arm'd with a Spear not less than 18 feet in length. I was lead into these reflections, by not being able to recollect the face of any one person I had seen here three years ago, nor hath it appear'd that any one of them had the least knowlidge of me or any other person with me that was here at that time, it is therefore not very improbable but[1] that the greatest part of the Inhabitants that were here in the beginning of the year 1770 are drove out of it or have on their own accord removed some were else; certain it is that not one third the people are here now that were then. Their Strong hold on the point of Moutara hath been some time deserted and we find many forsaken habetation in all parts of the Sound, however we are not wholy to infer from this that this place has been once very populous for each family may, for their own conveniency when they move from place to place, have more hutts than one or two. It may be ask'd, that if these people had never seen the Endeavour or any of her crew, how they became acquainted with the Name of Tupia or to have in their possession[2] such articles as they could only have got from that Ship, to this it may be answered that the Name of Tupia was at that time so popular among them that it would be no wonder if at this time it is known over great part of *New Zealand*, the name of Tupia may be as familiar to those who never saw him as to those who did, had a Ship of any other Nation whatever arrived here they would equally have enquired for him, by the same way of reasoning the Articles left here by the Endeavour may be now in possession of those who never saw her. I got from one of the people I am now with an Ear ornament made of glass very well form'd and polished.[3]

After spending about an hour on Motuara with these people and having distributed among them some presents and shew'd the Chief the gardens we had made, I return'd aboard and spent the remainder of our Royal Masters Birth Day in Festivity, having the company of Captain Furneaux and all his officers[4] and double allowance enabled the Seamen to share in the general joy.

Both Sloops being now ready to put to Sea I gave Captain Furneaux an account in writing of the rout I intended to take which

[1] *not very improbable but:* highly probable . . .—f. 72.

[2] . . . (which many of them had)

[3] . . . the glass they must have got from the Endeavour.

[4] '. . . all the Superior Officers of both Ships dined with Capt Cook & we spent the afternoon very cheerfully.'—Bayly. They also fired 21 guns (Log, 5 June), which may have given the Maoris general joy.

was to proceed immidiately to the East between the Latitudes of 41° and 46° untill I arrived in the Longitude of 140° or 135° West and then, providing no land was discovered,[1] to proceed to *Otaheite*, from thence to return back to this place by the Shortest rout, and after takeing in wood and Water to proceed to the South and explore all the unknown parts of the Sea betw^n^ the Meridian of New Zealand and Cape Horn and therefore in case of seperation before we reach'd Otaheite I appointed that Island for the place of Rendezvouz where he was to wait untill the 20th of Augt. Not being join'd by me before that time he was then to make the best of his way back to Queen Charlottes Sound and there remain untill the 20th of Novr after which[2] he was to put to Sea & carry into execution their Lordships Instructions. It may be thought by some an extraordinary step in me to proceed on discoveries as far South as 46° in the very depth of Winter for it must be own'd that this is a Season by no means favourable for discoveries. It nevertheless appear'd to me necessary that something must be done in it, in order to lessen the work I am upon least I should not be able to finish the discovery of the Southern part of the South Pacifick Ocean the insuing Summer, besides if I should discover any land in my rout to the East I shall be ready to begin with the Summer to explore it; seting aside all the[se] considerations I have little to fear, having two good Ships well provided and healthy crews.[3]

Mr Bayley commun[i]cated to me the Astronomical observations he had made in this place for determining its situation and other Nautical purposes: he made his observations on the SW point of *Motuara* the Latitude of which is 41°5′35″ S. Longitude 173°48′55½″ East. Variation of the Compass 13°33′ E. Dip of the South end of the needle 64°45′. High-Water at the full and change of the Moon at 9 o'Clock & the greatest rise 6½ feet perpendicular; the Latitude, Variation and Tides are confirmable enough to the like observations I made when I was here in Jan^ry^ 1770, but the Longitude differs considerably more than might be expected; in my Chart[4] I have

[1] The relevant observation of Forster (I, p. 233) is probably a just one: 'Many among our fellow-voyagers proceeded on this dangerous expedition in the firm belief that we should speedily find the coasts we went in quest of, whose novelty and valuable productions would amply reward our perseverance and fatigues. But captain Cook, and several others, judging from what had been done in the former voyage, and what they had already experienced on this, were far from expecting to discover new lands, and greatly doubted the existence of a southern continent'.

[2] . . . (if not joined by me) . . .—f. 72v.

[3] . . . where than could I have spent my time better, the least I shall do will be to point out to posterity that these Seas are to be navigated and that it is practical to go on discoveries, even in the very depth of Winter.

[4] . . . constructed at that time.

place'd [it] in 184°51′ West or 175°9′ East, deduced from observations of the ⊙ & ☽ and is 1°20′ more East than Mr. Baylies which we must allow to be nearer the truth, because deduced not only from a greater number but a variety of observations, they also corispond with Mr Wales's observations made in Dusky Bay reduced to this place by the Watches,[1] the Meridian distance in my Chart between these two places are conformable to these observations, therefore sence parts agree with parts it should seem that the whole of New Zealand is laid down too far East, but when I consider the great number of obser^{ns} I had to settle the p^{t} in question I cannot think the error so great as these two Astronomers have made it, but supposing it is it will not much effect either Geography or Navigation but for the benifit of both I thought proper to mention it though few I beleive will look upon it as a capital error.[2]

During our short stay in this Sound I have observed that this Second Visit of ours hath not mended the morals of the Natives of either Sex, the Women of this Country I always looked upon to be more chaste than the generality of Indian Women, whatever favours

[1] But in H Cook writes into the margin, 'Mr Wales does not agree with Mr Bayley in the Long. of this place.'

[2] The conflict between the longitudes deduced from Bayly's observations and from the earlier ones gave Cook much thought and led to much drafting and re-drafting. In his Log, 7 June, he merely remarks, of the 1770 results, 'errors as great as this will frequently be found in such nice observations as these, Errors I call them tho' in reality they may be None but only differences which cannot be avoided'. In A, p. 66, and B, f. 73, he has, in place of the passage in the text beginning 'deduced from observations of the ⊙ & ☽', passages fairly identical as follows: 'As it was settled by a great number of observations of the Sun and Moon, made by Mr Charles Green and others on board the Endeavour on the 16th 17th 18th 19th and 20th of Jan^{ry} 1770 and which observations differ from Mr Baylies 1°20′ being so much more east. It must however be allowed that the Longitude by Mr Bayly appears to be nearer the truth because deduced, not only from a greater number of observations but a variety & some of them such as are less liable to error than those of the Sun & Moon; they also corrispond with Mr Wales's observations made in Dusky Bay reduced to this place by the Watches. The difference of Longitude in my Chart between these two places is agreable enough to the differences of these gentlemens observations; sence therefore parts agree with parts it should seem that the whole of New Zealand is laid down too far East.' To the words in this, 'less liable to error than those of the Sun & Moon', A has a footnote: 'It has been found that this Sound lies 40′ more to the East than these Observations of Mr Baily's placeth it; if he has made no mistake, we here find that Observations for finding the Longitude, made even by Astronomers, may differ one from another 1°40′ for so much is the difference between Mr Green and Mr Baily; however I think, nay I am sure that this will very seldom happen'. But to the words 'reduced to this place by the Watches' B has a footnote, 'this subject wants revising as these points were afterwards better settled'. The revision is perhaps given in a further passage in a still further draft of B (it seems the final one), f. 75: 'At first they appeared to agree with the observations made by Mr Wales in Duskey Bay and reduced to this place by the Watch, but it was found that she had altered her rate of going between the two places so much as to make this a doubtfull point. Upon the whole it should seem that New Zealand is laid down too far East, but when I consider the great number of observations we had to settle it by I cannot think the error so great as Mr Bayly makes it'.—After all this painful cogitation and writing not a word on the subject appeared in the published account of the voyage except when Cook records Wales's final results, *Voyage*, *II*, p. 161.

a few of them might have granted to the crew of[1] the Endeavour it was generally done in a private manner and without the men seeming to intrest themselves in it, but now we find the men are the chief promoters of this Vice, and for a spike nail or any other thing they value will oblige their Wives and Daughters to prostitute themselves whether they will or no and that not with the privicy decency seems to require, such are the concequences of a commerce with Europeans and what is still more to our Shame civilized Christians, we debauch their Morals already too prone to vice and we interduce among them wants and perhaps diseases which they never before knew and which serves only to disturb that happy tranquillity they and their fore Fathers had injoy'd. If any one denies the truth of this assertion let him tell me what the Natives of the whole extent of America have gained by the commerce they have had with Europeans.

SATURDAY 5*th*, SUNDAY 6*th*. Both these days the Wind was at SE and blew a fresh gale so that we neither could sail or have any communication with our friends the natives.

MONDAY 7*th*. At 4 o'Clock in the morning the Wind coming more favourable we unmoor'd and at 7 wieghed and put to Sea with the Adventure in company, as soon as we had got out of the Sound we found the Wind at South so that we had to ply through the Straits. At Noon the two Brothers[2] which lie off Cape Koamaroo bore West distant one mile, the Tide of ebb was now makeing in our favour[3] so that we had some prospect of geting through before night.

TUESDAY 8*th*. At 5 o'Clock in the PM Cape Pallisser on the Island of Eahei-namauwe bore ESE½S and Cape Koamaroo on Tavai poenammoo bore NBW¾W, in this situation we had no ground with 75 fathoms of line; the Tide of flood now made against us and being little Wind next to a Calm we were drove fast back to the Northward but at middnight a light breeze afterwards freshen'd which together with the Tide of Ebb carried us by 8 o'Clock in the morning quite clear of the Strait, Cape Pallisser at this time bearing ENE and at Noon NBW distant 7 Leagues. From this Cape I take my departure allowing it to lie in the same Latitude and Longitude as laid down in my Chart of the Islands. To day when we attended the Winding up of the Watches the fusee of Mr Arnolds would not turn round and

[1] *the crew of:* some few people in . . .—f. 73v.
[2] . . . two small Islets
[3] . . . and enabled us to make good boards

after several unsuccessfull tryals we were obliged to let it go down, this is the second of this gentlemans Watches that hath fail'd, one of those on board the Adventure stop'd at the Cape of Good Hope and hath not gone sence.[1]

WEDNESDAY 9*th. Winds West to NNW. Course S* 54°30′ *E. Distce Sail'd* 95 *Miles. Lat. in South* 42°52′. Gentle gales and pleasent Weather. At 5 pm Shorten'd Sail, at 4 am made all Sail and betwen 8 and 12 exercized the people at great guns & Sm[l] Arms. Swell from SE, several Port Egmont Hens seen.

THURSDAY 10*th. Winds NNW to WNW. Course S* 51°30′. *Distce Sail'd* 101 *Miles. Lat. in South* 43°55′. *Long. in East* 179°41′ *Accot.* 179°50′ *Obsn. Long. made E of C. Pallisser* 3°38′. D[o] Weather. At 6 PM shorten'd sail and at day light made sail again. A great irregular swell, several peices of Weed and Port Egmont Hens seen this 24 hours. Lon[g] in p[r] ☉ & ☽ at 10 am 179°45′ E which exactly corresponds with the Longitude of Queen Charlottes Sound as it is laid down in my chart.[2]

FRIDAY 11*th. Winds WNW to North. Course S* 56° *E. Distce Sail'd* 89 *Miles. Lat. in South* 44°35′. *Longitude in West* 178°40′. *Long. made E of C. Pallisser* 5°17′. First part D[o] Weather, middle little and some times foggy, latter fresh gales and hazy with rain. At 5 PM shorten'd Sail, at 7 AM made Sail, at a 11 took in the Studding sails. Rock Weed and Port Egmont Hens seen as before.

SATURDAY 12*th. Winds North to West, WNW. Course S* 64°15′ *E. Distce Sail'd* 119 *Miles. Lat. in South* 45°26′. *Long. in West* 176°18′. *Long. made E of C. Pallisser* 7°49′. Fore and middle parts fresh gales and hazey with sm[l] rain; latter little wind and hazy, at 3 PM took a reef in each Top-sail. At 7 am made all Sail. Swell from the Northward, Weed seen as before.

SUNDAY 13*th. Winds West, SW, Easterly. Course S* 40° *E. Distce Sail'd* 47 *Miles. Lat. in South* 46°2′. *Long. in West* 175°36′. *Long. made E of C.*

[1] . . . the other aboard the Adventure hath hitherto been found to answer extremely well.—f. 74.—The Cape stoppage is that described by Wales, p. 47, n. 1 above.

[2] . . . After geting clear of the Straits I directed my Course SEBE having a gentle gale, but variable between the North and West. The late SE winds had caused a swell from the same quarter which did not go down for some days, so that I had little hopes of meeting with land in that direction. On the 10th at Noon we were in the Latitude of 43°55′ S. Longitude 179°50′ East by observations of the Sun and Moon made two hours before these observations exactly corresponds with our run from the land both by the reckoning and Watch. As we shall presently pass the Meridian of 180° after which I shall count my Longitude West of Greenwich, that it may be more consonant to the situations or Longitude of places mentioned in my former Voyage on which I counted my Longitude west . . . —f. 74.

Pallisser 8°31′. Little Wind and hazy with small rain all the fore and middle parts, latter fresh breeze and dark gloomy weather, at 3 PM shortend sail for the night and in the morning made sail again. Swell still continues to come from the Northward and Weed seen as usual.

MONDAY 14*th. Winds East to South and to West. Course S* 69½° *E. Distce Sail'd* 43 *Miles. Lat. in South* 46°17′. *Long. in West* 174°38′.[1] *Long. made E of C. Pallisser* 9°29′. First part moderate and Clowdy, remainder little wind with drizling rain. At 4 PM carried away the Fore Topg[t] Yard in the Slings, bore down to Adventure, Tack'd to the NE and shorten'd sail; in the AM rigg'd another topg[t] yard and made sail. Swell from NE.

TUESDAY 15*th. Winds WSW, NW. Course S* 56° *E. Distce Sail'd* 51 *Miles. Lat. in South* 46°46′. *Long. in West* 173°27′. *Long. in by the Watch* 173°2′. *Long. made E of C. Pallisser* 10°30′. *Variation of the Compass* 11°25′ *E.* Little Wind and hazy with rain at times. Swell from NE. Var. 11°25′ E.

WEDNESDAY 16*th. Winds NE to SEBE. Course S* 37° *E. Distce Sailed* 42 *Miles. Lat. in South* 46°56′. *Long. in West* 172°49′. *Long. made E of C. Pallisser* 11°8′. Little Wind and Clowdy all the Fore and middle parts, latter fresh gales and hazy. Stood to the SE and South with the Wind at NE & East till 7 am being then in the Latitude of 47°7′ we tack'd and Stood NE having a great head swell and the Wind at SEBE. Took a reef in each Topsail. Saw some weed.

THURSDAY 17*th. Winds SE. Course NE. Distce Sail'd* 55 *Miles. Lat. in South* 46°18′. *Long. in West* 172°48′. *Long. made E of C. Pallisser* 11°49′. First and middle parts strong gales and hazy with rain. In the PM close reef'd and at last handed the Topsails and got down top g[t] yards.[2] At 8 AM being more moderate, set the Topsails close reef'd.

[1] B f. 76v, 15 June (civil time) gives this longitude as 174°00′, to which it has the note: The Longitude was deduced from observations made 2 hours before and were agreeable to the Longit. of our departure as laid down in my Chart, but not with M[r] Bayleys observations.—There is a pencil note in the margin, 'omit this'.

[2] 'A very hollow sea caused the Ship to labour much, and a sudden jerk of the Tiller carried the man at the wheel clear over it. Luckily the Officer of the watch caught it, replaced him, & put a man on the Lee side to assist him. They had been there scarce 10′ before another Jerk carried the man on the weather side over again. The Tiller staid not a moment a-weather, but returned with such Velocity as brought the man on the lee-side over to windward. At this moment the Lieu[t] catched it again; which was very fortunate, for the latter man had got his leg jambed between a spoke of the Wheel and the Standard which supports it, so that if the helm had had time to return it must have been broke to pieces. The Care of Providence, in fitting the Back to the Burthen, was never more conspicuous than in this circumstance. The man who went over to leeward, and of course had much the greater fall, resembled much a seal in substance and make, and accordingly

Squally unsettled weather. A large piece of rock weed seen: a great Sea from NE.

FRIDAY 18*th. Winds SE. Course N* 75°45′ *E. Distce Sail'd* 89 *Miles. Lat. in South* 45°54′. *Long. in West* 170°5′. *Long. made E of C. Pallisser* 13°52′. Strong gales and Squally, at 7 AM loosd two reefs out of the Top-sails having no longer a head Sea to go against, having shifted to SE.

SATURDAY 19*th. Winds SE to South. Course ENE. Dist. Saild* 84 *Miles. Lat. in South* 45°22′. *Long. in West Reck.g* 168°13′. *Long. made from C. Pallisser* 15°44′ *East.* First part fresh gales and hazy, remainder moderate and clowdy. At 5 PM close reef'd the Topsails, at 7 am out all reefs, got Top-gall[t] yards across and made all sail. Swell from SE, some rock Weed seen.

SUNDAY 20*th. Winds SSW to SSE. Course ENE. Dist. Saild* 114 *Miles. Lat. in South* 44°38′. *Long. in West Reck.g* 165°45′. *Long. made from C. Pallisser* 18°12′ *East.* Moderate gales and Clowdy. In the evening shorten'd sail and at Day light made sail again. At noon had a great irregular swell from South. Some weed seen.

MONDAY 21*st. Winds SSE to WBS. Course N* 80° *E. Dist. Saild* 68 *Miles. Lat. in South* 44°26′. *Long. in West Reck.g* 164°11′ *Watch* 164°27′. *Long. made from C. Pallisser* 19°46′ East. Gentle breezes and Clowdy weather and a very high Swell, first from the South and then from SW so that no land can be expected between these two points but what must be at a great distance.

TUESDAY 22*nd. Therm.r* 48 *to* 50. *Winds WSW. Course S* 77° *E. Dist. Saild* 67 *Miles. Lat. in South* 44°41′. *Long. in West Reck.g* 162°39′ *Watch* 162°47′. *Long. made from C. Pallisser* 21°18′ *East. Varn. Compass* 10°19′ *E.* Gentle breezes and pleasent weather. AM Variation 10°19′ East. A very great Swell from the South such as makes it probable that no land can be near in that direction at least not on this side 50° Latitude.

WEDNESDAY 23*rd. Therm.r* 52. *Winds WNW and West. Course East. Dist. Saild* 51 *Miles. Lat. in South* 44°41′. *Long. in West Reck.g* 161°27′. *Long. made from C. Pallisser* 22°30′ *East. Varn. Compass* 11°23′ E. Little Wind and fair Weather. PM Variation 9°7′ East. AM hoisted out a boat for M[r] Wales to go a board the Adventure to compair the Watches.[1] The SW swell still continues as high as ever.

his fall on the deck made exactly the same squash that a Bag of Blubber would have done; on the contrary, the other was a poor raw-boned Lad, whose every bone rattled with the fall he got, and must have been broke to pices had he gone over to Leeward.'—Wales.

[1] . . . which he found to agree.—f. 74v.

THURSDAY 24*th. Winds E, ENE. Course N½W. Dist. Saild* 65 *Miles. Lat. in South* 43°36′. *Long. in West Reck.g* 161°37′. *Long. made from C. Pallisser* 22°20′ *East.* Calm untill 4 am when a breeze sprung up at East with which we stood to the Northward. Variation in the PM 11°23′ E p^r^ Az^th^. At 8 double reefed the Topsails and handed the Mizen Top-sail, the wind blowing a fresh gale and afterwards increased in such a manner as to bring us under our two courses and obliged us to strike Top-gallant yards. Some rock weed seen to day, indeed we have generally seen some every day sence we left the land and now and then a Port Egmont Hen or two and some few other Birds. Sea from East Northeast.

FRIDAY 25*th. Therm.r* 55½. *Winds ENE. Course NW. Dist. Saild* 48 *Miles. Lat. in South* 43°3′. *Long. in West Reck.g* 162°24′. *Long. made from C. Pallisser* 21°33′ *East.* Very hard gale and squally with a high Sea from NE. At 2 pm handed the Main-sail and laid to under the fore-sail and Mizen Staysail. At 8 am being more moderate set the Mainsail.

SATURDAY 26*th. Therm.r* 56. *Winds ENE to NNE. Course SW. Dist. Saild* 11 *Miles. Lat. in South* 43°11′. *Long. in West Reck.g* 162°34′, 162°45′ *pr.* ☉ *&* ☽. *Long. made from C. Pallisser* 21°23′ *East.* Fresh gales with showers of rain in the pm, remainder fair. At 2 pm set the Top-sails close reefed, at Middnight made the Signal and Wore being then in Lat. 42°33′ S, Longitude 162°40′ W. At 7 am loosed a reef out of each Topsail and set the Mizen Topsail. NE sea still continues.[1]

SUNDAY 27*th. Therm.r* 54. *Winds Easterly. Course N* 20′ *E. Dist. Saild* 42 *Miles. Lat. in South* 42°33′. *Long. in West Reck.g* 162°14′. *Long. made from C. Pallisser* 21°43′ *East.* Fresh gales and variable Weather. At 4 PM being in Latitude 43°20′ wore and stood to the Northward. At 8 am Loosed two reefs out of the Top-sails. Soon after pass'd a piece of rock Weed. Swell from ENE.

MONDAY 28*th. Winds SE to West. Course East. Dist. Saild* 33 *Miles. Lat. in South* 42°33′. *Long. in West Reck.g* 161°29′. *Long. made from C. Pallisser* 22°28′ *East.* First part fresh breeze, remainder little wind and hazey. PM saw a Port Egmont Hen, in the AM Loosed all the reefs out of the Top-sails and got Top-gallant yards aCross and set the Sails Swell from ESE.

TUESDAY 29*th. Winds WSW, NW, NE. Course SEBE. Dist. Saild* 26 *Miles. Lat. in South* 42°46′. *Long. in West Reck.g* 160°59′, 159°56′ *pr.*

[1] ADV '... we have very little to Amuse us but Reading'.—Bayly.

☽ *and* ☆, 160°40′ *pr.* ☽ and ⊙. *Long. made from C. Pallisser* 22°58′ *East.* Most part little wind, hazey and clear at times. Swell from the East.

WEDNESDAY 30*th. Winds East to South. Course S* 72° *E. Distce Sailed* 71 *Miles Lat. in South* 43°7′. *Long. in West Reck.g* 159°25′. *Long. made C. Pallisser* 24°32′. Fore and middle parts little wind and Clowdy, remainder fresh gales and clear. At 9 am Variation pr Azmth 7°59′ E. Saw a Port Egmont Hen. Swell from ESE.[1]

[JULY 1773]

THURSDAY 1*st. Winds SEterly. Course East. Distce Sailed* 74 *Miles. Lat. in South* 43°7′. *Long. in West Reck.g* 157°44′. *Long. made C. Pallisser* 26°13′. First and latter parts little wind and Clowdy, Middle little wind. Swell from South.

FRIDAY 2*nd. Winds SBE. Course N* 86°30′ *E. Distce Sailed* 64 *Miles. Lat. in South* 43°3′. *Long. in West Reck.g* 156°17′. *Long. made C. Pallisser* 27° 40′. Gentle breezes and fine Weather. PM Variation pr Azths 6°65′ E. AM 9°2′ E. Swell from South.

SATURDAY 3*rd. Winds South to West & NBW. Course S* 75° *E. Distce Sailed* 58 *Miles. Lat. in South* 43°18′. *Long. in West Reck.g* 155°30′. *Long. made C. Pallisser* 28°47′. PM Light airs next to a Calm. AM gentle breezes with some Showers. At pm Variation pr Azmth 8°2′ E and 8 am 7°16′ E. Swell from SSW.

SUNDAY 4*th. Winds NE to EBS. Course S* 56°15′. *Distce Sailed* 37 *Miles. Lat. in South* 43°58′. *Long. in West Reck.g* 154°18′. *Long. made C. Pallisser* 29°39′. Fresh gales with some Showers. At 4 PM took a reef in each Top-sail. Saw a Port Egmont Hen and a piece of Rock Weed. Variation pr Azth 8°11′ E. At 9 am Tacked and stood to the Northward, took the Second Reef in the Fore & Main Top-sail and handed the Mizen Top-sail. Swell from the Eastward.

MONDAY 5*th. Winds SEterly. Course NEBE½E. Distce Sailed* 101 *Miles. Lat. in South* 43°10′. *Long. in West Reck.g* 152°15′. *Long. made C. Pallisser* 31°42′. Fresh gales and clear till the AM when it became very squally with rain and obliged us to strike Topgallant yards and double reef the Fore Topsail. Swell from SE.

TUESDAY 6*th. Therm.r* 50. *Winds ESE and SEBE. Course N* 43°45′ *E. Distce Sailed* 79 *Miles. Lat. in South* 42°7′. *Long. in West Reck.g* 150°47′.

[1] ADV 'This morning Capt Furnx obsd for Longd by No 1: this being the first obsn of the Kind made by him'.—Bayly. 'No 1' was the number of the chronometer; and the entry casts a little light on the incuriosity of Furneaux's temperament.

Long. made C. Pallisser 33°10′. Fresh gales and squally. AM Loosed two reefs out of the Topsails and set Mizen Topsail being more moderate. Several Birds about the Ship such as Blue Piterls, Pintadoes &c[a]. Swell from ESE.

WEDNESDAY 7*th. Winds East to South. Course N* 30° *E. Distce Sailed* 52 *Miles. Lat. in South* 41°22′. *Long. in West Reck.g* 150°12′. *Long. made C. Pallisser* 33°45′. First part fresh gales remainder little wind and fair Weather, At 4 AM Loosed all the reefs out of the Topsails and got Topg[t] yards across. At 9 hoisted a Boat out to carry M[r] Wales aboard the Adventure to compare the watches and which was found to agree, a proof that they have both kept to their rate of going sence we left Queen Charlottes Sound, and yet all the observations for Longitude sence we came out hath generally been one degree to the East of the Watches, another proof that M[r] Bayly's Longitude of that place is too far west.[1] Swell from ESE.

THURSDAY 8*th. Winds South to WNW. Course S* 60°45′ *E. Distce Sailed* 80 *Miles. Lat. in South* 42°1′. *Long. in West Reck.g* 148°37′. *Long. made C. Pallisser* 35°20′. PM Gentle breeze and Clowdy, remainder fresh gale with some squalls attended with Showers of rain. At 2 AM set Studding sails and soon after carried away the Fore-top-mast studding sail boom. Swell from West.

FRIDAY 9*th. Therm.r* 50. *Winds WBN to SBW & to WSW. Course S* 64°15′ *E. Distce Sailed* 90 *Miles. Lat. in South* 42°40′. *Long. in West Reck.g* 146°51′. *Long. made C. Pallisser* 37°6′. First part fresh gales and Squally with Showers of rain, latter little wind and fair weather. At 4 pm Shorten'd sail and at 4 am made sail. At 10 one of our goats fell over board, hoisted a boat out and took it up alive but it died soon after. A Long hollow Sea from SW.

SATURDAY 10*th. Winds WSW to NW & back again to WSW. Course S* 60° *E. Distce Sailed* 132 *Miles. Lat. in South* 43°46′. *Long. in West Reck.g* 144°13′. *Long. made C. Pallisser* 39°44′. First part moderate breeze and fair, remainder fresh gales and Squalls attended with Showers of rain, in the evening handed the Mizen Top-sail and at 9 am double reefed the Main and fore topsails. Saw a Water spout and a Port Egmont Hen. Variation p[r] Az[th] 3° E. A great Sea from west.

[1] *a proof . . . west:* allowing for the difference of their rates of going, proof that they had gone well since we had been at Sea, and yet all the Lunar observations we had sence we left Queen Charlottes Sound generally gave our Longitude one, and never less than half a degree, more to the East than M[r] Kendals watch, by which the Longitude is carried on agreeable to M[r] Bayleys observations made in the Sound.—f. 77v.—In this passage the words 'and yet . . . Sound' are marked in the margin, 'omit'.

SUNDAY 11*th*. *Winds West, South, Variable. Course E* 7° *N. Distce Saild* 100 *Miles. Lat. in South* 43°34′. *Long in West Reck.g* 141°56′. *Long. made C. Pallisser* 42°1′. *Variation* 4°59½′. First part fresh gales and hazey with some showers of rain, remainder gentle breeze and clear pleasent weather. In the AM loosed all the reefs out and set all the small sails. At 9 Variation p[r] Az[th] 4°5′ E. At the same time the observed Longitude p[r] ☉ and ☽ was ° ′ West. A great swell from West South West.[1]

MONDAY 12*th*. *Therm.r morn*. 49, 47½. *Winds SSW. Course S* 78°15′ *E. Distce Saild* 79 *Miles. Lat. in South* 43°16′. *Long. in West Reck.g* 140°9′. *Long. made C. Pallisser* 43°48′. *Variation* 5°18′. Gentle breezes and fair Weather: at 3 pm Variation p[r] Az[th] 5°56′ E and at 9 am 5°31′ E. At the same time the Longitude p[r] Several observations of the ☉ and ☽ was 140°24′17½″ West being the Mean result of the observations made by M[r] Clerk, Gilbert, Wales and my self. Swell from SW.

TUESDAY 13*th*. *Winds SSW to NW. Course N* 72°15′ *E. Distce Saild* 46 *Miles. Lat. in South* 43°2′. *Long. in West Reck.g* 139°10′. *Long. made C. Pallisser* 44°47′. *Variation* 5°37′. Gentle breezes and fair Weather. At 4 pm Variation p[r] Az[th] 5°5′ E. In the night lost sight of the Adventure which occasioned us to burn some false fires by which she was discovered. At 9 AM Longitude in p[r] Observations as follows: Self 138°45′30″. M[r] Wales 138°48′, D[o] 139°48′. M[r] Clerk 139°12′ West the Mean is 139°23′. Variation at the same time 5°37′ E. A great Swell from SW.

WEDNESDAY 14*th*. *Winds NWBN, Calm, NNE to NE. Course East.*[2] *Distce Saild* 43 *Miles. Lat. in South* 43°2′. *Long. in West Reck.g* 139°9′. *Long. made C. Pallisser* 45°46′. Had light airs next to a Calm for some hours in the pm, which was succeeded by a breeze from the Northward which increased to a fresh gale and blew in squalls attended with dark gloomy unsettled weath[r] and a great hollow swell from

[1] ADV '. . . last night M[r] Scott: the Lieu[t] of Marines seemed to be out of his mind, as he ran about Almost Naked talking a great deal of Incohearent stuff: The 8th in the Evening M[r] Scott came into my Cabbin, & Told me he had something to intrust me with, Viz that he had that Evening Asked Doctor John (meaning the Surgeons first Mate) to drink Tea with him, (they frequently drank Tea together being very intimate) & that there was a Pill in his Tea, which he said that D[r] John put there in order to Poison him, he immagined; but that luckily he did not Swallow it; & that he had told me of it that I might remember it in case he did otherwise than well, He likewise told the Surgeon the same, But it soon appeared that he was Mad & that there was nothing in his Tea.'—Bayly.

[2] . . . The Calm [of the 7th] was succeeded by a Wind from the South, between which point and the NW it continued for the Six Succeeding Days but never blew strong, it was however attended with a great hollow swell from SW and West, a sure indication that no large land was near in these directions. We now Steered East. . . .—f. 77v.

SWBS, so that no land could be near in that direction. Saw a Port Egmont Hen.

THURSDAY 15*th. Therm.r* 52. *Winds NE & ENE. Course N* 20° *E. Dist. Saild* 25 *Miles. Lat. in South* 42°39′. *Long. in West Reck.g* 137°58′. *Long. made C. Pallisser* 45°59′. First part fresh gales and gloomy weather. At 2 pm single reefed the Top-sails and presently after the Clew of the fore top-sail gave way which obliged us to unbend the sail and bring a nother to the yard. At half past 5 being then in the Lat of 43°15′ S, Long 187°39′ West Tacked and stood to the North. At 8 double reefed the Top sails and handed the Mizen Top-sail. The gale kept increasing in such a manner as to oblige us at 2 am to hand the Fore Top-sail and some time after the Main Topsail and to strike Top gallant yards, the Fore Top-mast stay-sail being split we unbent it and bent a nother.[1] The gale was attended with rain and thick hazy weather, so that at 8 o'Clock we could not see the Adventure, judging she must be a stern we bro[t] to to wait for her, some time after we saw her to leward, bore down and joined her and then made sail under the Course's, towards Noon set the Top-sails close reefed, the gale being more moderate. A very high sea from NE.

FRIDAY 16*th. Therm.r* 46. *Winds SSW. Course N* 50° *E. Dist. Saild* 115 *Miles. Lat. in South* 41°25′. *Long. in West Reck.g* 135°58′. *Long. made C. Pallisser* 47°59′. Presently after noon the wind flatened to a Calm, weather foggy with drizling rain and a Prodigious high Sea from NE. At 5 am a breeze sprung up at SW, increased to a strong gale and fixed at SSW and was attended with fair weather; I now directed the Course NE, during the night we run under an easy sail but in the morn made more sail. Sea from SSW. A little before Noon pass'd a Billet of wood which appeared to be covered with barnacles.[2]

SATURDAY 17*th. Winds SSW. Lat. in South* 39°44′. *Long. in West Reck.g* 133°32′. *Long. made C. Pallisser* 50°25′. First part Strong gales and fair weather, the latter Squally showers of rain. At 4 pm close reef'd the Top-sails and handed the Mizen Top-sail. In the Morning loosed them out again but was obliged to reef again before Noon at which time we had run down the whole of the Longitude I at

[1] ADV 'N.B. I have observed since we left New Zealand, whenever we have had an alteration of wind from any quarter, into the NE quarter, it has always blown very hard with thick dirty weather.'—Kemp.

[2] . . . so that there was no judgeing how long it might have been there, or from whince or how far it had come.—f. 78.

first intended[1] and being nearly midway betwixt my track to the north in 1769 and return to the South the same year as will appear by the Chart,[2] I steer'd N½E having the Advantage of a strong gale at SSW, with a view of exploring that part of the Sea between the two tracks just mentioned down as low as the Latitude of 27° S in which space no one has been that I know of. A Great Swell from SW.

SUNDAY 18*th. Therm.r* 50. *Winds SSW, South. Course N* 5°30′ *E. Dist. Sailed* 109 *Miles. Lat. in South* 37°56′. *Long. in West Reck.g* 133°18′. *Long. made C. Pallisser* 50°39′. *Variation* 5°29′. First part very strong gales and Squally attended with Showers of hail and rain. Middle more moderate, latter gentle breeze and clear weather. At 6 AM out all reefs and made sail, at half past 8 Variation p[r] Az[th] 6°4′ E. A great swell from SSW.

MONDAY 19*th. Winds D°. to WNW & back to South. Course N* 5° *E. Dist. Sailed* 82 *Miles. Lat. in South* 36°34′. *Long. in West Reck.g* 133°7′. *Long. made C. Palliser* 50°50′. Gentle breezes with some Showers in the night, at 3 pm Var[n] 4°54′ E. Carpenters employed painting the Boats, sail-makers repairing the Sails. Swell from South.

TUESDAY 20*th. Winds SWBS to SEBS. Course N* 6° *W. Dist. Sailed* 72½ *Miles. Lat. in South* 35°22′. *Long. in West Reck.g* 133°17′. *Long. made C. Pallisser* 50°40′. First part gentle breezes and Clear; latter fresh gale and clowdy, at Noon the Southerly swell was partly gone down.

WEDNESDAY 21*st. Winds SE, East & SEBE. Course N* 6° *W′. Dist. Sailed* 156 *Miles. Lat. in South* 32°47′. *Long. in West Reck.g* 133°37′. *Long. made C. Pallisser* 50°20′. First part fresh gales, remainder strong gales and squally, hazy wea[r] with rain. At 2 AM Single reefed the Fore and Main Top-sails and handed the Mizen Top-sail. Great Swell from SE.[3]

THURSDAY 22*nd. Winds East, ENE, SE, South, SW. Course N* 16°30′ *W. Dist. Sailed* 105 *Miles. Lat. in South* 31°6′. *Long. in West Reck.g* 134°12′. *Long. made C. Pallisser* 49°45′. *Variation* 5°21′. First part fresh breeze and hazy, remainder gentle breezes and mostly clear, some Showers

[1] B f. 78–8v says this position 'was a degree and a half further East than I had intended to run'. Cf. Furneaux, Add. MS 27890, f. 13, who, recording that after leaving New Zealand the ships made 50° of longitude between the latitudes of 47° and 43° S, continues, 'We found a very hollow Sea from the Eastern quarter, so I believe there is no Land in that quarter before you reach the main Land of America, as we were not above 200 Leagues to the Westward of former Voyages'.

[2] See Fig. 1.

[3] 'Punish'd John Keplin Seaman 1 dozen for throwing an old Chew of Tobacco amongst Victuals dressing, which infamous proceedings have frequently before been practiced by persons unknown.'—Cooper.

in the night. In the PM set the Mizen Top-sail, AM loosed all the reefs out of the Top-sails and made sail. No birds to be seen to day for the first time sence we left New Zealand, having every day seen some Albatroses, Sheer waters, Pintadoes, Blue Peterls &c[a] but never many at one time nor has there been a single Bird seen that could in the least indicate the vicinity of land, for as to the Port Egmont Hens we have seen they can no longer be looked upon as such.[1] Employed repairing and painting our boats, repairing sails, &c[a].[2]

FRIDAY 23*rd. Winds WSW to NWBN. Course North. Dist. Sailed* 104 *Miles. Lat. in South* 29°22′. *Long. in West Reck.g* 134°12′. *Long. made C. Pallisser* 49°45′. *Variation* 5°34′. First part gentle breezes and fair, middle Squally with rain, latter fair wea[r] PM Variation 5°21′ E. AM 5°34′ E. At Noon the Wind having veer'd to NWBN, Tacked and stood to the westward, and took a reef in each Top-sail.[3]

SATURDAY 24*th. Winds NWBN to NNW. Course S* 72° *W. Dist. Sailed* 77 *Miles. Lat. in South* 29°46′. *Long. in West Reck.g* 135°36′. *Long. made C. Pallisser* 48°21′. PM Fresh gales and hazy with small rain, which in the night increased to a hard gale, blew in squalls attended with rain. At 7 pm double reefd the Top-sails. AM handed Mizen Top-sail and close reefed the Fore and M[n] Top-sail, soon after they were both split as well as the M[n] top-mast staysail, unbent them and bent others. Towards Noon more moderate.[4]

SUNDAY 25*th. Therm.r* 63. *Winds NW, North, WBN, NW. Course N* 85°15′ *W. Dist. Sailed* 37 *Miles. Lat. in South* 29°43′. *Long. in West Reck.g* 136°18′. *Long. made C. Pallisser* 47°39′. Very unsettled weather with rain. PM set the Mizen Top-sail, at 8 AM Tacked in Latitude 29°51′ S, Long[de] 136°28′ W and stood to the NE.

[1] *&c[a] . . . as such:* and Port Egmont Hens, but these are Birds that frequent every part of the Southern Ocean in the higher Latitudes.—f. 79.

[2] . . . The Weather was now so warm that it was necessary to put on lighter Clothes: the Mercury in the Thermometer at noon rose to 63, it had never been lower then 46 and seldom higher then 54 at the same time of the day sence we left New Zealand.—f. 78v.

[3] ADV 'Departed this Life Murduck Mahony Ship's Cook:—Furneaux, Log. Furneaux has no previous mention of the health of his crew either in his log or in his journal. This man was a natural prey for scurvy: cf. Bayly, 23 July (civil time): 'This morning was committed to the Deep the remains of Murdoch Mahoney Ship's Cook; he died Yesterday Evening of the Scurvy, he being so ver[y] indolent & dirtily inclined there was no possability of making him keep himself clean, or even to come on Deck to breath the fresh air'.

[4] 'At Noon a decreasing Gale with cloudy, hazey, Wet disagreeable Wea[r].—It has now for some hours blown fresh from the N.W[d] and the water is still smooth; this is very different from what we've experienc'd before since our departure from New Zealand—for we've no sooner had a 4 hours Gale but a large Sea has immediately attended it—Query whither this proceeds from the vicinity of Land to windward, or that these winds extend but a small distance and so blow in Veins.'—Clerke.

MONDAY 26*th. Winds NBW to WNW. Course N* 45° *E. Distce. Sailed* 69 *Miles. Lat. in South* 28°53′. *Long. in West Reck.g* 135°30′ *pr.* ☉ *&* ☽ 135°30′, *Watch* 135°40′. *Long. made C. Pallisser* 48°27′. *Variation* 5°3′ *E.* Soon after noon the sky cleared up and the weather became fair and clear and continued so the remainder of the 24 hours, with a gentle breeze of wind. In the evening saw a Tropick Bird[1] being the first we have seen in this Sea. AM loosed all the reefs out of the Top-sails and set small sails. Swell from W.

TUESDAY 27*th. Winds NWBW to WSW. Course N* 11° *E. Distce. Sailed* 61 *Miles. Lat. in South* 27°53′. *Long. in West Reck.g* 135°17′. *Long. made C. Pallisser* 48°40′. Gentle breezes and clear weather. In the PM Longitude in p^r^ the mean of Several Distances of the Sun & Moon made by my self, Mr Wales, Clerk and Gilbert 135°30′ W,[2] by Mr Kendals watch at the same time 135°40′. Var^n^ 5°3′ E. Swell still continues to come from WSW.[3]

WEDNESDAY 28*th. Therm.r* 69. *Winds SW, Calm, NBE, NBW. Course N* 62°15′ *W. Distce. Sailed* 20 *Miles. Lat. in South* 27°43′. *Long. in West Reck.g* 135°37′. *Long. made C. Pallisser* 48°20′. *Variation* 6°19′ *E.* PM Little Wind and Calms, AM gentle breezes and pleasent weather. PM had Several Observations of the Sun and Moon the results of which were consonant with yesterdays. AM spoke the Adventure as was told that her crew were sickly.[4] Swell from the Westward.

THURSDAY 29*th. Winds North to NWBW. Course N* 61° *W. Distce. Sailed* 26 *Miles. Lat. in South* 27°30′. *Long. in West Reck.g* 136°14′. *Long. made C. Pallisser* 47°43′. Gentle breezes with some Showers in the night. Stood to the Westward till 4 AM when we Tacked to the NE being then in Latitude 27°49′, Long^de^ 136°49′. Being a fine day I

[1] 'PM this Afternoon I saw a Tropic Bird who I believe has lately been as unfortunate in his Breeze as ourselves, for he had got confoundedly to Leeward of that part of the World these Birds in general chuse for their habitation, I never before met with one so far from the Equator.'—Clerke. Tropic or bo'sun birds are typical of low latitudes. This one was probably the Red-tailed Tropic Bird, *Phaëthon rubricauda melanorhynchos* Gm., which has been seen as far south as lat. 36°44′—about 650 miles further than its usual habitat.

[2] ... My reckoning at the same time was 135°27′ and which I have not had an occasion to correct sence I lift the land.—f. 79.

[3] There were now signs, not at all serious, of scurvy in the *Resolution*, and Cook took the appropriate steps.—'Brew wort & gave to those people who have the least symptoms of the scurvy which is to be cont^d^ (likewise the marmulet of Carrot.)'—Mitchel. See also Cook, 29 July below.

[4] ADV '20 Men Sick with the Scurvy & Flux.'—Furneaux log. 'Our People have complaind of a violent purging these 4 days past . . .'—Burney log. But Bayly (29 July) notes 22 men on the sick list, 'Mostly with Rumatic complaints; & two or three bad in the Scurvey'. In the *Resolution* Cooper writes, 'We at this time have but one Man ill, who has been ailing since our departure from England in a decline & now bad of the Dropsy'. This was Isaac Taylor, marine, who died just as the ships reached Tahiti.

hoisted a boat out and sent aboard the Adventure to inquire into the state of her crew when I learnt that her cook was dead and about Twenty more were attacked with the Scurvy and Flux;[1] at this time we had only three men on the Sick list and only one of them of the Scurvy, several more however began to shew some symptoms of it and were accordingly put upon the Wort, Marmalade of Carrots, Rob of Lemons and Oranges. I appointed one of my people Cook of the Adventure[2] and wrote to Captain Furneaux proposing such methods as I thought would tend to stop the spreading of the disease among his people. The methods I proposed were to Brew Beer of the Inspissated juce of Wort, Essence of Spruce and Tea plants (all of which he had aboard) for all hands, if he could spare Water, if not, for the Sick, to inlarge their allowance of Sour Krout, to boil Cabbage in their Pease, to serve Wine in lieu of spirit and lastly to shorten their allowance of Salt Meat. Swell from WSW.

*I know not how to account for the Scurvy raging more in the one Ship than the other, unless it was owing to the Crew of the Adventure, being more Scorbutic when they arrived in New-Zealand than we were[3] and their eating few or no Vegetables while they lay in Queen Charlottes Sound, partly for want of knowing the right sorts and partly because it was a New diet which alone was sufficient for Seamen to reject it. To interduce any New article of food among Seamen, let it be ever so much for their good, requires both the example and Authority of a Commander, without both of which, it will be droped before the People are Sencible of the benifits resulting from it; was it necessary, I could name fifty instances in support of this remark.[4] Many of my People, officers as well as seamen, at first, disliked Celery, Scurvy grass &c[a] being boiled in the Pease & Wheat and some refused to eat it, but as this had no effect on my

[1] The boat brought back Kemp to report, Furneaux himself being on the sick-list—with gout in his right foot, we learn from Bayly. Apart from sickness, Bayly reports a social visit: '. . . this morning the resolutions boat came on board with M[r] Foster Sen[r] M[r] Hodges & M[r] Pickersgill, M[r] Foster brought M[r] Wales's watch. . . . The Gentlemen of the Resolution staid on board all day & some of our Gent[n] went on board the Resolution to dinner, & all returned on board their own Ships in the Evening'.

[2] 'This day Capt[n] Cook appointed W[m] Chapman one of our Seamen, who is Aged & having lost the use of 2 of his fingers to be Cook of the Adventure the former deceas'd, a great act of humanity as well as Charity.'—Cooper. It is not quite clear where the benefit of this humanity and charity fell, on William Chapman or on the crew of the *Adventure*.

[3] But Burney, Ferguson MS, on arriving at Queen Charlotte Sound, 7 April 1773, gives a good report on health: only five men sick, and only one of those sick with scurvy—'we have been all very hearty thank God, since we left the Cape'.

[4] One instance is given in I, p. 74. See also Clerke, p. 38, n. 2 above. Michael Lewis, *The Navy of Britain* (1948), p. 296, gets the sailor, from this viewpoint, into a nutshell: 'Like most primitive people, he was intensely conservative and suspicious of all change; and, once his confidence was lost, very obstinate and difficult to handle'.

conduct, this obstinate kind of prejudice, by little and little, wore off and they began to like it as well as the others and now, I believe, there was hardly a man in the Ship that did not attribute our being so free of the Scurvy to the Beer and Vegetables we made use of at Newzealand.[1] I appointed one of my Seamen to be Cook of the Adventure and wrote to Captain Furneaux, disiring him to make use of every method in his Power to stop the spreading of the disease amongst his people and proposed such as I thought might tend towards it, but I afterwards found all this unnecessary, as every method had been used they could think of.[2]*—ff. 79v–80.

FRIDAY 30*th. Winds NW to NNE. Course N* 66° *E. Distce. Sailed* 69 *Miles. Lat. in South* 27°4′. *Long. in West Reck.g* 135°15′. *Long. made C. Pallisser* 48°42′. First and latter parts gentle breezes and fair weather, Middle Squally with rain, Winds Variable between NNE and NWBW which occasioned us to tack several times. Swell still continues to come from W.

SATURDAY 31*st. Winds NNW to SW and back to NWBW. Course N* 27° *E. Distce. Sailed* 51 *Miles. Lat. in South* 26°19′. *Long. in West Reck.g* 134°49′. *Long. made C. Pallisser* 49°8′. First part gentle breezes, Middle little wind and Calm with much rain, latter fair and Clowdy. In the evening saw a Tropick Bird and in the Morning another. Fixed light Tacks and sheets to the Courses.

[AUGUST 1773]

SUNDAY 1*st. Therm.r* 68. *Winds West to NW & WNW. Course N* 64° *E. Distce. Sailed* 87 *Miles. Lat. in South* 25°1′. *Long. in West Reck.g* 134°6′. *Long. made C. Pallisser* 49°51′. PM gentle gales, remainder fresh gales and which blew in squalls attended with some showers of rain and dark clowdy weather. AM cleaned and smoaked between Decks. Took in the Topg[t] sails and a reef in each Topsail. Swell still continues to come from the Westward.

MONDAY 2*nd. Therm.r* 68. *Winds NW to SW. Course North. Dist[n]. Sailed* 107 *Miles. Lat. in South* 23°14′. *Longde. in West Reck.g* 134°6′. *Long. C. Pallisser* 49°51′. First part fresh gales and Clowdy remainder

[1] 'After this, I seldom found it necessary to order any of my people, to gather Vegetables, when ever we came where any was to be got and if scarce, happy was he who could lay hold of them first.'—Note by Cook.

[2] 'It would be proper to examine the Surgeon of the Adventure's Journal to know when and in what quantity the wort was given to these Scorbutic people, for if it was properly applyed, we have a proof that it alone will nither cure nor prevent the Sea Scurvy.'—Note by Cook.

gentle breeze and clear weather.[1] Being in the Latitude of *Pitcair*[*n*]*s* Island discovered by Captain Carteret in 1767 we looked out for it but could see no thing excepting two Tropick birds, we undoubtedly left this Island to the East of us.[2] Having now crossed or got to the north of Captain Carteret's Track, no discovery of importance can be made, some few Islands is all that can be expected while I remain within the Tropical Seas. As I have now in this and my former Voyage crossed this Ocean from 40° South and upwards it will hardly be denied but what I must have formed some judgement concerning the great object of my researches (viz) the Southern Continent. Circumstances seem to point out to us that there is none but this is too important a point to be left to conjector, facts must determine it and these can only be had by viseting the remaining unexplored parts of this Sea which will be the work of the remaining part of this Voyage.[3] I shall now collect into one View such general remarks as hath occured to me sence we left New Zealand. After leaving the Coast[4] we dayly saw Rock Weed floating in the Sea for the space of 18° of Longitude. In my passage to New Zealand in 1769 we saw the same sort of Weed and in greater quantities between the Latitudes of 37° and 39° for the space of 12° or 14° of Longitude before we discovered the land, this Weed is undoubtedly the produce of New Zealand because the nearer we are to this Coast the

[1] 'Reev'd small Tacks and Sheets to our Courses for y[e] convenience of working lighter and more readily during our stay in these fine weather Countries'.—Clerke.

[2] Cook changed his mind about this later. B f. 85 (the original version) repeats the dogmatic opinion, 'we undoubtedly left this Island to the East of us'. But for the whole sentence 'Being . . . East of us', f. 80, the version revised (as one assumes) in England, reads, 'The Situation we were now in was nearly the same as Captain Carteret assigns for Pitcairns Island, discovered by him in 1767, we accordingly looked well out for it, but saw nothing, according to the Longitude he has placed it, we must have past about 15 Leagues to the west of it'. G goes on '. . . but as this was uncertain, I did not think it prudent, considering the Situation of the Adventures people, to lose time in looking for it; a sight of it would however [have] been of use in verifying or correcting, not only the Longitude of this Isle, but the others which Captain Carteret discovered in this neighbourhood, as his Longitude was not corrected, I think, by Astronomical observations, and therefore liable to errors which he could have no method to correct'. The position given in Hawkesworth (I, p. 561) is lat. 20°2′ s (which may be a typographical error), long. 133°21′ w; in the accompanying chart, lat. 25°02′, long. 133°30′. The correct position is lat. 25°04′ s, long. 130°06′ w. The *Resolution* passed to the west of the island; the *Endeavour*, on the first voyage, to the east.

[3] *which will . . . Voyage:* which must be the work of the Insuing summer agreeable to the plan I had laid down.—f. 81v. This is part of a second re-casting of the entry for this date, the original B version, f. 85, being closer to the words of the text.

[4] *As I have now . . . Coast:* I had now, that is on this and my former Voyage, crossed this ocean in the Latitude of 40° and upwards, without meeting any thing, that did in the least induce me to think, I should find what I was in Search after, on the contrary every thing conspired to make me beleive there is no Southern Continent, between the Meridian of America and New zealand, at least this passage has not produced any indubitable signs of any as will appear by the following remarks. After leaving the coast of New Zealand'—f. 80v.

greater is the quantity of weed we see, what we see at the greatest distance is always in small pieces and generally covered with Barnacles and rotten; it was necessary to mention this otherwise conjectors might arise that some other large land lay in this neighbourhood. I say large land because it cannot be a small extent of Sea Coast that can produce such a quantity as to spread over such a large space of Sea. After leaving the land we continued for some days to have a large hollow [swell] from the SE untill we arrived in the Latitude of 46° Long^{de} 177° W where we had large billows from the North and NE[1] and which continued for the space of 5° of Longitude more to the East altho the wind generally blue from a contrary direction, this was a Strong indication that there was no land between us and my Track to the West in 1769. In short the wind never blew a fresh gale but what it brought before it a long hollow swell which never ceased with the wind which first put it in motion, which plainly shewed that we were never in the neighbourhood of any large land and this opinion I hold to this hour for this day at Noon we had a large western swell higher than usual which convinced me that there was no land between us and my former Track to the South from which we were distant 230 Leagues.[2]

TUESDAY 3*rd. Therm.r* 71. *Winds SW, West, WBN. Course North. Distce Sailed* 66 *Miles. Lat. in South* 22°8′. *Long. in West Reck.g.* 134°6′. *Long. made C. Pallisser* 49°51′. Gentle Breezes and clear pleasent Weather, got up all the Boatswains stores, cleaned and aired the Store rooms. Westerly swell much gone down. Variation p^{r} Azth 4°24′ E.

WEDNESDAY 4*th. Therm.r* 74. *Winds WBN to NW. Course NBE* ½ *E. Distce. Sailed* 53 *Miles. Lat. in South* 21°18′. *Long. in West Reck.g.* 133°48′. *Long. made C. Pallisser* 50°9′. PM Little Wind and clear weather, in the night had a few hours Calm which was succeeded by a breeze from the old quarter. Some Tropick Birds, and a bird like a land bird, seen.[3]

THURSDAY 5*th. Therm.r* 77. *Winds NWBN, NBW to NW. Course N* 60°30′ *E. Distce Sailed* 77 *Miles. Lat. in South* 20°40′. *Long. in West*

[1] ... for five days successively ... f. 81.

[2] *and this ... Leagues:* and that there is no Continent to the South, unless in a very high Latitude ... ff. 81, 85.

[3] 'This Morning a Bitch litter'd onboard when a young New Zealand Whelp fell too and had devour'd the best part of one of the Pups (very Characteristically) before he was detected, and then 'twas with many hard thumps that he was prevail'd upon to spare the Rest'.—Clerke. Clerke rewrites, but does not improve, this passage in Add. MS 8952, where however he adds, after 'Characteristically', 'as the New Zealanders are certainly Cannibals'.

Reck.g. 132°36′. *Long. made C. Pallisser* 51°21′. First and middle parts gentle gales and Clear weather, latter a brisk gale and clowdy. In the AM saw some flying fish.[1]

FRIDAY 6*th*. *Therm.r* 78. *Winds NW and WNW. Course N* 38° *E. Distce Sailed* 62 *Miles. Lat. in South* 19°46′. *Long. in West Reck.g.* 131°51′. *Watch* 132°30′. *Long. made C. Pallisser* 52°6′. PM gentle breezes and clear weather. Saw a gannet, some Egg birds and flying fish. AM Clowdy, hoisted out a boat and sent on board the Adventure, Captain Furneaux dined with us from whom I learnt that his people were much better, the flux having left them and Scurvy was at a stand, he having put in practice some of the methods I had proposed.[2]

SATURDAY 7*th*. *Winds NWBW, SW, Variable, Calm, SE. Course N* 58°30′ *W. Distce Sailed* 106 *Miles. Lat. in South* 18°51′. *Long. in West Reck.g.* 133°26′. *Long. made C. Pallisser* 50°31′. PM little wind and dark Clowdy weather till Six o'Clock when it fell calm with rain, the Calm at 8 o'Clock was succeeded by a fresh trade wind at SE[3] before which we steer'd WNW till 8 AM, then WBN½N as well to keep in the Strength of the trade wind as to get to the north of the Isles discovered by me last Voyage, that if any thing new laid in the way I might have a chance to discover it. Hazy weather with some showers of rain.[4]

[1] 'Nothing Remarkable has occurr'd these 24 hours, we begin to think the Winds use us rather hardly, and grow very anxious for the trade, more particularly upon account of our Fellow Adventurers in the other Ship who are very sickly.'—Clerke.

[2] . . . which together with Cyder and some other things he gave to the Scorbutick people had the desired effect.—f. 86. Later revision, f. 81v, deletes the words 'he having . . . proposed', and substitutes 'some Cyder, which he happened to have and which he gave to the Scorbutic people contributed not a little to this happy change'. Cf. Furneaux: 'we tried all the remedies that could be invented but found none of them to have any great effect, except the Wort, which if it did not cure prevented from growing worse'.—Add. MS 27890, f. 13v. Dr James Lind (1716–94) the great pioneer in the treatment of scurvy at sea, spoke well of cider in his *Treatise on Scurvy* (1754, 2nd ed. 1762), and it may well be that Furneaux had read the book.

[3] *PM . . . SE:* The Weather to day was cloudy, the Wind unsettled and seemed to announce the approach of the so much wished for Trade Wind which at 8 oClock in the Evening, after two hours Calm and some heavy showers of rain, we actually got at SE being at the time in the Longitude of 133°32′ West and in the Latitude of 18°46′ South, the not meeting with the SE trade Wind sooner is no new Thing in this Sea, I have had occasion more than once before now to make this observation.—f. 86. Cook's judgment about the winds was better than that of his shipmates, who expected the change from westerlies and north-westerlies rather earlier. The ship had been for some days in a rather uncertain area, but to pick up the steady south-east trade at this time in August was about normal. See Vol. I, Fig. 5. Some impatience, however, may be understood.

[4] 'About 8 [pm] in the midst of hard Rain thick Clouds &c &c the Trade wind paid us a visit—never was there a more welcome Guest.'—Clerke 8952.—ADV 'The Trade wind, gave much pleasure, having long expected it; and more so on acct of sickness on board.'—Kemp.—Burney, Ferguson MS, mentioning the arrival of the trade, goes on, 'Our Sickness is, I believe chiefly owing to our ships being greatly Lumber'd, the people have scarce room to stir below, & this is more sensibly felt, coming from a cold climate to

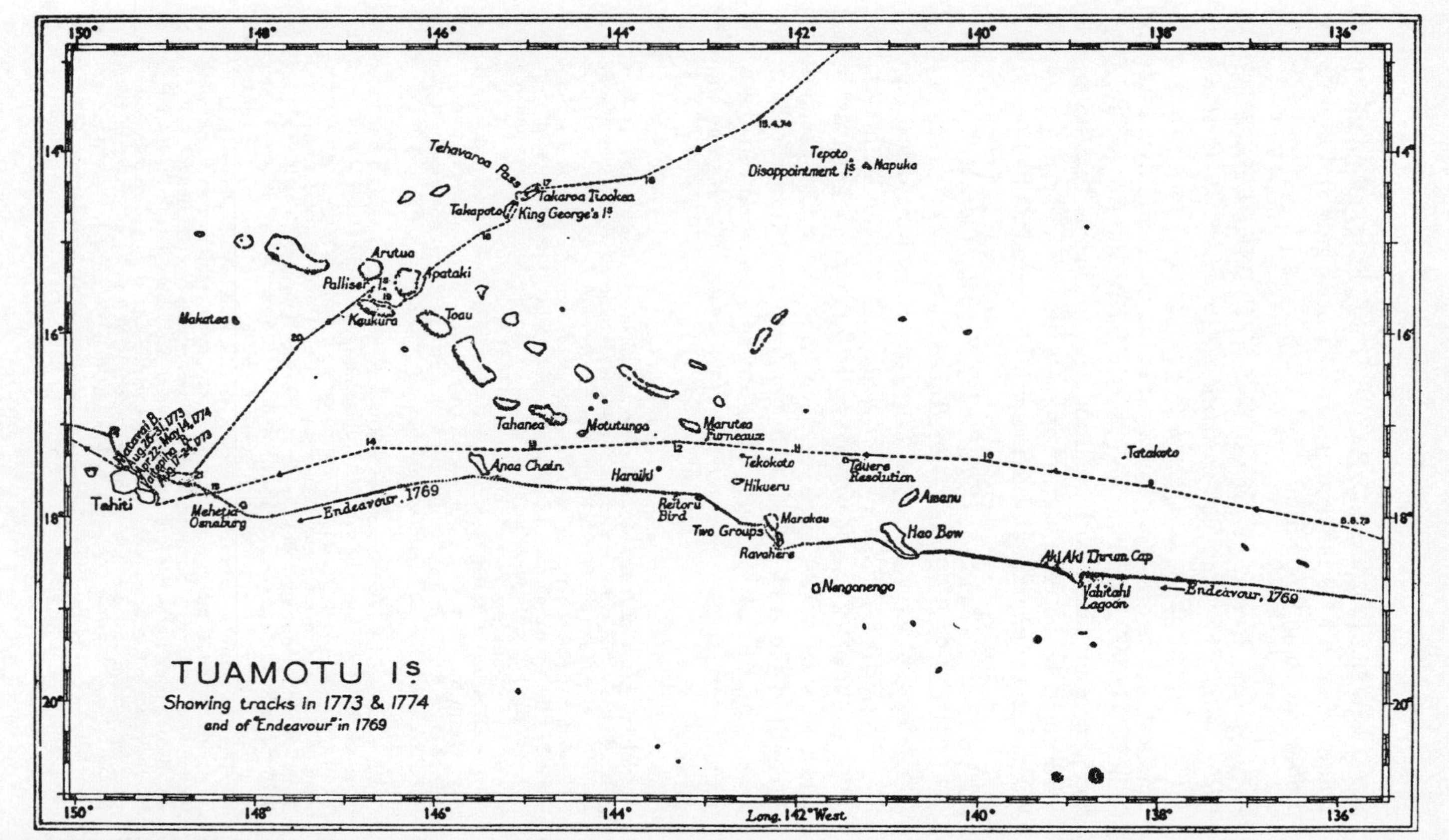

TUAMOTU Is.
Showing tracks in 1773 & 1774
and of "Endeavour" in 1769

SUNDAY 8*th. Winds SE. Course N* 72° *W. Distce Saild* 150 *Miles. Lat. in South* 18°5′. *Long. in West Reck.g* 135°57′. *Long. made C. Pallisser* 48°0′. Fresh Trade and pleasent weather with a following Sea.[1]

MONDAY 9*th. Winds ESE and EBS. Course N* 79° *W. Distce Saild* 126 *Miles. Lat. in South* 17°40′. *Long. in West Reck.g* 138°7′. *Long. made C. Pallisser* 45°50′. Do Weather, at 8 pm made the Signal for bringing to and brought too accordingly till 12 when the moon appear'd and then bore away under our Top-sails. At Day light made all sail. Saw many fish about the Ship but could catch none.[2] Bent the Cables and unstow'd the Anchors.

TUESDAY 10*th. Winds ESE and EBS. Course N* 80½ *W. Distce Saild* 106 *Miles. Lat. in South* 17°23′. *Long. in West Reck.g* 139°56′. *Watch* 140°19′. *Long. made C. Palliser* 44°1′. Fresh Trade with some showers of rain. Shortned sail during the night. Fish about the Ship as usual.[3]

WEDNESDAY 11*th. Winds East. Course N* 87½ *W. Distce Saild* 122 *Miles. Lat. in South* 17°18′. *Long. in West Reck.g* 142°3′ *Watch* 142°29′. *Long. made C. Pallisser* 41°54′. Gentle gales and fair weather. At 6 o'Clock in the morning land was seen to the Southward, we soon discovered it to be an Island about 2 Leagues in extent NW & SE, low and cloathed with wood above which the Cocoa-nutts shew'd their lofty heads. I beleive it to be one of the Isles discovered by M

a hot one. Our tedious passage has greatly contributed to depress their Spirits, especially as this was proposed when we left New Zealand, as a Cruize for refreshment. But the Trade Wind will, I hope be a good Doctor, & Otaheite an excellent Medicine Chest that will set us all to rights again. One of the Resolution's gentlemen says Nothing hurts him more than this Cruize being mentioned as a party of Pleasure, if, says he, they had put it down to the account of hard services, I had been content & thought myself well off, but to have it set down under the Article of Refreshment is d—d hard.' It is obvious that Cook, in ordering the ships away from Queen Charlotte Sound for a winter cruise in the south, had stressed not the uncomfortable part of the passage, but the pleasanter prospects at the end of it.

[1] 'The much wished for, and long-expected Trade-Winds seem now to have joined us. Our hopes began to grow very sanguine yesterday fore-noon for about 10 oClock AM a thick haze began to rise in the Eastern quarter, and by noon was so thick & high that I could not see the sun at times. We had had exceeding fine clear weather all the time that the NW winds prevailed.'—Wales. Perhaps it was the strain of the wind that caused the casualty to which Cooper refers: 'The foretopmt Steerings[l] yard broke which tore off the head of the Sail. Reeft & Set the Maintopmt Steeringsail forward'.

[2] *At Day light . . . none:* During the day time we made all the Sail we could but in the night either run under an easy sail or lay too, we daily saw flying fish Albacores Dolphins &ca but could catch none neither by striking nor with hook and line, it requires some art to catch these fish which none of us were masters of.—ff. 81v–2, 86.

[3] 'Spoke the Adventure & Bore away, they gave us the disagreeable information of their people being much worse.'—Cooper. ADV 'The Number of the Sick daily increases—there are now 28 in the List—which is more than one third of the Ships Company'.—Burney log.

de Bougainville (Latitude 17°24′ Longitude 141°39′ West).[1] The Scorbutic state of the Adventures Crew made it necessary for me to make the best of my way to Otaheite where I was sure of finding refreshments for them, concequently I did not wait to examine this Island which appear'd too small to supply our wants.

THURSDAY 12*th. Therm.r* 78. *Winds East. Course N* 85°30′ *W. Distce Sailed* 90 *Miles. Lat. in South* 17°11′. *Long. in West Reck.g* 143°38′ *Watch* 144° 4′. *Long. made C. Pallisser* 40°19′. Gentle breezes and clear weather. At 6 o'Clock in evening land was seen from the Mast head bearing west and by South, probably this was a nother of M. de Bougainville's isles.[2] We steer'd more to the north in order to avoid it and stood on under an easy sail all night, at day break in the morn, land was seen right a head not farther from us than two miles, this proved to be another low Island or rather a large shoal of about 20 Leagues in circuit, the firm land occupied but a small part of this space and laid in little Islets along the north side and connected to each other by the reef as is usual with these low Islands, this reef extended out from each extreme of the Islets in a circular form encircling a large Bason of Water in which was a Canoe under sail. As this Island which is situated in the Latitude 17°5′ s, Longitude 143°16′ w has no place in the Maps I named it .[3]

*[4]At Day break the next Morning We discovered land right a head, distant about two miles a proof that day light advised us of our

[1] 'it hath no reef or shoal off it as we could see, probably these as is usual lay on the south side consequently hid out of sight as we pass'd at the Distance of six miles north of it.'—Log. In the printed *Voyage* (I, p. 141) it is called Resolution Island: it is in fact Tauere, lat. 17°23′s, long. 141°30′w. Its first discoverer was not Bougainville, but Don Domingo de Boenechea, in the *Aguila*, on the Spanish voyage to Tahiti, 28 October 1772 (Corney, I, pp. 286–7). Cf. Clerke: '. . . this Sea abounds in these little paltry Islands from the latitudes of 8° or 10° to those of 18° or 20°. We saw many of them in the Dolphin and some in the Endeavour nearly in this Longitude. We landed upon some of them in the Dolphin and found abundance of Cocoa Nuts which I think is the only fruit they produc'd; they are very low and render the Navigation here in the Night dangerous, for there are Coral Reefs about them which wou'd with great difficulty be discover'd by Night, unless exceedingly well enlighten'd by the Moon'. See Fig. 33.

[2] . . . and lies in the Latitude of Longitude . I was sorry I could not spare time to haul to the North of Mr Bougainvilles discoveries, but the geting to a place where we could procure refreshments, was more an object at this time than discovery.—f. 82–2v.—In the printed *Voyage* (I, p. 141) this is called Doubtful Island. It is Tekokoto, and Cook was the first discoverer.

[3] No name is given in B; in the printed *Voyage* (I, p. 142) it is called Furneaux Island. It is Marutea, lat. 17°15′s, long. 143°04′w, one of the most dangerous atolls in the Tuamotu archipelago. Cook's description is accurate: cf. *Pacific Islands Pilot*, III, p. 103, 'the reef on the south-western side is almost entirely submerged, and on the north-eastern side there are only a few places where the reef is sufficiently above water to support any vegetation'.

[4] There are two versions of the following passage from B, ff. 82v–3 and ff. 86v–7v. I print the first, as probably the earlier written; it has passages not in the second, and corresponds quite closely with G.

danger but just in time. This proved another of these low or half drowned islands, or rather a large Coral Shoal of about 20 Leagues in Circuit a very small part of which was land, which consisted of little islots ranged along the North side and connicted to each other by Sand banks and breakers. These islots were cloathed with wood among which the Cocoanutt trees were only distinguishable. We ranged the South side of this isle, or Shoal, at the distance of one or two miles from the Coral bank, against which the Sea broke in a dreadfull surf; in the Middle is a large lake or inland Sea in which was a Canoe under sail. This Isle lies in the Latitude of 17°5′, Longitude 143°16′ W. The Situation is nearly the same as is assigned for one of those discover'd by Bougainville.[1] I must here observe, that amongst these low and half drowned isles, (which are numerous in this part of the ocean) Mr Bougainville's discoveries cannot be known to that degree of accuracy which is necessary to distinguish them from others, we are obliged to have recourse to his Chart for the Latitudes and Longitudes of the isles he saw and Otaheite, the only one he saw whose Situation is will known, is laid down 15 or 20 Miles too far to the North.[2] I cannot say if this error is in the original Chart, I have only had an oppertunity to consult the one in the English Edition. Be this as it will, what excuse can M. de Bougainville have for not once mentioning the Situation of any one place in his whole run through this Sea: this is what he seems carefully to have avoided, for reason[s] which can only be known to himself. Had he continued to make the same judicious Nautical remarks he has done in the Straits of Magelhanes, which he seems to have been very capable of, his narrative would, not only, have been the most entertaining, but the most usefull of any yet published. Without waiting to examine this isle, we continued to steer to the West all Sails set, till 6 oClock in the evening when we shortned Sail to the three Top-sails and at 9 brought-to.

FRIDAY 13*th*. At 4 AM made sail and at day-break, saw a nother of these low isles, situated in the Latitude of 17°04′, Longitude 144°36′ W. M. de Bougainville very properly calls this cluster of low over-flowed Isles, the dangerous Archipelago, the smoothness

[1] . . . and if it be one of them than it could not be land which we saw last night indeed we were very doubtfull about it at the time it was supposed to be seen.—f. 86v.

[2] The text of the MS here is confused, through incomplete deletion, or deletion over which Cook changed his mind. I print the version copied in G. In this Cook deletes the words 'saw and . . . known, is' but not the remainder of the sentence (which comes at the head of f. 83), so that the MS reads, 'the isles he discovered as neither the one nor the other is mentioned in his Narrative laid down 15 or 20 Miles too far to the North'. On f. 87 he goes back to his original, with the difference of a word or two.

of the Sea sufficiently convinced us that we were surrounded by them, and how necessary it was to proceed with the utmost caution, especially in the night.*—ff. 82v–83.

FRIDAY 13*th. Winds East. Course S* 86° *W. Lat. in South* 17°16′. *Long. in West Reck.g.* 144°54′ *Watch* 145°20′. *Long. made C. Pallisser* 39°3′. *Varn.* 6°48′. We continued to advance to the West all sails set till 6 o'Clock in the pm when we shortne'd sail to the three Top-sails, at 9 we brought too with our heads to the South[1] till 4 AM when we bore away under our Top-sails and at day-light discovered a nother low Island bearing N½W distant 3 or 4 Leagues.[2] It was lucky we brought too in the night for if we had not we must have been embarrass'd with this Island which is situated in the Latitude of 17°4′ south Longitude 144°36′ West and appear'd to be of too little concequence to devert me from my intended course. We have had a smooth sea sence we came among the Islands.[3]

SATURDAY 14*th. Winds East. Course W* 0°30′ *N. Distce Sailed* 102 *Miles. Lat. in South* 17°15′. *Long. in West Reck.g.* 146°41′ *Watch* 147°8′. *Long. made C. Pallisser* 37°16′. At 5 o'Clock in the pm saw land extending from WSW to SW dist[t] 3 or 4 Leagues. I judged it to be Chain Island discovered in my last Voyage.[4] Fearing to fall in with some of these low Islands in night and being desirous of avoiding the delay which lying too occasions I hoisted out the Cutter, equiped her properly and sent her a head to carry a light with proper signals to direct the Sloops in case she met with danger,[5] in this manner we

[1] '. . . it being too dark to run when we had reason to apprehend ourselves in the neighbourhood of some of those confounded low Islands.'—Clerke.

[2] The naming of this inconsiderable atoll seems to have given Cook considerable thought. H: 'as I looked upon this to be a new discovery I nam'd it *Stephens Isle,* in honour of *M[r] Stephens Secretary to y[e] Admty*'—the italicized words being supplied by Cook in blank spaces left for the purpose. B f. 87 first alters this to '. . . I named it Sandwich Isle, in honour of my Noble patron'; which version then becomes, by a process of imperfect deletion and addition, '. . . Harveys Isle, in honour of my Honourable friend Capt Harvey [Hervey]'. In f. 83 there is no mention of a name; nor in G. In the printed *Voyage* (I, p. 142) it is called Adventure Island. Wales has a neat little chart, in which it is named, more romantically, The Devil's Girdle. It is Motu Tunga or Tu'a—depending on one's dialect.

[3] *We have . . . Islands:* M de Bougainville very properly called this cluster of low and overflowed islands the dangerous archipelago, the smoothness of the Sea sufficiently convinced us that we were surrounded on every side by them and how necessary it was to proceed with the utmost caution especially in the night.—f. 87–7v.

[4] Anaa, lat. 17°21′ S, long. 145°31′ W; I, p. 72.

[5] *Fearing . . . danger:* extending from SW to WSW distant 4 Leagues. I believe this to be the most western isle in this archipelago of low Islands in the lattitud[e] we were now in (viz) 17°15′, but as I was not sure of it and being disireous of avoideing the delay which lying by in the night occasioned, I hoisted out the Cutter, maned her with a Lieutenant midshipman and Seven men and ordered her to carry a light at her mast head and to keep as far a head of the Sloops as signals could be distinguished which she was to make in case she met with danger . . .—f. 87v. These nights were moonless, as Clerke notes, 14 August.

proceeded all night without meeting with any thing, at 6 in the morning I called her on board and hoisted her in as it did not appear that she would be wanted again for this purpose, as we had now a large swell from the South a sure indication that we were clear of the low Islands.[1]

SUNDAY 15*th*. *Winds EBN. Course S* 71°45′ *W. Distce Sailed* 95 *Miles. Lat. in South* 17°45′. *Long. in West Reck.g.* 148°16′ *Watch* 148°34′. *Long. made C. Pallisser* 35°41′. *Varn.* 5°10′. Gentle breezes and pleasent weather. At 5 am saw Osnaburg Island bearing SBW½W.[2] At 9 o'Clock I sent for Captain Furneaux on board to acquaint him that I intended to put into Oaiti-peha Bay in the SE end of Otaheite[3] in order to get what refreshment we could from that part of the Island before we went down to Matavai Bay. At Noon Osnaburg Island bore ESE distent 5 or 6 Leagues. Swell from the Southward still continues.

At 6 PM saw the Island of Otaheite extending from WBS to WNW distant about 8 Leagues.[4] We stood on till midnight then brought too till 4 o'Clock when we made sail in for the land. I had given directions in what possision the land was to be kept but by some mistake it was not properly attended to for when I got up at break of day I found we were steering a wrong course and were not more than half a league from the reef which guards the South end of the Island. I immidiately gave orders to haul off to the Northward and had the breeze of wind which we now had continued we should have gone clear of every thing, but the wind soon died away and at last flatened to a Calm. We then hoisted out our Boats but even with their assistance the Sloops could not be kept from nearing the reef, but the current seem'd to be in our favour, we were in hopes of geting round the point of the reef into the Bay. At this time many of the natives were on board the Sloops and about them in their canoes, bring[ing] off

[1] . . . and therefore Steered for Otaheite without being apprehensive of meeting with any danger.—f. 83v.

[2] . . . This isle was first discovered by Captain Wallis, it is called by the Natives Maitea. —f. 83v., note. Now Mehetia.

[3] Strictly speaking, and thinking in terms of a large-scale chart, on the NE corner of the peninsula of Taiarapu or Tahiti-iti, which forms the south-eastern part of Tahiti.

[4] It should be noted that this was at 6 p.m. on *Monday* 16th, ship time, Cook having omitted the day and date.—ADV '. . . in the evening we made the east end of Otaheite, being so sickly we were obliged to have men from the Resolution to work the Ship.'—Furneaux, Add. MS 27890, f. 14. Furneaux's journal for 16 August notes '30 Men in the Sick List with the Scurvy and but few others without Scorbutic complaints'; 'very few,' says Burney, 15 August. Bayly, 13 August, has it 'tho' only 3 or 4 that are very bad the rest being lightly afflicted': not so lightly, as we gather from Furneaux, that they were of much use in the ship.

with them some fruit and fish which they exchanged for Nails, Beeds, &c^a^.[1]

TUESDAY 17*th*. About 2 o'Clock in the PM we came before an opening in the reef by which I hoped to enter with the Sloops as our situation became more and more dangerous, but when I examined the natives about it they told me that the Water was not deep and this I found upon examination,[2] it however caused such an indraught of the Tide

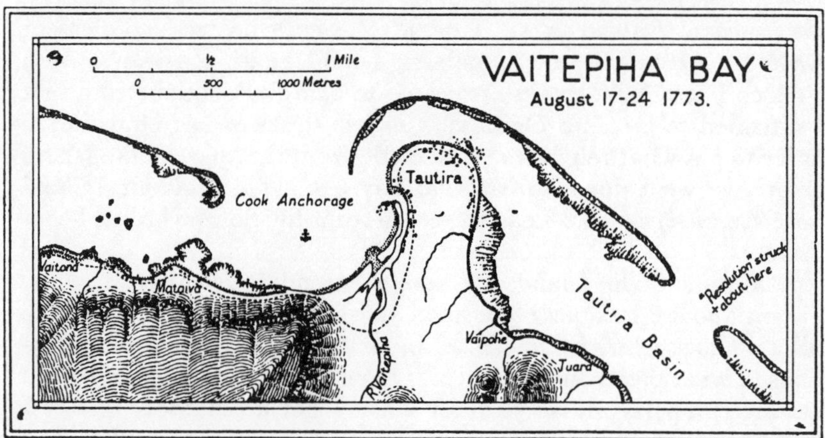

FIG. 34

as was very near proving fatal to both the Sloops, the Resolution especially, for as soon as the Sloops came into this indraught they were carried by it toward the reef at a great rate; the moment I preceived this I order'd one of the Warping Machines which we had in readiness to be carrid out with about 3 or 4 hundred fathoms of rope to it, this proved of no service to us, it even would not bring her head to Sea. We then let go an anchor as soon as we could find bottom but by such time as the Ship was brought up she was in less then 3 fathom water[3] and Struck at every fall of the Sea which broke

[1] . . . The most of them knew me again and many enquired for Mr Banks and others who were with me before, but not one asked for Tupia.—f. 84.—'An incredible number of the Natives round the Ship in their boats all loaded with Cocoa-Nuts, Plantains, Apples and other fruits, which we purchased for Beads, nails &c. It is impossible to express how agreeable these fruits are to us who had not tasted any thing of the kind since we left the Cape of Good Hope.'—Wales.

[2] '. . . there being an Opening in the Reef, Captn Cook sent a Boat in to See if there was a passage Navigable for the Ships to get through within the Reef, but found no more than 12 foot depth . . .'—Burney.

[3] *We then . . . water:* The horrors of ship-wreck now stared us in the face, we were not more than two Cables length from the breakers and yet we could find no bottom to anchor, the only means we had left us to save the Ships; we however droped an anchor but before it took hold and brought us up, the Ship was in less than 3 fathom water.—ff.

with great violence against the reef close under our stern and threatened us every moment with ship-wreck, the Adventure anchored close to us on our starboard bow and happily did not touch.[1] We presently carried out a Kedge Anchor and a hawser and the Coasting Anchor with an 8 inch Hawser bent to it, by heaving upon these and cuting away the Bower Anchor we saved the Ship; by the time this was done the currant or Tide had ceased to act in the same direction and then I order'd all the Boats to try to tow off the Resolution, as soon as I saw it was practical we hove up the two small anchors. At that moment a very light air came of from the land which with the assistance of the Boats by 7 o'Clock gave us an offing of about 2 Miles and I sent all the Boats to the assistance of the Adventure, but before they reached her she had got under sail with the land wind, leaving behind her three anchors, her coasting Cable and two Hawsers which were never recovered: thus the Sloops were got once more into safety after a narrow escape of being Wrecked on the very Island we but a few days ago so ardently

84–4v, 88–8v. A G and H have this same passage, except that they read 'Sloop' for 'Ship'; the trivial alteration was made—one supposes merely for consistency with the rest of the journal—from the original reading of B f. 88v.

[1] We may now attempt to localize more precisely wha had happened. On Monday morning when Cook came on deck the ship must have been off the reef somewhere on the east side of Taiarapu or Tahiti-iti; because this part of it ends—at least visibly—just beyond the islet of Tiere (see I, p. 109); and it does not emerge again till beyond the cliffs of Pari, round the SE point of the island. Forster (I, p. 258), though no one else, says Cook sent a boat to sound the Vaiurua or Aiurua passage, which is not far north of this point. This is where the Spanish *Aguila* entered in 1772. By 2 p.m. on Tuesday (still Monday 16th, civil time, as in the printed *Voyage*) he had worked north beyond the Vaionifa passage, which would have given him a fairly safe entry into the 'Tautira Basin'—if he had then been worried about his position—to a break in the reef something under two thirds of the way up from the Vaionifa passage to Tautira Point. This is unnamed; it is truly a break in the reef and not a passage through, though about 400 yards wide; and this is the opening Cook refers to and sent the boats to look at. It has mostly about 10 feet of water on it, but 13 or 14 at its southern edge; and here it was, at this depth, that the *Resolution* probably struck. Forster writes as if the ship remained outside the Vaiurua passage, and struck there (pp. 258–61), and, later (p. 269) says specifically 'The launches of both ships were sent to *o Whai-urua*, to fetch the anchors which we had left there when we struck on the reef'. I find this, like his account of the boat attempting to trade ashore (p. 258) difficult to reconcile with Cook, or with Pickersgill's 'in this manner we continued driveing along the reef . . .'. Cf. also Corney, III, p. 94, n. 2. Wales adds some vividness to the predicament when the ship did strike: 'To add to our Misfortune the Adventure was not above a Cable's length of setting directly down upon us at a great rate. . . . All this time the ship continued to strike so hard that it was [with] difficulty some times that we kept on our legs, and continued to do so all the time we were heaving on the stream Cable, untill it was almost directly up and down, when she ceased to do so. We were obliged to ride so for some time, expecting every moment the stream anchors would come home, and turn our attention to, if possible a more allarming circumstance than the former. The Adventure who was now not 20 Yards from us had let go her Anchors, and yet drove; but fortunately, when she was not more than Ten Yards from the Resolution She brought up and did not swing aboard of us; the two Ships riding along side of each other so near that a tolerable Plank would have reached from her Gunnel to ours.' I conclude from Corney, III, p. 156, n. 2, that the name of the district off which the break in the reef lay was then Araheru.

wished to be at.[1] We spent the night[2] making short boards and in the morning stood in for Oaiti-peha Bay where we anchor'd about Noon in 12 fathom water about 2 Cables length from the shore and moor'd with our stream anchors,[3] both Sloops being by this time surrounded by a great number of the natives in their Canoes, they brought with them Cocoa-nutts, Plantans, Bananoes, Apples, yams and other roots which they exchanged for Nails and Beeds. To Several who call'd themselves *arree's* (Chiefs) I made presents of Shirts, Axes and various other articles and in return they promised to bring me Hogs and Fowls, a promise they neither did nor never intended to perform.

WEDNESDAY 18*th*.[4] In the PM I landed in company with Captain Furneaux in order to examine the Watering place and sound the disposision of the Natives. The latter I found to behave with great Civility and the latter[5] as convenient as could be expected, we also got of some Water for present use, having scarce any left on board. Early in the morning I detached the two Launches and the Resolutions Cutter under the command of Mr Gilbert to endeavour to recover the Anchors we had lost, they return'd about noon with the

[1] We get a prim little paragraph from Sparrman: 'Even in my anxiety . . . I drew no small satisfaction from remarking the celerity and the lack of confusion with which each command was executed to save the ship. . . . I should have preferred, however, to hear fewer "Goddamns" from the officers and particularly the Captain, who, while the danger lasted, stamped about the deck and grew hoarse with shouting. I have sailed with captains capable of imposing the most perfect obedience and the most delicate manoeuvres without swearing, and I am convinced that under the circumstances in which we found ourselves the same results could have been achieved with fewer oaths'. He distributed speaking trumpets 'to those officers who appeared to me most efficient in handling the vessel. They thanked me for my idea which, indeed, had been the means of doing them a great service, but that'—he adds modestly—'was the only active part I played in the operations'.—Sparrman, pp. 51–2. He gives us another interesting side-light on Cook: 'As soon as the ship was once more afloat, I went down to the Ward Room with Captain Cook who, although he had from beginning to end of the incident appeared perfectly alert and able, was suffering so greatly from his stomach that he was in a great sweat and could scarcely stand. It was, indeed, hardly remarkable that, after so great a responsibility and so prodigious a strain on both his mental and physical capacities, he should be completely exhausted'. Sparrman got him to try 'an old Swedish remedy'—a good dose of brandy, and he rapidly recovered.—ibid., p. 52.

[2] . . . which proved squally and rainy . . .—f. 89.

[3] The reef runs parallel with the outer line of Tautira Point, to break off where the point curves into the bay and the influence of the Vaitepiha river is felt. The break, of about 1200 yards, gives a deep as well as wide entrance to this bay; Cook's anchorage—still shown on the French chart as *mouillage de Cook*—was on the eastern side of the bay. Cook got his name for the bay from the river; and he must have marked it down as a promising anchorage when he passed that way on his circuit of Tahiti, 27 June 1769 (see I, p. 108). See Fig. 34.

[4] 'Dyed Isaac Taylor a Marine of a consumptive disorder having been unwell ever since we left England.'—Gilbert. The body was taken out to sea and buried next day at sun-set; a melancholy parallel with Buchan's death and burial on the arrival of the *Endeavour* in 1769.

[5] *sic;* i.e. former

Resolutions Bower Anchor but could not recover the Adventures. The Natives crowded about us as yesterday with fruits &c[a] but in no great quantity. I had also a party tradeing on shore under the Protection of a Guard,[1] nothing however but fruit and roots were offered to us tho many Hogs were seen (as I was told) about the Habitations of the natives, the cry was they all belonged to *Oheatooa* the Arree dehi or King[2] and him we could not see or any other Chief of note, many however came on board who call'd themselves Arrees partly with a view of obtaining presents and partly to have an oppertunity to pilfer whatever came in their way, one of these sort of Arrees I had most of the day in the Cabbin, made him and all his friends, which were not a few, presents, at last he was caught takeing things which did not belong to him and handing them out of the quarter Gallery, many complaints of the like kind were made to me against those on deck which induced me to turn them all out of the Ship; my Cabbin guest made good haste to be gone, I was so exasperated at his behaver that after he had got a good distance from the Ship I fired two Musquet balls over his head which made him quet his Canoe and take to the Water. I then sent a boat to take up the Canoe, as soon as she came near the shore the people from thence began to pelt her with stones, the Boat still persuing the Canoe and being unarm'd I began to be in pain for her safety and went my self in another boat to protect her and order'd a 4 pounder to be fire'd a long the Coast, this made them all retire back from the shore and suffered me to bring away two Canoes without the least shew of opposision[3] and in a few hours after the People were as well reconciled as if nothing had happen'd. The Canoes I return'd to the first person who ask'd for them.[4] It was not untill the Evening of this

[1] ADV 'Read to the Ship's Company an order from Cap[t] Cook, prohibiting any person to trade with the Natives, without his knowledge, whome he may Appoint, & them not give Knives Nails or hard Ware . . .'—Lightfoot. This order, though not very lucidly expressed by Mr Lightfoot, is yet plain enough in its intention. Burney, Ferguson MS, has the text. The natives were to be shown 'every kind of civility and regard'; iron tools and nails were to be exchanged only for provisions; no curiosities were to be bought before the need for provisions was satisfied; and (one of Cook's cardinal principles) 'All provisions and other refreshments procured by any person whatever & not consumed on shore, shall be brought publickly on the Quarter Deck & afterwards distributed out in such a manner as circumstances shall make appear most equitable'. To what extent Cook thought these rules would be obeyed, after his *Endeavour* experience, is doubtful, but no doubt they would have some effect, and were therefore essential.

[2] i.e. Vehiatua the *arii rahi* or *arii nui*, 'high chief' of the Seaward Teva clan of Taiarapu.

[3] . . . in one of the canoes was a little boy who was much frightened but I soon dissapated his fears by giving him beads and puting him on shore.—ff. 89v–90.

[4] We get a 'shore view' of all this excitement from Bayly, who was delighted to walk on dry land once more: 'After dinner I went on shore again & walked along Shore a great way in Comp[y] with too of our Gent[n]—at about 4 PM heard a Musket fired from on board the Ships, & a second & the Natives on the beach seemed in great Consternation & talking

day[1] that any one enquired after Tupia[2] and as soon as they learnt the cause of his death they were quite satisfied, indeed it did not appear to me that it would have caused a moments uneasiness in the breast of any one had his death been occasioned by any other means than by sickness; as little enquiry was made after *Aotourou* the man M. de Bougainville to[ok] away with him, but they were constantly asking after Mr Banks and many others of the Gentlemen and people that were with me last voyage. These people informed us that *Toutaha*, King of the greater Kingdom of Otahiete was kill'd in a Battle which happen'd between the two Kingdoms about five months ago and that Otou was now the Reigning Prince. Tiboura and several more of our principal friends about Matavai fell in the same Battle and likewise a great number of Common people, at present a peace subsisted between the two Kingdoms.[3]

THURSDAY 19*th*. Gentle breezes with some smart showers of rain. Early in the morning I sent the Boats again to take up the Adventures anchors, but they return'd after as little success as the day before and we ceased looking for them any longer.[4] In an excursion

to each other in great disorder & begun to arm them-selves with sticks, but soon after the report of a 4 Pounder together with the whistling of the Shot right up the shore where I was, terified the Indians so much that they all fled for the Mountains in the greatest terror Immaginable, & as we were returning we met great Numbers of them which endeavoured to avoid us as much as possible, frequently laying down among the reeds til we had passed them & then get up & run as fast as possible towards the hills . . . when I came down to the beach I learned that the Indians had stole many things on board the Resolution, & in particular An Aree or Chief had siezed some Silver spoons ['a knife and a pewter spoon' says Forster] & immediately leaped over board with them, & swam a shore but his Canoe which was a large double one was Siezed & some of his Attendance, but were all released soon, & the Canoe given them again the next Morning.'

[1] Here, it appears, Cook has slipped insensibly into civil time, unless he has leapt right back to the 'PM' with which this entry begins—which seems unlikely. In the next entry he goes over deliberately to civil time, beginning with the employment of the morning—and maintains it till 17 September; after which, on sailing from Raiatea, he reverts to ship time.

[2] . . . and then but two or three;

[3] The misapprehensions in this passage will be plain to the reader of the Note on Polynesian History in I, pp. clxxvii ff. Tuteha ('Toutaha') had not been king of the 'greater kingdom', nor was Tahiti divided into two 'kingdoms': an important and influential chief, he had virtually run the affairs of Tu ('Otoo'), whose rank, though not ability, was higher than his own. The battle against Vehiatua of Taiarapu (Tahiti-iti or 'Little Tahiti') was in March 1773. 'Tiboura' (B 'Toubourai Tamaide') was Tepau i Ahurai Tamaiti, another extremely important chief of the western districts of Tahiti-nui ('Greater Tahiti'). The death of this man and Tuteha gave scope to Tu, who got away alive; although not yet 'Reigning Prince', except in his own district, he may already have begun to dream of the aggrandisement which did make him a 'king' before he died.

[4] '. . . at noon ye boats returnd not being Able to recover one of ye Anchors, our loss on this Occasion was only a few fathms of Cable & about 150 fathm of 3 Inch rope ye Adventures loss was greater being her coastg Anchor and cable two Kedge Anchors and as Many Hawsers. When I consider ye Dangerous situation we were in I cannot but think my self happy in coming off so well. Ceased serving Bread, peas & Wheat to ye Ships Company'.—Log.

I made along shore to the SW accompanied by Cap^n^ Furneaux we met with a Chief who entertained us with excellent fish and fruit, in return for his hospitality we made him sever^l^ presents[1] and he afterwards accompanied us to the Ship where he made but a short stay. Fruit and roots sufficient for both Sloops[2] but no Hogs, those that were lately in the adjacent house are carried off.

FRIDAY 20*th*. Nothing worthy of note happened till the Dusk of the evening when one of the Natives made off with a musquet belonging to the Guard,[3] I was present when this happen'd and sent two or three of our people after him, this would have signified but little had not some of the natives themselves pursued the thief, knock'd him down and took from him the Musquet and return'd it to us; fear in this affair certainly actuated more with them than principle, they however deserve to be apploaded for this act of Justice for if the Musquet had not been recovered by them in the manner it was it would not have been in my power to have recovered it by any gentle means whatever.[4]

SATURDAY 21*st*. Wind at North a fresh breeze. A Chief whose name was made me a viset this morning and brought with him a present of fruit a mong which were a number of Cocoa nutts we had drawn the Water from and then threw them over board, which he had picked up and tyed in bundles,[5] when he was told that he had imposed on me, he without betraying the least emotion and as if he was perfectly ignorant of the cheat opened two or three himself, signified that it was so[6] and then went on shore and sent off a quantity of Plantans and Bananoes. Having got on board a supply of fruit, roots and Water, I determined to sail in the morning for Matavai Bay as I found it was not likely I should get an interview of King Oheatooa without which I found it not possible for us to get any Hogs, two of the natives knowing my intintion slept on board board with a view of going with us to Matavai.

SUNDAY 22*nd*. The Wind blowing a fresh gale at NW right into the Bay made it impractical for us to get to sea, I therefore sent the trading party a shore to purchase refreshments as usual. In the

[1] *made . . . presents:* made him a present of an ax and other things . . .—f. 90v.

[2] 'AM ceas'd serving Bread, Pease, Wheat & Oyl to the Ship's Comp^y^ on Account of the great Quantities of Fruit got here'.—Willis.

[3] . . . on shore

[4] *for . . . whatever:* for if they had not given their immidiate assistance it would hardly have been in my power to have recovered it by any gentle means whatever & by makeing use of any other I was sure to loose more than ten times the value of the musquet.

[5] . . . so artfully that we did not at first preceive the cheat

[6] *that it was so:* to us that he was satisfied it was so

Evening I was inform'd that Oheatooa was come to this Neighbourhood and wanted to see me, in concequence of this information I determined to wait one day longer in order to have an interview with this prince.

MONDAY *23rd.* Accordingly early the next morning I set out accompanied by Captain Furneaux some of the Gentlemen and several of the Natives, we met the Chief about a mile from the landing place towards which he was advancing to meet us but as soon as he saw us coming he halted in the open field not so much as under a tree. I found him seated upon a stool with a circile of People round him. I knew him at first sight and he me, having seen each other several times in 1769 at which time he was but a boy,[1] after the first salutation was over he seated me on the same stool with him self, the other gentlemen on the ground by us, and began to enquire after M[r] Banks and the other gentlemen he knew, he next enquired how long I would stay and when I told him no longer than the next day he seem'd sorry and ask'd me to stay some months and at last Five Days, promissing in that time I should have Hogs in plenty, but as we had been here a week without geting one I could not put much faith in this promise.[2] I presented him with a sheet, Broad Ax, several Spike Nails, Knives, Looking Glasses, Beeds, &c[a] and in return he sent a Hog[3] down to the Boat. We stayed with him all the Fore-noon and kept me constantly with him, we walked arm in arm, when he was seated I was seated on the same stool which was carried about from place to place by one of his attendance. We at length took leave of him to return on board to dinner, after which we Viseted him again, made him more presents, for which he gave Captain Furneaux and me each of us a large Hog, these together [with those] got by purchase were sufficient to give the crews of both Sloops a fresh meal.[4]

[1] When he was 13 or 14. Vehiatua was of course a titular name, and this young man was the son of the 'very old man with a white beard' of Cook's visit to Tautira in June 1769, and Banks's 'little olive liped boy Tiaree who called himself son of Waeatua and seemed to have much influence'. The date of the old man's death is uncertain—Corney (II, p. xxxv) argues with some cogency for 1771 or early 1772. His personal names we do not certainly know (cf. Corney, II, p. 335, n. 1); but the young man's name was Ta'ataurarua. He was a gentle amiable person, who was to live for only two years after this interview.

[2] . . . and yet I beleive if I had stayed we should have faired much better than at Matavai.—f. 91–IV.

[3] *a Hog:* a pretty good Hog

[4] '. . . got information of a Ship being in Owhaiurua Harbour about 4 Months ago were she stayed Twenty days she left one of her Men behind her who was seen to day by some of our people but he made off as soon as he found himself discovered they took him for a frenchman.'—Log. There had indeed been a ship at Vaiurua, Boenechea's *Aguila*,

TUESDAY 24*th*. In the Morning I put to Sea with a light land breeze which soon after we got out came to the Westward and blew in squals attended with heavy showers of rain. I left Lieutenant Pickersgill with the Cutter in the Bay to purchas Hogs as several had been promised to day.[1] Many Canoes followed us out to Sea with Cocoa-nutts and other fruits and did not leave us till they had disposed of their cargoes. The fruits we got here contributed greatly towards the recovery of the Adventures Sick many of whom were so weak when we put in as not to be able to get on deck without assistance were now so far recovered as to be able to Walk about of themselves, they were put ashore under the care of the Surgeons mate every morning and taken aboard in the evening. When we put in here the Resolution had only one Scorbutic person on board and a Marine that had been long ill and who died the 2nd day after our arival of a complication of disorders without the l[e]ast touch of the Scurvy.

WEDNESDAY 25*th*. This day was spent at sea by reason of variable light winds and Calms. A little before Noon Lieut^t^ Pickersgill Return'd with Eight Pigs which he got in Oaiti-peha the same morning we left it, he spent the night at [Ohidea] and was well entertained by [Ereti] the Chief of that district,[2] he let him know that he had no Hogs, but any thing else was at his service, it was remarkable that this Chief never once asked after Aotourou nor did he take the least notice when Mr Pickersgill mentioned his name.[3]

THURSDAY 26*th*. At 4 o'Clock in the PM we anchored in Matavai Bay after which I sent our Boats to assist the Adventure who got in about two hours after. At the time we anchored many of the natives came of to us, several of whom I knew and almost all of them me, a

which lay there from 19 November to 20 December 1772; Boenechea called his anchorage *Puerto de Santa Maria Magdalena*. But no man was left behind. See Wales's more extended account, pp. 792–3 below.

[1] *several . . . to day:* several had promised to bring some down to day and I was not willing to loose them.—f. 91v.

[2] See p. 768 below.

[3] . . . and yet this is the very chief which M. de Bougainville says presented Aotourou to him, which makes it the more extraordinary that he should neither enquire after him now or when he was with us at Matavai, especially as they beleived that M. Bougainville came from the same Country as we did, that is from Brittanee for so they call our Country for they had not the least knowlidge of any other European Country—nor probably will they unless some of those men should return who had lately gone from the isles of which mention shall be made by and by. We told several of them that M. de Bougainville came from France a name they could by no means pronounce nor could they that of Paris much better, so that it is not likely that they will remember either the one or the other long, whereas Pretane [altered from Brittanee] is in every childs mouth and will hardly ever be forgot.—f. 92

great crowd were got together on the shore among whom was King [Otoo].[1] I was just going to pay him a visit when I was told he was mataou'd[2] and gone to Oparre.[3] I could not conceive the reason of this Chief being frightned as every one seem'd pleased to see me, a chief whose name was Marritata[4] was at this time aboard and advised me to put of my Viset till the next morning when he would accompany me. Accordingly in the morning, after having given directions about erecting Tents for the reception of the Sick, Coopers and guard, I set out for Oparre accompanied by Captain Furneaux, some of the gentlemen, Maritata and his Wife, as soon as we landed we were conducted to Otoo who we found seated on the ground under the shade of a tree with a crowd[5] of People round him. After the first salutation was over I made him a present of such things as were in most esteem with them with which he seem'd well pleased,[6] I likewise made presents to several of his attendance and was offer'd in return a large quantity of Cloth which I refused giving them to understand that what I had given was for Tiyo[7] (friendship), the King inquired after Tupia and all the gentlemen that were with me last Voyage by name, altho I do not know that he was personally acquainted with any one or that he had ever been seen by any of us. He promised that we should have Hogs the next day, but I had a good deal to do to perswaid him to come to the Ship, he said he was Mataou Poupoue,[8] that is afraid of the Guns, indeed all his actions shew'd him to be a timerous Prince, he is about 30 or 35 years of age, six feet three inches high and is as fine a person as one can see. All his subjects appeared uncovered before him, even his Wife and Father[9] were not excepted.[10] When I return'd from Oparre I found the Tents set up on the same ground we had occupied when I was here before. Mr Wales and Baily also set up their

[1] The MS has a blank for the name of Otoo, or Tu, throughout the entries from this date to 1 September. To avoid clogging the text with a multiplicity of square brackets, I make this note, and hereafter omit them. For Tu's portrait, see Fig. 62*a*.

[2] *matau*, to fear, be frightened.

[3] Pare, to the west of Matavai.

[4] Maraetaata: probably an *arii* from Anuhi, the present district of Pueu. Cf. I, p. 107.

[5] *a crowd:* an immense crowd . . .—f. 92v.

[6] *as were . . . pleased:* as I knew were most valuable in his eyes, well knowing that it was my Intrest to gain the friendship of this Man.

[7] *taio*, friend.

[8] *matau no* [or *i*] *te pupuhi*.

[9] *Wife and Father:* Father.—A has a note to 'Wife', in Cook's hand: 'We afterwards found that this Woman was his Sister'. In B the words 'Wife and' are deleted; G 'his Father'. Tu had no full sister though three half-sisters; this may have been one of them or even a cousin. Forster gives her name as 'Tedua Towrai'—i.e. Tetua i te Ahurai, 'The Lady' te Ahurai, which was not the primary name of any of the half-sisters.

[10] .. . what is meant by uncovering is the bareing the head and shoulders or wearing no sort of cloathing above the breast.—f. 92v.

Instruments at the same place, I had the Sick land, Twenty from the Adventure and one from the Resolution, landed a sufficient number of men to guard the Whole and left the command to Lieut[t] Edgcombe of the Marines.[1]

FRIDAY 27*th*. Early in the Morning Otoo with a numerous trane paid me a Viset, he first sent into the Ship a quantity of cloth, a Hog, two large fish and a quantity of fruit and after some perswasions came in himself with his wife[2] a younger Brother and many others, to all of them I made presents and after breakfast[3] took the King[4] and as many of his attendance as I had room for in the Pinnace and carried them to Oparre the place of their residance. I had no sooner landed than I was met by a venerable old Lady mother of the late Toutaha, she seized me by both hands and brust into a flood of tears saying Toutaha Tiyo no Toute matte[5] (Toutaha the friend of Cook is dead). I was so much affected at her behavour that it would not have been possible for me to refrain mingling my tears with hers had not Otoo come and snatched me as it were from her, I afterwards disired to see her again in order to make her a present but he told me she was Mataou and would not come, I was not satisfied with this answer and desired she might be sent for, soon after she appeared I went up to her, she again wept and lamented the death of her son. I made her a present of an Ax and other things and then parted from her and soon after took leave of Otoo and return'd aboard. Captain Furneaux who was with me gave to the King two fine goats male and female which if properly taken care of[6] will no doubt multiply.

SATURDAY 28*th*. At 4 o'Clock in the morning I sent Lieut[t] Pickersgill with the Cutter as far as Attahourou[7] to endeavour to procure Hogs

[1] . . . Maritata and his Wife remained with me the most of the day, this Lady wanted neither youth nor beauty, nor was she wanting in useing those charms which nature had given her to the most advantage, she bestowed her caresses on me with the utmost profusion and before I could get clear of her I was obliged to satisfy all her demands, after which both she and her husband went away and I was never troubled with either the one or the other afterwards, she no doubt thought I should expect some other favours for the presents I had made her than bare caresses and this was what she never meant to bestow. —f. 93.

[2] wife *deleted* Sister *substituted*.

[3] 'The King paid great attention to our breakfast, which was a mixture of English and Tahitian provisions, and was much surprised to see us drink hot-water, and eat breadfruit with oil.'—Forster, I, p. 333. With an excess of pedantry, he identifies the hot water as tea, and the oil as butter. The Tahitians, says Sparrman (p. 66) enjoyed tasting the butter spread upon slices of roasted breadfruit; but it must have been pretty rancid stuff.

[4] and Queen *deleted* his Sister *substituted*.—Similar alterations are made in the next entry.

[5] *Tuteha taio no Tute mate*.

[6] *if . . . care of:* if taken care of or rather if no care attall is taken of them . . .—f. 93v.

[7] Atehuru: see I, pp. clxxx–xi. He seems to have gone to Punaauia.

and a little after Sunrise I had a nother Viset from Otoo he brought me more cloth, a Pig, a large fish and some fruit. The Queen who was with him and some of his attendance came aboard, but he and others went to the Adventure with the like present to Captain Furneaux, it was not long before he left the Adventure and came with Captain Furneaux on board the Resolution when I made him a hansome return for the present he brought me and dress'd the Queen out as well as I could, she, the King's brother and one or two more appear'd covered before him to day. When Otoo came aboard [Ereti][1] and one or two of his friends were siting in the Cabbin covered, the moment they saw the King enter they undress'd themselves in great haste, that is they put off their ahows[2] or clothes from of their Shoulders, seeing I took notice of it they said it was because the Arree was present, and this was all the respect they paid him for they never rose from their seats or paid him any other obeisence. When the King thought proper to depart I carried him again to Oparre in my Boat and entertained him with the Bag-pipes of which musick he[3] was very fond, and dancing by the Seamen; he in return ordered some of his people to dance also which dancing consisted chiefly in strange contortions of the Body, there were some of them that could however immitate the Seamen tollerable well both in Country dances and Horn pipes. While I was here I had a present of cloth from Toutaha's Mother, this good old Lady could not look upon me without sheding tears, tho she was more composed to day than before. When I took leave the chief[4] told me he shou'd viset me tomorrow but that I must come[5] to him. In the evening Mr Pickersgill return'd empty but with a promise of some in a few days.

SUNDAY 29*th*. After breakfast I took a trip to Oparre in my Boat accomp^d^ by Cap^n^ Furneaux and some of the Officers to viset Otoo as he had requested, we made him up a present of such things as he had not seen before, one article was a large Broad sword at the very sight of which he was so intimidated that I had enough to do to perswaid him to have it buckled upon [him] where it remaind but a short time before he asked permission to take it off and send it away,[6]

[1] This was Bougainville's Ereti (Reti, O Reti), of Hitiaa, whom Cook may have met in June 1769 (I, p. 105). Pickersgill had brought him to Matavai Bay. But Forster (p. 317) says it was Ereti's brother 'Tarooree'. Taruri was Ereti's wife's brother (Corney I, p. 315).

[2] *ahu*, a cloak or mantle.

[3] *he:* they

[4] *chief:* King

[5] *must come:* must first come

[6] . . . out of his sight . . .—f. 94.

after which we were conducted to the Theatre where we were entertain'd with a Dramatick Heava or Play in which were both Dancing and Comedy, the performers were five Men and one Women, which was the Queen,[1] the Musick consisted of three Drums only, it lasted about an hour and a half or two hours and upon the whole was well conducted; it was not possible for us to find out the meaning of the Play, some parts of it seem'd to [be] adapted to the present time as my name was mentioned several times, other parts were certainly wholy unconnected with us. It apparently differed in nothing, at least the manner of acting, from those we saw at Ulietea in my last Voyage, the dancing dress of the Queen[2] was more elegant than any I saw there by being set off or decorated with long [tasles] made of feathers hanging down from the waste. As soon as the whole was over the King himself desired me to depart and ordered into the Boat different sorts of fruit and some dress'd fish with which we took leave and return'd aboard.

MONDAY 30*th*. The next Morning he sent me more fruit and several small parcells of fish. About 10 o'Clock in the evening we were alarmed by a great noise a Shore near the Bottom of the Bay at some distance from our incampment. I suspected that it was occasioned by some of our people and sent an Officer with an Arm'd Boat a shore to know what was the matter and to bring off such of our people as he should find their. I also sent to the Adventure and to the Post on shore to know what people were missing,[3] the Boat soon return'd with three Marines and a Seaman who belonged to the party on shore, some others belonging to the Adventure were also taken, all of them put in Irons and the next morning I ordered them to be punished according to their [deserts].[4]

TUESDAY 31*st*. I did not find that any Mischief was done, our people would confess nothing altho some of them were heard to call out Murder several times,[5] the Natives were however so much allarmed

[1] *which . . . Queen:* and this was no less than the King's sister

[2] *Queen:* Lady

[3] . . . for none were absent from the Resolution but those whose duty laid on shore.—f. 94v.

[4] . . . ye Officer I had sent on shore returned with Geo: Woodward, John Buttall Marines Em^{l} Peterson seaman & David Ross a Marine belonging to ye Adventure, I order'd them all in Irons & ye next morning punished ye Marines with 18 lashes each & ye seaman with one dozen & order'd Captn Furneaux to punish such of his people as were concern'd in this riott.—Log 31 August. The charge, says Clerke, was absenting themselves from duty and quarrelling with the natives. Cooper gives the note for the afternoon before, 'Punish'd John Marra Gunner's Mate with 6 lashes for Insolence'.

[5] . . . I believe this disturbance was occasioned by their makeing too free with the Women, be this as it will . . .—f. 94v.

that they fled from their habitations in the dead of the night and[1] when I went to viset Otoo in the morning by appointment I found him many Miles removed from the place of his aboad and it was some time[2] before I could see him attall and when I did he complain'd of the last nights riot. As this was intended to be my last Viset I had taken with me a present suteable to the occasion in which were three Cape Sheep, Axes Cloath and several other articles, the Sheep he had seen before and asked for them (for these people never loose any thing for want of asking) he was pleased at geting them tho they were of little Value to either him or us, to us because they were very poor, to him because they were of a sort that could not breed.[3] The presents he got at this interview intirely removed his fears and opened his heart for he sent for three Hogs for us one for me, one for Captain Furneaux and one for M[r] Forster, this last was small of which we took notice calling it ete ete,[4] presently after a man came into the circle and spoke to the King with some warmth and in a very peremptory manner something or other about Hogs, we at first thought that he was angery with the King for giving us so many especially as he took the little Pig away with him; the contrary however seem'd to be the true cause of his displeasure for presently after he was gone a Hog larger than either of the other two was brought us.[5] I acquainted the King when I took leave that I should leave the Island the next day at which he seem'd moved and embraced me several times. We embarqued in our Boat to return aboard and he directed his March back to Oparre. Yesterday I sent M[r] Pickersgill again to Attahourou for the Hogs he had promised him.[6]

[SEPTEMBER 1773]

WEDNESDAY *1st.* The Sick being all pretty well recovered, our Water Casks repaired and fill'd and the necessary repairs of the Sloops compleated I determined to put to sea without Loss of time, accordingly I ordered every thing to be got off from the Shore and the Sloops to be unmoor'd.[7] At 3 o'Clock in the afternoon the Boat return'd from Attahourou with my old friend Potattou the chief of

[1] *and:* the alarm spread many miles along the Coast for when
[2] *it . . . time:* I was obliged to wait some hours
[3] *they . . . breed:* he will be but little benifited by them as they were all weathers a thing he was made acquented with.—f. 95.
[4] *iti iti*, little, little.
[5] . . . in lieu of the little one.
[6] ADV 'Tradeing with the Natives for Cloths which we gave them in return Nails & Beeds they would reather have Glass Beed then any other'.—Constable.
[7] . . . on this work we were employed the most of the day . . .—f. 95v.

that district[1] his Wife and some more of his friends, they brought me a present of two Hogs[2] and Mr Pickersgill had got two more by exchanges from *Oamo* for he went in the Boat as far as Paparra where he saw old *Obarea*, she seem'd to be much altered for the worse, poor and of little concequence: the first words she said to Mr Pickersgill Arree Mataou ina Boa[3] (the aree is frightned, you can have no Hogs) from this it should seem that she had little or no property and was her self subject to the Aree which I believe was not the case when I was here before. The wind which had blowen Westerly all day shifted at once to the East with which we put to sea, on this account I was obliged to dismiss my friends sooner then they wished to go loaded with presents and well satisfied. Some hours before we got under sail a young man whose name was Poreo came to me and desired I would take him with me. I consented thinking he might be of service to us on some occasion, many more would have gone if I would have taken them. He beg'd a hatchet and a Nail for his father who was on board as we got under sail, he had them and gave them to his father after which they parted more like two strangers than father and son which gave me reason to think that this man was not his father, but that he had only call'd him so with a view of geting the Ax and Nail; as we were standing out of the Bay a Canoe conducted by two men came a long side and demanded him in the name of Otoo. I now saw that the whole was a trick to get some thing from me[4] and ask'd if they had brought the Hatchet and Nail with them, they said that was ashore, I told them to go and bring them and then he should go, this they said they could not do and so went away, the young man seem'd satisfied. He however could not refrain from Weeping when he view'd the land a stern.[5] We will now leave the sloops proceeding for the Island of Huaheine and take a short view of Otaheite. Soon

[1] Potatau was the familiar name of the gigantic but good-humoured *arii* of Punaauia, whose titular names were Pohuetea and Tetuanui Marua i te rai. His wife was called Purutihara or Purutifara, and often referred to by Banks in his journal as Polotheara. As Potatau was an 'old friend', it is curious that Cook does not once mention him by name in his first journal. See Fig. 63*b*.

[2] . . . and some fish

[3] *arii matau, aina puaa.*

[4] . . . well knowing that Otoo was not in the neighbourhood and could know nothing of the matter, Poreo seemed however at first undetermined whether he should go or stay, but he soon inclined to the former.—f. 95v.

[5] 'A young Otahitean whose name was Porio having a curiosity to know a little more of the World than he cou'd experience in Otahite, came on board and desir'd to be admitted as a Volunteer; he met with a cordial reception and very chearfully set out upon his Travels tho' notwithstanding his spirit & resolution when he saw the Dear Isle sinking in the Horizon he cou'd not refrain the tribute of a few Tears. Poor Porio's are not the only tears I've seen rous'd upon leaving this good Isle by some hundreds, tho' I've been in a condition myself at the time not to see a great way.'—Clerke.

after our arrival we were informed that a Ship about the seize of the Resolution Commanded by one Opeppe had put into Owhaiurua Harbour near the South end of the Island, various were the accounts the natives gave us concerning this Ship, from what I could learn she stayed here about three Weeks, that she had been gone near three when we arrived and that four of the Natives had gone away in her whose names were Debbe-de-bea, Pa-a-oodoo, Tanadoue and Apāhiāh;[1] probably this was one of the two French Ships that were fited out at the Mauritius and touched at the Cape of Good Hope in March 1772 in their way to this Sea having Aotourou on board the man M[r] Bougainville took from this Island and who died while the Ships lay at the Cape as was reported,[2] be this as it may we are sure that he is not return'd and now seems to be quite forgot by his Countrymen as well as Tupia who came away much later.

This fine Island which in the years 1767 and 8 swarmed as it were with Hogs and Fowls is now so scarce of these Animals that hardly any thing will induce the owners to part with them, the few that are now remaining seem in a great measure to be at the disposeal of the King, for while we lay in Oaiti-peha Bay in the Kingdom of Tiarrabou and at any time saw a Hog they never fail'd to say it belonged to Oheatooa, the same while we lay in Matavai in the Kingdom of *Opoureonu*[3] they there all belonged to Otoo. During the Seventeen days we were at the Island we got but 25 Hogs and one Fowl, half the Hogs were had from the two Kings and I beleive most part of the other half were sold us by their permission. We were however abundantly supplyed with all the fruits the Island produceth, except Bread fruit of which we got but little this not being the Proper season for it. I every day had a trading party on Shore by which means we got sufficient for present consumption and to take to Sea. The scarcity of Hogs and Fowls may be owing to two causes, first to the number which have been consumed and carried off by the Shiping which have touched here of late years and secondly by their frequent wars which not only distroy great numbers but does not

[1] This story of course refers to the visit of the Spanish *Aguila*. 'Opeppe' as the name of the commander is obviously founded on the conjunction of the Tahitian nominative prefix O with the common Spanish name Pepe, which the natives must frequently have heard. O Whaiurua: O Vaiurua. The ship stayed for a month; and on Cook's arrival had been gone for almost eight months. The four young natives who were taken away were called Tipitipia, Pautu, Tetuanui, and Oheiau—'Apahiah' is a rendering of a presumably alternative name for the last: perhaps Paaia or Paea?

[2] Cook makes a wildly wrong guess. The two French ships were the *Mascarin* and *Marquis de Castries* of Marion du Fresne. But Ahutoru died of smallpox at Madagascar, not the Cape; and Marion never saw Tahiti.

[3] Te Porionuu; see I, pp. clxxx–xi.

allow time to breed others.[1] Two distructive Wars hath happen'd between the two Kin[g]doms sence they ear 1767, at present they are at Peace but doth not seem to entertain much friendship for each other. I never could learn the cause of the late War or who got the better in the conflict in the Battle which I think put an end to the dispute, many were kill'd on both sides, on the side of Opoureonu fell Toutaha their Chief and several other chiefs which have been mentioned to me by name. Toutaha lies entar'd in the family Marai at Oparre,[2] his mother and several other Women that were of his family seem to be taken care of by Otoo the present *Arree de hi.*[3] I have already observed that he seems to be a timorous Prince, I know but little of Oheatooa of Tiarrabou, this prince altho he is not above 16 or 18 years of age appears with the Sedateness of a man of fifty, his subjects do not appear uncovered before him as the subjects of Otoo do before him, what I mean by uncovering is baring the body as low as the waist,[4] in other respects he seemed to appear in rather more state and had full as much respect paid him, he was attended by two or three middle-aged

[1] Cook's guess here is as good as any later one. With the exception of the *Aguila*, however, there had been no European shipping at Tahiti since the *Endeavour's* visit in 1769. No doubt the Spaniards warned the natives against the British, as Corney suggests, but though such talk might have some temporary effect in Taiarapu, it could have no effect at all at Matavai Bay. Probably the inroads of the recent war were largely responsible for the shortage in both parts of the island; and it is again not impossible that a *rahui* or general prohibition had been imposed on the consumption of pigs and fowls, for the purpose of building up stock again, which only the chief who had imposed it could break. —Corney, II, pp. 196–7 n. Corney's other suggestion that there may have been a *rahui* in connection with young Vehiatua's succession to power breaks down before his earlier argument that old Vehiatua died in 1771 or 1772, and not (as Forster reports) shortly after the war of 1773; and the fact that there was a shortage as well in Tahiti-nui, where part of the country had certainly been laid waste. It must also be remembered that pigs were never so plentiful in the island that they were a common article of consumption by any but chiefs.

[2] This was the *marae* at Point Utuhaihai, where the unlovely tomb of the last Pomare, the fifth of the name, now stands. The *marae*, as Forster reports (I, p. 325) was now no longer known as Tuteha's, but as Tu's *marae*—from which he draws the appropriate sentiment: 'A fine moral for princes, daily reminding them of mortality whilst they live, and teaching them that after death they cannot even call the ground their own which their dead corse occupies!' The *marae*, however, as Cook has it, was a family *marae*, and though Tuteha while he lived managed Tu and kept him in the shade, Tu now, as head of the family, would naturally have his name conferred upon the family property.

[3] *Otoo . . . Arree de hi:* A 92 Otoo, the reigning prince, a man, by all appearance, of no great talent. . . . A has a footnote, 'It will be seen in another place that this judgment was too hastily form'd'. B and G both characterize Tu in this context as does A; but neither has the footnote. The printed version (*Voyage*, I, p. 184) is 'Otoo the reigning prince—a man, who, at first, did not appear to us to much advantage'. Wales's journal has something to do with these alterations.

[4] Vehiatua did not have the special sacredness of the *arii rahi* who wore the red or yellow feather girdle, but though his subjects might not bare themselves to the waist, we must take Forster's testimony that they did, as we might expect, pay proper observance to his dignity: e.g. of the meeting of 23 August, 'A great croud coming down towards us, those who surrounded us pulled off their upper garments, so as to uncover their shoulders, which is a mark of respect due to the king'.—Forster, I, p. 304. Also Sparrman, p. 54.

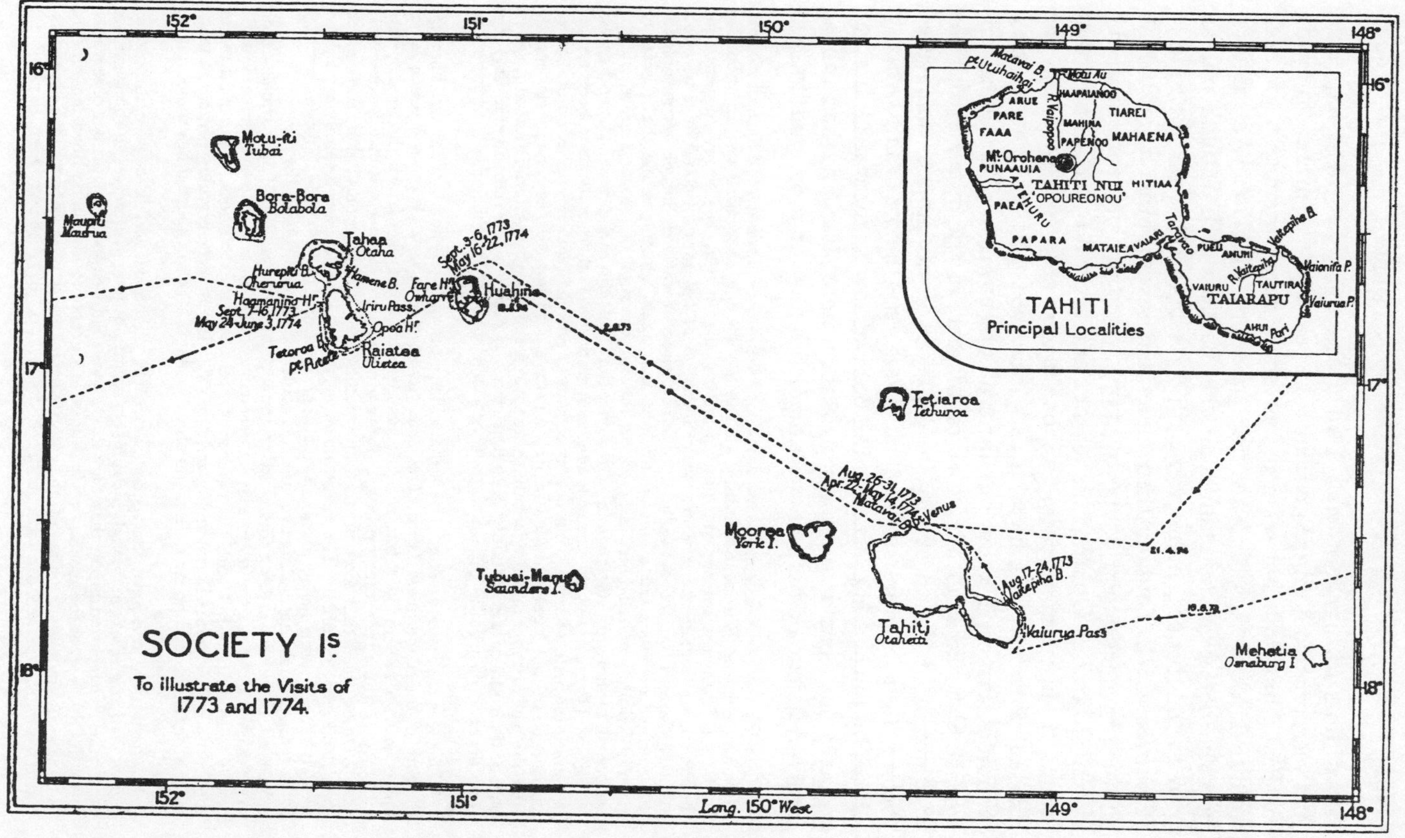
SOCIETY I^s.
To illustrate the Visits of
1773 and 1774.
TAHITI
Principal Localities
Motu-iti
Tubai
Bora-Bora
Bolabola
Maupiti
Maurua
Tahaa
Otaha
Hurepiti B.
Oherurua
Hamene B.
Haamanino H^r.
Sept. 7-16, 1773
May 24-June 3, 1774
Iriru Pass.
Opoa H^r.
Tetoroa B.
P^t. Piteata
Raiatea
Ulietea
Fare H^r.
Owharre
Huahine
Sept. 3-6, 1773
May 16-22, 1774
Tetiaroa
Tethuroa
Aug. 26-31, 1773
Apr. 22-May 14, 1774
Matavai B.
P^t. Venus
Moorea
York I.
Tubuai-Manu
Saunders I.
Aug. 17-24, 1773
Vaitepiha B.
Tahiti
Otaheiti
Vaiurua Pass
Mehetia
Osnaburg I.
Matavai B.
P^t. Utuhaihai
Motu Au
ARUE
R. Vaipopoo
HAAPAIANOO
TIAREI
PARE
MAHINA
FAAA
PAPENOO
MAHAENA
M^t. Orohena
PUNAAUIA
TAHITI NUI
'OPOUREONOU'
HITIAA
PAEA
TEHURU
PAPARA
MATAIEA
VAIARI
Taravao
PUEU
ANUHI
Vaitepiha B.
R. Vaitepiha
Vaionifa P.
VAIURU
TAUTIRA
TAIARAPU
Vaiurua P.
AHUI
Pari
152°
151°
150°
149°
148°
16°
17°
18°
Long. 150° West

FIG. 37

men who seemed to be his counsellors.[1] The Veneral disease which was so common in this Isle in the year 1769 is now far less so, they say they can cure it and it fully appears so for altho most of our people made pritty free use of their Women and these of the common sort, not more than   were affected by this disease in both Sloops and this in such a gentle manner as was easy to remove.[2] They complain of a disease communicated to them by Opeppe's Ship (as they say) they told us that it affected the head, Throat and Stomach and at last kills them, they dread it much and constantly enquiring if we had it, they call it by the name of the communicator Apa no Peppe.[3] I am however of opinion that it was some Epidemical disease that broke out among them at the time the Ship was there without her contributing in the least towards it. Some of our people pretend to have seen some who have had the Pox in a high degree.[4]

THURSDAY *2nd.* After leaving the Bay of Matavai as before mentioned I directed my course for the Island of *Huaheine* and at 6 o'Clock the following evening we were with[in] two or three Leagues of its northern point where we spent the night laying too and makeing short boards, and on Friday morning at day light made sail round the point for the Harbour Owharre[5] where we anchored at 9 o'Clock in 24 fathom water, as the wind blew out of the Harbour I choose to turn in by the southern channell, the Resolution turn'd in very well, but the Adventure missing stays got a shore on the reef on the north side of the channell.[6]

FRIDAY *3rd.* I had the Resolutions Launch in the Water ready in

[1] Forster gives more attention to these, particularly to the man he calls 'E-Tee', 'the fat chief' (I, pp. 305, 308–9): the influential Ti'i-torea, second husband of old Vehiatua's wife Purahi, and hence the young man's step-father.

[2] Cf. I, p. 99, n. 4.

[3] *Epohe no Pepe*, the sickness of Pepe. To judge from the description given, this was perhaps some sort of gastric influenza, which the Spaniards could certainly have transmitted with fatal results to the islanders.

[4] Scientific interest may again be noted in Clerke, on leaving Matavai Bay: '. . . the Watch makes this place to be in Longitude 209°59′ E^{t} or 150°01′ W^{t}, which is certainly great correctness for a Watch, but I think cannot be held in competition with the result of the Various Observations made in this Bay by Mr Green in '69 which gave the Longitude 149°36′ W^{t} or 210°24′ E^{t}—Lat^{de} 17°29′ S^{o}—Difference 00°25′.'—Add. MS 8952, 1 September. The *Pacific Islands Pilot* gives the position of Point Venus as 17°29′ s and 149° 29′ w, which is extremely close to Green.

[5] H Lat. 16°43′47″ s. Longit. 151°7′10″ w.—Figs. 35, 40.

[6] Cook went into the harbour of Fare, on the west side of Huahine, by the southern or Arapeihi passage, 'as being the widest', according to B, f. 96; but there is not much to choose in width between it and the northern or Avamoa passage. In both the shelving edges of the reef reduce the fairway to about 150 yards in width. The *Adventure* seems to have gone on to a spit which runs out westward from the end of the reef on the northern side of the channel.

case of an axcedent of this kind, and sent her immidiately to the Adventure by this timely assistance she was got off without receiving any damage.[1] As soon as the Sloops were in safety I landed[2] and was received by the natives with the utmost cordiality. I distributed some presents among them and presently they brought down Hogs, Fowls and fruit[3] which they exchanged for Hatchets, Nails, Beeds, &c[a], a like trade was soon opened aboard the Sloops, the natives bring[ing] them off in their Canoes so that every thing promised us a plentifull supply of fresh pork and Fowls which to people who had been living Ten months on salt meat was no unwelcome thing. I learnt that my old friend Oree was still living and chief of the Island and that he was hastning to this part to see me.

SATURDAY 4*th*. Early in the morning I sent Lieutenant Pickersgill with the Cutter on a tradeing party towards the South end of the Island and also a nother on shore near the Sloops, with this I went my self in order to see it was properly conducted at the first seting out, a very necessary point to be attended to, this being settled to my mind I went to pay my first Viset to Oree the Chief who I was told was waiting for me, accompanid by Captain Furneaux and M[r] Forster. We were conducted to the place by one of the natives, but we were not permitted to go out of the Boat without going through the following ceremony usual at this Isle on such occasions. The Boat being landed before the chiefs Housc which was close by the Water side Five young Plantan trees, which are their Emblems of Peace, were brought seperately and with some ceremony into the Boat. Three small Pigs[4] accompanied the first three and a Dog the fourth, each had its particular name and purpose rather too mysterious for us well to understand,[5] lastly the Chief sent me the Inscription engraved on a small peice of Pewter which I left with him when [I saw] him in 1769, it was in the same bag I had made for it together with a peice of counterfeit English coin and a few Beads given him at the same time,[6] this shews how well he had taken care of the whole. After they had done sending the things above mentioned to the Boat, our guide who still remained in the Boat with us desired us to decorate three young Plantan plants with Nails, looking glasses

[1] . . . Several of the Natives by this time had come off to us bringing with them some of the productions of the Island and . . .—f. 96.

[2] . . . with Captain Furneaux

[3] *Fowls . . . fruit:* Fowls, Dogs and fruit

[4] *Three small Pigs:* Three young pigs with their ears ornamented . . .—f. 96v.

[5] Cf. Forster I, pp. 375–6, where the ceremony is treated in more detail. Cook, I, p. 141, describes the corresponding ceremony of 17 July 1769, when he first met Ori.

[6] See I, p. 143.

Medals, &c[a] &c[a], which was accordingly done, we landed with these in our hands and walked up towards the Chief a lane being made by the people between us and him for here were a vast crowd. We were made to sit down before we came to[1] the chief, our Plantains were then taken from us one by one and laid down by him, one was for Eatoua[2] or God, the Second for the Arree or King and the third for Tyo or friendship. This being done Oree rose up came and[3] fell upon my neck and embraced me, this was by no means ceremonious, the tears which trinckled plentifully down his Cheeks sufficiently spoke the feelings of his heart. All his friends were next interduced to us among whome was a beautifull Boy his grandson. The whole ceremony being now over I made him the present I had prepared consisting of the most Valuable articles I had for this purpose[4] and in return he gave me a Hog and a quantity of Cloth and promised that all our wants should be supplied and it will soon appear how well he kept his word, at length we took leave and return'd aboard to dinner and some time after the Cutter arrived with 14 Hogs, many more were purchased on shore and a long side the Sloops.[5]

SUNDAY 5*th.* Early in the morning Oree made me a visit accompanied by some of his friends, he brought me a present of a Hog and some fruit for which I made him a suteable return, this good old Chief never faild to send me every day for my Table the best of ready dress'd fruit and roots and in great plenty. Lieut[t] Pickersgill was again detatched to the South end of the Island with both Cutter and Launch, he returned the same day with Twenty-eight Hogs and about four times as many more were got a shore and along side the Sloops.[6]

MONDAY 6*th.* In the morning I sent the tradeing party[7] a shore as usual and after breakfast went my self when I found that one of the natives had been a little troublesome,[8] this fellow being pointed out to me compleatly equiped in the War habit with a club in each hand, as he seem'd to be intent on Mischief I took from him the two

[1] *before . . . to:* a few paces short of

[2] *e atua.*

[3] *Oree . . . and:* I wanted to go to the King, but was told that he would come to me, which he accordingly did . . .—f. 97.

[4] . . . for I regarded this old man as a father, . . .—Cf. Log: 'this brave old chief who receiv'd me more like a son he had not seen these four years than a friend . . .'

[5] . . . besides fowls and fruit in abundance.

[6] 'People at no allowance [i.e. the ship's food was cut off entirely] they abound most plentifully in Pork and Yams.'—Clerke.

[7] . . . consisting of only two or 3 people

[8] *a little troublesome:* very troublesome and insolant

clubs and broke them and with some difficulty forced him to retire from the place, they told me that he was an Aree which made me the more suspicious of him and occasioned me to send for a guard which before I had thought unnecessary. About this time Mr Sparman being out alone[1] botanizing was set upon by two men who striped him of every thing he had but his Trowsers, they struck him several times with his own hanger but happily did him no harm, as soon as they had accomplished their end they made off after which a man came to him, gave him a piece of cloth to cover himself and conducted him to me. I went immidiately[2] to Oree to complain of this outrage takeing with me the man who came back with Mr Sparman to confirm the complaint,[3] as soon as the chief heard it he wept a lowd as did several others and after the first transports of his grief was over expostulated with the people shewing them how well I had treated them both in this and my former voyage or some thing to this purpose,[4] he then promised to do all in his power to recover what was taken from Mr Sparman and took a very minute account of every article after which he rose up and went to the Boat desiring me to follow, his people seeing this and being apprehensive of his safety they opposed his going into the Boat, he step'd in notwithstanding their opposision and intreaties. When the people saw their beloved chief wholy in my power they set up a great outcry and with Tears flowing down their cheeks intreated him once more to come out of the Boat.[5] I even joined my intreaties to theirs, it was to no purpose,[6] he insisted of my coming into the Boat and as soon as I was in ordered her off him self, his Sister with Spirit equal to her Royal Brother was the only person that did not oppose his going: as his intention for coming into the Boat was to go with us in search

[1] *being . . . alone;* having imprudently gone out alone . . .—f. 97v.

[2] *he . . . immediately:* the trading place where were a great number of the Natives, the very instant Mr Sparman appeared in the condition I have just mentioned, they fled to a man with the utmost precipitation, my first conjectures were that they had stolen something, but we were soon undeceived when we saw Mr Sparman and the affair was related to us. As soon as I could recall back a few of the Natives and had made them sencible that I should take no step to injure those who were innocent, I went . . .

[3] Taking also Sparrman and Forster, we learn from Sparrman. Poor Sparrman of course treats his misadventure in some detail (pp. 78–81), and inclines to blame Tubai, the bravo whose clubs Cook had broken. He adds ruefully, 'I had undertaken this unfortunate expedition by myself without any misgivings, since Captain Cook had often told us that the Society Islands were as safe and as peaceful as Otaheite . . . Captain Cook declared my solitary botanical excursion to have been imprudent, and, if indeed it were so, then many similar expeditions made on that voyage must be so considered'.

[4] *or . . . purpose:* and how base it was in them to commit such actions

[5] *and . . . Boat:* the grief they showed was inexpressable every face was bedewed with tears, they prayed, intreated and even attempted to pull him out of the boat,—ff. 97v–8.

[6] *it . . . purpose:* for I could not bear to see them in such distress, all that could be said or done availed nothing

of the Robbers we put off and proceeded accordingly as far as we could by Water, then land and entered the Country and traveled some miles, the chief leading the way inquiring of every one he saw, at length he step'd into a house which was by the road side and order some Cocoa-nutts to be brought for us to drink. After we had refreshed ourselves he wanted to proceed farther, this I opposed[1] and insisted upon his returning back which he was obliged to comply with when he saw I would not follow him. I disired him to send some people for the stolen things for I saw it was to little purpose going farther for the thieves had already got so much start of us that we might have pursued them to the very remote part of the Island,[2] besides as I intended to sail the next day, this occasioned a loss to us by puting a stop to all manner of trade for the natives were so Allarmed that none came near us but those that were about the chief, the accedent which befell Mr Sparman was first made known to us at the tradeing place by the precipitate retiring of all the people without my being able to conceive the meaning till Mr Sparman appeard, it became therefore the more necessary for me to return to endeavour to restore things to their former state, accordingly we return'd to our boat where we found the chief's sister and several more people who had traveled by land to the place. We immidiately embarqued in the Boat in order to go aboard without so much as asking the Chief to accompany us, he however insisted on going with us in spite of the opposission he met with from those about him, his Sister followed his example contrary to the tears and intreaties of her Daughter a young woman about 16 or 18 years of age. The Chief sit at Table with us and made a hearty meal, his sister sit behind us as it is not the custom for the Women to eat with the men. After dinner I made them both presents and in the Evening carried them a shore to the place were I first took him in where some hundreds waited to receive him many of whome imbracced him with tears of joy in their eyes, all was now harmony and Peace, the people crowded in from every part with Hogs, Fowls and Fruit so that we presently loaded two Boats, the Chief himself made me a present of a large Hog and some fruit, the hanger, the only thing of value Mr Sparman had lost, and part of his waist coat was brought us and we were told we should have the others the next day. Some of the officers who were

[1] . . . thinking that we might be carried to the very farther part of the island after things the most of which, before they came into our hands again, might not be worth the bringing home; the chief used many arguments to persuade me to proceed tilling me that I might send my boat round to meet us or that he would get a Canoe to bring us home if I thought it too far to travel;—f. 98.

[2] . . . without so much as seeing them

out on a Shooting party had some things stolen from them which were returned in like manner, thus ended the transactions of this day which I have been rather particular in enumerating because it shews what great confidence this Brave old Chief put in us, it also in a great degree shews that Friendship is Sacred with these people. Oree and I were profess'd friends in all the forms customary among them and he had no idea that this could be broke by the act of any other person, indeed this seem'd to be the great Argument he made use on to his people when they opposed his going into my boat, his words were to this effect: Oree (for so I was always calld) and I am friends, I have done nothing to forfeit his friendship, why should I not go with him. We however may never meet with a nother chief who will act in the same manner on any semiliar occasion.[1]

TUESDAY *7th*. Early in the morn we began to unmoor, while this was doing I went to take my leave of the chief accompanied by Captain Furneaux and Mr Forster. I tooke with me such things for a present as I knew were most useful and valuable to him. I also left with him the Inscription plate he had before in keeping and another small copper plate on which was engraved these words: Anchor'd here His Britannic Majestys Ships Resolution and Adventure September 1773, together with some Midals all put up in a Small Bag, the chief promised to take great care of the whole and to produce them to the first Ship that should come to the Isle. He next gave me a Hog and after trading for six or eight more and loading the boat with fruit we took leave at which the good old Chief imbraced me with Tears in his eyes. At this interview nothing was said about the remainder of Mr Sparmans Clothes. I judged they were not brought in and for that reason did not mention them least I should give the chief pain about a thing I did not give him time to recover.[2] When I came aboard I found the Sloops crowded round with Canoes full of Hogs, Fowls and Fruit as at our first arrival. Soon after Oree himself came aboard to inform me (as we at first understood him) that the robbers were taken and wanted me to go on Shore either to punish or see them punished, but this could not be done as the Resolution was just under sail and the Adventure already out of the Harbour. I likewise understood from him that four or five of his people were

[1] . . . It may be asked what he had to fear, to which I must answer nothing, for it never was my intention to hurt a hair of his head or to detain him one single moment longer than he disired, but how was he or the people to know this, they were not ignorant that if he was once in my power, the whole force of the isle could not take him from me, and that let my demands for his ransom been [*sic*] ever so high they must have comply'd with it; thus far their fears both for his and their own safety were justly founded.—f. 99.

[2] . . . for this was early in the morning

gone away in the Adventure and that he wanted to have them return'd, but in this the chief had either been misinformed or we misunderstood him for I immidiately sent ~~on~~ board Captain Furneaux for them, when the Boat returned she brought only one[1] no more being on board and as this man had been on board the Adventure from the first hour of her arrival at the Isle and it being known to all the natives that he intended to go away with us, without being once demanded[2] and as Captain Furneaux being desireous of keeping [him][3] I did not think it was necessary to send him on Shore for the Chief was now gone, he stayed aboard till we were a full half League out at Sea then went away in a small Canoe conducted by one man and himself.[4] While we lay in this Port several of the common people frequently desired me to Kill the Bolabola men (the people of a neighbouring isle). Oree probably heard of this and took an oppertunity when he was left aboard to disire that I would not, teling me that Opoone their King was his Friend, the Common people in general seem to bear an implacable hatred against the Bolabola men nor is this to be much wondred at sence they have made a conquest of most of the neighbouring iles, the little Island of Huaheine under the brave and wise conduct of Oree still preserves its independancy, not a Bolabola man have yet been able to get a footing there tho' we have been told some attempts have been made but of this we have no absolute certainty, from the great plenty of everything on the Isle one might conclude that it had injoyed the b[l]esings of Peace for many years, during our short stay we procured not less than 300 Hogs to both Sloops, besides Fowls[5] and Fruit and had we made a longer stay might have got many more for neither Hogs nor Fowls were apparently diminished but every where appeared as numberous as ever, such is the state of the little but fertile Isle of Huaheine.[6] My friend Oree was no sooner gone[7] than we made sail for Ohamaneno[8] Harbour on the West side of Ulietea where I intended to stop a few days to procure an addition of Fruit to our present stock:

[1] . . . whose name was Omiah

[2] . . . besides we were now some distance from the shore

[3] '. . . one of the Natives a young man who expressed the greatest desire to go to *Britania*'.—Furneaux. See Fig. 43.

[4] . . . all the others being gone long before. I was sorry that it was not convenient for me to go on shore with him to see in what manner these people would have been punished for I am satisfied that this was what brought him on board.—f. 99v.

[5] 'At Huahine we have got by purchase & presents in both sloops about 400 Hoggs & half as many Cocks.'—Log.

[6] A *note*. We met with a man at this Isle who measured 6 feet 3 inch & $\frac{9}{10}$.—B . . . and was the tallest man I ever saw in the isles.

[7] . . . and our boat returned from the Adventure

[8] Haamanino, inside the Rautoanui passage. Cook had anchored there, 2–9 August 1769.

in going round the South end of the Island I had an oppertunity to discover an error in my Chart of the Isle constructed in my former Voyage. The Harbour and Isle O-aihate which was laid down from the information of Tupia a little to the East of the South point of the Island, lies a little to the north of the said point, that is, there is one harbour more on the West side of the Isle than what is laid down in the Chart and one less on the SE side.[1] We got off the Harbour of Ohamaneno[2] at dark the close of the day where we spent the night makeing short boards. The night was dark but we were sufficiently guided by the many fishing lights that were on the reefs and Shores of the Islands.

WEDNESDAY 8*th*. At Day light the next morning after making a few trips we gained the Harbours mouth, the wind blowing right out we borrowed on[3] the South side of the Channell and with all our sails set shoot into anchoring ground and came too in 17 fathom water, we then carried out anchors and Hawsers to warp in by and as soon as the Resolution was out of the Way the Adventure anchored in like manner and warped in by the Resolution. The warping in and mooring the Sloops took us up the whole day. We were no sooner at

[1] . . . at least thier is a ha[r]bour and an isle in this place not taken notice of in the Chart.—f. 100.—The general sense of this is clear, but to follow the argument precisely one needs to have Cook's Chart IX (which, to complicate matters further, is drawn with south at the top) side by side with the modern chart and the *Pacific Islands Pilot*. Chart IX, though it gets the essential shape of Raiatea, is not very good in detail; for example, on the south side of the island it has what should be two separate islets, Nao Nao and Haaio, half a mile apart, joined together as part of the main island. Between the projection thus formed and Point Putete ('the South point of the Island') lies on this chart what Cook calls Oaehuti Harbour, the O-aihate of the present text—one of three harbours marked and named on the south side. Cook now proposes to move this harbour about five miles round the coast to the west side of the island, to the anchorage inside the Punaeroa passage, which he had failed to notice on his previous voyage. He had rowed down inside the reef from Rautoanui on 5 August 1769, but could not have come as far as this (I, pp. 149, 151–2) though his name is derived from Vaihuti, the bay inside this passage. He is now both correct and incorrect. It is true that his chart had one harbour too few on the western side, and that he had now discovered the missing one, and joined it up to its right name. But to make the sum right, he took it away from the wrong place: there is in fact good anchorage on either side of Haaio islet—the 'Oaehuti' and the 'Ohetuna' harbours of the chart, 'Ohetuna' apparently standing for Faatemu bay. He should have subtracted his easternmost harbour, 'Oninamu', which does not exist—though probably the name had some local connotation. As the whole island of Raiatea is so small, this discussion may seem needlessly pedantic; but the error, even if derived from Tupaia—for Cook himself does not seem to have had a close view of the southern end of the island at all—illustrates very well the difficulties of a rapid coastal survey under the conditions with which Cook was faced.

[2] H Lat. 16°45′25″ s. Longit. 151°34′30″ West. [Insertion by Cook.]

[3] *we borrowed on:* I sent a boat to lay in sounding that we might know when to anchor; as soon as the Signal was made by the boat we borrowed close to . . .—f. 100. To 'borrow' was to sail close to the land or the wind. Corney points out that Cook's skill as a practical seaman is observable from this account, 'in which he graphically yet simply describes the evolution of "borrowing" close to the reef and successfully shooting his vessel well into the passage with all sail set, right in the wind's eye'. (Corney II, p. 305, n. 1.)

Anchor at the entrance of the Harbour than the Natives crowded round us in their Canoes bringing with them Hogs and fruit the latter of which they exchanged for Beads and Nails, the former we refused to take as we had already as many on board as we could dispence with, some however we were obliged to take as several of the principal People brought off little Pigs[1] and put them into the Ship and Boats lying a longs[ide] together [with] Plantain Plants[2] by way of welcoming us to their Country & to shew their friendly disposission.

THURSDAY *9th.* In the Morning we paid a formal Viset to the Chief of this part of the Isle whose name is Oreo, the same as when I was here before.[3] We went through no sort of ceremony at landing but were conducted to the Chief at once who was seated in his House which stands close to the Water side. The Chief and his friends received us with great Cordiallity, express'd much satisfaction at seeing me again, desired that he might be call'd Cook (or Toote) and I Oreo which was accordingly done,[4] he then ask'd after Tupia and several other gentlemen by name who were with me last voyage. Now I have mentioned Tupia it is necessary to observe that scarce a person here or at Huaheine that did not enquire after him and the occasion of his death and like true Philosophers were perfectly satisfied with the answers we gave them, indeed as we had nothing but the truth to tell the story was always the same by whomsoever told. After I made the Chief and his friends the necessary presents we return'd aboard with a Hog and some fruit which the Chief gave me in return; in the after-noon he gave me a nother Hog still larger without asking for the least return. Fruit in abundance were brought off to the Sloops and exchanged for Nails &c[a].[5]

FRIDAY *10th.* In the Fore-noon Captain Furneaux and I paid Oreo a Viset and made him some returns for what he gave me yesterday. The Chief entertain'd us with a Comedy or Dramatick Heava such as is usually acted in the Isles, the Musick consisted of three Drums, the actors were Seven Men and one Woman, the chief's Niece,[6] the

[1] . . . Pepper or Eavaa [*ava*] root,

[2] . . . whether we would or no, for if we refused to take them on board they would throw them into the boats

[3] But in his first journal Cook does not record this man's name, Orio. Nor does Banks in his journal. The chief who then received their attention was Puni, the conqueror from Borabora.

[4] . . . I believe that this is the strongest tie of friendship they can shew to a stranger.—f. 100v.

[5] . . . Exchanges for fruit &c[a] were chiefly carried on along side the Ships, I attempted to trade for these articles on shore but did not succeed, as the most of them were brought in Canoes from distant parts and carried directly to the Ships.

[6] neice *deleted* Daughter *substituted.* Pickersgill seems to have got on extremely well with this charmer, 'Miss Poedua': see p. 771 below.

Play seemed to be nearly if not quite the same as was acted at Otaheite. The only entertaining part in it was a Thift committed by a man and his accomplice, this was done in such a manner as sufficiently desplayed the Genius of the people in this art.[1] The Thift was discovered before the thief had time to carry of his prize and a scuffle essued between him his accomplice and those set to guard it and altho' they were four to two they were beat off the Stage and the others carried off their prise in triumph. I was very attentive to the whole of this part in expectation that it would have had a quite different end, for I had before been told that Teto,[2] that is the thief, was to be acted and had understood that the Theift was to be punished with death or with a good Tiparrahying[3] (beating) but I found my self misstaken in both. We are however told that this is the punishment they inflict on those who are guilty of this crime, be this as it may strangers certainly have not the Protection of this Law, them they rob with impunity at every oppertunity. As soon as the Play was over we return'd aboard to dinner after which went ashore again where we spent the remainder of the day.[4] Learnt from one of the Natives that Nine Islands laid to the Westward at no great distance from hence, they are all small and two of them uninhabited.[5] Brisk trade for fruit &c[a].

SATURDAY 11*th*. Early in the Morn I had a Viset from Oreo and his Son, a youth about 12 or 13 years of age, the latter brought me a Hog, a piece of Cloth and some fruit for which I gave him an Ax, dress'd him out in a Shirt and other things which made him not a little proud of him self. After a Stay of two or three hours they went a shore and I followed soon after in Company with some of the gentlemen, the Chief hearing that I was on shore came to seek me, put a large Hog and some fruit into the boat and he together with some of his friends came aboard and dined with us. After dinner we were Viseted by his Brother [Oo oorou] the principal chief on the Island,[6] he brought me as a present a large Hog for which I made

[1] *art:* vice

[2] *tito*, 'to go softly on tiptoe, as a thief' (Davies).

[3] *taparahi*, to beat

[4] *after . . . day:* and in the cool of the evening we took a walk ashore.—f. 101.

[5] It is difficult to know what, if anything, is meant by this. The three atolls Mopihaa (with a number of low islets on its reef), Fenua Ura and Motu One, are something like 100–150 miles to the westward: beyond them, somewhat to the south, are the Lower Cook islands Aitutaki and its smaller scattered companions; but 'at no great distance', one would think, could hardly apply to these.

[6] . . . he was interduc'd to us by Oreo and . . . f. 101v. Orio was the dispenser of authority on the island, as representative of Puni, the conqueror, from Borabora (I, pp. 149–50, 153); but the *arii rahi* or 'high chief', Uru, had been left in possession of his formal dignity and status, though without power. 'Oo ourou' seems to be O [nominative predicative] Uru. Nor could the two chiefs have been brothers: Orio was a Borabora man. See Cook's own text, p. 429 below.

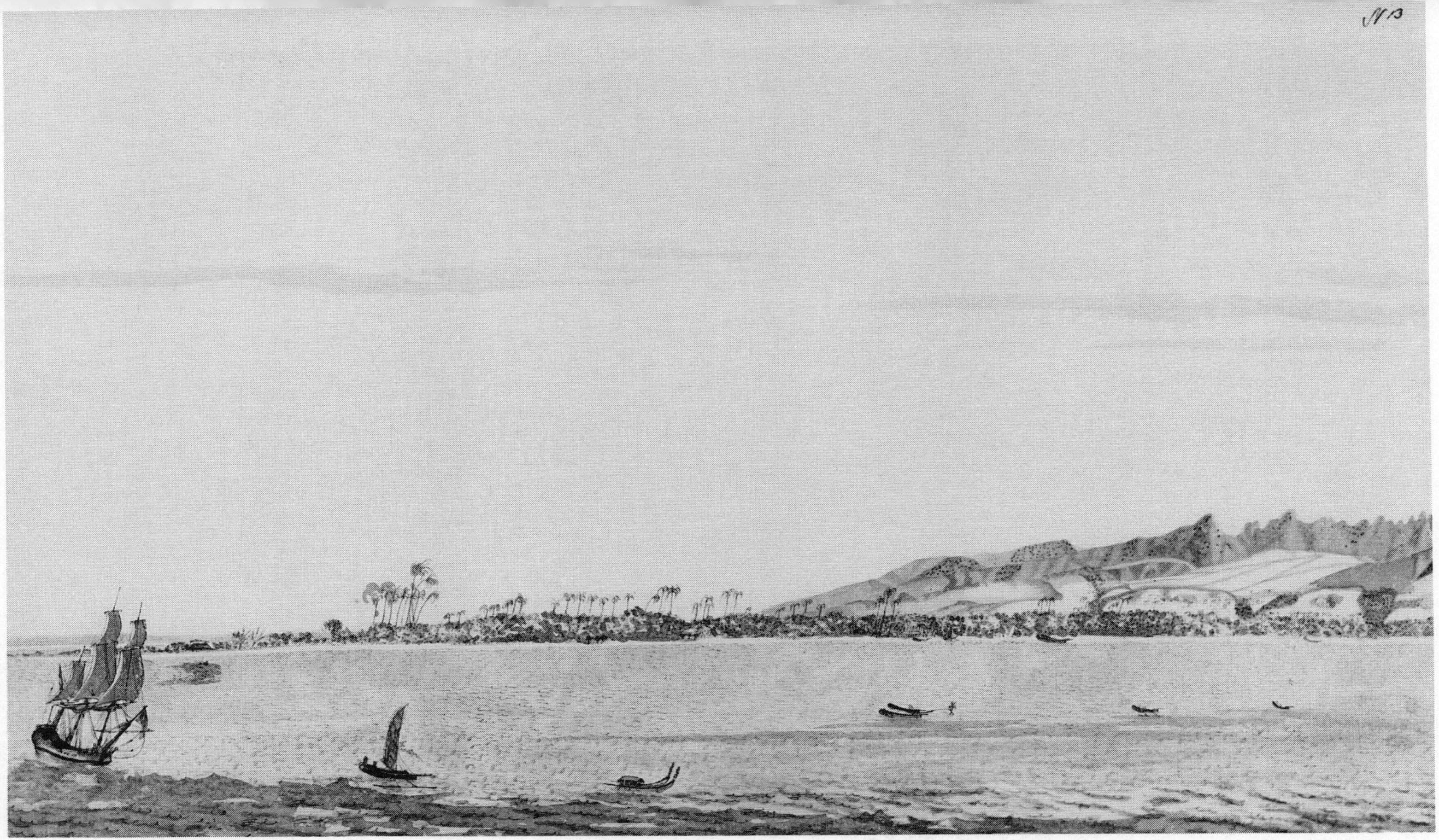

FIG. 36. View of Matavai Bay and Point Venus, Tahiti

Wash drawing by Hodges.—Mitchell Library, D11, no. 13

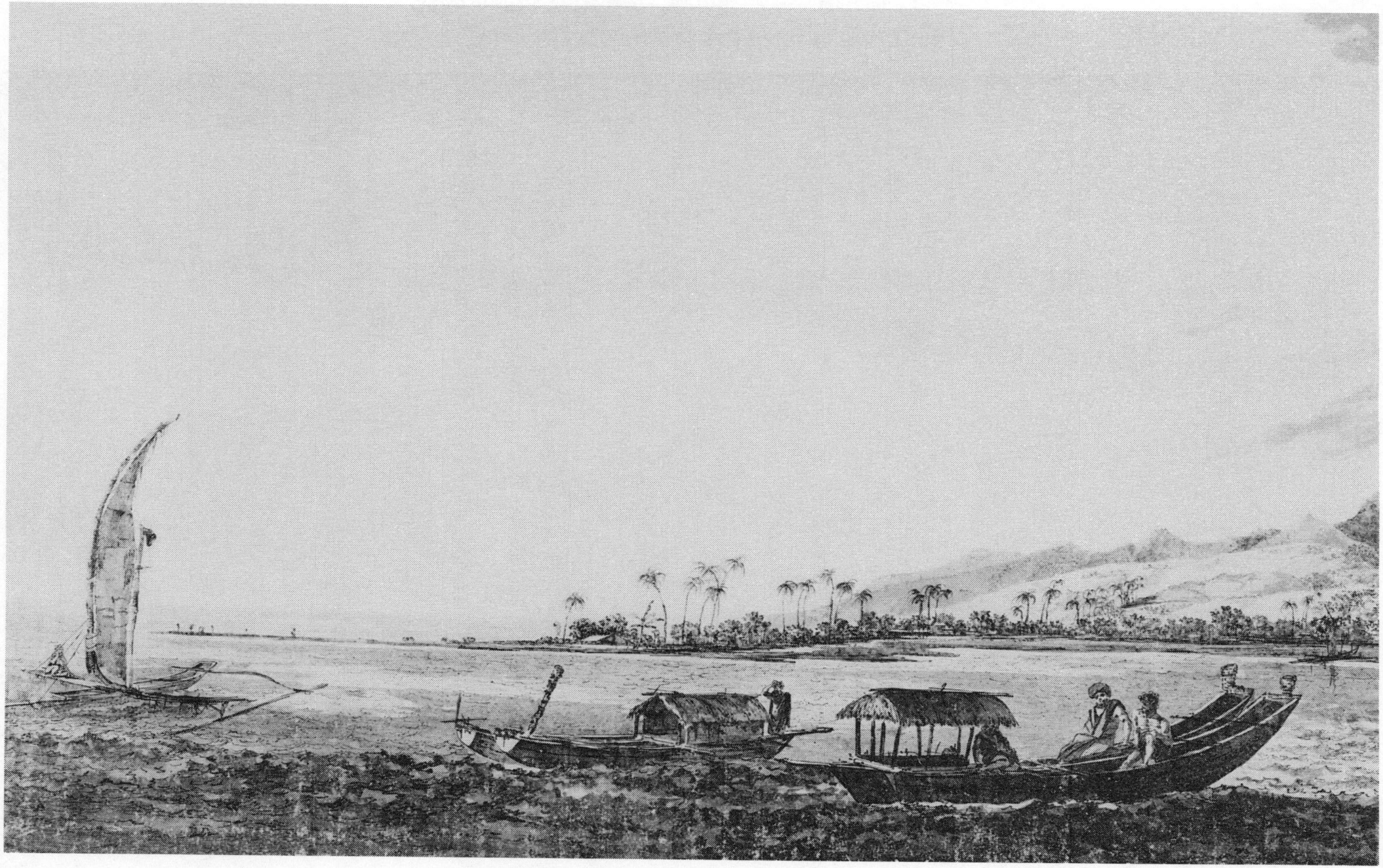

FIG. 37. Tahitian canoes in Matavai Bay

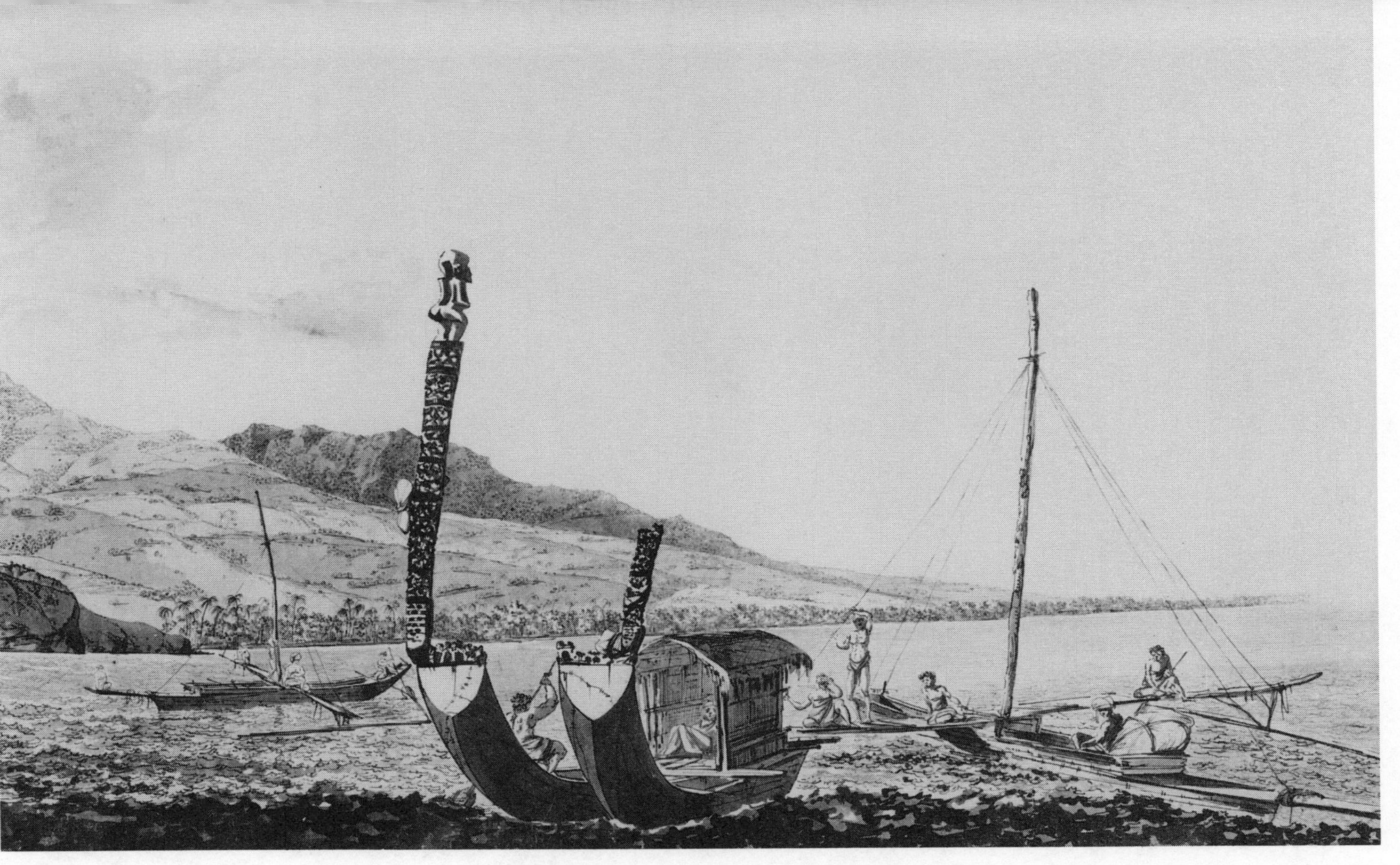

FIG. 38. Tahitian canoes in Matavai Bay

Detail of wash drawing by Hodges.—B.M., Add. MS 15743.

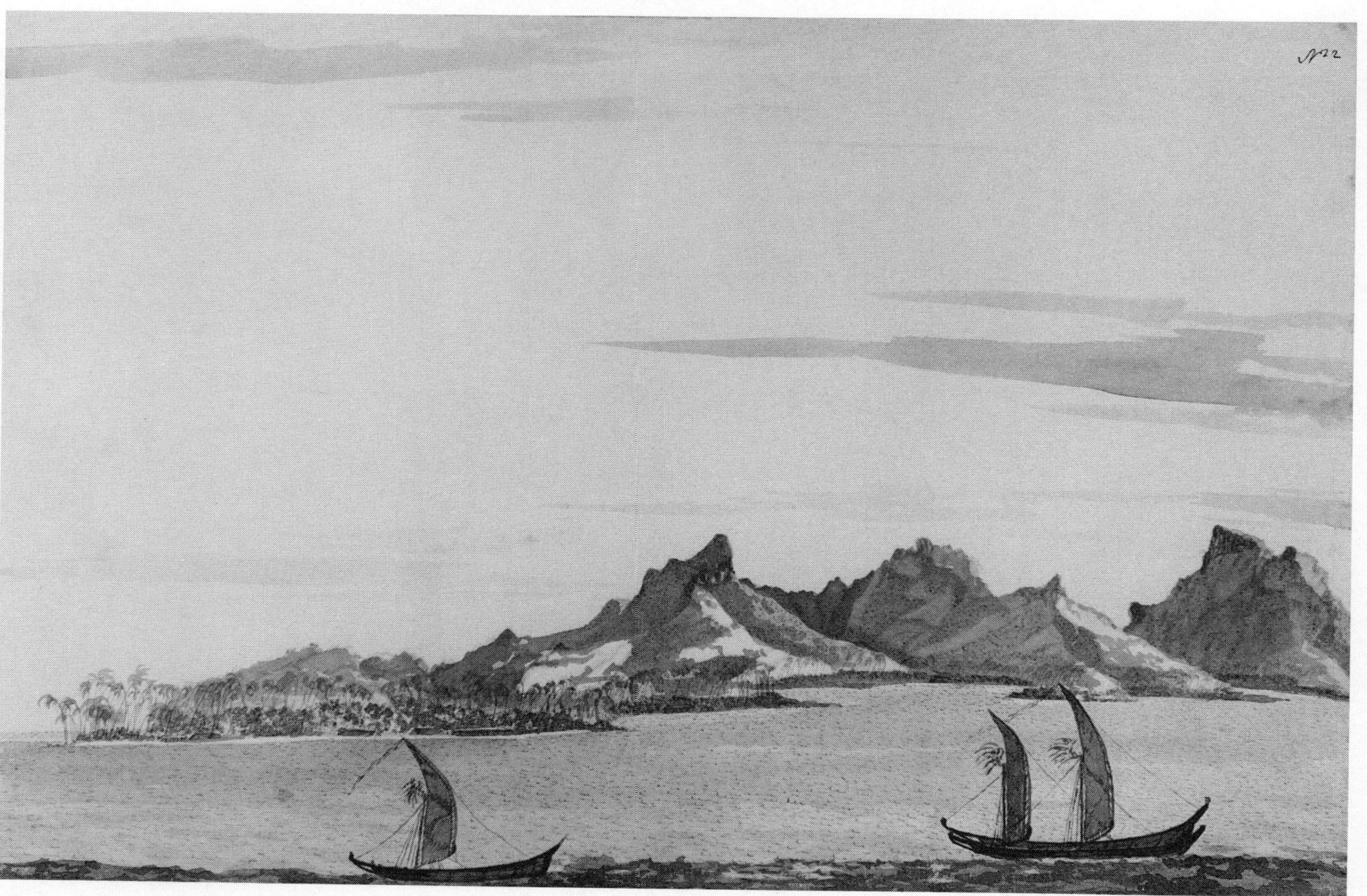

Fig. 39. View of Huahine

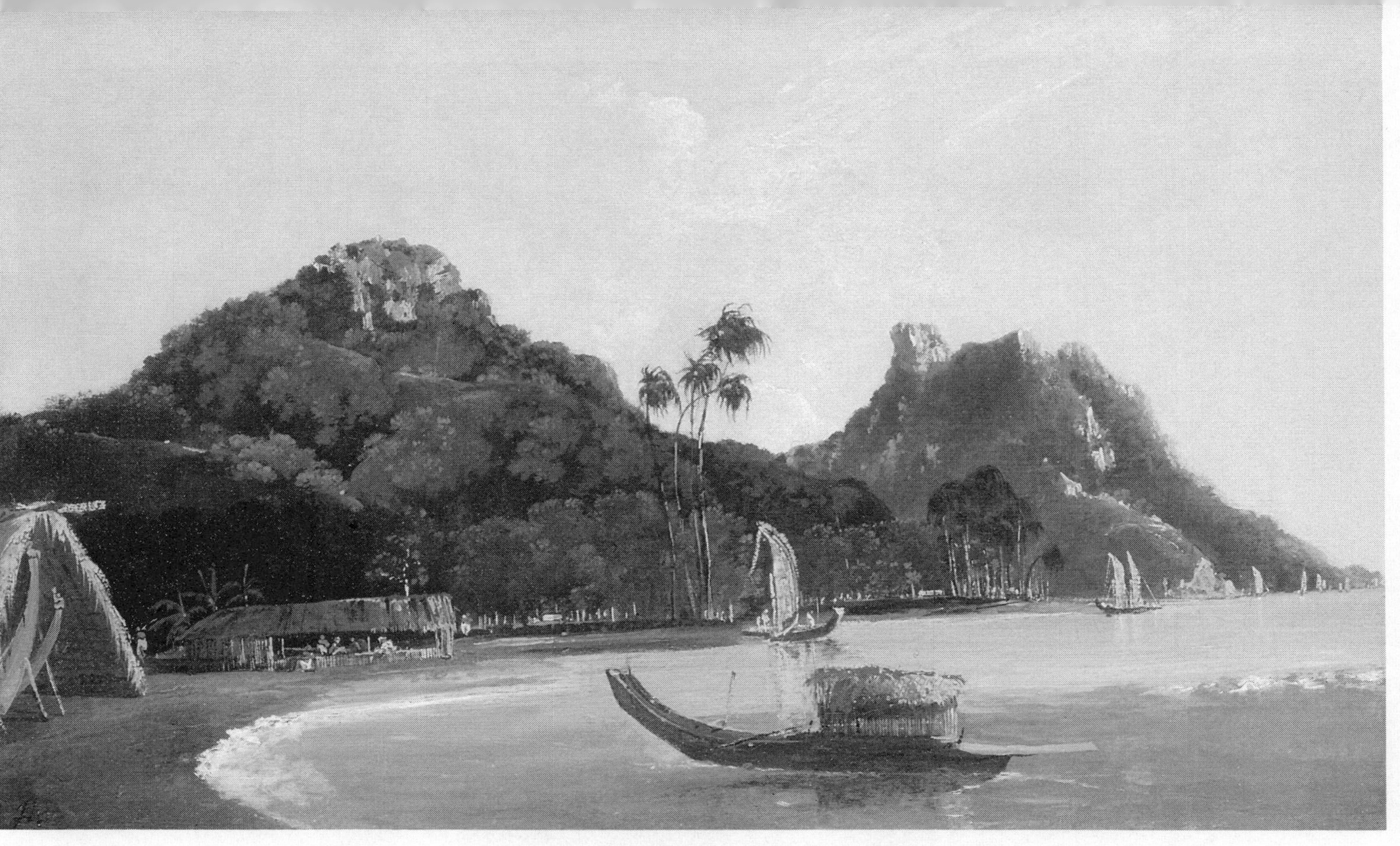

FIG. 40. The harbour of Fare, Huahine

Oil painting by Hodges, in Admiralty House

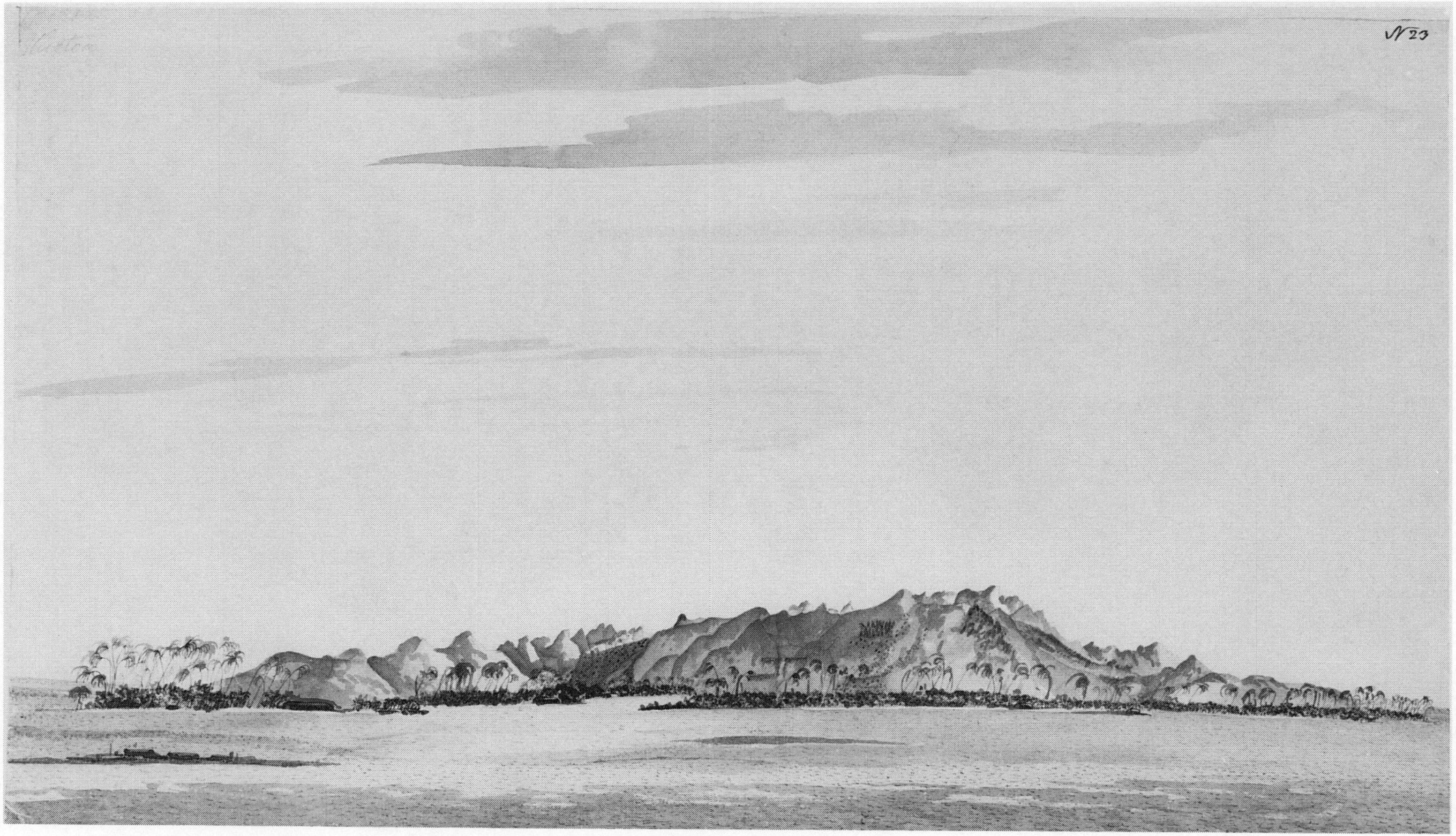

FIG. 41. View of Raiatea

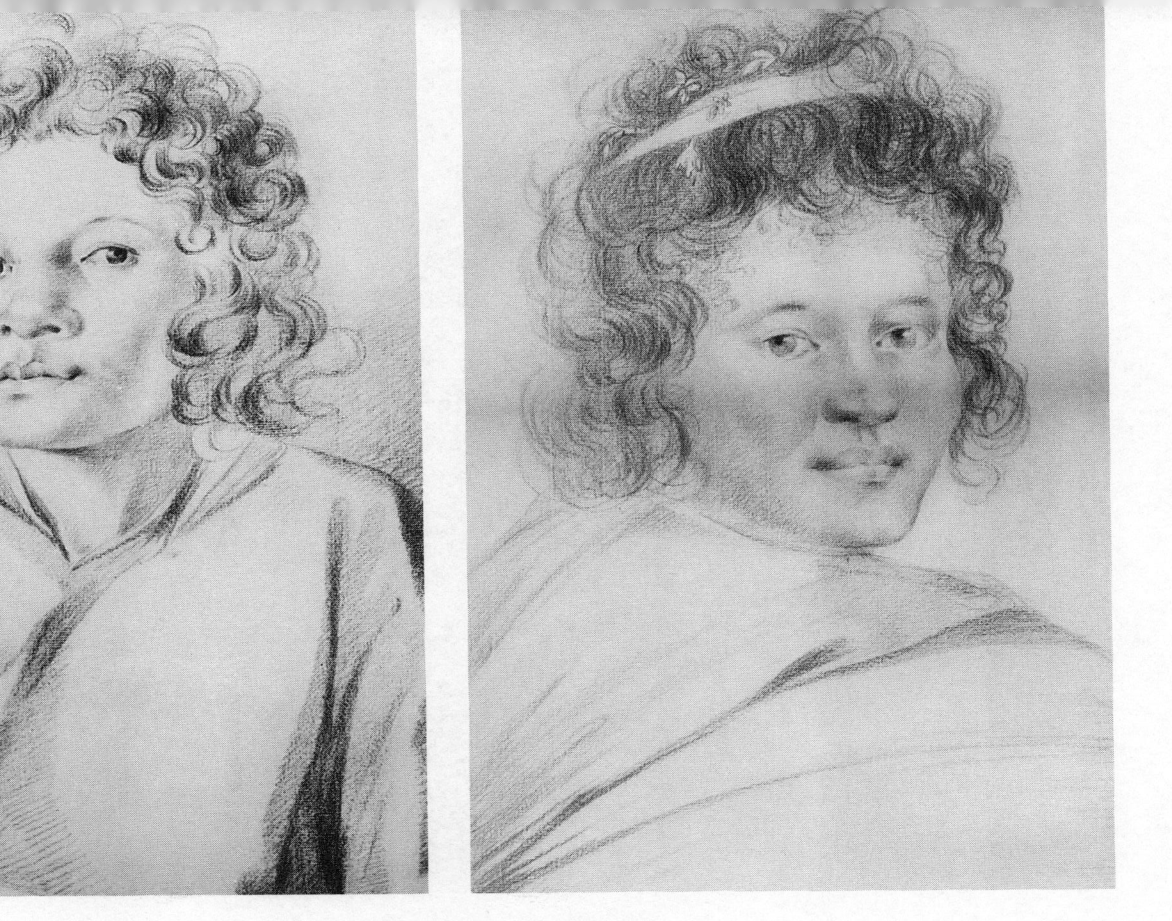

FIG. 42. Portrait heads of Raiateans

(*left*) Hiti-hiti, or 'Oedidee'; (*right*) 'Tynai-mai', a young woman. Crayon drawings by Hodges.—Commonwealth National Library

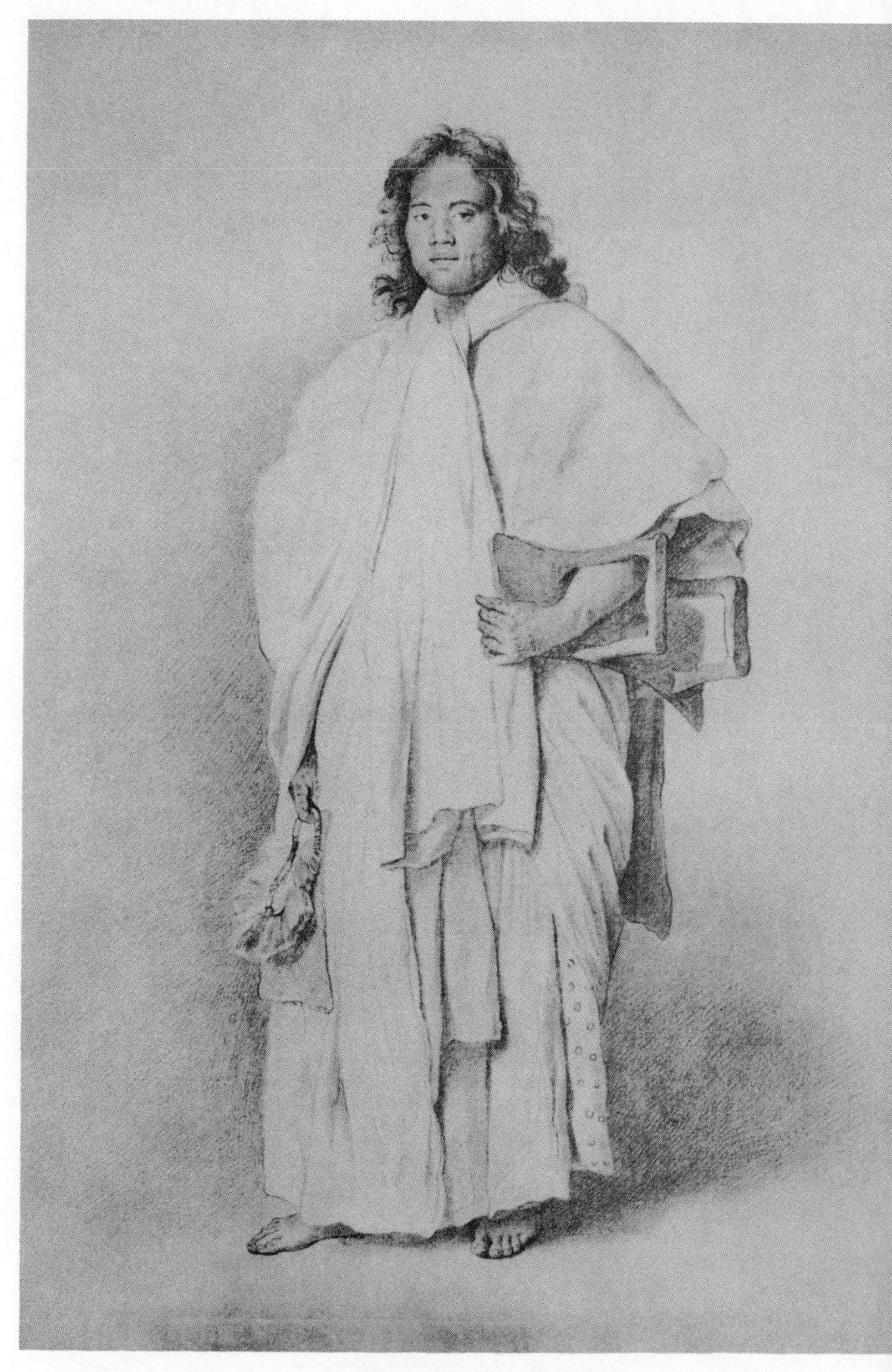

FIG. 43. Portrait of Omai, by Nathaniel Dance, 1775
Public Archives of Canada, Ottawa

him a handsom return. Oreo interduced into the Ship and presented to me three pretty young Women his relations,[1] this was done with a View of shewing them the Ship and to obtain presents in which I believe they were not disapointed;[2] This good natured Chief also purchass'd sever[l] Hogs for me[3] and made such bargins as I had reason to be sati[s]fied with. At length he and all his friends departed, first makeing me promise to go and see him in the morning.

SUNDAY 12*th*. Viseted Oreo according to promise, who entertain'd us with a Heva some what different from the one we saw before,[4] he after wards came aboard and dined with us together with two of his friends. Many of the Gentlemen and Seamen were on Shore to day rambling about the Country and met every were with sevel treatment from the Natives.

MONDAY 13*th*. Nothing happen'd worthy of note.

TUESDAY 14*th*. Early in the Morning I sent Lieutenant Pickersgill with the Resolutions Launch and the Adventures Cutter to Otaha to procure fruit, especially Plantains, for a Sea Store.[5] Had a Veset from Oreo and some of his Friends, acquainted the Chief that I should dine with [him] a Shore and desired he would order two Pigs to be dress'd for us in their own way,[6] giving him the Value of the Pigs before hand, but this was not absolutely necessary, he accordingly went a shore to prepare the dinner and about one o'Clock I and the officers of both Sloops went to pertake of it, when we came to the Chiefs house we found the Cloth already laid, that is green leaves were laid thick on the floor round which we seated our selves, the chief then asked me if the Victuals should be brought. I told him yes and presently after one of the Pigs came over my head souce

[1] In H Cook writes in the margin, 'one was his Daughter'.

[2] *Oreo . . . disapointed:* Oreo at this time interduced into the ship two very pretty young women [his neices *deleted*], these two beauties attracted the notice of most of the officers and gentlemen who made love to them in their turns, the ladies very obligingly received their addresses, to one they gave a kind look to a nother a smile, thus they distributed their favours to all, received presents from all and at last jilted them all.—f. 101v.

[3] . . . (for we now began to take of them).—'We get great plenty of fruits &c from our good Friends here and might have as many Hogs as we pleas'd but absolutely the Ship is fairly full of them and we cannot find stowage for any more. We live at present a very jolly life, we have the gratification of not only every necessitous but of every luxurious call of Nature'.—Clerke.—'Started the Water out of the Provision Cask Emp[d] filling of them again'—Smith.

[4] . . . Oreo ordered a Heava to be acted for our entertainment, in which the two young women above mentioned were the Actress's: this Heava was somewhat different from the one I saw before and not so entertaining.

[5] . . . for we could get little more of these articles at Ulietea than what served us for present consumsion

[6] i.e. cooked in an 'earth oven' or *umu*.

upon the leaves[1] and immidiatly after the other, both so hott that it was scarce possible to touch them, the dish was garnished with hot bread fruit and Plantains and a quantity of Cocoa-nutts were brought for drinks. There were several Women at table and no doubt some of them might be in a longing condition but as it is not the Custom here for the Women to eat with the men, we were not delayed or the victuals suffered to cool by carving out their longing bits.[2] Each man being ready with his knife in his hand we turn'd to without ceremony. Never was Victuals cleaner or better dress'd, the Pigs were dress'd whole, one wieghed between 50 and 60 pound the other about half as much and yet all the parts were equally well done and with all its juces in it and eat by far sweeter than it would have done had it been dress'd by any of our methods. The Chief his Son and some other of his Male friends eat with us and pieces were handed to siveral others who sat behind for we had a vast crowd about us.[3] The Chief never faild to drink his glass of Madeira when ever it came to his turn not only now but at all other times when he dined with us without ever once being the least affected by it. As soon as we had dined the Boats crew took the remains to the Boat where by them and the people about them the whole was consum'd. When we rose up many of the Common people rushed in to pick up the Crums which fell from our Table,[4] this led me to think that as plenty as Pork is at these Isles but little falls to the share of the Common people. Some of our gentlemen being present when these two Pigs were dress'd and kill'd saw the chief divide the intrails, lard &c[a] into ten or twelve equal parts and serve it out to certain people. Several dayly attended the Sloops and assisted the butchers for the sake of the intrails of the hogs we kill'd: probably little else falls to the share of the Common people, it must however be owned that they are ex-

[1] 'souce [souse] upon the leaves'—suddenly, thump upon the leaves. Johnson defines 'souse' (adv.) as 'With sudden violence. A low word'.

[2] *by carving . . . bits:* or the Ladies put to the blush by forcing each to name her longing bit as is the custom at most of the polite tables in Europe . . .—The sentence beginning 'There were several women . . .', but altered thus, was first written but then deleted in B f. 102, and was accordingly not printed. 'Longing condition', 'longing bits': I can find no trace of this vivid idiom in the dictionaries; was it perhaps peculiar to the East Riding?

[3] . . . so that it may be truely said we dined in publick.—f. 102.—'M[r] Foster Senior was not at this feast, there being some Misunderstanding between him & Cap[t] Cook relative to M[r] Fosters shooting an Indian in the back with Shot, for catching hold of M[r] F Junier's Gun; whither with a design to wrest it from him, or to prevent M[r] Foster's shooting him (as he thought) does not appear, but Circumstances seem to favour the latter.—but happily there was no great harm there being only 8 or 9 Shots in one side of the Mans back.' [and a note] 'M[r] Foster was gone to Otaha with the Boats'.—Bayly. There was later a sharp exchange of argument over this incident, and another concerning Forster senior, between George Forster (who does not advert to it in his book) and Wales: Wales, *Remarks*, pp. 97–8; Forster, *Reply to Mr. Wales's Remarks*, pp. 36–8.

[4] . . . and for which they searched the leaves very narrowly

ceeding carefull of all their Provisions and waste nothing that can be eat by man, flesh and fish especially. In the afternoon we were entertained with a Play with which ended the principal transactions of the day, Plays have indeed generally been acted every day sence we have been here either to entertain us or for their own amusement. Many fine large Hogs were offered us to Day for Axes and Hatchets which we were obliged to refuse having already got more than we know what to do with.[1]

WEDNESDAY 15*th*.[2] The Natives not coming off to the Sloops this morning as usual gave us reason to fear that some thing had happened and as two of the men belonging to the Adventure remained on Shore last night I judged it might be on their account,[3] in order to be fully informed Captain Furneaux and I went a Shore to Oreo's house which we found quite empty and he and all his family gone, the two people belonging to the Adventure made their appearence unhurt[4] nor could till what caused the precipitate retreat of the Natives for the whole neighbourhood was in a manner quite disarted, all that we could learn from the few who came to us was that several of them were killed and others wounded by our guns, pointing out to us where the Balls went in and out of the body &c[a] and as we understood them this happened on the Island of Ulietea, but as I knew this could not be I was uneasy for the safety of our Boats, fearing that some disturbance had happened at Otaha where they were gone, in order to know more of the matter I determined to see Oreo if possible, with this view we imbarked in our Boat and proceeded towards the north end of the Island were we were told he was gone, takeing one of the natives along with us. We soon came in sight of the Canoe in which he was but before we came up with her he landed, we landed presently after and found him fled still farther,

[1] 'Our friends here begin to grow confoundedly nimble finger'd, we gave one of them today 2 dozen for appropriating to his own use what did by no means belong to him.'—Clerke. Bayly also has something to say under this date about the nuisance from theft, but he undoubtedly overdoes the constancy of punishment, or Clerke would not have remarked on this particular instance as he does (cf. also Cook, pp. 388–9 below): 'The Natives cannot withstand thieving even from the King to the Towtow or servants, great Numbers of them constantly coming on board & going about the Ship & riging they frequently steal things, & whenever catched or the thing lost found on them, we immediately sieze them up to the Shrouds & give them a dozen or two according to the nature of the Theft, without any respect to rank or distinction, & let them loose & flock them out of the Ship & make them swim on shore, as no Canoe takes in the Teeto or Thief—notwithstanding there is few of them can Avoid thieving when an opportunity offers.'

[2] . . . This morning produced some circumstances which will fully shew the timerous disposission of these islanders; . . .—f. 102v.

[3] *I judged . . . account:* contrary to orders, my first conjectures were that the natives had striped them and were now affraid to come near us, least we should take some step to revenge this insult

[4] *unhurt:* and informed us that they had been very civily treated by the natives,

many people however remained behind[1] who wanted me to follow him, one man even offered to carry me on his back but I did not choose to seperate my self from the Boat as we were all unarmed and the whole story appearing rather more mysterious than ever, we therefore imbark'd again and rowed after him, we soon came before the house where our guide told us he was and put in the Boat accordingly, the boat grounded at some distance from the Shore, here we were met by a venerable old Laidy the Mother[2] of the cheif, she threw her self into my arms and wept bitterly, in so much that it was not possible to get one plain word from her, with this old laidy in my hand I went a shore[3] and walked up [to] the Chief who was seated under a shade before a large area without which were a great crowd of people, he took me in his arms and wept as much as his Mother had done before, all the Women and some of the men round us joined in the general lamentation,[4] it was some time before we could get a word from any one, at length all our enquiries gave us no other information than that they were allarm'd on account of our Boats and people being absant thinking that they had disarted from us and that I should take some violent measures to recover them for when we assured them that they would return back they seemd cheerfull and satisfied, and they to a man denied that any one was hurt either of their own or our people, it after wards proved to be a false allarm without the least foundation whatever.[5] After a stay of about an Hour I took leave of the Chief and return'd aboard to dinner, Three of the Natives coming with us who made it known to the people we met in our way that all matters were reconciled.

THURSDAY 16*th*. This Morning the Natives came off to the Sloops in their Canoes as usual, after breakfast Captain Furneaux and I paid the Chief a Viset, we found him at his house perfectly easy and satisfied in so much that he and some of his friends came a board and dined with us. In the after noon the Boats return'd from Otaha pretty well laden with Plantans an article we most wanted, they made the circuit of the Island, one of the Arree's whose name is Boba accompanied them, they were every were sivily treated by the natives (if we except a little thieving) and the first night they were

[1] *many . . . behind:* An immense crowd however waited our landing . . .—f. 103

[2] Mother *deleted* Wife *substituted.*

[3] . . . contrary to the advice of my Otaheite young man who seemed more afraid than any of us, he probably beleived every word the people had told us.—f. 103.

[4] . . . astonishment alone kept me from joining with them

[5] . . . nor could we ever find out by what means this general consternation first took its rise—f. 103v.—Cf. the story told by Pickersgill, p. 774 below, about the episode in which the Gunner and one of the young Gentlemen' were concerned, and of which Cook never heard. This may be the truth of the matter.

out entertained with a Heva. Having got a board a large supply of refreshments I determined to put to Sea in the morning and made the same known to the chief who promised to come and take leave of me on board the Ship.

Whilest I was with him [Oreo] yesterday, my Otaheite young man Porio took a sudden resolution to leave me, I have mentioned before that he was with me when I followed Oreo, and of his advising me not to go out of the boat, and was so much affraid at this time that he remaned in the boat till he heard all matters were reconciled, then he came out and presently after met with a young woman for whom he had contracted a friendship, he having my powder horn in keeping came and gave it to one of my people who was by me and then went away; I, who knew that he had found his female friend, took no notice thinking that he was only going to retire with her on some private buisness of their own, probably at this time he had no other intention, she however had prevailed upon him to remain with her for I saw him no more and to day I was told, that he was married and did not intend to go with us. In the after noon our boats returned from Otaha pretty well laden with Plantains an article we were most in want of, they made the Circuit of the isle, conducted by one of the Aree's whose name was Boba, and were hospitably entertained by the people who provided them with victuals lodgeing and bed fellows according to the custom of the Country; the first night they were entertained with a Play, the second night their repast was disturbed by the Natives stealing their military Chest, which put them upon making reprisals by which means they recovered the most of what they had lost.[1]—ff. 103v–4v.

FRIDAY 17*th*. At 4 o'Clock in Morning we began to unmoor and as soon as it was light Oreo and some of his friends came to take leave, many Canoes also came off with Hogs and fruit, the former they even beged of us to take from them, calling out, Tyo Boa Atoi[2] which was as much as to say, I am your friend take my Hog and give me an ax, but our decks were already so full of them that we could hardly move, having on board the Resolution about 230 and on board the Adventure about 150. The increase of our Stock together with what we have consumed[3] sence we came to this Isle I judge we have got here about 500[4] Hogs, big and little, some were only roasters, others

[1] See Pickersgill's account, pp. 773–4 below.

[2] *Taio! Puaa! Toi!*—No doubt a shout with gesticulation—'Friend! Pig! Axe!'

[3] *consumed:* salted and consumed

[4] H four hundred or upwards . . .—I print 500. Cook first writes 1500, and then smudges out the last 0, when what he obviously intended was to delete the 1.

wieghed 100 lb and upwards,[1] it is not easy to guess how many we might have got could we have dispenced with all that were offered us.

The Chief and his friends did not leave us till the Anchor was a weigh. At parting I made him a present of a Broad Ax and several other things with which he went away well satisfied. He was extremely desirous to know if, and when I would return, these were the last questions he asked me. After we were out of the Harbour and had made sail we discovered a Canoe conducted by two men following us, upon which I brought to and they presently came a long side with a present of fruit from Oreo, I made them some return for their trouble, dismissed them and made sail to the Westward with the Adventure in company.[2] The young man I got at Otahiete left me at Ulietea two days before we saild being inticed away by a young Woman for whom he had contracted a friendship. I took no methods to recover him as their were Volanteers enough out of whome I took one, a youth about [17 or 18] years of age who says he is a relation of the great Opoony and is a great advocate for Bolabola of which Island he is a native, his name is Oediddee,[3] he may be of use to us if we should fall in with and touch at any isles in our rout to the west which was my only montive for takeing him on board.[4]

*The Chief and his friends did not leave us till the anchor was a weigh, at parting I made him a handsome present; he took a very

[1] . . . but the greatest run was from forty to sixty . . .—The Log mentions also 'many Fowles and a great quantity of plantains & Bananoes'.

[2] ADV 'Punish Will.m Sanderson (Seaman) for uttering prophane Oaths and being Insolent'.—Wilby. This note is included as a curiosity of maritime history; for although insolence was more than once punished in Cook's ships, the uttering of 'prophane Oaths' was (as we know from Forster and Sparrman) more lightly looked upon; so either Furneaux was more easily shocked or the profanity of William Sanderson was of a deep and unexampled nature. Burney, log 18 September, gives us additional information on this ship: 'The fresh Provisions & Refreshments we have found at these Islands have Set our People to rights again'.

[3] 'It may be necessary to observe that our friend Porio took a french leave of us at Uliateah; when a Lad from thence whose name was Odiddy a native of Bolo Bolo being very desirous to see Britannia as he express'd himself desir'd to supply his place, which was readily granted him—the parting cost poor Odiddy and his freinds many tears but the good Lad adher'd to his resolution with a manly and commendable perseverance and attended us with an aching heart but apparently a chearfull spirit'.—Clerke, 19 September. 'Odiddy' or 'Oediddee' = O Hitihiti; Hitihiti, or alternatively, and originally, Mahine (as Forster always insists on calling him) was the youth's name—'he having exchanged [Mahine] for that of Hedeedee with a chief in Eimeo, a custom which is common in all these islands'.—Forster, I, p. 420. See Fig. 42*a*.

[4] 'I must own that 'tis with some reluctance I bid adieu to these happy Isles, where I've spent many very happy days, both in the Years 69 & 73; in the first place (for we must give this consideration the preference after a long Sea passage) you live upon, and abound in, the very best of Pork & the sweetest and most salutary of Vegetables; in the next place, the Women in general are very handsome and very kind, and the Men civil and to the last degree benevolent, so that I'm sure whenever we get among them we may with very great safety say, We've got into a very good Neighbourhood—in short, in my Opinion, they are as pleasant & Happy spots as this World contains.'—Clerke.

affectionate leave and asked me if, and when I would return, these were his last words; questions which have been very often put to me by many of these islanders, and when ever this happened they never failed to tell me to bring my Sons with me, for they would frequently ask me how many children I had and whether they were boys or Girls &c[a]. My friend Oree of Huaheine was very desireous for me to return to his isle; but as he did not expect this could be done till the expiration of the same time as I had been absent before, he one time very justly observ'd that both him and I might be dead, but says he, 'let your Sons Come they will be well received'. . . .

We will now leave the Sloops for a while and take a short View of the isles we have lately touched at, for although I have been pretty minute in relating our transactions while among them, some things rather intresting have been omitted. Soon after our arrival at Otaheite, we were informed that a Ship about the seize of the Resolution, commanded by one Opep-pe (as the natives call'd him) had put into Owhaiurua Harbour near the South end of the island. . . . . Probably this was one of the two French Ships that were fitted out at the Mauritius and touched at the Cape of Good Hope in March 1772,[1] as hath been allready mentioned.[2] What route she took after leaving Otaheite is not known, the Natives of Huaheine and Ulietea had no knowlidge of her.

The Otaheiteans complain of a disease communicated to them by the people in this Ship, they say that it affects the head, throat and stomack and at length kills them; they dread it much and were constantly enquiring if we had it. They call it by the name of the communicator Apa no opep-pe, just as they call the veneral disease Apa no Britannia or Brit-tanee, notwithstanding they to a man say that it was first communicated to them by M. de Bougainville, but I have already mentioned that they thought M. de Bougainville as well as we came from Britannia and that they have not the least knowlidge of any other European Country. I mention this as a fact which accrued to me and not with any view of exculpating the English from bringing this disease to the isles and fixing it on the French; the name the natives have given it together with what M. de Bougainvill has said on this subject will, in my opinion, for ever father it upon the English, howsoever innocent they may be.[3] Be

[1] Properly December 1771.

[2] . . . At this time we conjectured this was a French Ship, but on our arrival at the Cape of Good Hope we learnt she was a Spaniard which had been sent out from America.—f. 105v.

[3] Bougainville's remarks were as follows: 'I am yet ignorant, whether the people of Taiti, as they owe the first knowledge of iron to the English, may not likewise be indebted to them for the venereal disease, which we found had been naturalized among them, as

this as it will it is now far less common a mong them then in the year 1769, they even say they can cure it and so it fully appears, for altho' most of our people made pritty free use of the Women but few were affected with this disease and those in so slight a manner as was easy removed, but when ever it turns to a pox it is incurable, that is amongest the natives; some of our gentlemen pretend to say that they have seen some who have had the pox in a high degree but this wants confirmation, the Surgeon, who made it his business to enquire could never be satisfied in this point. These people are, and were when the Europeans first visited them very subject to eruptions of every kind, so that one may easily mistake one disease for a nother.[1] . . .

Cocoa-nutts, Bananoes and Plantains were what we got the most of at all the isles, the two latter together with the few yamms and other roots we got, were to us a substitute for Bread. At Otaheite we got plenty of apples[2] which proved of great service to our Scorbutick people. The fruit called by them Aheiya[3] which is something like an Nectrain both in shape and taste with a large stone in it, was now in season at all the isles which was not the case when I was here before. I did not even at that time see one. Pumpkins are now at all the isles and are the only thing which have succeeded of all the seeds that have been brought to these isles by Europeans, at least we have not seen the produce of any other[4]. . . . The other isles[5] have undergone no sort of Revolution but appear to be in the same state they were four years ago, whilest we lay at Huaheine, several of the common people frequently desired me to kill the Bolabola men. . . . One of the largest double Canoes I have any where seen was here, it was

will appear in the sequel.'—pp. 273–4. And 'At the same time there appeared in both ships several venereal complaints, contracted at Taiti. They had all the symptoms known in Europe. . . . Columbus brought this disease from America; here it is on an isle in the midst of the greatest ocean. Have the English brought it thither?'—pp. 285–6.

[1] 'The more I have enquired into and considered this subject, the more I am led to believe, that these people had the veneral disease among them long before they had any commerce with Europeans or at least some disease which is very near a kin to it, for I have heard them speaking of people who have died of the disorder, which we interpreted to be the Pox, long before that time. This note is founded partly from the information I had from Odiddy and partly from what I could pick upon on this subject the last time I was at these isles.'—Cook's note, f. 108, A91. Instead of this note, Cook writes on f. 106, 'These people are, and were before the Europeans visited them, very subject to Scrofulous diseases, so that a Seaman might easily mistake one disorder for another'. 'Scrofulous diseases' in that era covered a multitude of less closely defined ills, many characterized by skin eruptions. For a note on syphilis and the island disease of yaws, see I, p. 99.

[2] The Tahitian *vi*, the 'yellow apple' or Brazilian plum, *Spondias dulcis*.

[3] The Tahitian *ahia*, the Mountain-apple or Rose-apple, *Eugenia malaccensis*.

[4] *Pumpkins . . . other:* Of all the seeds that have been brought to these isles by Europeans, none have succeeded put [*sic*] Pumpkins and these they do not like a thing that cannot be wondered at.—f. 106v. Evidently Cook did not like pumpkins either.

[5] i.e. other than Tahiti.

built to row with 144 Paddles and was capable of carrying a far greater number of men.

The Islands of Ulietea and Otaha are in some measure under the dominion of Opoony the King of Bolabola who made a conquest of them some years ago, sence that period they have enjoyed the blessings of peace and the natives seem now to be as happy as any people under Heaven and have all the necessaries and some of the luxuries of life in the greatest profusion.[1] I saw Opoony in 1769 who was then very old, he was now at Maurua a neighbouring isle under his Juridiction so that we did not see him; he must be now very old and we are told walks almost double a very uncommon thing in these isles. The successor to this great man, who has made all the Nations round him tremble, is a young woman his daughter; we are told she is very handsome and has the same outward respect paid to her as Otoo of Otaheite.

My young man tells me that Hogs fruit &c[a] are in as great plenty at Bolabola as at any of the other isles a thing that Tupia would never allow, it must be observed that the one was predjuiced against, and the other in favour of this isle.

I shall not in this Journal take any notice of the gener[l] produce of these isles, the manners and Customs of the Natives &c[a] as these subjects have been treated at large in the Published account of my former Voyage. But as M de Bougainville in his Voyage round the world has mentioned some customs being amo[n]gst them not taken notice of by me in the said published account, and as they were to me rather doubtfull they became the object of my enquirey. He mentions, page 268,[2] human sacrifices; in order to satisfie my self in this point, I went one day to a marai in Matavai in company with Captain Furneaux, having a long with us, as I had upon every other occasion a marine who was with me last voyage and who spoke the language tolerable well.[3] Several of the Natives were with us one of whome appeared to be an intelligent sencible man. In the marai laid a Corps upon a Watarau,[4] some viands &c[a] so that every thing promised success to my inquireys. I began with asking questons relating to the several objects before us: if the Plantans &c[a] were for the Eatua;[5] if they sacrificed to the Eatua Hogs, Dogs

[1] *Deleted* They are also governed by their own Kings, or Chiefs for they are not stiled Aree de hi but Aree; Opoony reserves this title to himself and as far as I can find this is all he has got by the conquest.—f. 109v. There is a cross at 'Chiefs' for a footnote, but Cook gives this neither here nor in G. A refers to further discussion of the subject later on.

[2] An editor should correct Cook as Cook corrects longitudes; this figure should be 269.

[3] He at first wrote 'indifferent well'. This marine was Gibson, who gave such trouble on the first voyage by trying to desert at Tahiti.

[4] *fatarau*, properly an altar.

[5] *e atua*, a god

Fowles &c^a to all of which he answered in the afformative. I then asked if they sacrificed men to the Eatua, he answered Taata eno[1] they did, that is bad men, first Teparrahy or beating them till they were dead;[2] I then asked him if good men were put to death in this manner, he answer'd no Taata eno, I asked if any Aree's he said no and said these had Hogs &c^a to give to the Eatua and again repeated Taata eno. I next asked him if Towtows,[3] that is servants or slaves, who had nither Hogs, Dogs or fruit, but yet good men if they were sacrificed to the Eatua, his answer was no only bad men. I asked him several more questons, and all his answers seemed to tend to this one point that men for certain crimes were condemn'd to be sacrificed to the gods provide[d] they have not wherewithall to redeem themselves which I think implies that on certain occasions human sacrifices are necessary, when they take such men as have committed crimes worthy of death and such will generally be found amongest the lower class of people.[4] The man of whom I made these inquir[i]es as well as some others took some pains to explain the whole of this Custom to us but we were not masters enough of their language to understand them.[5] Thus far then M de Bougainville is right but he is wrong when he says, that the kind of wood, which is burnt for people of distinction is not the same with that which the common people are allowed to make use of;[6] that 'their Kings alone are allowed to plant before their houses the tree which we call the weeping-willow, or Babyloion Willow (Arbre du grand Seigneur)';[7] and that, 'the Grandees have liveries for the Servants, in proportion as their Masters rank is more or less elevated, their servants

[1] *taata ino*, mean or evil folk.

[2] *taparahi*, to beat; the doomed man was killed by a heavy blow on the back of the head.

[3] *teuteu*, hereditary retainers, not slaves.

[4] Cf. I, p. clxxviii. A further paragraph on this matter will be found on p. 238 below.

[5] There is an interesting echo of this remark in Boswell, who dined at the Mitre on 18 April 1776 with Sir John Pringle and other members of the Royal Society, including Cook. 'I placed myself next to Captain Cooke, and had a great deal of conversation with him; but I need not mark it, as his Book will tell it all. Only I must observe that he candidly confessed to me that he and his companions who visited the south sea islands could not be certain of any information they got, or supposed they got, except as to objects falling under the observation of the senses; their knowledge of the language was so imperfect they required the aid of their senses, and any thing which they learnt about religion, government, or traditions might be quite erroneous.' Boswell rather fancied going to one of the islands for three years to learn the language and bring home a full account, 'if encouraged by Government by having a handsome pension for life'.—*Private Papers of James Boswell*, II, pp. 256–7.

[6] 'I have not the least Idea of what sort of wood he means: the principal people and others without distinction are lighted at nights with a kind of oily nutts, which when stuck upon small sticks burn like a toarch.'—Cook's note, f. 115; Bougainville, p. 269. These 'oily nutts' were from the Candle-nut tree or Tutui, *Aleurites triloba*.

[7] 'There is no such distinction as this, nor know I what tree he means—unless it be the Etoe tree which is generally planted in the Maraies.'—Cook's note, f. 115; Bougainville, p. 269.

wearing their sashes more or less high'.[1] Such distinctions as these were never observed by us and are most certainly wholy unknown to them. He further says that the whole Nation wear Mourning for their Kings which may be, but it cannot be the Mourning he discribes for we know there are but few such dresses in the whole island and from this Custom of Mourning he certainly draws a wrong conclution. He is again very much misstaken when he says, P. 25, that 'every one gathers fruit from the first tree he meets with or takes some in any house on to which he enters'; he likewise seems to think there is no personal property among them. So far from it being so, that I much doubt if their is a fruit tree on the whole island that is not the property of some individual in it. We are even told that whoever takes fruit &c[a] the property of any other person is punished with death or a good beating Indeed it is highly obsurd to suppose every thing in Common in a Country where almost every article is raised by cultivation, it is true some things require but little labour, but others again require a good deal, such as roots of every kind and Bananas and Plantains will not grow spontaneously but by proper cultivation, nor will the Bread and Cocoa nutt trees come to perfection without. These are not the only Mistakes M. Bougainville has committed in his account of the Customs of these people[2] nor can I See how it could be otherwise, a stay of ten days was by no means sufficient for such a task. The love of truth alone obliges me to mention these things and not with a view of finding fault with M[r] Bougainville's Book, on the Contrary I think it the most usefull as well as entertaining Voyage through these Seas yet published. When I was at Ulietea in 1769, we thought the people but little addicted to thieving, probably they were at that time restrain'd by their countryman Tupia, for we now found them as expert thieves as the Otaheitians; the temptations were indeed now far greater and occured oftener, as being more of us and less upon our guard, though very little attention would have been sufficient as my self and some few others experienced while others less on their guard had their Pockets Picked every day. A forced restitution is all that

[1] 'M. de Bougainville has probably seen the Ari dehi, or King without knowing it, and has observed all the people about him uncovered, that is with their cloathes, or sashes as he calls them, worn no higher then their breasts; at other times he has seen the attendance of a Chief with nothing on but the marra or sash round their loins, without considering, that men of all ranks frequently wear nothing else.'—Cook's note, f. 115; Bougainville, p. 270.

[2] 'M. B. Page 256, says Polygamy seems established among them; I cannot recolect what is said on this subject in the account of my former Voyage, therefore shall now take upon me to say they have no such Custom, each man can only have one wife let h[is] rank be ever so much elevated.'—Cook's note.

can be expected, but unless this can be done immidiately or what you have lost be of some Value or concequence, it will be better to put up with the loss, for one no sooner attempts to force a restitution than the whole country is alarmed and a total stop put to all manner of supplies till all matters reconciled. One ought not to be too severe upon these people when they do commit a thieft sence we can hardly charge them with any other Vice, Incontency in the unmarried people can hardly be call'd a Vice sence neither the state or Individuals are the least injured by it. Maried Women are perhaps as faithfull to their husband[s] as any others whatever, at least I have not seen an instance to the contrary; upon the whole I think the women in general were less free of their favours now than formerly, none but common women would yeild to the embraces of our people; not one of the gentlemen were able to obtain such favours from any women of distinction, though several attempts were made, but they were always jilted in the end.[1] In short the more one is acquainted with these people the better one likes them, to give them their due I must say they are the most obligeing and benevolent people I ever met with. I had almost forgot to mention the Avā root a kind of Pepper plant on which they make a liquor which is intoxicating. I do not remember of seeing it used last Voyage which is the reason of my takeing notice of it now. The manner of Brewing or preparing the liquor is as simple as it is disgusting to a European and is thus; several people take of the root or stem adjoining to the root and chew it into a kind of Pulp when they spit it out into a platter or other Vessel, every one into the same Vessel, when a sufficient quantity is done they mix with it a certain proportion of Water[2] and then strean the liquor through some fiberous stuff like fine shavings[3] and it is then fit for drinking which is always done immidiately; it has a pepperish taste rather flat and insipid and intoxicating but I saw but one instance where it had this effect, as I have generally seen them drink it with great moderation and but little at a time; some times they chew this root in their mouths as Europeans do Tobacco and swallow the spittle, at other times I have seen them eat it wholy. At Ulietea they cultivate great quantities of this Plant, at Otaheite but little, I believe there are but few isles in this Sea but what produceth more or less of it and the Inhabitants apply it to the same use as appears by Le Maires account of Horn Island wherein

[1] For further meditations on this matter see pp. 238–9 below.

[2] *is done . . . Water:* is chewed, more or less Water is put to it, according as it is to be strong or Weak . . .—f. 112.

[3] The inner bark of the hibiscus.

he makes mention of the Natives makeing a liquor from a Plant in the manner above mentioned. Dalrymple's Voyages Book 2 P. [45].[1]

I shall conclude this account of the isle with a few remarks on the Astronomical observations made at Otaheite. Supposeing Queen Charlottes Sound to be in the Longitude of 186°11′ West as settled by Mr Baily, Mr Kendalls Watch will place Otaheite about half a degree more west than it was settled by us in 1769; but as their is reason to think Queen Charlottes Sound lies more East,[2] the error of the Watch may be little or nothing.

I have already observed that Messrs Wales and Baily made their observations on the same Spot which the Transit of Venus was Observed in June 1769, the Latitude of which they found to be, by their observations, 17°29′13″ s which is two Seconds less than it was settled by us at that time. It may not be amiss to observe that this is the most northern point of the isle, the Longitude of which is 149°35′ West.

Before I quet this subject I cannot help takeing notice of a remark which Mr Maskelyne has thought proper to affix to the observations made here in 1769, for finding the Latitude of the observatory; published in the Philosophical transactions for 1771, Number 43, page 406. He there says, that the results differ more from one another than they ought to do, and cannot account for it in no other way than the want of care and address in the observers. Mr M. might have assigned a nother reason, he was not unacquainted with the quadrant having been in the hands of the Natives, pull'd to peices and many of the parts broke which we had to mend in the

[1] Ava or Kava (*Piper methysticum* Forst.) is a shrub that grows on the volcanic islands, not the atolls; it has a large and knotted root, prepared in olden days as Cook describes but now bruised and battered without the aid of the human teeth. It can even be bought at the village store, on up-to-date islands—such is the decline of ancient custom—in a powdered form. It is not alcoholic and, in spite of what Cook says, not intoxicating; but if drunk in sufficient quantity is said to take away temporarily the use of the legs. As Corney pleasantly writes (III, pp. 248–9), 'excessive or habitual indulgence in *ava* tends to induce cerebral hyperaemia, evidenced by blood-shot eyes, drowsiness, apathy, and neglect of the toper's daily obligations. If persisted in, emaciation and free desquamation of the cuticle ensue'. Kava-drinking as a ceremony on some islands reached a very high degree of elaboration indeed, which can still be witnessed in Samoa, one of the few groups that Cook did not visit. Mariner describes it for Tonga in detail, II, pp. 150–67. The taste is curious, and many Europeans besides Cook have tried their hands at defining it—the classic, if vulgar, description having it a combination of quinine and dish-water. This is unjust. It is not a drink that one lingers over or is supposed to linger over, but it is refreshing and leaves one quite ready for the next cup. Enlightened pro-consuls nowadays give it to their visitors instead of morning tea. Le Maire's account, referred to by Cook, does not describe the chewing process, and calls the plant 'Acona' (Fijian *yaqona*); Schouten, in the same volume of Dalrymple, p. 54, is much more circumstantial, and uses the name *kava*.

[2] A *note* 'It has been found to lie 40′ more East therefore the error of the Watch did not exceed 10′ of Longitude, which is only 45 Seconds in time.'

best manner we could before it could be made use of.[1] Mr M. should have considered, before he took upon him to censure these observations, that he had put into his hands the very original book in which they were written in pencel only, the very moment they were taken and I appeal to Mr M. himself, if it is not highly probable that some of them might from various causes, be so doubtful to the observer, as either to be wholy rejected or to be marked as dubious and which might have been done had Mr Green taken the trouble to enter them in the proper book. Mr M should also have considered, that this was, perhaps, the only true original paper of the kind ever put into his hands; does Mr M. publish to the world all the observations he makes good and bad or did he never make a bad observation in his life.—ff. 107–10v, 115–16v.

I have sence learnt from Omai, that they offer Human Sacrifices to the Supreme Being. According to his account the Man so sacrificed, depends on the Caprice of the High Priest who, when they are assembled on any Solemn occasion, retires alone into the House of God and stays there some time. When he comes out, he informs them, that he has seen and conversed with their great God (the High-Priest alone having that power) and that he has asked for an human Sacrifice, and tells them that he has desired such a person, names a man present, whom most probably the Priest has an Antipathy against; he is immediately kill'd and so falls a Victim to the priests resentment, who no doubt, if necessary, has address enough to persuade the people that he was a bad man. If I except their Funeral Ceremonies all the knowlidge that has been obtained of their Religion, has been from information, and As their language is but imperfectly understood, even by those who pretend to the greatest knowlidge of it, Very little on this head is yet known with certainty.[2]—f. 113v.

Sence we can hardly charge them with any other vice great Injustice has been done the Women of Otaheite and the Society Isles, by those who have represented them without exception as ready to grant the last favour to any man who will come up to their price. But this is by no means the case; the favours of Maried women and

[1] See I, pp. 87–9.

[2] I print this paragraph in this place, rather than incorporate it in the foregoing general description of Tahiti, as is done in the printed *Voyage*, I, p. 186, because it is so obviously not a part of the original journal, but added during the later revision for publication. The same remark applies to the paragraph that follows, which is drafted on a separate page, on the other side of which is the passage 'I have sence learnt from Omai . . .' I have reversed the two paragraphs for the sake of logical order. It may be added that Omai's account of priestly resentment is rather fanciful, like a good deal of the other information he imparted.

also the unmarried of the better sort, are as difficult to obtain here as in any other Country whatever.[1] Neither can the charge be understood indiscrimenately of the unmaried of the lower class. Much the greater part of these admit of no such familiarities. That there are Prostitutes here as well as in other Countrys is very true, perhaps more in proportion and such were those who came on board the Ship to our people and frequented the Post we had on shore. By seeing these mix indiscriminately with those of a different turn, even of the first rank, one is at first inclined to think that they are all disposed the same way & that the only difference is in their price. But the truth is, the Women who becomes a Prostitute, do not seem on thier opinion to have committed a crime of so deep a die as to exclude her from the Esteem and Society of the Community in general.[2] On the whole a stranger who visits England might with equal justice draw the Characters of the women there, from those which he might meet with on board the Ships in one of the Naval Ports, or in the Purlieus of Covent Garden & Dury [*sic*] lane.[3]*—f. 113.

SATURDAY 18*th. Winds EBS. Course S* 69° *W. Dist. Sailed* 75 *Miles. Lat. in S.* 17°17′. *W. Longd. Greenwich pr. Reck.g.* 153°10′. *Longd. West of Ulietea* 1°31′. Having left Ulietea as before related, I directed my Course to the West inclining to the South as well to avoid the tracks of former Navigators as to get into the Latitude of Amsterdam Island[4] discovered by Tasman in 1643, my intention being to run as far west as that Island and even to touch there if I found it convenient before I proceeded to the South.[5] In the PM we saw the Island of Maurua,[6] one of the Society Isles bearing NBW distant 10 Leagues. A little after Sun set shorten'd Sail to single reefed Top-sails and brought to during the night, but in the day made all the sail we could. This we continued to do for several suceeding nights.

[1] as difficult . . . whatever *altered from* not to be purchased, but by consent of their Husbands or friends. It is possible that instances of this kind may some times happen, tho' undoubtedly very rarely, but than it cannot with justice be charged to the Womens account.

[2] By seeing these . . . in general *altered from* These are not less skilfull in their profession than Ladies of the same stamp in England, nor does a man run less risk of injuring his health and constitution in their Embraces.

[3] To this paragraph the *Voyage*, I, p. 188, adds the following, not found in the MSS: 'I must, however, allow that they are all completely versed in the art of coquetry, and that very few of them fix any bounds to their conversation. It is, therefore, no wonder that they have obtained the character of libertines'.

[4] Tongatapu.

[5] *proceeded to the South:* hauled up for New Zealand. We generally laid to every night in order that we might neither meet with or pass any land in the dark.—f. 121.

[6] Now called Maupiti; lat. 16°27′ S, long. 152°15′ W.

SUNDAY 19*th. Winds East. Course S* 69° *W. Dist. Sailed* 67 *Miles. Lat. in S.* 17°41′. *W. Longd. Greenwich pr. Reck.g.* 154°21′. *Longd. West of Ulietea* 2°42′. *Varn.* 7°50′ *E.* Gentle Trade and pleasent weather.

MONDAY 20*th. Winds E½N. Course S* 70¼° *W. Dist. Sailed* 69 *Miles. Lat. in S.* 18°4′. *W. Longd. Greenwich pr. Reck.g.* 155°29′. *Longd. West of Ulietea* 3°50′. Clowdy weather, Men of War, Tropic and Egg Birds seen.

TUESDAY 21*st. Winds East, NE & NNW. Course S* 68¼° *W. Dist. Sailed* 54 *Miles. Lat. in S.* 18°24′. *W. Longd. Greenwich pr. Reck.g.*

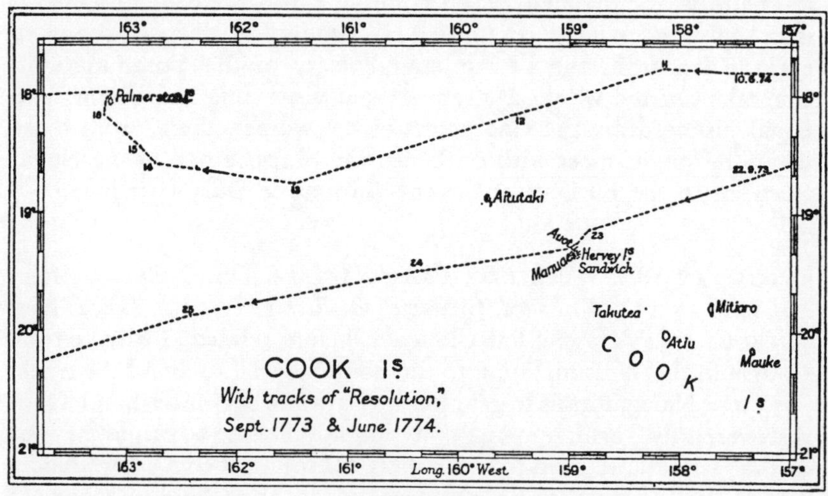

FIG. 44

156°22′. *Longd. West of Ulietea* 4°4′. *Varn.* 7°26′. Gentle breezes and variable Hazy weather with Thunder lightning and rain.[1] Several Sharks followed the Ship three of which we caught also several of the above mentioned Birds and a small Sea Bird which never by choise goes far from land.[2] A large swell from SSE.

WEDNESDAY 22*nd. Winds NWBW to SSE & East. Course S* 73½° *W. Dist. Sailed* 74 *Miles. Lat. in S.* 18°40′. Gentle breezes with some showers of rain in the night. A great swell from the South. Var. pm 7°26′ E. AM 7°56′ E.

[1] 'Much thunder & lightening: ran up the Conductor'.—Wales.

[2] 'This Afternoon there were a remarkable number of Sharks about the Ship—we caught several with Hooks & Lines. We reckon'd at one time eleven about us. We saw also a Land Bird a good deal resembling a Snipe. I've seen many of them along the shores of these S° Sea Islands. . . . Here's been more Tropic Birds about us for these 2 or 3 days past than I ever remember to have seen before, I saw this morning some Men of War Birds.' Clerke, who however gives the date 22 September.

THURSDAY 23*rd. Winds East to SE. Lat. in S.* 19°18′. *W. Longd. Greenwich per Reck.g.* 157°58′. *Longd. West of Ulietea* 5°40′. Fresh Trade with some Showers of rain. At 10 o'Clock AM saw land from the mast head and at Noon from the Deck extending from SBW to SWBS, hauld up in order to discover it plainer.

FRIDAY 24*th. Winds SE. Course S* 76½° *W. Saild* 90 *Miles. Lat. in S.* 19°29′ *W. Longd. Greenwich per Reck.g.* 160°22′. *Longd. West of Ulietea* 8°43′. PM gentle gales and Clowdy. At 2 o'Clock pass'd the Land above mentiond at the distance of one League which proved to be three small Islands connected together by a reef of rocks in which they were incircled and which might be about 18 miles in circuit.[1] They are low and cloathed with wood among which the Cocoa-nutt trees were the most conspicious, we saw no people or signs of inhabitants. I named them Sandwich in honour of my noble Patron the Earl of Sandwich.[2] (Latitude 19°18′ S. Longitude 158°54′

[1] These were the Hervey islands, in the Lower Cooks. They are two, not three, small islands, Manuae and Te Au o Tu or Auotu, in a deep lagoon which is full of coral patches. It would have been presumably possible to make three out of them, and Cook seems not to have been quite sure. Chart XXX*a* has quite unambiguously two; but Pl. XII in the published *Voyage* leaves the question open. In B, f. 121v 'they lie in a triangler form'; in f. 117, his rewritten version, they are 'connected together by breakers like most of the low isles in this sea'; in the printed *Voyage* (I, p. 190) they are 'two or three small islots', so connected. The position of Manuae is lat. 19°21′ S, long. 158°58′ W. Cook comes very close. See Fig. 44.

[2] In B we get some interesting and amusing rewriting of this sentence, in the course of which Sandwich's name is once again jettisoned for Hervey's—or perhaps Hervey came in as Sandwich was elevated to a more important island. H: 'I afterwards altered the name of this isle, and called it Herveys isle and gave the name of Sandwich to one of the Hebrides'. On f. 121v Cook first writes, 'As these three islots are like most others in this Sea included within one reef or Shoul, may without any great impropriety be accounted as one island which I have named Sandwich, in honour of my Noble Patron the Earl of Sandwich'. He then deletes this and substitutes the following: 'The Situation of the isle is nearly the same as Dalrymple has assin'd for La Dezena discovered by Quiros, but as I cannot reconsile my self to the rout Mr Dalrymple has given this Navigator, I believe this isle was never seen before and that Quiros's discoveries in this Latitude lies many degrees farther to the East, probably La Dezena is one of those isles seen by Captain Wallis. I named it Harveys Isle, in honour of my honourable friend Capt Harvey'.—In f. 117–7v we have his final version, a shortened form of the foregoing one; his 'honourable friend Capt Harvey' in this becomes: 'the Honble Captain Harvey of the Navy and one of the Lords of the Admiralty'—to which the printed page adds, 'and now Earl of Bristol'. G is intermediate: 'I named it *Herveys Island* in honor of Captain Hervey of the Navy and one of the Lords of the Admiralty'.—Augustus John Hervey (1724–79), 3rd Earl of Bristol, was so much a contrast to Cook in character and life that friendship between them seems almost the attraction of opposites. A person of great 'interest', he entered the navy in 1736, was a lieutenant when he secretly became the first husband of the celebrated Miss Chudleigh in 1744, and was a post-captain at the age of 23. In action he was a dashing and sometimes brilliant commander, and saw much Mediterranean, Channel and West Indian service. His active life at sea ended in 1763. He was in the House of Commons from 1757 to 1775, when he succeeded to his peerage, and a lord of the Admiralty 1771–5; rear-admiral 1775, vice-admiral 1778. He spoke much in parliament and wrote much in the newspapers; after his retirement from the Admiralty he became the personal enemy of Sandwich, for whose dismissal from office he moved in 1779.—The identity of Quiros's La Dezena is hard to settle: it must have been one of the

West). Having no time to loose to attempt a landing altho' this seemed Practical on the NW side, we reassumed our course to the West. In the night had a few hours Calm which was succeeded by a fresh trade wind at SE attended with some showers of rain.

SATURDAY 25*th. Winds SE. Course S* 79° *W. Dist. Sailed* 119 *Miles. Lat. South* 19°52′. *West Longd. Greenwich Reck.g.* 162°26′ *Watch* 162°26′. *West Longd. Ulietea* 10°47′. Fresh gales and Clowdy with some flying showers. To day we began again to use of our Sea Bisket, the fruit which has served as a substitute (viz Plantans and Bananoes) Sence our arrival at Otaheite being all expended, but our stock of Pork still continues each man having as much every day as he can consume. Swell from SSE.

SUNDAY 26*th. Winds SEBE. Course S* 73° *W. Dist. Sailed* 107 *Miles. Lat. South* 20°23′. *West Longd. Greenwich Reck.g.* 164°15′. *West Longd. Ulietea* 12°36′. Fresh gales and Clowdy with some few sho[we]rs of rain. Saw some Tropic Birds and a Small Sea Bird which by choise we believe cannot go far from land.[1] A great Swell in the direction of the Wind.

MONDAY 27*th. Winds ESE. Course S* 81° *W. Dist. Sailed* 110 *Miles. Lat. South* 20°40′. *West Longd. Greenwich Reck.g.* 166°12′. *West Longd. Ulietea* 14°33′. *Var.* 11°41′ *E.* Fresh gales and fair weather. Saw some Tropic Birds.[2]

TUESDAY 28*th. Winds ESE. Course S* 80° *W. Dist. Sailed* 130 *Miles. Lat. South* 21°3′. *West Longd. Greenwich Reck.g.* 168°29′. *West Longd. Ulietea* 16°50′. Fresh trade and pleasent Weather & Moon light most part of the night.

WEDNESDAY 29*th. Winds E & ESE. Course S* 76¼° *W. Dist. Sailed* 110 *Miles. Lat. South* 21°29′. *West Longd. Greenwich Reck.g.* 170°18′ *Watch* 170°18′. *West Longd. Ulietea* 18°38′. *Var.* 10°45′. Gentle Trade and pleasent weather. Swell as before.

Tuamotus, possibly Niau, the approximate position of which is lat. 16°15′ S, long. 145°20′ W —well to the east and north of the Herveys. Quiros's discoveries anywhere near the latitude of these islands did lie about 17 or 18 degrees to the east. Wallis may have seen one of them, but he certainly did not see La Dezena-Niau; his landfalls, apart from Mehetia, were to the south and east. For Dalrymple's chart, see I, p. clxiii, Fig. 18.

[1] *by choise . . . land:* is seldom seen but about the shores of the isles.—f. 121v. Cook virtually repeats himself from 21 September. Forster (I, pp. 421–2) says that this bird resembled a sandpiper in its flight and note; it actually settled in the rigging but was not identified.

[2] ADV 'The Indian that came with us from Huaheine is in high Spirits he being well of the Sea-sickness common at first going to sea—& has forgot his country in some Measure.'—Bayly.

THURSDAY 30*th. Winds ESE to SE. Course N* 81½° *W. Dist. Sailed* 128 *Miles. Lat. South* 21°10′. *West Longd. Greenwich Reck.g.* 172°33′ *Watch* 172°35′. *West Longd. Ulietea* 20°53′. Fresh Trade and Clear Weather. Being by observation 9 miles to the South of Amsterdam Island we steer'd W ½ North in order to get into the Latitude of the Said Island. At 5 pm being in the Latitude of 21°26′ Longitude W the variation was 10°45′ E. In the am got all the Bread out of Bread room upon deck to sift and air. Saw one of those small birds which we look upon to be a sign of the vicinity of land.

[OCTOBER 1773]

FRIDAY 1*st. Ther.r* 70. *Winds SE to East. Course S* 82°30′ *W. Dist. Sailed* 85 *Miles. Lat. South* 21°21′. *West Longd. Greenwich Reck.g.* 174°4′. *West Longd. Ulietea* 22°36. First part fresh gales remainder gentle gales and Clowdy. At Sun set the People at the mast head said they saw land to the westward, this occasioned us bring[ing] to during the night. Day light shew us our misstake when we again made sail to the West.

SATURDAY 2*nd. Winds Easterly.* Fresh gales and fair Weather. At 2 pm Saw the Island of Middleburg[1] bearing WSW. At 6 o'Clock we were about 12 miles from the East side the extreams bearing from SWBW to NW and another land bearing NNW, at this time we hauled to the Southward in order to get round the South end of the Island. At 8 o'Clock we discovered a small Island lying WSW from the South end of Middleburg,[2] not knowing but these two Islands might be connected to each other by a reef the extent of which we must be ignorant of and in order to guard against the worst, we haul'd the wind and spent the night makeing short boards under an easy sail.

At the return of Day-light we made Sail and bore up for the SW side of the Island, passing between it and the little Island above mentioned where we found a Channell of 2 miles broad. We rainged the SW side of the Island[3] at the distance of half a mile from shore on which the Sea broke with great [violence] as to leave us no hopes of finding Anchorage[4] this continuing till we came to the most western point of the Island (from which the land trend NNE and NEBN) we bore up for the Island of Amsterdam which we had in sight but before we had time to trim our sails the Shore of Middleburg assumed

[1] Eua.

[2] This is the islet Kalau, 2½ miles off the coast of Eua; in spite of the fact that in B Cook calls it a 'small low Island' it is 120 feet high.

[3] *Island:* greater Island

[4] *Anchorage:* either anchorage or a landing place ...—f. 122.

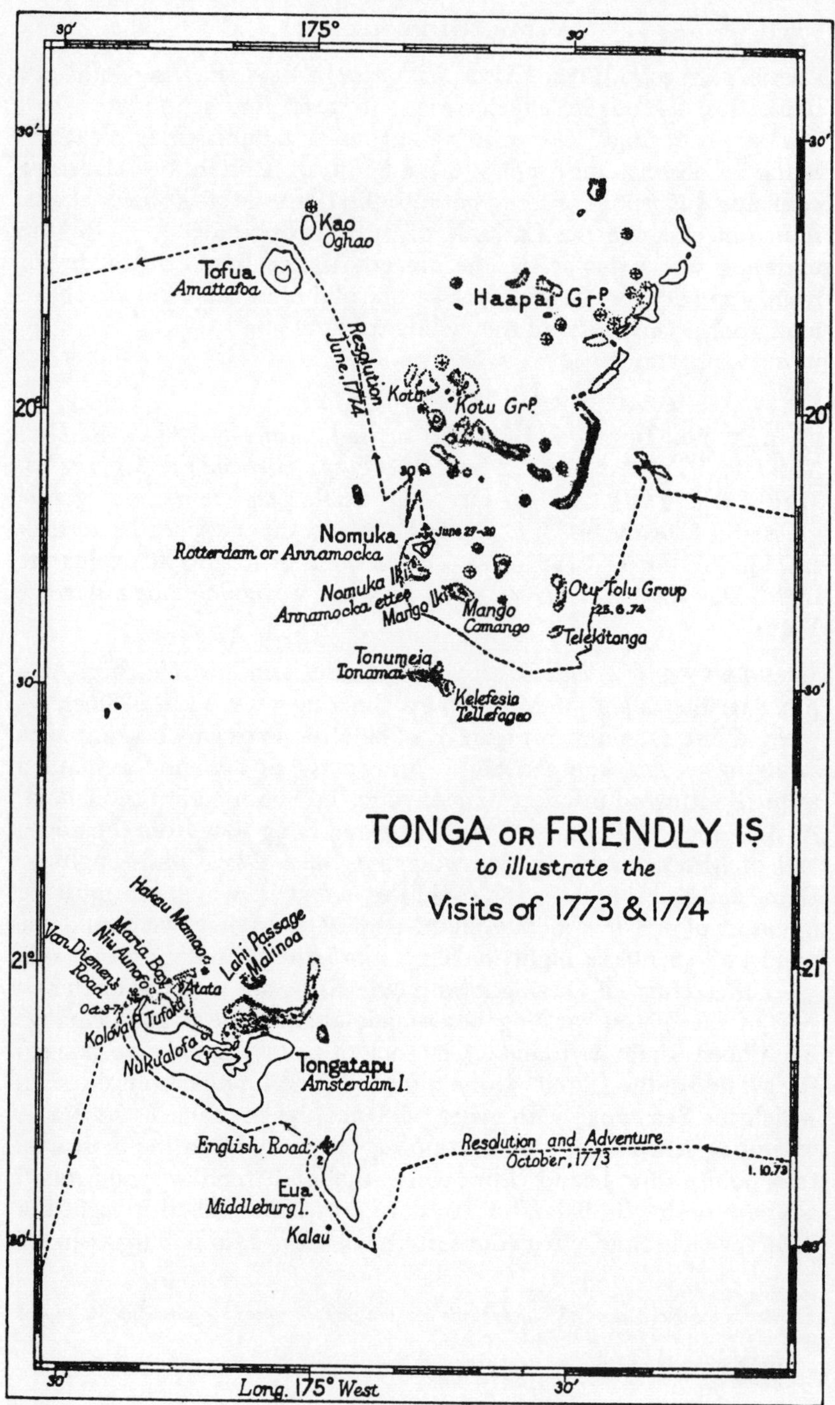
TONGA OR FRIENDLY Is
to illustrate the
Visits of 1773 & 1774
175°
Long. 175° West
Kao
Oghao
Tofua
Amattafoa
Haapai Grp
Resolution
June, 1774
Kotu
Kotu Grp
Nomuka
Rotterdam or Annamocka
June 27-30
Nomuka Iki
Annamocka ettee
Mango Iki
Mango
Comango
Otu Tolu Group
25.6.74
Telekitonga
Tonumeia
Tonamai
Kelefesia
Tellefageo
Hakau Mamao
Maria Bay
Niu Aunofo
Van Diemens Road
Lahi Passage
Malinoa
Atata
Tufaka
Kolovai
Nuku'alofa
Tongatapu
Amsterdam I.
English Road
Eua
Middleburg I.
Kalau
Resolution and Adventure
October, 1773
1.10.73

FIG. 45

another asspect and promised fair to afford Anchorage, upon this I hauled the wind again in order to get under the land. Soon after two Canoes, each conducted by two or 3 men came along side and some of the people into the Ship without the least hesitation, this mark of confidence gave me a good opinion of these Islanders and determined me to anchor if I found a convenient place and this we soon met with and came to in 25 fathom water about 3 Cables length from the shore and before a small creek formed by the Rocks which made landing in Boats easy,[1] the highest land on the Island[2] bore from us SEBE, the north point NE½N distant   miles, the West point SBW½W distant   miles and the Island of Amsterdam extending from NBW½W to NW½W.[3] By this time we had a great number of Canoes about the sloops and many of the Islanders aboard, some bringing with them Cloth and other Curiosities which they exchanged for Nails &c^a^. There was one man aboard who from the authority he seem'd to have over the others I discovered to be a chief and accordingly made him a present of a hatchet, Nails and several other things with which he seemed will pleased, thus a frienship between this chief, whose name is Tioonee,[4] and me commenced. Soon after we had come to an Anchor, I went a shore with Captain Furneaux and some of the officers and gentlemen, having in the Boat with us Tioonee who conducted us to the proper landing place where we were welcomed a shore by acclamations from an immence crowd of Men and Women not one of which had so much as a stick in their hands,[5] they crowded so thick round the boats with Cloth, Matting, &c^a^ to exchange for Nails that it was some time before we could get room to land, at last the Chief cleared the way and conducted us up to his house which was situated hard by in a most

[1] This anchorage, on the north-west side of Eua, Cook called English Road: Chart XXXV. By a stroke of luck or good observation he was anchored off the only possible landing-place on this side of the island, an anchorage which is itself unsafe with a westerly wind or swell. The 'small creek' is not more than sixty feet across, and leads directly to the shore, the reef here being very close in. The land rises immediately in a pleasant ascent from what beach there is, though there is also a narrow flat piece on its south side. The present village, Ohonua, straggles up and about the grassy slope, looking rather unlike the eighteenth century; but, perhaps because the ground is relatively clear, it is possible to visualise the incidents of the landing more clearly than at most places.

[2] The highest point, towards the south end, rises to 1078 feet.

[3] Cook does not give these distances in B, but they were all small—Eua itself being a small island, no more than about 11 miles on its longest side, from north to south. The distance between it and Amsterdam or Tongatapu is 10 miles.

[4] Taioni or Taione? Tongan tradition does not know the chief by this name: he is said to have been called Tavui. Cook on the third voyage, curiously enough, refers to him as Taoofa (Ta'aufa'a). He may by then have changed his name. Taione is still a chiefly name in Vava'u.

[5] *stick . . . hands:* stick or any other wepon in their hands, a strong proof of their good intention . . .—f. 122v.

delightfull spot, the floor was laid with Matting on which we were seated, the Islanders who accompanied us seated themselves in a circle round the out sides. I ordered the Bag-pipes to be played and in return the Chief ordered three young women to sing a song which they did with a very good grace. When they had done I gave each of them a necklace, this set most of the Women in the Circle a singing, their songs were musical and harmonious, noways harsh or disagreeable.[1] After we had sat here some time I disired to see the adjoining Plantations which were fenced in on every side,[2] accordingly we were conducted into one of them through a door way, the door was hung in such a manner as to shut of itself. In this Plantation the Chief had a nother house into which we were interduced, Bananas and Cocoa nuts were brought to us to eat and a bowl of liquor, made in our presence of the Plant,[3] to drink of which none of the gentlemen tasted but my self, the bowl was however soon emptied of its Contents of which both men and Women pertook, by this time it was noon when we return'd aboard to dinner with the Chief in our company, he sat at table but did [not] eat any of our victuals. In the after-noon went a shore again and was received by the crowd as before. M[r] Forster and his party and some of the officers walked into the country as soon as we landed, Captain Furneaux and I were conducted to the Chiefs house where we had fruit brought us to eat, afterwards he accompanied us into the Country through several Plantations Planted with fruit trees, roots &c[a] in great tast and ellegancy and inclose by neat fences made of reeds.[4]

[1] Forster (I, p. 429) gives us a specimen of these songs, or rather its tune, taken down by Burney, who records it himself in Ferguson MS.

[2] *which . . . side:* as the elegant and judicious manner they seemed to be laid out and fenced in rendered them worth the looking into; . . .—f. 123.

[3] *of . . . Plant:* of the juice of Wawavouru or Pepper root . . .—f. 123. The 'Pepper root' was of course *kava*, which no Tongan or other Polynesian ever called 'wawavouru'. Cook may have heard some descriptive phrase—e.g. in Maori *ua* meant the underground branches of the *kumara*, and may have had some more general significance in Tongan; and one of the meanings of Tongan *ulu* was thick or bushy, which is a fair description of the *kava* root. But this is pure speculation. Cf. p. 237, n. 1 above.

[4] Bayly, who 'walked into the country' with Forster and the officers, gives us an interesting description of these fences, which we get nowhere else. He speaks of what we may call the Tongan 'roading system', a series of 'walks', with small ones intersecting longer ones about every quarter-mile, and so breaking up the plantations. 'The sides of these walks are made of Bambo canes of the bigness of a mans little finger these are about 10 & 12 feet high in general; the method of making is this. Along the sides of these walks are trees planted very regular, at every 3 or 4 feet there is bambo canes of the Size of a mans thumb lashed horizontal one over each other, then the small canes are taken & the lower end stuck into the ground to make an angle of 45 degrees, & 3 or 4 Inches from each other these are carried on to the whole extent of the fence, & then there is another row of canes stuck into the ground in the same manner only to incline the contrary way so that the fence is composed of two rows of Bambo canes which makes it in dimonds, these are lashed to the horizontal canes, with fine line made of Cocoa nut rind, & are the neatest fences I ever beheld.'—3 October.

*. . . it was some time before we could get room to land; they seemed to be more desireous to give than receive, for many who could not get near the Boats threw into them over the others heads, whole bales of Cloth and then retired without either asking or waiting to get any thing in exchange. At length the Chief caused them to open to the right and left and make room for us to land, he then conducted us up to his house which was situated about 300 yards from the Sea, at the head of a fine lawn and under the shade of some Shaddock trees, the Situation was most delightfull, in front was the Sea and the Ships at Anchor, behind and on each side where pla[n]tations in which were some of the richest productions of Nature; . . . After siting here some time we were at our own request conducted into one of the adjoining Plantations where the Chief had another house into which we were conducted; Bananoes and Cocoanuts were set before us to eat and a bowl of liquor prepared in our presence of the Juice of Eava for us to drink; pieces of the root was first offered to us to chew, but as we excused our selves from assisting in the opperation it was given to others to chew which done it was put into a large wooden bowl and mixed with Water in the manner already related and as soon as it was properly streaned for drinking, they made cups of Green leaves which held near half a pint and presented to each of us a Cup of the liquor, but I was the only one who tasted of it, the manner of brewing had quenished the thirst of every one else; the bowl was however soon emptyed of its contents, of which both men and women pertook, I observed that they never filled the same Cup twice, nor did two persons drink out of the same, each had a fresh Cup and fresh liquor.

This house was situated at one corner of the Plantation, had an Area before it on which we were Seated, the whole was planted round with fruit and other trees whose spreading branches afforded an agreeable shade and the air was perfumed by their fragrancy. Before we had well viewed the plantation it was Noon and we returned on board to dinner with the Chief in our Company, he sat at Table but eat nothing, our dinner was fresh Pork roasted which made it a little extraordinary. After dinner we landed again and were received by the Crowd as before. Mr F. with his Botanical party, some of the officers and gentlemen walked into the Country, Captain Furneaux and my self were conducted to the Chiefs house, where fruit and some Greens which had been stewed, were set before us to eat, as we had but just dined it cannot be supposed we eat much, but Odidde and Omiah, the man on board the Adventure, did honour to the feast.*—ff. 118v–19.

In the lanes and about their house[s] were runing about Hogs and large fowls which were the only domistick Animals we saw and these they did not seem desireous to part with, nor did they during this day offer to exchange any fruit or roots worth mentioning, this determined me to leave the Island in the morning and go down to that of Amsterdam where Tasman in 1643 found refreshments in plenty. In the evening we all returned aboard every one highly dilighted with his little excursion and the friendly behaver of the Natives who seem'd to [vie] with each other in doing what they thought would give us pleasure.

SUNDAY *3rd.* Early in the morning while the Sloops were geting under sail I went a shore in company with Captain Furneaux and Mr Forster to take leave of the Chief and to carry him an assortment of garden seeds and to make him some other presents.[1] I gave him to understand that we were going away at which he neither seem'd pleased nor sorry, he[2] came into our boat with an intent to accompany us aboard and came off about half way, but when he saw that the Resolution was already under sail he call'd to a Canoe to come and take him in together with a nother or two of his friends who were in the boat. As soon as I was aboard we bore away for the Island of Amsterdam all sails set, we ran a long the South Side of the Isle half a mile from shore and had an oppertunity with the assistance of our glasses to view the face of the Country every acre of which was laid out in Plantations,[3] we could see the natives in different parts runing a long the shore, some having little white flags in their hands which we took for signs of Peace and answered them by hoisting a St Georges Ensign.[4] The people were as little afraid of us as those of Middleburg, while we were but middway between the Isles we were met by 3 or 4 Canoes, each conducted by 2 or 3 men, who strove hard to get aboard, but this was not to be done as we were runing at the rate of 5 or 6 Knots, we threw the end of a lead-line into one which they held fast till it brok, they afterward made the like but unsuccessfull attempt to get aboard the Adventure who was a stern of us. After we had opened the West side of the Isle we were met by severl more Canoes with two and 3 men in each, they

[1] ... he received us at the landing place and would have conducted us up to his house had we not excused our selves—f. 123v.

[2] ... and two or three more

[3] ... not an acre of waste land was to be seen

[4] ... Three men belonging to Middleburg, which had somehow or other been left on board the Adventure now left her and swam for the shore, not knowing that we intended to stop at the isle and having no inclination as may be supposed to go away with us.—f. 120.

brought with them and presented to us some of the [Pepper] root after which they came a board without farther ceremony.[1] After makeing a board or two we anchored in Van diemens Road in 18 fathom water about a Cables length from the Rocks or breakers off the shore and moored with the Coasting Anchor and Cable out to sea to prevent the Ship from tailing ashore in case of a shift of wind or a Calm,[2] by this time we had a great number of the Islanders aboard and about the sloops, some coming off in Canoes and others swiming off, bringing little else with them but Cloth and other curiosities, things which I did not come here for and for which the Seamen only bartered away their clothes.[3] In order to put a stop to this and to obtain the refreshments we wanted, I gave orders that no Curiosities should be purchassed by any person whatever either aboard or along side the Sloops or at the landing place on shore; this had the desired effect for in the morning the Natives came off with Bananas and Cocoa-nutts in abundance and some Fowls and Pigs which they exchanged for Nails, and peices of Cloth.[4]

MONDAY 4*th*. After breakfast I went a shore with Captain Furneaux, Mr Forster and several of the officers, a chief, or man of some note, to whom I had made several presents was in the Boat with us, his name was Hātago[5] by which name he desired I might be called and he by mine (Otootee). We were lucky in having[6] anchored before a narrow creek in the rocks which just admitted our Boats within the breakers where they laid secure and at high water we could land dry on the shore;[7] into this place Hatago conducted us, there [were] on the

[1] . . . and invited us by all the signs of friendship thev could make to go to their island a thing we had already determined upon—f. 124.

[2] . . . this last anchor laid in 48 fathom water, so steep is the bank on which we anchored. —ff. 120, 124.—Cook thought his anchorage was in what Tasman called Van Diemens Road, but so far as one can tell from Tasman's not very satisfactory chart, it was a good deal closer to the north-west end of Tongatapu, though off the coast of the same Hihifo district.

[3] . . . the effects of which it was probable they would soon feel.—f. 120.—'. . . a great number of the inhabitants on board many in their Canoes alongside a great many swimming off both men and women promiscuously together and some thousands assembled on the shore opisite to the ships'.—Gilbert.

[4] . . . even old raggs of any sort was enough for a Pigg or a Fowl.

[5] Cook tries this name in various ways—Hātago, as here, Attago, and finally settles for Otago. Forster 'Attahha or Attagha'. He was Ataongo—not to be confused with a later Ataongo, the son of Mumui the Tui Kanokupolu from 1793 to 1797. See Fig. 50*a*.

[6] *lucky in having:* lucky, or rather we may thank the Natives for having . . .—f. 120v.

[7] The western shore of the Hihifo district generally is of coral rock a few feet high, iron-hard, irregular and knife-sharp, cut here and there by little gulleys between the sea and the vegetation a few yards off. The beach on which Cook landed—according to Tongan tradition, which there seems no reason to doubt—is the more northern of two, and is called Pokula; it is a short distance from the present village of Ha'atafu, the last on the road which runs from Nuku'alofa almost to the north-west point of the island. There are two small breaks in the reef, through either of which the boats might have come.

shore an immence crowd of men Women and children who Welcomed us in the same manner as those of Middleburg and were like them all unarm'd. All the officers and gentlemen set out into the Country as soon as we land, excepting Captain Furneaux who stayed with me on the shore, we two Hatago seated on the grass and ordered the People to set down in a circle round us[1] which they did, never once attempting to push themselves upon us as the Otahieteans and the people of the neighbouring Isles generally do. After distributing some trifles among them we signified our desire to see the Country, this was no sooner done than the chief shewed us the way, conducting us along a lane which led us to an open green on the one side of which was a house of Worship[2] built on a mount which had been raised by the hand of Man about 16 or 18 feet above the common level, it had an oblong figure and was supported by a Wall of Stone about three feet high, from the top of this Wall the mount rose with a gentle slope and was covered with a green turf, on the top of the mount stood the house which was of the same figure as the mount about 20 feet long and 14 or 16 broad. As soon as we came before this place every one seated him self on the ground about 50 or 60 yards from the house, presently after came three elderly men and seated them selves between us and the house and began to speak what I understood to be a prayer, their discourse being wholy directed to the house, this lasted about ten minutes and then the three priests, for such we took them to be, came and sit down with us and the rest of the people when both Captain Furneaux and I made them presents of Nails, Medals &c[a] giving them to understand that we did it to shew our respect to that house which I now desired leave to examine, the chief contrary to my expectations immidiately

[1] B f. 120v enlarges the foregoing passage, from the beginning of the entry, as follows: 'Matters being thus established and proper persons apointed to trade under the direction of the officers, to prevent disputes, after breakfast, I landed, accompaned by Captain Furneaux, M[r] F. & several of the officers, having along with us a Chief or person of some Note whose name was Attago and who had attatched himself to me from the first moment of his coming on board which was before we had anchored. I know not how he came to discover that I was the Commander but certain it is, he was not long on deck before he singled me out from all the other gentlemen and made me a present of some Cloth and other things he had about him and as a greater testimony of Friendship we now exchanged names, a Custom which is practised at Otaheite and the Society Isles. . . . As soon as we were landed all the gentlemen set out into the Country, accompaned by some of the Natives, but the most of them remained with Captain Furneaux and me who amused our selves some time in distributing presents amongst them, especially to such as Attago pointed out, which I observed were not many and such as we afterwards found were of superior rank to himself, at this time he however appeared to us to be the principal person and seemed to us to be obeyed as such. After we had spent some time on the beach we complained of the heat. Ottago immidiately conducted us off the beach and seated us under the shade of a tree & ordered the people [to] form a circle round us

[2] It was a *faitoka* or chiefly burial place. (*Faitoka* is now the Tongan word for any cemetery.) Ataongo had led them over the narrow neck of land towards Maria Bay.

went with us without shewing the least backwardness and gave us full liberty to examine every part of it. In the front were two steps leading up to the top of the wall, after which the assent was easy to the house round which was a fine good Walk, the house was built in all respects like to their common dwelling houses (viz) with Posts and rafters and the Covering of Palm thatch, the eves came down to within 3 feet of the ground which space was fill'd up with strong Matting made of Palm leaves which formed a kind of Wall, the floor of the house was laid with gravel, except in the middle where it was raised with fine blew pebbles to the height of about Six Inches and had the same form as the house that is oblong. At one corner of the house stood a rude image and on one side laid a nother, each about two feet in length, I who had no intention to offend either them or their gods, did not so much as touch them, but asked the chief as well as I could if they were Eatua's; whether he understood me or no I cannot say, but he immidiatly turned them over in the doing of which he handled them as roughly as he would have done any other log of wood, which raised a doubt in me that they were representations of the Divinity.[1] I was curious to know if their dead were enterr'd in these Mounts and asked my friend several questions relating thereto but I was not certain that he understood any of them, at least I did not understand the answers he made.[2] Before we queted the house we laid[3] upon the blue Pebbles some Medals, Nails and other things which my friend took up and carried away with him.[4] The Stones on which the wall was made that inclosed the Mount were like flags, some of them 9 or 10 feet by 4, and about Six inches thick, it is difficult to conceive how they could cut such stones out of the coral rocks.[5] This Mount stood in a kind of grove open only on one side which fronted the high road and green on which the people

[1] *raised . . . Divinity:* convenced me that they were not there as representations of the Divinity.—f. 125v. What they were is not absolutely certain, but it is not impossible that they were purely decorative.—E. W. Gifford, *Tongan Society* (B. P. Bishop Mus. Bull. 61, Honolulu 1929), p. 318.

[2] *understood . . . made:* understood me well enough to satisfy my enquiries, for the reader must know that at our first coming among these people we hardly could understand a word they said, even my Otahiete youth and the man on board the Adventure were equally at a loss, but more of this by and by.—f. 125v.

[3] *we laid:* we thought it was necessary we should make our offering at the alter, accordingly laid down

[4] *which . . . him:* which we had no sooner done, than my friend took them up and put in his pocket.—ff. 125v–6.

[5] The limestone of the coral reef was indeed difficult to quarry, and was used only for the largest structures of the sort Cook is describing—generally royal tombs or *langi*. But the most commonly used limestone, found stratified in quarries ashore, or even to be found sometimes lying in slabs on the beach, was much more easily cut out with basalt tools.

were seated, at this green[1] was a junction of five roads and two or three of them appeared to be very publick ones: the grove was composed of several sorts of trees among which was the Eatua tree or [2] and a kind of low Palm which is very common in the northern parts of New Holland.[3] After we had [d]one examining this place of worship which in their Language is called *Afiā-tou-ca*,[4] we desired to return, but instead of conducting us directly to the Water side they struck into a road leading into the Country, this road which was a very publick one, was about [16] feet broad and as even as a B[owling] green, there was a fence of reeds on each side and here and there doors which opened into the adjoining Plantations; several other Roads from different parts joined this, some equally as broad and others narrower, the most part of them shaded from the Scorching Sun by fruit trees. I thought I was transported into one of the most fertile plains in Europe, here was not an inch of waste ground, the roads occupied no more space than was absolutely necessary and each fence did not take up above 4 Inches and even this was not wholy lost for in many of the fences were planted fruit trees and the Cloth plant, these served as a support to them,[5] it was every were the same, change of place altered not the sene. Nature, assisted by a little art, no were appears in a more florishing state than at this isle. In these delightfull Walks we met numbers of people some were traveling down to the Ships with their burdthens of fruit, others returning back empty, they all gave us the road[6] and either sit down or stood up with their backs against the fences till we had pass'd. At several of the cross Roads or at the meeting of three[7] or more roads, were generally an Afiā-tou-cā, such as above discribed with this difference, that the Mounts were Palisaded round in stead of a stone wall.[8] At length[9] we came to one larger than common, near to which was a large House belonging to a Chief[10] which was with us, here we were desired to stop which we

[1] . . . or open place

[2] *Eatua tree or* : Etoa tree, as it is called at Otahiete, of which is made clubs &c[a] . . . —f. 126. 'Eatua' is of course a slip: in B, Cook having written it, he erases it and substitutes 'Etoa'. Toa or ironwood, *Casuarina equisetifolia*.

[3] Forster refers to pandanus and the wild sago-palm—which would certainly not be wild but cultivated, if there at all. The palm, however, was probably the 'cabbage tree' or Ti, *Cordyline terminalis*, a tree of sacred associations all over the Pacific.

[4] *faitoka*.

[5] *fruit trees . . . them:* some usefull trees or plants . . .—f. 126.

[6] . . . by turning either to the right or left and siting down

[7] *three:* two

[8] These mounds seem to have been *esi* or resting-places for chiefly persons on a journey; they would generally command a pleasant view, to which Tongans were very partial.

[9] . . . after walking several miles . . .—f. 126v.

[10] *a Chief:* an old Chief

accordingly did and had some Cocoa-nutts brought us; we were no sooner seated in the house than the oldest of the Priests began a speach or prayer which was first directed to the Afiā-tou-cā and then to me and it altarnetly, when he adress'd me he paused at each sentance, till I gave a nod of approbation. I however did not understand one single word he said. At times the old man seem'd to be at a loss what to say, or perhaps his memory fail'd him, for every now and then he was prompt by a nother[1] who sat by him. Both during this Prayer and the one before mentioned the people were silent but not attentive. At this last place we made but a short stay, our guides conducted us down to our Boat and returned with my friend Ata-go aboard to dinner. We had but just got aboard when an old gentleman came a long side who I understood from Atago was some King or great man, he was according interduced into the Ship when I made him a present of some red Cloth, Nails &c[a] [2] and seated him at Table to dinner, we now saw that he was certainly a man of some concequence for Ata-go would not sit down and eat before him, but as the old gentleman was almost blind, he got to the other end of the table and sat and eat with his back towards him,[3] the old gentleman eat a bit of fish and drank a glass of Wine and then returned a shore. After Ata-go had seen him out of the ship he came and took his place at Table finished his dinner and drank about two glasses of wine. As soon as dinner was over we all went a shore again were we found the old Chief who presented me with a Hog and he and some others took a Walk with us into the Isle,[4] our rout

[1] *a nother:* one of the other priests

[2] *according . . . &c[a]:* accordingly ushered on board when I presented him with such things as he most valued (being the only method to make him our friend) . . .—f. 128.

[3] It was forbidden to eat in the presence of a superior. Turning the back was a sort of fictitious absence, sometimes practised.

[4] . . . Before we set out I happened to go down with Attago to the landing place and there found M[r] Wales in a laughable, tho distressed situation. The Boats which brought us on shore, not being able to get near the landing place for want of a sufficient depth of Water, he pull'd of his Shoes and Stockings to walk through, and as soon as he got on dry land he put them down betwixt his legs to put on again, but they were instantly snatched away by a person behind him, who immidiately mixed with the Crowd. It was impossible for him to follow the Man bare footed over the sharp coral rocks, which compose the shore, without having his feet cut to pieces. The Boat was put back to the Ship, his Companions had each made his way thro' the crowd and he left in this condition alone. Otago soon found out the thief, recovered the Shoes and Stockings and set him at liberty.—f. 127. —This is an insertion in the text of B (and not in G), which from the ink and writing looks as if it were later reminiscence; or Cook may have been reminded of it by his perusal of Wales's journal; see p. 812 below. The story, one feels, is probably the origin of the later Christ's Hospital schoolboy legend, as related by Leigh Hunt in his *Autobiography*—'. . . Mr Wales, a man well known for his science who had been round the world with Captain Cook; for which we highly venerated him. . . . When he was at Otaheite, the natives played him a trick while bathing, and stole his small-clothes; which we used to think a liberty scarcely credible'.

was by the first mentioned Afiā-tou-ca before which we again seated our selves, but had no praying[1] on the contrary here the good natured old Chief interduced to me a woman and gave me to understand that I might retire with her, she was next offered to Captain Furneaux but met with a refusal from both, tho she was neither old nor ugly. Our stay here was but short. The Chief, probably thinking that we might want water on board the Sloops conducted us to a Plantation hard by and there shewed us a pool of fresh Water without our makeing the least enquiry after such a thing. I believe it to be the same as Tasman calls the Washing place for the King and his nobles,[2] from hence we were conducted down to the shore of Maria Bay or NE side of the Isle, where in a Boat house the old chief shewed us a large double Canoe not yet launched and did not fail to make us sencible that it belonged to him, here we left him and returned aboard.[3] Mr Forster and his party spent the day in the Country botanizing and several of the officers were out Shooting, every one met with sevel treatment from the natives and found the Country just as I have described. We had also a brisk trade for Bananas, Cocoa-nutts, yams, Pigs and fowls all of which were purchass'd with nails and pieces of Cloth, a Boat from each Sloop was employed tradeing a shore bring[ing] off their cargo as soon as they were loaded which was generally in a short time, by this method we got a good quantity of fruit as well as other articles[4] from people who had no canoes to bring them aboard, bought them cheaper and with less trouble.[5]

TUESDAY 5*th*. Pretty early in the morn my friend Otago came off and brought me a Hog and some fruit for which I gave him a Hatchet and some Cloth,[6] I also sent the Pinnace with a petty officer to trade with the People, she soon return'd before she was quite loaded, the officer informed me that the natives were very troublesome and were for takeing the oars and every thing out of the boat,[7] the day before they had stolen the grapling whilest she was riding by it and carried it off undiscovered, having first dived and unbent the rope

[1] *praying:* prayers although the old Priest was with us

[2] In B f. 128 Cook here gives a reference to 'Dalrymple's Collection of Voyages Vol 2. Page 80.' This page includes a key to the engraving of a diagrammatic picture of 'Amsterdam', taken from Tasman's journal, where 'L' marks a little pond inside a palisade, which contains also a number of coconut palms and a house where the 'king' received the Dutch.

[3] *here . . . aboard:* Night was now approaching, we took leave of the old Chief and returned on board, being conducted by Attago down to the Water side.—f. 128v.

[4] *articles:* refrishments

[5] With the result that in the *Resolution* they 'stop'd serving bread'.—Clerke.

[6] *and some Cloth:* a Sheet and some Red Cloth

[7] . . . and in other respects very troublesome

from it.[1] From this report I judged it necessary to have a guard on shore to protect the Boats and people whose business made it necessary for them to be there and accordingly sent Lieutenant Edgcomb with the Marines for that purpose. Soon after I went myself with my freind Otā-go, Cap. Furneaux and several more of the gentlemen, at landing we found the old King who presented me with a Pig which I desired might remain there till I went aboard as Mr Hodges was then going with me into the country to make drawings of such places and things as were most intresting; when these were done we returned aboard to dinner with Otago and two other Chiefs one of which sent a Hog a board the Adventure for Captain Furneaux several hours before without stupelating for the least return the only instance we had of this Kind. My friend took care to put me in mind of the Hog the old Chief gave me in the morning and for which I now gave him a chequed Shirt and a piece of Red Cloth, I had tyed them together for him to take a shore, but he was not satisfied till he had them put on, which was no sooner done than he went on deck and shew'd himself to all his Countrymen that were in and about the Ship, he did the very same thing in the Morning with a clean white sheet I had given him, Captain Furneaux friend was complimented with an Ax which was what he wanted. In the evening we went ashore again and saw the old chief who took to himself every thing my friend and the others had got. The different tradeing parties were so successfull to day as to procure for both Sloops a tollerable supply of refreshments[2] in concequence of which I gave the next morning every one leave to purchass what curiosities and other things they pleased,[3] after this it was astonishing to see with what eagerness every one catched at every thing they saw, it even went so far as to become the ridicule of the Natives by offering pieces of sticks stones and what not to exchange, one waggish Boy took a piece of human excrement on the end of a stick and hild it out to every one of our people he met with.

*To day a man got into the masters Cabbin through the out side

[1] The grapnel, says Bayly, weighed nearly 100 lb, so the exploit was no mean one; they 'then attempted to sieze the Pinnes but the people beat them off without firing but 2 or 3 of them were cut with cutlashes. . . .'—p. 98.

[2] All this while it was fine pleasant weather, we learn from Clerke (6 October), and trade was good: 'a cheap and plentifull Market—a happy Climate with friendly Benevolent People, who are anxious to oblige and give you welcome'.

[3] Forster (I, pp. 458–9) notes one disappointment of the sailors. They had enjoyed themselves thoroughly cock-fighting with fowls bought at Huahine; and now, finding at Tongatapu a large race of bird, with highly decorative plumage, hastened to buy more to carry on the contests. Alas! the Tongan cocks would not fight, and had to be eaten; they were, however, 'extremely well-tasted'.

scuttle and took out some Books and other things, he was discovered just as he was geting out into his Canoe and pursued by one of our boats which obliged him to quet his Canoe and take to the Water, the people in the boat made several attempts to lay hold of him but he as often dived under the Boat and at last, unship'd the rudder which rendered the boat ungovernable by which means he got clear of;[1] some other very daring thefts were committed at the landing place, one fellow took one of the Seamens Jackets out of the Boat and carried it off in spite of all they could do, nor would he part with it till he was both pursued and fired at by our people in the boat nor would he have done it then had not his landing been intercepted by some of us who were on shore. The rest of the Natives who were very numerous took very little notice of the whole transaction, nor were they the least alarmed when the Man was fired at.[2*]
—f. 129v.

WEDNESDAY 6*th*. My friend Otago viseted me this morning as usual, brought with him a Hog and assisted me in purchassing several others, after this I wint a shore, viseted the old Chief where I stayed till noon and then returned aboard to dinner with my friend who never quited me. As I intended to sail the next day, I made up a present for the old Chief whom I proposed to take leave of in the Evening, when I landed for this purpose I was told by the officers on shore that there was a far greater Chief no less than the King of the whole Island, come to viset us; he was first seen by Mr Pickersgill and some others of the officers who were in the Country and found him seated in a lane with a few people about him and soon saw that he was a man of some concequence by the extraordinary respect paid him, some when they approached him fell on their faces and

[1] Forster, giving instances of theft, begins by remarking, 'The harmless disposition of these good people could not secure them against those misfortunes, which are too often attendant upon all voyages of discovery'; and goes on to this incident, describing how a nimble fellow, 'luckily slipping into the master's cabin stole from thence several mathematical books, a sword, a ruler, and a number of trifles of which he could never make use'. Seen escaping, he displayed wonderful agility diving and doubling in the water, until he was caught under the ribs with a boat-hook, which caused some loss of blood. He then escaped again, and altogether. 'It is remarkable that even such a disposition for cruelty, as had been displayed in the pursuit of this poor wretch, did not deprive us of the confidence and affection of his countrymen.' I, pp. 464–5. The heightened tone of this account was another reason for Wales's later onslaught on Forster's book: *Remarks*, pp. 32–4.

[2] Forster (I, p. 464) remarks that the firing was without the captain's orders, and agrees that the natives 'heard with unconcern the balls whistling about their ears'. But 'several innocent people were wounded'. Bayly is rather more dramatic: '. . . one of the Natives took a mans Coat out of the Boat & walked off with it, there was two muskets fired at him but missed him when the first Lieut of the Resolution hit him in the Jaw with a ball he threw down the Coat but run off holding his Jaws with his hands & Several more cases of the like kind happened wherein several of them were wounded but none killed so that at last they were in fear of a Gun'.—Bayly, p. 98.

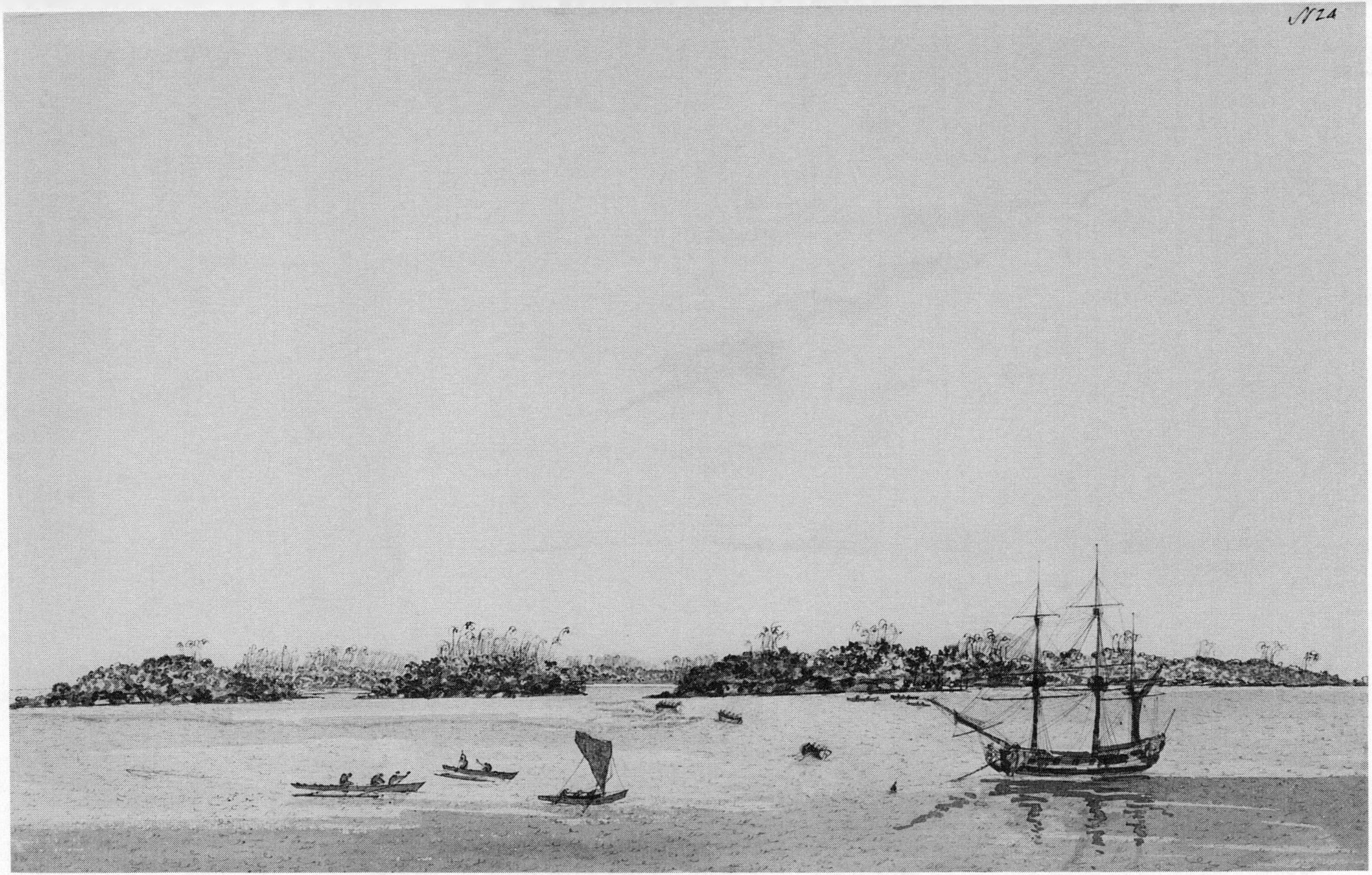

FIG. 46. View of the 'Bay of Amsterdam' (Tongatapu)

Wash drawing by Hodges.—Mitchell Library, D11, no. 24

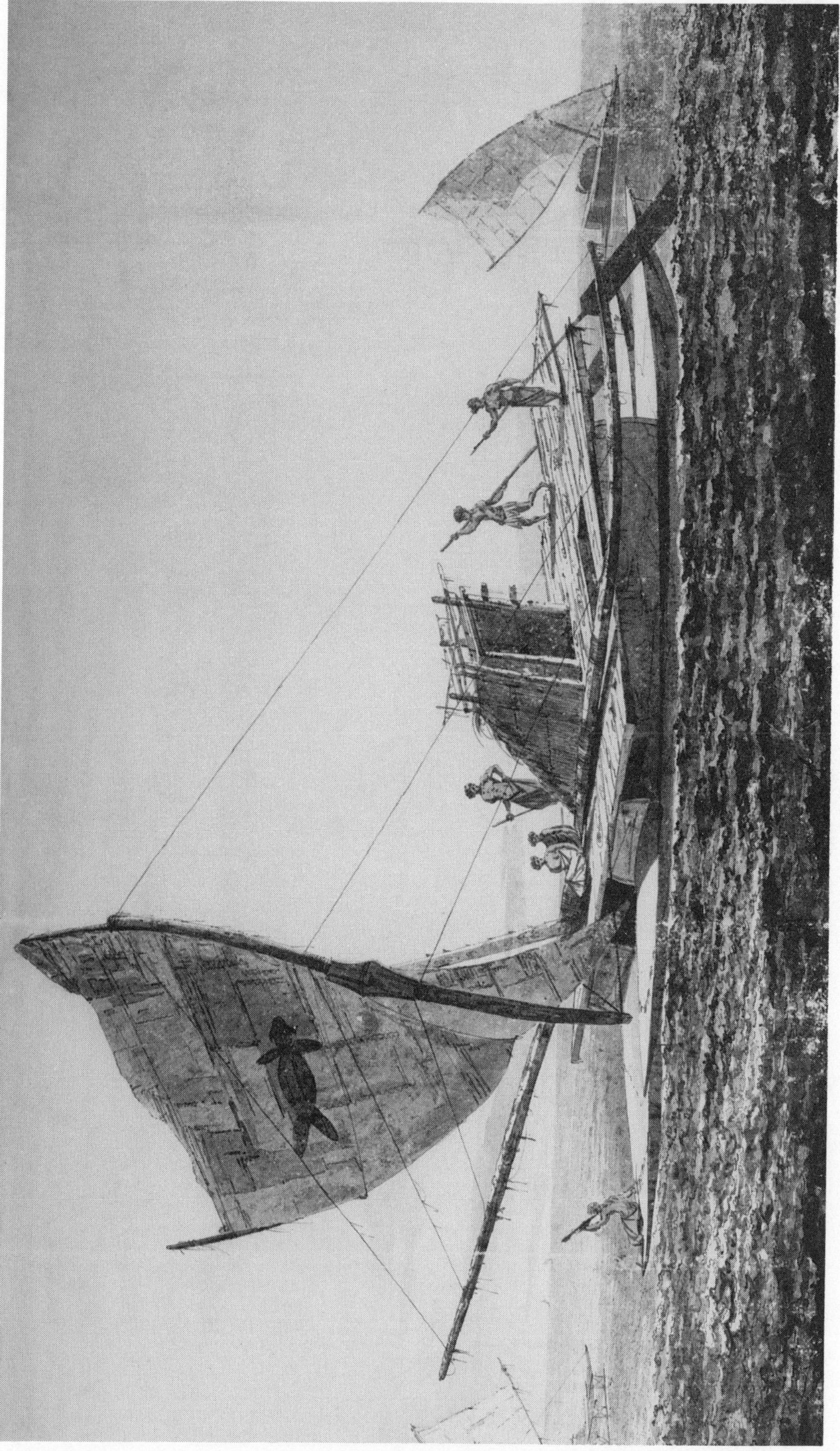

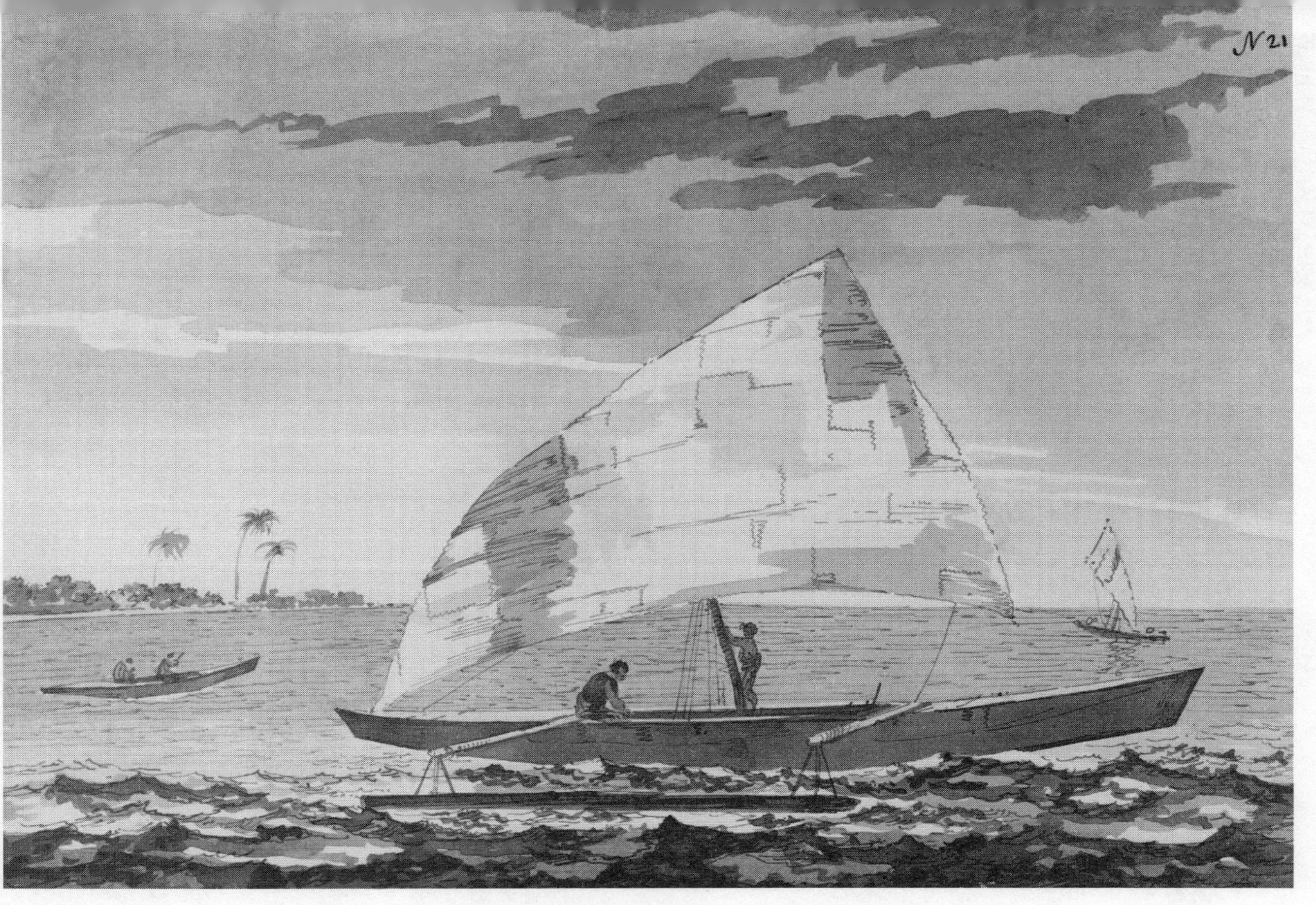

Fig. 48. Fishing canoe of Tongatapu

Wash drawing by Hodges.—Mitchell Library, D11, no. 21

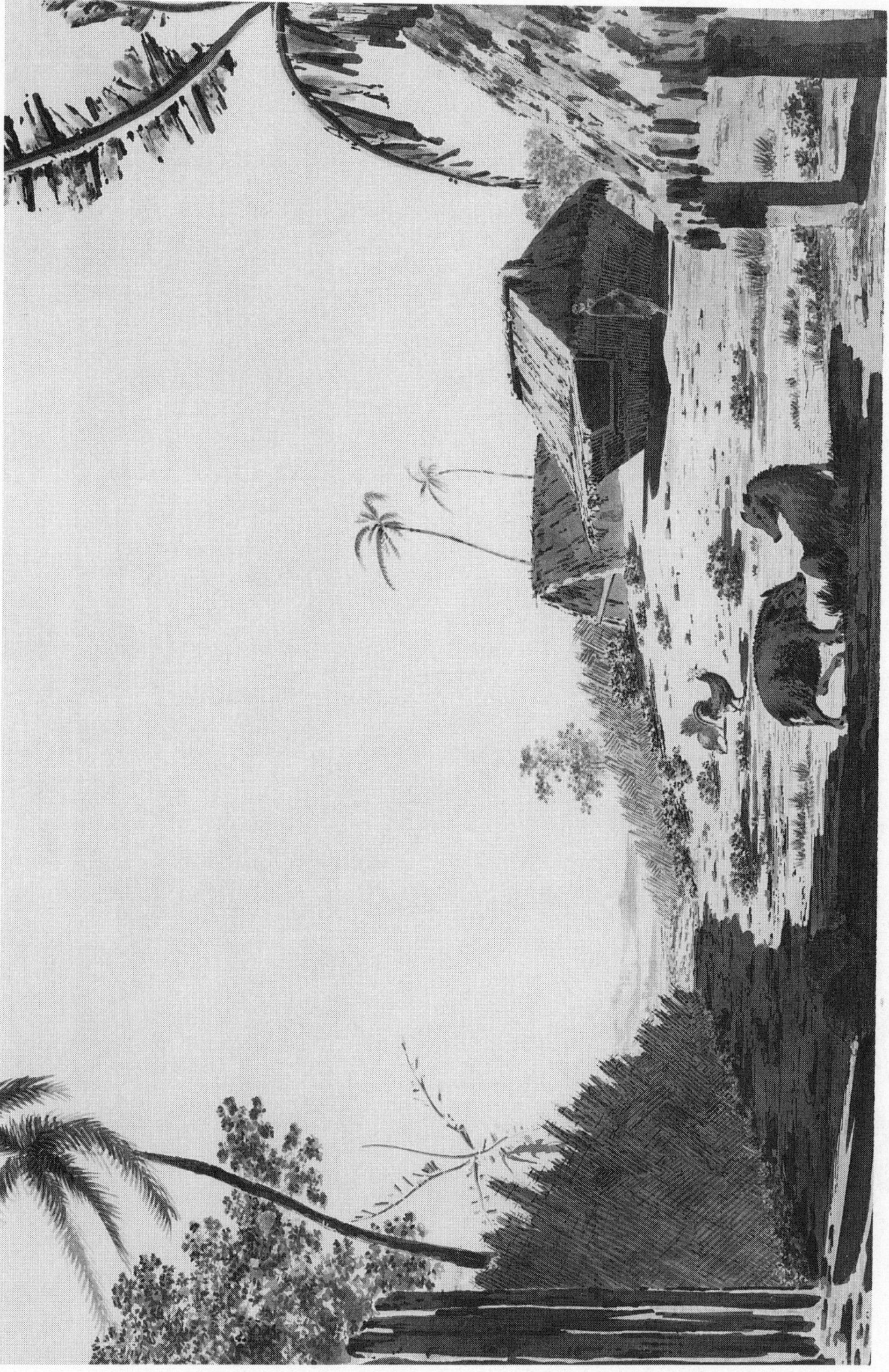

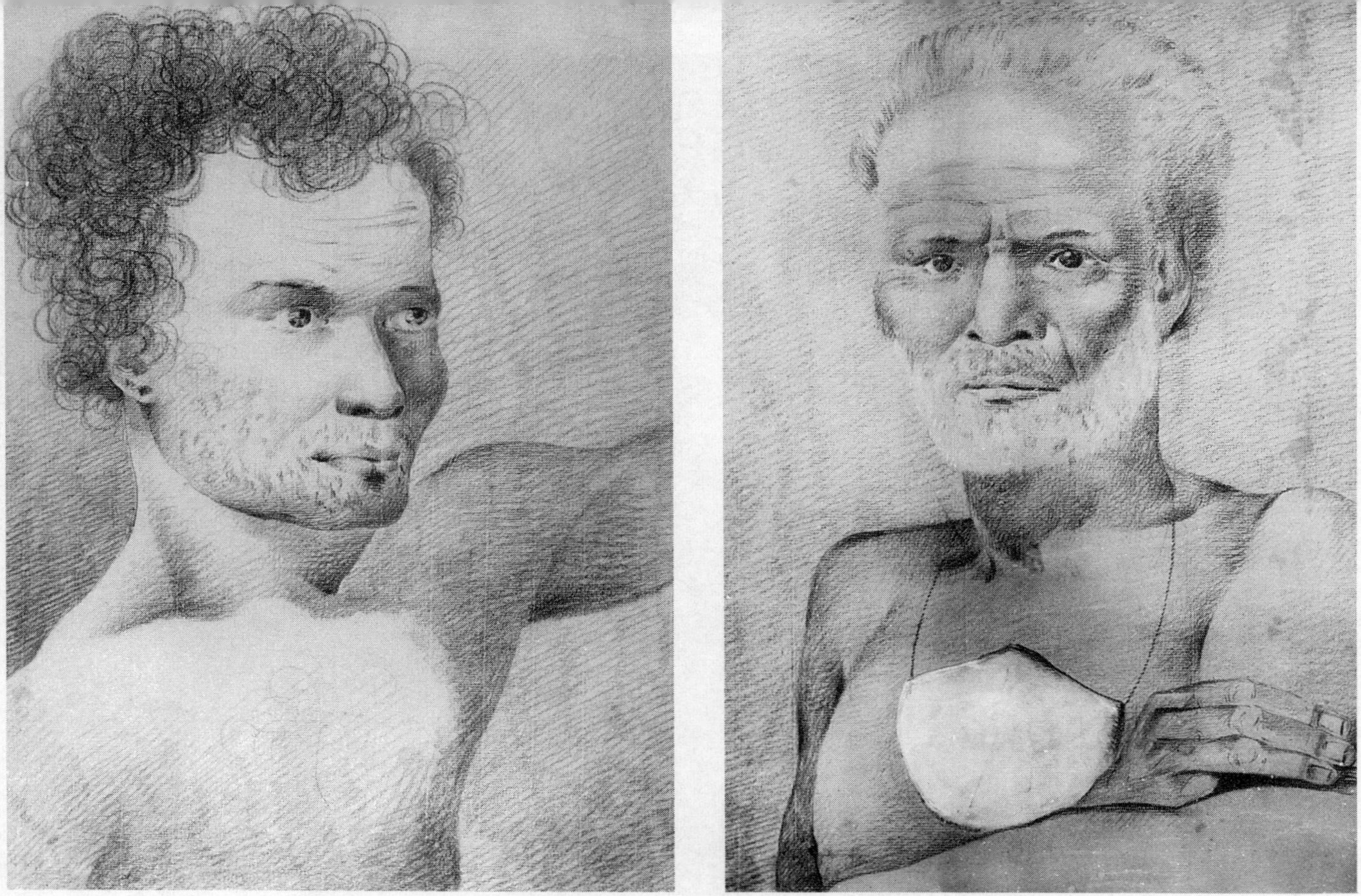

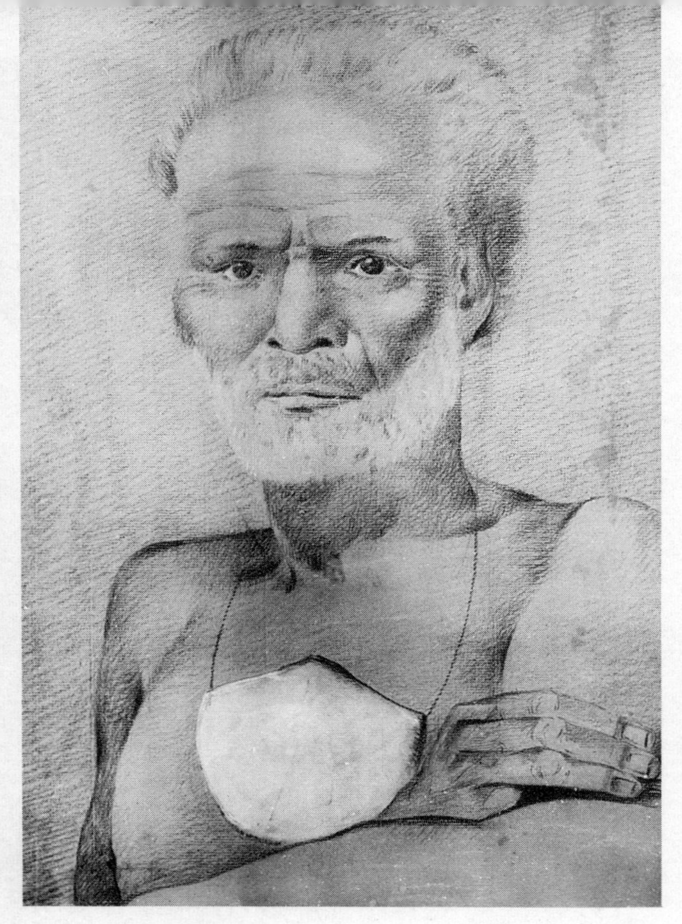

FIG. 50. Portrait heads of Tongans, by Hodges

(*left*) Ataongo. Red chalk drawing.—Mitchell Library, D11, no. 24a. (*right*) An old man of Tongatapu. Crayon drawing.—Commonwealth National Library

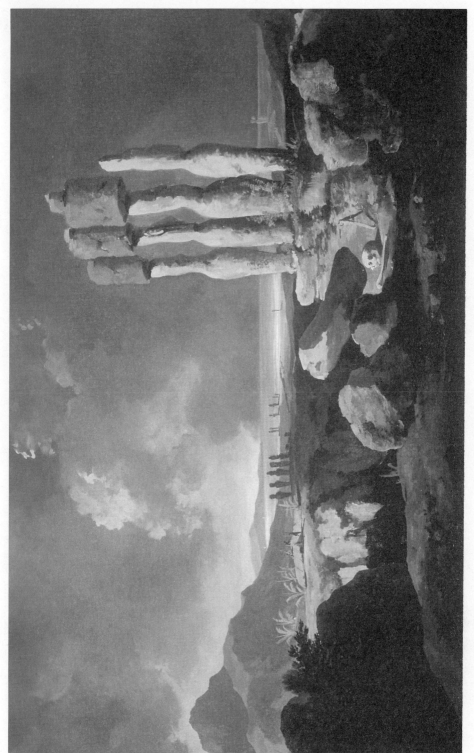

FIG. 51. Monuments of Easter Island

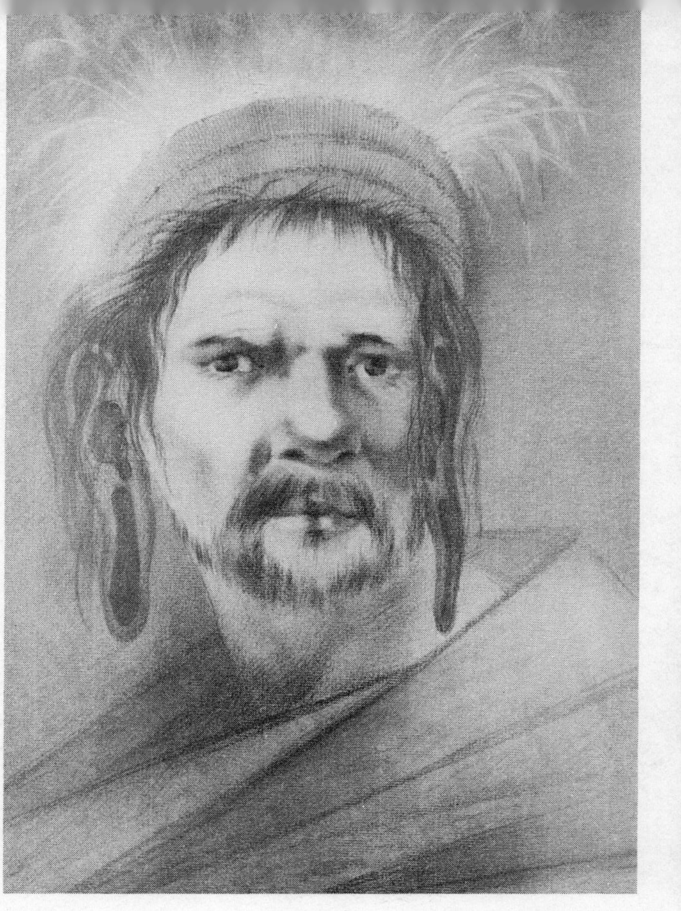

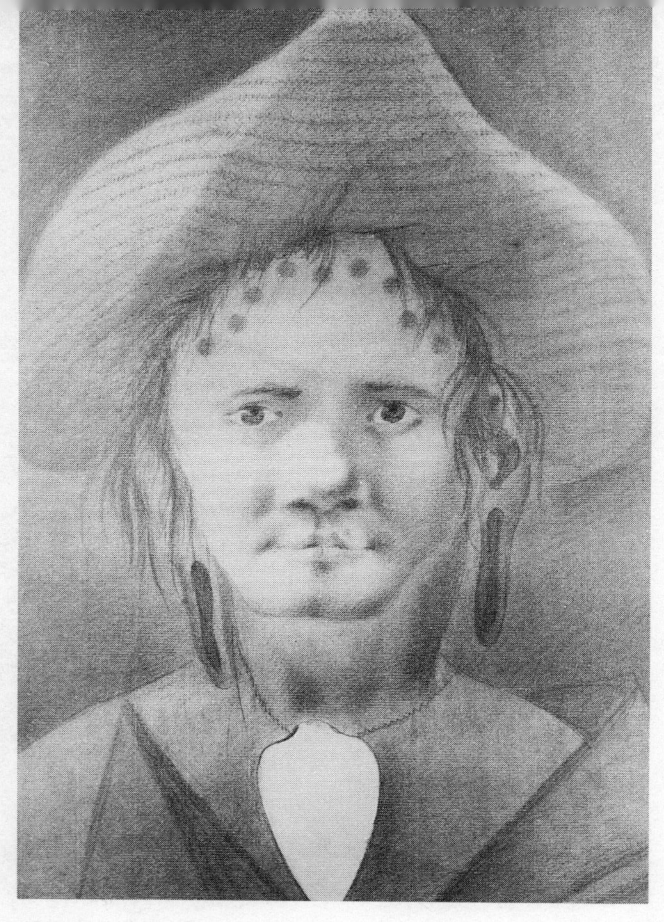

FIG. 52. Portrait heads of Easter Islanders

(*left*) Man; (*right*) Woman. Crayon drawings by Hodges.—Commonwealth National Library

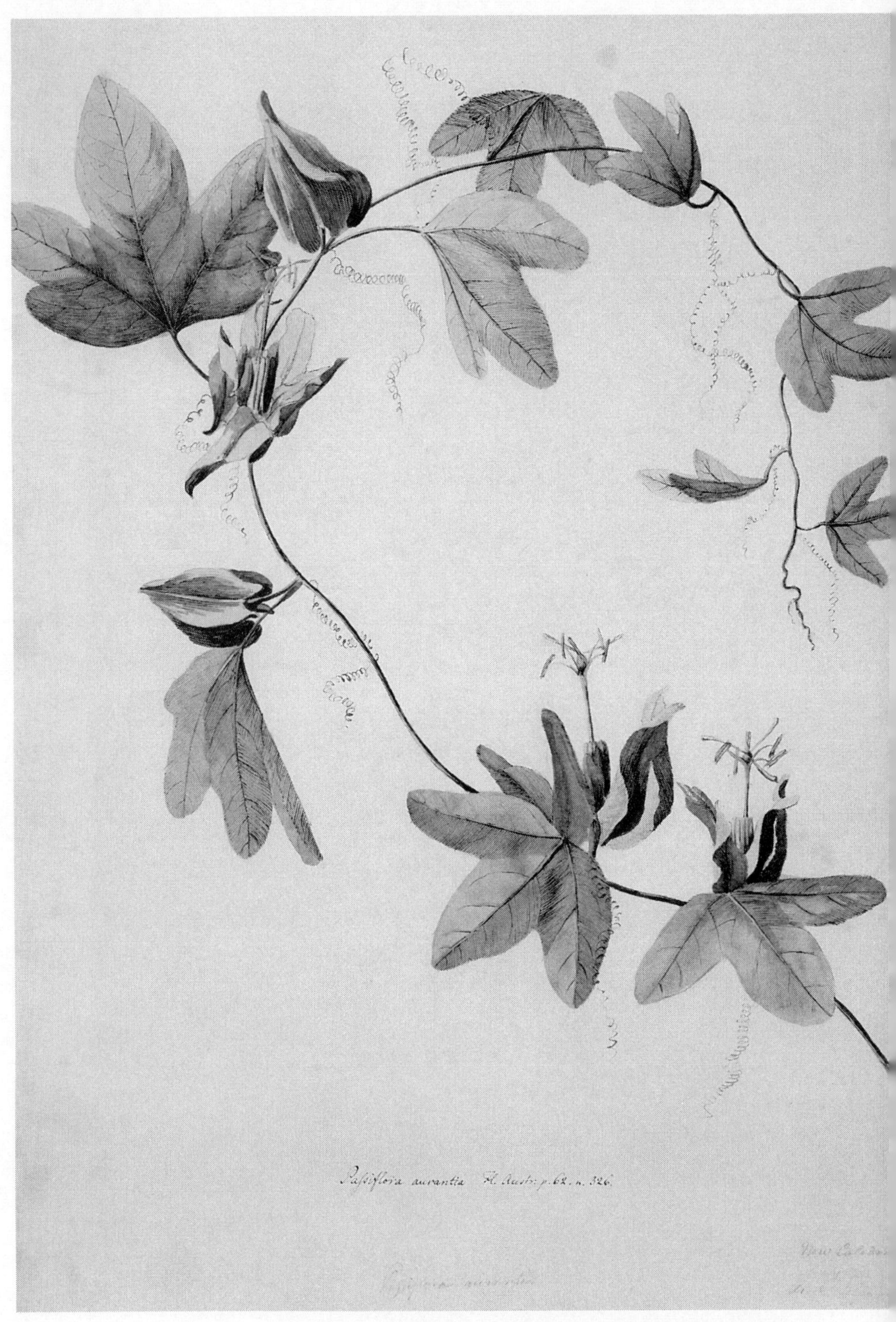

Fig. 53. Passion flower of New Caledonia (*Passiflora aurantia*)

Drawing by George Forster in B.M. (N.H.)—'Botanical Drawings', II, pl. 248

put their heads between his feet[1] and what was still more no one durst pass him till he gave them leave. Mr Pickersgill took hold of one arm and a nother of the gentlemen the other and conducted him down to the landing place where I found him seated with so much sullen and stupid gravity that[2] I realy took him for an ideot which the people were ready to worship from some superstitious notions, I salluted him and spoke to him, he answered me not, nor did he take the least notice of me or alter a single feature in his countenance, this confirmed my former opinion and [I was] just going to leave him when one of the natives an intelligent youth under took to undeceive me which he did in such a manner as left me no doubt but that he was the principal man on the Island, accordingly I gave him the present I had intended for the old chief which consisted of a Shirt, An axe, a piece of Red Cloth, a looking glass & some Medals and Beeds, he still preserved his sullen gravity, I got not one word from him nor did he so much as turn his head or eyes either to the right or left but sit like a Post stuck in the ground just as I found him so I left him and soon after he retired.[3] I had not been long aboard before word was brought me that a quantity of Provisions was sent me from this chief, a boat was sent to bring it aboard, it consisted of about 20 baskets containing roasted Bananas, sour bread and yams and a Pig of about twenty pound weight. Mr Edgcumb with his party was just imbarking when these came down to the Water side, the bearers thereof told him that it was a present from the King of the Island to me,[4] that is the same person as I have been speaking of, after this I was no longer to doubt his dignity.

THURSDAY *7th*. Early in the Morn while the Sloops were unmooring I went a shore with Captain Furneaux and Mr Forster in order to make some return to the King for his present, we were met at our landing by my friend Otā-go, we asked for the King whose name is [Kohagee-too-Fallangou] or [Latoo-Nipooroo].[5] Otago undertook to

[1] This was the ceremony of *moemoe*, obeisance to one's hereditary chief.

[2] ... notwithstanding what had been told me ...—f. 130.

[3] *he still ... retired:* He received these things or rather suffered them to be put upon him and laid down by him without loosing a bit of his gravity, speaking one word or turning his head either to the right or left but sat the whole time like [a] statue in which situation I left him to return on board and he soon after retired.—f. 130. This may be taken as an example of revision wherein Cook's writing lost its original force.

[4] *from ... me:* from Areike that is King of the Island to the Areike of the Ships ...—f. 130v.

[5] I take the first of these names from B, the second from Forster, I, p. 466. It is possible to work out a plausible equivalent for 'Kohaghee-too-Fallangou', but none known otherwise to Tongan history; the name, whatever it was, has sunk out of sight. 'Latoo-Nipooroo' (given elsewhere as 'Latooliboula') is Latunipulu, the personal name of a male Tamaha—a man of very great importance, though not a king; it is of Fijian origin.

conduct us to him but whether he misstook the man we wanted or he did not know where he was I know not, he certainly took us a wrong road, but we had but gone a little way before he stoped and after a little conversation between him and a nother, we return'd back and presently after the King appeared[1] when Otā-go sat down under a tree and desired us to do the same, the King seated him self on a peice of elivated ground about 12 or 15 yards from us, and appeared with all the Sullen gravity he had done the day before; here we sat faceing each other for some minutes, I waited for Otago to shew us the way, but seeing that he did not offer to rise I got up my self and went to the King and saluted him, Captain Furneaux did the same and then we sat down by him and gave him a White Shirt which we put upon him, a few yards of Red Cloth, a brass Kettle, a Saw, two large spikes, three looking glasses and put about his neck about a Doz[n] Medals and some strings of beads, all this time [he] preserved his former gravity, he even did not seem to see or know what we were about, his arms appeared immoveable at his sides, he did not so much as raise them when we put on his shirt. I told him both by words and signs that we were going to leave his Island, he scarce made me any answer to this or any other thing we said or did, we therefore rose up but I yet remained near him.[2] At length he entered into some conversation with Otago and an old woman whom we took for his Mother. I did not understand any part of the conversation it however made him laugh in spite of his assumed gravity. I say assumed because I think it could not be his real disposission unless he was an idiot indeed, as they are, like all the Islanders, a people of a good deal of levity and he was in the prime of life; at last he rose up took french leave and retired with his Mother and two or 3 More. Otā-go who remained with us conducted us to another circle where was seated the old Chief and several respectable old people of both sex among whom was the old priest seated at the chiefs right hand, this reverend Father seemed to be troubled with a disease that is not very uncommon, we observed that in a morning he could Walk as well as any other man but in the evening he was obliged to be led home between two people, we supposed that the juce of the [Pepper root] plant had the same effect upon him as Wine and other strong liquors has upon people in Europe who drink a large portion of them, it is very certain that these old gentlemen seldom sit down without preparing a Bowl of this Plant,[3] I believe with an intent to

[1] . . . with very few attendance
[2] . . . to observe his actions.—f. 131.
[3] *plant:* liquor which is done in the same manner as at Ulietea. . . .

treat us, the greatest part however generally fell to their share. I was not well prepared to take my leave of this old chief having exhausted almost all our store on the other and those about him, however by rumageing our Pockets and Trade Bags (for my treasurer constantly attended me where ever I went) we made up some tolerable presents for him and his friends. This old chief had an air of dignity about [him] which commanded respect that the other had not, he was grave but not sullen, he would crack a joak, talk on different subjects and endeavour to understand and be understood, for it must be observed that we knew but little of their language nor could the two Islanders we had on board understand them which surprised [me] as the difference between the two Languages is certainly not very great.[1]

At length[2] we took leave of the old people who express'd niether sorrow nor joy at our departure. Otāgo and some others accompanied us aboard, stayed breakfast, after which I made them presents and then they departed. Otā-go was very desirous for me to return again to the isle and to bring with me Cloth, Axes, Nails &c[a] telling me that I should have Hogs, Fowls, Fruit and roots in a bundance, he particularly desired me[3] to bring him such a sute of Cloths as I had then on and which was my uniform. This good natured Islander was very serviceable to me on many occasions, during our short stay he constantly came aboard every Morning soon after it was light and never quited me during the remainder of the day, he was always ready either aboard or a shore to do me all the service that lay in his power, his fidelity was rewarded at small expence and I found my account in having such a friend. In unmooring the Coasting Cable parted about the middle of its length, by this accident we lost the anchor[4] which laid [in] 40 fathom Water without any Buoy to it. We also found the Cable of the Bower Anchor much rubed by the Rocks where it had laid upon the ground, by this a judgement may be formed of the sort of anchoring ground we laid in.

At 10 o'Clock we got under sail but as our decks were very much lumbered with fruit &c[a] [5] we kept plying with our Top sails under the land till they were cleared. The Supplies we got at this Island were

[1] *for it must . . . great:* During this viset the old preist repeated a short prayer or speach, the purport of which we did not understand, indeed he would frequently at other times break out in prayer, but I never saw any attention paid him by any one present.—f. 131v.

[2] *At length:* After a stay of near two hours

[3] . . . more than once,

[4] *the anchor:* the other half together with the anchor

[5] ADV '. . . Came to sail In Company with the Resolution who as well as ourselves were very well stored with Plantens &c which we hung round our Taphrail & Awning.— Falconer.

about 150 Pigs, double that number of fowls, Bananas and Cocoa-nutts as many as we could dispence with and a few yams and had we stayed longer we might no dought have got a great deal more, this in some degree shews the fertillity of the isle which together with the neighbouring isle of Middlebourg I shall now give a more particular account of.

These Islands were first discovered by Captain Tasman in Jan^ry^ 1643 who named them Amsterdam and Middleburg, but the former is called by the Natives *Ton-ga-tabu* and the latter *Ea-ōō-we*. They are situated between the Latitude of 21°29′ and 21°3′ s and between the Longitude of 17[4°40′] and 17[5°15′][1] West, deduced from Observations of the Sun and Moon made on the spot. Mr Kendals Watch places them 34′ more westerly.

They lie in the direction of NW and SE from each other distant four Leagues. Ea-oo-we which is the Southermost is Ten leagues in circuit and of a height sufficient to be seen 12 leagues. The skirts of this isle, that is from the Sea to about a Mile inland appeared to be mostly occupied with Plantations, the SW and NW sides were at least so,[2] the interior parts were but little cultivated, tho' very proper for it; here we see[3] groves of Cocoa-nutt and other trees and Launs cover with the finest Grass, here and there Plantations and Paths leading to every part of the Island in such beautifull disorder as greatly heightens the prospect.[4] The Anchorage, which I named English Road as we were the first who ever Anchored there, is on the NW side in Latitude 21°20′30″ s, the bearings we took when at Anchor (which are already mentioned) together with the Chart will be more than sufficient to find this anchorage, the small creek before it makes it safe landing for Boats at all times of the Tide which here as well as at Tonga tabu rises about [4 or 5] feet, the Bank is coarse Sand and extends two miles from the land whereon is from 20 to 40 fathom Water. The Island of Tonga-tabu is shaped something like an Isos-

[1] These figures and the other insertions between square brackets for the next few pages are from M A H; in the last some blanks are filled by Cook himself.

[2] *were ... so:* A especially

[3] *it; ... see:* M however the want of it added greatly to the beauty of the Isle, for here are agreably dispers'd,

[4] All the journals display enthusiasm over the prospect of Eua. 'The little hills along the sea shore well cover'd with fruit trees of different kinds, the land within them gently rising to a moderate hight, affording large plains interspers'd with little wood[s] and plantations the whole Island having the appearence of one intire Garden laid out with great Design the verdant hills and plains making the most pleasing prospect immaginable ...' —Gilbert, 7 October. '[It] affords, without exception, the most beautiful & varigated Prospect I ever beheld. What a lovely Scene would the Pen of a *Bougainville* make of this who would say so many fine things of *Otahitee!*'—Wales, 1 October.—ADV 'Middleburgh affords the most delightfull prospect that can be seen, & which I shall leave to a more able pen to discribe what is due to that pleasing spott.'—Kemp, 3 October.

celes Triangle[1] the longest sides whereof are 7 Leagues each and the shortest four, it lies nearly in the direction of ESE and WNW; it is all of an equall height which is rather low, no where exceeding [Sixty or Eighty] feet above level of the Sea.[2] Van Diemens Road where we Anchored is under the NW point of the Island midway between the most Northern and Western point, a Reef of Rocks over which the Sea constantly breaks bearing NWBW. The bank does not extend more than three Cables length from the Shore, without that is an unfathomable depth, sufficient proofs that the bottom is not to be relied on,[3] there is however on the East side of the North point of the isle (as Mr Gilbert informed [me] who I sent to survey these parts) a very Snug Harbour of one mile or more in extent wherein is 7, 8 and 10 fathom Water, Coarse[4] Sandy bottom, the Channell by which he went in and out of this Harbour lies close to the point in which is only three fathom water but he believes that farther to the NE is a Channell of a much greater depth which he had not time to examine, indeed it would have taken up more time than I could spare to have surveyed these parts Minutely as there are a number of small Islots and reefs of rocks extending to the NE even farther than we could see.[5] The Variation of the Compass was here [10°45′] East.

The Island of Tonga-tabu and the skirts of Ea-oo-we are as I have before observed wholy laid out in Plantations in which are some of the richest Productions of Nature, in these plantations are the greatest part of the Houses of the Inhabitants built[6] with no other order than conveniency requires, paths leading from one to a nother and

[1] Triangle is not a shape that very readily leaps to the mind of one scrutinizing the modern chart, or even the one engraved in the printed *Voyage*; but Chart XXX*b* will show readily enough what Cook means.

[2] M This Island and also that of Eaoowe, is guarded from the Sea by a reef of coral rocks extending out from the shore one hundred fathoms, more or less, on this Reef the force of the Sea is spent before it reaches the land or shore; indeed this is in some measure the Situation of all the Tropical isles in this Sea which I have seen; thus Nature has effectually secured these Isles (many of which are mere points when compared to this Vast Ocean) from the incroachments of the Sea.—The highest point of Tongatapu, at the southern extremity, is higher than Cook thought—about 250 feet.

[3] *not . . . on:* M none of the best

[4] *Coarse:* M a clean

[5] To judge from the anchorage marked on the engraved chart, *Voyage* I, pl. XIV, Gilbert's 'very Snug Harbour' lay within Tasman's Maria Bay, formed by the inward curve of the western part of the north coast of the island (not simply the opening in the reefs at the western approach to Egeria channel, one of the channels leading to the anchorage off the modern Tongan capital of Nuku'alofa, which is now called Maria Bay). The 'North point of the isle' is called Niu'Aunofo; Gilbert's channel farther to the north-east seems to have been the opening into Maria Bay itself, on the western side of the islet of Atata, which lies 3¾ miles ENE of Niu Aunofo. 'The small Islots and reefs of rocks extending to the NE' are Tufaka, Atata, Malinoa, and reefs named and unnamed, which stretch round to the Lahi passage. It would certainly have taken time to explore the whole complex 'minutely'.

[6] *in these . . . built:* M Here are no Towns or Villages, most of the houses are built in the Plantations. . .—At this time Tongans did not build in villages. These sprang up later than Cook's visit, as a development in mutual defence, in the period of wars

publick lanes which open a free communication to every part of the Island.[1]

The Chief Productions of these isles are Cocoa-nutts, Bread fruit, Plantains or Bananas, Shaddocks, Lemons,[2] a fruit like an Apple called by them Feghega and in Otaheite Aheiya,[3] Sugar Cane, Yams and several other Roots and fruits which are common in the other Isles.[4] In general M[r] Forster has found the same sort of Plants here as are at Otaheite besides several others which are not to be found there and I probably may have added to their Stock of Vegetables by leaving at both the isles an assortment of Garden Seeds, Pulse &c[a]. Bread fruit as at all the other isles was now out of Season, Shaddocks and Lemons the same, of the former we got but a few at Ea-o͞o-we[5] and as to the latter we found only the tree nor was this the Season for roots. We saw no other Domistick Animals among them but Hogs and Fowls, the former are of the same sort as at the other isles, but the latter are far superior being as large as any we have in Europe and full as well tasted.[6] We belive that they have no Dogs as they were exceeding desirous of those we had on board, their desire was satisfied so far as a Dog and a Bitch would do it,[7] the one was from New Zealand and the other from Huaheine or Uliatea. The name of a Dog in their Language is [Kooree or Gooree] the same as at New Zealand, this shows that they are no strangers to the name what ever they may be to the Animal. The land Birds found here are of the same sort as at Otaheite and the neighbouring isles (viz) Pigeons,[8] Turtle Doves,[9] Parrots,[10] Perrokeets[11] and several

described by Mariner; and after the era of fortifications they remained. A village arrangement is the normal modern one.

[1] 'Fresh water is a Scarce Article at both these Islands I saw only one pool or small pond at Amsterdam which was in a plantation not far from y[e] North point of y[e] Island, at Middleburg I saw no more than what was sufficient to Convince me that such an Article was on y[e] Island, as we were not in want of any it was not much look'd for, I am however of opinion that there is not a running stream on either of these Isles, and yet for fertility they may vie with any two in y[e] World. . . .'—Log. He might have found one small stream up in the hills in Eua, if he had explored so far.

[2] M deletes 'Lemons'. A *note*: It is a doubt with me if they have Lemons, all the authority I had for mentioning them was from Capt[n] Furneaux saying he had seen the trees but no one of us ever saw any of the fruit.

[3] Tongan *fekika* and Tahitian *ahia*, the Mountain or Malay Apple, *Syzygium amicorum*.

[4] *and several . . . Isles:* M in short here are most of the Articles which the other Islands produce besides some which they have not.

[5] *Ea-oo-we:* M Middleburg; the produce and cultivation of this isle is the same as at Amsterdam with this difference that a part only of the former is cultivated, whereas the whole of the latter is.

[6] *and full . . . tasted:* M and their flesh is very whit as good if not better

[7] *their . . . it:* M My friend Atago was complimented with a Dog and Bitch

[8] The Pacific Pigeon, *Ducula pacifica* (Gm.).

[9] A small fruit pigeon, *Ptilinopus porphyraceus porphyraceus* (Temm.).

[10] The Red-breasted Musk Parrot, *Prosopeia tabuensis* Gm.

[11] The Blue-crowned Lory, *Vini australis* (Gm.). Forster mentions (I, p. 447) the pur-

other small Birds, here are also Both in abundance Bald Couts of a blue Plumage[1] and a pretty sort of an Owl[2] which I have not seen at any of the other Isles, the latter Oediddee informs me is to be found at Tupi.[3] We have seen no other wild Animals in these isles excepting a small sort of a Lizard.[4] We know no more of their fishery than that[5] they have the same instruments for Catching fish as at the other isles, Hooks made of Mother of Pearl, gigs with two, three or more prongs and netts made with a very fine threed and the mashes worked exactly like our[s]; but nothing shews their ingenuity so much as the manner in which their Canoes are built and constructed; they are long and narrow with out-riggers and built of several pieces which are curiously[6] sew'd together with platting made of the out side fibers of Cocoa-nutts. The sewing is all in the inside, they work a sort of kant on the insides edges of the pieces to be joined together in which they make holes through which they pass the platting so that no part of it is to be seen on the outside[7] and the Seams are so closely fitted to each other as hardly to admit in any Water altho' they are neither caulked nor payd.[8] The Common Canoes are about [30] feet in length and [two] in breadth,[9] the body nearly round, the Stern terminates in a point and the head some thing like a wedge which has

chase of 'several beautiful parroquets, pigeons and doves, which they brought to us perfectly tame'.

[1] The Purple Gallinule, *Porphyrio porphyrio* Linn.

[2] The Pacific representative of the Barn Owl, *Tyto alba lulu* Peale.

[3] 'Tupi' is presumably Tubuai-manu, about 40 miles west of Moorea, lat. 17°38′ s, long. 150°37′ w; Wallis's Saunders Island, Cook's Tapoamanau of the first voyage (I, p. 140; but Tubai, p. 293). A adds to this list of birds, 'and large Batts in abundance'. Cook must here refer to the colony of fruit-bats or flying foxes a little south of the *faitoka* he described, hanging like thick black fruit to the casuarinas on the edge of the present village of Kolovai, and sacred to the Ata clan. Bayly (pp. 95–6) gives a picturesque description: '. . . a great number of Bats near the size of an English Pigeon, their wings when extended measure from 16 to 22 or 24 Inches, they hang on the trees by the hooks or claws at [the] Joint of the wing, with their bodies between them the head resting on the breast, & the back downwards this way they hang swing-swang to the branches of the tops of high trees & sleep all day; they have a head and nose like a dog & brest like a woman, they suckle their young like Animals'. He adds (p. 97), 'we saw no venomous Creature among them except the Santopee [centipede], of which we saw many'; and on the islets and rocks off Maria Bay 'we saw great Numbers of small snakes'.

[4] *We have seen . . . Lizard:* M We saw no Ratts in these isles or any other wild quadrupede except small Lizards. A [alteration by Cook] Besides Hogs and Ratts, here are no other. . . Lizards.—This lizard may have been the pretty little skink called *pili*, very common about the houses. On La Pérouse's voyage a large green lizard was collected, the iguana *Brachylophus fasciata* (Brongniart).

[5] *We know . . . that:* M The produce of the Sea we know but little of, it is reasonable to suppose that the same sort of fish is found here as at the other isles,

[6] M and neatly

[7] *in which . . . outside:* M in which the holes are made for sewing the planks together just in the manner a Shoe-maker would sew together two pieces of leather, so that no part of the Sewing is to be seen on the outside;

[8] *nor payd:* M or cover'd with any coating.

[9] M consequently long and narrow

its edges rounded: neither the one nor the other is raised above the common level of the Gunwale, over each is a kind of deck about ¼ part the length of the Canoe, the middle of these decks in some are decorated with a row of whiete shells stuck on little pegs which are worked out of the same piece as composeth the deck; the middle is open[1] where there are thwarts secured to each gun[wale] which serve as seats to the rowers and a security to the Canoe, they are rowed by Paddles the blades of which are short and broadest in the middle, some are fitted with a mast and sail, we however saw but one of these small Canoes thus equiped, the generallity of those that are intended for sailing are a great deal larger,[2] but constructed in the very same manner with the addition of a riseing in the middle round the open part of the Canoe in the form of a long trunck or trough which is open longitudinally at the uper and under sides, it is composed of boards closely fitted together and well secured to the boddy of the Canoe. Two such Canoes they fasten together alongside of each other (leaving a space of about [6] feet between them) by means of strong beams secured to the upper parts of the riseing above mentioned. The ends of these beams project but very little without the off sides of the Canoes, over them is laid a boarded platform the ends of which project considerably over the beams, at the one end it preserves its breadth and is supported by sta[n]tions fitted to the body of the Canoe and the other end the projecting part is no broader than the space between the Canoes and is supported by longitudinal spars fasten'd to the beams. I have already observed that the risings are open at the uper part, nor are the[y] covered by the platform concequently remain as hatchways leading into the Canoes from off the platform[3] and as all the parts which compose these two bodies are made as tight[4] as the nature of the work will admit, they may be immerged in Water to the very platform without being in danger of filling nor is it possible under any circumstances whatever for them to sink so long as they hold together. Thus they are not only made Vessels of burdthen but fit for distant Navigation, they are rigged with one mast which steps upon the Platform and can easily be raised or taken down, a long one not being necessary as they are sailed with a Lateen-sail, or a triangular sail extended by a long yard which is a little bent or crooked, the sail is made of Matting,

[1] *the . . . open:* M the Middle of the Cannoe is open about half its length

[2] M 69 feet in length and of a proportional breadth,

[3] *nor . . . platform:* M The way into the hold of the Canoes is from of the platform down a sort of uncovered hatch-way in which they stand to bail out the Water.

[4] *tight:* A light.—But this must be a slip of the clerk, evidently repeated elsewhere, for it somehow got as far as the printed *Voyage*, I, p. 216, 'strong and light'. MGH tight.

some of the rope necessary for rigging of these vessels is 4 or 5 Inches thick and made exactly like ours. They fix a little hut or shed (for it is open on one side) on the Platform in which they keep their provisions &c[a], it also serves to screen them from the Sun and shelter them from the Weather;[1] they carry likewise a[2] Fire-hearth which is a square trough of Wood about 8 Inches deep[3] fill'd with Stones, for the conveniency of making a fire to dress their Victuals. I think these Vessels are navigated either end foremost and that in changing tacks they only shift the Sail, but of this I am not certain as having seen none under sail, or with the Mast and sail on end but what were at some distance off.[4]

Their Houses are no less neatly constructed but do not however exceed those of the other isles, the materials on which they are built are the same and some little variation in the disposission of the framing is all the difference in their construction. The floor is a little raised and coverd with thick strong Matts, the same sort of matting serves to inclose them on the windward side, the other being open, thire are little area's before the most of them generally planted round with trees and Shrubs of Ornament whose fragrancy perfume the very air in which they breathe. Their whole household furniture consists in a wooden platter or two, a few Cocoa-nutt Shells and some neat wooden Pillows shaped like little Stools.[5] We got from them two earthen Vessels, which [were] all that were seen among them, the one was in the shape of a Bom-shell with two holes in it the one opposite to the other, the other was a little Pipkin which would contain about [five or Six] pintes and had been in use on the fire, I am of opinion that those were the Manufactory of some other isle, for if they had been of their own make we ought to have seen more than these two, nor am I to suppose that they came from Tasmans ship, the time is too great for britle Vessels like these to be preserved.[6] The

[1] M and serves for other purposes

[2] *a:* M a Moveable

[3] *square . . . deep:* M square, but shallow trough of wood

[4] M All those Canoes which go single, by sails or paddles, have out-riggers without which they would over-set.—In the printed *Voyage*, I, pl. XVI shows the lines of both a double and a single canoe. Mariner says that the Tongans learnt much about the building and rigging of canoes from the Fijians, who had better wood, though the Tongans were the better navigators. 'All their large canoes, therefore, are either purchased or taken by force from the natives of Fiji'.—Mariner, II, p. 194. See Figs. 47, 48.

[5] M their common cloathing with the addition of a Matt serves them for Beding;

[6] The question whether the Tongans ever made pottery for themselves does not seem to have been dogmatically resolved, though the finding of some 1600 potsherds is recorded by W. C. McKern (*Archaeology of Tonga*, B. P. Bishop Mus. Bull. 60, Honolulu 1929). McKern (p. 118) inclines to the opinion that pots were made in Tonga as well as brought from Fiji. Mariner (II, p. 199) says definitely, 'They perform the process of boiling in earthen pots, of the manufacture of the Fiji Islands . . .' Tasman's ship as a source can certainly be ruled out.

only piece of Iron we saw among them was a small tool like a bradawl and which had been made of a small nail.[1] What tools we saw among them which were but few were made of stone, bone, shells &c[a] as at the other Isles, when we view the works which are perform[d] with such tools we are struck with admiration at the ingenuity[2] of the workman. Their knowlidge of the utillity of Iron was just sufficient to make them prefer Nails to Beads and such like Trifles, some, but very few, would exchange a Pig for a large Nail or a Hatchet, old Jackets, Shirts, peices of Cloth and even old rags were in more esteem with them than the best edge tool we could give them concequently they got but few axes from us but what were given as presents, but if I take together the Nails that have been given in exchange for Curiositys by the officers and crews of both Sloops and those given for Refreshments, they have not got less than three or four[3] hundred weight from the largest spike down to a Sixpeny Nail.

They make the same kind of Cloth as at Otaheite and of the same Materials, they have not such a Variety nor do they make it so fine, but as it is all die'd with a thick gummy glossy Colour it is perhaps more durable, these Colours are black, Brown, Purple, yellow and Red, I am unacquainted with the material with which they are made, a kind of Red and Yellow pigment we have seen.[4] They also make various sorts of Matts of a very fine texture which serve them both for Cloathing and beding. Their Dress is a piece of Cloth or Matting wraped round their Middle reaching from the breast down below the knee, they seldom wear any thing over their Shoulders or

[1] M and is now in the possession of M[r] Forster as a great curiosity.—'. . . they possessed some nails, which must have been brought to the island in Tasman's time. We purchased one of these nails, which was very small and almost consumed with rust, but had been carefully preserved by being fixed on a wooden handle, probably to serve the purposes of a googe or borer, and is now deposited in the British Museum'.—Forster, I, pp. 470–1. It has more than once been suggested that this nail could not have survived from Tasman's time and must have been a relic of Wallis's visit to Niuatoputapu in 1767; but if Forster's description is correct, a Tasman origin does not seem at all impossible.

[2] M and patience

[3] *three or four:* M five

[4] *I am . . . seen:* M all made from vegetables.—'Bark-cloth' in Tonga was called *tapa* only when not dyed or stained. In its finished, decorated form it was known as *ngatu*. The colours commonly used came from a variety of plants. The *tuitui* (Tongan form of the Tahitian *tutui*) or candlenut gave a black or dark brown dye; turmeric yellow; mangrove a red; the *koka* (*Bischofia javanica*) red-brown. The juice of the *hea*, says Mariner, gave a brilliant red varnish:—'The hea tree is only plentiful at Vavaoo' (p. lxx). This was *Parinarium insularum* A. Gray, says T. G. Yuncker, in his valuable *Plants of Tonga*, B. P. Bishop Museum Bull. 220, Honolulu, 1959. I do not know precisely what colour, or combination of colours, Cook defined as purple. Mariner gives an interesting account of the whole process of cloth-making and dyeing, pp. 202–6; it is fundamentally the same today, and on the southern islands the sharp sound of the tapa-mallet comes continually over the air as in the eighteenth century.

upon their heads. The dress of the Men and Women are the same. With respect to their persons and colour I neither think them ugly nor handsome,[1] there are none so fair, so tall or so well made as some of the natives of Otaheite and the neighbouring isles: on the other hand they are not so dark, so little or ill shaped as some we see at these isles, nor is there that disproportion between the Men and Women.[2] Their hair in general is black, and they all wear it croped short. I saw but two people that were an exception to this rule; many of them paint or Colour it Red and some few we saw who had their hair coloured blue;[3] the men Cut or shave their Beards quite short, this I have been told is done with two Shells.[4] The same Custom of Tattowing (inlaying the Colour of black in the skin in such a manner as to be indelible) prevails here as at the other isles, the men are tattowed from the Middle of the thigh up to above the hips, even their gentiles, I am told do not escape. The Women are not tattowed in this manner, they have it only slitely done on the Arms hands and fingers. Both sex have their Ears pierced but do not seem fond of ear-rings, their chief ornaments are Necklaces and Bracelets made of Bones, shells &c[a], they have also a kind of worked apron which is curious on account of the time it must take to make one.[5] It seems to [be] a Custom with them to anoint their heads and all the upper part of the body that is exposed to the Sun, every morning, at least I found my friend Attā-go had done it every morning before he visited me, perhaps it might be done out of respect to his friend.[6]

[1] *With respect . . . handsome:* M In their persons and Colour they differ but little from the other islanders, that is they are of a common size with Europeans and their colour is uniformly Brown inclining to copper.

[2] B [some of our] Gentlemen were of opinion, these were a much handsomer race of people, the Women especially, others again were of a contrary opinion of which number I was one; New faces and new favours adds charms to the fair sex which a little acquaintance wears of; be this as it will they are certainly proportionate and well shaped, have good features, are active brisk and lively.—f. 132.—Bayly says of Eua (p. 97), 'The Women from 5[F] 4[I] to 5[F] 7[I] or 8[I] in general & many of them very regular fetures & they are fat & Jolly in general'.

[3] B f. 132 *note*: They comb or manage it so as to make it grow upright like hogs bristles. —So also A G. The 'red' probably came from powdered turmeric—Forster mentions 'an orange powder'; the blue from some local earth. Lime—powdered coral—was also used, partly to clean the scalp. Cf. p. 445, n. 1 below.

[4] . . . which are substitutes for better instruments. Their teeth are white and perfect to an advanced age.—f. 132v.

[5] 'Among their other manufactories I ought to have mentioned worked Baskets made of the fibers of Cocoa-nutts twisted, some are long others round &c[a] all equally curious, beautifull and lasting; they have many little nick nacks among them which shew they neither want taste nor ingenuity or skill to execute whatever they take in hand.'—f. 132. The 'worked apron', says Mariner, was the chief distinction of the female dress; it was about a foot in breadth.

[6] *perhaps . . . friend:* whether out of respect to his friend or Custom I know not.—f. 132v. —This oiling was generally done all over, and followed the morning bath as a matter of routine.

It is not the custom here as at Otaheite for the men and women to have seperated Messes, here they eat at the same table. I have seen the women tip of their Cup of the liquor made of [the pepper] root in their turn[1] with the men without the least ceremony, nay I have even seen the men so genteel as to help the Ladies first. Most of the people of these Isles wanted either one or both of their little fingers, little children, some few young people and two or three aged persons were the only exceptions, we could not learn the cause of this mutilation with any degree of certainty, but judged it to be on account of the death of their parents.[2] This Custom and for this reason I am told prevails a mong the Hottantots, the New Zealanders cut and scar themselves on the same account. They either burn or make incisions in their cheeks near the Cheek bone, in some these wounds were quite fresh in others heald, but the marks were remaining,[3] if this is not done with a view of curing some disorder they may be afflected with I know not what it is done for, they however seem to be as free from diseases as any Nation what ever, I neither saw a sick or lame person among them, all appeared healthy and strong a proof of the goodness of the Climate in which they live. As we had yet some Venereal complaints on board I took all possible means to prevent its being communicated to the Natives by not suffering a Man to go on shore on whom there was the least suspicion nor did I permit that any women should be allowed to come on board the Sloops. I cannot tell if the women are so free of their favours as at Otaheite, I think not and yet I believe incontinency to be no great crime among them, with the unmarried especially.[4]

[1] *eat . . . turn:* Eat and Drink as well as sleep together and can tip of their Cup of Wawavouru . . .—For 'Wawavouru' here H reads 'Pepper juice'.

[2] . . . or some other near relation . . . f. 132v.—The amputation of part of a finger was not a sign of mourning, but a sacrifice to some god for the recovery of a sick relation superior in rank to the victim—if victim is the right word when the deprivation was so common. See the portrait of 'Otago' in the printed *Voyage*, pl. XL. It was called *tutu nima—tutu*, to cut off; *nima*, the hand. Mariner, II, pp. 178–9.

[3] *They either . . . remaining:* They also, either burn or make incisions in their Cheeks near the Cheek bone, the reason of this was equally unknown to us: in some the wounds were quite fresh, in others it could only be known by the mark which remained or the colour of the skin which was changed: there can be no set time or age when these ceremonies or customs must be performed as we saw by the green wounds that both had been lately performed on persons of almost all ages.—f. 132v.—What Cook saw was the result of the mourning ceremony of *tuki* (from the word for a blow): the mourner beat his cheeks continually, and rubbed off the skin with coconut husk or some other harsh substance wound round the hand. Actual burning, a less painful process, was also common—Mariner, I, pp. 319–20.

[4] *I cannot . . . especially:* Incontinency, is I beleive, in the unmaried people no crime with them and I beleive the women are as free of their favours as at any of the other isles the lower glass [*sic*] especially. . . .—f. 132v.—It is clear from this, as well as from Cook's more recent conclusions on Tahitian behaviour, that he was getting at the truth in the matter of sexual morality. Apparently the *Adventure* could not keep her deck free, but

Their Common method of Saluting or embracing one a nother is by join[in]g or touching Noses the same as in New Zealand and their Signs of Peace seems to be the displaying a white flag or flags, at least such were displayed on the Shore in several places as we rainged along the Coast and before the place where we Anchored, but those people who came first off to us in their Canoes brought with them some [of the pepper] Root on which they make their drink which they sent aboard before they came in themselves. One would not wish for a better sign of friendship than this; can we make a friend more welcome than by seting before him the best liquor in our posession or that can be got? In this manner did those friendly people receive us; I never Viseted the old Chief but he ordered some of the root just mentioned to be brought me and would also set some of his people to chew it and prepare the Liquor, notwithstanding I seldom tasted any,[1] he even carried his hospitality farther by procuring me a Woman as I have before related.

Every thing you give them they apply to their heads by way of thanks, this Custom they are taught from their infancy, when I have given things to little children the mother has lifted up the child's hands to its head just as we in England teach a child to pay a compliment by kissing its hand. They also made use of this Custom in the exchanges between us, whatever we gave them for their goods was applied to the head, just the same as if we had given it for nothing, some times they would take our goods and examine them and if not liked return them back, but when ever they applied them to the head the bargin was infallibly struck.[2] I have also seen when I have given any thing to the Chief which was to them curious that it has been handed about from one to a nother, every one into whose hands it came has put it to their heads, and the women have very often when I have been a mong them taken hold of my hand Kiss'd it and then laid it to their heads. From all this it should seem that this Custom has various significations accordingly as it is applyed, all however complimental: their manner of paying obeisance to their King by bowing their heads to his feet[3] has a tendancy to this Custom. I ought not to forget to mention that the King did not pay me any

Cook's other precaution had some effect: 'Virtue is held in little esteem here', writes Bayly of Eua (p. 97), 'the women gladly jumping out of their canoes & swiming to the ships sides and getting on board for the sake of a Nail or a bit of old cloth, but there was none suffered to have any but thos[e] that were pronounced clean by the Surgeon'.

[1] *notwithstanding . . . any:* but the manner of Brewing was generally sufficient to quench my thirst . . .—f. 133.

[2] Forster picked up the word for 'thanks'—*fakafetai*, but applied it to the whole little ceremony; e.g. 'performed the *fagafetai*' (I, p. 464).

[3] . . . that is putting their heads betweer his feet . . .—f. 133v.

of the Compliments I have just mentioned for the articles I gave him, at least not the last time which was quite a Viset of Ceremony, his behavour on this particular the time before partly escaped my notice, he however return'd the compliment in a manner more becoming the dignity of a Prince as he probably would have done the other had I given him time.[1] I have here mentioned a King which implies the goverment being in a Single person, without knowing whether it is so or no with any degree of certainty, we were however told by some that the Man I have just been speaking on was their King or the first Man on the Island, from this and other circumstances I am led to beleive that their Goverment is much like that of Otahiete,[2] that is in a King or Chief whom they call [Areeke] with other Chiefs under him who are Lords and perhaps sole proprietors of certain districts, to whom the people seem to pay very great obedience, there are people again of no little authority[3] under them, of this third sort was my friend Atta-go. I am likewise of opinion that all the lands on the Islands, Especially on Tonga-tabu, is private property and that there are among them, as at Otaheite Servants or Slaves who can have no share in it,[4] indeed it would be obsurd to suppose every thing to be in Common in a Country so well cul[t]ivated as this. Intrest is the great Spring which animates the hand of industry, few would toil themselves in cultivating and planting the land if he did not expect to injoy the fruits of his labour, if every thing was in common the Industerous man would be upon a worse footing than the Idle Sluggard.[5] M. Bougainville is vastly misstaken where he says, page 252, that the people of Otahiete gathers fruit from the first tree they meets with or takes some in any house into which they enters &c[a]. I queston if there is a fruit tree on that whole island that is not the property of some individual in it, Oediddee tells me that he who takes fruit &c[a] in the Manner just mentioned is punishable with death; be these things as they will, no one seems to want the Common necessaries of life, joy and Contentment is

[1] *had . . . time:* had we not sail'd so soon after

[2] . . . and the neighbouring isles . . .—For all this discussion of kingship and authority see Introduction, pp. lxxiv–lxxvi above.

[3] . . . over the common people . . .—f. 134.

[4] There was no class of slaves in Tonga; the lowest social class was the *tua* or 'peasants'. There seem to have been a relatively few slaves, properly speaking—prisoners of war, and those guilty of crimes, who were enslaved instead of being summarily knocked on the head.

[5] . . . I have frequently seen parties of six eight or ten people, bring down various articles to the landing place where one person, a man or a woman has superintended the sale of the whole, no exchanges have been made but with his or her consent and whatever we gave in exchange was always given to them which plainly shewed they were the owners of the goods and the others no more than their servants.—f. 134.

painted in every face and their whole behaviour to us was mild and benevolent, were they less addicted to thieving we should not, perhaps, be able to charge them with any other vice, they are however far less addicted to this vice than the people of Otahiete,[1] indeed when I consider their whole conduct towards us and the manner in which the few arts they have among them are executed I must also allow them to be in a higher state of civilization.

*Both men and Women are of a Common size with Europeans and their Colour is that of a lightish Copper and more uniformly so than the Inhabitants of Otahiete and the Society Isles. Some of our gentlemen were of opinion these were a much handsomer race, other again mentioned a contrary opinion of which number I was one, be this as it will, they have a good shape and regular features and are active brisk and lively; the Women in particular, who are the merriest creatures I ever met with and will keep chattering by ones side without the least invitation, or consideration whether or no they are understood provide one does but seem pleased with them. In general they appeared to be modest, though there were no want of those of a different stamp. . . . Their hair in general is black, but more especially that of the Women; different Colours was found among the men some times on the same head, caused by some thing they put upon it which stains it white, Red and Blue. Both sex wear it short, I saw but two exceptions to this custom, and the most of them Combed it upwards. Many of the Boys had it cut quite close except a single lock on the top of the head and a small quantity on each side which was quite long. . . . They have fine eyes and in general good teeth, even to an advanced age. . . . The Dress of both Sex, consists of a piece of Cloth or Matting wraped round the Waist and hangs down below the knee, and from the waist upwards they are generally naked and it seemed to be a custom to anoint these parts every Morning, my friend Attago never failed to do it, but whether out of respect to his friend or from Custom, I will not pre-

[1] But cf. M: they were full as expert in [pilfering] as the Otahieteans.—B Like the other islanders they have a strong propensity to pilfer strangers and like them their only vice; their beheavour to us was mild and Benevolent beyond conception.—f. 132.—Cf. also Gilbert's summary on leaving Tonga: '. . . The Inhabitants exceedingly Hospitable and ready to part with the products of the Island; but so anxious to get any of our commodities that if any thing lies in their way they can't help pilfering having no laws to restrain them from it I believe for otherways they are a mighty agreeable people . . .'. Bayly has the same story about constant flogging as at Tahiti—which cannot, however, be true, or the Forsters would have moralized at length upon it. He adds (p. 98), 'they seemed not to have the least Compassion for a Thief: & even rejoiced to see them flogged'. This is in line with Mariner's report: 'Theft is considered by them an act of meanness rather than a crime; and although some of the chiefs themselves have been known to be guilty of it on board ships, it is nevertheless not approved of'.—Mariner, II, p. 138.

tend to say, but I rather think the latter as he was not the only one. Their Ornaments are Amulets, Necklaces and Bracelets, of Bone Shells and Beads of Mother of pearl, Tortise Shell &c[a] these are worn by both sex, the Women also wear on their fingers neat rings made of tortise shell and pieces in their ears about the size of a small quill, but ear ornaments are not commonly worn, they all have their ear's pierced. They have also a curious apron, made of the out side fibers of the Cocoanut shell and composed of a number of small pieces sewed together in such a manner as to form stars, half Moons, little squars &c[a] and studed with beads of shells and covered with red feathers, so as to have a pretty effect.

They make the same kind of Cloth and of the same materials as at Otaheite, but they have not such a variety nor make they any so fine, but as they have a method of glazing it, it is more durable and will resist rain for some time which Otahiete cloth will not. Thier Colours are black, brown, purple, yellow and red, and all made from Vegetables. They make various sorts of Matting and some of a very fine texture, this is generally used for cloathing and the thick and strong sort is used to Sleep on and to make sails for thier Canoes &c[a]. Among other useful utentials they have various sorts of Baskets, some made of the same materials as their matts, others are made of the twisted fibers of Cocoanuts, these are not only durable but beautiful, being generally composed of different colours and studed with beads. They have many little Nick nacks amongst them, which shews that they neither want taste to design nor skill to execute whatever they take in hand. . . . Not only their voices but their music also was very harmonious and they have a considerable compass in their notes. I saw but two Musical Instruments amongst them one was a large Flute made of a piece of bamboo, which they fill with their noses as at Otaheite, but these have four holes or stops, whereas those at Otaheite have but two, the other was composed of 10 or 11 small reeds of unequal lengths, bound together side by side, as the Doric Pipe of the ancients is described to have been done; the open ends of the reeds are of equal height or in a line into which they blow with their mouths.—M.

Benevolent Nature has certainly been very bountifull to these isles, nevertheless the inhabitants cannot be said to be wholy exempt from the curs[e] of our forefathers, part of their Bread must be earnd with the sweat of their brows, the high state of cultivation these isles are in must have cost them immense labour and this is now amply rewarded by their vast produce of which every one seems to partake, no one wants the common necessaries of life, joy and contentment is painted in every face; indeed how can it be otherwise, here an easy freedom prevails among all ranks of people, they injoy every blessing of life and live in a climate where the extremes of heat and cold is unknown, the Thermometer at noon during our stay was from 71 to 76, on our passage from Ulietea from [79°] to [70°].[1] If nature has been wanting in any thing it is in the article of fresh water which is shut up in the bowels of the Earth and for which they are obliged to dig wells, of these we saw only one, so that it is probable there are but few. At Middleburg we saw none, nevertheless they are not without.[2]*—f. 134–4v.

We are in a manner wholy unacquainted with their diversions, the women have now and then entertained us with a song which they some times accompany with a snaping of the fingers in such a manner as appears gracefull enough and some have tolerable good voices; their musical instruments is a kind of flute made of Bamboo with four holes on which they play Notes, they blow into it through one Nostrel in the same manner as at the other isles, and an Organ made of ten or eleven small reeds or pipes; they have also a drum which without any great impropriety may be compaired to a hollow log of wood about [6] feet in length and in girt, it is hollowed out by means of a longitudal slit or open place about inches broad from the one end to the other, they beat on the side of this instrument with two sticks made of hard wood.[3] From the high cultivated state of the isles and the friendly manner we were received by these islanders one may venture to conjector that they are seldom disturbed by either domistick or foreign troubles, they are however not without arms, such as Bows and Arrows, Spears, Darts and clubs, these last are from 3 to 5 or 6 feet long and of various shapes some having square ends others flatish, others like Paddles, Spades &c[a] they are all made with surpriseing neatness, and of the hard wood which is common in all the isles.[4] I have been told that they never use more than one arrow which as soon as it is shott off they quit the Bow and take to their other weapons, this seems very probable

[1] The figures in square brackets are taken from Table IV, *Voyage*, II, p. 302.

[2] *dig wells . . . without:* M dig, a runing stream was not seen and but one well at Amsterdam: at Middleburg no Water was seen but what the Natives had in Vessels, but as it was sweet and cool I had no doubt of its being taken upon the isle and probably not far from the spot where I saw it.

[3] *two . . . wood:* two short sticks and produce a hollow sound not quite so musical as that produced from an empty cask.—f. 135. Such drums or *lali* still form part of the pattern of Tongan life on a number of islands. They give time to the dance; they summon worshippers to church, in lieu of a bell; and small ones, as a sort of tuning-fork, set the note for singing.

[4] M Some of their spears have many barbs and must be very dangerous Weapons where they take effect. . . . By their having such offensive Weapons we must suppose them to have sometimes wars.

for on the back of the bow is a groove just big enough to lodge the arrow and which is its place when the bow is unstrung, the arrows are made of a kind of reed and pointed with hard wood.[1] They have breast plates made of the bone of some large sea animal.[2]

We know so little of their Religion that I hardly dare mention it,[3] the building called *Afiā-tou-ca* before spoke of is undoubtedly set apart for this purpose. Mr Forster and one or two of the officers think that they understood for certain that their dead was entarred in them, this is even probable enough as we saw no other place so likely; I however could by no means satisfy my self on this point, but one thing I am certain of, which is, that they are places to which they direct their prayers for this I have both seen and heard in the manner already related, but to whome or on what account the prayer is made I know not, it was from thence I concluded that there are priests or men among them who exercise the sacret function: the old chief which I have had occasion more than once to mention was constantly attended by one of the Reverand fathers, he seemed to be the head of the church and was distinguished by us by the name of Canterberry, this man would frequently when seated in my presence speak a prayer or make a speach, but I always understood the former because he would break out as it were just when the spirit moved him, no one made him any answer, nor indeed seemed to take much notice of what he said; he was also one of those who attended on Captain Furneaux and me the first day we landed to the two principal Afiā-tou-cas in the neighbourhood. It should seem that this was a necessary ceremony for us two commanders to go through for no other person saw any thing that had the least tendancy to shew that these Afia-tou-cas were places of worship and yet it seems as if they were frequently resorted to for some purpose or a nother, for the Areas or open places before them being covered with a green sod on which the grass was not above an inch or two in lengh, it did not appear to me to be reduced or cut by the hand of man but to be hindred from growing by being frequently trod and sit upon, this however is only a conjecture of my own. It cannot be expected that we could know much either of their civil or religious policy in so short a space as three days, especially as we knew but little of their Language notwithstanding many words are exactly the same as at

[1] Plate XXI in the published *Voyage* shows an 'organ', bow and arrow, spear, and club, the latter decorated in the typical Tongan fashion of multitudinous patterned incision.

[2] These were of whale-bone: the jaw-bone of the sperm-whale seems to be indicated. Such 'breast plates' were more characteristic of Fiji than of Tonga, but the two cultures were linked.

[3] M but do not think they worship Idols.

Otahiete, others nearly so, but their are others again which differ very much and these occured so often that even the two Islanders we had on board could not understand a single sentance they spoke, nay they were worse of than we were for by a little application and attention we could in some measure both understand and be understood in most common occurrences.

... even the two island[er]s we had with us could not understand them and yet we shall find by the vocabulary the difference is not so great as we at first thought and lies more in the pronunciation than in the words. Mr Forster who is well acquainted with Languages is of opinion that the difference is so very little that it may without any impropriety be said to be the same, this is no more than confirmable to what Tupia allways told us, which was that the same language was spoke in all the isles. Our two islanders not understanding these people is no proof against this assertion of Tupias no more than their Countryman Aotourou not understanding the People of the isle of navigators as mentioned by Bougainville.[1] These three men had never before been from their Native isles, consequently wholy unacquainted with the Provincial dialect of the different isles, which Tupia who had traveled much was; besides he had perhaps more understanding than all these three put together. Tupias assersion is greatly Strengthened by the Vocabulary in Mr Dalrymples Collection of Voyages to the S.S. where it appears that the Inhabitants of Cocos & Horn Islands speake the Same Language as at these and other isles we have touched at, at least many words are the very same and others differ but little. By carefully perusing the Voyages of former Navigators, I find such an affinity in the Language, Manner[s] & Customs of the different Islanders that I am led to believe they have all had one Origin.[2]—ff. 135v–6.

FRIDAY *8th. Winds Easterly. Course S 17° W. Dist. sailed 63 Miles. Lat. in South 22°3′. Longde in West Reckg. 175°30′. Longde. made Amsterdm 0°19′ West.* It was 5 o'Clock in the PM before we were in a condition to make sail at which time Van Diemens Road, Lat 21°40′, Longd 275°11′, from whence I take my departure, bore NE distt two miles, at this time a Canoe conducted by four Men came along side with one of those Drums already mentioned on which one man kept continually beating, thinking no doubt that we should be charm'd with his musick. I gave them a piece of Cloth and a Nail for their Drum and took this oppertunity to send to my friend Attago some

[1] Bougainville, p. 280. The 'isle of navigators' was Samoa.
[2] Cf. Cook's reasoning in I, p. 286; and below, pp. 354–5.

Wheat, Pease & Beans which I had forgot to give him when he had the other seeds. After this Canoe was gone we stretched to the Southward with a gentle gale at SEBE, it being my intention to make the best of my way to New Zealand and there take in Wood and Water and then proceed to the South.[1]

SATURDAY 9*th. Winds Southerly. Course SE½E. Dist. sailed* 40 *Miles. Lat. in South* 22°28′. *Longde in West Reckg.* 174°56′. *Longde. made Amsterdm* 0°15 *E.* In the pm had a few hours Calm after which a light breeze sprung up at SW. At 8 PM saw the Island of Pilstart bearing SWBW½W Distant 7 or 8 Leagues. This Island, which is[2] situated in the Latitude of 22°26′ South, Longitude 175°59′ West, seemed to be of small extent and forms two Hills of considerable height, the Southermost is the highest,[3] it lies from the South end of Middleburg [S 52° W] Distant [32] Leagues.

SUNDAY 10*th. Therm.* 70. *Winds South to SE. Course S* 65° *W. Dist. sailed* 66 *Miles. Lat. in South* 22°46′. *Longde. in West Reckg.* 176°13′. *Longde. made Amsterdm* 1°2′ *West.* Fresh breeze and fair Weather. At 4 pm Tack'd and Stretched to the Westward, the wind veering more and more to the East. At 6 o'Clock in the AM saw again the Island of Pilstart bearing NW½N Dist[t] 5 or 6 Leagues, and had it in sight most part of the day.

MONDAY 11*th. Winds SE & ESE. Course SW. Dist. sailed* 90 *Miles. Longde in West Reckg.* 177°23′. *Longde. made Amsterdm* 2°12′ *W.* Fresh breeze and Clowdy, Swell from the South. Saw an Albatross.

TUESDAY 12*th. Winds ESE. Course SSW. Dist. sailed* 112 *Miles. Lat. in South* 25°36′. *Longde in West Reckg.* 178°12′. *Longde. made Amsterdm* 3°1′ *West.* Fresh gales and Clowdy. Swell as yesterday.

WEDNESDAY 13*th. Winds SEBE. Course SSW¼W. Dist. sailed* 100 *Miles. Lat. in South* 27°11′. *Longde in West Reckg.* 179°6′. *Longde. made Amsterdm* 3°55′ *West.* Pleasent Weather. At 6 pm Shortned Sail to

[1] *to the South:* on farther discoveries to the South and East.—f. 140.

[2] *which is:* which was also discovered by Captain Tasman is

[3] *seemed . . . highest:* it is more conspicuous in height than circuit, having in it two considerable Hills, seemingly disjoined from each other by a low vally.—f. 140. The figures in square brackets are inserted by Cook in blanks in H. Cook is not entirely accurate about this island, 'Ata or Pylstaert. Its position is lat. 22°20′ s, long. 176°13′ w; it lies 85 miles south-westward of Tongatapu. It is the northern hill, 1,165 feet, that is the higher, though only by 6 feet. Nor are the two 'disjoined . . . by a low vally'; there is simply a moderate dip in the land between them. Tasman sighted the island 19 January 1643, on his track north-east from New Zealand, and called it Pylstaert after the tropic-birds he saw flying about it—'Pylstaert literally signifying arrow-tail, alludes to the two long feathers in the tail of this bird. . .'—Forster, I, p. 480.

Single Reef'd Topsails and in the Morning made all sail again. AM a Gannet and Egg birds seen.

THURSDAY 14*th. Therm.* 66½. *Winds ESE. Course SSW. Dist. sailed* 94 *Miles. Lat. in South* 28°38′. *Longde. in West Reckg.* 179°47′. *Longde made Amsterdm* 4°36′ *West. Varn.* 11°11′ *East.* Moderate breezes and pleasent Weather. Variation 11°11′ East.

FRIDAY 15*th. Winds Easterly. Course S¾W. Dist. sailed* 98 *Miles. Lat. in South* 30°15′. *Longde in East Reckg.* 179°54′. *Longde made Amsterdm* 4°55′ *West.* Fresh gales and clear weather, Some peices of Sea Weed and Birds daily seen.

SATURDAY 16*th. Winds Easterly. Course SBW. Dist. sailed* 88 *Miles. Lat. in South* 31°41′. *Longde in East Reckg.* 179°32′. *Longde made Amsterdm* 5°17′ *West. Varn.* 11°22′ *East.* Winds and Weather as yesterday. Variation p[r] Az[th] 11°22′ E.

SUNDAY 17*th. Winds ENE. Course South. Dist. Sailed* 60 *Miles. Lat. in South* 32°41′. *Longde. in East Reckg.* 179°32′. *Longde. made West* 5°17′. First part gentle breeze, remainder little wind, pm Variation 10°42′ East, pass'd some rock weed and saw some albatroses, Sheer-waters &c[a].

MONDAY 18*th. Therm.r. Noon* 67. *Winds ENE to N. Course S½E. Dist. Sailed* 63 *Miles. Lat. in South* 33°48′. *Longde. in East Reckg.* 179°49′. *Longde. made West* 5°10′. *Varn.* 10°49′ *East.* PM Little wind and fair weather, in the AM the wind increased to a fresh gale. Variation p[r] Morning and Evening Az[ths] 10°49′ East.

TUESDAY 19*th. Winds Northerly, North to Westerly. Course S¼E. Dist. Sailed* 131 *Miles. Lat. in South* 36°58′. *Longde. in East Reckg.* 179°48′. *Longde. made West* 5°0′. Fresh gales and Clowdy. At midd-night Shortned Sail to Single reefed Top-sails for the Adventure to come up and at day-light made sail again.

WEDNESDAY 20*th. Winds Northerly, North to Westerly. Course S½W. Dist. Sailed* 110 *Miles. Lat. in South* 37°48′. *Longde. in East Reckg.* 179°38′. *Longde. made West* 5°11′. First part frish gales and fair weather, at 7 in the evening it blew in squalls attended with rain, the Adventure being about 3 Miles a stern I shortned sail to the three Top-sails for her to come up. At 8 o'Clock the wind Veered to NBW upon which I altered the Course from South to SWBS[1] and made the

[1] . . . in order to fall in with Cape East [East Cape, the easternmost point of the North Island of New Zealand] . . .—f. 140v.

same known to the Adventure by Signal. About 11 o'Clock I was informd that land was seen extending from the South to the West and that we were very near it, when[1] I got on deck I soon saw that it was only a black clowd forming in the Horizon which soon broke in a very heavy shower of rain, the Wind too shifted to the same quarter were it remained unsettled for some houres and then fixed at West and blew a fresh gale with which we stretched to the Southward. The night was so obscure that we were frequently obliged to fire guns and burn false fires to prevent being seperated.[2]

THURSDAY 21*st. Winds Westerly. Course S* 27° *W. Dist. Sailed* 87 *Miles. Lat. in South* 39°6′. *Longde. in East Reckg.* 179°22′. *Longde. made West* 6°11′. Fresh gales and fair Weather. At 3 o'Clock in the PM our Longitude by observations of the Sun and Moon was 180°11′ West. At 5 o'Clock in the AM we saw the land of New Zealand extending from NWBN to WSW. At Noon Table Cape bore West distant 8 or 10 Leagues.

FRIDAY 22*nd. Winds Variable.* We stretched in for the land with a fresh gale at North and NW. I was desirous of having some communication with the Inhabitants of this Country as far north as possible[3] in order to give them some Hogs, Fowls, Seeds, roots &c[a] I had provided for the purpose, we fetched in with the land a little to the Northward of the Isle of Portland and stood as near the shore as we could with safety do, we saw several people on the Shore but none attempted to come off to us, seeing this I bore away under Portland[4] were we lay to some time as well to give time for the Natives to come off as to wait for the Adventure which was some distance a stern, the wind blew fresh from off the land which might be the reason why no boddy came off therefore as soon as the Adventure was up with us I made Sail and Steered for Cape Kidnappers, having a moderate breeze at SW and West, hazy dirty weather. At middnight the Sky cleared up and the wind fixed at NW. At 5 o'Clock[5]

[1] *it, when:* it, I was a little surprised at this, knowing that we could not be near the coast of New Zealand, but when ...—f. 140v.

[2] Cooper notes seeing the flashes of the *Adventure's* guns, and hearing the reports. At 9 p.m. 'burnt a false fire, not answer'd'. He adds, 'This is the last day of serving the people Fresh Pork, which they have had every day since the 2[d] of September, & now have several Puncheons in Corn'—i.e. several puncheons of the island pork that they had salted.

[3] ... that is about Poverty or Tolaga Bay where I look upon them to be more civilized than at Queen Charlottes Sound;

[4] 'The Shambles SBW½W at which time we bore away & sailed between them and Portland'.—Wales. For the Shambles, see I, p. 175. It might there have been pointed out that the name was taken, obviously, from the similar dangerous place off the Bill of Portland on the south coast of England.

[5] ... the next morning ...—f. 141.

we passed the above mentioned Cape and at half past 9 o'Clock (being about 3 Leagues short of Black head)[1] we saw some Canoes put off from the Shore upon which I brought to in order to give them time to come on board and made the Signal to the Adventure to continue her Course.[2] It was not long before three Canoes reached us in which were about 18 people, the first that came were fishers and exchanged some fish for Cloth and Nails, I was not over desireous of geting any of the Men in this Canoe aboard because in one of the other two I expected to find a Chief, nor was I misstaken for in the Second Canoe which came was one or two as appear'd by their dress and manner of acting, the principal of these two came aboard without hesitation and was soon after followed by the other. I conducted him into the Cabbin and presented him with several large nails which he coveted so much that he seized hold of all he could cast his eyes upon and with such eagerness as plainly shewed that they were the most Valuable things in his eyes in our posession. I also gave him a peice of Cloth and a looking glass and then brought before him the Piggs, Fowls, Seeds and roots I intend'd for him, the Piggs and Fowls he at first took but little notice of till he was given to understand that [they] were for himself, nor was he then in such raptures as when I gave him a spike nail half the length of his arm, I however took notice that at going away he very well remember'd how many were brought before and took care that he had them all and kept a watchfull eye over them least any should be taken away; he made me a promise not to kill any, if he keeps his word and proper care is taken of them there were enough to stock the whole Island in due time, there being two Boars, two Sows, two Cocks and four Hens; the seeds and roots were such as are most usefull (viz) Wheat, French and Kidney Beans, Pease, Cabages, Turnips, Onions, Carrots, Parsnips, Yams &c[a] &c[a],[3] with these Articles I dismissed my two chiefs and made sail again but by this time the wind had Shifted from NW to WSW with which we stretched off to the Southward. At

[1] ADV 'All this Land is high and Chiefly Barren—and not unlike the Sea beaten Shore of N. America'.—Wilby. The likeness is not one usually pointed out; evidently Wilby had seen American service.

[2] . . . as I was willing to loose as little time as possible.

[3] Maori tradition kept the memory of this encounter. Colenso the missionary wrote a hundred years later, 'This chief, of whom a portrait is given in Cook's Voyages [possibly pl. LV, Vol. II of this *Voyage*], I have ascertained to be Tuanui, the ancestor of the present Henare Matua, of Porangahau, so well known among us. Tuanui put off from Poureerere, and Cook's gifts to him were well remembered and circumstantially related. From some of these "garden seeds" sprang the "Maori cabbage" of the coast, which, thirty years ago, grew very thickly there and on to Palliser Bay, and often served me, when travelling, for breakfast'.—William Colenso, 'Notes on the ancient Dog of the New Zealanders', *Trans. N.Z. Institute*, X (1877), p. 146 n. Tuanui in his turn gave Cook a *taiaha*.

Noon our Latitude was 4 ° ′ s [Cape Turnagain] bearing distant Leagues. It was evidant that these people had not forgot the Endeavour being on their Coast for the first words they said to us was we are affraid of the guns [Mataou no te poupou][1] probably they were no strangers to the affair which happened of Cape Kidnappers.[2]

SATURDAY 23*rd*. In the PM the wind blew fresh at West and WBN and in squals. I carried a press of sail in order to keep the land aboard which occasioned the loss of our fore-top-gallant mast which went away close to the cap. At half passed 7 we tacked and stretched in shore, Cape Turnagain at this time bore about NW½N, 6 or 7 Leagues distant, the Adventure being too far to leeward to distinguish any Signal was seperated from us, the Squals increasing and obliged us to Double Reef the Main Top-sail and to single-reef the Fore and Mizen Top-sails, the latter was no sooner set than it split in two from the one leach[3] to the other. We spent the night stretching off and on, at 6 o'Clock in the Morning we found our selves about 7 Leagues from the land which we now stood in for under our Courses the gale having increased in such a manner as not to admit of carrying more sail, the wind too had veered to SW and SSW and was attend with rainy weather. At 9 o'Clock the sky began to clear up and the gale abated so as to admit of our carrying close reefed Top-sails. At 11 o'Clock we were close in with Cape Turnagain accordingly Tacked and Stood off. At Noon it bore West a little northerly distant 6 or 7 miles, our Latitude by observation was 40°30′ s.

SUNDAY 24*th*. Soon after noon the Wind flat'ned almost to a Calm and we were in hopes that it would be succeeded by one more favourable, according we got up a nother Topgall[t] Mast loosed the reefs out of the Top-sails and got topg[t] yards a Cross. At 4 o'Clock a breeze sprung up at WBN with which we stretched along shore to the Southward as near the wind as we could lay, which began to increase in Such a manner as to oblige us to close reef our topsails and strike top-gallant yards. We continued to stretch to the Southward all night under two Courses and two close reef'd Top-sails, having a very strong gale attended with heavy Squals, towards day-light the gale abated and we were again tempted to shake out the reefs and get

[1] *mataku no te pu*. Cook must have been drawing on his Tahitian for *matau*, but possibly Tuanui's dialect did not accentuate the *k*. To the Maori in pre-European days, *pu* was any hollow stick that could be blown through—hence its application to the musket. Cf. p. 206 above.

[2] . . . experience had taught them to have some regard to these instruments of death.—f. 141v.—For 'the affair which happened of Cape Kidnappers' see I, pp. 177–8.

[3] i.e. side. The leech is the vertical side of a sail.

topgall[t] yards a Cross, this was again all labour lost for before 9 o'Clock we were reduced to the same sail as before, the wind was at WNW and blew as hard as ever attended with very heavy squalls. Soon after the Adventure joined us and at Noon Cape Palliser the Northern[1] point of *Eaheinomauwe* bore west distant 8 or 9 Leagues.

MONDAY 25*th*. The gale continued without the least variation for the better till middnight when it fell little wind and shifted to SE. Three hours after it fell Calm, during this time we loosed the reefs out of the Top-sails and rigged top-g[t] yards with the vain hopes that the next wind which came would be favourable, we were misstaken, the wind only tooke this little repose in order to gain strength to fall the heavier upon us, for at 6 o'Clock a gale sprung up at NW with which we attempted to stretch to the SW. Cape Palliser at this time bore NNW distant about 8 or 9 Leagues, as the gale increased we reduced our sails till about 11 o'Clock when it came on in such fury as to oblige us to take in all our sails with the utmost expedition and to lay-to under our bare poles with our heads to the SW. The brails[2] of the Mizen giving way the wind took hold of the sail and tore it in several places, we presently lowered down the yard and bent a nother sail. The Sea rose in proportion with the Wind so that we not only had a furious gale but a mountainous Sea also to incounter, thus after beating two days against strong gales and arriving in sight of our Port we had the mortification to be drove off from the land by a furious storm;[3] two favourable circumstances attended it which gave us some consolation, the Weather continued fair[4] and we were not apprehinsive of a lee-shore.

TUESDAY 26*th*. The Storm continued all the PM without the least intermission. At 7 o'Clock the Adventure being to leeward and out of

[1] A curious slip, in this context, for 'southern'; but it got through to the printed page.

[2] Brails were small ropes fastened to the outermost leech or edge of certain sails by which to truss them up close in the process of furling.

[3] This was the occasion which led Forster to one of his almost classic observations on the British seaman. Adding to his description of the mountainous seas and general uproar, he writes (I, p. 488), 'To complete this catalogue of horrors, we heard the voices of sailors from time to time louder than the blustering winds or the raging ocean itself, uttering horrible volleys of curses and oaths. Without any provocation to serve as an excuse, they execrated every limb in varied terms, piercing and complicated beyond the power of description. Inured to danger from their infancy, they were insensible to its threats, and not a single reflection bridled their blasphemous tongues'. From the *Adventure* we get a more cheerful report: 'Our Uaheine Man was much terified having never seen the like before but our ship being an excellent sea boat soon convinced him that he had little to fear as she rowled very easy with the Sea he cryed out with rapture "Pie Miti Middidehay am na Matti," that is "it was a good Ship & the Sea could not sink her".'—Bayly. Omai's Tahitian, as rendered here, seems both simplified and garbled. Possibly what he cried out was *Pahi maitai, miti tihae aina mate:* 'a good ship, angry sea [can]not destroy!'

[4] i.e. clear overhead. Cf. the entry of 1 November below, 'clear and fair'.

sight we bore down to look for her and after runing the distance we supposed her to be off, brought to again without seeing her, it being very hazey in the horizon[1] occasioned in a great measure by the spray of the Sea which was lifted up to a great height by the force of the wind. At middnight the gale abated so that we could bear the Mizen stay sail and soon after it fell little wind and at 4 o'Clock shifted to SW when we wore, set the Courses and close reefed Top-sails and stood in for the land. The Wind soon after freshned and fixed at South but as the Adventure was some distance a stern we lay-by[2] for her to come up till 8 o'Clock when we made all the sail we could and steered NBW½W for the Straits. At Noon our Latitude by observation was 42°27′ S. Cape Palliser by judgement bore North distant 17 Leag[s].

WEDNESDAY 27*th*. Our favourable wind was not of sufficient duration, it fell by degrees and at last at 7 in the evening flatned to a Calm which at 10 was succeeded by a fresh breeze from the North with which we stretched to the Westward till 3 in the Morning when being near the land of Cape Campbel we tacked and stretched over for Cape Pallisser under our Close reef'd Top-sails and Courses, being as much sail as we could carry. At day-light we could but just see the Adventure from the Mast head to the Southward. At Noon the last mentioned Cape bore West distant 4 or 5 Leagues, we now Tacked and stretched to the SW having a strong gale and fair weather.

THURSDAY 28*th*. Wind and weather continues the same, the former rather increaseing for at 4 pm we were obliged to take in the Top-sails. At 6 Cape Pallisser bore NBW½W distant 6 Leagues. At middnight wore and stood to the Northward. At 6 am set the Top-sails close reefd, the Adventure in sight to the South. At 8 wore and Stretched to the SW, at Noon we were by Observation in the Latitude 42°17′ S the high land over Cape Campell west distant 10 or 12 Leagues. By this time the gale had increased so as to make it necessary to take in the Top-sails and main-sail and to lay too under the fore-sail and Mizen stay-sail, the Adventure 4 or 5 Miles to lee-ward.

FRIDAY 29*th*. We continued to lie to untill 4 o'Clock in the pm when the gale being some thing abated we wore and set the Main Top-sail close reefed, some time after set the main-sail, under these sails we stretched to the Northward all night with the wind at WNW and WBN,

[1] *it . . . horizon:* it being so very hazey and thick in the Horizon that we could not see a mile round us . . .—f. 142v.

[2] An equivalent of 'lay to'.

a strong gale attended with squalls which at 4 o'Clock in the morning began to abate so that we could bear the Fore top-sail. Soon after the wind shifted to SW and blew a gentle gale. We took immidiate advantage of it and set all our sails and stretched in for Cape Pallisser which at Noon bore WBN½N distant about 6 Leagues. Latitude Observed 41°44′ S.

SATURDAY 30*th*. The breeze continued between the SW and South till 5 o'Clock in the PM when it fell calm, we being about 3 Leagues short of Cape Pallisser. At 7 o'Clock a breeze sprung up at NNE which was as favourable as we could wish,[1] it proved however of short duration for about 9 the wind shifted into its old quarter NW and increased to a fresh gale with which we stretched to the SW under Courses and single-reefed top-sails. At Middnight the Adventure was two or three Miles a stern, soon after she disapeared nor was she to be seen at day-light, we supposed she had tacked and stood to the NE by which means we had lost sight of her; we however continued to stand to the westward with the wind at NNW and which increased in such a manner as at last to bring us under our two Courses, after spliting a new Main top-sail. At Noon Cape Campbell bore NBW distant 7 or 8 Leagues.

SUNDAY 31*st*. At 8 o'Clock in the pm the gale became somewhat more moderate and veered more to the north so that we fetched in with the shore under the Snowey mountains[2] about four or five leagues to windward of the Lookers on, where there was all the appearence of a large bay,[3] had the Adventure[4] been now with me I should have given up all thoughts of going to Queen Charlottes Sound to Wood and Water and sought for these articles farther South as the wind was now favourable for rainging a long the coast but as we were now seperated I was under a necessity [of] going to the Sound as being the place of rendezvouz. As we drew near the land[5] we sounded and at the distance of 3 Miles found 47 fathom which decreased in such a manner that at the distance of 1 Mile there was 25 fathom, we then wore and stood to the Eastward, under

[1] . . . so that we began to reckon what time we should reach the sound next day . . .—f. 143.

[2] The Kaikoura ranges. In the journal of his first voyage Cook refers to their highest peak, Tapuaenuku, as the 'Snowey Mountain'. See also Chart XIX *b*.

[3] The appearance of a large bay here would be caused by the curve of the coast in from, and north of, the Kaikoura peninsula; added to which, the land close to the sea may have been invisible under the weather conditions.

[4] *had the Adventure:* I now regreted the loss of the Adventure, for had she . . . f. 143v.

[5] *As . . . land:* As we approached the land we saw smoke in several places along the shore a sure sign that the Coast was inhabited: . . .—f. 143v.

the two Courses and Close reefed Top-sails, but these last we were soon put past and at 7 o'Clock in the Morning we wore and brought to under the Fore-sail and Mizen Stay sail the wind being now at NNW and blew with great fury[1] till 9 when it abated a little and we set the Main Sail and two close reef'd Top-sails but the latter we were obliged to take in again at Noon at which time the snowey mountains bore WNW distant 12 or 14 Leagues. Our Latitude by observation was 42°22′ S.

[NOVEMBER 1773]

MONDAY 1*st*. The gale continued without the least variation till 6 o'Clock in the evening when it fell little wind. I susspected that it would be of short duration and therefore did not make any more sail. I was right in my conjector for in less than a quarter of an hour it began to blow with greater fury than ever, in so much that we were obleged to lie to under the Mizen Stay-sail. At middnight the gale abated and we made sail under the Courses, two hours after it fell Calm, at 4 the Calm was succeeded by a breeze from the South which increased to a fresh gale and was attended with hazey rainy weather, which gave us great hopes that the NW gales were quite over for it must be observed that they were attended with clear and fair weather. We took immidiate advantage of this favourable wind by steering north for Cape Campbell under all the sail we could set. At Noon the said Cape bore north distant 3 or 4 Leagues.

TUESDAY 2*nd*. Fresh gales with rain. At two pm pass'd Cape Campbel at the distance of one league[2] concequently entered the Straits with a fresh gale at South so that we thought of nothing but reaching Queen Charlottes Sound the next flood tide. Vaine were our expectations, at 6 o'Clock our favourable wind desserted us and was succeeded by one from the north which veered to the NW and increased to a fresh gale; we were at this time off Clowdy Bay, we spent the night plying; our tacks were disadvantageous and we lost more on the Ebb than we had gained on the flood.

In the Morning I stretched over to the coast of Haeinomauwe where on the east side of Cape Teerawhitte we discovered a new inlet which had all the appearence of a good Harbour. Being tired

[1] *being . . . fury:* having increased to a perfect storm . . .—f. 144.

[2] At 3 p.m., says Wales, Cape Campbell was SW about 3 miles, and they unstowed the anchors. He goes on, 'A long Shore runs off from Cape Campbell: It was so shallow even where we passed that it was doubtfull with some whether or no we should not touch.' It is curious that Cook does not mention anything of this sort. Mariners are warned not to approach too close to Cape Campbell, a low sandy feature of the coast. There are reefs off the cape, and it seems likely that Wales was referring to some part of these.

with beating against the obstinate NW winds I resolved (if I found it practical) to put into this place or to anchor in the Bay which lies before it, having the flood tide in our favour we by noon got far enought to windward to stretch in. In the morning we had a clear horizon out to sea and looked well out for the Adventure without seeing any thing of her and therefore concluded she had got into the Sound.

WEDNESDAY *3rd.* In stretching into the Bay, that is after we were within the two points which form the entrance, we found from 35 to 12 and 10 fathoms, the bottom every were fit for anchoring. At 1 o'Clock we reached the entrance[1] of the inlet just as the Tide turned against us[2] and obliged us to anchor in 12 fathom water the bottom a fine sand the eastermost of the black Rocks which lie on the larboard hand going in bore NBE distant one mile Cape Teerawhitte or the w[t] point of the land, west distant about 2 Leagues and the Eastermost land NBW distant 4 or 5 Miles.[3] This inlet runs in north and seems to incline to the West and to be covered from all winds.

Soon after we had anchored several of the Natives came off to us in three Canoes, two from the one shore and one from the other, it required but little address to get three or four aboard to whom I distributed midals and nails, the latter they were extravigantly fond of,[4] I also gave to one man two cocks and two hens, these he recieved with such indifferency as gave me little hopes that proper care would be taken of them. The shore between Cape Teerawhitte and

[1] *the entrance:* the narrow entrance . . .—f. 144v.

[2] . . . The wind being likewise against us

[3] *Eastermost . . . Miles:* East point of the bay NBE 4 or 5 Miles.—f. 144v. This is a little puzzling. It is clear enough where Cook was—at the entrance to Port Nicholson or Wellington harbour; and the Wellingtonian must bitterly regret the turning of the tide that kept him from going in. The 'black Rocks' were the fangs of Barrett's Reef. But from his anchorage the projection he called on his first voyage Cape Terawhiti (see Chart XVIII) did not lie 'west distant about 2 Leagues'. This is the bearing and distance of Sinclair Head, the south-east point of the sort of high blunt isthmus which runs south beyond the western side of the harbour and falls to the sea in steep and barren slopes which take the full force of the southerly winds. Cape Terawhiti is the south-west end of this tangle of hills, about seven miles north-west of Sinclair Head in a direct line. Cook may for the moment have thought of this whole isthmus as Cape Terawhiti. He slips again over the bearing of the 'Eastermost land': in B, as we have seen, he alters NBW to NBE, but this is absurd, and would produce a line, roughly, to the other end of the harbour; he has simply given his own bearing from the land, and thus reversed the proper direction, which should be SBE. The farthest land he could see to the eastward was Baring Head, where the main guiding light to the harbour now stands; and this was in fact SBE 'distant 4 or 5 Miles' from the point where he was anchored. See Fig. 32, p. 166.—The harbour remained unvisited by Europeans for another half-century. Captain Herd, of the first New Zealand Company's ship *Rosanna*, seems to have been the first man in, in 1826; he charted it, and called it Port Nicholson after the harbour-master at Sydney. D'Urville was kept out by the wind at the end of January 1827.

[4] . . . above every other thing

Cape Pallisser forms two deep Bays or Inlets both of which extend in north inclining to the west,[1] I should have made myself better accquainted with one of these Bays had the Adventure been with me, but now it was necessary for me to go for Queen Charlottes Sound in order to join her, nor was it long before an oppertunity offered, for at 3 o'Clock the wind shifted to NE a light breeze with which we got under sail, the Anchor was no sooner up than we got a fresh gale at South, stretched round Cape Teerawhitte and then bore away for the Sound under all the sail we could bear, having the advantage or rather disadvantage of an increaseing gale which already blowed too hard; we hauled up for the Sound just at dark and after makeing two boards, in which most of our sails were split, anchored in 18 fathom water.[2] It continued to blow excessive hard and in Squalls till towards the Morning when it began to abate, at 6 o'Clock we wieghed in order to turn up to Ship Cove, soon after it fell Calm and obliged us to drop an anchor again in 40 fathom. At 9 the Calm was succeeded by a breeze at NW, with which we wieghed and ran up to Ship Cove where we moored with the two Bowers and afterwards unbint all our sails not having one but what wanted considerable repairs.[3] We did not find the Adventure here as I expected.

We had no sooner anchored than several of the Natives made us a Viset, among whom were some that I knew when I was here in the Endeavour.[4]

THURSDAY *4th.* Gentle breezes and clear pleasent weather. Sent on shore all our empty Casks in order to be repaired cleaned and fill'd with Water, set up tents for the reception of the Sail-makers, Coopers and others whose business made it necessary for them to be on Shore, began to caulk the decks and sides, Overhaul the rigging, to cut firewood and set up the forge to repair the Iron work all of which were absolutely necessary occupations. In the Morning I made some hauls with the seine but got no fish, the natives in some measure made up for this difficiency by bring[ing] us a good quantity which they exchang'd for pieces of cloth[5] &c[a].

[1] Port Nicholson and Palliser Bay. But Palliser Bay inclines to the east, if anything. D'Urville visited it, 29 January 1827, and called it *Baie Inutile*—which it was, for a seafarer's purposes.

[2] . . . between the White Rocks and the NW shore.—f. 145.

[3] . . . Indeed both our sails and riging had sustained a good deal of damage in beating off the Straits mouth.

[4] . . . particularly the old man Goubiah who was one of our best friends at that time.—f. 145. 'Goubiah' perhaps represents 'Ko [it is, he is] Paea'.

[5] *cloth:* Otaheite cloth.—Cf. Clerke: 'this Afternoon some of the Natives brought us onboard great plenty of Fish which they barter'd for any trifle or bauble whatever, but they were most attach'd [to] the white Cloath we got at the Society Isles half a yard of

FRIDAY 5*th.* PM fair weather, AM clowdy with rain which hindered us from finishing boot-toping[1] the Starboard side which we had begun. In opening some of our Bread Casks we found to our irrepairable loss a good deal of the bread very much damaged, owing as we supposed to the Casks being made of green Wood.[2] I ordered the Oven to be set up to bake or dry such as was damp and not so bad but that it might be eat. This mor[n]ing some of the natives stole from out of one of the tents some of our peoples Cloaths,[3] as soon as I was informed of it I went to their habitations in an adjoining Cove and demanded them again and after some time recovered the most of them,[4] here I saw the youngest of the two Sows Cap[t] Furneaux left in *Canibal Cove*, it was lame in one of its hind legs otherwise in good case;[5] if we understood these people right, the Boar and other Sow was also taken away and the one carried towards the East and the other to the west,[6] we have also been informed that the two Goats have likewise been caught killed and eat,[7] thus all our endeavours for stocking this Country with usefull Animals are likely to be frusterated by the very people whom we meant to serve; our gardens had faired some thing better, every thing in them excepting the Potatoes, they had left intirely to nature who had acted her part so well that we found most articles in a florishing state,[8] the Potatoes they had dug up, some few, however remained and were growing.[9]

SATURDAY 6*th.* PM hard rain so that no work could go forward. AM fair weather. In the morning I went to the cove where the natives resided to haul the Seine and took with me a young boar and a sow, two Cocks and two hens I had brought from the Isles and gave them to the Natives who seemed as if they would take proper care of them, at least I had good reason to think so sence they had kept Captain Furneaux's young sow near five month for I must suppose that it fell into their hands soon after we left the place.

which wou'd purchase a very excellent dish of fish'. Again, Clerke, 6 November: 'Natives supply us with great Plenty of Excellent Fish and are very Moderate in their Price—A Peice of Cloath that cost a Nail at the Islands wou'd here purchase at least 300 Weight of as good Fish as I ever tasted in my Life'.

[1] Cleaning the upper part of the ship's bottom, and smearing it all over with tallow and sulphur, or some such mixture.

[2] *owing . . . Wood: deleted on* f. 145v, *which adds* To repair this loss in the best manner we could we had all the Casks opened & the Bread picked . . .

[3] *some . . . Cloaths:* a bag of Cloathes belonging to one of the Seamen . . .—f. 145v.

[4] *recovered . . . them:* in a friendly application recovered them. Sence we were among thieves and had come off so well I was not sorry for what had happen'd as it taught our people to keep a better look out for the future.

[5] . . . and very tame

[6] . . . but not killed

[7] *have . . . eat:* I put on shore up the Sound had been killed by that old Rascal Goubiah

[8] . . . a proof that the winter must have been mild.—f. 146.

[9] . . . I think it probable they will never be got out of the ground.

We had no better success with the Seine than before, nevertheless, we did not return on board empty, having purchased a large quantity from the Natives: when we were upon this traffick they shew'd a great inclination to pick my Pockets and to take away the fish with one hand wich they had just given me with the other, an evil which one of the chiefs undertook to remove, and with fury in his eyes made a shew of keeping the people at a proper distance, I apploaded his conduct but at the same time kept so good a lookout as to detect him in picking my Pocket of a handkerc[h]ief, which I suffered him to put in his bosom before I seem'd to know any thing of the matter and then told him what I had lost, he seemed quite ignorant and inicent, till I took it from him, and then he put it of with a laugh, and he had acted his part with so much address that it was hardly possible for me to be angery with him, so that we remained good friends and he accompanied me on board to dinner, about which time we were visited by several Strangers in four or five Canoes, bring[ing] with them fish and other articles which they exchanged for cloth &c[a].—f. 146–6v.

Towards Noon several Indians came from up the Bay in four or five Canoes, these together with what might be in the Cove before made up about one hundred and fifty, these new commers took up their quarters near us but very early the next morning moved off with Six of our small water-casks and with them all the others that we found here upon our arrival, the precipitate retreat of these last we supposed was owing to the theeft the others had committed, they left behind them some of their dogs and the boar I had given them and which I now took back again,[1] our Casks will be the least loss we shall sustain by these people leaving us as they were very usefull in providing us with fish which they were far more expert in catching than we.

MONDAY 8*th*. Hazy weather with drizling rain which proved rather unlucky as it hindered us from working upon our Bread, but the next day proved very favourable for this as well as our other works,[2] the wind too was at NE which gave us some hopes of seeing the Adventure but these hopes vanished in the after-noon when the Wind shifted to the West. Pretty early this morning some of our friends the Natives paid us a viset and brought with them a quantity of fish which they exchanged for two hatchets.

[1] ... as it was the only one I had.—f. 146v.

[2] 'PM fair weather. AM hazy with drizling rain. Sail-makers repairing the Main Top-sail Carpenters Caulking the Sides, Seamen employed in the hold and overhauling the rigging.—Log.

WEDNESDAY 10*th*. Showery most part of the day and the wind variable.[1]

THURSDAY 11*th*. Wind Southerly with Showery weather.

FRIDAY 12*th*. Wind as yesterday but fair weather which gave us an oppertunity to finish over hauling the bread [4292] pounds of which we found Mouldy and rotten and totally unfit for men to eat [3000] pounds more that few would eat but such as were in our circumstances, this damage our bread had susstained was wholy owing to the Casks being made of green wood and not well seasoned before the Biscuit was packed in them for all the biscuits that were in co[n]tact or near the insides of the Casks were damaged while those in the middle were not the least injured.[2] Mr Forster and his party in the Country botanizing.

SATURDAY 13*th*. Clear pleasent weather. Early in the Morning the Natives brought us a quantity of fish which they exchanged as usual for Cloth &ca but their greatest branch of trade is for the green-talk or stone (called by them Poenammoo)[3] a thing of no sort of Value, nevertheless it is so much sought after by our people that there is hardly any thing that they would not give for a piece. Great part of our Coals being expended we took into the Main hold two launch loads of ballast after taking out all the Coals.

SUNDAY 14*th*. Weather as yesterday. In the Morning had a plentifull supply of fish from the Natives, who remained with us the most part of the day.

MONDAY 15*th*. Fair weather winds notherly a gentle breeze. In the Morng I went in the Pinnace over to the East Bay, accompanied by some of the officers and gentlemen; as soon as we landed we went upon one of the hills in order to take a view of the Straits, to see if we could discover any thing of the Adventure, we had a fatiguing walk to little purpose for when we got to the top of the hill we found the Eastern horizon so foggy that we could not see above two or three miles. Mr Forster who was one of the party profited by this excursion in collecting some new plants; as to the Adventure I dispair[4]

[1] 'First and middle parts fine weather latter showery—Employed as before—Condemn'd the old messenger and coverted it to okam.'—'We're all much surpriz'd that our Consort the Adventure does not make her appearance, nor are we able to form any idea what can have detain'd Her so long.'—Clerke.

[2] *this damage . . . injured: deleted* f. 147. A has a footnote to 'buisquet was pack'd in them': 'We afterwards found that this was not the cause of the Bread being damaged, see Page 142'—p. 142 referring to the entry for 3 May 1774. G retains the passage and has no note.

[3] *pounamu.*

[4] *I dispair:* I now begin to dispair . . .—f. 147.

of seeing her any more but am totally at a loss to conceive what is become of her till now. I thought[1] that she might have put into some port in the Strait when the wind came at NW the day we Anchor'd in Ship Cove and there stayed to compleat her wood and Water; this conjector was reasonable enough at first, but the elapsation of twelve days has now made it scarce probable.[2] The hill we were upon is the same as I was upon in 1770[3] on which we then built a tower of Stones which was now leveled to the very ground, done no doubt by the Natives with a view of finding some thing hid in it. When we returned from the hill we found a number of the natives collected round our boat, we made some exchanges with them and then returned on board and in our way viseted some others.[4]

TUESDAY 16*th*. Gentle breezes Northerly and fair weather, very busy in geting ready for Sea.

WEDNESDAY 17*th*. Fresh gale at NW and Clowdy weather. Our friends the Natives employed themselves most of the day in fishing in our neighbourhood and as they caught the fish came and sold them to us.[5]

THURSDAY 18*th*. Strong gales at NW with heavy squalls from off the high-land and clowdy rainy weather, so that little work could be done.

FRIDAY 19*th*. Wind Westerly strong gales with rain.

SATURDAY 20*th*. Wind Southerly fair weather, several of the Natives came into our neighbourhood and brought us some fish.

SUNDAY 21*st*. Strong gales and Clowdy with some showers of Rain. Bent all the Sails, and cleaned the Sloop.[6]

[1] *her . . . thought:* her: till now I thought

[2] *but . . . probable*: as the Southerly wind which brought us into the Sound was of sufficient duration to have brought her into the Strait if she had even been blown 20 Leagues farther off the Coast than we were, which was scarce possible under any circumstances whatever, but it is now hardly probable she could be Twelve days in our neighbourhood without our either hearing or seeing some thing of her.—f. 147v. On this day the *Adventure* was lying in Tolaga Bay, preparing to leave it for the second time.

[3] . . . when I had the Second view of the Strait . . .—26 January 1770; see I, p. 240.

[4] . . . by whom we were kindly received.

[5] . . . insomuch that we had more than we could dispence with. From this day to the 22nd nothing remarkable happened: we were employed in geting every thing in readiness to put to Sea, being resolved to wait no longer than the Assign'd time for the Adventure. —f. 147v.—'We're all much surpriz'd at the long absence of our fellow travellers.'—Clerke.

[6] The Log for 17–22 November has much longer and more detailed entries than these in the Journal, which give a good picture of the state of the ship and the work necessary to be done on her. The following specimens may be given. 17th: 'First part gentle breezes latter fresh gales and Clowdy. PM got on board all our Water excepting such Cask as wanted repairs AM lowered down and striped the main yard in order to over haul the

MONDAY *22nd.* Clear pleasent Weather, winds variable. Early in the morning we were visited by several of the Natives, some of whom were Strangers, these last offered us various curosities in exchange for Otahiete cloth and Red Baze &c[a]. At first the exchanges were in our favour till an old man, who was no stranger to us, came and assisted his countrymen with his advice and in a moment turned the exchanges above a thousand per cent in their favour. After they were gone I took four Hogs, three sows and one boar, two hens and three cocks and carried them a little way into the woods in the very bottom of West Bay where I left them with as much food as would serve them a week or ten days.[1] This I did in order to keep them in the woods, least they should come down to the shore in search of food and be discovered by the natives, indeed their is not much fear of this as there was not the least appearence of any having been their for a very long time or within some miles of it. We shall also leave some cocks and hens in the woods at Ship Cove, but these will have a chance of falling into the hands of the Natives whose wandering way of life will prevent them from breeding even Should they take proper care of them. When I return'd aboard I found our good friends the Indians had been out fishing of which they brought us a good supply. Some of our gentlemen having made them a viset at their habitations and got from them some thigh bones the meat of which had been lately picked off, the gentlemen had reason to believe that at this time they had some human flesh by them. I am of opinion that those men whom we took to be strangers are of the same tribe or family and have been out on some war expedition,[2] indeed we had some information of this sort yesterday morning, for about 4 o'Clock a number of women and children came off in a Canoe from whom we learnt that a party of men were then out for whose safety they were under some apprehension, but this report had little credit with us from a supposission that we did not understand them.[3] Having now

Blocks, the Straps of most of them being decayed, found the jeers stranded which are repaired by knotting, lifted the main stay to repair the service of the Colour [collar?] and to look at the Shrouds under it'.—18th: '... AM employed in overhauling the Runing riging, condemning such as was quite wore out, converting to the best advantage from one use to another and makeing up the deficiency with new—Armourers makeing bolts to secure the tops, Caulkers caulking the sides, Cooper repairing Casks and Sailmakers repairing the Sails.'—21st: 'Fresh gales and Clowdy, Bent all the sails, got on board all our water casks and afterwards gave the people liberty to go on shore'.—22nd: '... AM got on board all the spare sails that were ashore repairing, the sail-makers tent, the astronomers observatory and Instruments and sent a party of men to cut Brooms, Caulkers and smiths still at work.'

[1] *a week ... days:* ten or twelve days.

[2] ... and those things they sold us were the spoils of thier Enemies

[3] *from ... them:* as we soon after saw some Canoes come in from fishing which we judged to be them.—f. 149.

got the principal parts of the Sloop caulked, the rigging over hauled and in other respects in a condition for Sea,[1] I ordered the tents to be struck and every thing to be got on board.

The Boatswain with a party of men being in the wood cuting brooms, some of them found a private hut of the Natives [in] which were part of the treasure they have had from us with some other articles of their own, soon[2] after they came and took them all away, but missing a hatchet and some other articles they came in the evening when the brooming party came on board, and made their complaint to me and pitched upon one of the party as the person who had taken the things and for which I ordered him twelve lashes[3] after which the complaintant went away seemingly satisfied altho he did not recover any of his things nor could I find what was become of them though nothing was more certain than they had been taken away by some of the party if not by the very man the natives had pitched upon.

It has ever been a maxim with me to punish the least crimes any of my people have commited against these uncivilized Nations, their robing us with impunity is by no means a sufficient reason why we should treat them in the same manner, a conduct we see they themselves cannot justify, they found themselves injured and sought for redress in a legal way. The best method in my opinion to preserve a good understanding with such people is first to shew them the use of fire arms and to convince them of the Superiority they give you over them and to be always upon your guard; when once they are sencible of these things, a regard for their own safety will deter them from disturbing you or being unanimous in forming any plan to attack you, and Strict honisty and gentle treatment on your part will make it their intrest not to do it.—f. 149v.

TUESDAY 23*rd*. Calm or light airs from the Northward so that we could not get to sea as I intended, some of the officers went on shore to amuse themselves among the Natives where they saw the head and bowels of a youth who had lately been killed, the heart was stuck upon a forked stick and fixed to the head of their largest Canoe, the gentlemen brought the head[4] on board with them, I was on shore

[1] . . . and to incounter the Southern Latitudes,

[2] *own, soon:* own, it is very probable some were set to watch this hutt, as soon

[3] The criminal was Richard Lee, seaman, as we learn from the other journals.

[4] *the gentlemen . . . head:* One of the gentlemen bought the head, brought it . . . f. 150.—'Bought a human head onshore, (for two nails) might have had the liver &c—)but found that sufficient . . .'—Mitchel. It was Pickersgill who bought the head, according to his own journal.

at this time but soon after returned on board when I was informed of the above circumstances and found the quarter deck crowded with the Natives. I now saw the mangled head or rather the remains of it for the under jaw, lip &c[a] were wanting,[1] the scul was broke on the left side just above the temple, the face had all the appearence of a youth about fourteen or fifteen, a peice of the flesh had been broiled and eat by one of the Natives in the presince of most of the officers.[2] The sight of the head and the relation of the circumstances just mentioned struck me with horor and filled my mind with indignation against these Canibals, but when I considered that any resentment I could shew would avail but little and being desireous of being an eye wittness to a fact which many people had their doubts about, I concealed my indignation and ordered a piece of the flesh to be broiled and brought on the quarter deck where one of these Canibals eat it with a seeming good relish before the whole ships Company which had such effect on some of them as to cause them to vomit. [Oedidee] was [so] struck with horor at the sight that [he] wept and scolded by turns, before this happened he was very intimate with these people but now he neither would come near them or suffer them to touch him, told them to their faces that they were vile men and that he was no longer their friend,[3] he used the same language to one of the officers who cut of the flesh and refused to except, or even touch the knife with which it was cut, such was this Islanders aversion to this vile custom.[4] I could not find out the reason of their undertaking this expedition, all I could understand for certain was that they had gone from hence into Admiralty Bay[5] and there fought with their enemies

[1] . . . lying on the Tafferal

[2] *most . . . officers:* all the officers and most of the crew.—f. 150. Clerke 8952, 24 November, gives us the circumstantial details: '. . . I ask'd him if he'd eat a peice there directly to which he very chearfully gave his assent. I then cut a peice of carry'd [it] to the fire by his desire and gave it a little broil upon the Grid Iron then deliver'd it to him—he not only eat it but devour'd it most ravenously, and suck'd his fingers ½ a dozen times over in raptures: the Captain was at this time absent, he soon after came on board, when I cut & dress'd my friend the other steak which he Eat upon the Quarter Deck before Cap[t] Cook and both were before the Ships Crew.'

[3] The foregoing passage, from 'a seeming good relish', is one that Cook worked over in B, f. 150, a great deal, presumably to get the greatest possible dramatic effect. The page is a mass of correction and rewriting, including the final red ink. In the end we get this: '. . . surprising avidity. This had such effect on some of our people as to make them sick who came on board with me. Oediddee was so affected with the sight as to become perfectly motionless and seemed as if metamorphosed into the Statue of horror: it is, utterly impossible for Art to depict that passion with half the force that it appeared in his Countenance when roused from this state by some of us, he burst into tears, continued to weep and scold by turns; told them they were Vile men, and that he neither was nor would be no longer their friend he even would not suffer them to touch him. . .'. We have here some direct transcription from Wales.

[4] . . . and worthy of imitation by every rational being.

[5] . . . (the next inlet to the West) . . .—f. 150v.

many of whom they killed, they counted to me fifty a number which exceeded all probabillity by reason of the smallness of their own number, I think I understood them for certain that this youth was killed there and not brought away a prisoner, nor could I learn that they had brought away any more which increased the improbabillity of their having killd so many. We had reason to beleive that they did not escape without some loss, a young woman was seen, more than one, to cut and scar herself as is the custom when they loose a friend or relation.

That the New Zealanders are Canibals can now no longer be doubted, the account I gave of it in my former Voyage was partly founded on circumstances and was, as I afterwards found, discredited by many people. I have often been asked, after relateing all the circumstance, if I had actualy seen them eat human flesh my self, such a queston was sufficient to convence me that they either disbelieved all I had said or formed a very different opinion from it, few considers what a savage man is in his original state and even after he is in some degree civilized; the New Zealanders are certainly in a state of civilization, their behavour to us has been Manly and Mild, shewing allways a readiness to oblige us; they have some arts a mong them which they execute with great judgement and unweared patience; they are far less addicted to thieving than the other Islanders and are I believe strictly honist among them-selves.[1] This custom of eating their enimies slain in battle (for I firmly believe they eat the flesh of no others) has undoubtedly been handed down to them from the earliest times and we know that it is not an easy matter to break a nation of its ancient customs let them be ever so inhuman and savage, especially if that nation is void of all religious principles as I believe the new zealanders in general are and like them without any settled form of goverment; as they become more united they will of concequence have fewer Enemies and become more civilized and then and not till then this custom may be forgot,[2] at present they seem to have but little idea of treating other men as they themselves would wish to be treated, but treat them as they think they should be treated under the same circumstances. If I remember right one of the arguments they made use on

[1] . . . i e in the same tribe, or such as are at peace one with another.—f. 152.

[2] . . . especially if that Nation hath no manner of connections or commerce with strangers for it is by this, that the greatest part of the human race has been civilized, an advantage which the New Zealanders, from their Situation, never have had: an intercourse with Foreigners would reform their manners and polish their Savage minds, or were they more united under a settled form of Government, they would have fewer enemies concequently this Custom would be less in use, and might in time be in a manner forgot.—f. 152.

against Tupia who frequently expostulated with them against this custom, was that there could be no harm in killing and eating the man who would do the same by you if it was in his power, for said they 'can there be any harm in eating our Enimies whom we have killed in battle, would not those very enimies have done the same to us?' I have often seen them listen to Tupia with great attention, but I never found that his arguments had any weight with them or[1] that they ever once owned that this custom was wrong and when [Oediddee] shewed his resentment against them they only laughed at him,[2] indeed it could not be supposed that they would pay much attention to a youth like him. I must here observe that [Oediddee] soon learnt to convirse with these people tolerable well as I am perswaided he would have done with those of Amsterdam had he been the same time with them.[3]

WEDNESDAY 24*th*. At 4 o'Clock in the Morning we unmoored with an intent to put to Sea, but the wind being Northerly or NE without and blew in strong pufs into the Cove so that we were obliged to lay fast. While we were unmooring, some of our old friends the Natives came to take their leave of us and after wards took all their effects into their Canoes and left the Cove, but the party which had been out on the late expedition remained, these some of the gentlemen viseted and found the heart still remaining on the Canoe and the bowels and lungs lying on the beach, but the flesh they believed was all devoured.[4]

THURSDAY 25*th*. At 4 o'Clock in the Morning we weighed with a light breeze out of the Cove which carried us no farther than betwen Motuara and Long-island where we were obliged to anchor, pre-

[1] ... or with all his Rhetorick could persuade any one of them that this custom was wrong, and when Oediddee and several of our people shew'd their abhorrence against it they only laughed at them.

[2] B f. 151 is a separate slip of paper, which, though it is similar to the paper of the rest of the journal, from the ink and the writing appears to be an afterthought, probably added in England when Cook was preparing the journal for publication. It is keyed to a red cross at 'when Oediddee and several of our people shewed. . . . laughed at them'. It runs as follows: 'Among many reasons which I have heard assigned for the practice of this horrid custom, the want of animal food has been one; but how far this is deducible from either facts or circumstances, I shall leave those to find out who advanced it, as [in] every part of New Zealand which I have been in, Fish have been found in such plenty that the Natives have generally caught as much as served both themselves and us; they have also plenty of Dogs, nor is there any want of wild fowl, which they know very will how to kill. So that neither this nor the want of food of any kind, can in my opinion, be the reason, but whatever m[a]y be it, I think it was but too evident that they have a great liking for this kind of food.'

[3] *the same . . . them:* a little longer with them, for he did not understand the New Zealanders at first no more or not so much, as the Amsterdamers.—f. 152v.

[4] *but . . . devoured:* Liver and Lungs were now wanting probably they had eat them after the carcase was all gone

sently after a breeze sprung up at North with which we weighed and turned out of the Sound by 12 o'Clock.[1] During our stay in this place we were well supplyed with fish which we purchased of the Natives at a very easy rate and besides the Vegetables our own gardens produced we found every were plenty of Scurvy grass and sellery which I caused to be dressed every day for all hands, by this means they have been mostly on a fresh diet for these three months past and at this time we had neither a sick or scorbutic person on board. I have now[2] some Pork on board that was salted at Ulietea, it is as well tasted and as well cured as any I ever eat, the manner we did it is thus, in the cool of the evening the Hogs were killed and dressed, then cut up the bones taken out and the Meat salted while it was yet hot, the next Morning we gave it a second Salting, packed it in a Cask and put to it a sufficient quantity of Strong Pickle, great care is to be taken that the meat be well covered with pickle other wise it will soon spoile.

I have made mention of the Natives of Queen Charlottes Sound geting the three Hogs which Captain Furneaux put on shore; the young sow we know is in their posession but it is by no means certain that they got the old sow and boar, but even suppose they did by their own accounts they are yet alive and great reason to believe that they will take care of them and as to those I put on shore I have great reason to think they will never find. More Cocks and Hens are left behind than I know of as several of our people had of these as well as my self, some of which they put on shore and others they sold to the Natives, whom we found took care enough of them. The two goats however I believe were killed. I should have replaced them with two others, but had the missfortune to loose the ram a few days after we arrived.

*The sow Pig we have not seen sence the day they had her from me, we are however told she is still alive as also the old Boar and Sow of Captain Furneaux's so that there is still reason to hope they may succeed. It will be unfortunate indeed if every method I have taken to provide this Country with usefull animals should be frustrated. We have likewise been told that the two Goats are still alive and runing about, but I give more credit to the first Story than this. I should have replaced them by leaving behind the only two I had left, but had the missfortune to loose the Ram sence we have been here, in a manner we could hardly account for; they were both put on shore at the Tents soon after we arrived, where they seemed to thrive

[1] *by 12 o'Clock:* and stood over for Cape Teera-whitte.

[2] *I have now:* It is necessary to mention, for the information of others, that we have now

very well, at last the ram was taken with fitts boardering on madness, we were at a loss to tell whether it was occasioned by any thing he had eat or by being Stung with Netles which were in plenty about the place, but supposed it to be the latter and therefore did not take the care of him we ought to have done; One night while he was lying by the Centinal, he was seized with one of these fitts and ran headlong into the Sea, but soon came out again and seemed quite easy, presently after he was seized with a nother fit and ran a long the beach and the she goat after him; some time after she returned but the other was never seen, more dilligent search was made for him in the woods to no purpose, we therefore supposed he had run into the Sea a Second time and been drown'd, after this accident it was to no purpose to leave the she goat, as she was not with kid, having kided but a few days before we arrived and the both of them died immidiately after. Thus the reader will see how every method I have taken to stock this Country with Sheep and Goats have proved ineffectual.*—ff. 148–9.

The morning before we sailed I wrote a memorandum seting forth the time we arrived last here, the day we sailed, the rout I intended to take & such other information as I thought necessary for Captain Furneaux to know and buried it in a bottle under the root of a tree in the garden in the bottom of the Cove in such a manner that it must be found by any European[1] who may put into the Cove.[2] I however have not the least reason to think that it will ever fall into the hands of the person I intended it for, for it is hardly possible that Captain Furneaux can be in any part of New Zealand and I not have heard of him in all this time, nevertheless I was determined not to leave the country without looking for him where I thought it was

[1] *any European:* him or any European . . .—f. 153.

[2] Furneaux sets forth the memorandum in his journal, 1 December 1773: 'On the root of a large tree at the watering place was this inscription "Look underneath" upon digging I found the Following note sealed up in a bottle.

"Queen Charlotte's Sound New Zealand 24th Novr 1773

"His Britannic Majesty's Sloop Resolution Captain Cook arrived last in this Port on the 3d instant and sailed again on the date hereof, Captain Cook intended to spend a few days in the east enterance of the straits in looking for the Adventure Captain Furneaux who he parted company with in the night of the 29th of last month, afterwards he will proceed to the South and Eastward. As Captain Cook has not the least hopes of meeting with Captain Furneaux he will not take upon him to name any place for a Rendezvous; he however thinks of retiring to Easter Island in Latd 27°6′ so Longitude 108°0′ West a [*sic*] Greenwich in about the latter end of next march, it is even probable that he may go to Otaheite or one of the society Isles but this will depend so much upon circumstances that nothing with any degree of certainty can be depended upon

Jas Cook" '.

The copy of this note given in Furneaux's log shows a number of inconsiderable differences, and the signature is 'Jams Cooke'. Cook's ordinary signature and what he no doubt wrote, was 'Jams Cook'.

most likely for him to be found; accordingly as soon as we were clear of the Sound I hauld over for Cape Teerawhitte and ran along the shore from point to point to Cape Pallisser fireing guns every half hour without seeing or hearing the least signs of what we were in search after. At 8 o'Clock we brought too for the night, Cape Pallisser bearing SEBE distant 3 Leagues, in this situation we sounded and had 50 fathom water. I had now an oppertunity to make some observations on the Bay[1] which lies on the West side of Cape Pallisser which forms the most eastern point, the bay does not appear to run so far inland to the Northward as I at first thought, the deception being caused by the land in the bottom of it being low, it however is not less than 5 Leagues deep and full as wide at the Entrance, the two points being NWBW and SEBE from each other, it seems to lie wholy exposed to the Southerly and SW winds, it is however probable that there may be places in the bottom of the Bay better sheltered.[2] The Navigation of this side of the Strait is by far safer than the other, the tides do not run near so strong and their is not the least danger but what shews it self and lies nearer the shore than any Ship would wish to come. The Course from Cape Pallisser to Cape Terawhitte is N 69° W[3] distant about [10] Leagues, between these two Capes are two Bays, the one just mentioned and the one on the East side of the last mentioned Cape in the entrance of which we anchored before we put into the Sound. From Cape Terawhitte to Cape Ko[amaroo] the Course is NW½N distant   Leagues and to the two brothers [16 miles]. To the north of Cape Terawhitte, between it and entry Island is an Island lying pretty near the Shore, I judged this to be an Island when I was here last voyage but not being certain I left it as undetermined in my chart of the strait.[4] All the Land adjoining to the Sea between Cape Terawhitte and Cape Pallisser is exceeding barren, probably occasioned by its being so much exposed to the Cold southerly winds.

The next Morning at day-light we made Sail round Cape Pallisser

[1] *on the Bay:* on the coast between Cape Teera Whittee and Cape Palliser; the Bay . . .—f. 153v.

[2] *it is . . . sheltered:* Log 956 'but there may be places in the bottom of it, sheltered from even these winds. The Bay, or Inlet, on the East side of Cape Teerawhitte, before which we anchored lies in the direction of North inclining to the West and seemed to be well sheltered. The Middle Cape or Point [the two points Baring Head and Turakirae] which disjoins these two Bays, is of a considerable height, especially in land, for close to the Sea is a skirt or low-land off which lie some pointed rocks; but so near the shore as to be no ways dangerous . . .' This is added to the original log entry in a different ink after Add. MS 27887 was copied. The passage is copied in B f. 153v.

[3] . . . and S 69° East

[4] . . . which is the reason of my mentioning it now, as also the Bays &c[a].—f. 153v. This was the small flat-topped island called Mana.

fireing guns as usual but saw not the least signs of the Adventure and therefore bore away[1] for Cape Campbell on the other side of the Strait having a light breeze at NE. Soon after we discovered a smoak to the NE a little way in-land, it was improbable enough that this should be made by any of the Adventures crew, I however determined to put it out of all manner of doubt and accordingly hauled the wind again, we kept plying till 6 o'Clock in the evening, several hours after this smoke and every other sign of people disapeared. All the officers being unanimous of opinion that the Adventure could neither be stranded on the Coast or be in any of the Ports in this Country determined me to spend no more time in search of her, but to proceed directly to the Southward. I am under [no] apprehensions for the safety of the Adventure nor can I even guess which way she is gone, the manner she was seperated from me and [not] coming to the rendezvouze has left me no grounds to form any conjectors upon, I can only suppose that Captain Furneaux was tired with beating against the NW winds and had taken a resolution to make the best of his way to the Cape of good hope, be this as it may I have no expectation of joining him any more.

*I was however under no sort of Anxiety for her safety on the other hand the manner she was seperated from us and afterwards not coming to the rendezvous has hardly left me any room even to conjecture which way she has gone; I can only suppose, that Captain Furneaux being tired with beating against the NW winds had taken a resolution to make the best of his way to Cape Horn or perhaps to the Cape of Good Hope; be this as it will it is not likely we shall join again, as no rendezvous was absolutely fixed upon after leaving New Zealand. Nevertheless this shall not discourage me from fully exploring the Southern parts of the Pacific Ocean in the doing of which I intend to employ the whole of the insuing season and if I do not find a Continent or isle between this and Cape Horn in which we can Winter perhaps I may spend the Winter within the Tropicks or else proceed round Cape Horn to Faulkland Islands, such were my thoughts at this time, the execution of which will depend in a great Measure on circumstances which at this time it was not possible for me to fore see.

On our quiting the Coast and consequently all hopes of being joined by our consort, I had the satisfaction to find that not a man was dejected or thought the dangers we had yet to go through were

[1] *as usual . . . away:* as usual as we ran along the shore; in this manner we proceeded till we were 3 or 4 Leagues to the NE of the Cape when the wind shifted to NE and we bore away . . .—f. 154.

in the least increased by being alone, but as cheerfully proceeded to the South or wherever I thought proper to lead them as if she or even more Ships had been in our Company.*—f. 154–4v.

SATURDAY 27*th. Ther.r* 62. *Winds Northerly. Course S* 14°45′ *E. Dist. Sailed* 107 *Miles. Lat. in* 43°27′. *Long. in West Reck.g.* 184°1′. *Long. mde C. Pallisser* 0°38′ *East. Varn.* 12°52′ *East.* Fresh gales and fair weather. At 8 o'Clock in the pm I took my departure from Cape Pallisser, which at that time bore NW½N dis[t] Six Leagues, and directed my Course S½E, having a light moon and a known Sea the night did not retard us; in the Morning we set the Studing sails, not long after the Main Top-gallant yard broke in the Slings,[1] and as we had never a nother or a spar that would make one I orderd the Carpenter to make one out of the boom belonging to the boat in frame.[2]

SUNDAY 28*th. Ther.r* 54. *Winds Variable. Course S* 25°15′ *E. Dist. Sailed* 57 *Miles. Lat. in* 44°18′. *Long. in West Reck.g* 183°28′. *Long. mde C. Pallisser* 1°11′ *East. Varn* 13°58′ *East.* First part fresh gales and fair weather, remainder little wind and gloomy weather. At 6 pm, being in Latitude 44°00′ S the Variation was 12°52′ East. In the AM saw some Seals and Sea Weed.

MONDAY 29*th. Ther.r.* 55. *Winds Variable. Course S½E. Dist. Sailed* 20 *Miles. Lat. in* 44°38′. *Long. in West Reck.g.* 183°21′. *Long. mde C. Pallisser* 1°18′ *East.* Some times gentle breezes and other times light airs next to a Calm and fair weather. A billet of wood, Seals, Albatroses, Sheer-waters and Port Egmont hens seen.

TUESDAY 30*th. Ther.r.* 49. *Winds SW. Course S* 43° *E. Dist. Sailed* 96 *Miles. Lat. in* 45°50′. *Long. in West Reck.g* 181°47′. *Long. mde C. Pallisser* 2°52′ *East.* Fresh gales and Clowdy weather. In the evening double reefed the Top-sails. In the night the clew[3] of the Fore sail broke which occasioned the spliting of the sail and obliged us to bend a nother. The Sprit-sail some hours after went in the same manner. Seals &c[a] seen as yesterday. A Swell from SW.

[1] Smyth, *Sailor's Word-Book*, defines slings as 'The rope or chain used to support a yard which does not travel up and down a mast. The slings of a yard also imply that part on which the slings are placed'.

[2] The *Resolution*, it will be remembered, carried the parts of a small vessel, to be put together for use where she could not go herself. See p. 16 above.

[3] The clew or clue of a square sail (like the foresail, as here) was one of its lower corners, reaching down to where the tacks and sheets were made fast to it.

[DECEMBER 1773]

WEDNESDAY *1st. Ther.r* 49. *Winds SW. Course S* 40° *E. Dist. Sailed* 94 *Miles. Lat. in* 47°4′. *Long. in West Reck.g.* 180°30′. *Long. mde C. Pallisser* 4°9′ *East.* Weather as yesterday, first part fresh gales, latter moderate so as to carry single reef'd Top-sails. Sail-makers repairing Sails. SW Swell.

THURSDAY *2nd. Ther.r* 46 *to* 48. *Winds SWBW. Course S* 31°45′ *E. Dist. Sailed* 93 *Miles. Lat. in* 48°23′. *Long. in West Reck.g.* 179°16′. *Long. mde C. Pallisser* 5°23′ *East.* Gentle gales and Clowdy weather. A great Swell from SW. Rock Weed, Seals, Penguins with red bills,[1] Grey Albatroses, Pintadoes and other Petrels and Port Egmont Hens seen.

FRIDAY *3rd. Ther.r.* 47. *Winds SWBW to NW. Course S* 14° *E. Dist. Sailed* 34 *Miles. Lat. in* 48°56′. *Long. in West Reck.g.* 179°2′. *Long. mde C. Pallisser* 5°27′ *East.* Little [wind] and mostly foggy weather. Loosed all the reefs out of the Top-sails and in the Morning got Top-gallant yards aCross, set the Sails and likewise the Studding sails. Seals, Penguins &c[a] seen as yesterday. A great Swell from the Southward.

SATURDAY *4th. Winds NNW to NBE. Course SBW. Dist. Sailed* 60 *Miles. Lat. in* 49°55′. *Long. in West Reck.g.* 179°16′. *Long. mde C. Palliser* 5°23′ *East.* First part gentle breezes and hazey, remainder little wind and foggy. Took in the Studding sails during night. A great Swell from the Southward. Seals and Penguins yet to be seen.

SUNDAY *5th. Ther.r* 47. *Winds Variable, SSE. Course S* 62° *W. Dist. Sailed* 43 *Miles. Lat. in* 50°15′. *Long. in West Reck.g.* 180°16′. *Watch* 180°16′. *Long. mde C. Palliser* 4°23′ *East. Varn.* 18°25′ *East.* First part little wind, foggy rainy weather, Remainder gentle breezes and fair weather. Cleaned and Smoak'd betwixt decks. Several Seals and Penguins. A great hollow swell from SW.

MONDAY *6th. Ther.r.* 49. *Winds SSE, EBN. Course South. Dist. Sailed* 35 *Miles. Lat. in* 50°50′. *Long. in West Reck.g.* 180°16′. *Long. mde C. Pallisser* 4°23′ *East.* Fore and Middle parts light airs and Clowdy, latter a fresh breeze with drizling rain. pm Var p[r] Az[th] 18°25′ E. Seals, Penguins, Albatroses, Petrels and a Whale seen. SW Swell.

TUESDAY *7th. Ther.r* 49. *Winds NBE to NW. Course S* 15° *E. Dist. Sailed* 140 *Miles. Lat. in* 55°7′. *Long. in West Reck.g.* 179°46′. *Watch*

[1] Possibly *Megadyptes antipodes* (Homb. and Jacq.), the Yellow-eyed Penguin, which breeds in the South Island of New Zealand and in the islands further south.

179°46′. *Long. mde C. Pallisser* 4°53′ *East.* Frish gales and hazey foggy weather with rain at times. At 8 pm Shortned Sail and hauled the wind to the Eastward till 3 am when we bore away and made sail. Seals, Sea Weed and Birds as usual. At half past 8 pm Antipodes to London.[1]

WEDNESDAY 8*th. Winds NW and WNW. Course SBE. Dist. Sailed* 155 *Miles. Lat. in South* 55°39′. *Long. in West Reck.g.* 178°53′. *Long. E. from C. Palliser* 5°46′. Strong gales and hazey. At pm took in the Top-sails and Main sail till the Morning when they were set again, but before Noon we shifted the Top-sails to repair. The SW swell hardly yet gone down, a proof beyond a doubt there can be no land in that direction but what must be at a vast distance, for we have had no wind from that quarter these five days past, on the contrary have had a steady and strong gale for these last two days from the North and NW: hence I conclude that there can be no land under the Meridian of New Zealand but what must lie far to the South of 60°.[2] Neither Seals or Penguins to be seen, hence we conjectured that those we had seen were Natives of New Zealand, or retur[n]ed there when nature made it necessary for them to be on land.

THURSDAY 9*th. Winds WNW, NNW, and North. Course S* 146. *Dist. Sailed* 158 *Miles. Lat. in South* 58°2′. *Long. in West Reck.g* 177°43′. *Watch* 177°42′. *Long. E from C. Pallisser* 6°56′. Strong gales and Squally hazey weather. At 8 pm handed the Main-sail,[3] at 11 close reef'd and handed the Top-sails and brought to under the fore sail and Mizen Stay-sail with her head to SW. At 2 am bore away under the Fore-sail and close reef'd Top-sails. Towards noon the gale abated and we loosed all the reefs out and set the Main-sail. A great swell from NW. A piece of Weed, Albatroses and Peterels seen.

FRIDAY 10*th. Winds NW to SW. Course S* 46°30′ *E. Dist. Sailed* 102 *Miles. Lat. in South* 59°12′. *Long. in West Reck.g.* 175°22′. *Long. E from C. Pallisser* 9°17′. Strong gales and Squally with showers of sleet and Snow and a great Sea from the West and NW. Stood to the Southward till 8 pm when being very thick we took in the Top-sails and

[1] *At half . . . London:* At half an hour past 8 oClock the next evening [civil time], we reckoned our Selves Antipodes to our friends in London consequently as far removed from them as possible.—f. 155.—'Between 7 & 8 oClock, passed directly opposite to London, & drank to our friends on that side of the Globe: The good People of that City may *now* rest perfectly satisfied that they have no Antipodes besides Pengwins and Peteralls, unless Seals can be admitted as such; for Fishes are absolutely out of the question.'—Wales.

[2] This was a quite valid conclusion: the nearest land in that direction was the north coast of Victoria Land; its Cape North is in lat. 70°33′ S, long. 75°33′ E.

[3] To hand a sail was to furl it.

Courses, wore and lay-to under Mizen Stay-sail till middnight, then wore and made Sail to the SE under the Courses and close-reef'd Top-sails, the weather being some thing clearer. At 5 loosed a reef out of each Top-sail.

SATURDAY 11*th. Winds SW to NW. Course S* 37½° *E. Dist. Sailed* 113 *Miles. Lat. in South* 60°42′. *Long. in West Reck.g.* 173°4′ *Watch* 173°2′. *Long. E from C. Pallisser* 11°35′. *Var.* 17°18′. Fresh gales and hazey with some Showers of rain. At 4 AM loosed the 2nd reef out of the Top-sails and some time after saw a piece of Weed.

SUNDAY 12*th. Therm.r* 32. *Winds WBS to SWBS. Course S* 31° *E. Dist. Sailed* 146 *Miles. Lat. in South* 62°46′. *Long. in West Reck.g.* 170°26′ *Watch* 170°24′. *Long. E from C. Palliser* 14°13′. PM Fresh gales and Clowdy. Loosed all the reefs out, and found the Var[n] by several Az[ths] to be 17°18′ E being then in Lat 61°15′ S. At 8 o'Clock the weather became Squally with thick Showers of Snow and hail which continued till near noon. Double reef'd the Top-sails and handed the Mizen Top-sail. At 4 am Saw an Island of Ice in Latitude 62°10′ S which is 11½° farther South than the first Ice we saw after leaving the Cape of Good Hope. Grey Albatroses, Pintados, Blue Pitrels and one Antartic Petrel seen.

MONDAY 13*th. Therm.r.* 32. *Winds SW to NNE. Course S* 52½° *E. Dist. Sailed* 92 *Miles. Lat. in South* 63°42′. *Long. in West Reck.g.* 167°44′. *Long. E from C. Pallisser* 16°55′. First part fresh gales and Clowdy. Middle little wind, Latter fresh gales and thick hazey weather with Snow. In the pm found the Variation to be 19°13′ E. We stood to the SE with the Wind at SW and as the wind backed to the West we hauled more and more to the South, keeping the wind allways upon the beam till 9 am, when the wind veered to the North and being thick weather we hauled the wind to the Eastward under double reefd Top-sails and Courses. By sailing with the Wind on the Beam we had it in our power to return back over that space of Sea we had in some measure made our selves acquainted with, in case we had met with any danger. Split the Main Topmast stay-sail all to raggs, it being an old sail the greatest part blew away.

TUESDAY 14*th. Therm.r. Noon* 32. *Winds North to WNW. Course S* 57½° *E. Dist. Sailed* 136 *Miles. Lat. in South* 64°55′. *Longde. in West Reck.g.* 163°20′. *Long. made from C. Pallisser* 21°19′. *Varn.* 14°12′ *E.* Fresh gales. First part a thick Fog attended with Sleet, Middle hazey, latter fair and tolerable clear. At 3 am loosed all the Reefs out and at 8 got Topg[t] yards a Cross and set the Sails. Saw in this 24 hours four

Ice islands, a quantity of loose ice, Albatroses, Pintadoes, Blue Petrels and Fulmers.

WEDNESDAY 15*th. Therm.r. Noon* 31. *Winds WBN, NNW, & West. Course S* 60°15′ *E. Dist. Sailed* 116 *Miles. Lat. in South* 65°52′. *Longde. in West Reck.g.* 159°20′. *Long. made from C. Pallisser* 25°19′. Fresh gales and thick Foggy weather with snow, except in the pm when we had some intervals of clear Weather in one of which we found the Variation to be 14°12′ E. At 6 o'Clock double reefed the Top-sails and handed the Main sail and Mizen Top-sail. The Ice begins to increase fast, from Noon till 8 o'Clock in the evening we saw but two islands, but from 8 to 4 am we passed fifteen,[1] besides a quantity of loose Ice which we sailed through, this last increased so fast upon us that at 6 o'Clock we were obliged to alter the Course more to the East, having to the South an extensive feild of loose ice; there were several partitions[2] in the feild and clear water behind it, but as the wind blew strong the Weather foggy, the going in among this Ice might have been attended with bad concequences, especially as the wind would not permit us to return. We therefore hauled to the NE on which course we had stretched but a little way before we found our selves quite imbayed by the ice and were obliged to Tack and stretch back to the SW having the loose field ice to the South and many large islands[3] to the North. After standing two hours on this tack the wind very luckily veered to the westward with which we tacked and stretched to the Northward (being at this time in Lat 66°0′ S) and soon got clear of all the loose ice but had yet many huge islands to incounter, which were so numerous that we had to luff for one and bear up for a nother,[4] one of these mases was very near proving fatal to us, we had not weather[ed] it more than once or twice our length, had we not succeeded this circumstance could never have been related.[5] According to the old proverb a miss is as good as a

[1] *fifteen:* H seventeen

[2] *there . . . partitions:* The ice in most part of it laid close packed together, in other places there appeared partitions . . .—f. 156.

[3] . . . which made it the more necessary for us to get clear of this loose ice, which is rather more dangerous than the great islands

[4] *but . . . a nother:* but not before we had received several hard knocks from the larger pieces, which with all our care we could not avoid. After clearing one danger we still had a nother to encou[n]ter, the weather remained foggy and many large islands laid in our way, so that we had to luff for one and bear up for a nother . . .—f. 156.—'To bear up . . . a nother', i.e. the ship had to sail nearer the wind to get clear of one iceberg, which meant simultaneously sailing towards another.

[5] This was undoubtedly the occasion referred to by Elliott, in one of his most vivid passages. Forster, in an unusually brief passage where danger is concerned (I, p. 531), agrees on the detail 'whilst the people were at dinner', on 15 December. 'But I will here observe that while amongst the Ice Islands, we had the most *Miraculous* escape from being every soul lost, that ever men had; and thus it was; the officer of the Watch on deck,

mile, but our situation requires more misses than we can expect, this together with the improbability of meeting with land to the South and the impossibility of exploreing it for the ice if we did find any, determined me to haul to the north. This feild or loose ice is not such as is usually formed in Bays or Rivers, but like such as is broke off from large Islands,[1] round ill-shaped pieces from the size of a small Ship's Hull downwards, whilest we were amongest it we frequently, notwithstanding all our care, ran against some of the large pieces, the shoks which the Ship received thereby was very considerable, such as no Ship could bear long unless properly prepared for the purpose. Saw a great number of Penguins on an ice island and some Antartick Petrels flying about.[2]

THURSDAY 16*th. Therm.r. Noon* 31 *to* 33. *Winds West, Calm, SE. Course N* 19½° *E. Dist. Sailed* 102 *Miles. Lat. in South* 64°16′. *Longd. in West Reck.g.* 158°0′. *Longd. made from C. Pallisser* 26°39′. Continued to stretch to the Northward with a very fresh gale at west which was attended with thick snow showers till 8 pm when the weather began to clear up and the gale to abate. At 6 o'Clock in the am it fell Calm and continued so till 10 when a breeze sprung up at SEBS with which we stretched to the NE. Weather dark and gloomy and very cold our sails and rigging hung with icicles for these two days past. At present

while the people was at Dinner, had the imprudence to attempt going to windward of an Island of Ice and from the ship not going fast, and his own fears making her keep too much near the Wind, which made her go slower, he got so near that he could get neither one way, nor the other, but appeard inev[itably?] going right upon it, and it was Twice as high as our Mast Heads: In this situation He call[ed] up all hands, but to discribe the horrour depicted in every persons face at the Awful situation in which we stood is impossible, no less in Cooks, than our own; for no one but the officer, and a few under his orders, had notic'd the situation of the ship. In this situation, nothing could be done but to assist the ship, what little we could with the Sails, and wait the event with awful expectation of distruction, Captn Cook order'd light spars to be got ready to push the ship from the Island if she came so near, but had she comd within their reach, we should have been Overwhelm'd in a Moment and every Soul drown'd; the first stroke would have sent all our Masts overboard, and the next would have knock'd the Ship to pieces, and drown'd us all. We were actualy within the *back surge of the Sea*, from the Island: But most providentially for us, she when [i.e. went] clear; her stern just trailing within the Breakers from the Island. Certainly never men had a more narrow escape, from the jaws of death'.—Elliott *Mem.*, ff. 24v–26. It may be thought that Elliott, writing years later, would be prone to ornament his narrative; but this is precisely the sort of thing that would be riveted in every detail on the memory of a young man.

[1] *but . . . Islands:* and near shores but such as breaks off from large islands and may not improperly be called the pareings of the large pieces or the Rubbish or Fragments which breake off when the great islands breake loose from the place where they are formed.—f. 156.

[2] 'AM at 5 saw a large field of Pack'd Ice and a great many Islands—haul'd to the Eastward—at 7 found ourselves confoundedly entangle'd with loose and field Ice—the surface of the water was nearly cover'd with it—haul'd to the N'ward and work'd to windward as fast as we cou'd. At Noon a great deal of field Ice and a vast number of Islands about.'—Clerke.

but few ice islands in sight but have past a great many this last 24 hours.

FRIDAY 17*th. Therm.r. Noon* 33¾. *Winds East to North. Course S* 67° *E. Dist. Sailed* 64 *Miles. Lat. in South* 64°41′. *Longd. in West Reck.g.* 155°44′. *Longd. made from C. Pallisser* 28°50′. Gentle gales attended with Frost, snow showers and thick hazey weather. At 4 pm, the wind veering more to the East, tacked and Stood to the North till 5, then wore brought to and hoisted out two boats to take up some loose ice to serve as fresh water. But after the boats had made one trip in which they got but little, we hoisted them in again and made sail to the East with the wind at North and NNE: the Sea run high and the pieces of ice were so large as made it dangerous for the Boats to lay along side of them. We continued to stand to the East till 8 o'Clock AM when falling in with a quantity of loose ice as well as several large Islands, circumstances being favourable for takeing some on board we accordingly hoisted out two Boats which by noon took up as much as we could dispence with, it was none of the best for our purpose, being composed chiefly of frozen Snow, was poras and had imbibed a good deal of Salt Water, this however dreaned of after it had laid some time, after which the ice yeilded sweet water.[1] Grey Albatross, Sheer-waters and blue Petrels &c[a].

SATURDAY 18*th. Winds NBW to NE. Course East. Dist. Sailed* 95 *Miles. Lat. in South* 64°41′. *Longd. in West Reck.g.* 152°1′. *Longd. made from C. Pallisser* 32°33′. *Varn.* 10°18′ *East.* Moderate breezes thick foggy weather with snow and sleet which froze to the Rigging as it fell so that every thing was cased with ice.[2] At 1 pm hoisted the Boats in and stretched away to the East, falling in every now and then with large ice islands of near two miles in circuit.[3]

SUNDAY 19*th. Winds Northerly. Course S* 83° *E. Dist. Sailed* 69 *Miles. Lat. in South* 64°49′. *Longd. in West Reck.g.* 149°19′. *Longd. made from C. Pallisser* 35°15′. *Varn.* 13°25′ *East.* Thick foggy weather, continued

[1] 'All Hands very busy in recieving and stowing away Ice—Cold Weather—the rigging cover'd with Ice which falls about the Decks whenever we have occasion to trim sails or any ways handle it.'—Clerke. What was taken up from the sea was rotten ice rather than frozen snow.

[2] 'Employ'd Night and day Melting that which we took up yesterday, which affords but a small quantity of Water it being nothing but congeal'd Snow instead of Solid Massy Ice.'—Cooper. Marra, p. 114, details the hardships and the cold, adding, 'yet under all these hardships, the men chearful over their Grog; and not a man sick but of old scars.'

[3] . . . We continued to Stretch to the East with a piercing cold Northerly wind attended with a thick fog, snow and Sleet which decorated all our rigging with icicles; we were hourly meeting with some of the large ice island[s] which in these high Latitudes render Navigation so very dangerous.—f. 157.

to stand to the Eastward without seeing any ice till 7 o'Clock pm when we fell close aboard one. Being exceeding Foggey we wore and stood back to the west. At 10 o'Clock the weather being some thing clearer we again reassumed our Course to the East. At Noon the weather cleared up, the Sun appeared and our Latitude was determined by an Ob^{n}.[1]

MONDAY 20*th. Therm.r.* 33. *Winds NW to NE. Course S* 20° *E. Dist. Sailed* 68 *Miles. Lat. in South* 65°57′. *Longd. in West Reck.g.* 148°23′. *Longd. made from C. Pallisser* 36°11′. PM Clear weather which afforded an oppertunity to know our Longitude both [by] observation of the Sun and Moons distance and the Watch, by the former it was 149°19′ West and by the Latter 148°36′ W, and by my Reckoning 148°43′ W. The Variation of the Compass by several Az^{ths} taken at the same time and after was 14°25′ E. Latitude 64°48′ S. The wind veering to the NW and the clear weather tempted me to stand to the South which we accordingly did till 7 am when the wind veered to the NE and the sky became clowded, we hauled to the S East. Pass'd at different times 24 large ice islands besides innumerable small peices. Sails and rigging cased with ice.[2]

TUESDAY 21*st. Therm.r. Noon* 33. *Winds NE. Course S* 41° *E. Dist. Sailed* 70 *Miles. Lat. in South* 66°50′. *Longde. in West Reck.g.* 66°50′.[3] *Long. made C. Pallisser* 38°11′. In the pm the wind increased to a strong gale attended with a thick fogg sleet and rain which constitutes the very worst of weather, our rigging was so loaded with ice that we had enough to do to get our Top-sails down to double reef. At 7 o'Clock we came the second time under the Polar Circle and stood to the SE till 6 o'Clock in the am when being in Lat 67°5′ South, Longitude 145°49′ West, the fogg being exceeding thick we came close aboard a large Island of ice and being at the same time a good deal embarrass'd with loose ice we with some difficulty wore[4] and stood to the NW untill Noon when the fogg being some what disipated we resumed our Course again to the SE. The ice islands we fell in with in the morning, for there were more than one, were very high

[1] '... the Ice upon the rigging thaws and falls in large lumps upon the Deck which renders it rather disagreeable.'—Clerke.

[2] 'PM this Afternoon we beat the Ice off the shrouds and melted it with the rest which prov'd no inconsiderable addition to our water ... Melting Ice all Night ... Clean'd ship and smoak'd Her with fire Balls.'—Clerke.

[3] Error for 145°49′.

[4] 'Discovered a very large Island of Ice directly a head and scarce more than 100 yards distant: the Ship luckily wore clear of it; but before she was half round, another large one was discovered, at about the like distance on the lee bow. The Lieu^{t} had therefore no resource but to put the helm up again, and endeavour to drive her through a large field of loose Ice which lay betwixt them, and as soon as she was clear of them Tacked and stood Northward.'—Wales.

and rugged terminating in many Peaks, whereas all those we have seen before were quite flat at top and not so high.[1] A great Sea from the North. Grey Albatroses and a few Antarctick Petrels.[2]

WEDNESDAY 22*nd. Therm.r. Noon* 31 *to* 33. *Winds Northerly. Course S* 70°15′ *E. Dist. Sailed* 109 *Miles. Lat. in South* 67°27′. *Longde. in West Reck.g.* 141°55′. *Long. made C. Pallisser* 42°39′. Fresh gales the most part of this day, at times very thick and hazey and other times tolerable clear. Saw not fewer than twenty ice islands, some grey Albatroses and a few Antarctick Petrels. In the PM a squall of wind took hold of the Mizen Top-sail and tore it all to pieces, and rendered it for ever useless.[3]

THURSDAY 23*rd. Therm.r. Noon* 33. *Winds Northerly. Course N* 80°15′ *E. Dist. Sailed* 94 *Miles. Lat. in South* 67°12′. *Longde. in West Reck.g.* 138°00′ *Watch* 137°41′. *Long. made C. Pallisser* 46°39′. Moderate gales and Pirceing cold, very thick and hazey at times. At Noon Twenty three ice islands were seen from the Deck and twice that number from the mast head.

FRIDAY 24*th. Therm.r. Noon* 32. *Winds Northerly. Course S* 40° *W. Dist. Sailed* 9 *Miles. Lat. in South* 67°19′. *Longde. in West Reck.g.* 138°15′. *Long. made C. Pallisser* 46°24′. At 4 o'Clock in the PM as we were standing to the SE, fell in with such a vast quantity of field or loose ice as covered the whole Sea from South to East and was so thick and close as to obstruct our passage, the wind at this time being pretty moderate, brought to in the edge of this feild, hoisted out two boats and sent them to take some up, and in the mean time we slung several large pi[e]ces along side and hoisted them in with our tackles;[4] by such time as the Boats had made two trips it was Eight o'Clock when we hoisted them in and made sail to the westward under double reef'd Top-sails and Courses, with the wind notherly a strong gale attended with a thick fog Sleet and Snow which froze to the Rigging as it fell and decorated the whole with icicles.[5] Our ropes were like

[1] . . . and yet many of them were between two and three hundred feet in height and between two and three miles in circuit, whose perpendicular clifts or sides were astonishing to behold. Most of our winged companions had left us . . .—f. 157v. The flat-topped bergs were the ones now classed as 'tabular'.

[2] 'Compleated melting our Ice today, which render'd us 7 Ton which is a Fortnights Water.'—Clerke 8952.

[3] . . . At 6 oClock in the Morning the wind veering toward the West, our course was East Northerly. At this time we were in the Latitude of 67°31′ which was the highest we have yet been in, Longitude 142°54′ West.—f. 157v.—'The Weather these 24 hours has been much more favourable than the last—it has every now and then so far clear'd up that we cou'd see 3 or 4 miles around us, and by that means avoid these confounded Ice Isles which render the Navigation here very disagreeable in hazey Foggy Wea^r.'—Clerke.

[4] . . . The takeing up ice proved such cold work that . . .—f. 158.

[5] *decorated . . . icicles:* made the ropes like wires.

wires, Sails like board or plates of Metal and the Shivers[1] froze fast in the blocks so that it required our utmost effort to get a Top-sail down and up; the cold so intense as hardly to be endured, the whole Sea in a manner covered with ice, a hard gale and a thick fog: under all these unfavourable circumstances it was natural for me to think of returning more to the North, seeing there was no probability of finding land here nor a possibility of get[ting] farther to the South and to have proceeded to the East in this Latitude would not have been prudent[2] as well on account of the ice as the vast space of Sea we must have left to the north unexplored, a space of 24° of Latitude in which a large track of land might lie, this point could only be determined by makeing a stretch to the North. While we were takeing up the ice two of the Antarctick Petrels so often mentioned were shott; we were right in our conjectures in supposeing them of the Petrel tribe; they are about the size of a large pigeon, the feathers of the head, back and part of the upper side of the wings are a lightish brown, the belly and under side of the wings white, the tail feathers which are 10 in number are white tiped with brown. At the same time we got another new Petrel smaller than the former, its plumage was dark grey.[3] They were both casting their feathers and yet they were fuller of them than any birds we had seen, so much has nature taken care to cloath them sutable to the climate in which they live. At this time we saw two or three Chocolate coloured Albatrosses with yellowish Bills,[4] these as well as the Petrels above mentioned are no were seen but among the ice.[5] The bad weather continuing without the least variation for the better which made it necessary for us to proceed with great caution and to make short boards over that part of the Sea we had in sóme measure made our selves accquainted with the preceeding day, we were continually falling in with large ice islands which we had enough to do to keep clear of.

SATURDAY 25*th. Therm.r. Noon* 34. *Winds NW. Course N* 48¼° *E. Dist.*

[1] i.e. sheaves.

[2] *would . . . prudent:* must have been wrong

[3] Very probably this was the Mottled Petrel, the Rain-bird of New Zealand, *Pterodroma inexpectata* (Forster). In *Descr. An.*, p. 204, J. R. Forster notes that this was found with the Antarctic Petrel in the Antarctic Ocean.

[4] Probably the Giant Petrel.

[5] . . . hence one may with reason conjecture that there is land to the South, if not I must ask where these Birds breed, a quiston that perhaps will never be determined, for hitherto we have found these lands, if any, quite inaccessible. Besides these birds, we saw a very large Seal, which kept playing about us some time, one of our people who had been at greenland called it a Sea Horse, but every one else who saw it took it for what I have said. Sence our first falling in with the ice the Mercury in the Thermometer has been from 33 to 31 at Noon day.—ff. 158v–9. The 'sea horse' was the walrus, which is not found in the Antarctic; the animal must have been, as Cook said, a large seal.

Sailed 84 *Miles. Lat. in South* 66°23′. *Longde. in West Reck.g.* 135°7′. *Long. made C. Pallisser* 49°32′. In the PM the wind veer'd more to the West, the gale abated and the sky cleared up and presented to our view the many islands of ice we had escaped during the Fog. At 6 o'Clock being in Latitude 67°0′ S, Long^{de} the same as yesterday at noon, the variation was observed to be 15°26′ East. As we advanced to the NE with a gentle gale at NW the ice increased so fast upon us that at Noon no less than 90 or 100 large islands were seen round us besides innumberable smaller pieces.[1]

SUNDAY 26*th. Therm.r.* 37. *Winds NNW, Calm, WSW. Course N* 66° *E. Dist. Sailed* 20 *Miles. Lat. in South* 65°15′. *Longde. in West Reck.g.* 134°22′. *Long. made C. Pallisser* 50°17′. *Varn.* 16°2′ *East.* At 2 o'Clock in the pm it fell calm,[2] we had before preceived this would happen and got the ship into as clear a birth as we could where she drifted along with the ice islands and by takeing the advantage of every light air of wind was kept from falling foul of any one; we were fortunate in two things, continual day light and clear weather, had it been foggy nothing less than a miracle could have kept us clear of them,[3] for in the morning the whole sea was in a manner wholy covered with ice, 200 islands and upwards, none less than the Ships hull and some more than a mile in circuit were seen in the compass of five miles, the extent of our sight, and smaller peices innumberable.[4] At 4 in the AM a light breeze sprung up at WSW and enabled us to Steer north the most probable way to extricate our selves from these dangers.[5]

[1] [Midnight] 'The Ice Isles increase upon us confoundedly. AM at 5 we reckon'd 53 Ice Isles about us—These have been 24 hours of very good Wea^{r} which is a very fortunate circumstance just at this time, for we are fairly beset with these divilish Ice Isles; at Noon we reckon'd from the Deck 90 stout fellows, besides innumerable peices vastly larger than this Ship which wou'd a good deal damage her were we unfortunate enough to get foul of any of them.'—Clerke.

[2] 'On the 25th, the weather was clear and fair, but the wind died away to a perfect calm. . . . This being Christmas-day, the captain according to custom, invited the officers and mates to dinner, and one of the lieutenant's entertained the petty-officers. The sailors feasted on a double portion of pudding, regaling themselves with the brandy of their allowance, which they had saved for this occasion some months before-hand, being sollicitous to get very drunk, though they are commonly sollicitous about nothing else.'—Forster, I, p. 535. Sparrman (p. 111), less the critic, though a sober man enough, transmits a bit of tipsy conversation that has the authentic ring: 'Sailors and marines . . . joked about the voyage, and vowed that, if they were wrecked on any of the 168 masses of ice surrounding us, they would certainly die happy and content, with some rescued keg of brandy in their arms.'

[3] *kept . . . them:* saved us from being dashed to pieces, . . .—f. 159.

[4] '. . . By observation we found that the Ship had drifted or gone about 20 Miles to the NE or ENE whereas by the ice islands it appeared that she had gone little or nothing, by which we concluded that the ice drifted in nearly the same direction and at the same rate.'

[5] 'These have been 24 hours of very fine Wea^{r} and smooth Water—the Ice Islands fairly too thick to be accurately counted—this morning we attempted it upon the Quarter

MONDAY 27*th. Therm.r. Noon* 35. *Winds SW, NW & NE. Course N* 36° *E. Dist. Sailed* 27 *Miles. Lat. in South* 65°53′. *Longde. in West Reck.g.* 133°42′ *Watch* 133°22′. *Long. made C. Pallisser* 50°57′. We continued to steer to the north with light airs from the west till 4 o'Clock in the AM when meeting with a quantity of small Ice we hoisted out two Boats and took on board sufficient to fill all our empty Casks and for several days present expence; this done we hoisted in the Boats again and made sail to the NW with a gentle breeze at NE, clear pleasent frosty weather.[1]

TUESDAY 28*th. Therm.r. Noon* 33¼. *Winds Easterly. Course N* 5°30′ *W. Dist. Sailed* 94 *Miles. Lat. in South* 64°20′. *Longde. in West Reck.g.* 134°4′. *Long. made C. Pallisser* 50°35′. The same Weather continued till the AM when the wind increased to a fresh gale attended with thick Snow Showers and sharp frosty weather. Ice Islands not half so thick or so many as before.[2]

WEDNESDAY 29*th. Winds SE. Course N* 6° *E. Dist. Sailed* 116 *Miles. Lat. in South* 62°24′. *Longde. in West. Reck.g.* 133°37′. *Long. made C. Pallisser* 51°2′. *Varn.* 13°46′. Continual Snow and Sleet and a fresh gale at SE and SSE with which we steer'd North Easterly till Noon then NWBN.[3]

THURSDAY 30*th. Therm.r. Noon* 33¾. *Winds South to West. Course N* 30° *W. Dist. Sailed* 85 *Miles. Lat. in South* 61°5′. *Longde. in West Reck.g.*

Deck and made them to be 238; they were several times counted and this is the Mean, so I'm sure it's very near the truth. Many of these Islands are at least 200 feet above the surface of ye Water.'—Clerke.—'The greatest number of Ice Islands about that I ever saw. They are all small ones, and resemble much the Pieces which used to break off from the shores about Churchill River in the spring of the year that I wintered there, from whence I cannot avoid thinking we are not far from Land, whose shores are not so high as those where large Islands are found.'—Wales. The nearest land was the even now still somewhat conjectural Hobbs Coast, east of the Ross Sea, over 550 miles to the south.

[1] 'Very fine wear and smooth water these 24 hours—the Ice Isles thin very fast which is a matter of much satisfaction to us—we can count now but 65 from the Deck.'—Clerke. Forster (I, p. 538) gives a report on the general health at this time: 'My father, and twelve other persons were again much afflicted with rheumatic pains, and confined to their beds.' There were a few slight symptoms of scurvy, treated with wort. 'A general langour and sickly look however, manifested itself in almost every person's face, which threatened us with more dangerous consequences. Captain Cook himself was likewise pale and lean, entirely lost his appetite, and laboured under a perpetual costiveness'.

[2] 'Fourteen Islands of ice in Sight . . . Employed Melting and filling the Casks in the hold with ice'.—Log.—'PM this Afternoon I saw a Large Pyeball'd Whale, the first of the kind I ever saw in these Seas—at the same time I saw another Whale of the Common sort —both remarkably large'.—Clerke. The 'Pyeball'd' whale had probably been attacked by squids, whose suckers had left the white marks on its surface. Cf. p. 581, n. 2 below.

[3] 'These 24 hours have been one continued snow Shower, with thick hazey disagreeable Wr. We've seen but two Ice Isles—however we may have pass'd many, for the Weather has been too thick to discern them or anything else at any distance. I've seen no fowl but 2 Or 3 black Albetrosses'.—Clerke 8952.—'Passed very near another large Island of Ice. The Pitcher is not yet broken!'—Wales.—Clerke's 'black Albetrosses' may have been the Giant Petrel, *Macronectes* sp., or—more likely—the Sooty Albatross, *Phoebetria* sp.

134°12′. *Long. made C. Pallisser* 50°27′. The same weather continued till 3 pm when the wind abated and the weather cleared up and became fair, soon after found the variation to be 13°46′ E. Lat 62°12′, Longde 133°52′ W. In the am had little wind at SW and dark Clowdy weather. Several Whales seen,[1] but few birds. A Swell from WNW. Pass'd Several islands of ice.

FRIDAY 31*st. Therm.r. Noon* 34½. *Winds Westerly. Course N* 19° *W. Dist. Sailed* 90 *Miles. Lat. in South* 59°40′. *Longde. in West Reck.g.* 135°11′ *Watch* 135°11′. *Long. made C. Pallisser* 49°28′. *Varn.* 13°9′. PM little wind with showers of snow and Sleet, Middle fresh gales, latter gentle breeze and clear pleasent weather; this gave us an oppertunity to air the spare Sails and to clean and smoak the Ship betwixt decks. At Noon we found our selves 20 Miles North of account having had no observation the three preceeding days; it is natural to suppose there must be a Current from the South which bring along with it, tho' with a slow motion, the many ice islands[2] we daily see.

[JANUARY 1774]

SATURDAY 1*st. Therm.r. Noon* 36½. *Winds NW to East & SSE. Course N* 16° *W. Dist. Sailed* 32 *Miles. Lat. in South* 59°9′. *Longde. in West Reck.g.* 135°29′. *Long. made C. Pallisser* 49°10′. In the PM had a few hours calm which was succeeded by a breeze from the East and enabled us to reassume our NWBN Course, but have little hopes of meeting with land in that quarter as we have had a long hollow swell from WNW and NW the three preceeding days. Piercing cold weather, frequent snow showers, many ice islands.

SUNDAY 2*nd. Therm.r* 38¼. *Winds SW, Westerly, Calm, East. Course N* 23° *W. Dist. Sailed* 78 *Miles. Lat. in South* 57°58′. *Longde. in West Reck.g.* 136°27′. *Long. made C. Pallisser* 48°12′. *Varn.* 11°12′. The wind increased to a fresh breeze and veered to the SW and west attended with some snow Showers. At 5 o'Clock in the AM it fell calm, being then in Lat. 58°2′ S Longde 136°12′ W the variation was 11°12′ East. At 9 a breeze sprung up at East with which steered NWBW.[3] The swell still continues to come from this quarter, notwithstanding the wind has not blown from thence for some time past, one cannot have a better sign than this of there being no land in that direction. At 8

[1] . . . playing about the Ship

[2] *the . . . islands:* these huge masses of ice . . .—f. 159v.

[3] . . . my reason for steering this Course was to explore part of the great space of sea between us and our track to the South.—f. 160.

o'Clock in the PM past three ice islands in the Lat of 58°39′ and have seen none since.[1]

MONDAY *3rd. Therm.r. Noon* 36. *Winds NE round by the East to SW. Course NWBW. Dist. Sailed* 130 *Miles. Lat. in South* 56°46′. *Longde. in West Reck.g.* 139°45′ *Watch* 139°40′. *Long. made C. Pallisser* 44°54′. Fresh gales with Snow and Sleet, till towards noon when the weather became fair and the wind veered to SW. About this time saw two small Divers of the Petrel Tribe, such as are usally seen near land[2] and two pieces of Sea weed. A great number of Blue Petrels and sever[l] Albatrosses of the large white or grey kind.

TUESDAY 4*th. Therm.r. Noon* 46¼. *Winds Westerly. Course NBE. Dist. Sailed* 114 *Miles. Lat. in* 54°55′. *Longd. in West Greenwich Reck.g.* 139°4′, *East C. Pallisser* 45°45′. Fresh gales and Clowdy with some Showers of Sleet. In the PM saw a few more of the small divers, and some small pieces of weed which appeard to be old and decayed and not as if it had lately been broke from rocks. I can not tell what to think of the divers, had there been more of them I should have thought them signs of the vicinity of land,[3] as I never saw any so far from known land before, probably these few may have been brought out thus far to Sea by some Shoal of fish, such were certainly about us by the vast number of Blue Petrels and Albatrosses,[4] all of which left us before the evening. As the wind seems now fixed in the western board, we shall be under a necessity of leaving unexplored to the west a space of Sea containing 40° of Longitude and 20° or 21° of Latitude, had the wind been favourable I intended to have run 15° or 20° of longitude to the west in the Latitude we are now in and back

[1] An omission by Cook for this date, from a document which was designed to go to his masters at the Admiralty, is eloquent of his character. This was one of the painful incidents arising from the unstable character of the 'young gentleman' called Charles Loggie, at this time only nineteen, whose conduct got him a flogging. Cooper is brief and simply mentions 'Drunkenness and Rioting' as the cause. Clerke 8952 gives a fuller account: 'This Morning read the Articles of War and punish'd Cha[s] Logie with a dozen lashes for abusing, drawing his knife upon, & cutting 2 of the Midshipmen—this Logie was formally a Midshipman of this ship, but for repeated ill behaviour the Captain thought proper to dismiss him the Quarter Deck—he has since more than once behav'd ill, and now had proceeded to such lengths that y[e] Common safety of the Ship['s] Company render'd it necessary to disgrace him with Corporal punishment'. Elliott supplies us with some of the background, in which, it may be remarked, that 'Hypocritical canting fellow' Maxwell is concerned. 'M[r] Maxwell, M[r] Loggie & some others, of the Gentlemen, having made an agreement amongst themselfs to make merry; A Quarrel arose between the two Pervious mention'd, which was the Occation of the former's Striking M[r] Loggie, He in Return opend his knife & swore he'd stab him; For which he was Punished with a Dozen Lashes having done his Duty before the Mast'.

[2] . . . especially in the Bays and on the Coast of New Zealand.

[3] *I should . . . land:* I should have been ready enough to believe that we were at this time not very far from some land, . . .—f. 160.

[4] . . . and other birds, such as are usually seen in the great Ocean

again to the East in the Latitude of 50° or near it, this rout would have so intersected the space above mentioned as to have hardly left room for the bare supposission of any large land lying there.[1] Indeed as it is we have no[2] reason to suppose that there is any for we have had now for these several days past a great swell from west and NW, a great sign[3] we have not been covered by any land between these two points.[4] In the AM saw some Pie bald porpuses.[5]

WEDNESDAY 5*th. Therm.r.* 46¾. *Winds Westerly. Course N* 34° *E. Dist. Sailed* 87 *Miles. Lat. in* 53°43′. *Longde. in W. Greenwh. Reck.g.* 137°40′ *Watch* 137°46′, *East Cape Pallisser* 46°59′. In the PM the wind increased to a Storm and blew in squalls attended with showers of rain, obliged us at last to take in the Top-sails, the Fore top-sail being Split unbent it to repair. At 3 am, being more moderate, set the Main Top-sail close reefed and some time after bent the fore top-sail and set it in like manner. A Prodigious high Sea from WNW. At Noon saw a small piece of weed.

THURSDAY 6*th. Therm.r.* 47. *Winds West, NW, & WSW. Course N* 36°45′ *E. Dist. Sailed* 128 *Miles. Lat. in* 52°0′. *Longde. in W. Greenwh. Reck.g.* 135°32′ *Watch* 135°38′, *East Cape Pallisser* 49°7′. Very strong gales and excessive heavy squalls attended with rain. At 8 pm took in the Top-sails till 8 am when the gale being some what abated set them again close reef'd. At Noon loosed all the reefs out and bore away NE with a fresh gale at WSW, fair weather, the distance between us now and our rout to Otahiete being little more than two hundred leagues in which space it is not probable there can be any land,[6] and it is less probable there can be any to the west from the vast high billows[7] we now have from that quarter.

FRIDAY 7*th. Therm.r.* 50. *Winds WSW to NW. Course N* 44°40′ *E. Dist. Sailed* 117 *Miles. Lat. in* 50°36′. *Longde. in W. Greenwh. Reck.g.* 133°19′ *Watch* 133°25′, *East Cape Pallisser* 51°20′. *Varn.* 6°26′. Fresh gales and fair weather, pm got Topg[t] yards aCross and set the Sails.

[1] Cook did 'intersect' all this space in his passage from New Zealand to Cape Horn, at the end of this year 1774.

[2] *no:* little

[3] *NW . . . sign:* NW, when at the same time the wind has blown from a contrary direction great part of the time, which is a great sign . . .—f. 160v.

[4] . . . While we were in the high Latitudes, many of our people were attack'd with a slight Fever, occasioned by colds, it happily yeilded to the simplest remidies and was generally removed in a few days and at present we have not above two or three on the sick list.

[5] Probably Hector's Dolphin, *Cephalorhynchus hectori* (Van Beneden).

[6] *Here . . . land:* all circumstances considered, there is any extensive land . . .—f. 161.

[7] 'A Prodigious Long hollow Sea from the West'.—Log.

At 8 AM observed several distances of the Sun and Moon, the results were as follows, Mr Wales 133°24′, Mr Gilbert 133°10′, Mr Clerk 133°00′,[1] and Self 133°37′ West Longitude. Mr Kendals watch at the same time gave 133°44′ W. Variation 6°26′ E.

SATURDAY 8*th. Therm.r. Noon* 49¾. *Winds NW & West. Course NE. Dist. Sailed* 126 *Miles. Lat. in South* 49°7′. *Longde. W. Greenwh. Reck.g.* 131°2′ *Watch* 131°8′. *Long. E C. Pallisser* 53°37′. Fresh gales with now and then showers of rain. In the PM found the variation to be 6°2′ E and in the AM 6°26′ East. At 9 o'Clock had again several Observations of the Sun and Moon the results were confirmable to yesterday and determined our Longde beyond a doubt. Indeed our error can never be great so long as we have so good a guide as Mr Kendalls watch. At Noon altered the Course to ENE Easterly.

SUNDAY 9*th. Therm.r. Noon* 51¼. *Winds Westerly. Course N* 72° *E. Dist. Sailed* 161 *Miles. Lat. in South* 48°17′. *Longde. W. Greenwh. Reck.g.* 127°10′ *Watch* 127°16′. *Long. E C. Pallisser* 57°59′. Fresh gales and clear pleasent weather. A great Westerly swell.[2]

MONDAY 10*th. Therm.r. Noon* 52½. *Winds Westerly. Course N* 84° *E. Dist. Sailed* 97 *Miles. Lat. in South* 48°7′. *Longde. W. Greenwh. Reck.g.* 124°40′. *Long. E C. Pallisser* 59°53′. PM Fresh gales and pleasent weather. In the am little wind and clowdy weather: hoisted out a small boat in which some of the officers went and Shott several Birds which made us a fresh meal, they were all of the Petrel tribe no others being to be seen and any other thing what ever that can shew the least sign of the Vinicity of land.

TUESDAY 11*th. Therm.r. Noon* 50. *Winds Westerly. Course N* 81° *E. Dist. Sailed* 103 *Miles. Lat. in South* 47°51′. *Longde. W. Greenwh. Reck.g.* 122°12′ *Watch* 122°17′30″. *Long. E C. Palliser* 62°27′. Little wind continued most part of the PM. In the night it began to freshen, blew in Squalls attended with rain, afterwards the weather became clear and the wind sittled. At Noon being little more than two hundred Leagues from my track to Otaheite in 1769 in which space it was not probable any thing was to be found, we therefore hauled up SE with a fresh gale at SWBW.[3]

[1] ... Mr Smith 133..37..25 Mean 133..21..43

[2] 'Many Albatrosses about the Ship & other sea Birds. The Albatrosses are all very large & grey like those we used to see at, and after leaving the Cape of Good Hope. One was catched with a Hook & line which measured near 10 ft from the tip of one wing to that of the other.'—Wales. Only the Wandering Albatross has a wing span of this extent, but these birds are not grey, although the immatures are mottled.

[3] This must be the occasion to which Elliott refers, though the new course was not due South: 'At this time we all experienced a very severe mortification, for when we were

WEDNESDAY 12*th. Therm.r. Noon* 56. *Winds SWBW to NWBN. Course S* 42°30′. *Dist. Sailed* 138 *Miles. Lat. in South* 49°32′. *Longd. W. Greenwh. Reck.g.* 119°52′ *Watch* 119°57′. *Long. E. C. Pallisser* 64°47′. Fresh gales and pleasent weather. In the pm found the variation 2°34′ East.[1] The Westerly swell still continues. Very few birds seen and these such as are found all over the Ocean in these Latitudes. At Noon hauled more to the Southward.

THURSDAY 13*th. Therm.r. Noon* 53½. *Winds NWBN to North. Course N* 18°30′ *E. Dist. Sailed* 158 *Miles. Lat. in South* 52°0′. *Longd. W. Greenwh. Reck.g.* 118°33′. *Long. E. C. Pallisser* 66°6′. Fresh gales and fair weather. In the PM being in the Latitude of 50°5′ S[2] the variation was 4°30′ East. At Noon had a great northerly swell a sign we had left no land behind us in that direction.

FRIDAY 14*th. Therm.r. Noon* 51¼. *Winds NW. Course S* 23°15′ *W. Dist. Sailed* 124 *Miles. Lat. in South* 53°54′. *Longd. W. Greenwh. Reck.g.* 119°55′. *Long. E. C. Pallisser* 64°44′. Fresh gales and very foggy in the night.[3] In the PM saw a piece of weed. At 8 handed[4] the Main-sail, Fore and Mizen Top-sails and hauled to the SW under the Fore-sail and double reef'd Main Top-sail. At 2 am set the Fore Top-sail double reef'd and towards Noon the mainsail.

SATURDAY 15*th. Therm.r. Noon* 51. *Winds NW to North. Course S* 29° *W. Dist. Sailed* 148 *Miles. Lat. in South* 56°4′. *Longd. W. Greenwh. Reck.g.* 122°1′. *Long. E. C. Palliser* 62°38′. Strong gales and thick hazy weather with rain. At 6 pm the Fore Top-sail being split, unbent it to repair and handed the Mizen Top-sail and soon after the Main-sail. In the Morning set them again, bent the Fore Top-sail and loosed the Reefs out of the Main Top-sail. At Noon, the Wind being

steering East, we had all taken it into our heads that we were going streight for Cape Horn, on our roud [*sic*] home, for we began to find that our stock of Tea, Sugar &c began to go fast, and many hints were thrown out to Capt[n] Cook, to this effect; but he only smiled and said nothing, for he was close and secret in his intentions at all times, that not even his first Lieutenant knew, when we left a place, where we should go to next. In this respect, as well as many others, he was the fit[test] Man in the world for such a Voyage; In this instance all our hopes were blasted in a Minuite, for from steering East, at Noon, Capt[n] Cook orderd the Ship to steer due South, to our utter astonishment, and had the effect for a Moment, of causing a buz in the Ship but which soon subsided.'—Elliott *Mem.*, f. 24–4v. This trait in Cook was not one that appealed to the Forster mind: 'It must be owned, however, that nothing could be more dejecting than the entire ignorance of our future destination, which, without any apparent reason, was constantly kept a secret to every person in the ship'.—Forster, I, p. 540. But Cook did not wholly ignore his officers; see p. 328 below.

[1] ... which is the least Variation we had found without the Tropick.—f. 161v.

[2] ... Longitude 119½° W.

[3] ... a strong gale with a thick Fogg and rain, which made it unsafe to steer large, ... —f. 161v. To steer large: 'to go free, off the wind' (Smyth).

[4] i.e. furled.

at North a hard gale with very thick weather, I did not think it safe to run to the South and therefore hauld the wind to the East under double reefed Top-sails & Courses.

SUNDAY 16*th. Therm.r. Noon* 47¾. *Winds North to WNW. Course S* 70° *E. Dist. Sailed* 88 *Miles. Lat. in South* 56°19′. *Longde. in West Reck.g.* 119°24′ *Watch* 119°27′. *Long. E. C. Pallisser* 65°15′. *Varn. East* 9°28′. First part Excessive hard gales and thick hazy weather. At 8 pm took in the Sails and brought-to under the Mizen Stay-sail. A very high Sea from NW. Saw a small piece of Weed. At 8 am, wore and stood to the Southward under the Courses and double-reef'd fore Top-sail, the Main-top-sail being unbent to repair, the gale being a good deal abated but the NW Sea ran prodigeous high.[1]

MONDAY 17*th. Winds Westerly. Course S* 15°30′ *E. Dist. Sailed* 140 *Miles. Lat. in South* 58°34′. *Longde. in West Reck.g.* 118°14′. *Long. E. C. Pallisser* 65°25′. PM fresh gales and clear weather. At 5 found the Variation as p[r] Column, Lat 56°48′, Long[de] p[r] Distance ☉ and ☽ 118°51′ W. Night squally with rain and Sleet. Morning moderate and fair, loosed all the reefs out. A great swell from Westward.[2]

TUESDAY 18*th. Therm.r. Noon* 40. *Winds Westerly. Course S* 15°15′ *E. Dist. Sailed* 145 *Miles. Lat. in South* 60°54′. *Longde. in West Reck.g.* 116°58′. *Long. E. C. Pallisser* 67°41′. First part fresh gales and fair, remainder thick and hazy with rain; pm double reef'd the Top-sails. Not the least signs of land.

WEDNESDAY 19*th. Winds Southerly, North, & NE. Course South. Dist. Sailed* 58 *Miles. Lat. in South* 61°52′. *Longde. in West Reck.g.* 116°58′. *Long. E. C. Pallisser* 67°41′. PM Moderate gales and hazy, Wind veering to the South and SSE; at 8 being in the Latitude of 61°9′, Long[de] 116°7′, Tacked and stood to the SW. At 10 it fell Calm and continued

[1] 'At nine o'clock a huge mountainous wave struck the ship on the beam, and filled the decks with a deluge of water. It poured through the sky-light over our heads, and extinguished the candle, leaving us for a moment in doubt whether we were not totally overwhelmed and sinking into the abyss.'—Forster, I, pp. 540–1.

[2] 'AM this morning I saw a Whale and many Pyeball'd Porpusses'.—Clerke. Small piebald dolphins of the genus *Cephalorhynchus* are abundant in high latitudes in the Southern Ocean. The Forsters were too uncomfortable at this time to make observations in natural history, and George draws a dismal picture of the prevailing conditions (I, pp. 541–3). 'A gloomy melancholy air loured on the brows of our shipmates, and a dreadful silence reigned amongst us.' Salt meat had become loathsome, and the bread had again gone rotten—added to which, for economy, it was on a two-thirds allowance. On this day the first mate as spokesman came to Cook to complain, and full allowance was restored. This is borne out by Mitchel: 'Served whole allowance of bread, it being so bad (being the damp and indifferant baked at Charlottes sound) which situation it has been these three weeks past—application being at last made'. George Forster notes that 'The captain seemed to recover again as we advanced to the south', which could hardly have been much comfort to George's rheumatism-afflicted elder.

so till 2 am when a breeze sprung up at North and afterward veered to NE, with which we stood to the South. Thick hazy weather with rain and a vast swell from the westward.

THURSDAY 20*th. Therm.r.* 40. *Winds NE & Easterly. Course S* 21° *E. Dist. Sailed* 45 *Miles. Lat. in South* 62°34′. *Longde. in West Reck.g.* 116°24′. *Long. East C. Pallisser* 68°15′. First part fresh gales and hazey with rain, remainder little wind and Mostly fair. At 7 PM saw a large piece of Weed. In the AM two ice islands one of which was very high terminating in a peak or like the Cupala of St Pauls Church, we judged it to be 200 feet high.[1] A great Westerly swell still continues a probable certainty there is no land[2] between us and the Meridian of 133½° which we were under when last in this Latitude.[3]

FRIDAY 21*st. Therm.r.* 37. *Winds S.Easterly. Course S* 38° *W. Dist. Sailed* 10 *Miles. Lat. in South* 62°26′. *Longde. in West Reck.g.* 116°38′. *Long. East C. Pallisser* 68°1′. PM light airs next to a Calm till 3 o'Clock when a fresh gale came at SSE attended with thick snow Showers and piercing cold weather. The Wind remaining unsittled in the SE quarter, caused us to make frequent tacks, the most of them disadvantagous, so that our situation this day at Noon differed but little from yesterday.

SATURDAY 22*nd. Therm.r.* 37. *Winds SBE & SE. Course N* 80°45′ *E. Dist. Sailed* 106 *Miles. Lat. in South* 62°9′. *Longde. in West Reck.g.* 112°54′. *Long. East C. Pallisser* 71°51′. *Varn. East* 10°59′. Fresh gales with Showers of Sleet at times. Saw an Antarctick Petrel but very few other birds.[4]

SUNDAY 23*rd. Therm.r.* 38½. *Winds Southerly. Course S* 79°30′ *E. Dist. Sailed* 71 *Miles. Lat. in South* 62°22′. *Longde. in West Reck.g.* 110°24′. *Long. East C. Pallisser* 74°15′. *Varn. East* 11°55′. Moderate gales and Clowdy, with now and then Showers of rain or Sleet. PM found the Variation by several Azths to be 10°59′ E.[5]

[1] Obviously a berg which had melted away under water, and then overturned.

[2] *a probable . . . land:* which made it improbable any large land should lie

[3] . . . In all this rout we have not seen the least thing that could induce us to think we were ever in the neighbourhood of any land. We had indeed frequently seen pieces of Sea Weed but this I am well assured is no sign of the vicinity of land, for weed is seen in every part of the ocean.—f. 162.

[4] . . . In this situation saw an ice island an antarctick Peterel, several Blue Peterels and some other known birds, but no one thing that could give us the least hope of finding land.—f. 162.—'. . . the Sea does not rise with this Southerly wind in the Manner it has done with the Winds from any other Quarter of the Compass—it has now blown fresh 24 Hours from ye S.ward and we have very little Sea Going, which I think must be owing to a large quantity of Ice or possibly Land, so near to windward as to prevent the waters regular Course.—Clerke 8952. Cf. Wales: 'An ugly short jerking Sea something like what is usually met with in the Chops of the English Channel'.

[5] 'Not a Bird of any sort to be seen these two Days past'.—Wales, who thus conflicts with Cook.

MONDAY 24*th. Therm.r. Noon* 39. *Winds South to WNW. Course S* 53°30′ *E. Dist. Sailed* 97 *Miles. Lat. in South* 63°40′. *Longd. in W. Greenwh. Reck.g.* 108°17′, *East C. Pallisser* 76°22′. Fresh gales and dark clowdy weather. At 3 o'Clock in the PM pass'd by an ice island and two hours after found the Variation to be 11°53′ E. Being at this time in Latitude 62°36′ S, Longitude 109°32′ W. In the am saw a nother ice island. The wind abated and veer'd to West and WNW with which steer'd South all reefs out, having a great swell from SSW and several blue Petrels about us.

TUESDAY 25*th. Therm.r. Noon* 42. *Winds WNW to North. Course SBW½W. Dist. Sailed* 109 *Miles. Lat. in South* 65°24′. *Longd. in W. Greenwh. Reck.g.* 109°31′, *East C. Pallisser* 75°8′. *Varn. East* 19°27′. First part fresh breeze and clowdy, Middle hazy with Sleet and rain, latter a gentle breeze and pleasent weather and the air very warm considering the Latitude. Not a bit of ice to be seen, which we who have been so much used to it think a little extraordinary and causes various opinions and conjectures.[1]

WEDNESDAY 26*th. Therm.r. Noon* 40. *Winds Northerly. Course South. Dist. Sailed* 72 *Miles. Lat. in South* 66°36′. *Longd. in W. Greenwh. Reck.g.* 109°31′, *East C. Pallisser* 75°8′. *Varn. East* 18°20′. Gentle breezes and Clowdy mild weather. At 6 PM Latitude 65°44′ S. Variation p^r Azm^uths 19°27′ E and at 7 AM being then in Latitude 66°20′ the Variation was 18°20′ East. At this time saw Nine Ice islands, the most of them small, several Whales and a few blue Petrels. At 8 o'Clock we came the third time within the Antarctick Polar Circle. Soon after saw an appearence of land to the East and SE, haul'd up for it and presently after it disapeared in the haze.[2] Sounded but found no ground with a line of 130 fathom. A few whales & Petrels seen.

THURSDAY 27*th. Therm.r.* 37½. *Winds NE. Course S* 21°15′ *E. Dist. Sailed* 83 *Miles. Lat. in South* 67°52′. *Longd. in W. Greenwh. Reck.g.* 108°15′, *East C. Pallisser* 76°24′. Little wind and foggy with rain and Sleet, at intervals fair and tolerable clear. Continued to stretch to the SE till 8 o'Clock am by which time we were assured our supposed land was vanished into clowds[3] and therefore resumed our Course to the

[1] *and causes . . . conjectures:* as it is but a month ago and not quite 200 leagues to the East that we were in a manner blocked up with large Islands in this very latitude. Saw a single Pintado Peterel, some blue Peterels and a few brown Albatrosses.—f. 162.

[2] 'a remarkably strong appearance of Land . . .'—Wales.—'. . . At Noon the Haze cover'd our suppos'd Land, we're confoundedly afraid its nothing more, mere supposition'. —Clerke.

[3] . . . or a Fog bank.—f. 162v.—'PM by 8 we were convinc'd to our sorrow that our Land was nothing more than a deception of the sight'.—Clerke.

South. A smooth Sea, what little swell we have is from the NE. A few Blue Petrels, Black Sheer-waters[1] and Mother Caries Chickens are all the Birds we see.

FRIDAY 28*th. Therm.r.* 36. *Winds N.Easterly. Course South. Dist. Sailed* 103 *Miles. Lat. in South* 69°35′. *Longd. in W. Greenwh. Reck.g.* 108°15′, *East C. Pallisser* 76°24′. A gentle breeze of Wind, attended with a thick Fogg and snow and then Showers of Snow and Sleet. Continued our Course to the South till 11 o'Clock PM, when falling in with Some Ice Islands and the fog being very thick we hauled the wind to the Eastward, on which Course we stood but one hour before we resumed our Course to the South, the fog being something thiner. At 4 o'Clock past four Ice Islands, after which the fog was so thick that we could not see a quarter of a Mile round us. A few Blue Petrels and Pintadoes seen, but nothing that could give us the least hopes of finding land.

SATURDAY 29*th. Therm.r.* 36½. *Winds NE, NW, & NNE. Course S* 33° *E. Dist. Sailed* 30 *Miles. Lat. in South* 70°00′ *Obn. Longd. in W. Greenwh. Reck.g.* 107°27′ *Watch* 107°36′, *East C. Pallisser* 77°12′. *Varn. East* 22°41′. At 1 o'Clock in the PM fell in with some loose ice, brought-to, hoisted out two Boats and took a quantity on board; which done made sail to the NW not daring to stand to the South in so thick a fog which hindered us from seeing the extent or quantity of ice we were among. The wind was Variable between NW and North and but little of it. At Midnight Tacked to the Eastwards.[2] At 4 o'Clock the Sky cleared up, the wind fixed at NNE and we bore away SSE passing several large Ice islands. Betwixt 4 and 8 o'Clock found the variation by several trials to be 22°41′ E. Latitude at this time about 69°45′ S. Clear pleasent Weather, Air not cold.[3]

SUNDAY 30*th. Winds ESE. Course S* 20° *E. Dist. Sailed* 51 *Miles. Lat. in South* 70°48′. *Longd. in W. Reck.g.* 106°34′. Continued to have a gentle gale at NE with Clear pleasent weather till towards the

[1] In such a latitude these would almost certainly be Cape Hens, *Procellaria aequinoctialis*.

[2] *took a quantity . . . Eastwards:* took up as much as yielded about ten tons, this was cold work but it was now familiar to us. As soon as we had done we hoisted in the Boats and after wards made short boards over that part of the Sea we had in some measure made our selves acquainted with, for we had now so thick a Fog that we could not see 200 yards round us, and as we knew not the extent of the loose Ice, I dar'd not steer to the South till we had clear weather. Thus we spent the night or rather that part of the 24 hours which answered to night for darkness we had none but what was occasioned by fogs.—f. 162v.

[3] 'Fine pleasant wea^{r}—a very extraordinary incident in this part of the World—its the first day I can by any means denominate pleasant that I ever met with either within, or near the Antartick Circle. This morning we saw a Port Egmont Hen, some Pintada's, Albetrosses and Peterels.'—Clerke.

evening, when the Sky became Clowded and the air Cold atten[d]ed with a smart frost. In the Latitude of 70°23′ the Variation was 24°31′ East; some little time after saw a piece of Rock Weed covered with Barnacles which one of the brown Albatroses was picking off. At 10 o'Clock pass'd a very large Ice island which was not less than 3 miles in circuit, presently after came on a thick fog, this made it unsafe to stand on, especially as we had seen more Ice Islands ahead; we therefore tacked[1] and made a trip to the North for about one hour and a half in which time the fog dissipated and we resumed our Cou[r]se to the SSE, in which rout we met with several large ice islands. A little after 4 AM we precieved the Clowds to the South near the horizon to be of an unusual Snow white brightness which denounced our approach to field ice, soon after it was seen from the Mast-head and at 8 o'Clock we were close to the edge of it which extended East and West in a streight line far beyond our sight; as appear'd by the brightness of the horizon; in the Situation we were now in just the Southern half of the horizon was enlightned by the Reflected rays of the Ice to a considerable height. The Clowds near the horizon were of a perfect Snow whiteness and were difficult to be distinguished from the Ice hills whose lofty summits reached the Clowds.[2] The outer or Nothern edge of this immence Ice field was compose[d] of loose or broken ice so close packed together that nothing could enter it; about a Mile in began the firm ice, in one compact solid boddy and seemed to increase in height as you traced it to the South; In this field we counted Ninety Seven Ice Hills or Mountains, many of them vastly large.[3] Such Ice Mountains as these are never seen in Greenland, so that we cannot draw a comparison between the Greenland Ice and this now before us: Was it not for the Greenland Ships fishing yearly among such Ice (the ice hills excepted) I should not have hisitated one moment in declaring it as my opinion that the Ice we now see extended in a solid body quite to the Pole, and that it is here, i.e. to the South of this parallel, where the many Ice Islands we find floating about in the Sea are first form'd, and afterwards broke off by gales of wind and other causes,[4] be this as

[1] '... at 12 the Weather was so thick we cou'd scarcely see the Ship's length, so wore and stood upon the other Tack.'—Clerke.

[2] '... A long way within y[e] field (which we could not see over) was the appearance of a long ridge of very high mountains [of] Ice; but I am of opinion this was nothing more than a strong Fog bank, illuminated by the rays of light which were reflected from the Ice. I[t] seems, to me, improbable that it should be Ice or Snow, unless land was under it, of which we had no other signs.'—Wales. The illumination was ice-blink; cf. p. 61, n. 3.

[3] '... a vast number of exceeding large and high Ice Islands ... we counted 90, then found our endeavours to numerate fruitless, for they were totally innumerable'.—Clerke.

[4] This theory of the formation of icebergs Cook later rightly discarded; see pp. 644–5 below.

it may, we must allow that these numberless and large Ice Hills must add such weight to the Ice feilds, to which they are fixed, as must make a wide difference between the Navigating this Icy Sea and that of Greenland: I will not say it was impossible anywhere to get in among this Ice, but I will assert that the bare attempting of it would be a very dangerous enterprise and what I believe no man in my situation would have thought of. I whose ambition leads me not only farther than any other man has been before me, but as far as I think it possible for man to go, was not sorry at meeting with this interruption, as it in some measure relieved us from the dangers and hardships, inseparable with the Navigation of the Southern Polar regions. Sence therefore we could not proceed one Inch farther South, no other reason need be assigned for our Tacking and stretching back to the North, being at that time in the Latitude of 71°10′ South, Longitude 106°54′ w.[1] We had not be[en] long tacked before we were involved in a very thick fog, so that we thought our selves very fortunate in having clear weather when we approach'd the ice. I must observe that we saw here very few Birds of any kind; some Penguins were heard but none seen, nor any other signs of land whatever.

*SUNDAY 30*th.*[2] At 4 oClock in the Morning we preceived the C[l]ouds over the horizon to the South to be of an unusual Snow white brightness which we knew denounced our approach to field Ice; soon after it was seen from the Top-mast head and at 8 oClock we were close to the edge of it, it extended east and west far beyond the reach of our sight. In the situation we were in just the Southern half of our horizon was illuminated by the rays of light which were reflected from the Ice to a considerable height.[3] Ninety Seven Ice hills were distinctly seen within the feild, besides those on the outside and many of them were very[4] large and looked like a ridge of

[1] This was not merely Cook's farthest south, but the farthest south anyone has ever attained by sea in this longitude. It is probable that the 'firm ice' Cook saw did at that time extend 'in a solid body quite to the Pole'. He was now only about 120 miles from the nearest land, which lay roughly to the south-west—the Walgreen coast of Marie Byrd Land, the line of which is still conjectural, discovered by Admiral Byrd from the air in 1929. See Introduction, pp. lxxxv–vi above.

[2] Though the following version of this famous passage is largely repetitive of what appears above, it has so many small additions, and is so characteristic of Cook's rewriting, in his effort to get clarity and vividness, but at the same time not to overstate, that it has seemed worth while to print it here in full. A further comparison of this with the printed page (*Voyage*, I, pp. 267–9) will show how closely Douglas, in his editing, followed the words of the MS.

[3] *Deleted* the Clouds were of a perfect Snow white brightness and difficult to be distinguished from the Ice hills whose lofty summits were lost in them.

[4] very *altered from* vastly

Mountains rising one above another till they were lost in the clouds.[1] The outer or Northern edge of this immense field, was composed of loose or broken ice close packed together, so that it was not possible for any thing to enter it, this was about a mile broad, within which was solid Ice in one continued compact body; it was rather low and flat (except the hills) but seemed to increase in hieght as you traced it[2] to the South in which direction it extended beyound our sight. Such Mountains of Ice as these were, I believe, never seen in the Greenland Seas, at least not that I ever heard or read of, so that we cannot draw a comparison between the Ice here and there; it must be allowed that these prodigeous[3] Ice Mou[n]tains must add such additional weight to the Ice fields which inclose them as must make a great difference between the Navigating this Icy sea and that of Greenland. I will not say it was impossible any where to get farther to the South, but the attempting it would have been a dangerous and rash enterprise and what I believe no man in my situation would have thought of. It was indeed my opinion as well as the opinion of most on board, that this Ice extended quite to the Pole or perhaps joins to some land, to which it had been fixed from the creation and that it here, that is to the South of this Parallel, where all the Ice we find scatered up and down to the North are first form'd and afterwards broke off by gales of Wind or other cause and brought to the North by the Currents which we have always found to set in that direction in the high Latitudes. As we drew near this Ice some Penguins were heard but none seen and but few other birds or any other thing that could induce us to think any land was near; indeed if there was any land behind this Ice it could afford no better retreat for birds or any other animals, than the Ice it self, with which it must have been wholy covered. I who had Ambition not only to go farther than any one had done before, but as far as it was possible for man to go, was not sorry at meeting with this interruption as it in some measure relieved us, at least shortned the dangers and hardships inseparable with the Navigation of the Southern Polar Rigions; Sence therefore, we could not proceed one Inch farther to the South, no other reason need be assigned for my Tacking and Standing back to the north, being at this time in the Latitude of 71°10′ s, Longitude 106°54′ w. It was happy for us that the Weather was Clear when we fell in with this Ice and that we discovered it so soon as we did for we had no sooner Tacked then we were involved in a thick fog. The Wind was

[1] and looked . . . clouds *interlinear insertion.*
[2] as you traced it *altered from* as it lay advanced
[3] prodigeous *altered from* vast

at East and blew a fresh breeze, so that we were inabled to return back over that space we had already made our selves acquainted with. At Noon the Mercury in the Thermometer stood at 32½ and we found the air exceeding cold.*—f. 163–3v.

MONDAY 31*st. Therm.r. at Noon* 34. *Winds ESE to ENE. Course NBE. Dist. Sailed* 96 *Miles. Lat. in South* 69°13′. *Longd. in W. Reck.g.* 105°39′. Fresh breezes and thick foggy weather with Showers of Snow, piercing cold air; the Snow and Moistness of the fog gave a Coat of Ice to our riging of near an Inch thick. Towards noon had intervals of tolerable clear weather.

[FEBRUARY 1774]

TUESDAY 1*st. Therm.r. at Noon* 35. *Winds Easterly. Course NBE. Dist. Sailed* 74 *Miles. Lat. in South* 68°1′. *Longd. in W. Reck.g.* 105°00′. In the PM the Fog dissipated after which the weather was gloomy and Clowdy, the air very Cold, yet the Sea was pretty clear of ice.

WEDNESDAY 2*nd. Therm.r. at Noon* 37. *Winds ESE. Course N* 27°30′ *E. Dist. Sailed* 61 *Miles. Lat. in South* 67°7′. *Long. in W. Reck.g.* 103°46′. Gentle breezes and Clowdy. At 2 o'Clock in the PM faling in with a few pieces of Ice, which had brok from an Island to windward, we hoisted out two Boats and took up as much as yeilded five or Six Tons of Water, and then hoisted in the Boats and made sail again to the Northward with a gentle breeze at East and ESE and a Swell from ENE. At Noon only two Ice islands in Sight and but very few Birds have been seen for some days past.

THURSDAY 3*rd. Therm.r. at Noon* 33. *Winds SE. Course N* 56° *E. Dist. Sailed* 75 *Miles. Lat. in South* 66°25′. *Long. in W. Reck.g.* 101°8′. Gentle breezes and Clowdy with some Showers of Snow. In the PM pass'd an Island of Ice, but nothing else worthy of note.

FRIDAY 4*th. Therm.r. at Noon* 34½. *Winds SE to NE. Course N* 38° *E. Dist. Sailed* 55 *Miles. Lat. in South* 65°42′. *Long. in W. Reck.g.* 99°44′. Little Wind and Clowdy. PM Variation 22°33′ E, AM 24°49′. AM clear pleasent Weather, but the air very cold.

SATURDAY 5*th. Therm.r. at Noon* 38½. *Winds NE to E, ENE. Course North. Dist. Sailed* 96 *Miles. Lat. in South* 64°6′. *Long. in W. Reck.g.* 99°44′. First part Little wind and pleasent Weather. In the PM found the Variation to be 26°35′ E. In the night the wind increased to a fresh gale and in the AM it blew in Squalls attended with Showers of Snow which at Noon obliged us to take a reef in our Top-sails. Saw a

Grampuss or small whale, but very few birds or any other signs of land.

SUNDAY 6*th.*[1] At 1 pm took the second reef in the Top-sails and got down Top g[t] yards which was no sooner done than it fell Calm and soon after had variable breezes between the NW and East, attended with Snow and Sleet. In the AM we got the wind from the South, loosed all the reefs out,[2] got top-g[t] yards and set the Sails and steered North-Easterly, with a resolution to proceed directly to the North as there was no probability of finding Land in these high Latitudes, at least not on this side Cape Horn and I thought it equally as improbable any should be found on the other side, but supposing the Land laid down in M[r] Dalrymples Chart to exist or that of Bouvets, before we could reach either the one or the other the Season would be too far spent to explore it this Summer, and obliged us either to have wintered upon it, or retired to Falkland Isles or the Cape of Good Hope, which ever had been done, Six or Seven Months must have been spent without being able in that time to make any discovery what ever, but if we had met with no land or other impediment we must have reached the last of these places by April at farthest when the expedition would have been finished so far as it related to the finding a Southern Continent, mentioned by all authors who have written on this subject whose assertions and conjectures are now intirely refuted as all there enquiries were confined to this Southern Pacific Ocean[3] in which altho' there lies no continent there is however room for very large Islands, and many of those formerly discover'd within the Southern Tropick are very imperfectly explored and there situations as imperfectly known. All these things considered, and more especially as I had a good Ship, a healthy crew and no want of Stores or Provisions[4] I thought I cou'd not do better than to spend the insuing Winter within the Tropicks: I must own I have little expectation of makeing any valuable discovery, nevertheless it must be allowed that the Sciences will receive some im-

[1] In H Cook inserts the observations for this day: *Therm.* $39\frac{3}{4}$. *Winds Northerly. Course NE. Miles 17. Lat. 63°54′ S. Long. R. 99°16′ W. Long. C.P. 85°22′.* He inserts additional figures for the other dates 1–8 February, but they need not be printed.

[2] The discipline of the young gentlemen was still tight. 'M[r] Maxwell in unbending the Main topsail, Cut it in several Places; for which he was Order'd off the Quarter Deck to do Duty before the Mast'.—Elliott.

[3] This is not entirely true: the traditional Terra Australis had never been confined to the Pacific ocean, and Gonneville was supposed to have discovered it in the South Atlantic. Dalrymple had it circling the world. But it is true that most of the discussion was in terms of the Pacific.

[4] 'no want of . . . Provisions'—the result of careful husbandry, which had led to the revolt referred to above, p. 317, n. 2.

provement therefrom especially Navigation and Geography. I had several times communicated my thoughts on this subject to Captain Furneaux, at first he seem'd not to approve of it, but was inclinable to get to the Cape of Good Hope, afterwards he seem'd to come into my opinion; I however could not well give any Instructions about it, as at that time it depended on so many circumstances and therefore cannot even guess how Captain Furneaux will act; be this as it will, my intintion is now to go in search of the Land said to be discovered by Juan Fernandas in the Latitude of 38° s, not finding any such Land, to look for Easter Island, the situation of which is so variously laid down that I have little hopes of finding [it].[1] I next intend to get within the Tropicks and proceed to the west on a rout differing from former Navigators, touching at, and settling the Situation of such Isles as we may meet with, and if I have time, to proceed in this manner as far west as Quiros's Land or what M. de Bougainville calls the Great Cyclades.[2] Quiros describes this Land, which he calls Tierra Austral[3] del Espiritu Santo, as being very large, M. de Bougainville neither confirms nor refutes this account. I think it a point well worth clearing up; from these isles my design is to get to the South and proceed back to the East between the Latitudes of 50 and 60°, designing if Possible to be the Length of Cape Horn in November next, when we shall have the best part of the Summer before us to explore the Southern part of the Atlantick Ocean. This I must own is a great undertaking and perhaps more than I shall be able to perform as various impediments may. . . .[4]

*SUNDAY 6th. After a few hours Calm we got a breeze at South which soon after freshened and fixed at wsw and was attended with Snow and Sleet. I now came to a resolution to proceed to the North and to spend the insuing Winter within the Tropick, if I met with no employment before I came there I was now well satisfied no Continent was to be found in this Ocean but what must lie so far to the South as to be wholy inaccessable for Ice and if one should be found in the Southern Atlantick Ocean it would be necessary to have

[1] Cook is referring both to the theory that Easter Island was in reality Davis's Land—which did mean a violent change in the position of Davis's Land as first reported—and to positions laid down by Dalrymple and others (lat. 27° s, long. 106°30′ w) and Pingré (lat. 28°30′ s, long. 123° w). See I, pp. lxxii, 289; and below, pp. 336, n. 7, 348–9.

[2] The New Hebrides, discovered by Quiros in 1606, rediscovered by Bougainville in 1768.

[3] i.e. Austrialia.

[4] The paragraph breaks off at 'may', as if Cook had been interrupted in his writing, or perhaps had come for the time being to the end of his thought. This is the last entry in the fourth section of the MS, a page and a half (or rather more) being left blank, as if he had every intention to resume and finish; but when he did resume this topic it was to redraft the entry for B, as given in the next paragraph on this page.

the whole Summer before us to explore it, on the other hand, if it proves that there is no land there, we undoubtedly might have reached the Cape of Good Hope by April and so have put an end to the expedition, so far as it related to the finding a Continent, which indeed was the first object of the expedition. But for me at this time to have quited this Southern Pacifick Ocean, with a good Ship, expressly sent out on discoveries, a healthy crew and not in want of either Stores or Provisions, would have been betraying not only a want of perseverance, but judgement, in supposeing the South Pacific Ocean to have been so well explored that nothing remained to be done in it, which however was not my opinion at this time; for although I had proved there was no Continent, there remained nevertheless room for very large Islands in places wholy unexplored and many of those which where formerly discovered, are but imperfectly explored and there Situations as imperfectly known; I was of opinion that my remaining in this Sea some time longer would be productive of some improvements to Navigation and Geography as well as other Sciences. I had several times communicated my thoughts on this Subject to Captain Furneaux but as it then wholy depended on what we might meet with to South, I could not give it in orders without runing the risk of drawing us from the Main Object. Sence now nothing had happened to prevent me from carrying them into execution, my intention was, first to go in Search of the land, said to have been discovered by Juan Fernandes above a Century ago,[1] in about the Latitude of 38°; if I failed of finding this land, then to go in Search of Easter Island or Davis's land, whose Situation is known with so little certainty that the attempts lately made to find it have miscarried.[2] I next intended to get within the Tropick and then proceed to the West, touching at and settling the Situations of Such isles as we might meet with till we arrived at Otaheite where it was necessary I should touch to look for the Adventure. I had also thoughts of runing as far West as the Tierra Austral del Espiritu Santo, discovered by Quiros and which M. de Bougainville calls the Great Cyclades. Quiros Speaks of this land as being large or lying in the neighbourhood of large lands, and as this is a point which Bougainville has neither confirm'd nor refuted, I thought it well worth clearing up. From this Land, my design was

[1] This is not the actual island Juan Fernandez, discovered by that celebrated pilot in 1563, which was perfectly well known—lat. 33°36′ s, long. 78°45′ w; but the continent he was alleged to have found some years later. See note, p. 332 below, where Cook has more to say on the subject.

[2] Presumably he refers to the searches carried out by Carteret in 1767 and Bougainville in 1768. He knew nothing of the Spanish expedition of 1770–1.

to Steer to the South and so back to the East between the Latitudes of 50° and 60° intending if possible to be the length of Cape Horn in November next, when we should have the best part of the Summer before us to explore the Southern part of the Atlantick Ocean. Great as this design appeared to be, I however thought it was possible to be done and when I came to communicate it to the officers[1] I had the satisfaction to find that they all heartily concur'd in it. I should not do my officers Justice if I did not take some oppertunity to declare that they allways shewed the utmost readiness to carry into execution in the most effectual manner every measure I thought proper to take. Under such circumstances it is hardly necessary to say that the Seamen were always obedient and alert and on this occasion they were so far from wishing the Voyage at an end that they rejoiced at the Prospect of its being prolonged a nother year and soon enjoying the benefits of a milder Climate.*—ff. 164–5.

MONDAY 7*th.* [*Therm.*] 40. [*Winds*] *South to West.* [*Course*] *NBE.* [*Dist.*] 171 *Miles.* [*Lat.*] 61°6′. [*Long.*] 98°13′. The Wind veered in the PM to the SW and at last fixed at West and blew a hard gale Attended with snow and sleet.[2] At 11 o'Clock as we were takeing in the Top-sails, a Squall of wind took hold of them and tore them all to pieces, this loss was not great as they had already done much service and were worn to the very utmost: it was not long before others were bent and set close reef'd and we continued to advance to the North at a good rate.[3] Towards Noon the wind was more moderate and the weather fair. Saw a sm[l] diver and yesterday a nother.

TUESDAY 8*th.* [*Therm.*] 41½. [*Winds*] *West* & *SW.* [*Course*] *N* 6° *E.* [*Dist.*] 184 *Miles.* [*Lat.*] 58°5′. [*Long.*] 97°24′. Fresh gales and fair weather; except in the night when the Wind blew in Squalls attended with both Snow and Sleet. A prodigious Swell from SW.

WEDNESDAY 9*th.* [*Therm.*] 47. [*Winds*] *West.* [*Course*] *North.* [*Dist.*] 146 *Miles.* [*Lat.*] 55°39′. [*Long.*] 97°24′. Fresh gales and Squally hazy weather with some rain. AM saw many birds, Sheer-waters, blue Petrels &c[a].

THURSDAY 10*th.* [*Therm.*] 47. [*Winds*] *Westerly.* [*Course*] *North.* [*Dist.*]

[1] *Deleted* (who till now thought we were bound directly to the Cape of Good Hope)

[2] 'In this storm, the service bearing hard upon the mariners, the captain, to ease them as much as possible, very humanely ordered the officers mates before the mast.'—Marra, p. 128. The officers' (i.e. warrant officers') mates may have thought less highly of the captain's humanity.

[3] 'AM at daylight we find the two Topsails abovemention'd most confoundedly shatter'd and torn, great part of the Canvass blown overboard so the Captain order'd one to be cut up to mend the other'.—Clerke.

124 *Miles.* [*Lat.*] 53°37′. [*Long.*] 97°24′. The same Wind and Weather continued in some degree till the AM when we had fair Weather and a great Swell from the Westward.

FRIDAY 11*th.* [*Therm.*] 51. [*Winds*] *West to NW.* [*Course*] *N* 39° *E.* [*Dist.*] 150 *Miles.* [*Lat.*] 51°46′. [*Long.*] 94°47′. PM fresh gales and fair Weather. AM had strong gales and hazy with rain, which brought us under double reef'd Top-sails.

SATURDAY 12*th.* [*Winds*] *NW to SW.* [*Course*] *N* 12° *W.* [*Dist.*] 93 *Miles.* [*Lat.*] 50°15′. [*Long.*] 93°18′. In the Evening the gale abated, after which had fair but Clowdy wea^{r}. In the AM Loosed all the reefs out, got Top g^{t} yards aCross and set the Sails.

SUNDAY 13*th.* [*Therm.*] 52. [*Winds*] *NW.* [*Course*] *N* 86° *W.* [*Dist.*] 23 *Miles.* [*Lat.*] 50°15′. [*Long.*] 96°1′. PM had Light airs next to a Calm, put a Boat in the Water in which some of the officers went and shott several Birds,[1] Albatroses and Sheer-waters, and one of those we call Port Egmont Hens, they are of the gull kind,[2] all of a dark brow[n] Plumage except the wings where there is a little white.[3] At 6 o'Clock in the Evening being in Lat 50°10′ S, the Variation was 12°58′ East; a few hours after a breeze sprung up at NW with which we stretched to NE till midnight then Tacked & stood SW, having a vast Swell from the same quarter. In the AM a piece of Wood, a piece of Sea Weed and a small Diver was seen.

MONDAY 14*th.* [*Therm.*] 53. [*Winds*] *NW.* [*Course*] *N* 46° *W.* [*Dist.*] 45 *Miles.* [*Lat.*] 49°42′. [*Long.*] 95°11′. Continued to stretch to the SW with a fresh gale at NW till 8 o'Clock pm when we tacked and stretched to ye North or NE under single reef'd Top-sails and Courses, having a fresh gale and thick Misty weather with small rain.

TUESDAY 15*th.* [*Therm.*] 54. [*Winds*] *SW, NNE to NW.* [*Course*] *N* 29° *W.* [*Dist.*] 37 *Miles.* [*Lat.*] 49°10′. [*Long.*] 95°38′. In the PM had light Airs next to a Calm and Clear Weather. In Lat 49°38′ S, same Longitude as on the preceeding Noon, the Variation was 13°42½′ East. At 4 AM a breeze sprung up at NNE with which we stood to the Westward till noon, then Tack'd, the wind having veered to NW attended with thick weather.

WEDNESDAY 16*th.* [*Therm.*] 56. [*Winds*] *NW.* [*Course*] *N* 31°45′ *E.* [*Dist.*] 100 *Miles.* [*Lat.*] 47°45′. [*Long.*] 94°19′. PM Thick Misty

[1] . . . on which we feasted the next day . . .—f. 165v.

[2] . . . about the size of a raven

[3] *except . . . white:* except the underside of each wing where there are some white feathers.

Weather with small rain and a great swell from SW. AM fair weather, but hazy, swell mostly from NW.[1]

THURSDAY 17*th*. [*Therm.*] 55. [*Winds*] *NW*. [*Course*] *N* 12½° *E*. [*Dist.*] 91 *Miles*. [*Lat.*] 46°16′. [*Long.*] 93°52′. PM Fresh gales and hazy with a very great swell from WNW and NW. In the Evining handed the Mizen Top-sail, double reef'd the Fore and Main Top-sails and got down Top-g[t] Yards. In the night had frequent Squalls with rain. In the AM had fair weather and a Moderate gale, Loosed the 2nd reefs out of the Top-sails, set the Mizen Top-sail, got Topg[t] yards a cross and set the Sails.

FRIDAY 18*th*. [*Therm.*] 50⅓. [*Winds*] *NW to SW*. [*Course*] *N* 2° *W*. [*Dist.*] 126 *Miles*. [*Lat.*] 44°11′. [*Long.*] 93°55′. Very fresh gales and Squally, with Showers of rain in the night, towards noon had fair and clear weather, and a very great swell from SW. Some Albatros's and other Birds about the Ship.

SATURDAY 19*th*. [*Therm.*] 58½. [*Winds*] *SW to W*. [*Course*] *N* 25° *W*. [*Dist.*] 139 *Miles*. [*Lat.*] 42°5′. [*Long.*] 95°20′. Fresh gales and fair Weather. At 3 o'Clock in the PM our Longitude p[r] Mean of Several Lunar Observations[2] was 94′19′30″ West, the watch at the same time gave 94°46′ W.[3] We are now nearly upon the Track of the Dolphin Captain Wallis, having cross'd that of the Endeavour two days ago, my intention was to have kept more to the West, but the winds prevailing in that quarter has unavoidably force'd me on the Tracks of these two Ships.[4]

SUNDAY 20*th*. [*Therm.*] 66. [*Winds*] *WNW*. [*Course*] *N* 14° *E*. [*Dist.*] 131 *Miles*. [*Lat.*] 39°58′. [*Long.*] 94°37′. Fresh gales and clear pleasent weather. Swell from west.[5]

MONDAY 21*st*. [*Therm.*] 67½. [*Winds*] *WNW*. [*Course*] *NBE*. [*Dist.*] 128 *Miles*. [*Lat.*] 37°54′. [*Long.*] 94°5′. Fresh breezes and fine pleasent weather, a Number of Grampuses playing about the Ship, but very few birds to be seen.

TUESDAY 22*nd*. [*Therm.*] 69. [*Winds*] *WNW to SW*. [*Course*] *N* 21°30′

[1] 'It is a little remarkable that in all our track to the Southward, this Season, we have never once seen the least Glimpse of the Southern Lights; Indeed I don't, at present, recollect that we have had one night, in all the time, clear enough for their appearance.'—Wales.

[2] . . . by M[r] Wales, Clerke, Gilbert and Smith,

[3] . . . As we advanced to the North we felt a most sencible change in the weather.

[4] See I, Figs. 5, 10.

[5] . . . The day was clear and pleasent and I may venture to say the only summers day we had had sence we left Newzealand.—f. 166.

W. [*Dist.*] 112 *Miles.* [*Lat.*] 36°10′. [*Long.*] 94°56′.[1] Fresh gales and pleasent weather,[2] Being now in the Latitude in which most Geographers place the discovery of Juan Fernandes. Mr Dalrymple places the Eastern side of this Land under the meridian of 90° and Mr Pengre in 111°, and in a note quotes the Authority from whence he has it, by which indeed it appears, they are two different discoveries or Else the same land discovered at two different Periods. I think it can'ot lie to the East of the Situation Mr Dalrymple has given it and if it lies in that situation it can have no great extent East and west, for if it has we ought either to see it or some signs of it. Mr Pengres situation falls under the like observation for the Endeavour cross'd these Latitudes in the Meridian of 112°; and Captain Wallis in about 98 or 100 without seeing the least signs of land; it is therefore plain that it can be no more than a small Island but I think it as probable that the whole is a fiction and that no such discoveries were ever made. See what is said on this Subject in Mr Dalrymple's Col. of Voyage[s] to the S. S.[3]

*We still continued to Steer to the North as the Wind remained in its old quarter and the next day at Noon we were in the Latitude 37°54′ s, which was the same as Juan Fernandes's discovery is said to lie in, we however had not the least signs of any land being in our neighbourhood. The next day at Noon Tuesday 22nd We were in Latitude 36°10′ s, Longitude 94°56′ w. Soon after the Wind veered to South South East and inabled us to Steer wsw which I thought the most probable direction to find the land we were in search after, and yet I had no hopes of Succeeding as we had a large hollow swell from the same point. We however Continued this Course till the 25th when the Wind having veered again round to the Westward, I gave it up and stood away to the North in order to get into the Latitude of Easter Island: our Latitude at this time was 37°52′ Longitude 101°10′ w: Var. 6°31′ E: I was now well assured that this discovery of Juan Fernandes, if any such was ever made, can be nothing

[1] In H Cook has written further observations for the dates 22 February–11 March, and all the observations for 7–11 March are in his hand. The additional figures note the longitudes by watch, except on five days, and the longitudes made from Cape Palliser. Those by watch are ahead of those by observation, as here printed, by amounts varying from 26½′ (25 February) to 1°5′ (8 March).

[2] 'Punish'd Jno Ennel [Innell] with a dozen, Jno Leverick and Richd Lee with a ½ dozen each for drunkenness and neglect of duty'.—Clerke. The question is, where did these men get the liquor to become drunk on? It could only have been by theft; perhaps they tapped the wine in the hold according to the traditional habit and made themselves stupid. There is a further question, where Leverick and Lee came from, for their names are not in the muster books.

[3] Cook's expansion of this entry is printed in the following paragraph, to which is attached the necessary annotation.

but a small Island, there being hardly room for a large land as will fully appear by the tracks made by Captain Wallis, Bougainville, the Endeavour and this of the Resolution. Whoever wants to see an account of the discovery in question I must refer them to Mr Dalrymples Collection of Voyages to the South Seas. This gentleman places it under the Meridian of 90° where I think it cannot be for M de Bougainville seems to have run down under that Meridian and we have now examined the Latitude in which it is satd to lie from the Meridian of 94° to 101°; it is not probable it can lie to the East of 90 because if it did, it must have been seen at one time or a nother by Ships bound from the Northern to the Southern parts of America. Mr Pengre in a little Treatise concerning the Transit of Venus published in 1768, gives some account of land having been discovered by the Spaniards in 1714, in the Latitude of 38° and 550 Leagues from the Coast of Chili, which is in the Longitude of 110° or 111° w and which is within a degree or two of my track in the Endeavour, so that this can hardly be its situation; In short the only probable situation it can have must be about the Meridian of 106° or 108° and then it can only be a small isle as I have allready observed.[1]*—f. 166–6v.

[1] The 'discovery of Juan Fernandes' referred to in this entry has nothing to do with the island now known by his name, but refers to what Dalrymple calls his 'great discovery about 1576'. This 'discovery' is first described in the memorial of Dr Juan Luis Arias that Dalrymple prints in his *Collection*, I, pp. 53–4. (A modern version of the famous document will be found in Markham's *Voyages of Pedro Fernandez de Quiros* [Hak. Soc., 1904], II, pp. 517–36.) At the end of this *Collection*, II, Dalrymple reprints from his *Account* of 1767 the 'Investigation of what may be farther expected in the South Sea'; on p. 19 of which he writes, 'In the first place must be mentioned the discovery of Juan Fernandes, who in the passage from Lima to Chili, having stood to the westward a certain distance, for the advantage of a fair wind, steered south till he discovered land, which he supposed to be the Southern Continent, as he saw on the coast the mouths of very large rivers, from whence, and from what the natives intimated, he formed his conclusion. The country was very fertile and agreeable, and appeared much better and richer than Peru. It was inhabited by white people, of our stature, very well disposed, and cloathed with very fine cloths'. It is in the *Account* that Dalrymple gives the position: 'The exact situation of this discovery is not distinctly related, but it appears to be about 40° s. long. about 90° w.' Cook deduces the 111° from Pingré, whose 'Authority' Dalrymple (p. 19 n.) also gives: Pingré quotes a '*Memoire pour la France, servant à la decouverte des Australes*, published by a *Mariner of St. Malo, named Bénard de la Harpe*', that 'in 1714 the Captain of a Spanish Brigantine going from Callao to the island of Chiloe, being in 38° s, at 550 leagues w a Chili; discovered a high country which he coasted a whole day; that he judged it inhabited from the fires which were seen in the night, and that the contrary winds obliging him to put into Concepcion, he found there the ship *Le François* of St. Malo commanded by Monsieur du Fresne,—Marion [Marion du Fresne, less celebrated than the later explorer of that name] who asserted that he had seen the Spanish captain's journal and found there the fact above recited'. Dalrymple suggests that the latitude should be 28° and not 38°; in which case, Corney suggests in his turn (II, p. 180 n.) the Spanish captain may have sighted Easter Island. In latitude 38° there is nothing but water between South America and New Zealand; but as late as 1785, in spite of Cook, La Pérouse was directed to search for the missing land. Pingré's pamphlet was published in 1767, not 1768; cf. I, p. 289.

WEDNESDAY 23*rd.* [*Winds*] *SE.* [*Course*] *S* 68°30′ *W.* [*Dist.*] 110 *Miles.* [*Lat.*] 36°40′. [*Long.*] 97°2′. At 2 pm the wind veer'd to SE blew a gentle gale attend with small rain, we now steer'd WSW in order to make a nother search for the land, being at this time in the Latitude of 36°39′, Long[de] 97°10′ W; circumstances gave us no hopes of finding what we were in search after, having continually a large swell from SW and West.[1]

THURSDAY 24*th.* [*Winds*] *NE to North.* [*Course*] *S* 61°30′ *W.* [*Dist.*] 94 *Miles.* [*Lat.*] 37°25′. [*Long.*] 98°44′. Gentle gales and fair weather. Set the Carpenters to work to repair the Boats. Sail-makers constantly at work repairing Sails.

FRIDAY 25*th.* [*Winds*] *North to NW.* [*Course*] *S* 78°15′ *W.* [*Dist.*] 118 *Miles.* [*Lat.*] 37°50′. [*Long.*] 101°8′. PM fresh gales and fair Weather. In the night squally with rain, AM fair weather, fresh gales with a great swell from westward.

SATURDAY 26*th.* [*Winds*] *SW.* [*Course*] *NNW½W.* [*Dist.*] 84 *Miles.* [*Lat.*] 36°37′. [*Long.*] 101°57′. At 1 o'Clock in the PM the wind shifting to SWBW we Tacked and stretched away to the NW giving over all farther search for Juan Fernandes land.[2] In the evening being in the Latitude of 36°7′ the Variation was 6°38′ East. Westerly swell still keeps up. At Noon steer'd NNW in order to get into the Long[de] of Easter Island.

SUNDAY 27*th.* [*Winds*] *SW to SSE.* [*Course*] *N* 15°30′ *W.* [*Dist.*] 108 *Miles.* [*Lat.*] 34°53′. [*Long.*] 102°33′. Gentle gales and Clear pleasent Weather. In the evening in Lat[de] of 36°1′ the Variation was 5°53′ E.

*I was now taken ill of the Billious colick and so Violent as to confine me to my bed, so that the Management of the Ship was left to M[r] Cooper my first Officer who conducted her very much to my satisfaction. It was several days before the most dangerous symptoms of my disorder were removed, during which time M[r] Patten the Surgeon was to me, not only a skilfull Physician but a tender Nurse and I should ill deserve the care he bestowed on me if I did not make this publick acknowledgement. When I began to recover, a favourate dog belonging to M[r] Forster fell a Sacrifice to my tender Stomack; we had no other fresh meat whatever on board and I could eat of this flesh as well as broth made of it, when I could taste nothing

[1] 'This day the Captain was taken ill, to the grief of all the ship's company.'—Marra, p. 134.

[2] 'Bore away for Easter Island there being but little probability of getting so far to the Westw[d] as Juan Fernandez land, provided there is such a place, as there is so great a swell from that Quarter'.—Cooper.

else, thus I received nourishment and strength from food which would have made most people in Europe sick, so true is it that necessity is govern'd by no law.[1]*—f. 166v.

MONDAY 28*th*. [*Winds*] *SE to NE*. [*Course*] *North*. [*Dist*.] 106 *Miles*. [*Lat*.] 33°7'. [*Long*.] 102°33'. Moderate breezes and clear pleasent weather. In the pm found the Variation to be 3°44' E. Latitude 34°28' S. AM saw some Egg Birds and Flying-fish.[2] The Birds were judged to be of that sort as seldom go above 60 or 80 Leagues from land, but of this we have no absolute certainty, no man yet knows to what distance the Aquatick Birds goes from land.[3]

[MARCH 1774]

TUESDAY 1*st*. [*Winds*] *Easterly to SW*. [*Course*] *N* 7° *W*. [*Dist*.] 60 *Miles*. [*Lat*.] 32°8'. [*Long*.] 102°47'. Gentle breezes and pleasent Weather. AM Variation 3°45' East. Same birds seen as yesterday.[4]

WEDNESDAY 2*nd*. [*Winds*] *WSW to WNW*. [*Course*] *N* 15° *E*. [*Dist*.] 58 *Miles*. [*Lat*.] 31°12'. [*Long*.] 102°29'. Gentle breeze and fine

[1] Forster, after reporting the beneficial effect of the warm weather on his father, continues (I, pp. 547–8): 'The warm weather . . . proved fatal to captain Cook's constitution. The disappearance of his bilious complaint during our last push to the south, had not been so sincere, as to make him recover his appetite. The return to the north therefore brought on a dangerous obstruction, which the captain very unfortunately slighted, and concealed from every person in the ship, at the same time endeavouring to get the better of it by taking hardly any sustenance. This proceeding, instead of removing, encreased the evil, his stomach being already weak enough before. He was afflicted with violent pains, which in the space of a few days confined him to his bed, and forced him to have recourse to medicines. He took a purge, but instead of producing the desired effect, it caused a violent vomiting, which was assisted immediately by proper emetics. All attempts however to procure a passage through his bowels were ineffectual; his food and medicines were thrown up, and in a few days a most dreadful hiccough appeared, which lasted for upwards of twenty-four hours, with such astonishing violence that his life was entirely despaired of. Opiates and glysters had no effect till repeated hot baths, and plasters of theriaca applied on his stomach, had relaxed his body and intestines. This however, was not effected till he had lain above a week in the most imminent danger'. On the 26th, Forster continues, Cook was recovering and in the following days was able to sit up and take a little soup. The sickness has been diagnosed as 'acute cholecystitis and complicating intestinal obstruction', by W. R. Thrower, 'Contributions to Medicine of Captain James Cook, F.R.S., R.N.', in the *Lancet*, CCXLI (1951, Vol. II), p. 218. In other words, Cook had an acute infection of the gall-bladder, with secondary paralysis of the bowel. As the sickness recurred slightly later, there may have been some underlying gall-stone trouble.

[2] . . . and Nodies.—f. 166v.

[3] . . . For my own part, I do not believe there is one in the whole tribe that one can rely on in pointing out the venicity [*sic*] of land.—f. 167. Marra (p. 135) reports on Cook: '. . . the captain this day much better, which each might read in the countenance of the other from the highest officer to the meanest boy on board the ship'.

[4] Forster now (I, p. 550) records the appearance of scurvy, with which he himself was badly afflicted. A number of other people 'crawled about the decks with the greatest difficulty'. Their stomachs were too weak, he adds, 'through abstinence from an unwholesome and loathed diet,' to take the wort in sufficient quantity for a cure. Cf. Wales, next note below.

Weather. Variation 4°34′ E. Egg birds still about the Ship and many fish which kept mostly under the Ships bottom so that we could catch none.[1]

THURSDAY 3*rd.* [*Winds*] *NW & NNW.* [*Course*] *N* 47° *E.* [*Dist.*] 51 *Miles.* [*Lat.*] 30°37′. [*Long.*] 101°45′. Light breezes and pleasent weather. pm Variation 4°38′ East. AM Saw some Tropic and Man of War birds.[2]

FRIDAY 4*th.* [*Winds*] *NNW, WNW.* [*Course*] *N* 46° *E.* [*Dist.*] 57 *Miles.* [*Lat.*] 29°56′. [*Long.*] 100°59′. Gentle breezes and fair weather. In the AM came on a great swell from SW.

SATURDAY 5*th.* [*Winds*] *NW & Calm.* [*Course*] *NE.* [*Dist.*] 17 *Miles.* [*Lat.*] 29°44′. [*Long.*] 100°45′. Light and Calm PM. Variation p^r Az^th 4°50′ E. AM Saw some Tropick and Egg birds, had a prodigeous swell from SW[3] so that no large land can possibly be in that quarter but from the many birds we see, which generally frequent the shores of land, we are in hopes of meeting with Davis or Easter Island.

SUNDAY 6*th.* [*Winds*] *NE.* [*Course*] *N* 38° *W.* [*Dist.*] 27 *Miles.* [*Lat.*] 29°23′. [*Long.*] 101°3′. PM Light airs and fine weather. Morning rain, towards noon fair weather and a gentle breeze at NE with which we steer'd NW. Several Petrels or Sheer waters and Eaggs Birds seen. The great SW Swell still continues.

MONDAY 7*th.* [*Winds*] *NEBE, East.* [*Course*] *N* 40°15′ *W.* [*Dist.*] 78 *Miles.* [*Lat.*] 28°20′. [*Long.*] 102°3′. Gentle breezes and pleasent weather. AM a large piece of Spung floated past the Ship. Variation 4°47′ E. In the AM caught four Albacores[4] about 25 or 30 pound each, which were very acceptable, they were about the Ship in vast numbers, but unfortunately we have no one on board who know the

[1] 'Omnium rerum Vicissitudo, say my brother Star-gazers; and though they have worn the expression thread-bare, I am fully convinced by experience it is not a jot the less true, for it's scarcely 3 weeks ago we were miserable on acc^o of ye cold: we are now wretched with ye heat: the latter is I think less supportable of ye two, as being attended with a sickly Appetite; but Salt Beef & pork, without vegetables for 14 weeks running, would probably cure a Glutton, even in England.'—Wales.

[2] 'This fore Noon saw a Tropic Bird, the first this trip to the N^oward—about 11 saw a Man of War Bird. We've seen but few of the Brown Egg Birds today I think its very probable we may have pass'd some spot of Land at no great distance, from seeing so many of those Birds, and now the Man of War Bird'.—Clerke.

[3] *a prodigeous* . . . *SW:* . . . we had a Calm for near two days together, during which the heat was intolerable, but what ought to be remarked was a very great swell from the SW.—f. 167. Cf. Wales: 'The South-west Swell considerably increased, which gives us some hopes of a wind from that quarter. We have much need of it, for the heat, this calm weather, is almost insupportable.—Wretched Sauce to salt Beef, and a bad Appetite!'

[4] A name generally applied to any large tunny-like fish.

art of catching them.[1] The SW swell as high as ever. Saw a Tropic and Man of War bird.

TUESDAY *8th.* [*Therm.*] 75½. [*Winds*] *Easterly.* [*Course*] *N* 52° *W.* [*Dist.*] 124 *Miles.* [*Lat.*] 27°4′. [*Long. by reckoning*] 103°58′. [*Long. by watch*] 105°3′. Gentle gales and fine pleasent weather. In the AM saw many Birds, such as Tropick, Men of War and Egg Birds of two sorts, grey[2] and White,[3] many sheer-waters or Petrels of two or three sorts, one sort small and almost all black, another sort much larger with dark grey backs and white bellies.[4] Swell not much and from the East.[5]

WEDNESDAY *9th.* [*Winds*] *Easterly.* [*Course*] *W* 2° *S.* [*Dist.*] 106 *Miles.* [*Lat.*] 27°7′. [*Long.*] 106°00′. Weather and winds as yesterday. Judgeing our selves by observation to be nearly in the Latitude of Davis's land or Easter Island we steer'd nearly due west meeting with the same sort of Birds as yesterday.[6]

THURSDAY *10th.* [*Therm.*] 76¾. [*Winds*] *Easterly.* [*Course*] *West, Southly.* [*Dist.*] 102 *Miles.* [*Lat.*] 27°9′. [*Long.*] 107°55′. In the evening took in the Studding Sails and ran under an easy sail during night, at day-light made all sail again, meeting with the same sort of Birds as yesterday and abundance of Albacores & flying fish not one of which we could catch.

FRIDAY *11th.* [*Therm.*] 75. [*Winds*] *Easterly.* [*Course*] *W* 2° *S.* [*Dist.*] 60 *Miles.* [*Lat.*] 27°11′. [*Long.*] 109°2′. Gentle breeze and pleasent weather. At Middnight brought to till day-light then made sail and soon after saw the Land from the Mast head bearing West.[7] At Noon it was seen from the deck extending from W¾N to WBS. Distant about 12 Leagues.[8]

[1] *In the AM . . . them:* We also saw plenty of fish, but we were such bad fishers that we caught only four albacores, which were very aceptable, especially to me who was just recovering from my late illness.—f. 167. Wales calls the fish caught bonitos: 'Catched five & ought to have got many More if our Tackling had not been bad'.

[2] These were almost certainly the Grey Noddy, *Procelsterna cerulea skottsbergii* Lönnberg.

[3] The White Tern, *Gygis alba royana* Mathews.

[4] These birds are unidentifiable: various migrating petrels might be in the vicinity of Easter Island at this time of year, and since the Forsters give no additional notes it is impossible to say which species were seen.

[5] 'Catched two more Bonitos, and lost several others through the badness of our Tackle.'—Wales.

[6] 'Several small pieces of Sponge went past the Ship & a small dryed leaf not much unlike a Bay-leaf . . . Many Men-of-War and Tropic Birds about the ship. Passed by a sea snake: it was speckled, black & white, & in every respect like those we used to see at Tonga and the Society Islands.'—Wales. Cook lifted most of this entry and incorporated it in his own for 8 March in B, f. 167—forgetting that Wales's 8th was his own 9th, ship time.

[7] 'The joy which this fortunate event spread on every countenance is scarcely to be described. We had been an hundred and three days out of sight of land. . .'.—Forster, I, p. 552.

[8] . . . I made no doubt but this was Davis Land or Easter Island, as its appearences from this situation corresponded very well with Wafers accou[n]t and we expected to

SATURDAY 12*th*. At 7 o'Clock in the pm being about 5 Leagues from the island which extending from N 62° W to N 87° W we sounded but had no ground with a line of 140 fathoms; we now Shortned Sail

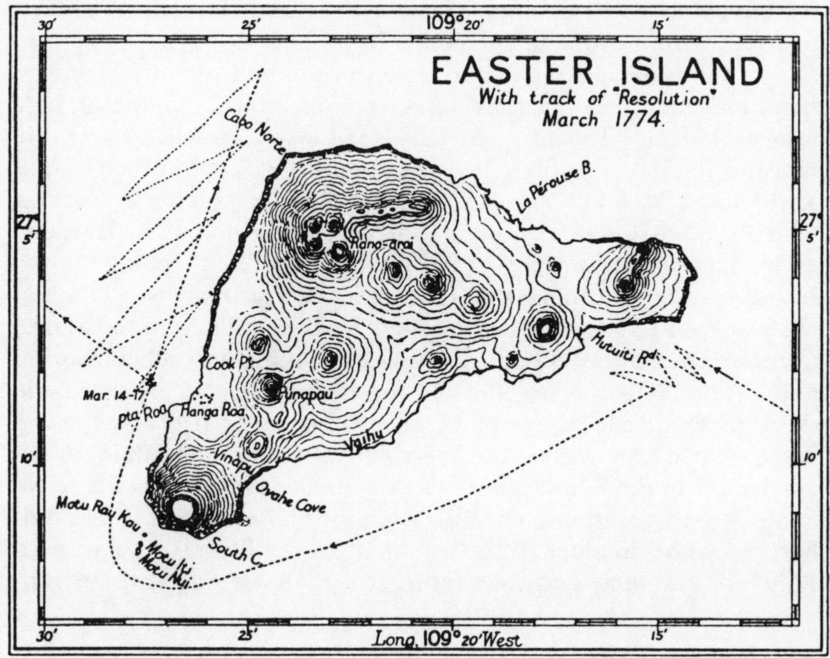

FIG. 54

and Stood off SE & SSE having but very little wind and at 2 am it fell quite calm, and continued so till 10 AM when a breeze sprung up at SW & WSW with which we stood in for the land the extremes of which at Noon bore from NW to west by North distant 4 or 5 Leagues. Lat ob^d 27° South.

have seen the low Sandy Isle which Davis fell in with, which would have been a confirmation, but in this we were disapointed.—f. 167–7v.—They were disappointed because of course Easter Island was not Davis Land. Wafer's account (in his *New Voyage*, 1699), as printed by Dalrymple (*Collection*, II, p. 123), runs, 'We steered S and by E, half easterly, until we came to the lat. of 27°20′ S; when, about two hours before day, we fell in with a small, low, sandy island, and heard a great roaring noise, like that of the sea beating upon the shore, right a-head of the ship. . . . we plyed off till day and then stood in again with the land; which proved to be a small flat island, without the guard of any rocks. We stood in within a quarter of a mile of the shore, and could see it plainly, for it was a clear morning, not foggy nor hazy. To the westward, about twelve leagues by judgment, we saw a range of high land, which we took to be islands, for there were several partitions in the prospect. This land seemed to reach about fourteen or sixteen leagues in a range; and there came hence great flocks of fowls'.

SUNDAY 13*th*. In stretching in for the land we discovered[1] people and those Moniments or Idols mentioned by the Authors of Roggeweins Voyage[2] which left us no room to doubt but it was Easter Island. At 4 o'Clock we were within about half a League of the NE point, bearing NNW where we found 35 fathom a dark sandy bottom. We plyed to windward in order to get into a Bay which appeared on the SE side of the isle,[3] but night put a stop to our endeavours, which we spent makeing short boards, Soundings from 75 to 110 fathoms, bottom dark Sand. During night the wind was variable, but in the morning it fixed at SE, blew in squals attended with rain which ceased as the day advanced. The wind now blowing right on the SE shore on which the Sea broke very high and there being no bay or Harbour as we had immag[in]ed, I steer'd round the South point[4] of the Island in order to explore the western side, accordingly we ran along the western and NW side at the distance of one mile from the Shore, untill we open'd the nothern point without seeing any safe anchoring place. The Natives were collicted together in several places on the shore in small companies of 10 or 12. The most likely anchoring place we had seen was on the West side of the isle [5] miles to the northward of the South point before a small sandy beach where we found 40 and 30 fathoms one mile from the Shore, Bottom dark sand, here a Canoe conducted by two Men came off and brought us a Bunch of Plantans[6] and then returned a shore.[7] Seeing no better an-

[1] *we discovered:* by the help of our glass we discovered

[2] By 'the authors of Roggeweins Voyage' Cook certainly means the authors quoted in Dalrymple's *Collection*, vol. II. Dalrymple uses, first, the French translation (1739) of the German account of Behrens (Leipzig 1738), who commanded Roggeveen's marines (pp. 89–95); and second, an anonymous Dutch account, printed at Dordrecht in 1728 and reprinted in 1758 (pp. 111–15). Of the first, he says (p. 85), it is 'a very poor performance, written with much ignorance, though with the parade of knowledge'; of the value of the second he also has his doubts. Both accounts refer to 'idols', pp. 94–5, 114–15.

[3] From the look of the chart, XXXI*a*, this was the cove or anchorage of Hutuiti, but as Cook found next morning, there was nothing there in the nature of a harbour.

[4] The text of B here varies without adding anything, except that 'South point' is followed by 'off which lies two small Islots, the one nearest the point is high and peaked and the other low and flatish'.—f. 167v. The first, a rock 230 feet high, was Motu-kaukau (or Rau Kau); the second was really two rocks, Motu-iti and Motu-nui, Motu-nui being larger than the others; these two are steep though flattish, and the highest point is 174 feet—hardly 'low', except by contrast. Cook could easily miss seeing Motu-iti, which lies behind Motu-nui. The South Cape is itself high and conspicuous. See the view, Chart XXXI*a*.

[5] The distance is not mentioned in B. It is about three miles.

[6] . . . which they sent into the Ship by a rope . . . f. 168.—'Some Hours before we Anchor'd a couple of the Natives came off and brought us a Bunch of ripe Plantins (a most gratefull Present) then return'd again to the shore seemingly exceedingly pleas'd and happy with a couple of Medals which they got in return.'—Clerke, account of Easter Island, following 16 March.

[7] . . . This gave us a good opinion of the Islanders and inspired us with hopes of geting some refreshments which we were in great want of.—f. 168.

chorage than the one just mentioned we Tacked and Plyed back to the South in order to gain it.

MONDAY 14*th*. At half past 6 o'Clock pm Anchored at the place before mentioned in 36 fathom Water, the bottom a fine dark sand.[1] Having sent the boat in shore to sound one of the natives swam off to her, came on board and remained with us all night and next day, this confidence gave us a favourable Idea of the rest of the Natives.[2] At 3 am a breeze from the land drove us of the bank, which after the Anchor was up we plyed in for again and in the mean time I went a shore[3] to inform my self if any refreshments or Water were to be got. We landed at the sandy beach where about 100 of the Natives were collected who gave us no disturbance at landing,[4] on the contrary hardly one had so much as a stick in their hands. After distributing among them some Medals and other trifles, they brought us sweet Potatoes, Plantains and some Sugar cane which they exchanged for Nails &c[a]; after having found a small Spring or rather Well made by the Natives, of very brackish Water, I returned on board and anchored the Ship in 32 f[m] Water, the bottom a fine dark sand, something more than a mile from the Shore.[5]

TUESDAY 15*th*. PM Got on board a few Casks of Water and Traded with the Natives for some of the produce of the island which appeared in no great plenty and the Water so bad as not to be worth carrying on board, and the Ship not in safety determined me to shorten my stay here. Accordingly I sent Lieutenants Pickersgill and Edgcumb with a party of Men, accompanied by M[r] Forster and several more of the gentlemen, to examine the Country; I was not sufficiently recovered from a fit of illness[6] to make one of the party.

[1] The anchorage was off the south point of Hanga-roa bay, Punta Roa. It is about 1¾ miles from here to the north extreme of the bay, Cook point. From this point to Cabo Norte, the north-western extremity of the island itself, is 4¾ miles; Cook had this cape visible from his anchorage. The island is not big; its longest direct distance, from west to east, is only 13 miles.

[2] *one of . . . natives:* one of the Natives swam off to her and insisted on coming on board the ship where he remained two nights and a Day. The first thing he did after coming on board, was to measure the length of the Ship by fathoming her from the Tafferl to the Stern and as he counted the fathoms we observed that he called the Numbers by the same names as they do at Otaheite, Nevertheless his Languish [*sic*] was in a manner wholy unintillegible to all of us.—f. 168. Forster describes this man at length (I, pp. 560–2), and gives his name as 'Maroowahai'.

[3] . . . accompaned by some of the gentlemen

[4] *where . . . landing:* where some hundreds of the Natives were assembled and who were so impatient to see us, that many of them swam off to meet the Boats.—f. 168.

[5] '. . . the women (which seem very few) soon came in the boats & settled their matters'. —Mitchel.

[6] The reader will note that this is Cook's first mention of his illness in this MS.

At the Ship employed geting on Board Water and tradeing with the Natives.

WEDNESDAY 16*th*. About 7 in the evening the exploaring party returned and the next morning Mr Pickersgill made me the following report.

' Remarks '

' Sir,

' At ½ past 9 o'Clock we left the beach, and took to a Path leading a cross the Isthmus,[1] as we advanced we pass'd some few Plantations (chiefly Potatoes) but the Country had much the same barren appearence as near where the Ship lays, being full of Stones Rocks and dry hard clay; but when we came about the Middle of the Isthmus the land towards the South hills seem'd more fertile, bore a longer grass and was free from stones tho' as we came towards the eastern shore we again got amongst the Stoney ground.

' At ½ past 10 we got to the Eastern Sea side where we found a row of Stone Images whose names we got from the Natives and by what I could understand from them, they were errected to the memory of their chiefs; for they had all different Names and they allways call'd them *Areekes*[2] which I understood to be King or chief; and they did not seem to pay that respect to them, that I should think they would to a Deity; they bore the same figure as the rest and wheather they are Sement or Stones I'm sure I cannot tell only from their appearence they seem'd to be the latter.[3]

' The East shore is all steep clifts and the shore so rocky, which with the great surf I think renders it impossible for a boat to land;[4] here we search'd for water but could find none nor could the Natives tell us of any. We had many of the Natives went with us a cross the Isthmus and one man constantly kept a head of us carrying a white flag who seem'd to direct the crowd.[5]

[1] i.e. the south-west corner of the island, from Hanga-roa to Ovahe cove.

[2] *ariki*, a chief, nobleman.

[3] A *note* I have not the least doubt but it is stone. . .—They were, of course, stone, but the rough surface of the trachyte, the volcanic stone out of which they were hewn, might perhaps convey an impression that they were moulded out of some cement mixture—and thus, to use Cook's word, p. 358 below, 'factitious'.

[4] A *note*: This must depend on which way the wind blows, for when this is the lee side of the isle, it must be as good landing there as any where else. I believe it to have been on this side of the isle where Admiral Roggewein landed. . .—Cook is perfectly correct about landing; for Ovahe cove is the alternative anchorage to Hanga-roa in summer northerly gales. But he is wrong about Roggeveen, whose anchorage and landing were on the more eastern part of the northern coast, probably somewhere about La Pérouse bay, where there is a beach.

[5] This 'flag' was a sign of honour and friendship, such as was brought before the king.

' From this place we traveled about 3 miles further a long shore,[1] the man still carrying his flag and the Natives flocking round us to about 150 in Number; this part of the Country was very barren, hardly a house or Plantation to be seen and the rocks seem'd to contain Iron ore;[2] here the Path struck up a little from the Sea side and we pass'd some Plantations where the people behaved exceedingly civil, bring us dress'd Potatoes and plenty of Sug^r Cane but we could get no water but what was brackish. After passing this vally[3] we saw a number of men collected upon a hill some distance from us and some with spears but on the people which were with us calling to them they dispers'd except a few amongst [them] which was a man seemingly of some note, he was a stout made man with a fine open countenance, his face painted, his body tatowed and some thing whiter than the rest and he wore a better ah-hou,[4] he salluted us before we came to him by stretching out his arms with both hands clinch'd lifting them over his head, opening them wide and leting them fall gradually down to his sides, they told us he was the arreeke of the Island which they call'd *Wy-hu*, this they seem'd all to agree in.[5]

' Walking on further we stop'd on a hill to rest when one of the people taking off his bag to get some thing out, one of the natives catched it up and run off but Mr Edgecumb seeing him and being load^d with small shott fired at him on which he droped the bag and run off in the crowd, most of the rest run away tho' some few stayed and one man throwing off his ah-hou talked a good deal and then ran several times round us, and which they again spread their flag and we again went on passing by a number of very large Images many of them fallen down and broke the names of which I took going along, here we found a well of Midling water but very little of it and here the King came again to us and we persued our Journey to a hill from whence I saw all the East and North shores on which I could not see either Bays, places for boats to land or

[1] i.e. to the eastward.

[2] This was a bad guess: he may have been struck by the appearance of weathered lava. Pickersgill knew nothing about geology. Perhaps he got the idea from Wales: see p. 824 below.

[3] 'this valley': it is very difficult to guess what Pickersgill means by this, topographically, especially as he has not mentioned it before. He may mean that the path ran up a depression; Easter Island has no deep valleys.

[4] Tahitian *ahu*, cloak; the corresponding Easter Island word was *kahu*.

[5] 'Wy-hu' was Vaihu: the man may very well have been the *ariki* of the small district of this name, on the south coast, but not of the whole island. The 'king', the *ariki-mau*, would not have announced himself in that casual fashion. Nor did the island in general have a name at that time; the modern Polynesian name Rapa-nui seems to have been given some time in the nineteenth century. See Alfred Métraux, *Ethnology of Easter Island*, (B. P. Bishop Mus. Bull. 160, Honolulu 1940), pp. 33–6.

signs of Water, the flat land at the north end where we saw the num[r] of Images from the Ship seem'd to be better inhabited than the rest, from the number of houses and Images upon it. As we had no occasion to go farther we stop'd, dined and prepared to return over the hills, just as we were going away those few which were with us ran off and said there were bad men coming, and looking we saw a number of men coming in a body with the same flag they had before, but what terms they were coming upon we had not time then to wait to know, so takeing our road a Cross the hills for the ship the Natives left us except one man and a boy and Walking over a most desert barren country full of rocks and only three or four bushes not 5 feet high we arrived at the beach all heartily tired about 7 o'Clock having been by my estimation about 20 or 21 miles.

Rich[d] Pickersgill.'

This report of M[r] Pickersgills so far as it regarded the Produce of the Island was confirmed by the whole party and determined me to quit the island without further delay, a breeze of wind about 10 o'Clock Coming in from Sea, attended with heavy showers of rain made this the more necessary, accordingly we got under sail and stood out to Sea, but as we had but little wind I sent a boat a shore to purchase such refreshments as the Natives might have brought to the Water side.

*Not one of them had so much as a stick or a Weapon of any sort in their hands. After destributing a few trinkets amongst them, we made signs for some thing to Eat, on which they brought down a few Potatoes, Plantains and Sug[r] Cane and exchanged for Nails, Looking Glasses and pieces of Cloath. We presently discovered that they were as expert thieves and as trickish in their exchanges as any people we had yet met with. It was with some difficulty we could keep the Hatts on our heads, but hardly possible to keep any thing in our pockets not even what themselves had sold us, for they would watch every opertunity to snatch it from us, so that we some times bought the same thing two or three times over and after all did not get it. Before I sail'd from England, I was informed that a Spanish Ship had visited this isle in 1769,[1] some signs of it was seen among the people now about us. One Man had a pretty good broad brim'd European hat on; a nother had a Greko Jacket[2] and a nother had a

[1] The Spanish visit was in November 1770.

[2] A 'grego' was a sort of jacket with a hood, made of coarse stuff, and worn in the Levant—hence 'Greek'.

red silk handkerchief. They also seemed to know the use of a Musket (of which they stood in much awe) but this they probably learnt from Roggewein, who, if we are to believe the authors of that Voyage, left them sufficient tokens.[1] Near the place where we landed, were some of those Colossean Statues before mentioned, which I shall discribe in another place. The Country appeared barren and without wood, there were nevertheless several plantations of Potatoes, Plantains and sugar cane; we also saw some Fowls and found a well of Brackish Water. As these were articles we were in want of and as the Natives seemed not unwilling to part with them, I resolved to stay a day or two. With this view I repaired on board and brough[t] the Ship to an anchor in 32 fathom Water the bottom a fine dark Sand. Our Station was about a mile from the nearest shore, which was the South part of a small Bay in the bottom of which is the Sandy beach before mentioned, which bore ESE distant one and a half Mile. The two rocky islots lying off the South point of the Island were just shut behind a point to the North of them and bore S 6°30′ W four Miles distant, and the other extreme of the island bore N [25°][2] E Distant about Six Miles. But the best Mark for this anchoring place is the beach, because it is the only one on this side the island. In the after-noon we got on board a few Casks of Water and opened a trade with the Natives for such things as they had to dispose of, and some of the gentlemen made an excursion into the island to see what it produced and returned again in the evening with the loss only of a hat which one of the Natives snatched of the head of one of the party.[3]

TUESDAY 15*th*. Early in the Morning I sent Lieutenants Pickersgill and Edgecumb, with a party of Men, accompaned by several of the Gentlemen, to examine the Country; As I was not sufficiently recovered from my late illness to make one of the party, I was obliged to content my self with remain[g] at the landing place among the Natives. We had at one time a pritty brisk trade with them for Potatoes, which we observed they dig up out of an adjoining Plantation. But this trafick, which was very advantageous to us, was soon

[1] On 10 April 1722 Roggeveen was proceeding in elaborate military order to march into the country, but had hardly left the beach when the men in his rear, taking alarm at the behaviour of the 'Indians', fired without orders, and killed ten or twelve before he could stop them.

[2] The MS lacks the figure, which is supplied from the printed page.

[3] This was Hodges, who was sketching. Wales, who was standing by him with a musket, philosophically reflected that Hodges's hat was hardly worth a Polynesian life.—p. 822 below, and Forster, I, p. 573. The Easter Islanders had a special passion for headgear: Roggeveen, Gonzalez, Cook's men, La Pérouse, as well as later visitors, all report hat-snatching.

put a stop to, by the owner (as we supposed) of the plantation coming down and driving all the people out of it by this we concluded that he had been robed of his property and that they were not less Scrupulous of robing one another than they were us, on whome they practised every little fraud they could think on and generally with success, for we no sooner detected them of one than they found out another. About 7 o'Clock in the Evening, the party I had sent into the Country returned after having been over the greatest part of the island.

They left the Beach about 9 o'Clock in the Morning and took a path which lead across to the SE side of the island, followed by a great crowd of the Natives who pressed much upon them; but they had not proceeded far before a middle aged Man, punctured from head to foot and his face painted with a sort of white pigment,[1] appeared with a spear in his hand and walked along side of them, making signs to his Countrymen to keep at a distance and not to molest our people. When he had pretty well effected this, he hoisted a piece of White Cloth on his Spear, placed himself in the front and lead the way with his Ensign of Peace as they understood it to be. For the greatest part of the distance a Cross, the ground had but a barren appearence, being a dry hard Cley and every where covered with Stones; but notwithstanding this there were several large tracts planted with Potatoes and some Plantain Walks, but they saw no fruit on any of the trees. Towards the highest part of the South end of the island the Soil, which was a fine red earth, seemed much better, bore a longer grass and was not covered with stones as in the other parts; but here they saw neither house nor Plantation. On the East side of the Island near the Sea, they met with three Platforms of Stone work, or rather the ruins of them: on each had stood four of those large Statues, but they were all fallen down from two of them and also one from the third; every one except one were broken by the fall and otherways defaced.[2] Mr Wales measured this one and found it to be 15 feet in length and 6 feet broad over the Shoulders. Each Statue had on its head a large Cylindric Stone of a red

[1] The islanders painted themselves extensively with different-coloured volcanic earths dug from pits. The white pigment probably came from some unoxidised tuff.

[2] These platforms were *ahu*, which extended in some form or other all round the coast. They were used as burial vaults; and corresponded to the *marae* of other parts of Polynesia (e.g. Tahiti and the Society Islands, as Cook and Banks described them on the first voyage). Buck writes, 'Beyond the low inland curb a roughly paved area represented the paved court of the maraes of other groups. The entire enclosure was called *ahu*, a term used in central Polynesia to designate the raised platform at the end of the marae court'. —*Vikings of the Sunrise*, p. 234. The stonework of the facings of some of these platforms, says Métraux, 'are among the most perfect masonry work in Polynesia'; and 'The large image ahus are the masterpieces of Easter Island architecture'.—*Ethnology*, pp. 290, 284.

Colour worked perfectly round;[1] the one they measured, and that apparently not by the far the largest was 52 Inches high and 66 in diameter. In some the upper Corner of the cylinder was taken off in a sort of Concave quarter-round; but in others the Cylinder was intire. From this place they followed the direction of the Coast to the NE the man with the flag still leading the way. For about three Miles they found the Country very barren and in some places striped of the soil to the bare Rock, which seemed to be a poor sort of Iron Ore. Beyond this they came to the most fertile part of the island they saw; it being interspersed with large Plantations of Potatoes, Sugar Cane and Plantain trees and these not so much incumbered with Stones as those which they had seen before but they could find no Water, except what the Natives twice or thrice brought them, and although brackish and Stinking, their thirst was so great as to make it very exceptable. They also passed some Huts, the owners of which met them with roasted Potatoes and Sugar Canes and placed themselves ahead of the foremost of the party, (for the[y] Marched in a line in order to have the benefit of the path) gave to each man as he passed by one. They observed the same method in distributing the Water which they brought and were particularly carefull that the foremost did not drink too much, least none should be left for the hindmost. But at the very time these were relieving the thirsty and hungry, there were not wanting others who endeavourd to steal from them at every oppertunity and even to snatch from them the very things which had been given them by others. At last to prevent worse consequences, they were obliged to fire a load of small shott at one, who was so audacious as to snatch the bag which contained every thing they carried with them, from the Man who carried it. The shot hit him on the back, on which he droped the bag, ran a little way and then droped himself; but he afterwards got up and walked, and what became of him afterwards they knew not, or whether he was much wounded or no.

As this affair occasioned some delay, and drew the Natives together, they presently saw the Man who had hitherto led the way and one or two more coming runing towards them, but instead of

See also his *Easter Island*; and Heyerdahl, *Aku-aku*. The images faced inwards from the sea. The travellers seem to have been at Vinapu, where stood the finest *ahu* in the island. The prone statues may have been pushed over in the course of inter-tribal wars, or have fallen simply through neglect, their family owners having died out. Wars were certainly responsible for wholesale levelling of images.

[1] perfectly round *substituted for* so truly round that some thought they must have been turned into that form, but I think the size alone will . . .—The most persuasive theory about these cylinders is that they were formalized topknots or *pukao*. Heyerdahl sees in them the red hair of his Inca people; Métraux thinks they were a late innovation that did not have time to become universally adopted.

stoping when they came up, they continued to run round them repeating in a kind manner a few words, untill our people set forwards again, when thier old guide hoisted his flag and led the way as before and none ever attempted to steal from them the whole day afterwards. As they passed along they observed on a hill a number of People collected together, some of which had spears in their hands, but on being called to by their countrymen, they dispersed except a few, amongst which was one seemingly of some note. He was a stout well made man with a fine open Countinence, his face was painted, his body punctured and he wore a better Ha-hou or Cloth than the rest; he Saluted them as he came up, by stretching out his arms with both hands clinched, lifting them over his head, opening them wide and then leting them fall gradually down to his sides. To this man, which they understood was the Chief of the Island, their other friend gave his white flag, and he gave it to another who carried it before them the remainder of the day.

To wards the eastern end of the Island, they met with a well whose water was perfectly fresh, being considerably above the level of the Sea, but it was very dirty owing to filthyness, or cleanliness (call it which you will) of the Natives, who never go to drink without washing themselves all over as soon as they have done, and if ever so many of them are together the first leaps right into the Middle of the hole, drinks and washes himself without the least ceremony, after which another takes his place and does the same.

They observed that this side of the Island was full of those gigantic Statues so often mentioned, some placed in groups on Platforms of masonry, others single and without any, being fixed only in the Earth and that not deep; these latter are in general much larger than the others; They measured one which was fallen down and found it very near 27 feet long and upwards of Eight feet over the breast, or shoulders and yet this appeared considerably short of the size of one which they saw standing: its shade a little past two oClock, being sufficient to shelter all the party, consisting of near 30 persons, from the rays of the Sun.[1] Here they stoped to dine after which they repaired to a hill from whence they saw all the East and North shores of the isle, on which they could not see either Bay or Creek, not even fit for a Boat to land in, nor the least signs of fresh

[1] The isolated statues provide another puzzle. What evidence there is for a solution is marshalled by Métraux, *Ethnology*, pp. 297–8. They may have belonged to *ahu* that have disappeared; or marked boundaries, like the Tahitian *tii*; or, it has been suggested, have bordered some important road. The monster in the shade of which the party dined was, so Forster says (I, p. 591), called Mango-toto—i.e. Maunga Toatoa; he picked up other names (p. 587).

water. What was brought them here by the Natives was real Salt water, but they observed that some of them drank pretty plentifully of it; so far will necessity and custom get the better of Nature. On this account they were obliged to return to the last mentioned Well, where after having quenched their thirst, they directed their rout a Cross the Island towards the Ship, as it was now four o'Clock. In a small hollow, on the highest part of the island, they met with several of such Cylinders as are placed on the heads of the Statues, some of which appeared larger than any they had seen before, but it was now two late to stop to measure any of them. M[r] Wales from whom I had this information, is of opinion that this had been a quarey where these stones had formerly been dug, from whence he thinks it would have been no difficult matter to rol them down the hill after they were formed.[1] I think this a very reasonable conjecture and have no doubt but that it has been so. On the declivity of the Mou[n]tain towards the West, they met with another well; but the Water was a very strong Mineral, had a thick green scum on the top and stunk intolerably. Necessity however obliged some to drink of it, but it soon made them so sick that they threw it up the same way it went down.

In all this excursion as well as the one made the preceding day only two or three shrubs were seen, the leafs and seed of one (call[ed] by the Natives Torromedo)[2] was not much unlike those of the common Vetch, the pod indeed was more like that of a Tamarind in its size and shape. The Seeds have a disagreeable bitter taste and the Natives when they saw our people chew them, made signs to spit them out, from whence it was concluded that they think it poisonous. The wood is pretty hard of a redish Colour and rather heavy; but very crooked, small and short, not exceeding six or seven feet high. At the sw Corner of the island they found another small Shrub whose leafe was not much unlike that of an ash. The wood was white and brittle and in some measure resembling that of the asp.[3] They also saw in several places the Otaheite Cloth Plant[4] but it was poor and weak and not above 2½ feet high at most. They saw not an Animal of any sort and but very few Birds, or indeed any thing which can induce Ships, that are not in the utmost destress, to touch at this island. This account of the excursion I had from M[r]

[1] Wales was right; this was the quarry of red tufa, on the hill called Punapau. But the highest part of the island was Rano-aroi, in the northern corner.

[2] Toro-miro, *Sophora toromiro*. Forster called it a mimosa.

[3] It was the Marikuru, *Sapindus saponaria*. The asp is a poplar, *Populus tremula*; the printed *Voyage*, I, p. 285, makes it 'ash'. Cf. Wales, p. 827 below.

[4] Tahitian Aute, the paper mulberry, *Broussonetia papyrifera*.

Pickersgill and M[r] Wales, men on whose veracity I could depend and therefore I determined to leave the island the next Morning. Sence nothing was to be got that could make it worth my while to make a longer stay, for the Water which we had taken on board was not much better than if it had been taken up out of the Sea.

WEDNESDAY 16*th*. We had a Calm till 10 o'Clock in the Morning at which time a breeze sprung up at West accompaned with heavy showers of rain which lasted about an hour, the weather than cleared up and we got under sail and stood out to Sea, and kept plying to and fro while an officer was sent on Shore with two boats to purchas such refreshments as the Natives might have brought down; for I judged this would be the case, as they knew nothing [of] our sailing and the event proved that I was not misstaken, for the Boats made two trips before night when we hoisted them in and made sail to the NW with a light breeze at NNE.*—ff. 168v–72v.

THURSDAY 17*th*. PM Plying off the Island with variable light winds and had a boat and people on Shore tradeing, in the evening they return'd on board when we hoisted the boat in and made Sail NW with the wind at NNE. At Noon the body of the Island bore ESE½S distant 15 Leagues. Lat Ob[d] 26°48′ S.

This is undoubtedly the same Island as was seen by Roggewein in Ap[l] 1722 altho' the descriptions given of it by the authors of that voyage do's by no means correspond with it now;[1] it may also be the same as was seen by Captain Davis in 1686, but this is not altogether so certain, and if it is not than[2] his discovery cannot lie far from the

[1] 'This island is very convenient to touch at for refreshments; the whole of it is cultivated and tilled, it is full of woods and forests.'—Dalrymple, *Collection*, II, p. 95. This is from Behrens. Roggeveen's own journal conveys quite the opposite impression, one of 'extraordinarily sparse and meagre vegetation'.—Corney, *Voyage of Captain Don Felipe Gonzalez* (Hakluyt Society, 1908), p. 10.

[2] Cook is very much exercised over the Davis Land problem, and finds it difficult to shape his thought satisfactorily. Curiously enough, he does not take into consideration, as a factor, the distance of Easter Island from America. Here in the MS (f. 194v) he first writes, and then deletes, the following passage: 'I shall mention some reasons both for and against it and leave the reader to judge for himself. In the first place we did not see the low-Island said to lie to the East of it, and if any island had laid in that situation we must have seen it. Wafer the Author of Davis's Voyage, says the low Island lies in the Latitude of 27°20′ S, in this situation its possible we might have pass'd it unseen; but then he says, the high land laid to the westward of it, but, this might be WNW or even NW. It must be allowed that Easter Island seen from the Eastward corresponds very well with what Wafer has said on the subject; besides for some days before we made the land, we saw vast flocks of Birds which came in the Mor[n]ings from the West and return'd back in the Evenings, and as we saw few birds about the Island, it seems probable that there is some uninhabited i[s]le in the neighbourhood where they resort to; In short if this is not the land discovered by Davis,'. For all this he substitutes merely 'and if it is not than'; and in B, f. 173 changes the preceding words 'but this . . . certain' to 'for when seen from the East it answers very well with Wafer's discription'.

continent of America, for this Latitude seems to have been very well explored between the Meridian of 80 and 110, Captain Carteret carries it much farther, but his Track seems to be a little too far to the South. Had I found fresh Water on this isle I intended to have determined this point by looking for the low sandy isle mentioned by Wafer, but as I did not, and had a long run to make before I was assured of geting any and being at the same time in want of refreshments, I declined it, as a small delay might have been attended with bad consequences.[1] No Nation will ever contend for the honour of the discovery of Easter Island as there is hardly an Island in this sea which affords less refreshments and conveniences for Shiping than it does;[2] Nature has hardly provided it with any thing fit for man to eat or drink, and as the Natives are but few and may be supposed to plant no more than sufficient for themselves, they cannot have much to spare to new comers. The produce is Potatoes, Yams, Taro or the Eddy root,[3] Plantains and Sugar Cane, all excellent in its kind, the Potatoes are the best of the sort I ever tasted; they have also Gourds[4] and the same sort of Cloth Plant as at the other isles but not much, Cocks and Hens like ours which are small and but few of them and these are the only domistick Animals we saw a mong them, nor did we see any quadrupedes, but ratts which I believe they eat as I saw a man with some[5] in his hand which he seem'd unwilling to part with.[6] Land Birds we saw hardly any and Sea Birds but a few, these were Men of War birds, Noddies, Egg Birds, &c[a].[7] The Sea seems as bar-

[1] *consequences:* consequences to the Crew many of whom began to be more or less affected with the scurvy.—f. 173v. This passage occurs also in A and G; in A p. 128, but not elsewhere, it has the following footnote appended: 'It was afterwards found, that the few Roots &c[a] we got at this isle proved of infinate service to us and made us once more relish salt Beef and Pork, for which most of the Officers and some of the Crew had quite lost all appetite, nor is this to be wonder'd at, sence we had had no other flesh Meat for near four months.'

[2] . . . here is no safe Anchorage no wood for fuel nor no fresh water worth the takeing aboard.—f. 173v.

[3] 'Eddy root' seems to be derived from a Gold Coast word 'Eddoes', for the tuberous root of the taro, which came into the language (says *O.E.D.*) in 1685. It is a phrase Cook never uses in his first journal, and he may have picked it up from the Forsters, with whom it was habitual.

[4] . . . but so very few that a cocoa nut shell was the most valuable thing we could give them.—f. 173v. This is a red ink addition. The gourd, Hue (*Lagenaria vulgaris*) was invaluable as a container. Coconut trees did not grow on the island.

[5] *some:* some dead ones

[6] . . . and gave me to understand they were to eat.—f. 173v. The native Polynesian rat was in due course exterminated on Easter Island, as elsewhere, by the European rat. Gilbert, in his description of Easter Island (following his entry for 16 March), gives a brief commentary on Cook's remarks: 'Coconut shells and Otaheita cloth are the best comodities for traid, old hats rags and Bottles are not bad things. fish seems very scarce we caught none, no Quadruped Animals except ratts. Providence has even denigh'd them the pleasing services and companionship of the faithfull dog'.

[7] The *Resolution* was at the island at the wrong season for sea-birds. In the spring Cook could not have failed to notice the hundreds of thousands of terns that settled on Motu-nui, Motu-iti, and Motu-kaukau, and were (or whose eggs were) the centre of the bird-man

ren of fish for we could not catch any altho we try'd in several places with hook and line and it was very little we saw a mong the Natives. Such is the produce of *Easter* Island[1] which is situated in the Latitude of 27°6′ South and the Longitude of 109°51′40″ W,[2] it is about 10 Leagues in circuit and hath a hilly Rocky surface,[3] the hills are of such a height as to be seen 15 or 16 Leagues; off the South end are two rocky Islots, the one nearest the Point is high and Peaked, the other lower and flatish, the north and South points of the isle rise directly from the Sea to a considerable height, between them on the SE side is a sort of Bay in which there appear'd to be safe Anchorage with westerly and NW Winds and it was here, I believe, where the Duch anchored.[4] We anchored, as hath been already mentioned, on the West side of the Isle Three miles to the northward of the South point, with the Sandy beach bearing East and the two rocky Islots just shut behind the South point, this is a very good road with Easterly winds but a dangerous one with westerly as the other must be with an Easterly: for this and other ilconveniences already mentioned, nothing but necessity will induce any one to touch at this isle which affords but little refrishments, no safe anchorage, no wood for fuel, no fresh water but what must be got by a great deal of trouble and Labour, as we saw but two springs on the Island, the one on the SE side about ¾ of a mile from the shore and the other up in the center of the isle, this was so strongly impregnated with Iron ore that it made some sick who drank of it.[5]

The Inhabitants of this isle from what we have been able to see of them do not exceed six or seven hundred souls and a bove two thirds of these are Men, they either have but few Women among them or else many were not suffer'd to make their appearence, the latter seems most Probable.[6] They are certainly of the same race of

festival of the island, an important part of the cult of the god Makemake. See Métraux, *Easter Island*, (1957), pp. 130–9.

[1] ... or Davis's land ...—f. 174.

[2] *Voyage*, I, p. 288, gives lat. 27°5′30″, long. 109°46′20″; Cook may have got this from Wales. The modern reckoning for Hanga-roa is 27°09′ and 109°26′.

[3] ... and an Iron bound shore [*red ink*]

[4] See p. 340, n. 4 above.

[5] *which affords ... drank of it:* unless it can be done without going much out of the way, in this case touching here may be advantageous, as the people willingly and readily part with such refreshments as they have got and at an easy rate. We certainly received great benifit from the little we got, but few Ships can come here without being in want of Water and here is none to be got worth the takeing on board the little we took in we could not make use of, it was only Salt water which had filtrated through a stony beach into a stone well the Natives had made for the purpose a little to the Southward of the Sandy beach so often mentioned, and in which the water ebbed and flowed with the Tide.—f. 174–4v.

[6] Cook's guess at population does not seem to be a particularly good one; and the estimates of all early visitors seem to be unreliable. But when La Pérouse landed at Hanga-roa in 1786, he was faced there by a crowd of 800, and thought the total population

People as the New Zealanders and the other islanders, the affinity of the Language, Colour and some of thier customs all tend to prove it, I think they bear more affinity to the Inhabitants of Amsterdam and New Zealand, than those of the more northern isles which makes it probable that there lies a chain of isles in about this Parallel or under, some of which have at different times been seen.[1]

I did not see a Man in this Isle that measured Six feet;[2] in generall they are [a] very Slender race but very Nimble and Active, well featured with agreeable countenances,[3] but as much addicted to thieving as any of their Neighbours;[4] Tattowing that is inlaying the Colour of black in the Skin is much used here, the Men are coloured in this manner from head to foot, the figures they mark are all nearly alike only some give them one direction on the boddy and some a nother according to fancy,[5] they also make use of Red and White Paint, to their faces and sometimes to other parts of their bodies, the former is made of Tamrick[6] but what the latter is made of I know not. Their Hair in general is black, the men wear both it and their beards croped Short and the women wear it long. Their cloathing is a piece of Quilted Cloth 5 feet by 4 made of the Bark of the same sort of plant

was about 2000. Métraux, after considering the available evidence (*Ethnology*, pp. 20–22), puts the population c. 1840 at between three and four thousand; so whether La Pérouse under-estimated or not, Cook certainly did. Métraux adds, 'As Cook suggested, the natives were undoubtedly frightened by the arrival of foreigners and hid their women in inland caves as was done in wartime'. The women who rushed the sailors—who, to quote Mitchel, 16 March, 'are always at our command', and whom Forster describes with appropriate references to Messalina and Cleopatra—it may be assumed, were not the sort that can be kept hidden; or else, being unmarried or of low class, were virtually detailed for the work.

[1] Easter Island lies at the extreme eastern point of the 'Polynesian triangle'; but the 'chain of isles in about this Parallel' theory must be given a pretty liberal interpretation to tally with geography. The island, thinks Métraux (*Easter Island*, chap. XIV) was undoubtedly colonized from the Marquesas, the last expiring wave of the great Polynesian migration from the west; Heyerdahl believes (*American Indians in the Pacific*, 1952, and *Aku-aku*, 1958) that the statues were the work of a white-skinned, red-haired people ('long-ears') from Peru, who were joined only a thousand years later by his North-west American Polynesians ('short-ears')—possibly as late as 1600. This latter hypothesis still leaves some room for the Marquesas.

[2] . . . so far are they from being giants as one of the Authors of Roggeweins Voyage asserts.—f. 175.

[3] . . . are friendly and hospitable to strangers,

[4] A *note:* When our people were a Shore Watering, they oblig'd the Natives to keep at a proper distance from them, least they should steal any thing; One man fairly out wited them, by tumbling, as it were by accident down a bank under which the Cooper was at work, our people ran to his assistance, help'd him up & led him off, as they thought much hurt, but as soon as he was out of their hand[s] he made haste to be gone, carrying with him the Coopers Adze.—Gilbert says, 'The Natives of a middle stature well made of a copper colour complexion with a brisk and lively countanence very active and audacious'.

[5] . . . The Women are but little punctured,

[6] i.e. turmeric. A mixture of powdered turmeric root and sugar cane juice was rubbed on the skin, but the colour it gave was yellow or orange. The red like the white paint came from an earth. Forster (I, p. 564) describes a reddish-brown undercoat, with the turmeric orange to finish off with.

as is used for the same purpose at all the Nothern isles[1] but the men as often go in a manner naked having only a slip of cloth fastened between their legs by means of a small cord tyed round their waist; this piece of cloth does by no means answer the end it seems to be intended. They have enormous holes in their Ears, but what their Chief ear ornaments are I cannot say. I have seen some with a ring fixed in the hole of the Ear, but not hanging to it, also some with rings made of some elastick substance roled up like the Spring of a Watch, the design of this must be to extend or increase the hole.[2]

Their Arms are wooden Patta pattows and Clubs very much like those of New Zealand and spears about 6 or 8 feet long which are pointed at one end with pieces of black fli[n]t.[3]

Their Houses are low long and narrow and have much the appearence of a large boat turned bottom up whose keel is curved or bint, the largest I saw was 60 feet in length, 8 or 9 high in the middle and 3 or 4 at each end, its breadth was nearly the same; the door was in the middle of one Side, built like a Porch so low and narrow as just to admit a man to creep in upon all fours. The framing is made of small twigs and the covering of the tops of Sugar Cane and Plantains leaves and extends from the foundation to the roof so that they have no light but what the small door admits. These people dress their Victuals in the same mann[r] as at the other Isles.

Not more than three or 4 Canoes were seen upon the whole Island and these very mean, made of many pi[e]ces of Boards sew'd together with small line, they are about 18 feet long,[4] head and Stern curved, are very narrow with outriggers, and Seem not to be able to carry above 3 or 4 men and are by no means fit for any distant navigation: as small and mean as these Canoes were it was a matter of wonder to us where they got the wood to build them on, for in one Canoe was a board 14 Inches broad at one end, but not so much at the other, and Six or Eight feet long whereas we did not see a stick on the

[1] *5 feet . . . isles:* Six feet by four, or a Matt, one piece wraped round their loins and another over their Shoulders make a compleat dress . . .—f. 175.

[2] Sugar-cane leaf; or a strip of bark could be used, or feathers. These extraordinary ears, minus the ornaments, are portrayed in the engravings from Hodges, in the *Voyage*, pls. XLVI and XXV. See also Fig. 52 in this volume.

[3] The 'wooden Patta pattows' (Maori *patu*) were called *paoa*; the handle end was carved with a human face or lizard head. By 'clubs' Cook may have meant either the same thing or a 'long club', called *ua*, equivalent to the Maori *taiaha*, also decorated at one end with carved human heads; but below (p. 355) he says 'short wooden clubs'. The spear points (*mataa*) were of obsidian and made a fearful wound.

[4] This must be an overestimate: all other observers make what canoes there were much shorter. Forster (I, p. 558) says the length of the canoe that first came out to the ship 'might be about ten or twelve feet'—and that was probably a maximum.

Island that would have made a board one half this Size,[1] nor could we conceive it to be Possible in such Canoes to bring wood from any other Isle, suppose any lay in the neigherhood. One of the accounts of Roggeweins Voyage, in describing one of these Canoes, says the whole was patched together out of pieces of wood which could hardly make up the largeness of half a foot. The other account says every part of the Island which is not cultivated is full of Woods and Forests: how are we to reconcile these two accounts? Would the natives prefer such pieces of wood for building their Canoes to larger, or did this Forest produce no larger tree than would make a board of half a foot square? The first of these Authors (I believe) is right in his description of the Canoe, but in allmost every other thing seems to have written with no other view but to impose upon the world and the other has asserted many things at random or else the State of this Isle is very different now to what it was then.

Of their Religion, Goverment &c[a] we can say nothing with certainty. The Stupendous stone statues errected in different places along the Coast are certainly no representation of any Deity or places of worship; but most probable Burial Places for certain Tribes or Families. I my self saw a human Skeleton lying in the foundation of one just covered with Stones, what I call the foundation is an oblong square about 20 or 30 feet by 10 or 12 built of and faced with hewn stones of a vast size, executed in so masterly a manner as sufficiently[2] shews the ingenuity of the age in which they were built. They are not all of equal height, some are not raised above two or three feet, others much more,[3] and seems to depend on the nature of the ground on which they are built. The Statue is errected in the middle of its foundation, it is about high and round[4] for this is its shape, all the appearences it has of a human figure is in the head where all the parts are in proportion to its Size;[5] the head is crow[n]ed with a Stone of the shape and full size of a drum, we could not help wondering how they were set up, indeed if the Island was once Inhabited by a race of Giants of 12 feet high as one of the Authors of Roggewein's Voyage tell us,[6] than this wonder

[1] This was perhaps driftwood; or perhaps, as Métraux suggests (*Ethnology*, p. 204), had been left by Gonzalez. Cook himself suggests the Spaniards, pp. 354, 359 below.

[2] *as sufficiently:* as to become a master piece of Indian Masonry and sufficiently . . .—f. 181.

[3] *much more:* are eight or ten

[4] *it is . . . round:* it is a huge stone from 15 to 30 feet high and from 16 to 24 round. . . .

[5] . . . except the ears which are out of all proportion large or long.

[6] Dalrymple's anonymous Dutchman recounts that a boat came out to meet Roggeveen's ship, managed by a single man, a giant of twelve feet high, whom the Dutch surrounded and took but afterwards let go, as conversation was impossible. He was painted dark brown. All the Easter Islanders proved to be giants, very well proportioned; but,

ceaseth and gives place to another equally as extraordinary, viz. to know what is become of this race of giants. Besides these Statues which are very numerous and no were but a long the Sea Coast there are many little heaps of stones here and there on the bank along the Sea Coast, two or three of the uppermost stones of these piles are generally white, perhaps always so when the pile is compleat: it can hardly be doubted but these piles of stones have some meaning tho' we do not know it.[1]

From the report of M[r] Pickersgill it should seem that the Island is under the goverment of one Man whom they stile Arreeke, that is King or Chief.[2]

Some pieces of Carving were found a mongest these people which were neither ill designed nor executed. They have no other tools than what are made of Stone, Bone, Shells &c[a]. They set but little value on Iron and yet they knew the use of it, perhaps they obtained their knowlidge of this Metal from the Spaniards who Viseted this Isle in 1769 some Vistiges of which still remained amongest them, such as pieces of Cloth &c[a].

*The Inhabitants of this Island do not seem to exceed Six or Seven hundred Souls and above two thirds of them were Males, they either have but few females amongst them or else many were not suffered to make their appearence during our stay and yet we saw nothing to induce us to believe the men were of a jealous disposission or the Women afraid to appear in publick, and yet something of this kind was certainly the case. In Colour, Features, and Language they bear such affinity to the people of the more Western isles that no one will doubt but that they have had the same Origin, it is extraordinary that the same Nation should have spread themselves over all the isles in this Vast Ocean from New Zealand to this Island which is almost a fourth part of the circumference of the Globe, many of them at this time have no other knowledge of each other than what is recorded in antiquated tradition and have by length of time become as it were different Nations each having adopted some pecular custom or

we are told, with a very Gulliver-like reasonableness, 'none of their wives came up to the height of the men, being commonly not above ten or eleven feet.' These ladies were painted scarlet.

[1] They signified an area made *tapu*, round about a body wrapped in a mat and left to decay, as a preliminary to the interment of the bones in a vault beneath an *ahu*. Only the top stones seem to have been painted white.

[2] . . . I think this probable enough, as it is agreeable to what we find at most of the isles, but what his power may be over each individual we know not.—f. 177v.—Pickersgill's report, as an argument for a king, was of no significance; but there was in fact a 'king', or *ariki-mau*, of Easter Island—a 'principal high chief', extremely *tapu* or sacred, and of great importance in social and religious matters. He had, however, no function in government in any political sense.

habit &c[a] never the less a carefull observer will soon see the Affinity each has to the other.[1] . . . Their Cloth is made of the same materials as at Otaheite, viz. of the bark of the cloth plant, but as the[y] have but little of it, our Otaheite cloth or indeed any sort of cloth came here to a good market. Their hair in general is black, the women wear it long and sometimes tied up on the Crown of the head, but the men wear both it and their beards crop'd short. Their head dress is a round fillit adorned with feathers and also a straw bonnet something like a Scotch bonnet, The former I believe is chiefly worn by the Men and the latter by the Women.[2] Both Men and Women have very large holes or rather slits in their Ears, extended to near three Inches in length, they some times turn this slit over the upper part and then the Ear looks as if the flap was cut off. The chief Ear Ornament is the white down of feathers and Rings which they wear in the inside of the hole made of some elastick substance, roll'd up like the spring of a Watch, I judged this was to keep the hole at its utmost extension. I do not remember seeing them wear any other ornaments excepting Amulets made of bone or shells.[3] As inoffensive and friendly as these people seem to be they are not without offensive weapons, such as short wooden clubs and Spears, the latter are crooked Sticks about Six feet long arm'd at one end with pieces of flint—they have also a weapon made of wood like the Patoo patoo of New Zealand. Their Houses are low miserable huts formed by seting sticks upright in the ground at 6 or 8 feet distance and bending them towards each other and tying them together at the top, forming thereby a kind of Gothic arch and shorter each way and at less distance asunder, by this means the Building is highest and broadest in the middle and lower and narrower towards each end. To these are tyed others horizontally and the whole is thatched over with the leaves of Sugar Cane. The Door way is in the middle of one

[1] On this see Buck, *Vikings*, chap. 17, particularly pp. 228–38. One can possibly draw out of Cook's words more than he meant to put into them, yet they summarize remarkably well both the link between the Polynesian peoples and the differences that grew up between them as they became adapted to different environments. The New Zealand *marae* differed from the Tahitian *marae* but was a *marae*; New Zealand and Tongan fortification was allied but weapon carving was quite different; the Tahitians, the other Society Islanders, the Marquesans, the Easter Islanders all built in stone; the Marquesans and the Easter Islanders carved in volcanic stone but in different styles; and nothing could be more different from the stone-carving developed in Easter Island than the wood-carving of the heavily-forested New Zealand. The Easter Islanders did carve small wooden figures, but they again were very different in style from anything in New Zealand. Yet, as Cook detected, the language 'affinity' was everywhere, to say no more.

[2] See Figs. 52*a* and *b*, and the engravings from Hodges in *Voyage*, I, pls. XXV, XLVI.

[3] *ornaments* . . . *shells*: A has 'ornament worth notice, excepting some who wore large bunches of feather[s]'. The words 'excepting . . . feather[s]' were added to the clerk's copy by Cook.

side formed like a Porch and so low and narrow as just to admit a man to enter upon all fours. The largest house I saw was about Sixty feet long, 8 or 9 hight in the Middle and 3 or 4 at each end, its breadth at these parts was nearly equal to the height. Some have kind of Vaulted houses built with Stone and partly under ground, but I never was in one of these.[1] I saw no household utensils amongst them except gourds and of these but a very few, but they were extravigantly fond of Cocoanut shells, more so than any thing we could give them.[2] They dress their victuals in the same manner as at Otaheite that is with hot stones in an Oven or hole in the ground. The Straw or tops of Sugar Canes Plantain lea[ves] &c[a] serve them for fuel to heat the stones; Plantains, which require but little dressing, they roast under fires of straw dryed grass &c[a], whole races of plantains[3] they ripen or roast in this manner,[4] we frequently saw ten or a dozen or more such fires in one place and most commonly in the Mornings and evenings. . . .—ff. 174v–7.

[*On wood for canoes*] There are two ways by which it is possible they may have got this large Wood; it might have been left here by the Spaniards, or it might have been drove on the shore of the island from some distant land. It is even possible that there may be som[e] land in the neighbourhood from which they might have got it. We however saw no signs of any, nor could we get the least information on this head from the Natives, although we tryed every method we could think of to obtain it. We were almost as unfortunate in our enquiries for the proper or native name of the Island for on compareing notes I found we had got three different Names for it, viz. Tamareki, Whyhu and Teapij.[5] Without pretending to say which, or that any of the three, is right, I shall only observe that the last was obtained by Odiddy, who understood their Language (tho' but very imperfectly) much better than any of us.

[1] These were caves, walled in at the entrance when necessary: either quite small, or what Métraux calls 'subterranean lava tubes' (*Ethnology*, p. 192). Forster says (I, pp. 570–1), 'Besides these huts [of sticks and thatch], we observed some heaps of stones piled up into little hillocks, which had one steep perpendicular side, where a hole went under ground . . . the natives always denied us admittance into these places'.

[2] Coconuts would not grow on Easter Island; but the people preserved their memory, and that of the uses to which the shells might be put.

[3] Cook here and elsewhere uses 'race', I think, in the sense of branch, meaning probably the whole produce of the plant. Johnson gives one meaning of 'race' as a root or sprig.

[4] After 'manner' Cook deletes the words, 'the heat of the sun being hardly sufficient to bring this fruit to perfection'. He was quite right to delete them; but green bananas were ripened quickly, not by 'roasting', but by covering them with earth for three or four days in a ditch where a fire had just been extinguished, also by a layer of earth; so that they underwent continuous gentle heat.

[5] The first and last of these names, like Vaihu, seem to have been those of districts, or even perhaps of places still more limited in extent.

It appears by the accounts of Roggeweins Voyage, that these people had no better Vessels when he first visited them. The want of Materials and not of Genius, seems to be the reason why they have made no improvement in this art. Some pieces of Carving was found amongst them, both well designed and executed.

Their Plantations are prettily laid out by line but are not inclosed by any fencing, indeed they have nothing for this purpose but stones. I have no doubt, but that all these Plantations are private property[1] and that there are here as at Otaheite Cheifs (which they call Areekees) to whome these Plantations belongs. But of the Power or authority of these Cheifs, or of the Goverment of these people, I confess my self quite ignorant. Nor are we better acquainted with their Religion;[2] The gigantic Statues so often mentioned, are in my opinion not looked upon as Idols by the present Inhabitants, whatever they might be in the days of the Dutch, at least I have not seen any thing that could induce me to think so, On the Contrary I rather think that they are Burying places for certain Tribes or Families, I as well as some others, saw a Human Skeleton lying in one of the Platforms just covered with stones. Some of these Platforms of Masonary are 30 or 40 feet long 12, or 16 broad[3] and from 3 to 12 in height; this last in some measure depends on the Nature of the ground on which they are built, which is generally on the brink of the Bank facing the Sea, so that this face may be 10 or 12 feet or more high and yet the other may not be above 3 or 4. They are built or rather faced with hewn stones of a very large size and the workmanship is not inferior to the best plain piece of Masonary we have in England. They use no sort of Cement, the joints are exceeding close and the Stones are mortised and Tenonted one into a nother in a very artfull manner. The side walls are not perpendicular, but inclining a little inwards in the same manner that Breast-works &c[a] are built in Europe;[4] yet had not all this care,

[1] ... one day when our boat was a shore taken in water the people brought down roots &c[a] to excha[n]ge, which as soon as they had disposed of they went into an adjoining plantation of Potatoes which they dug up and sold to our people for mere trifles, but this trafick so advantageous to us was soon put a stop to by the owner (as we supposed) of the plantation coming down in a great passion and driving the people away after which we soon found the difference between the price of stolen goods and those honestly come by.—f. 177v.

[2] ... Was it not necessary to say something of the Stupendous Stone statues, errected in different place[s] along the Coast, I should have pass'd over their Religion and Goverment in silence so little do we know of either.—f. 177v.

[3] It will be noticed that Cook has raised these figures from the '20 cr 30' and '10 or 12' given by him on p. 353 above, and one wonders why. Was even he, now and again, afflicted with the traveller's desire to enlarge his wonders? He had not seen much of these particular wonders himself.

[4] There were other sorts of *ahu* than these; see Métraux, *Ethnology*, pp. 283–8.

pains and sagacity been able to preserve these curious Structures from the ravages of all-devouring time.[1]

The Statues or at least many of them are erected on these platforms which serve as a foundation, they are as near as we could judge about half length;[2] ending in a sort of stump at the bottom on which they stand. The workmanship is rude but not bad, nor the features of the face ill formed, the Nose and chin, in particular, but the Ears are unconscionably long, and as to the body's there are hardly any thing like a human figure about them. I had an oppertunity to examine only two or three of these Statues, which were near the landing place, they were of a grey stone, seemingly of the same sort as the Platforms were built; but some of the gentlemen who traveled over the Island and had an oppertunity to examine a great many were of an opinion that the stone on which they were made was different from any other which they saw on the Island and had much the appearence of being factitious, We could hardly conceive how a nation like these wholy unacquainted with every mechanical power, could raise such stupendous figures and after wards place the large Cylindric Stones, before mentioned, upon their heads.[3] The only method I can concieve, is by raising the upper end by little and little, supporting it by stones as it is raisd and building about it till they get it erect, thus a sort of mount or scaffolding will be made up which they may roll the Cylinder and place it on the head of the statue after which the stones may be removed from about it. But if the Statues are factitious they might have been put together on the place and in the position they now stand and the Cylinder put on by building a mount round them as above mentioned. But let them have been made and set up by this or any other method, they must have been a work of immense time and sufficiently shew the Ingenuity and perseverence of the age in which they were built, for the present have most certainly had no hand in them, they do not even repair the foundations of those which are going to decay. They give different names to them such as Gotomoara, Marapoti, Kan a ro, Goway too goo, Matta Matta &c to which the[y] some times prefix the word Moi and some times annex Areekee: the latter

[1] One must not be taken aback by this sudden burst of metaphor: Cook was merely copying Wales.

[2] As Buck says (*Vikings*, p. 232), 'They are really busts'; or, to quote Heyerdahl (*Aku-aku*, p. 88), 'lengthened busts with complete torsos'.

[3] Cook, like other people baffled over the Easter Island figures, had never seen Polynesians handle really heavy weights, such as the trunks of huge forest trees in New Zealand, or the vast corner stones of a Tongan *langi*. He tends to underestimate the manpower that could be called on for transport. Heyerdahl, *Aku-aku*, describes and illustrates a method he actually saw practised of raising a statue and placing it on an *ahu*.

signifies Chief and the other burying or sleeping place[1] as well as we could understand. Bes[i]des the Monuments of Antiquity, which were pretty numerous and no where but upon or near the Sea-coast,[2] there were many little heaps of stones, piled up in different places along the Coast, two or three of the upermost stone[s] in each pile were generally white, perhaps always so when the Pile is compleat. It will hardly be doubted but these Piles of stones had some meaning or an other—probably they might mark the places where people had been buried and served instead of the large statues.

The working Tools of these people are but very mean, and like those of all the other Islanders, made of stone, bone, Shells &c^a^. They set but little Value on Iron or Iron tools, which was the more extraordinary as they knew the use of them; but the reason may be their having but little use for them.—ff. 178–80v.

I know not if they obtained their knowlidge of Iron from the Dutch or from the Spaniards; the latter, I have been told, Visited them in 1769, some vistiges of which still remain such as Hatts, old Cloathes pieces of Cloth &c^a^. Its probable they made a longer stay at this isle than we did and may favour the world with a better account of it than I can, a stay of two days was by no means sufficient for this task.

Names of the Images or Statues, mentioned by Mr Pickersgill[3]

Go-tomoara
Coo-hau
Mara-hine
Omo-reera } Standing in a row
Adrago
Co-more-mori-mouhuti
Quiperea
Go-way-too-goo
Matta Matta

[1] *moe*, to sleep; and in a secondary sense, to die.

[2] This is incorrect; there were many figures inland.

[3] The majority of the names in this list have not been printed before. Comparison with the names in the lists of kings given in Métraux, *Ethnology*, facing p. 90, does not get one very far. 'Adrago' may be identical with Atara[n]ga; Matte Matte may be Pickersgill's rendering of Makemake, the principal Easter Island god and creator; or there was an *akuaku* or spirit of the dead, ordinarily represented by one of the carved beak-nosed images, with prominent ribs and hollow stomach, called Mata-mata-pea. 'Kan-a-ro' may represent Nga-ara (*Ko* = it is), or possibly Kao-aroaro. 'Moui' may be Maui, the culture-hero known all over Polynesia. To quote Buck, 'Originally the stone images may have represented gods and deified ancestors but in the course of time they became more truly an expression of art' (*Vikings*, p. 234). And Métraux: 'If the statues are deified ancestors, they may be compared with Marquesan statues of deified ancestors who had become tribal deities' (*Ethnology*, p. 307).

Moui
Go-be-pau
Harre-awayaa
Mouhga
Heke-keoe
Coetica
Hangamahega
Koa-de-waū } Two which stood near the landing place
Kan-ā-ro }

The following short Vocabulry which I had from M[r] Pickersgill, will show the affinity of their Language to that Spoke in the other isles—

Numbers		Words, Easter Island	Otaheite	English
Ta hie	1	Mau-au	Manoo	a Fowl
Roua	2	An-no-ho	Anoho	Sit down
Toru	3	Ma-e-ca	Maiā	Plantains
Aha	4	Papa	Tata	a Man
Rema	5	Keno	E'no, Keno }	Bad
Hona	6		New Zealand }	
Hetu	7	Coo-marra	Coomallo, or }	Potaties
Wharrou	8		Coomarro }	
Heva	9	Moica	Moe	Sleep, or sleeping place
Co-behu	10			
Co-tu-eno	10	Arreeke	Aree	King
N.B. all the		Hu-hee	Aoowhe	Yams
numbers, except		E-kie	Eyā	Fish
10, is the same		Eipa	Aima, Aipa	No
as at Otaheite.		Eripa	Arapo	Dirty*

—f. 182–2v.

FRIDAY 18*th*. *Winds NNE to ENE. Course N* $47\frac{3}{4}°$ *W. Dist.* 64 *Miles. Lat.* 26°5′. *Long.* 111°32′.[1] Winds at NNE and ENE with which we steer'd NW & NNW. In the AM being in Lat 25°55′ the Variation was 2°38′ E.[2]

[1] In H, for this date and down to Wednesday 6 April, Cook inserts the longitude made from Easter Island. I do not print these figures.

[2] . . . After leaving Easter Island I steer'd NWBW and NNW with a fine Easterly gale, [*deleted* during day time had all Sails set, but in the night kept but little sail abroad.] Intending to touch next at the Marquesas, If I met with nothing before I got there. We had not been long at sea before the Bilious disorder made a nother attack upon me, but not so Violent as the former, I believe this second Visit was owing to my exposing and fatiguing my self too much at Easter Island.—f. 183. It was during this passage that the elder Forster's Tahitian dog was sacrificed to provide fresh food for Cook. Others were sick, including Patten the surgeon.—Forster II, pp. 1–3.

SATURDAY 19*th*. *Winds Easterly*. *Course N* 32½° *W*. *Dist*. 89 *Miles*. *Lat*. 24°50′. *Long*. 112°28′. First part little wind remainder fresh breezes. In the PM being in Latitude 25°15′, Longitude 111°36′ the Variation was 2°32′ E, both by the Az^th & Amplitude.[1]

SUNDAY 20*th*. *Winds Easterly*. *Course N* 14¼° *W*. *Dist*. 114 *Miles*. *Lat*. 23°0′. *Long*. 113°1′. Fresh gales and fair Weather, Shortned sail during night.

MONDAY 21*st*. *Winds Easterly*. *Course N* 24° *W*. *Dist*. 130 *Miles*. *Lat*. 21°1′. *Long*. 113°58′. Fresh breezes & Clowdy with some showers of rain.

TUESDAY 22*nd*. *Winds ENE, Variable, East*. *Course N* 25½° *W*. *Dist*. 112 *Miles*. *Lat*. 19°20′. *Long*. 114°49′ [*Watch* 115°37½′].[2] First part fair weather, Middle rain, latter fair & Clowdy. PM Variation 3°4′ E.

WEDNESDAY 23*rd*. *Winds East*. *Course N* 42° *W*. *Dist*. 97 *Miles*. *Lat*. 18°8′. *Long*. 115°57′. Moderate breezes PM Showery, remainder fair. Altered the Course to NW.

THURSDAY 24*th*. *Winds East, Var., East*. *Course N* 45° *W*. *Dist*. 84 *Miles*. *Lat*. 17°7′. *Long*. 117°0′. First and latter parts Moderate, Middle variable Light airs next to a Calm.

FRIDAY 25*th*. *Winds East*. *Course N* 52¾° *W*. *Dist*. 109 *Miles*. *Lat*. 16°1′. *Long*. 118°30′. Gentle gales and fine Weather. At 5 o'Clock pm being in Lat 16°55′ S, Long^de 117°12′ west the Variation was 1°56′ E. In the AM Saw Tropick Birds & flying fish.

SATURDAY 26*th*. *Winds SSE & E*. *Course N* 53¼° *W*. *Dist*. 122 *Miles*. *Lat*. 14°48′. *Long*. 120°11′. Gentle breezes and clear pleasent weather. At 6 o'Clock in the AM in Lat 15°13′, Long^de 119°45′ the Variation 1°1′ East. After this the Variation began to increase.

SUNDAY 27*th*. *Wind ESE*. *Course N* 42½° *W*. *Dist*. 132 *Miles*. *Lat*. 13°11′. *Long*. 120°57′. A Steady Trade and clear weather.

MONDAY 28*th*. *Wind Easterly*. *Course N* 47½° *W*. *Dist*. 129 *Miles*. *Lat*.

[1] We get at this time an interesting glimpse of the process of justice at sea, provided by Mitchel: 18 March PM 'Wm Wedgerborough marine confined, there being strong presumptive proof, of uncleanliness; by easing himself betwixt decks—and proof positive in point of Drunkeness.'—AM 'People &c turned aft in order to punish the above, when the Lieut^t of marines publicly declared he objected to it—which the Captn was made acquainted with (being ill at this time) the prisoner was again confined.'—19 March AM 'Read the articles of war & Punished Wm Wedgerborough marine with a dozen lashes—after his having another hearing, when their appear'd such proofs that no doubts could be left.' William Wedgeborough gave a good deal of trouble, one way or another.

[2] These last figures, and those corresponding for 29–31 March, I print from H

11°44′. *Long.* 122°34′. D° Wea[r]. Set up the Forge to repair the Iron work. Saw some Egg and other birds.[1]

TUESDAY 29*th. Wind Easterly. Course N* 47¼° *W. Dist.* 124 *Miles. Lat.* 10°20′. *Long.* 123°58′ [*Watch* 125°28′]. Fresh gales. Same Birds seen as yesterday. Altered the Course to west N west.

WEDNESDAY 30*th. Winds Easterly. Course N* 66° *W. Dist.* 133 *Miles. Lat.* 9°24′. *Long.* 126°1′ [*Watch* 127°35′]. Gentle Trade and pleasent weather. A Gannet, Men of War and Egg Bird seen. Altered Course to West.[2]

THURSDAY 31*st. Winds EBS. Course S* 86.½° *W. Dist.* 120 *Miles. Lat.* 9°17′. *Long.* 128°3′ [*Watch* 129°44′]. D° Gales. In the evening a Gannet kept some time about the Ship. In the AM saw more Birds.[3] In the Lat of 9°18′, Long[de] 127°39′ the Variation 3°23′ East being the most we have found it since the 26th.

[APRIL 1774]

FRIDAY 1*st. Winds EBS. Course S* 83¼° *W. Dist.* 112 *Miles. Lat.* 9°30′. *Long.* 129°56′. Gentle breezes and hot weather, Birds seen as usual.

SATURDAY 2*nd. Winds East. Course West. Dist.* 106 *Miles. Lat.* 9°29′. *Long.* 131°44′. D° Weather. pm Saw a large flock of Men of War birds and others.

SUNDAY 3*rd. Winds East. Course West Southerly. Dist.* 92 *Miles. Lat.* 9°32½′ *Long.* 133°18′. Gentle breezes, half past 7 am Long[de] p[r] Distance 132°45′ west, Latitude 9°32′ s and a little before the Variation was 4°40′ East.[4]

MONDAY 4*th.* [*Winds East. Course W. Southerly.* 92 *m.*][5] Steer'd West with the wind at East a gentle breeze. At Noon we were in the Latitude of 9°32½′ s. Longitude 134°52′ west.

TUESDAY 5*th.* [*Winds EBS. Course West.* 104 *m.*] PM clear weather

[1] 'Set the Forge up for the Armourer to make hatchets after the form of the stone ones of Otaheite, to trade with the Natives at the Marquesas'.—Cooper.

[2] ... Tuesday 29th ... Altered the Course to WNW and the next day to West, being then in Lat. 9°24′ which I judged to be the Parallel of the Marquesas where as I have before observed, I intended to touch in order to settle their situation, which I find different in different Charts. Having now a steady settled trade wind and pleasent weather I ordered the forge to be set up to repair and make various necessary articles in the Iron way, the Calkers had already been some time at work Calking the decks ...—f. 183.

[3] 'Men of War and Egg birds seen, flying fish and Mother caries chickings'.—Log.

[4] ... As we advanced to the west we found the Variation to increase but slowly ...

[5] This bracketed passage, and those corresponding for the next two days, I print from H.

AM gloomy weather. At 10 pm Brought to till the Moon was up then made sail to the West. At Noon our Latitude was 9°33′, Long^{de} 136°38′.

WEDNESDAY 6*th*. [*Winds East. Course N* 81° *W.* 83 *m.*] Gentle breezes at ENE and fine weather. At 6 brog^{t} to till day-light then made Sail again to the west and at Noon we were in the Latitude of 9°20′ s, Long^{de} 138°1′ west. Birds seen as usual.[1]

THURSDAY 7*th*. At 4 o'Clock in the PM after runing 4 Leagues West sence Noon, Land was seen bearing WBS distant about 9 Leagues, two hours after saw a nother land bearing SWBS and appeared more extensive than the first: hauld up for this land and kept under an easy Sail all night having Squally unsittled weather with rain.[2] At 6 am the Land first seen bore NW the other SW½W and a third West, I directed my Course for the Channell between these two last lands, under all the Sail we could set, having unsittled Squally Showery weather. Soon after we discovered a fourth land still more to the westward and were now well assured that these were the Marquesas discovered by Mendana in 1595.[3] At Noon we were in the Channell which divides St Pedro and La dominica.

FRIDAY 8*th*. Continued to rainge a long the SE Shore of La Dominica without seeing any signs of an Anchoring place, till we came to the Channell which divides it from St Christina through which we pass'd and haul'd over to the last mentioned Island and ran along the shore to the South westward in search of Mendana['s] Port. After passing Several Coves in which seem'd to be tollerable Anchorage, but a great Surff on the Shore; from some of these places came of some of the Natives in their Canoes, but as we had a fresh of wind and did not shorten Sail none came up with us. At length we came to the Port we were in search after,[4] into which we hauled and made an attempt to turn in, in the doing of which we were attacked by such

[1] John Innell, the ringleader in drunkenness of 22 February, was again flogged this day, for insolence.

[2] . . . which is not very uncommon in this sea when near high land.—f. 183v.

[3] . . . The first isle was a new discovery, which I named Hoods Island after the young gentleman who first saw it, the second was that of St Pedro, the third La dominica, and the fourth St Christina.—f. 183v. The young gentleman, Alexander Hood, was now sixteen; he was a first cousin of Admiral Lord Hood and became a captain at the age of 23. His island was the large rock Fatu Huku; San Pedro was Motane, a little larger but uninhabited; La Dominica was Hiva Oa; Santa Christina was Tahuata. These, with Fatu Hiva (Mendaña's La Madalena) formed the south-eastern group of the Marquesas. They are all high islands, from 1200 to 3500 feet, and are visible 50 or 60 miles away. Chart XXXII and Figs. 55, 56.

[4] Mendaña's Madre de Dios—Resolution or Vaitahu Bay. Chart XXXII, inset.

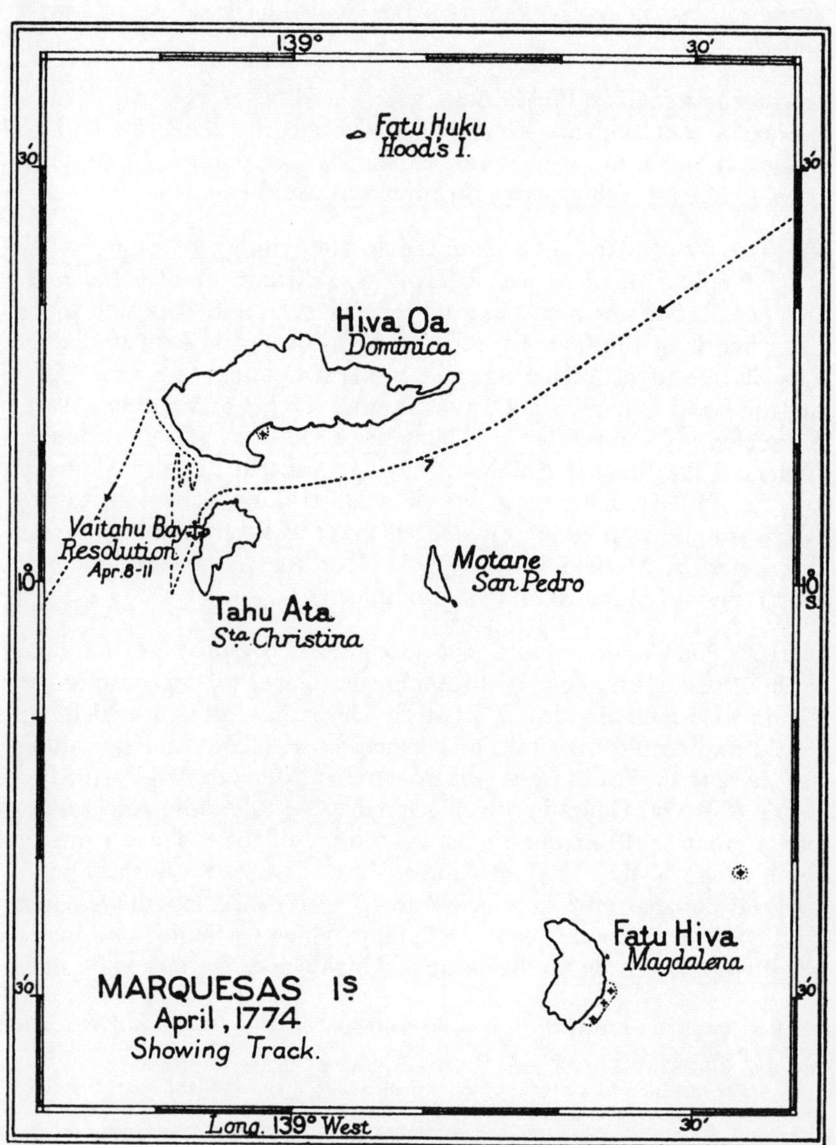
139°
30'
Fatu Huku
Hood's I.
30'
30'
Hiva Oa
Dominica
Vaitahu Bay
Resolution
Apr. 8-11
10°
Motane
San Pedro
10°
S.
Tahu Ata
Sta. Christina
Fatu Hiva
Magdalena
30'
30'
MARQUESAS Is.
April, 1774
Showing Track.
Long. 139° West
30'

FIG. 55

Violent Squalls from the high lands that we were[1] within a few yards of being driven against the rocks to Leeward. After escaping this danger we stood out again made a stretch to windward and then stretched in and Anchored in the Entrance of the Bay in 34 fathom water, sandy bottom, without so much as attempting to turn farther in, when Anchord with ⅔ of a Cable out the North point of the Bay bore   the South point   and the point in the middle of the Bay which divides the two Strands
dist[t] one Mile. We had no soon anchored then about 30 or 40 of the Natives came round us in a Doz[n] or fourteen Canoes, but it requir'd some address to get them along side, at last a Hatchet and some large Nails induced the people in one Canoe to put under the quarter gallery, after this all the others put along side and exchanged Bread fruit and some fish for small Nails and then retired a shore.[2] But came off again to us very early the next morning in much greater numbers bringing off Bread fruit, Plantains and one Pig which they exchanged for Nails &c[a] but in this Traffick they would frequently keep our goods and make no return, tell at last I was obliged to fire a Musquet ball Close past one man who had served[3] us in this manner after which they observed a little more honisty and at length several of them came on board. At this time we were prepairing to warp the Ship farther into the Bay and I was going in a Boat to look for the most convenient place to mo[o]r her in; observing so many of the Natives on board, I said to the officers, you must look well after these people or they certainly will carry off some thing or other, these words were no sooner out of my mouth and had hardly got into my Boat, when I was told they had stolen one of the Iron Sta[n]chions from the opposite Gang-way,[4] I told the officers to fire over the Canoe till I could get round in the Boat,[5] unluckily for the theif[6] they took better aim than I ever intend and killed him the third Shott, two others that were in the same Canoe jumped overboard but got in again just as I got to the Canoe, the one was a Man

[1] *lands . . . were:* lands one of which took us just after we had put in stays, payed the Ship of again and before she wore round, was . . .—f. 184. The bay is backed by a high and steep range of hills. 'When the Trade wind is blowing, violent squalls come down from the valleys at the head of the bay . . . it is advisable to anchor as near the northern shore as possible, to avoid being driven on to the southern entrance point.'—*Pacific Islands Pilot,* III, p. 186. There are rocks off this southern point, which provided the peril to the *Resolution.* See Fig. 57.

[2] . . . the Sun being already set We observed a heap of stones in the Bow of every Canoe and every man to have a Sling tied round his head.—f. 184.

[3] *had served:* had several times served

[4] . . . and were makeing off with it,

[5] . . . but not to kill any one, but the Natives made too much noise for me to be heard and . . .—f. 184v.

[6] *theif:* unhappy theif

and seem'd to laugh at what had happen'd,[1] the other was a youth about 14 or 15 years of age, he looked at the dead man with a serias and dejected countinance and we had after wards reason to believe that he was son to the disceas'd. This accident made all the Canoes retire from us with precipitation. I followed them into the Bay and prevaild upon the people in one Canoe to come along side the Boat and receive some Nails and other things I gave them.[2] When I returnd on board we carried[3] out a Kedge Anchor with 3 hawsers upon an end to warp in by and hove short on the bower. One would have thought that the Natives by this time were fully sencible of the effect of our fire Arms[4] but the event proved other wise for the boat had no sooner left the Kedge anchor than a Canoe put of from the Shore, took hold of the Buoy and attempted, as we supposed, to drag what was fast to the rope a shore, but fearing they would at last take away the Buoy[5] I ordered a Musquet to be fire[d] at them, but as the ball fell short they took no notice of it, but the 2nd ball that was fired pass'd over them on which they let go the buoy and made for the shore and this was the last shott we had occasion to fire and probably had more effect upon them than killing the Man as it shewed them that they were hardly safe at any distance for they afterwards stood in great dread of the Musquet, nevertheless they would very often exercize their tallant of thieving upon us, which I thought necessary to put up with as our stay was likely to be but short among them. The Natives had retarded us so long that before we were ready to heave up the anchor and warp in the wind began to blow in Squalls out of the Bay, so that we were obliged to lay fast where we were.

It was not long before the Natives ventured off to us again, in the first Canoe which came was a man who seem'd of some consequence, he advanced slowly with a Pig upon his Shoulder which he sold for a Spike nail as soon as he got a long side. I made him a present of a Hatchet and several other Articles which induced him to come into the Ship where he made a short stay and then retired;[6]

[1] *Canoe, . . . happen'd:* Canoe, the Sta[n]chion they had thrown over board, one of them was a Man grown and sat baling out the blood & Water out of the Canoe in a kind of Hysteric Laugh . . .—f. 184v.

[2] . . . this to some measure allay'd their fears.—f. 185.

[3] *When . . . carried:* After having taken a view of [the] Bay and found that fresh Water, which we most wanted was to be got I returned aboard and carried . . .

[4] *were . . . Arms:* would have been so sencible of the effect of our fire arms, as not to have provoked us to fire upon them once more

[5] *than a Canoe . . . Buoy:* than two men in a Canoe put off from the Shore, took hold of the buoy rope and attempted to drag it a shore, little considering what was fast to it, but lest, after discovering their mistake, they should take away the buoy, . . .—f. 185.

[6] *which . . . retired:* and speaking some thing which we did not understand; as soon as he got along side I made him a present of a Hatchet and several other Articles and in

his example was followed by all the other Canoes and trade was presently reestablished.[1] Things being thus Settled on board I went a shore with a party of Men to try what was to be done there, we were received by the Natives as if nothing had happened, traded with them for some Plantains and a few Sm[l] Piggs and after Loading the Launch with water returned on board to dinner.

SATURDAY *9th.* PM sent the boats and a guard a Shore again for Water; upon their landing the Natives all fleed but one Man and he seemed much frightned, he was disir'd to go and fetch some fruit which he did accordingly and after him one or two more came and these were all that were seen till 8 o'Clock in the AM at which time some made their appearence just as the Boats put off from the Watering place; after breakfast I went a Shore my self before the guard when the Natives crowded round me in great numbers but as soon as the guard landed I had enough to do to prevent them from runing off, at length their fears were dissipated and a trade opened for fruit and Pigs.[2] I beleive the reason of their flying from our people last evening was their not seeing me at the head of them, for they certainly would have done the same now had I not been present. Towards Noon a chief of some consequence, attended by a great number of People, came down to us, I made him a present of Nails and Several other Articles and in return he gave me some of his ornaments, after these Mutal exchanges a good under Standing Seemed to be settled between us and them so that we got by exchanges as much fruit as Loaded two boats and then return on board.[3]

SUNDAY 10*th.* PM Launch Watering and a party Trading with the Natives,[4] went my self into the Southern cove of the Bay where I procured five Pigs, and came to the House which we were told belonged to the Man we had kill'd; there were Six Piggs in it which we were told belonged to the deceased Son who had fled upon our

return he sent up his Pig and was at last prevailed upon to come himself up into the gangway, where he made but a short stay before he went away.

[1] Willis, journal, says the people 'soon return'd humbling themselves very much, laying their Heads down on the Deck & putting our Feet on them, & never made the least Attempt to steal any thing afterwards'; but as this is not behaviour noticed by anybody else it may have been a flight of fancy on Willis's part.

[2] Sparrman, p. 119, gives us a picture of the less formal side of this trade, at a nail for a coconut: 'Having made the bargain we would add a little rum to the coconut milk to improve its flavour and to render it more refreshing. After having drunk we would return this grog to the vendor, who would dip his fingers in the liquid and then repeatedly rub them over his tongue and nose and those of such of his fellows who happened to be present, appearing thus to render them a singular honour'.

[3] . . . to dinner but could not prevail on the Chief to accompany us.—f. 186.

[4] . . . the latter got but little as most of the Natives were retired into the Country.

approach. I wanted much to have seen him to have made him a present and by other kind treatment convinced him and the others that it was not from any bad design we had against the Nation we had kill'd his father; it would have been to no purpose my leaving any thing in the house as it certainly would have been taken away by others.[1] Strict honisty was seldom observed amongest them selves when the property of our things came to be disputed, I saw a Striking instance of this. I offered a man a Six Inch Spike for a Pig which he readily excepted of and hand'd the pig to a nother man to give me which was done and the Spike given in return, but in stead of giving it to the Man who sold the Pig he kept it him self and offered him in lieu a Sixpenny Nail, words of course arose and I waited to see how it would end, but as the man who had got possession of the Spike seem'd resolved to keep it I left them before it was desided.[2]

AM Emp^{d} as usual (viz) in Watering and Trading with the Natives. Some Canoes from more distant parts came and sold us some Pigs so that we had now sufficient to give all hands a fresh meal, the Pigs they bring us are so small that 40 or 50 are hardly sufficient for this purpose.[3]

MONDAY 11*th*. In the PM I made an expedition towards Southward[4] in which I collected 18 Pigs and I believe should have got more had I had more time,[5] in the Morning I went to the same places but instead of geting Pigs as I expected I found every thing quite changed, the Nails and other things they were Mad after the Evening before they now dispised and in stead of them they wanted they did not know what, the reason of this was, some of the young gentlemen having been a Shore the preceeding day and had given them in exchange various Articles such as they had not seen before and which took with them more than Nails, or perhaps they thought they had already enough of these and wanted some thing more curious, which I nor indeed any one else had to give them sufficient to supply us with refreshments, thus our market was at once spoil'd and I was obliged to return with 3 or 4 little Pigs which cost me more than a Doz^{n} would have done the evening before; when I got on board I found that the party at the water place had had no better success.

[1] . . . especially as I could not sufficiently explain to them my meaning.—f. 186v.

[2] . . . In the evening returned on board with what refreshments we had collected and thought we had made a good days work.

[3] . . . The trade on shore for fruit was as brisk as ever.

[4] . . . accompanied by some of the gentlemen

[5] . . . The people were exceeding obligeing wherever we landed and readily brought down whatever we desired.—ff. 186v–7.

When I got aboard I found the same thing had happened there and also at the tradeing place on shore; the reason was, several of the young gentlemen having been on shore the preceeding Day and had given away in exchanges various Articles, such as the people had not seen before and which took with them more than Nails or more usefull Iron tools, but what ruined our Market the most was one of them giving for a Pig a very large quantity of Red feathers he had got at Amsterdam, which these people much value and which the other did not know, nor did I know at this time that Red feathers was what they wanted, and if I had I could not have supported this trade in the manner it was begun one day. Thus, was the fine prospect we had of geting a plentifull supply of refreshments of these people frustrated, and which will ever be the case so long as every one is allowed to make exchanges for what he pleaseth and in what manner he please's.—f. 187–7v.

When I saw that this place was not likely to supply us with sufficient refreshments,[1] not very convenient for geting off wood and Water nor for giving the Ship the necessary repairs, I resolv'd forth with to leave it and seack for some place that would supply our wants better, for it must be supposed that after having been 19 Weeks at Sea (for I cannot call the two or 3 days spent at Easter Island any thing else) living all the time upon a Salt Diet, but what we must want some refreshments altho I must own and that with pleasure, that on our arrival here, it could hardly be said that we had one Sick Man on board and not above two or three who had the least complaint, this was undoubtedly owing to the many antiscorbutic articles we had on board and the great care and Attention of the Surgeon who took special care to apply them in time.[2]

TUESDAY 12*th*. At 3 o'Clock in the PM weighed[3] and Stood over for St Dominica in order to take a View of the West side of that Island but as we could not reach it before dark the night was spent Plying

[1] . . . such as we might expect to find at the Society Isles, . . .—f. 187v.

[2] Forster, II, p. 36, adds his tribute to Patten, though he thinks less highly of the condition of the crew than does Cook: 'our worthy surgeon, Mr Patton, took the best precautions possible to preserve the healths of all on board, by suggesting the proper methods to Captain Cook, and by watching over us with unremitting assiduity. I will venture to affirm, that it is to him alone, under Providence, that many of us are indebted for our lives. . . . Great commendations are likewise due to Captain Cook, who left no experiment untried which was proposed to him. . . .' In due time, of course, it became clear to John Reinhold Forster that the credit for all this was properly due to himself.

[3] From Sparrman, pp. 119–20, we get a quite vivid picture of the risk attendant on coming off to the ship. The last time the longboat left the beach it had in it Cook, the Forsters, and Sparrman himself. The sea got up, 'and no sooner had we taken our places in the boat than it was flung hither and thither and seemed on the point of being totally

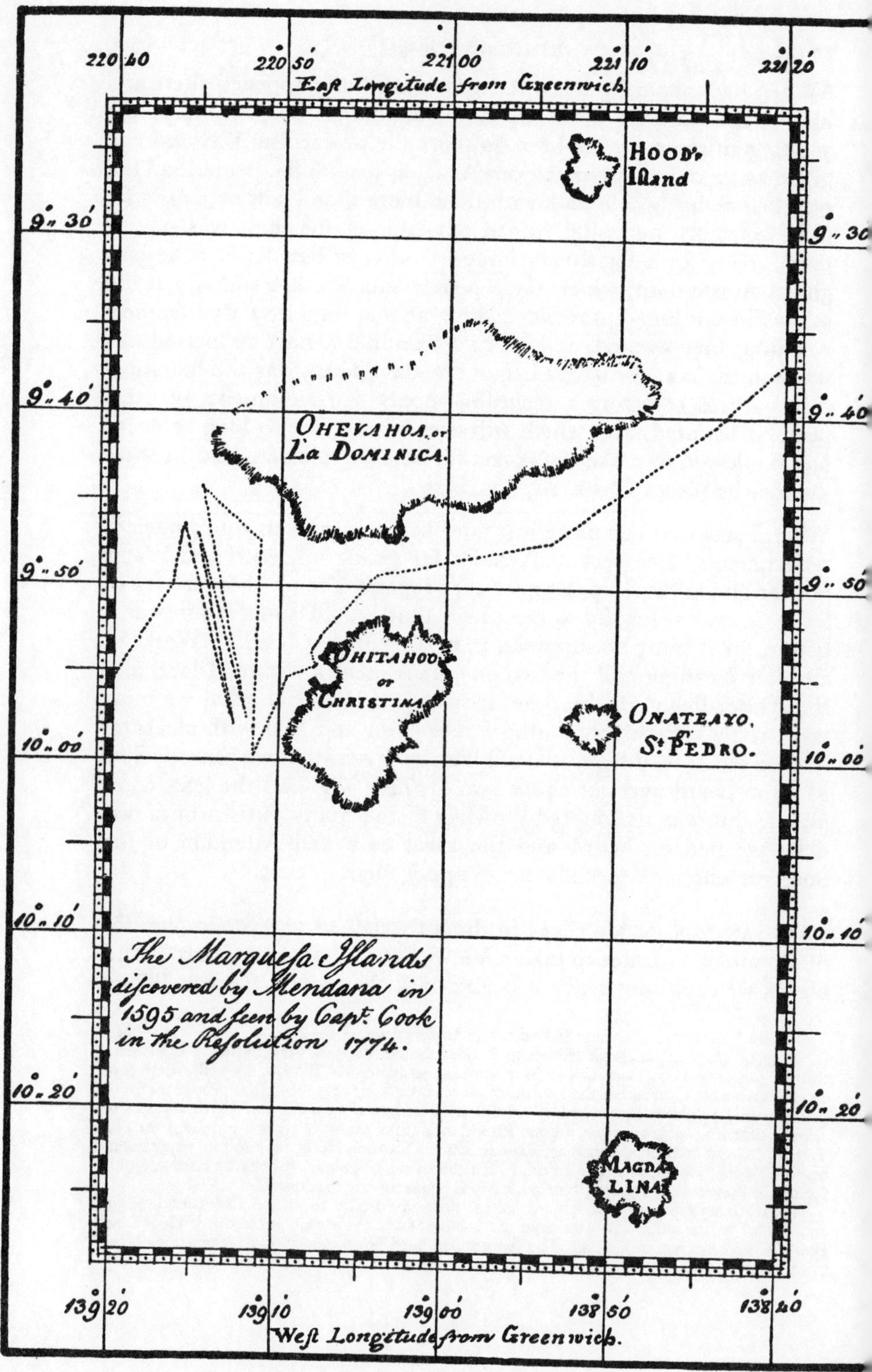

FIG. 56. William Wales, chart of the Marquesas

between the two Islands. In the morning we had a full View of the SW and western sides of the Isle neither of which seem'd to afford any Anchorage. At 8 o'Clock we were off the NW point from which the land trended NE Easterly, so that this side was not likely to have any safe Port as being exposed to the Easterly winds; we had now but little and that very variable with Showers of Rain: at length we got a breeze at ENE with which we steered to the South ward with a view of leaving these Isles altogether, which I shall now give a short, but rather more Particular account of.

These Isles as I have before observ'd were first discovered by *Mendana* and by him called *Marquesas*,[1] he likewise gave names to the different isles. The Nautical discription of them in M[r] Dalrymple['s] Collection of Voyages is diffecient in nothing but Situation and this was the chief point I wanted to settle and my reason for touching at them as it will in a great measure fix the Situation of all Mendana's other discoveries.[2] The Marquesas are five in number Viz La Magdalena, S[t] Pedro, La Dominica, S[t] Christina and Hoods isle,[3] this last was discovered by us and named after the young Gentleman who first saw it; we had but a very distant View of this isle, it appeared of a small curcuit, round and of a good height with some lower land or small islots on y[e] west side of it,[4] it is the most northermost Isle, situated in the Latitude of 9°26′ S and N 13° W, 5½ Leagues from the East Point of La Dominica, which is the largest of all the isles, extending East and west Six Leagues, is of an unequal breadth and 15 or 16 Leagues in circuit and Situated in the Latitude of

wrecked. . . . It was only the extraordinary address of our oarsmen and their prodigious efforts which finally saved us from the rocks where the waves broke so furiously'. The Forsters became 'paler than any living being upon whom I have ever set eyes, and I do not know why they never mentioned this perilous incident in their journal, which is so prolix in recounting every other occurrence'. If the danger was as imminent as Sparrman points out, one can hardly blame the Forsters for turning pale.

[1] Mendaña discovered the islands in July 1595; the name he gave them, in full, was Las Marquesas de Mendoza, after the friendly viceroy of Peru under whose aegis he had set out. The murder committed by his men at Resolution Bay was frightful. Three crosses were raised to commemorate the advent of Christianity.

[2] 'they are laid down full half a Degree too far to the South, this might be owing to the Instruments use'd in them days . . .'—Log.

[3] . . . which is the northermost.—f. 188. The Marquesas in fact lie in two groups (or rather three, geographically speaking, but the three most northerly islands are all inconsiderable). Neither Mendaña nor Cook sighted the north-west group, of which the largest is Nukuhiva; the most southerly, Ua Pou, lies about 55 miles WNW of Hiva Oa or La Dominica. This group was first sighted by the American merchant vessel *Hope*, Captain Ingraham, in 1791; and a good deal of European contact with the Marquesas thereafter became centred with whalers on Nukuhiva. Melville's *Typee* has made it, and not Cook's Marquesas, classic.

[4] There is no low land on the rock of Fatu Huku, though the summit, 1180 feet high, slopes from north to south; there is a rock on which the sea breaks to the NNW. Cook's latitude is correct.

9°44½′ South, it is full of Hills[1] which rise in ridges directly from the Sea to a considerable height,[2] these ridges are disjoined by deep Vallies which are cloathed with wood, and as well as the sides of some of the hills and ridges, most probably many of these are fruit trees, however the Country in general appears Barren, it is never the less Inhabited. *St Pedro* which is about 3 Leagues in circuit of a good height but not hilly[3] lies South 4 Leagues and a half from the East end of La Dominica, we know not whether or no it is inhabited, probably it is not as Nature seems not to have provided it with the necessary subsistance for Man. *St Christina* lies under the Same Parallel 3 or 4 Leagues more to the West: this isle lies North and South and is 7 Leagues[4] in circuit, a narrow ridge of hills of considerable hieght extends the Whole length of the isle, other ridges take their rise from the Sea and with an unequal assent join the Main Ridge, these form deep and narrow Vallies which generally terminate at the foot of the Main Ridge, these Vallies are full of fruit and other trees and afford Rivulets of fresh Water.[5]

La Magdalena we only saw at a distance, by the bearing we took of it and that mentioned by Quiros, its Situation must be nearly in the Latitude of 10°25′ s, Long^de^ 138°50′[6] so that these isles occupy one degree of Latitude and near half a degree of Longitude, viz from 138°47′ to 139°13′ w,[7] and as they are all of a considerable height and within sight of each other its impossible to misstake them. Mr Forster found nearly the same Shrubs, Plants &c^a^ as at Otaheite and the other isles. The Refreshments to be got here are Hogs, Fowls, Plantains, Yams and some other roots, Bread fruit and Cocoa-nutts, but these last are scarce. At first all these Articles were purchased with Small Nails but they soon loosed their Value of other articles, far less usefull.[8]

The Inhabitents of these Isles are without exceptions as fine a race

[1] *hills:* rugged hills.—f. 188.

[2] The highest point of Hiva Oa, 3,520 feet; its position is lat. 9°46′ s, long. 139°04′ w. In B, f. 188, Cook gives the latitude of the island as 9°44′30″, as here.

[3] Motane is 1640 feet in the south, but sinks gradually towards its northern end.

[4] *is 7 Leagues:* is 9 Miles long in that dire[c]tion and about 7 Leagues . . .—f. 188v.

[5] *are full . . . Water:* which are adorned with fruit and other trees and Water[ed] by fine streams of [crystal *deleted*] excellent Water.—f. 188. The description of Tahuata, which rises to 3,280 feet, is very accurate, though we here seem to see Cook sheering rather narrowly off a purple patch.

[6] The south-western extremity of the island, Fatu Hiva, is now given as lat. 10°30′ s, long. 138°41′ w. Cook's positions are extremely good.

[7] . . . which is the longitude of the West end of La Dominica . . .—f. 188v. The correct figures are more like 138°36′ to 139°9′ w.

[8] *with . . . usefull:* with Nails. Beads, looking-glasses and such trifles which are so highly valued at the Society isles, are in no esteem here; and even Nails at last lost their Value for other articles far less useful.—f. 189.

of people as any in this Sea or perhaps any whatever; the Men are Tattowed or curiously Marked from head to foot[1] which makes them look dark but the Women (who are but little Tattow'd) youths and young children are as fair as some Europeans, they cloath them Selves with the same sort of cloth and Matting as the Otaheiteans; they wear as Ornaments a kind of Fillit curiously oramented with Tortice and Mother of Pearl Shills, Feathers &c^a^. Round their Necks an Ornament of this form,[2] it is made with Wood on which are stuck with gum a great num^r^ of small red Pease,[3] they also wear bunches of human hair round their legs and arms &c^a^. The Men in general are tall that is about Six feet high, but we saw none so lusty as at Otaheite and the neighbouring isles, nevertheless they are of the same race of People, their language customs &c^a^ all tend to prove it.

They dwell in the Vallies and on the sides of the hills near their plantations, their Houses are built after the same manner as at Otaheite, but are much meaner and only covered with the leaves of the bread tree. They have also dwellings or Strong holds on the Summits of the highest Mountains, these we saw by the help of our Glasses, for I did not permit any of our people to go to them for fear of being attack'd by the Natives,[4] whose deposission we were not sufficiently acquainted with.

The Bay or Port of *Madre de Dios* so named by Mendana[5] is situated near the middle of the West side [of] St Christina under the highest land on the island in Latitude 9°55′30″ S, Longitude 139°8′40″ W and N 15° W from the West end of La Dominica. The South point of the Bay is a steep rock of considerable hieght forming at the Top a peaked hill above which you will see a path way leading a long a narrow Ridge to the summits of the hills where the Natives have their Strong holds; the North point is not so high and rises with a

[1] A note in B.M. Add. MS 27889, f. 79, runs 'Marquesas. Tattouing like a coat of Mail—'.

[2] There is a space left here in the MS, f. 203, for a drawing; but Cook left it unfilled. See the engraving from Hodges, *Voyage*, I, pl. XVII; in the notes on the plates it is called a gorget.

[3] 'These red seeds, embellished by a little black spot, are one and the same as those now [c. 1800] modish in Europe under the name of African seeds, out of which bracelets and necklaces are fashioned. Formerly they were used only for rosaries, and the botanists then named the tree *Arbus precatorius*.'—Sparrman, p. 119.

[4] Nevertheless George Forster, Sparrman, Patten 'and two other gentlemen' went up the heights behind the bay, following a native path, for three or four miles, but saw little beyond fruit trees, some houses, and hospitable natives. 'We were the more easily presuaded to desist from our purpose [to climb to the summit], as the heat of the day, our precarious state of health, and the fatigue of the ascent, had entirely exhausted us, and as we saw no prospect of reaching the summit.'—Forster, II, pp. 23–6.

[5] *so . . . Mendana:* which I named Resolution Bay . . .—f. 188v.

more gentle Slope, they are a mile from each other[1] and the Bay is near three quarters of a mile deep in which is from 30 to 12 fathom water a clear Sandy bottom, in it are two beaches divided from each other by a rocky point, in each of [them] is a River[2] of excellent Water, the one on the North side is the most comodious for wooding and Watering. Here is the little Water-fall mentioned by Quiros,[3] but there is no Town in this cove but in the other there is. There are Several other coves on this side of the isle and some of them especially to the Northward bear some likeness to this, therefore the best mark to know it by is the bearing of the West end of La Dominica.[4]

*The Inhabitants of these islands taken collectively are without exception the finest race of people in this Sea; for a fine shape and regular features, they, perhaps, surpass all other Nations,[5] nevertheless the affinity of their language to that spoken in Otaheite and the Society Isles, shew that they are of the same Nation; Oedidee could converse with them tolerable well, tho we could not, but it was easy to see that their Language was nearly the same.

The Men are Punctured or curiously Tattoued from head to foot, the figures are various and seem to be directed more by fancy than custom; these punctuations makes them look dark,[6] but the women who are but little punctured, youths and young children who are not attall are as fair as some Europeans. The men are in general tall, that is about 5 feet 10 inches or six feet, but I saw none that were fatt and lusty like the Arees of Otaheite nor did I see one that could be called Meager.[7] They make the same kind of cloth and matting

[1] ... in the direction NbE & sbw

[2] *River:* Rivulet

[3] ... Mendana's Pilot ...—Cook found this remark by Quiros in a footnote in Dalrymple, *Collection*, I, p. 66: 'there is a fine rivulet close to the beach, of very fine water; it falls from a hill about twice a man's height, above four or five fingers broad, and close to it is a small brook of water.'

[4] In H, at the end of his description of the Marquesas, Cook later inserts the note, 'There are no Dogs at these isles'.

[5] 'The Inhabitants to speak of them in general are the most beautiful race of People I ever beheld—of a great number of Men that fell under my inspection I did not observe a single one either remarkably thin or disagreeably Corpulent but they were all in fine Order and exquisitely proportion'd. We saw very few of their Women but what were seen were remarkably fair for the situation of the Country and very beautifull—the Men are punctuated or as they call it tattow'd from head to foot in the prettyest manner that can be conciev'd. . . .' Clerke, 12 April.—The women, says Mitchel, 'are very handsome & well made wearing their hair long & tied negligently behind, others wearing it in a club & are not marked in any part except a few strokes on the lips, was very shy, but however they was a little afterwards found to be women . . .'.

[6] Gilbert, when writing of Easter Island (following 16 March) goes on to discuss tattooing throughout the Pacific, and though he refers especially to Tahiti his remark may come in appropriately here, that the tattooing was 'curious and exceeding handsome Nay so becoming in those people that to an European they wou'd appear naked without it'.

[7] The following four sentences are on a 'Paper annexed'—i.e. a separate slip, which Cook, having added it to his text, nevertheless marks marginally 'omit'.

as at that Island and cloath themselves with it in the same manner, but they have it not in such plenty nor is it so good; little cloathing indeed is wanting, we seldom see the men with any thing more than what is sufficient to hide their Natural parts. Some wear their hair long and others short, there seems to be no establiged custom for this. When dress'd they wear on the fore head as an ornament a curious fillet of shell work decorated with feathers &c[a], round the neck a kind of Ruff made of Wood decorated with small red pease which are stuck on with gum and bunches of human hair fastened to a string and tyed round the legs and arms; in this manner was the chief who came down to visit us dress'd;[1] some wear necklaces and Amulets, I do not recolect of seeing any with ear ornaments, their ears are nevertheless pierced. They have a custom of hanging beads to their beards, at least some of those they got from us were applyed to this use.

Their Dwellings are in the Vallies and on the sides of the hills near their plantations, they are built after the same manner as at Otaheite, but are much meaner and only covered with the leaves of the bread tree, the most of them are built on a square or oblong pavement of Stone raised some height above the level of the ground; they likewise have of these pavements near their houses, on which they sit to eat and amuse themselves. In the article of eating these people are by no means so cleanly as the Otaheiteans, they are like wise equally dirty in their Cookery. Pork and Fowles are dress'd in an Oven of hot stones as at Otaheite but fruit and roots they roast on the fire, and after takeing off the rind or skin, put them into [a] Platter or trough with Water, out of which I have seen both men and Hoggs eat at the same time. I once saw them make a Batter of fruit and roots deluted with Water, in a Vessel that was loaded with dirt and out of which the hogs had been but that moment eating, without giving it the least washing, or even washing their hands, which were equally dirty, and when I express'd a dislike was laugh'd at. I know not if all are so, the actions of a few individuals are not sufficient to fix a Custom to a whole Nation, nor can I say if it is the Custom for men and Women to have separate Messes. I saw nothing to the Contrary, indeed I saw but few Women upon the whole. They seemed to have dwelings or strong hold[s] on the Summitts of the highest hills, these we only saw by the help of our glasses, for I did not permit any of our people to go there, as we were not sufficiently acquented with the disposission of the Natives which (I believe) is humane and pacifick.

[1] See the engravings in *Voyage*, I, pls. XVII, XXXIII, XXXVI.

Their Weapons are Clubs[1] and Spears alike to, but somewhat neater than those of Otaheite, the[y] have also Slings with which they throw stones with great velosity and to a great distance but not with a good aim. Their Canoes are made of wood and pieces of the Bark of a soft wood, which grows near the Sea in great plenty, and is very tough and proper for the purpose; They are from 16 to 20 feet long and about 15 Inches broad. The head and stern is made of two solid pieces of Wood, the Stern rises or curves a little, but in an irregular direction and ends in a point; the head projects out horizontally and is car[v]ed into some faint and very rude resemblance of a human face. They are rowed by Paddles and some have a sort of Latteen sail made of Mating.[2] Hogs were the only animals we saw and Cockes & Hens the only tame fowls, but the Woods seemed to abound with small birds of a very beautifull Plumage and fine Notes, but the fear of alarming the Natives hindered us from shooting so many of them as might otherwise have been done.*—ff. 189–90v.

WEDNESDAY 13*th. Winds NE to ESE. Course S* 36° *West. Distce Sailed* 75 *Miles. Latde in* 10°56′. *Longde in West* 139°54′. Gentle breezes with rain. At 5 o'Clock in the PM the Harbour of Madre de Dios bore ENE½E distant 5 Leagues and the body of the Island Magdalena SE about 9 Leagues; this was the only View we had of this last isle. From hence I directed my Course SSW½W for Otaheite and likewise with a view of falling in with Some of those isles discovered by former Navigators[3] whose Situations are not well determined.

THURSDAY 14*th. Winds ESE. Course S* 36°30′ *W. Distce Sailed* 110 *Miles. Latde in* 12°24′. *Longde in West* 141°1′. Fresh Trade and fine Weather. At 4 pm the Variation was 5°16′ East. At 6 Shortned Sail and brought to till day light when we made Sail again. In the am the Variation was 5°30′ East.

FRIDAY 15*th. Winds ESE. Course S* 48°30′ *W. Distce Sailed* 115 *Miles. Latde in* 13°40. *Longde in West* 142°29′. Winds and Weather as yesterday. Saw nothing remarkable.

SATURDAY 16*th. Winds East. Course S* 63°30′ *W. Distce Sailed* 83 *Miles. Latde in* 14°17′. *Longde in West* 143°43′. At 6 in the AM being in Lat Longde the Variation was East.

[1] The Marquesan clubs were heavy and deadly weapons, with characteristic carved heads or striking ends; see *Voyage*, I, pl. XVII.

[2] See Fig. 57, and *Voyage*, I, pl. XXXIII.

[3] . . . especially those discovered by the Dutch

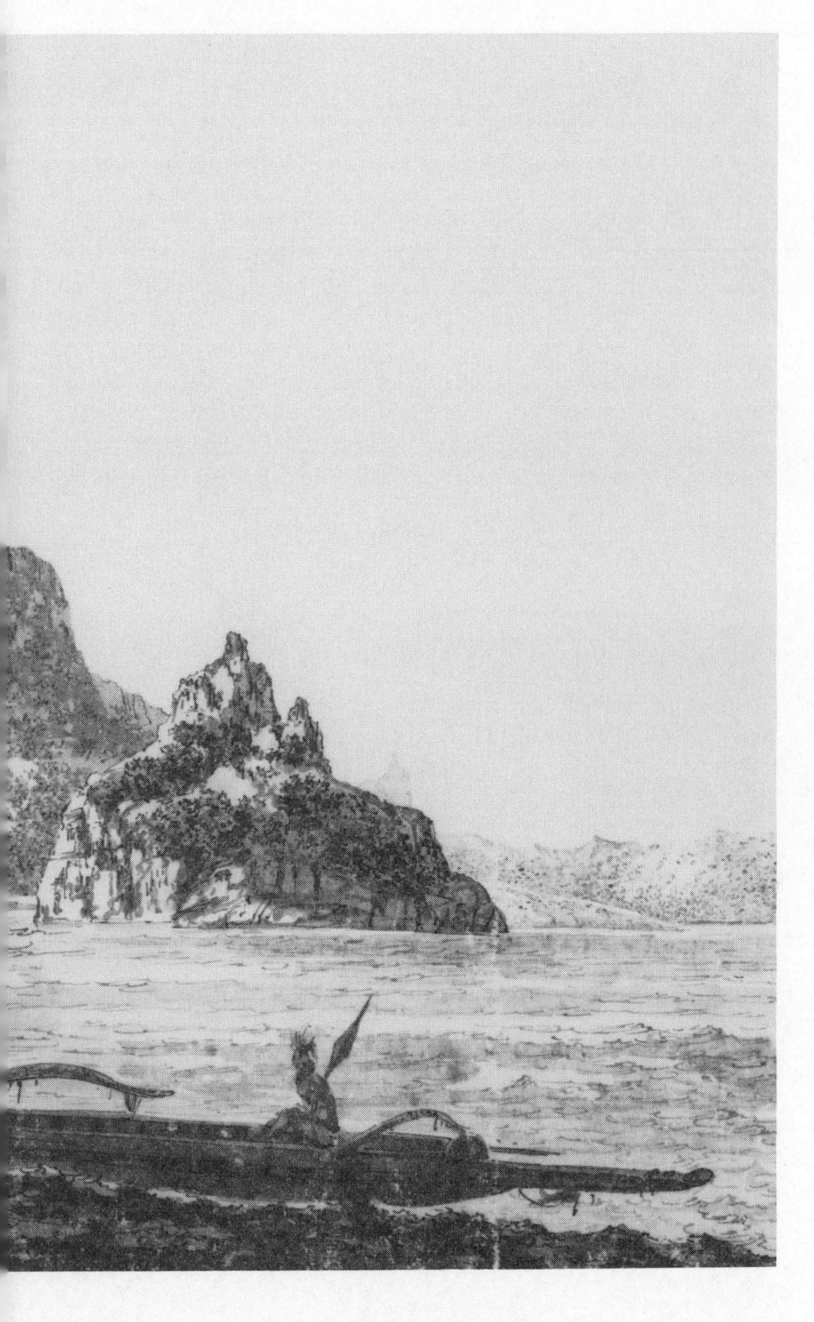

View of Resolution Bay (Vaitahu), Santa Christina (Tahuata) in the Marquesas

Wash drawing by Hodges—B.M., Add. MS 15743.4

SUNDAY 17*th. Winds EBS. Course S* 84° *W. Distce Sailed* 75 *Miles. Latde in* 14°25′. *Longde in West* 144°59′. Gentle breezes and pleasent Weather. At 7 AM Shortned Sail for the night as usual. At 10 AM saw land bearing W½N, which at Noon extended from S 71° W to N 56° West. Our distance from the Northern point was about 2½ M[ls].

MONDAY 18*th. Winds Easterly. Course S* 44° *W. Dist. Sailed* 44 *M. Lat. in* 14°55′. *Longde. in* 145°32′. Fresh breezes and pleasent Weather. As soon as we were the length of the north point of the isle hauld up a long the NW side at the distance of one mile from the Shore, at 3 o'Clock saw a creek or inlet which seemd to comunicate with the Inland Sea or lake. Bro[t] to, hoisted out a boat and Sint the Master to examine it;[1] Upon his return reported that there was no passage into the lake, that in the creek was sufficient Water for a Ship, that it was fifty fathom wide at the Entrance and 30 deep, farther in 30 fathom wide and 12 deep, and that the bottom was every were rocky and the Sides bounded by a Wall of Coral rocks.[2] I was under no necessity to put the Ship into such a place, but as the Natives had shew'd some signs of a friendly disposission by coming to the boat and takeing such things as were offered them I sent two Boats well Arm'd a Shore under the Command of Lieut[ts] Cooper and Pickersgill with a view of having some intercourse with them, to get some refreshments and to give M[r] Forster an oppertunity to Collect some Plants. The boats landed without opposission, a few of the Natives only met them on the beach, the rest kept in the Skirts of the Wood with their Arms (spears) in their hands; the presents which our people made them were received with great indifferency which plainly shew'd that we were unwelcome Visitors;[3] our people had not been long a shore before the natives were reinforced by 40 or 50 more all Arm'd, this was first observed from the Ship and therefore we hastned in Shore to Support our people in case they should be attack'd: however nothing of this sort happened, for when this party came up our people thought proper to imbark as the day was far spent and I had given orders not to fire upon the Natives if it was possible to avoid it. When they were in the boats

[1] *Bro[t] to . . . it:* as I wanted to obtain some knowlidge of the produce of these half drown'd isles, we brought to, and hoisted out a boat and sent the Master in to Sound, for without was no Soundings. As we ran a long the Coast the Natives appeared in several places arm'd with long Spears and Clubs, and some were now got together on one side of the creek.—f. 191.

[2] This must have been the Tehavaroa passage, which does not go right through the reef into the lagoon, except for a tricky narrow channel for small craft: hence Cook's words 'creek or inlet'. See Fig. 33, p. 192 above.

[3] 'Our Indian Adventurer from Uliateah cou'd understand no more of the Language of these people than Ourselves'.—Clerke.

some of the Natives were for pushing them off others for detaining them, at last they suffer'd them to go at their leasure: they brought on board five Dogs which they said were in plenty on the isle, they saw no fruit but Cocoa-nuts of which they got[1] two doz^{n}, indeed as they were never off the beach they could know but little of the produce, they gave to one of our people a dog for a Single Plantain which made us conjecture that they have none of this fruit. As soon as the boats were hoisted in I ordered two or three Guns to be fired over the little isle the Natives were upon in order to shew them that it was not their own Superior strength and Numbers which obliged us to leave their isle, this made them fly from it as fast as their legs could cary them,[2] this done we spent the night plying on and off in order to take a view the next morning of a nother isle we saw to the WSW.

The Island we have been upon is the same as was discovered and Visited by Commodore Byron and I think it was named by him Coral Island,[3] but its proper name is [Ti-oo-kea].[4] It is like most of the other low Isles in this Sea a narrow String of Small Islots lying in an Oval form & connected together by[5] a reef of coral rocks, the whole incloseing a lake of Salt water of 8 or 10 Leagues in circuit. The one I am speaking off lies WNW and ESE four leagues and is about 4 miles broad; It is situated in the Latitude of 14°27′30″ South, Longitude 144°56′ West. The Inhabitants of this isle and perhaps those of most of the other low isles are of a much darker Colour than those of the high isles and seem to have a more ferine

[1] *got:* got by exchanges . . .—f. 191v.

[2] 'Five shot were fir'd over the Natives from the ship which made them retire with much greater swiftness then they advanc'd leaving their Habitations and gardens (which I think are the most beautifull spots to appearence in nature) to the mercy of a people to whom they could not have the highest opinion from the treatment in 1764 being fir'd and severl kill'd in order to gain a canoe night coming on the Capt thought it necessary to leave the Island.'—Gilbert. Cf. n. 3 below.

[3] Byron discovered this island, Takaroa, one of the northernmost of the Tuamotus, on 9 June 1765; but he had been preceded by Roggeveen, in May 1722, who called it *Twee Gebroeder*. Byron called it, with its neighbour Takapoto, King George's Islands, which name remains. He tried a friendly approach, but found the inhabitants hostile, and finally forced a landing at the expense of two or three native lives. He took two fine canoes, and next day was able to load coconuts and scurvy grass; he also found a carved rudder-head and some small Dutch iron tools, which must have come from Roggeveen's *Afrikaansche Galei*.

[4] *is* : amongst the Natives is Ti-oo-kea.—f. 191v.—According to Forster, it was 'Odiddy' (or Mahine) who got this name, Teoukea as he spells it. But Clerke says, 'We got their Name for the Island I believe tolerably distinctly—they call it Taowhāar'; and Wales says it was Taoukaà. Whatever it was called then, it was the island now called Takaroa.

[5] The words 'lying in an Oval form and connected together by' are substituted for the deleted ones 'chained together, as it were, with'. The image of the chain is interesting, as it takes us back to Cook's 'Chain Island' (Anaa) of April 1769; and, as will be seen from Gilbert's Chart XXXIII*a*, is also a good one.

disposition,[1] our people observed they were stout well made men and had tattow'd on various parts of the bodies the figure of a fish.[2] At day-light in the Morning we bore down to the Island to leeward,[3] fell in with the NE point and ran along the SE side at the distance of one Mile from the Shore; we found it to be just like the former, extend[ing] NE and SW near 4 Leagues and from 5 to 3 miles broad, it lies SWBW 2 Leagues from the West End of Tiookea,[4] the Middle is situated in Lat 14°37′ S, Longitude 145°10′ west. This must be the same isle to which Commodore Byron gave the name of Georges Island;[5] the Longitude of these isles were determined by Lunar observation made near the Shores, and still farther corrected by the difference of Longitude carried on by the watch to Otaheite, whose Situation cannot be disputed; thus by knowing the Longitude of these two Isles I shall be able to correct all Mr Byron's discover[ie]s, the Correction wanting is only about and arises chiefly from his placeing the point of his departure too far and not from any imperfection in his Journal. After leaving these isles we steer'd SSW½W and SWBS[6] having still signs of the vicinity of land such as smooth Water &c^a^.

TUESDAY 19*th. Winds NE to East. Course S* 55° *W. Dist. Sailed* 73 *M. Lat. in* 15°38′. *Longde. in* 146°34′. A gentle trade and pleasent weather, Continued to Steer SWBS till 8 o'Clock in the PM when we shortned Sail and spent the night plying under our Topsails. At 7 o'Clock in the AM saw land to the westward and bore down to it; at 9 we were the length of the SE side and hauld up to the SW, this

[1] ... this may be owing to the isles on which they live where Nature has not bestowed her favours in that profusion she has done to some of the others, the Inhabitants of these low Islands are chiefly beholden to the Sea for thier subsistance conssequently are much exposed to the Sun and Weather and by that means become more dark more hardy and robust, for there is no doubt but they are of the same Nation.—f. 192.

[2] ... a very good emblem of their profession.—f. 192.—'Those people are large in stature indifferently made of a swarthy complexion their Countenances clouded there does not seem to be the least chearfullness about them like unto the adjacent Islanders going almost naked having Figurs punctuated on different parts of the body.'—Gilbert.

[3] *the Island to leeward:* a nother isle we had in sight to the westward

[4] The name is a later insertion in a blank space.

[5] Takapoto. It was on this island that Roggeveen lost his *Afrikaansche Galei* in May 1722; he called it *Schadelijk* or 'Pernicious'. Wales writes of both islands, 'I make no doubt of these being the Pernicious Isles of Roggewein as not only the Latit. but the Longit, also, from Easter Island, as put down in the Dutch Relation of that Voyage corresponds extreamly well: They are the Isles of Disappointment also of Capt Byron'. This last guess was wrong: Byron's Islands of Disappointment, which seemed to promise so much of fruit for scurvy-stricken men, and where he could not land, were Tepoto and Napuka, about 3½ degrees east of Takaroa, and a little north. The Takapoto people were friendly to Byron, but he could not find anchorage. Apart from other discoveries, Takapoto seems to have been Schouten's 'Bottomless Island'—*Eylandt Sonder Grondt*—of April 1616.

[6] ... with a fine easterly gale

proved to be another of those drowned isles,[1] extending NNE and SSW about 5 Leagues, breadth 3 Leagues, Situated in Lat 15°26′ S, Long^de^ 146°20′ West. As we approached the South end of this isle, we saw from the Mast head a nother Low Island bearing SE distant 4 or 5 Leagues,[2] this being to windward we could not fetch it; soon after we saw a third Land bearing SWBS for which we Steer'd.[3]

WEDNESDAY 20*th. Winds Easterly. Course S* 63° *W. Dist. Sailed* 58 *M. Lat. in* 16°4′. *Longde. in* 147°28′. PM Fresh breezes and fine Weather. At half an hour past 2 o'Clock reached the East end of the 3rd isle[4] and ran along the North side at the distance of half a mile from Shore, we found this isle to extend WNW and ESE Seven Leagues, in breadth about two, it was in all respects like those we had seen before only there are fewer isles and less firm land on the reef which incloseth the lake; As we ran a long shore we saw People, Hutts, Boats and places seemingly for drying of fish; they seem'd to be the same sort of people as those on Coral Island and were Arm'd with long pikes like them. The SE point of this Isle is situated in the Lat 15°47′ S, Longitude 146°30′ West.[5] In runing down the whole length of the N side of it, we saw not the least signs of Anchorage. Coming near the West end we discovered a nother or 4th Isle bearing NNE,[6] it seem'd to be low like the others and lies West from the first isle about Six Leagues.[7]

Here[8] we spent the night Plying under the Top-sails and at daylight hauld round the west end of the 3rd Isle and seeing no more land and finding a great Swell rolling in from the South, a certain

[1] *Those drowned isles:* these half over-flowed or drown'd Islands which are so Common to this part of the ocean, that is a number of little isles rainged in circlear form, connected together by a reef or Wall of Coral Rocks, for the Sea is in general, every where on the out side unfathomable. All the interior part of these isles or Keys is Water which I have been told abound with fish and Turtle on which the Inhabitants subsist and some times exchange the latter with the high Islanders for Cloth. These Inland Seas would be excellent harbours were they not Shut up from the access of shiping, which I believe is the case with the most of them, if we can believe the report of the Inhabitants of the other isles; indeed few of them have been well searched by Europeans, the little prospect of meeting with fresh water hath generally discouraged every attempt of this kind. I who have seen a great many have not seen yet an inlet into one.—f. 192v. This particular drowned isle was Apataki.

[2] Toau, lat. 16°02′ S, long. 145°56′ W.

[3] We learn from Cooper that this day the armourer, who had been making a new keel band for the pinnace, was at work on nails for trade at Tahiti. Later—so great was the run on trade goods—we find him making hatchets as well as nails.

[4] Kaukura.

[5] A much better position than that for Apataki. The modern reckoning is 15°49′ S, 146°28′ W.

[6] Arutua, lat. 15°22′ S, long. 146°37′ W.

[7] . . . These four isles I called *Palliser's Isles* in honour of my worthy friend Mr Pallisser Comptroller of the Navy.—f. 193. Chart XXXIII*b*, and Fig. 33 above.

[8] *Here:* Not chuseing to run farther in the dark . . .—f. 193.

Sign we were clear of these low Islands, We steer'd sw½s for Otahiete having a stout gale attended with Showers of rain.[1]

THURSDAY 21*st. Winds EBN. Course S* 38°45′. *Dist. Sailed* 113 *M. Lat. in* 17°32′. *Longde. in* 148°42′. First part fresh gales with rain, remainder fair and Clowdy. At 10 AM Saw the high land of Otahiete and at Noon Point Venus bore west-northerly distant 13 Leagues.

FRIDAY 22*nd. Winds Easterly. Lat. in* 17°29′. *Longde. in* 149°35′, [*watch*] 151°44′. PM Moderate breezes and Clowdy. At 7 Shortned Sail and spent the night plying of and on. AM Squally with heavy Showers of rain. At 8 Anchored in Matavai Bay in 7 fathom Water, which was no sooner done than we were viseted by several of our old friends, who express'd not a little joy at seeing us.[2]

As my reasons for puting in here was to give Mr Wales an oppertunity to know the error of the Watch from the known Longitude of this place and to determine a fresh her rate of going; the first thing we did was to land his Instruments &ca and to set up tents for the reception of a guard and such others as it was necessary to have on Shore. As to Sick we had none.[3]

SATURDAY 23*rd.* Showery rainy Weather. The Natives[4] begin to

[1] While they were still among the atolls Wales, that steady man, displayed a little petulance. 'The Islands [we] were now amongst were strenuously disputed by most of the Officers to be those which form the Labarynth of Roggewein; I cannot imagine how such a thought could Enter the head of Man since they do not correspond in any one particular except that of there being several: I saw but three; however some pretend a fourth was seen by somebody or other; ought it not then to have been Mentioned in the Log? . . . On the whole, I rather think these Islands have not been seen before; although I would be Cautious saying this, as I firmly believe Islands have been greatly multiplied, and Much Confusion has arisen in the Geography of these seas from a desire of being thought the first discoverers of any land that has been seen.' On this Cook (B, f. 193v) provides proper comment: 'It cannot be determined with any degree of certainty whither the groupe of iles we have lately seen, be any of those discovered by the dutch navigators or no as the situation of their discoveries [*deleted* especially those of Roggeweins] are far from being handed down to us with that accuracy necessary to determine this point. [*deleted* I, perhaps, may consider this subject in another place when I have more time to spare than at present] It is however necessary to observe that this part of the Ocean, that is from the Latitude of 20 down to 14 or 12 and from the Meridian of 138 to 148 or 150° is so strewed with these low Isles that a Navigator cannot proceed with too much caution'. Roggeveen appears to have sailed right through the Palliser group. See the map in Mulert, *De Reis van Mr Jacob Roggeveen* (Linschoten-Vereeniging, 1911).

[2] '. . . we were no sooner Anchor'd than viseted by several of our friends who seem'd glad to see us, but gave us to understand we were not to expect much refreshments till the arrival of Otoo who was at a distant part of the isle.'—Log.—'. . . a little after 9 o'Clock came to an Anchor in 7½ fathoms, and moored with a small Anchor to leeward; but it was not done before the Ship was crouded with our old friends, and if there be any truth in Physiognomy they were extreamly glad to see us, from what Motive I will not pretend to say.'—Wales.

[3] . . . the refreshments we got at the Marquases [*sic*] had removed every complaint of that kind.—f. 194.

[4] *The Natives:* Our very good friends the Natives

bring us in refreshments, such as fruit and Fish, sufficient for all hands.

SUNDAY 24*th. Otou* the King with a vast train and several Chiefs of distinction paid us a Viset and brought with them as presents Ten or a Doz^{n} Hogs which made them exceeding welcome. I was advertised of the Kings coming and met him at the Tents a shore, conducted him on board where he stay'd Dinner, after which he and his attendance were dismiss'd with Suteable presents.[1]

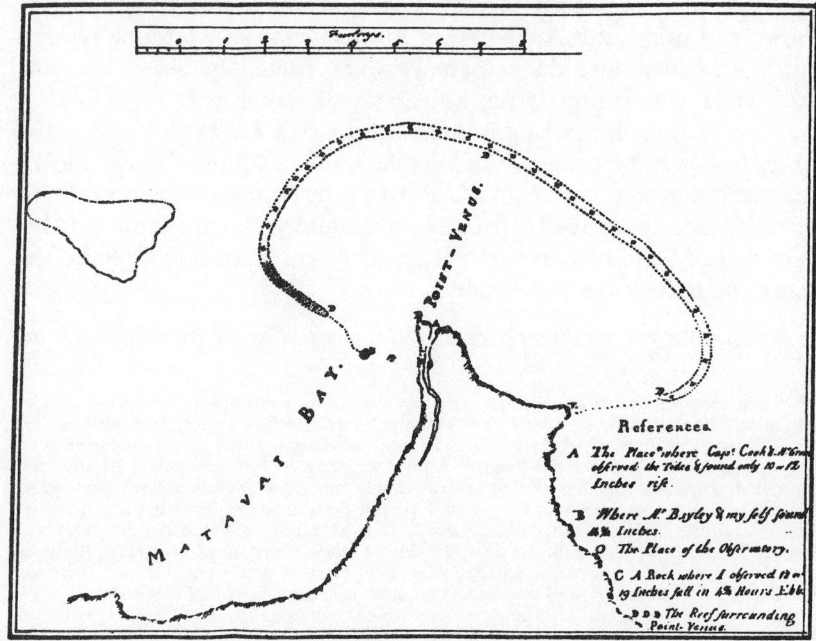

FIG. 58. William Wales, chart of Matavai Bay

MONDAY 25*th.* Much rain, Thunder and Lightning. Nevertheless I had a nother Viset from Otou who brought with him a quantity of refreshments &c^{a}. When we were at Amsterdam, among other Curosities we Collected some red Parrot Feathers[2] which were highly Valued by these people; When this came to be known in the isle all the Principal people of both Sex endeavour'd by every means in

[1] *I was . . . presents:* I was advertised of the Kings coming and looked upon it as a good omen, and knowing how much it was to my intrest to make this man my friend, I met him at the Tents and conducted him and his friends on board in my boat where they stayed dinner, after which they were dismissed with Suteable presents and highly pleased with the reception they met with.—f. 194.

[2] Probably those of the Red-breasted Musk Parrot.

their power to Ingratiate themselves into our favour in order to obtain these Valuable Jewels by bring[ing] us Hogs and every other thing the Island produced, and generally for Tiyo (Friendship) but they always took care to let us know that Oora[1] (red Feathers) were to be a part of the return we were to make. Having these Feathers was a very fortunate circumstance to us for as they were Valuable to the Natives they became so to us allso, for our Stock of trade was by this time greatly exhausted and if it had not been for them I should have found it difficult to have supplyed the Ships with the necessary refreshments.[2]

When I put in here my intention was to stay but a few days, that is no longer than M[r] Wales had made the Obser[ns] for the purpose already mentioned from a supposition founded on the reception we met with the last time we were here that we should get no Hogs; but the Number the Natives have already brought us and the few excursions we have made which have not exceeded the Plains of Matavai and Oparre hath convinced us of our error. We find at these two places built and building a great number of Canoes and houses both large and small, People living in spacious houses who had not a place to shelter themselves in Eight Months ago, several large hogs near every house and every other Sign of a riseing state.

Judging from these favourable circumstances that we should not mend our Situation by removeing to a nother island I therefore resolved to make a longer stay & to begin with the repairs of the Ship;[3] accordingly I ordered the empty Casks and Sails to be got on shore to repair, the Smiths Forge to be set up to repair our Iron work, the Ship to be Caulked and the rigging &c[a] to be overhauled, Works which the high Southern Latitudes had made highly necessary.

TUESDAY 26*th*. In the Morning I set out for Oparre accompaned

[1] *ura*, red; and compendiously, red feathers.

[2] 'So very solicitous & zealously desirous are our good friends here for the attaining of these red Feathers and so thoroughly convinc'd of their efficacy with their Sovereign Deities that they will very chearfully oblige us in good natur'd but rather unhallow'd rites for the possession of them to render back religious Ceremonies by way of Propitiation to their Jolly Gods.'—Clerke 8952 (folio inset after 14 May).—Red was a colour sacred to the great god Oro, and red feathers were an important part of his local cult—'talismanic mediums of divine power' (Handy, *Polynesian Religion*, p. 126). The sacred girdle that Tuteha snatched from Papara (I, p. clxxxiv) was the *maro-ura*, the red feather girdle. The 'good-natur'd but rather unhallow'd rites' referred to by Clerke in one particular instance upset the senior Forster. That great chief Potatau and his second wife 'Wainee-ou' (? Vahine-ou), took counsel together on the subject of *ura*, and accordingly she 'offered herself to Captain Cook, and appeared as a ready victim.—*Tunica velata recincta* . . . . my spirits were damped by this unexpected scene of immorality and selfishness, in a family where I least expected to hear of it'.—J. R. Forster, *Observations*, pp. 391–2. Cook however was, as usual, impregnable.

[3] . . . and Stores &c[a]

by the two M[r] Forsters and some of the officers to pay Otoo a formal Viset by appointment, as we approached Oparre we observed a number of large Canoes in Motion; but we were surprised when we got there to see upwards of three-hundred of them all rainged in good order for some distance along the Shore all Compleatly equip'd and Man'd, and a vast Crowd of Men[1] on the Shore; So unexpected an Armament collected together in our Neighbourhood in the space of one night gave rise to various conjectures: we landed however[2] and were received by a Vast Multitude some under Arms and some not, the cry of the latter was Tiyo no Otoo and the former Tiyo no Towha,[3] this Cheif as we soon after learnt was General or Admiral of the fleet. I was met by him presently after we landed, he received[4] me with great Courtsey and then took hold of my right hand. A Cheif whose name was Tee, Uncle to the King and one of his Prime Ministers, had hold of my left, thus I was draged along as it were between two parties, both declaring themselves our friends,[5] the one wanted me to stay by the fleet and the other to go to the King, at last coming to the general place of Audience a Mat was spread on the ground for me to sit down upon and Tee went to bring the King, Towha was unwilling I should sit down but partly insisted on my going to the fleet but as I knew nothing of this Chief I did not comply; presently Tee return'd and wanted to conduct me to the King and took me by the hand for that purpose, this Towha opposed so that between the one party and the other I was like to have been torn to pieces and was obliged to disire Tee to desist, and to go with the Admiral and his party to the fleet. As soon as we came before the Admirals Vessel two lines of Arm'd Men were drawen up on the shore before her to keep of the Crowd[6] and clear the way for me to go in, but as I was determined not to go (unless forced) I made the Water which was between me and the Canoe an excuse, this did not answer for a Man immidiately squated himself down at my feet and offered to carry me in and then I declar'd I would not go and that very moment Towha quited me without my seeing which way he went nor would any one inform me; I therefore turn'd back and in-

[1] *of Men*: of arm'd men

[2] . . . in the midst of them

[3] *Taio no Tu*, friend of Tu!—*Taio no Towha*, friend of Towha!

[4] *General . . . received:* Admiral or Commander of the Fleet and Troops present. The moment we landed I was met by a cheif whose name was Tee [Ti'i], Uncle to the King and one of his Prime Ministers, of whome I enquired for Otoo presently after we were met by Towha who recieved . . .—f. 195.

[5] *thus . . . friends:* and without my knowing were they intended to carry me, draged me as it were through the Crowd which was divided into two parties both of which profess'd themselves my friends by crying out Tiyo no Tootee, [friend of Cook!] . . .—f. 195.

[6] . . . as I supposed

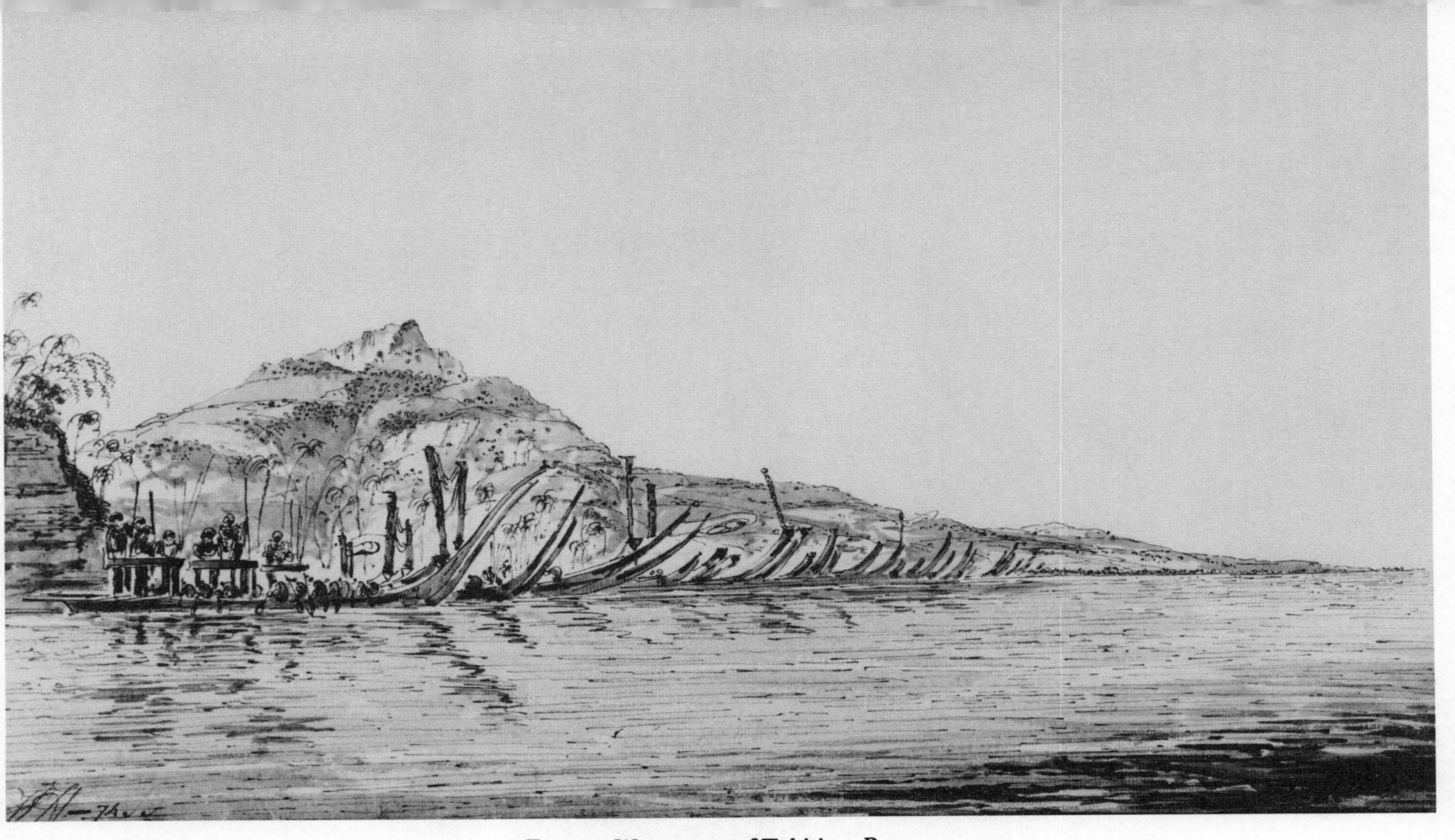

FIG. 59. War canoes of Tahiti, at Pare

Wash drawing by Hodges.—Mitchell Library, D11, no. 14

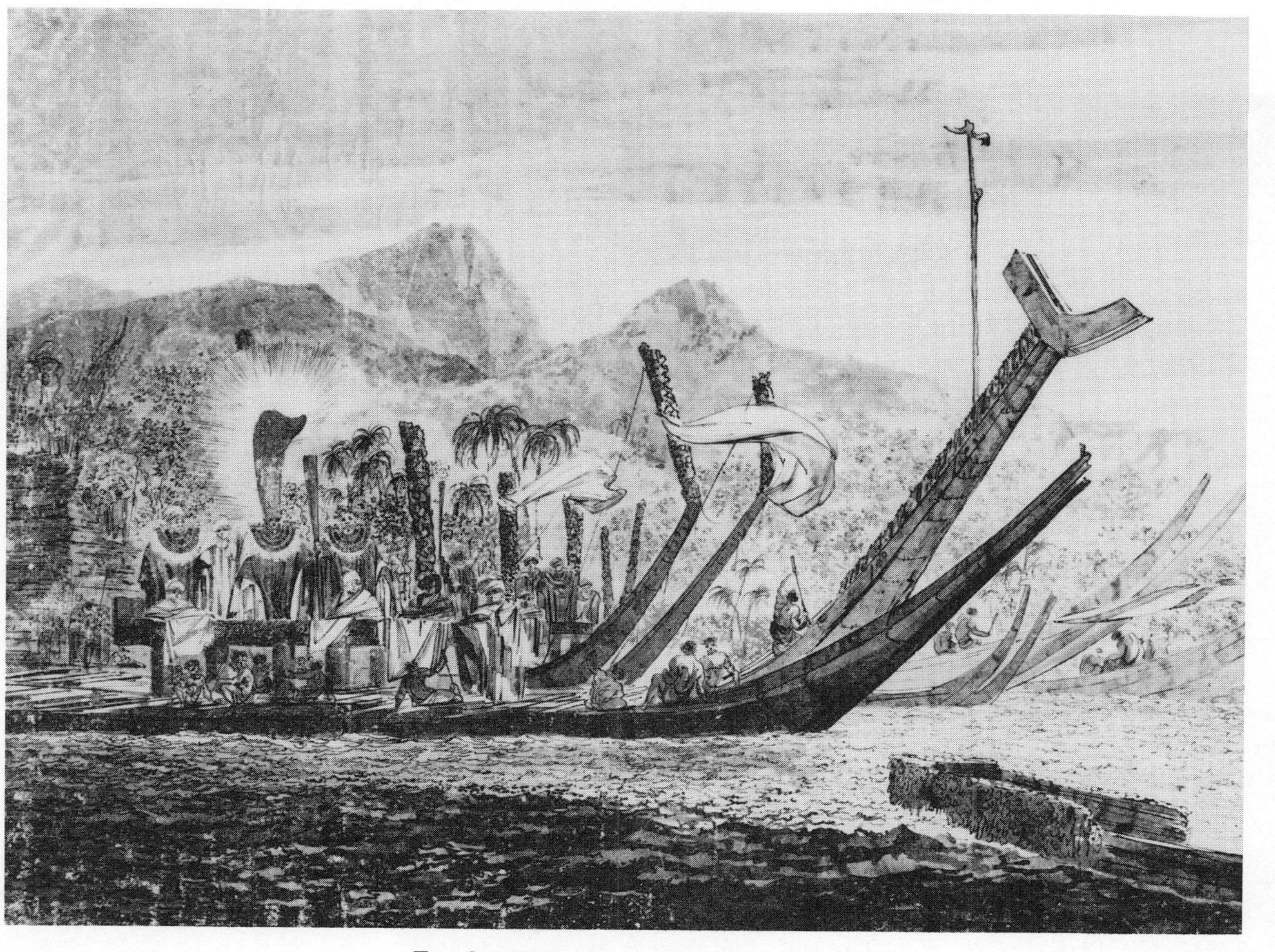

Fig. 60. War canoes of Tahiti, at Pare

quired for the King, Tee who I beleive never lost sight of me, came and told me he was gone into the Country Mataou[1] and advised me to go to my boat which we according did as soon as we got all together for Mr Edgcumb was the only gentleman that could keep with me, the others were jostled about in the crowd in the same Manner as we were. When we had got into our boat we took our time to view this fleet, the Vessels of War consisted of 160 large double Canoes,[2] very well equip'd, Man'd and Arm'd, altho' I am not sure that they had on board either their full compliment of Fighting men or rowers, I rather think not. The Cheifs ie all those on the Fighting Stages were drist in their War habits, that is in a vast quantity of Cloth Turbands, breast Plates and Helmmets, some of the latter are of such a length as to greatly incumber the wearer, indeed their whole dress seem'd ill calculated for the day of Battle and seems to be design'd more for shew than use, be this as it may they certainly added grandure to the Prospect, as they were complesant enough to Shew themselves to the best advantage, their Vessels were decorated with Flags, Streamers &ca so that the whole made a grand and Noble appearence such as was never seen before in this Sea,[3] their implements of war were Clubs, pikes and Stones. These Canoes were rainged close along side each other with their heads a Shore and Sterns to the Sea, the Admirals Vesel was, as near as I could guess, in the center. Besides these Vesels of War there were 170 Sail of Smaller double Canoes, all with a little house upon them and rigg'd with Masts and sails which the others had not; These Canoes must be design'd for Transporte or Victulars or both and to receive the wounded Men &ca; in the War Canoes were no sort of Provisions whatever. In these 330 Canoes I judged there were

[1] *matau*, frightened.

[2] B *note* What I call a double Canoe, is 2 Canoes fixed parallel to and about 4 feet from each other, by means of cross-beams.—f. 195v. Similarly AGH. The MS text has a space left for this footnote, which Cook forgot, or did not trouble, to supply.

[3] . . . nor what any one would [have] expected.—f. 196. See the engraving after Hodges, *Voyage*, I, pl. LXI. Hodges afterwards made a large painting of the scene, which now hangs in Admiralty House. For Clerke it seems to have been a sort of climax: 'Tho' we ever found ourselves at Home among these good People, their reception this visit was if possible more social than ever, I suppose owing to the happy state of tranquillity they were in, in respeet to each other; and probably in some measure to the report of our friend Odiddy who has been the last Campaigne with us. Nothing in Nature cou'd exceed the unbounded civillity and friendship with which they now treated us, and as to provision, whatever this fine Salutary Isle produc'd, we were most abundantly suppli'd with, and that in such plenty that all ye inconvenience we lay under, was to find room to stow it away. To say any thing of the properties of this good Isle after the publication of the Endeavours Voyage wou'd be tautology; but I was fortunately an eye witness to one circumstance during our present stay, which we never had an opportunity of seeing before'. He goes on to describe the fleet. This is in his notes on Tahiti, following his entry for 14 May. See the drawings by Hodges, Figs. 59, 60.

no less than 7760 Men a number which appears incredable, especially as we were told that they all belonged to the districts of Attahourou and Ahopatea;[1] in this computation I allow to each War Canoe one with a nother 40 Men, rowers and fighting Men, and to each of the Small Canoes eight, but most of the gentlemen who saw this fleet thinks the number of Men to the War Canoes were more than I have reckoned. I must own these Canoes in general are fitted to row with more Paddles than I have allow'd them Men, but at this time I beleive they were not compleat. Tupia inform'd us last Voyage that the whole Island raised only between Seven and Eight[2] Thousand Men, now we see two districts only raise that Number so that he must have taken his account from some old establishment or else he only meant fighting Men, Taata-o tai (Men trained to Arms)[3] and did not include the rowers and those in the other Vesels attending on the fleet, indeed this is most probable for Tupia, I think, he only spoke of this number as the Standing Troops or Militia of the island and not their whole force, tho we understood him so at that time. I shall leave this point to be discussed in a nother place and return to the subject.

When we had well view'd this fleet I wanted much to see the Admiral to have gone with him on board the Vesels, I enquired for him as we rowed past the Vesels to no purpose, we then put a shore and inquire'd for him, but the noise and Crowd was so great that no one attended to what we said, at last Tee came and whispered us in the ear that the King was gone to Matavai and advised us to go their also and not to land where we were, we took his advice put off and row'd for the Ship accordingly, this account and advice of Tee gave rise to new conjectures, in short we conclude that this Towha was some disaffected Chief upon the point of making War against

[1] Cook's 'district' names are most unreliable. Atehuru properly included three districts —Faaa, Punaauia, and Paea, which is their order from north to south. Cook's Attahourou, of which Tuteha had been the chief, was Paea. But on Chart V, drawn on the first voyage, we have, running from north to south, Tettahah (Faaa), Otaapoona (probably a place-name—it occupies part of what is properly Punaauia), Apoonawea, (Punaauia), Ahopatea, and Atahourou—which is nomenclatural confusion, tallying with neither Cook's text nor reality. Ahopatea occupies the place properly belonging to Paea: it may have been a place-name inside that district—a stream and valley not far from the Punaauia border are (or were) called Hopa. See Fig. 35, inset (above, p. 214).

[2] *Seven and Eight:* 6 and 7.—Since the first volume of this work was published, a note by Banks has been found, B.M. Add. MS 27889, f. 71, headed 'Forces of Otahite 6780', and listing numbers by 14 districts. The sum of these individual numbers, however, is 6280.

[3] *Taata-o'tai* (*Men trained to Arms*): Tatatoas, that is Wariors or men trained from their infancy to arms . . .—f. 196v.—Cook evidently picked up two different phrases. In Tahitian *tai* means sea; *taata o tai* may have signified seamen sailors ('men of the sea'). 'Tatatoas': *taata-toa; toa* is warrior[s], so that we have a reduplicated form, 'men [who are] warriers'. Similarly, in Tongan *tangata toa* signified warrior[s].

his King.[1] We had not long left Oparre before the whole fleet was in Motion and proceeded back to the westward from whence they came.

When we got on board the Ship, we were told that this fleet was a part of the armament intended to go against Eimeo whose Chief had revolted from Otou his Lawfull Sovereign.[2] I was also inform'd that Otou was not nor had been at Matavai, and therefore after dinner I went again to Oparre where I found him, I now learn that his fears and the reason of his not seeing us in the Morning was occasioned by some of his people stealing (owing to the neglect of the washerman) a quantity of my Clothes[3] and was fearfull least I should demand restitution,[4] when I assured him I should not disturb the peace of the isle on any such occasion[5] he was satisfied; I likewise understood that Towha was alarm'd partly on this account and partly by my not honoring him with my company on board his fleet when he desired it. I was Jealous at seeing such a Force in our neigherhood without being able to know any thing of its design; thus by misunderstanding one a nother I lost the oppertunity of examining more narrowly into a part of the Naval force of this Island and makeing my self better acquainted how it acts and is conducted. Such a nother oppertunity may never happen again as it was commanded by a brave, Sencible and intelligent Chief who no doubt would have satisfied us in all the questions we had thought proper to ask and as the Objects were before our eyes we could not well have mistook one another.[6] Matter[s] being Thus cleared up and mutual presents having pass'd between Otou and me we return'd on board in the evening.

WEDNESDAY *27th.* Morning, Received a present from Towha consisting of Two Large hogs and some fruit sent me by two of his Servants who had orders to receive nothing in return. Soon after I took a trip in my boat to Oparre were I found both this chief and the King, after a Short Stay I brought them both on board to dinner

[1] ... for we could not immagine Otoo had any other reason for leaving Oparre in the manner he did.—f. 196v.

[2] *had revolted . . . Sovereign:* had thrown off the yoke of Otahiete and assumed an independency.—f. 197. This alteration radically changes the sense. A chief of Aimeo (Moorea) might very well be tributary to Tu, but could not possibly throw off the yoke of Tahiti, which had no yoke. The error springs from the English persuasion that Tu was a king—a persuasion that was to have more serious consequences; cf. I, pp. clxxxii ff., and p. xcii above.

[3] ... which were on shore washing

[4] ... and asked me over and over again if I was not angry

[5] *when . . . occasion:* when I assured him I was not and that they might keep what they had got,

[6] ... It happened unluky [*sic*] Oediddee was not with us in the morning for Tee, who was the only man we could depend on, served only to perplex us.—f. 197–7v.

together with the Kings Brother,[1] they were shew'd all over the Ship, the Admiral who had never seen such a one before view'd every thing with great attention and express'd much surprise at what he saw.[2] After dinner he put a Hog on board the Ship and retired before I had time to make him any return either for this or what I had in the Morning and soon after the King and his Brother took leave. The King seem'd not only to pay the Admiral much respect himself but was desireous I should do the same, he was nevertheless certainly jelous of him, but on what account we knew not for it was but the day before he frankly told us the Admiral was not his friend. Both these Chiefs when on board to day Solicited me to assist them against the people of Tiarabou altho at this time the two Kin[g]doms are at peace and we were told go with their joint force against Eimeo. To this request of theirs I made an evasive answer which I believe they understood was not favourable to their request.[3]

THURSDAY 28*th*. Remaind on board all day. Had a Present of a Hog sent me by Oheatua the King of Tiarabou, for which in return he disired a few red feathers.[4] In the afternoon M[r] Forster and his party set out for the Mountains with an intent to Stay out the night.[5]

FRIDAY 29*th*. Early in the Morn Otoo, Towha and Several other Grandees came on board and brought with them not only provisions but some of the Most Valuable curiosities in the island which they gave to me and for which I made them such returns as they were well pleased with, I likewise took the oppertunity to repay the civilties I had received from Towha.

Last night one of the Natives made an Attempt to Steal one of our Water Casks from the Watering Place, he was caught, sent on board and put in Irons in which Situation he was found by the two Chiefs

[1] *together . . . Brother:* together with Tarĕvatoo the Kings younger brother and Tee.—f. 197v. 'Tarĕvatoo', Te-ari'i-fa'atau. Cf. p. 410, n. 1.

[2] *they were . . . saw:* As soon as we drew near the Ship the Admiral, who had never seen one before, began to express much surprise at so new a Sight; he was shewed all over the Ship every part of which he Viewed with great attention, on this occasion Otoo was the principle showman for by this time he was well acquainted with the different parts of the Ship.—f. 197v.

[3] . . . Whether this was done with a View of breaking with their Neighbours and Allies, if I had promised them assistance or only to sound my disposition I know not, probable they would have been ready enough to embrace an oppertunity which would have inabled them to Conquer that Kingdom and annexed it to their own as it was formerly; be this as it may, I heard no more of it, indeed I gave them no incouragement.—f. 198.

[4] . . . which were together with other things sent him accordingly.

[5] 'Fine weather Employed Watering, Airing and Picking the Bread, overhauling the Rigging &c[a] &c[a].'—Log.

to whom I made known his crime.[1] Otou beg'd he might be set at liberty which I refused tilling him it was but Just the Man should be punished,[2] accordingly I orderd him a shore to the Tent, where I went my self with the two Chiefs and others, here I ordered the Man to be tyed up to a Post, Otou his Sister and some others beg'd hard for the Man, Towha said not one word but was very attentive to every thing going forward; I expostulated with Otou on the conduct of this Man and his people in general tilling him that neither I nor any of my people took any thing from him or his people without first paying for it and innumirated the Articles we gave for such and such things and that he well knew that when any of my people broke through these rules they were punished for it and that it was but right this man should be punished also, besides I told him it would be the means of saving the lives of some of his people by detering them from commiting crimes of this nature in which some would be kill'd[3] at one time or a nother; I said more to the same purpose most of which I believe he pretty well understood as he was satisfied and only desired the Man might not be kill'd.[4] I then ordered the guard out to keep the Crowd which was very great at a proper distance and in Sight of them all ordered the fellow two dozen lashes with a Cat of Nine tails which he bore with great firmness, he was then set at liberty and Towha the Admiral began to Harangue the crowd for not a man left us on this occasion, he spoke for a full quarter of an hour and with seemingly great Perspicuity and he was heard with great Attention,[5] his speach consisted mostly of short Sentences, nevertheless I could understand but few words,[6] he recapitulated most of what I had said to Otou, named several Advantages they had received from us, condemn'd their present conduct and recommended a different one for the future.[7] Otou on this occa-

[1] Marra, pp. 180–3, gives an account of this incident, with the wrong date. The attention of the sentry and the watch was distracted, he says, by the sound of splashing in the water. Then the thief swam under water to the cask, made off with it on his back, and concealed it on a sedgy swamp, in a hole in the bushes which he had previously made for the purpose. The trouble given in such ways, it may be added, was partly due to the fact that in the Polynesian pattern theft from strangers was popularly regarded as a challenge to ingenuity and a game of skill, and not at all as a matter of moral obliquity.

[2] *it was . . . punished:* sence I punished my people when they commited the least offence against his, it was but just the Man should be punished also, and as I knew he would not do it I was resolved to do it my self.—f. 198v.

[3] *kill'd:* shot dead

[4] *kill'd:* Matteerou (killed).—'Matteerou' is probably *mate rava* (*rava* is an intensive, and the pronunciation of the *v* would lean to *w*): quite killed, killed stone dead.

[5] *and Towha . . . Attention:* after which the Natives were going away but Towha stepd forth called them back and Hara[n]gued them for near half an hour . . .—f. 199.—'. . . a speech which lasted about four or five minutes', says Forster (II, p. 79).

[6] . . . but from what we could gather

[7] . . . The gracefulness of his action when he spoke and the attention with which he was heard bespoake him a great Orator.—f. 199.

sion spoke not one word. As soon as the Chief had ended his speach I order'd the Marines to go through their exercise and to Load and fire which gave the Two Chiefs, especially the Admiral, much entertainment,[1] this done I invited them on board to dinner but they excused themselves took leave and retired with all their attendance.[2] In the evening M[r] Forster[3] return'd from the Mountains, where he found some new Plants[4] and from whence he saw Huaheine which lies to the westward, by this a judgment may be form'd of the height of these hills in Otaheite which I believe will not be found not less than

SATURDAY 30*th*. I had an oppertunity this Morn[g] at Matavai to see the people in Ten War Canoes go through their exercize in Padling, they were at the same time properly equip'd for war, the chiefs in their war habits &c[a]. I was present at their land[g] [5] and observed that the moment the Canoe touched the Shore all the padlers jump'd out and with the assistance of a few people on the shore draged her on the Strand when, without stoping the Canoe those on the Stage and in the Stern got out, all those on the Stage except one Walkd off with their Arms &c[c] but the one which remained walked between the two heads of the Canoe till She was in her proper place where she was left, every one carrying off his Padle, Arms &c[a] so that in Five minuets time you could not tell that any thing of this kind had been going forward. I had here an oppertunity to see those men on the Stage undress and was not a little surprised at the quantity and weight of Cloth they had upon them and how they could stand under it in the day of battle. I told them that when we fought in our Ships we took off our Clothes (throwing off my clothes at the same time) but they paid little attention to what I either did or said.

*... I thought these Vessels were thinly manned, with rowers especially, the most being not above thirty and the least Sixteen or Eighteen, I observed the Wariors on the Stage encouraged the

[1] *Load ... entertainment:* load and fire in Vollies with ball, and as the Marines were very quick in their Manouvres, it is easier to conceive than to describe the amazement the Natives were under the whole time, especially those who had not seen any thing of the kind before.

[2] ... scarcely more pleased than frightened at what they had seen.

[3] ... and his party.—The party was Sparrman, a sailor and a marine. Guided by Tahitians, they had climbed some steep hills and got wet to the skin, but from the heights had a good view of Huahine, Tetiaroa, and Tubuai-manu. On the way down the elder Forster slipped heavily in a rocky place, and both bruised his leg painfully and ruptured himself.—Forster, II, pp. 81–3.

[4] ... and some others which grow in New zeeland.

[5] *I was ... land[g]* they were put off from the shore before I was appriz'd of it, so that I was only present at their landing ...—f. 199.

rowers to exert their utmost. Some Youths sat high up in the curved Stern above the steersmen with white wands in their hands, I know not what they were placed here for unless it was to look out and direct or give notice of what they saw as they were elevated above every one else. Tarevatoo the Kings brother gave me the first notice of these Canoes being at Sea and knowing that Mr Hodges made drawings of every thing curious, desired of his own accord that he might be sent for, I being at this time ashore with Tarevatoo: Mr Hodges was therefore with me and had an oppertunity to collect some materials for a large drawing or Picture he intends to make of the fleet assembled at Oparre which will convey a far better idea of them than can be express'd by words.[1] I was present when the Wariors undress'd and was surpris'd at the quantity and weight of Cloth they had upon them and how it was possible for them to stand under it in time of battle; not a little was wraped round their heads as a Turband and made into a Cap, this indeed might be necessary in preventing a broken head; many had fix'd to one of these sorts of caps dryed branches of small shrubs which were cover'd over with white feathers, these however could only be for Ornament.*—G, pp. 191–2.

[May 1774]

SUNDAY May *1st.* Had a Vast Supply of Provisions sent and brought us by different Chiefs.

MONDAY *2nd.* Received a present consisting of a Boat Load of various Fruits and a Hog from Towha sent me by his Servants together with a Message that he would see me in two days, the like present I also had from Otoo, brought by Tarevatoo his Brother who stay'd dinner after which I went down to Oparre with him viseted Otou and return'd on board in the Evening.

TUESDAY *3rd.* In looking into the State of our Sea Provisions we found the Biscuit in a state of decay and that the Airing and Picking we had given it at New-zealand had not done it that service we intended and expected so that we were obliged to have it all a Shore here where it has under gone a nother airing and clencing, in which has been found unfit to eat [3420] pounds,[2] we cannot well

[1] These materials are perhaps the drawings reproduced in this volume as Figs. 59 and 60.

[2] *in which . . . pounds:* in which a good deal was found wholy rotten and unfit to be eat. —f. 200.—See Cook's order to the warrant officers of 28 April, 'Whereas Complaints are daily made unto me, that a part of the Bread on board, is Mouldy, rotten & unfit for men to eat' etc., p. 948 below. The bad bread was to be thrown into the sea. The figure in brackets is from the report signed by Gilbert the master, Gray the boatswain, and Isaac Smith the master's mate, 10 May 1774.

account for this decay in our Bread especially as it is pack'd in good casks and Stowed in a dry part of the hold, be which way it will[1] the loss to us is equal, it puts us to a scanty allowance and have bad bread to eat into the bargin.

WEDNESDAY *4th.* Nothing happen'd worthy remark.

THURSDAY *5th.* The King and Several other great Men paid us a Viset and brought with them as usual a quantity of Provisions. In the evening Mr Forster and his party set out for the Country with an Intent to stay all night.[2]

FRIDAY *6th.* In the Evening Mr Forster returnd having made some new discoveries in the Botanical way.[3]

SATURDAY *7th.* On going a Shore in the Morning I found Otou at the Tents and took the Oppertunity to ask his leave to cut down some trees for fuel, he not well understanding me I took him to some standing near the Shore and fit for nothing else, these he gave me leave to cut down, but as they were not Sufficient I desired he would let us know where we could get more, declaring at the same time that I should Cut down no trees which bore any fruit, he was so pleased with this declaration that he told it a loud three times to the people about us.

In the afternoon he and the whole Royal Family (Viz) his Father, Brother and three Sisters with their attendants, made me a Viset on board; His Father made me a present[4] of a compleat Mourning dress, curiosities we most valued, in return I gave him what ever he desired[5] and distributed red feathers to all the others and then conducted them a shore in my boat; Otou was so well pleased with the reception he and his friends had met with that he told me at parting, I might cut down as many and what Trees I pleased.

[1] *be . . . will:* we judged it was owing to the Ice we so frequently tooke in when to the Southward which made the hold damp and cold and the great heat which succeeded when to the North be it this or any other cause . . .—f. 200.—This cause was suggested by the warrant officers in their report, 10 May, p. 948 below.

[2] 'Mostly such weather as yesterday. PM Moor'd the Ship with the two Bowers and took up the Kedge Anchor: AM Lifted and repair'd the Main Rigging, airing the Bread &c[a].'—Log, 4 May. —' . . . the Carpenters very close at their Work caulking the sides, only when they're interrupted by the Showery wea[r].'—Clerke, 4 May.

[3] George Forster went up into the hills with his father and Sparrman this time, and enjoyed himself. He makes the expedition on the 6th and 7th, however, saying, 'in order to keep our plants dry, we hastened down, and at four o'clock reached the ship, where we found the whole royal family assembled . . .' This leads him to dilate for some pages, not with great accuracy, on Tahitian history.—II, pp. 91–6.

[4] *His Father . . . present:* this was properly his fathers Visit of Ceremony, he brought me a present . . .—f. 200v.

[5] . . . which was not a little

SUNDAY 8*th.* Last Night in the Middle Watch through the negligence of one of the Sentinels on Shore all our Friendly connections received an interruption, he having either slept or quited his Post gave one of the Natives an oppertunity to carry off his Musquet,[1] the first news I heard of it was brought me in the morning by Tee whom Otou sent for this purpose and to desire I would go to him for he was Mata-ou (frightned, alarmd &c). I did not fully understand the story of the Musquit till I got on shore and was inform'd of it by the Serj[t] who had the Command. I found the Natives were all alarm'd and the most of them fled, the Kings Brother slept on board all night and came a Shore with me, but having heard the whole story from Tee he gave me the Slip in a Moment before I knew well what was the matter.[2] I cross'd the River and went alone with Tee and some others into the Woods in search of Otou. As we went a long I endeavoured to allay the fears of the People but at the same time insisted on having the Musquet return'd. After traveling some distance in the woods, enquiring of every one we met where Otou was, Tee stop'd all at once and advised me to go back for that Otou was gone towards the Mountains, that he would go to him and tell him that I was still his friend[3] and that he would use his endeavours to have the Musquet return'd. I was satisfied by this time it was to no purpose my going farther, for altho' I was alone and without Arms, Otou's fears were such that he dar'd not see me and therefor took Tees advice and return'd. As soon as I got on board I sent Odiddy to Otou to let him know I only requird the return of the Musquet which I knew to be in his power to do. Soon after Odiddy was gone we Observed Six large Canoes coming round Point Venus seemingly Load[ed] with Baggage Fruit &c[a]. I presently[4] come to a resolution to intercept them and put off in the pinnace for that purpose and gave orders for a nother boat to follow. One of the Canoes which was some distance a head of the others came directly for the Ship, she I went a long side of, two or three women being in her

[1] The defaulting sentry was the marine Richard Baldy. Other things were taken, including some linen. Cook was obviously much annoyed by the incident, for it gave him a great deal of trouble, and most of the journals say something about it. 'Read the Articles of War and punish'd Rich[d] Baldie, Marine with a dozen for so far neglecting his duty as to have his Musquet stolen . . . [9 May] AM gave Rich'd Baldie the other dozen for his very extraordinary carelessness and neglect.'—Clerke. This was the severest punishment Cook meted out on this voyage.

[2] . . . and hardly any remained by me but Tee, . . .—f. 201.

[3] . . . a question which had been asked me fifty times by different people and if I was angry &c[a].

[4] *seemingly . . . presently:* some people I had sent out to watch the conduct of the Neighbouring Inhabitants informed me they were laden with Baggage Fruit, Hogs &c[a]. There being some reason to think that some person belonging to these Canoes had committed the thieft, I presently . . .—f. 201–01v.

whom I knew, they told me they were going on board the Ship[1] and that Otou was at the tents, pleased with this news I contridicted the orders I had given to intercept the other Canoes, thinking they might be coming on board also as well as this one: this Canoe I left within a few yards of the Ship and row'd aShore to speak to Otou, but when I came there was told he had not been their nor knew they any thing of him, but the Canoes that had just past were load[ed] with the effects of some of the Neghbouring Houses and upon my looking behind me saw they were every one makeing off in the utmost haste, even the one I had let in a manner close along side the Ship had evaded going aboard and was makeing her escape. Vex'd at being thus outwitted I resolved to pursue them and as I pass'd the Ship gave orders to send a nother boat for the same purpose, Five out of Six we took and brought on board, but the first which acted the Finesse so well got quite off, and so might one or two more if the people had not quited the Canoes upon the first Musquits I fired for the Shott did not reach above half way. When we got on board with our Prizes I learnt that the people in the Canoe which had deceived me used no endeavours to lay hold of the Ship on the side they were upon but let the Canoe drop past as if they meant to come under the Ships Stern, but as soon as they were past they Paddled off with all speed: thus this Canoe in which were only a few Women was to have amused us with false stories as they actually did while the others got past.

In one of the Canoes we had taken was a Chief (a friend of Mr Forster who had hitherto call'd himself an Arree)[2] and some Women, I think his Wife and Daughter, and the Mother of the late Toutaha, these together with the Canoes I resolved to detain and to send the Chief to Otou, thinking he would have so much weight with him as to Obtain the return of the Musquet as his own property was at stake, he was however very unwilling to go upon this Embassy and made Various excuses, one of which was his being of too mean a rank for this honourable Employment saying he was only a Manahouna and not an Aree[3] and therefore was not a fit person to go to him, that an Aree ought to be sent to speake to an Aree and as there were no

[1] . . . with something for me

[2] . . . and would have been much offended if any one had called his title in question, also . . .—f. 202.

[3] A *note*: We hardly ever met with a man of the least Note who did not call himself an Aree, nay even the very common fellows would now and then interduce themselves to us with this title. It gave them an air of importance, they could not have assum'd without, and was usefull to them in many other respects. Our very best friends, would suffer us to be impos'd upon by any fellow who had address enough to do it—nay whatever the fellow said they would confirm.

Arees but Otou and my self it would be much more proper for me to go. All his Arguments would have availed little if Tee and Odiddy had not at this time come on board and given a new turn to the affair, they both declar'd that the Man who Stole the Musquet was from *Tiarabou* and had carried it to that Kingdom and that it was not in the power of Otou to recover it. I very much suspected the truth of this till they offer'd, in Otou's Name, to go with some of my people in one of our boats to Oheatua the Chief of that Kingdom and get it, I asked why this could not be done without my sending a boat, they Answer'd, it would not be deliverd up to them without. This Story of theirs altho it did not quite satisfy me it nevertheless carried with it the probability of truth, therefore I thought it better to drop the affair altogether rather than to punish a Nation for a Crime I was not sure any of its Members were guilty of, therefore I suffer'd my new Ambassadour to depart with his two Canoes without executing his commission, the other three Canoes belong'd to Maritata a *Tiarabou* chief who had been some days near the tents and there was good reason to believe it was one of his people who had committed the theift, for this reason I intended to have detained them but Tee and Odiddy both declar'd that Maritata and all his men were quite innocent. I suffered them to go also and desired Tee to let Otou know I was now satisfied it was none of his people which had Stolen the Musquet, that I was as much his Friend as ever and should proceed no farther in the affair; thinking indeed that the Musquet was irrecoverably lost, but in the dusk of the evening it together with some other things which we knew nothing of and stolen at the same time were brought us by three Men who had pursued the thief and taken the things from him. I know not by whose orders this was done,[1] I rewarded the Men for their fidelity and made no father enquirey about it. It was now I learnt for certain[2] that it was one of Mariatata's Men who carried off the Musquet and other things, and I was not a little vex'd at having let his Canoes slip thro' my fingers. In this particular I believe both Tee and Odiddy willfully deceived me.[3]

[1] *by . . . done:* if these men did it of their own accord or by order of Otoo, . . .—f. 202v.

[2] *It . . . certain:* These men, as well as some others present, assured me that

[3] . . . When the Musket and other things were brought in, every one present or who came after, pretended to have had some hand in recovering them and claimed a reward accordingly; but there was no one who acted this Farce so well as *Nuno* a man of some note and well known to us when I was here in 1769, this man came with all the savage fury immaginable in his Countenance and a large Club in his hand which he beat about him with, in order to shew us how he, only, had killed the thief, at the very same time we all knew that he had not been out of his house the whole day. Thus ended this troublesome day.—f. 203.

MONDAY 9*th*. In the Morning Tee, Otou's fathfull Ambassadour, came again on board to acquaint me that Otou was gone to Oparre and desired I would send one of the Natives to let him know that I was still his friend. I asked why he had not done it as I desired, he made some excuse, I believe he had not seen him, in short I saw it was necessary for me to go my self, for while we thus spent our time with Messages we were without refreshments.[1] Accordingly I set out with Tee, Mr Forster and some of the Officers, we proceeded in our boat to the very utmost Limmits of Oparre where after waiting some time and Several Messages had passed to and fro, the King at last appeared. After we were seated under the shade of some trees as usual and the first salutations were over, he desired me to Parou,[2] make a speach, as we understood, to the People, but this was more than any of us could do, and be understood, therefore to cut the Matter Short, I began with blaming Otou for being Mataou, sence I had all along profess'd My self his friend and that I was not angry with him or any of his people but those of *Tiarabou* who had stolen the Musquet. I was then asked how I came to fire at the Canoes, Chance on this occasion furnished me with a very good excuse. I told them they belonged to Mariatata a Tiarabou Man one of whose men had occasion'd all this disturbance and if I had them now in my posession I would distroy them or any other belonging to Tiarabou, this declaration pleased them as I expected from the natural aversation the one Nation has to the other; what I said being inforced by a few presents (which had perhaps the greatest weight with them) restored things to their former state, Otou promised on his part that on the morrow we should be supplyed with provisions as usual.

We now return'd with him to the place of his residence where after Viewing some of his dock yards (for such they well deserve to be calld) and large Canoes[3] we return'd on board with Tee in our Company, who after dinner went to acquaint the Kings father who was in the Neighbourhood of Matavai, that all differences were accomodated. It should seem from what followed that this old gentleman was not pleased with the Conditions, for in the Evining all the Women which were not a few, were taken out of the Ship and Sentinals stationed on the beach to prevent any one from coming off to the Ship and the next Morning—

[1] *refreshments:* fruit, for a stop was put to all exchanges of this Nature, that is the Natives brought nothing to Market.

[2] *parau*, to speak, advise.

[3] . . . some lately built and others building two of which were the largest I had ever seen in this Sea or indeed any where else under that name.—f. 203v.—'that name': the name of canoe, presumably, or *pahi*.

TUESDAY 10*th.* No Supplies whatever was brought us, on enquiring the reason was told that Happi[1] meaning Otou's father, was *Mataou* and had forbid any supply's to be brought us. Chagrained as I was at this disapointment I forbore taking any step from a Supposision that Tee had not yet seen old Happi or that Otous orders had not yet reached Matavai: a supply of fruit sent us from *Oparre* and some brought us by our friends served us for the present and made me less anxious about it, thus Matters stood till the afternoon when Otou himself came to the Tents with a large supply, there I went to him and charged him with a breach of his promise in not permitting the People of Matavai to bring in the supplies as usual and insisted on him giving immidiate direction about [them], which I believe he did, if not done already, for presently after more was brought us than we could well purchas;[2] this must not be wonder'd at for the people had every thing in readiness to bring us the Moment they were permitted and I believe thought themselves as much injured by the restriction as we did.

Otou desired to see Some of the great guns Fired from the Ship, accordingly I ordered Twelve to be fired[3] all Shotted, which he viewed seemingly with more pain than pleasure. I believe he had never seen a Cannon fired before. In the Evening we entertained him with fire-works,[4] which gave him great satisfaction, thus ended the day and all our differences.

*. . . in the evening we entertained him with fireworks which gave him great satisfaction, thus ended all our defferences which occasioned the following remark. I had occasion some were in this Journal before to observe that these people are continually upon the lookout to rob us upon every occasion, which the Legislature[5] either encourage or have not power to prevent, but most probable the former, because the offender is allways screened; that they should commit such daring thiefts is the more extraordinary, as they are frequently done at the risk of being shott, and if the article they steal be of any consequence they know they will be obliged to make restitution; the moment a thieft of this kind is committed it spreads like the wind over the whole neighbourhood, they judge of the consequences from what they have got, if a trifle, and such things as we usually give them, little or no notice is taken of it, but if the con-

[1] Hapai, or Teu. Like so many *arii*, he had alternative or successive names; Hapai seems to have been the one used at this period.

[2] *purchas:* dispence with

[3] . . . towards the Sea

[4] The Tahitians' first experience of this joy: they called, and still call, the phenomenon *ahi-tiri*, lit. 'fire to throw' (or 'scatter').

[5] No doubt he means by this the chiefs.

trary than every one takes the alarm and begins to move off with their Moveables in all haste; the Chief is Mataou'd, gives orders to bring us no supplies and flies to some distant part; all this is some times done in so short a time that we have obtained by this means the first knowlidge of our being robed. Whether we obliged them to make restitution or no, the Chief must be reconciled before any of the people are permitted to bring in any refreshments—they know very well we cannot do without them, therefore never fail of strictly observing this rule, without ever considering that all their War Canoes, on which the strength of their Nation depends, thier houses and even the very fruit they refuse to supply us with are intirely in our power. It is hard to say how they would act was one to distroy any of these things; except the detaining some of their Canoes for a while, I have never touched the least article of thier property, of the two extremes I have allways chused that which appeared the most equitable and mild, a trifleing present to the Chief has always succeeded to my wish and very often put things upon a better footing than they were before. That they were the first aggressors had very little influence on my conduct in this respect, because no differences happened but when it was so, my people very rarely or hardly ever broke through the rules I thought proper to prescribe. Had I observed a different conduct I was sure to be the looser by it in the end, and all I could expect after distroying some part of their property was the empty honour of obligeing them to make the first overturne[1] towards an accommodation; but who knows if this would have been the event. Three things made them our fast friends, Their own good Natured and benevolent disposition, gentle treatment on our part, and the dread of our fire Arms; by our ceaseing to observe the Second the first would have wore of[f] of Course, and the too frequent use of the latter would have excited a spirit of revenge and perhaps have taught them that fire Arms were not such terrible things as they had imagined, they are very sencible of the superiority they have over us in numbers and no one knows what an enraged multitude might do.*—f. 204–4v.

WEDNESDAY 11*th*. In the Morning had a very large Supply of Fruit brought us from all parts, some of which came from Towha the Admiral, sent as usual by his Servants with orders to receive nothing in return, only desired to see me at Attahourou as he was ill and could not come to me; as I could not well undertake this Journey now I sent Odiddy along with his Servants with a present sutable to

[1] *sic;* no doubt for 'overture'.

those I had in so genteel a manner received from Towha. As the Most Essential repairs of the Ship were now nearly finished I resolved to leave the isle in a few days, accordingly ordered every thing to be got off from the Shore, that the Natives might see we were about to depart.

THURSDAY 12*th*. Showery Rainy weather. To Day we had a Viset from Old Obarea the Dolphins Queen[1] who looked as well and as young as ever. She presented me with two Hogs, some Cloth &c[a]. Presently after her came Otou with a great retinue and a great quantity of Provisions, to every one of them I made large presents thinking it might be the last time I should see them[2] and in the evening entertain'd them with fire works.

FRIDAY 13*th*. Winds Easter, fair Weather. Two things prevented our Sailing this Morning, first Odiddy was not yet return'd from Attahourou, Secondly Otou desired I would not sail till he had seen me again;[3] various were the reports about Odiddy, some said he was return'd, others that he was at Oparre and others said he would not return. In the evening a party of us went down to Oparre to learn more of the truth, here we found not only Odiddy, but Towha also who notwithstanding his ill state of health had resolved to see me before I went away and had got thus far on his Journey, he had got a swelling in his feet and legs which had intirely taken away the use of them; our Viset was short for[4] after seeing Otou we return'd with Odiddy on board, this youth I found was desirous of remaining at this isle and therefore[5] told him he was at liberty to remain here or at Ulietea and Frankly told him that if he went to England it was highly probable he would never return, but if after all he choosed to go I would take care of him and he must look upon me as his Father, he threw his arms about me and wept saying many people persuaded him to stay at the isle. I told him to go a Shore and speak with his friends and then come to me in the morning. He was

[1] . . . whom I had not seen since 1769 . . .—f. 205. ABG footnote: 'When the Dolphin was here in 1767, they took this woman to be Queen of the Island'. See I, pp. clxxxiii–iv, and the Tahitian portion of the Journal, *passim*. 'O-Ammo [Amo, Purea's ex-husband: the highest ranking chief, after his son, of the district of Papara, on the south of the island] likewise came to the ship about this time, but was still less noticed than his late consort; and being little known on board, was not permitted to come even into the captain's cabin. . . . These two royal personages are living examples of the instability of human grandeur.'—Forster, II, p. 101. The moral is uncalled for: Purea and Amo, though since their defeat of little account in the north, still enjoyed their powers and dignity at Papara.

[2] *them:* these good people who had so liberally relieved our wants . . .—f. 205.

[3] . . . and I had a present to make him which I reserved to the last

[4] *our Visit . . . for:* As the day was far spent we were obliged to Shorten our stay and

[5] *and therefore:* as I had before told him, as likewise many others that we should not return, I now . . .

very well beloved in the Ship for which reason every one was persuading him to go with us, telling what great things he wou'd see[1] and return with immence riches, according to his Idea of riches, but I thought proper to undeceive him,[2] thinking it an Act of the highest injustice to take away a person from these isles against his own free inclination under any promise whatever much more that of bringing them back again, what Man on board can make such a promise as this.[3] At this time it was quite unnecessary to persuade any one to go with us, there were many youths who Voluntary offered themselves to go with us and even to remain and die in Brit-tania.[4] The King importuned me very much to take one or two to collect red feathers for him at Amsterdam, willing to risk the chance of their returning or no; some of the gentle[men] on board were desirous of takeing some as Servants, but I refused all manner of Solicitations of this kind,[5] knowing from experience that they would be of no use to us in the course of the Voyage,[6] but what had the greatest weight with me was the thinking my self bound to see they were after wards properly taken care of as they could not be taken from their Native spot without my consent.

SATURDAY 14*th*. Early in the Morning Odiddy came on board with a resolution to stay at the Isle, but Mr Forster prevailed upon him to go with us to Ulietea. Soon after Towha[7] came a long side and also several more of our friends with fruit &c^a^. Towha was hoisted in and place'd in a Chair on the Quarter deck,[8] amongest the various articles I gave this Chief was an English Pendant, told him the use of it and instructed him in what manner and where it was to be hoisted in his Canoe, after which he seem'd highly pleased.[9] We had no sooner dis-

[1] *see:* see in England

[2] ... as knowing that the only inducement of his going was the expectation of returning and I could see no prospect of an oppertunity of that kind happening, unless a ship was expressly se[n]t out for that purpose, which [neither] I nor any one else had a right to expect.—f. 205v.

[3] *whatever ... this:* which was not in my power to perform.

[4] *Brit-tania:* Pritanee as they call our Country

[5] One of the gentlemen who was anxious to take a Tahitian to England, 'entirely at his own expence', was J. R. Forster. According to George Forster, Cook at first consented, but changed his mind the same day. Forster was not pleased: 'As it was intended to teach him the rudiments of the arts of the carpenter and smith, he would have returned to his country at least as valuable a member of society as O-Mai [the youth taken by Furneaux], who, after a stay of two years in England, will be able to amuse his countrymen with the music of a hand-organ, and with the exhibition of a puppet-show.'—Forster, II, pp. 90–1. Imagination blanches at the prospects of a Tahitian in England, living entirely at the expense of J. R. Forster.

[6] ... and farther my Views were not extended

[7] *Towha:* Towha, Poatatou, Oamo, Happi, Obarea

[8] ... his wife was with him

[9] *after ... pleased:* which pleased him more than all the rest,

patched our friends than we saw a Number of War Canoes coming round the point of Oparre, being desirous to have a nearer view of them I hastned down to Oparre (accompanied by some of the officers &c[a]) which we reached before the Canoes were all landed and had an oportunity to see in what manner they approached the shore which was in divisions consisting of three or four or more lashed close[1] a long side each other, such a division one would think must be very unwieldy, yet it was a pleasure to see how well they were conducted, they Paddled[2] in for the Shore with all their might conducted in so judicious a manner that they closed[3] the line a Shore to an inch, we landed with the last and took a view of them as they lay in along the Shore.[4] This fleet consisted of Forty sail, were equiped in the same manner as those we had seen before and belonged to the little district of Tettaha and were come to Oparre to be reviewed before Otou as those we had seen before had done, there were tending on this Fleet one or more Small double Canoes which they call'd Marai having on their fore part a kind of double bed place laid over with green leaves each just sufficient to contain one Man, these they told us was to lay their Slain upon, their Chiefs I suppose they meant, otherways their Slain must be very few. Otou who was present caused[5] some of the Troops to go through their exercize on Shore, Two parties first began with Clubs, but this was so soon over that I had no time to make observations upon it, they then went to Single Combat and went thro' the Various Mithods of fighting with great allertness and parried off the blows, pushes &c[a] each combatant intended the other with great dexterity; their Arms were Clubs and Spears which they also used as darts. In fighting with the Clubs, I observed all side-blows were parried with the Club except those intended the legs which were evaded by leaping over them, a downright blow on the head they evaded by couching a little and leaping on one side, thus the blow would fall to the ground: they parried off the Spear or dart by fixing the point of their spear in the ground and holding of it before them in an inclined posission more

[1] *close:* square and close . . .—f. 206.

[2] *they Paddled:* and then each division one after the other paddled

[3] *closed:* formed and closed

[4] *we landed . . . Shore:* The rowers were incouraged to exert their strength by their leaders on the stages, and directed by a man who stood with a wand in his hand in the fore part of the middlemost Vessel, this man by words and actions directed the paddlers when all should paddle when either the one side or the other should cease &c[a] for the steering paddles alone were not sufficient to direct them: all these motions they observed with such quickness as clearly shewed that they were expert in thier business. After M[r] Hodges had made a drawing of them as they lay ranged along the Shore, we landed and took a nearer view of them, by going on board several.—f. 206. For Hodges's drawing, see Fig. 59.

[5] . . . at my request

or less elivated, according to the part of the boddy they saw their antagonist intended to make a push or throw his dart, and by turning their hand a little to the right or left turn off[1] either the one or the other. I thought that when one combatant had parried the blows &c^{a} of the other, he did not take all the advantages which seem'd to me to accrue, as for instance, after he had parried of a dart he still stood on the defensive and suffered his Antagonist to take up another, when I thought their was time enough to have run him thro' the boddy, but by such a step they might have exposed themselves to more danger than I could see or be aware of.[2]

This being over the fleet depart as fast[3] as they were got afloat and I went with Otou to one of his large double Canoes which was building and nearly ready to launch. She was by far the largest I had seen at any of the isles,[4] he beged of me a grapling and grapling rope for her to which I aded an English Jack and Pendant, the use of which he had been before fully instructed in. I desired that these two Joint Canoes, ie what is understood as a double Canoe, might be call'd Britanne (Brit-tania) the name they have addopted for our Country, to which he very readily consented and she was Christened accordingly. After this he presented me with a Hog and a Turtle of about 60^{lb} weight, this last was put privately in to the boat, the giving it away not being agreeable to some of the great Lords about him who were thus disapointed of a feast.[5] The King[6] came on board with us and after dinner took a Most Affectionate leave, he hardly ever ceased to day Soliciting me to return and just before he went out of the Ship took a youth by the hand, presented him to me and disired I would take him on board to Collect red feathers, I told him I could

[1] . . . with great ease

[2] . . . The Combatants had no superfluous dress upon them, an unnecessary piece of cloth or two they had on when they begun were presently torn of by the by standers and given to some of our gentlemen present.—f. 206v.

[3] *as fast:* not in any order but as fast

[4] *one of . . . isles:* one of his Dockyards where the two large Pahies or Canoes were building, each of which was 108 feet long, [*deleted* built on the same Construction as the large pahies at Ulietea] they were allmost ready to launch and were intended to make one joint Double Pahie or Canoe.—f. 206v. The other MSS preserve the deleted words of this passage, with the footnote, 'The Ulietea Pahèes, or large Canoes, have a Sharp floor and round side, whereas, those of Otahiete have a flat floor and an upright side'. B has the note to the deleted words, marked marginally 'omit'; but rephrases the sentence as part of the text on Tahitian tactics, f. 210, (see p. 406, note 1 below), as follows: 'These War Canoes go always double and are of two sorts distinguishable from each other by the Construction but equiped alike, the one sort they call Ivahahs [*va'a*] and the other Pahies [*pahi*], I shall give a description of both when the drawings, for which we have got Materials, are finished'. Cook did not get round to this description. There is an elaborate draught, plan and section of the *Britannia*, (a *pahi*), in *Voyage*, I, pl. XV.

[5] . . . he likewise would have given me a large shark they had prisoner in a creek (some of his fins be[ing] cut off so that he could not make his escape) but the fine Pork and fish we had got at this isle had spoiled our palates for this food.—f. 207.

[6] . . . and his prime minister Tee.

not take him knowing he would never return, but that if any Ship should happen to come here again from Brit-tania I would take care to either bring or send him plenty of red feathers; this seem'd to satisfy him, but the youth was exceedinly disireous of going and had I not made a resolution to carry no one from the isles[1] I believe I should have taken him.

Otou remained along side of the Ship till we were under sail when he put off and we Saluted him with three guns. Our treatment at this isle was such as had induced one of our gunners mates to form a Plan to remain at it, he knew he could not execute it with success while we lay in the Bay, therefore took the oppertunity as soon as we were out[2] and all our Sails set to slip over board (he being a good swimer) but he was discov[er]ed before he had got clear of the Ship, we presently Broug[t] to, hoisted out a boat and sent and took him up:[3] a Canoe was observed about half way between us and the Shore seemingly coming after us, she was intended to take him in, but seeing our boat, kept at a distance, this was a preconcerted plan between the Man and the Natives with which Otou was acquainted and had incouraged. I kept the Man in confinement till we were clear of the isles then dismiss'd [him] without any other punishment,[4] for when I considered the situation of the Man in life I did not think him so culpable[5] as it may at first appear, he was an Irishman by birth, a good Seaman and had Saild both in the English and Dutch Service. I pick'd him up at Batavi in my return home from my last Voyage and

[1] . . . (except Odiddy if he chused) and had but just refused M[r] Forster the liberty of takeing a Boy,

[2] . . . the boats in

[3] Other notes on this incident seem worth printing. 'Weigh'd & Came to sail, soon afterwards John Marra Gunner's Mate jump'd over board & endeavour'd to get on shore, Bro't too, hoisted out the Cutter & sent after him, they took him up, he afterwards jump'd out of the Boat, dived & endeavour'd to get away, but again was taken up, Bro't on board & confin'd in Irons . . .'—Cooper, 15 May.—'And when under sail, and saluting the King one of our gunners Mates, slip'd overboard (being an exelent swimmer) intending to stay at Otaheite, they having promis'd a House, Land and a Pretty Wife: after much difficulty we got him a board again (for he would have been a great loss to us) and proceeded on our way.—Elliott *Mem.*, f. 28v. Marra's own account (pp. 235–6) ingeniously puts forward anthropological research as an advantage to be gained from his desertion: 'and pity it was that he happened to be discovered, as from him a more copious and accurate account of the religion and civil government of these people might have been expected after a few years stay among them, than could possibly be collected from a few short visits, by gentlemen who had the language to learn, and whose first business was to procure necessaries, in order to enable them to pursue more important discoveries'. This was very likely invented by his editor.

[4] Marra was put in irons at once. B f. 239 is a direct witness to Cook's clemency. It is a slip of paper, written in ink now very much faded, a sort of gaoler's report: 'John Mara Prisoner in Irons one Night 15th May 1774—J: Hamilton Serj[t]', and addressed on the verso 'To Cap[t] Cook Esq[r]'. Hamilton was the sergeant of marines. Marra himself says (p. 241) he was released from irons and made a prisoner at large with a sentinel to attend him, but returned to irons when the ship arrived at Raiatea.

[5] . . . or the resolution he had taken to stay here so extraordinary.—f. 207v.

he had remained with me ever sence. I never learnt that he had either friends or connection to confine him to any particular part of the world, all Nations were alike to him, where than can Such a Man spend his days better than at one of these isles where[1] he can injoy all the necessaries and some of the luxuries of life in ease and Plenty.[2] As soon as the Boat was hoisted in again we directed our Course for Huaheine in order to pay a Viset to our friends there, but it will be necessary first, to give some account of the present state of Otaheite especially as it differs very much from what it was Eight Months ago.

I have already mentioned the improvements we found in the Plains of Oparre and Matavai: the same was observed in every other part into which we came, it seem'd to us allmost incredable that so many large Canoes and Houses could be built in so short a space of time as Eight Months, the tools which they got from the English and other Nations who have touched here have no doubt greatly accelerated the work and according to the old Proverb many hands make light work, for I shall soon make it appear there are no want of these; the Number of Hoggs too was a nother thing which struck our attention, but this is more easy accounted for, they might and certainly had a good many when we were here before but not chusing to part with any had conve[ye]d them out of our Sight, be this as it will, we now got [not only] as many as we could consume during our Stay, but some to take to Sea with us.

When I was last here I conceived but an inddifferent Opinion of *Otou*'s Talents as a King, but the improvements he has sence made in the isles has convince'd me of my Mistake and that he must be a Man of good parts, he has indeed some judicious, sensible men about him who I beleive have a great share in the Goverment.[3] I was sorry to see a jealousy subsisting between him and other great Men, he publickly told us one day that neither Towha the Admiral nor Poatatou, two leading Chiefs,[4] were not his friends, this Shews that there are Divisions amongest the great people in this state as well as in Most others, probably this jealousy arose from their great power for

[1] . . . in one of the finest climates in the World

[2] . . . I know not if he might not have obtained my consent if he had applied for it in proper time.

[3] . . . Indeed we know not how far his power extends as King, nor how far he can command the assistance of the other Chiefs or is controllable by them: it should however seem that all have contributed towards bringing the isle to its present flourishing state.—f. 208.—This passage seems to show that if Cook had stayed longer continuously at Tahiti on this voyage, and visited other parts of the island, he might have got a truer idea of its political institutions.

[4] Neither of these chiefs, of course, was 'subject' to Tu.

Otou on all occasions seem'd to pay them much respect[1] and so far as we knew they raised by far the greatest Number of Boats and Men to go against Eimeo and were two of the Commanders on the expedition which we were told was to take place five days after we sail'd. Oheatoua of Tiarrabou was also to send a Fleet to join those of Otous to assist him in reducing to Obedience the Chief of Eimeo.[2] One would think so small an Island would hardly attempt to make head against the United force of the two Kingdoms but endeavour to settle Matters by Negotiation, but we heard of no such thing, on the Contrary every one spoke of nothing but fighting. Towha told us more than once that he should die there which in some Measure shew'd what he thought of it. Odiddy told me the Battle would be fought at Sea, in which case they must have a Fleet nearly if not quite equal to the one going against them and as this is not probable it is more likely they will remain on shore upon the defensive as we have been told they once did[3] when attack'd by the People of Tiarrabou whom they repulce'd. Five general officers were to command in this expedition of which number Otou was one and if they named them according to the Post they held he was only the 3rd in Command, this seems probable enough as being but a young man could not have the experience necessary to command such an Expedition where the greatest Skill and judgement is required.[4]

I must confess I would willingly have stayed five days longer had I been sure the expedition would then take place, but it rather seem'd that they wanted us to be gone first. We had been all along told it would be ten Moons before it took place and it was not till the evening before we sail'd that Otou and Towha told us it was to be in five days after we were gone, as if it was necessary to have that time to put every thing in order for while we lay their great part of their time and attention was taken up with us. I had observed that for several days before we Sail'd, Otou and the other Chiefs had cease'd to Solicit my assistance,[5] I had assured Otou that if they got their

[1] *for . . . respect:* for on every occasion he seemed to court their intrest.—f. 208. Tu, if he was then meditating greatness, might well have been jealous of Towha of Faaa and Potatau of Punaauia; for they were both important *arii,* and Towha was by no means Tu's admiral. Tu did not like them because they were urging him, a timorous man, to take part in a war, but he was afraid of them; and they did not like him because he was getting far too much attention from the English. Possibly they even had a certain contempt for him, because of his character. In the end he did not help them in the war. See Introduction, p. xcii above.

[2] . . . I think we were told that that young prince was one of the Commanders.

[3] *once did:* did about five or six years ago . . .—f. 208v.—This incident, if it ever took place, seems to be shrouded in obscurity.

[4] Nor, as we have seen, was he in any other way the principal leader in the campaign.

[5] . . . as they were continually doing at first . . .

fleet ready in time I would Sail with them down to Eimeo. After this I heard no more of it, they probably had taken it into consideration and concluded themselves safer without me, well knowing that it would be in my Power to give the Victory to which side I pleased and that at the best I might thwart some of their favourate Customs or run away with the spoils, be their reasons what it will, they certainly wanted us to be gone before they undertook any thing. Thus we were deprived of seeing the whole of this grand Fleet and perhaps too of being Spectators of a Sea Fight, a Sight, I am well convenced, well worth the seeing.[1] I took some pains to inform my Self in what manner they joined Battle and fought at Sea, but knowing but little of their Language and they none of ours, the account I got must be very imperfect,[2] it however gave me a tolerable Idea of it, which I shall endeavour to convey to the reader. I have before said that all their Vesels of War have a raised platform or Stage at the very fore part of them which will contain Eight or Ten Men, these are the Tata otai's or fighting Men. In forming the line of battle they draw up a breast of each other with their heads to the Enimy and as I understood in divisions as when they land, for the more readier closeing the line when the action begins:[3] the enimies fleet being drawn up in like manner, they rush with all their might upon each other, the Attack is first begun with Stones, but as soon as they Close they take to their other weapons for the stages of the one fleet will be as it were joind to those of the other; it seems that general Ship is here very necessary,[4] to take the advantages of winds, currents and various other circumstances which may accrue, and may make it necessary to put in practise other Manoeuvres besides these just mentioned, but their Manner of fighting must however be the same.[5] I have said that each fighting stage will contain Eight or ten Men but we cannot suppose this to be the Number of Troops in each Cannoe, but even this number

[1] *a Sight . . . seeing:* by that means gaining some knowlidge of the Manœuvres. In order to make up for this disappointment . . .—f. 208v. The passage that follows, to the end of the next paragraph, though rewritten in B, ff. 209–10, was excluded from the printed *Voyage*—for what reason we do not know: perhaps it was thought that Polynesian tactics would try the reader's patience too much. The rewritten version is marked 'omit', but not in Cook's hand (it is possibly Douglas's).

[2] . . . nor was every one on whom I enquired able to give me the information.—f. 209. A scrap of redrafting, Add. MS 27889, f. 70, adds that Cook could get no information from Odiddy, who 'knew very little of the matter, as he was but a youth'.

[3] . . . and to add greater weight to the whole

[4] *very necessary:* as necessary, as in the conducting of one of our large fleets,

[5] *and may . . . same:* I know not if the whole fleet joins battle at once, I rather think not and that a part lies out of the line in order to be ready to assist and support such as may be in danger of being over powered, for as they have niether Masts nor Sails but are Navigated by paddles only, this may easily be done; this may however in some measure depend on the conduct and judgement of the leaders and the Nature and situation of the place.—f. 209–9v.

cannot act on the stage at once,[1] on the Contrary I think we understood clearly from Tupia who made a drawing of one of these Vessels[2] that no more than one or at the Most two Fought at the same time and as they were Kill'd or wounded were relieved by others.[3]

Their Manner of landing in An Enimies Country must be in divisions in the same Manner as we saw them land at Oparre, these divisions must be formed with out the reach of the Enimies Stones, from what I have seen a division consists of no fixed number, if the shore is straight the divisions may be large, if Crooked they must be Small, otherways all cannot get close to the Shore;[4] when the divisions and[5] a resolution taken begin the attack they pull in for the shore, not directly in a line a breast, but each division upon the quarter of the other, in order the more readier to Close or form a line a Shore, at least it was something in this Manner they did it at Oparre; at this time the Padles exerted all their strength being incouraged by thier leaders on the Stage and directed by a Man who stood with a wand in his hand at the fore part of the divisions, this Man by words and actions directed the Paddlers when all should paddle, when either the one side or the other should cease &c[a], for the Steering Paddles a lone are not sufficient, all these Motions they observe'd with such quickness as shewed they were very expert in their business; the very Instant the division touches the ground all the rowers jump out and drag it on the Shore till it is fast grounded, thus they form a line abreast all along the Shore not only of Vessels but arm'd men also, for the troops being mounted on the Stages are ready to land in an Instant, if the enimy give them so much time, if not they are ready to force a landing. We have been told that the Enimy some times meet them up to the Middle in Water but they must be a Strong boddy of Men that can support themselves against the weight of one of these heavy divisions.[6] I never thought to ask how the Paddlers were imploy'd after the Troops were landed or in

[1] . . . for want of room

[2] . . . with the warriors in her . . .—f. 211v.

[3] . . . how far this may be true I will not pretend to say, but it seems to me to be too deliberate a way of fighting for people whose passions are Violent and are said to fight with great obstinancy; certain it is that the contest is never long and that a single battle desides the fate of the Nation for that time.—f. 209v.

[4] *close . . . Shore:* so close to it as to form a good line

[5] *sic,* for 'on'? But as the MS here is obviously fair copy, I imagine that Cook has omitted some of his intended words, which perhaps ran, 'When the divisions are formed and a resolution taken to begin the attack' etc. This would be in line with other versions of the passage, e.g. G H.

[6] *the more readier . . . heavy divisions:* the more easier to close and form a line a long the Coast. The reason of their going in in this manner is plain, for were they to go in in a line a breast, they must also be close and if one or more of the divisions were to strike or stick fast on any rock or Shoal, the line by that means would be broke whereas by the

an Engagement at Sea when the fleet had graple'd each other, but I believe they do nothing but attend their paddles.[1] This is the best account I can give of the Management and use of these Vessels of War on which the Strength and Power of these isles in a great measure depends: it was by these Opoone the King of Bolabola was inabled to conquor most of the neighbouring isles.[2]

They are the best calculated for landing in a Surf of any Vessels I ever saw, their high round sterns recives the force of the Sea in Such a manner that none ever enters the Vessel.

I cannot pretend to say what number of Vessels were to go on this expedition, we know of no more than 210 besides Transports &c[a] and the Fleet of Tiarabou, the strength of which we never learnt nor could I ever learn what number of men was necessary to man this fleet, when ever this queston was asked them their answer was Warou warou warou te Tata,[3] Many, many, many Men as if the number exceeded their Arethmatick. If we allow forty men to each War Canoe and but four to each of the others we shall find this fleet would require above 9 Thousand men an Astonishing number to be raised in four districts only and one of them (viz) Matavai did not equip one fourth part their fleet.[4] The whole Armament might be double or thrible this force for any thing we know to the Contrary, however I beleive the whole Isle did not Arm on this occasion for we saw not the least preparations makeing in Oparre. It appeared that the Chief of each district superintended the fiting out of the fleet belonging to his district, yet after they are equiped they must pass a review before the King and be approved of by him, by this means he knows the state of his whole fleet before they are Collected together to go on service, a very commendable institution and leads us to beleive that this is by no means a bad regulated state.[5]

other method it cannot, for if one division is by any accedent stoped the next can pass and close the line in its place, thus they form a Compact line a long the shore not only of Vesels but armed men also for the Troops being all mounted on the Stages are ready to engage and force a landing, if they make good the latter the Victory is thereby generally obtained, this the invaded are so Sencible of that I am told they generally meet the Canoes up to the middle in the Water, it must however be a very strong body of Men to resist the weight of one of these heavy divisions, I however have no doubt of the fact, as this is the only method they can have to breake the line and throw it into Confusion and there can be no doubt but it some times succeeds.—ff. 209v–10v.

[1] . . . and the Management of the Vessels.—f. 210.

[2] *it was . . . isles:* it was in Canoes they attacked Captain Wallis in the Dolphin of 20 Guns.

[3] *ua rau, ua rau, ua rau te taata. Rau* means literally a hundred; repetition is common in Polynesia to indicate great numbers.

[4] . . . the fleet of Tiarabou is not included in this account and many of the Districts might be arming which we knew nothing of.—f. 210–10v.

[5] Cook's assumption of a 'review' springs from his persuasion that Tu was a king. In fact the appearance of the canoes at Pare was more likely to have been for the purpose of overaweing him than of gaining his approval.

From this Equipment and their Naval force in general I shall make some attempt to calculate the Number of People in the whole Island. We find that Tettaha one of the smallest districts in it can equip forty war Canoes. Now there are twenty four districts in the Kingdom of Opoureonu and nineteen in the Kingdom of Tiarabou, the former according to the above computation can raise Nine hund^rd^ & Sixty Vesels of war and the latter Seven hundred & sixty which makes in the whole Seventeen hund^rd^ and twenty; but we are told that Tiarabou can raise as great a force as Opoureonu. If we allow forty men to each Canoe according to my former computation it will require Sixty eight Thousand able bodied men and as these cannot amount to One third part the number of both Sex the whole Island cannot contain less than two hundred and four thousand inhabitants.[1]

*This Island was formerly under one Kin[g]dom, how long sence it was formed into two I cannot say, but I believe not long. The Kings of Tearabou are a branch of the same family as those of Opoureonu and at present the two families are nearly related. I am not sure if the former is not in some measure dependant on the latter[2] and if Otoo is not stiled Arreedehi of both. We understood for certain that Oheatoua the King of Tiarabou must uncover before him in the same manner as the meanest of his Subjects.[3] This Homage is due to Otoo as Earee dehie of the isle, to Tarevatou his Brother and his second sister, to the one as heir and to the other as heir apparent his eldest Sister being married, is not intitled to

[1] . . . In this estimate I have made no account of the men necessary to man the Transports &c[a] which cannot require less than Two Thousand. We are told that Tiarabou can raise as many men as Opoureonu it is therefore probable I may have under rated that Kin[g]dom and that the whole isle may contain some thousands more Inhabitants than the number above mentioned.—f. 212v. For remarks on this calculation see I, pp. clxxiv–vii. Cook seems to have totally forgotten the size and topographical nature of the island, and the evidence of his eyes on his tour round it in 1769. He was quite misled in reckoning forty-three 'districts' in the whole island—an error he seems to have fallen into from regarding every place-name he picked up as being the name of a 'district' (see Chart V). Even if we accept the nineteen districts of Teiura Henry, we may certainly regard some of these, for 'political' or 'administrative' purposes, as sub-districts—e.g. Pare and Arue, which together made up Tu's Te Porionuu. Williamson, *Social and Political Systems*, I, map facing p. 170, illustrates this point very well. Cook is also in error in assuming each of his districts to be equivalent in canoe-numbers and hence population. Towha's small Faaa was much more important in every way than the north-east districts, larger in area though they were. One is forced to conclude that the Captain's statistical method was regrettably loose.

[2] Of course the island did not formerly make one kingdom; nor did the family of Taiarapu depend on that of Te Porionuu. But Tu and Vehiatua were related, through common descent from the Vehiatua-i-Mata'i who lived c. 1650; his daughter married an *arii* of Pare, whence in the fourth generation sprang Tu. This gave Tu, on the death without issue of the last Vehiatua in 1790, a chance to push a claim to succeed him, and he pushed it successfully.

[3] Tu, or fervent upholders of Tu's family, may have told Cook this, but it was not true. Nor was Tu styled *arii rahi* of the whole island; that claim was ridiculous.

this Homage.[1] The Eowa's and Whanno's,[2] we have sometimes seen covered before the King, but whether by courtesy or by Vertue of their office we never could learn; these men are the Principal persons about the King and form his Court and are generally, if not allways his relations. Tee whom I have so often mentioned was one of them; we have been told that the Eowas, who have the first rank attend in their turns, a certain number each day, which occasioned us to call them Lords in waiting, but whether this was realy so I cannot say, we seldom found Tee absent, indeed his attendance was necessary, as being the best able to negotiate matters between us and them, on which service he was allways imployed and which he executed, I have reason to think, to the satisfaction of both parties. It is to be regreted that we know little more of this goverment, than the general outlines of its Subdivisions, Classes, or orders of the constuent parts, how desposed or in what manner connected so as to form one body politic, we know but little; we however know that it is of the feudal kind and if we may judge from what we have seen, it has sufficient Stability and by no means badly constituted. The Eowa's and Whanno's allways eat with the King, indeed I do not know if any one is exempted from this privilege but the Toutous; for as to the Women they are out of the queston, as they never eat with the Men let their rank be ever so much elevated.

Notwithstanding this kind of Kingly Establishment, there is very little about Otoo's person or Court, by which a Stranger could distinguish the King from the Subject. I have seldom seen him dressed in any thing but a Common piece of Cloth wraped round his loins, so that he seems to pay the same homage to his Subjects which is due to him from them; he seems to avoide all unnecessary pomp and shew and even to demean himself, more than any other of the Earee's; I have seen him work at a Paddle, in coming to and going from the Ship, in common with the other Paddler[s] and even when some of his Toutous, were seting looking on. Every one has free access to him and speak to him where ever they see him without the least ceremony, such is the easy freedom which every endividual of this happy isle enjoys. I have observed that the Chiefs of these isles are more beloved by the bulk of the people than feared, may we not conclude from this that the goverment is mild and equitable? It

[1] This claim again was merely family 'build-up'. 'Tarevatou' (Te-ari'i-fa'atau, lit. 'the lazy chief') was the eldest of Tu's four brothers. The eldest sister, married to Teriirere of Papara, was Te-arii-na-vaho-roa; the second was named Arii-paea; there was a third sister, Vaii-o, for whom apparently no overweening claims were made.

[2] Eowa = *e Houa*; Whanno = *Fana*. They were officials who were sent on messages allegedly requiring speed; *houa* is, literally, to be in a state of perspiration; *fana* is a bow. The *houa* had apparently the greater dignity, and might be a sort of ambassador.

hath been said that Oheatoua of Tiarabou is related to Otoo, the same may be said of the Chiefs of *Eimeo*, *Tapamannoo*, *Huaheine*, *Ulietea*, *Otaha* and *Bola bola* for they are all related to the Royal family of Oteheite. It is a Maxim with the Earee's and others of Superior Rank never to inter marry with the Toutous or others of inferior Rank—probably this custom was one great inducement in forming the Societies called Arreoies;[1] it is certain that these Societies greatly prevent the increase of the Superior Classes of people of which they are Composed and do not attall interfere with the inferior or Toutou's, for I never hea[r]d of one of these being an Arreoy nor did I ever hear that a Toutou could rise in life above the rank he was born in. I have occasionally mentioned, the extraordinary fondness the people of Otaheite shewed for red feathers, which they call Oora and are as valuable here as Jewels are in Europe, especially, those which they call Ooravine[2] and grow on the head of the Green Paraquet,[3] all red feathers are indeed esteemed but none equal to these and they are such good judges as to know very well how to distinguish one sort from another; many of our people attempted to deceive them by dying other feathers, but I never heard that any one succeeded. These feathers they make up in little bunches consisting of eight or ten and fix them to the end of a small cord about three or four Inches long, which is made of the strong out side fibers of the Cocoanut, twisted so hard that it is like a piece of twisted wire and serves as a handle to the bunch. Thus prepared they are used as Symbols of the Eatua's or Divinities in all their religious ceremonies. I have very often seen them hold one of these bunches and some times only two or three feathers between the fore finger and thumb and say a prayer, not one word of which I could ever understand. Who ever comes to this isle will do well to provide himself with Red feathers, the finest and smallest that are to be got, he must also have a good stock of Axes and Hatchets, Spike Nails, Files, Knives, Looking Glasses, Beads &c[a]. Sheets and Shirts are much sought after, especially by the Ladies as many of our gentlemen found by experience.[4] The Two Goats which Captain Furneaux gave to Otoo when we were last here, seem to promise fair to answer the end for which

[1] Cook seems here to regard the *arioi* society as an exclusive aristocratic preserve, or as a haven for wifeless *arii*. On the Tahitian social structure and the *arioi* see I, pp. clxxvii–clxxix, clxxxviii–cxc.

[2] *ura vini*.

[3] This appears to be the extinct *Cyanoramphus zealandicus*, so named by Latham in 1790, from some confusion as to its origin.

[4] Burney, Ferguson MS, in his description of the Society Islands, notes that 'had we staid much longer at these Islands few of the Younkers in either ship would have had a shirt left'.

they were put on shore; the Ewe soon after had two feemale kids which were now so far grown as to be nearly ready to propagate and the old Ewe was again big with kid; the people seemed very fond of them and they seemed to like their situation as well, as they were in most excellent case: It is to be hoped that in a few years they will have some to spare their Neighbours and by that means they may in time spread over all the Neighbouring isles. The Sheep which we left died soon after, excepting one, which we understood was yet alive. We have also furnished them with a Stock of Catts, no less than twenty were given away at this isle besides what were left at Ulietea and Huaheine.*—ff. 212v–14v.

SUNDAY 15*th*. I have already mentioned that after leaving Otaheite we directed our Course for Huahine and at one o'Clock in the after noon of this day Anchor'd in the North entrance of Owharre Harbour, hoisted out the boats and Warp'd into a proper birth and there Moor'd the Ship.[1] While this was doing several of the Natives came on board amongest whom was Oree the Chief, he brought with him a Hog and some other Articles which he presented to me with the usual cerimony.

MONDAY 16*th*. In the Morning I return'd Oree's Visset and made my present in return, after which he put two Hogs into my boat and he and several of his friends came on board and dined, after dinner I gave to Oree Axes, Nails &c[a] and desired he would distribute them to his friends which he accordingly did seemingly to the satisfaction of every one.[2]

M[r] F. and his party being out botanizing his Serv[t] a feeble Man was set upon by five or Six fellows who would have strip'd him if they had not been prevented by a nother of the party.[3]

[1] . . . with the bower and Kedge Anchor, not quite a Cables length from the Shore.—f. 215.

[2] . . . Monday 16th Morning the Natives began to bring us fruit. I returned Orre's Visit and made my present in return, one article of which was red feathers, two or three of which the Cheif took in his right hand holding them up between the finger and thum, and said a prayer as I understood which was little notice'd by any present. Two Hogs were soon after put into my Boat and he and several of his friends came aboard and dined with us. After dinner, Orre gave me to understand what Articles would be most agreeable to him and his friends, which were cheifly axes and Nails, accordingly I gave him what he asked and disired he would distribute them to the others, which he did, seemingly to the Satisfaction of every one; a youth about 10 or 12 years of Age either his Son or grandson seemed to be the person of most note and had the greatest share. After the distribution was over, they all retired ashore.—f. 215.

[3] . . . after which they made off with a hatchet they had got from him.—f. 215. The Huahine men were altogether too lively: 'Two of the natives in a canoe endeavouring to cutt the buoy away where discovered—a musket was fired which occasioned them to jump overboard, bro[t] the canoe onboard & cutt her up, by way of example'.—Mitchel, 17 May PM.

TUESDAY 17*th*. Being on shore in the after-noon Oree sent for me to a large house where were collected a good number of people, here a kind of Councel was hild. I well understood it regarded us and that the Chiefs all declared they had no hand in asulting M^r F Servant and desired I would Matte the fellows who did. I assured Oree that I was satisfied neither he or any of the people present had any hand in it and that I should certainly do with the fellows as they desird but the Quiry was where and how I was to find them. After this the Councel broke up.

*TUESDAY 17*th*. I went a Shore to looke for the Cheif in order to complain of the outrage committed yesterday, but he was not in the neighbourhood. Being a shore in the after noon, a person came and told me Orre wanted to see me, I went with the man and was conducted to a large house where the Cheif and several other persons of note were assembled in Councel, as well as I could understand. After I was seated and some conversation had past among them, Orre made a Speach and was Answered by a nother, I understood no more of either than to know it regarded the robbery commited yesterday. The Chief then began to assure me that neigher he or any present (which were the principle Cheifs in the Neighbourhood) had any hand in it and desired me to kill with the guns all those which had: I assured him that I was satisfied that neither he or those present were attall concearned in the affair, and that I should do with the fellows as he desired, or any others who were guilty of the like crimes, and asked where the fellows were and to bring them to me that I might do with them as he had desired; his answer was, they were gone to the Mountains and he could not get them. Whether this was the Case or not I will not pretend to say, I knew fair means would never make them deliver them up and I had no intention to try others and so the affair droped and the Cou[n]cel broke up.

In the Eveng some of the gentlemen went to see a Dramatic Entertainment. The Piece represented a Girl as runing away with us from Otaheite and which was in some degree true as a young Woman had taken a passage with us down to Ulietea and happened now to be present at the Representation of her own adventures which had such an effect upon her that it was with great difficilty our gentlemen could prevail upon her to see the play out or to refrain from tears while it was acting. The Piece concluded with the reception she was supposed to meet with from her friends at her return which was not a very favourable one. These people can add little Extemporary pieces to their entertainments whenever they see occasion; is [it] not therefore reasonable to believe that this was intended as a Satire against this girl and to discourage others from following her steps.*—ff. 215–16.

WEDNESDAY 18*th*. Some Showers of rain. Morning Oree came with a present of fruit, stay'd dinner and in the after noon desired to see some great guns fired, Shotted, which I comply'd with and then he return'd a shore well satisfied.[1] Some of the Petty officers going out into the Country took two men as guides and to carry their money bags, containing hatchets, Nails &c[a] the Currant coin of these countries, but the fellows found means to move off with their burdthens and the Method they took was artfull enough, they pointed out to them some birds to shoot,[2] one of the two Musquets they had went of and the other miss'd fire several times, so that they saw they were secure from both and ran off immidiately and left the gentlemen gazeing at them like fools.

THURSDAY 19*th*. Showery all the morning, afternoon fair weather; little or no supplies from the Natives, or any thing else remarkable.

FRIDAY 20*th*. Early in the Morning three of the officers set out on a Shooting party,[3] about 3 o'Clock in the after-noon I received intelligence that they were Seized and stripd of every thing about them, immidiately upon this I went a Shore with M[r] F. and a boats crew and took possession of a large house with all the effects in it and two Chiefs, but in such a manner that they hardly knew what we were about being unwilling to alarm the neighbourhood. In this situation we were till the officers returnd safe and had had all their things restored; some insult[4] on their side induced the Natives (who perhaps

[1] . . . The reason of his makeing this requist, was his hearing from Odiddy and our Otahiete passingers, that we had so done at that island. The Cheif would have had us fired at the hills in the Country, but I did not approve of it, least the shott should fall Short and do some Misschief; besides the effect was better seen in the Water.—f. 215v.

[2] *they . . . shoot:* the gentlemen had with them two Muskets for shooting birds, the fellows after a shower of rain pointed out some for them to Shoot. . . .

[3] . . . rather contrary to my inclination as I found the Natives, at least some of them, were continually on the lookout watching an oppertunity to rob stragling parties, and were daily growing more and more daring.—f. 217.—The officers, says Forster (II, p. 122), were Cooper, Clerke, and one of the mates.

[4] *restored; some insult:* restored and then I quited the house and presently after every thing in it was carried off. When I got aboard I was informed of the whole affair by the officers themselves: some little insult . . .—f. 217. Forster, II, pp. 122–4, gives a circumstantial account; according to him, Clerke 'ingenuously confessed' that he and Cooper had been the aggressors, 'and had drawn upon themselves the severe revenge which the natives had taken'. One of them had bullied and beaten a native into acting as a retriever for the ducks he had shot, and when the man tried to escape with the ducks, shot at him with ball—luckily missing. This hardly seems a 'little insult'; and it seems quite out of Clerke's character, whatever Cooper was capable of. Possibly Forster exaggerated. Cook could hardly have regarded the prevention of murder as an 'outrage'—the word used by him a few lines below.

waited for such an oppertunity) to seize their guns, upon which a scuffle insued, some chiefs interfeer'd and took the officers out of the Crowd and caused what had been taken from them to be restored.[1] I wint to look for Oree to complain of those repeated outrages, but not being in the neghberhood did not see him, after I had got on board I was told he was come to his house and was much grieved at what had happen'd.

SATURDAY 21*st*. Early in the Morn sail'd from hence for Ulietea, upward of Sixty Canoes, we were told the people in them were Arioe's and were going to the neghbouring isles to viset thier Brethren of the same ferternity, one may almost compair these Men to free masons, they tell us they assist each other when need requires and they seem to have Customs amongest them which they either will not or cannot explain, Odiddy says he is one and yet he cannot give us hardly any Idea of them.[2]

Odiddy who generly sleeps on Shore came off with a Message from Oree desiring I would come on shore with 22 Men to go with him to Chastise the robers, the Messenger brought with him 22 pices of leaves least as I suppose he should forget his number, but this is one of their customs. Upon my receiving this extraordinary message I went ashore for better information; all I could learn from the Chief was these fellows were a sort of Banditi that had form'd themselves into a boddy with a resolution to seize and rob our people where ever they found them and therefore he wanted them chastized. I told him they would fly to the Mountains, he said no they had arm'd themselves to fight us.[3]

[1] . . . This was a place where we had before been told a set of fellows had formed themselves into a gang with a resolution to rob every one who should go that way. It should seem from what followed that the Chief could not prevent this or put a stop to those repeated outrages. I did not see him this evening as he was not come into the neighbourhood when I went on board, but I learnt from Odiddy that he came soon after and was so concearned at what had happened that he wept.—f. 217.

[2] *and yet . . . them:* Tupia was one, and yet I have not been able to get any tolerable idea of this set of men from either of them. Odiddy denies that the children they have by their Mistresses are put to death as we understood from Tupia and others.—f. 217v. At this point Cook writes into H, 'It is a well known fact that they are put to death'. A151 has a footnote: 'This assertion of Odiddies is of very little weight with me, I have found him but very little or hardly att all acquainted with many of their Customs of which this is one. Nuno an Arioe of Otahiete keeps a Mistress, a Sister of Odiddies, on asking him what became of the Children she might have by Nuno, he tells us she can have none, for that they have no other connections with each other than just sleeping together in the bed. Is it possible for any one to beleive this?' The text in both B and G are marked for a note, but B leaves inadequate space for it, and G no space at all. For the *arioi* see I, pp. clxxxviii–cxc.

[3] *no . . . fight us:* they were resolved to fight us, and desired I would distroy both them and their house, but desired I would spare those in the neighbourhood as Also the Canoes and the Whenooa, and by way of security for these, presented me with a pig as a peace offering for the Whenooa, it was too small to be meant for any thing but a cerimony of

When I got on board I acquainted the officers with what I had heard and desired to have their opinion of the Matter, in short it was concluded to go upon this consideration, that if we declined it as it was at the request of the cheif, these fellows would thereby be incouraged to commit greater acts of Violence and as these proceeding[s] would soon reach Ulietea, at which isle we intended to touch, the people there might treat us in the same manner or worse as being more numerous. Accordingly we landed 48 Men including my self, M[r] F. and officers, the Cheif join'd us with a few people and we set out on our march in good order, the Chiefs party gather'd like a snow ball as we marched thro' the Country, some arm'd and some not; Odiddy who was with us began to be alarm'd and told us that many of the people in our company were of the party we were going against and at last told us that they were only leading us to some place where they could attack us to advantage, whether there was any truth in this or only occasioned by Odiddies fears I will not pretend to say, he however was the only person we could confide in and we regulated our march accordingly; after we had march'd several miles we got intelligence that the people we were going against were fled to the Mountains, but I think we were not told this till I had diclar'd to the Chief that I would March no farther for we were then about crossing a deep Vally bounded on each side with Steep Rocks where a few men with stones only might have cut off our retreat supposeing their intention to be what Odiddy had said and what he still abided by; having therefore no business to proceed farther we return'd back in the same order as we went, and saw in several places people[1] come down from the sides of the hills with their arms in their hands, which they laid down[2] when ever they found they were seen by us, this shews that there must have been some truth in what Odiddy had said, but I must acquit Oree the Chief from having any hand in it. In our return Stoping at a house[3] to refresh our selves with Cocoa-nutts two Chiefs brought each of

this kind. This sencible old chief could see (which perhaps none of the others never thought of) that every thing in the Neighbourhood was at our mercy, and therefore took care to secure them by this method which I suppose to be of weight with them. When I returned on board I considered of the Chiefs request, which upon the whole appeared an extraordinary one.—f. 217v. 'Whenooa': *fenua*, the country; presumably it means here the district concerned. Cf. p. 422, n. 1.

[1] . . . who had been following us, . . .—f. 218.

[2] *laid down:* instantly quited and hid in the bushes

[3] *Stoping at a house:* we halted at a convenient place to refresh our selves with a few Cocoanutts which I ordered the people to bring us which they readily complied with; indeed by this time I believe many of them wished us on board out of the way, altho no one step was taken that could give them the least alarm, nevertheless they certainly were. [*sic*, and so G]—f. 218. The printed text reads 'were in terror'.

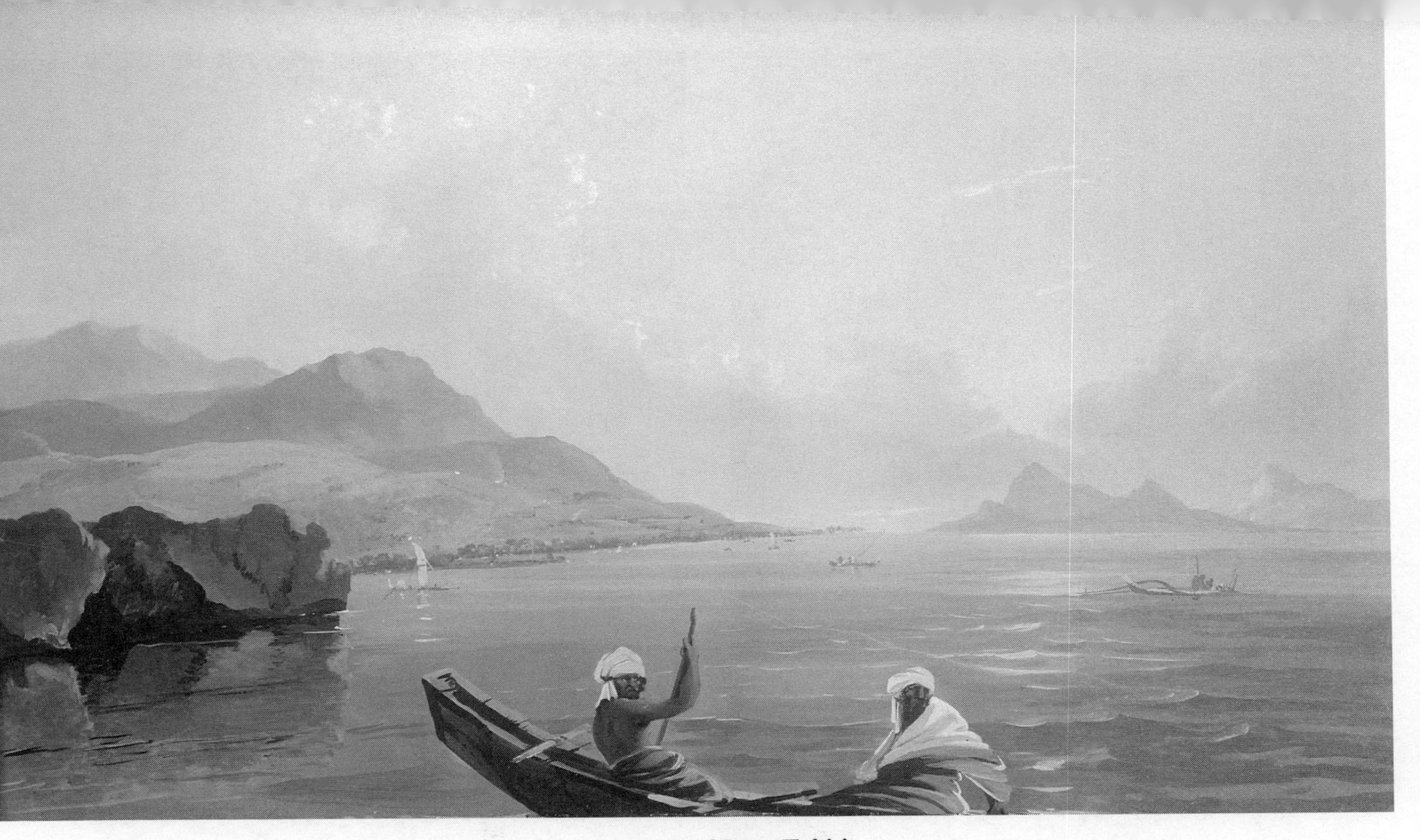

FIG. 61. View of Pare, Tahiti

Oil painting by Hodges, in the National Maritime Museum

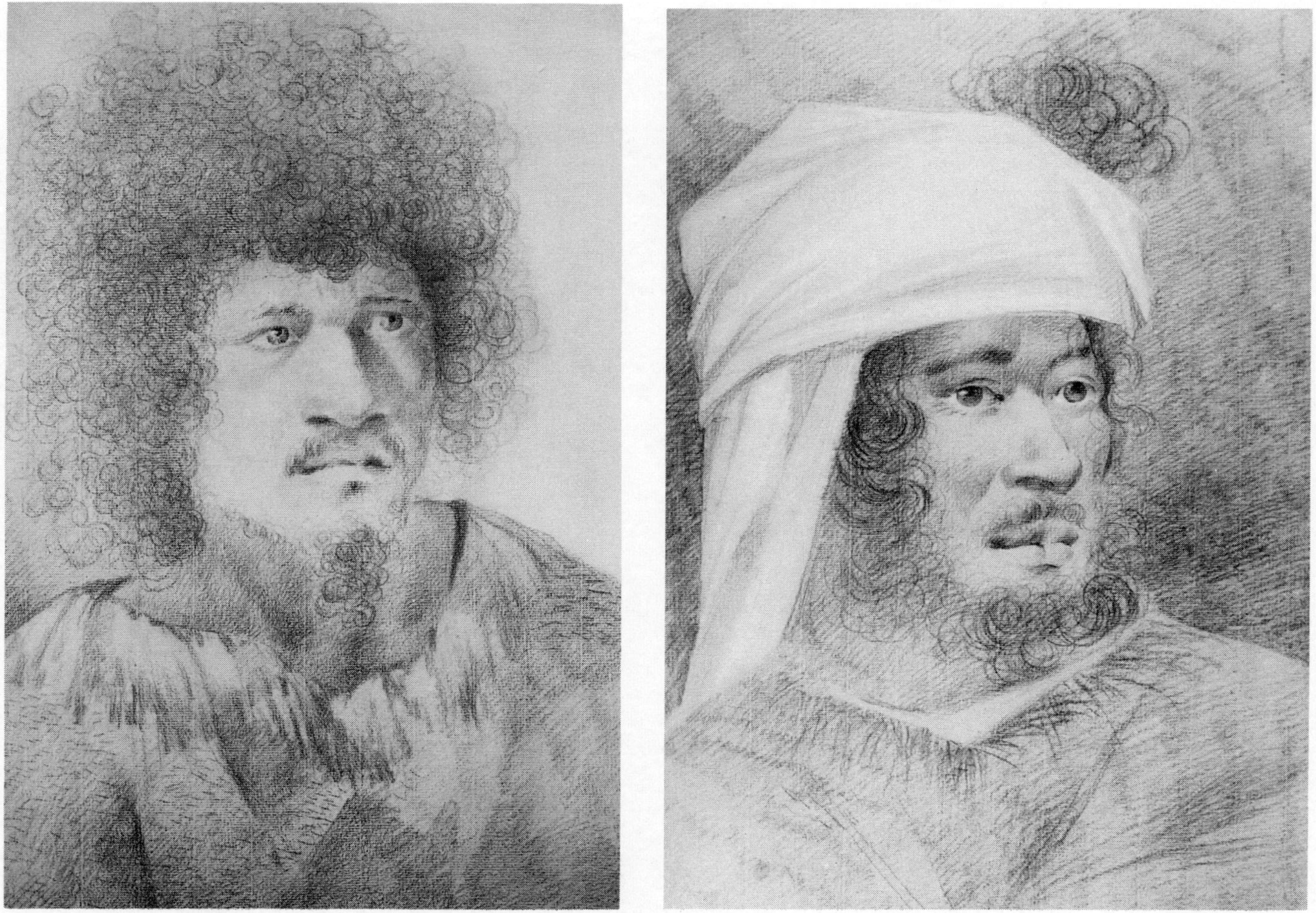

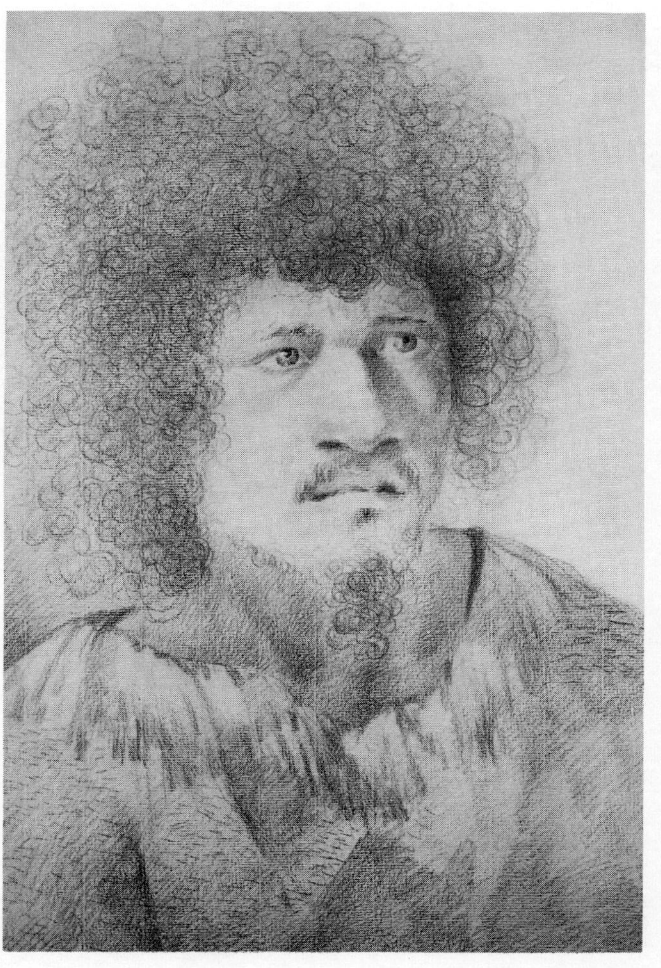

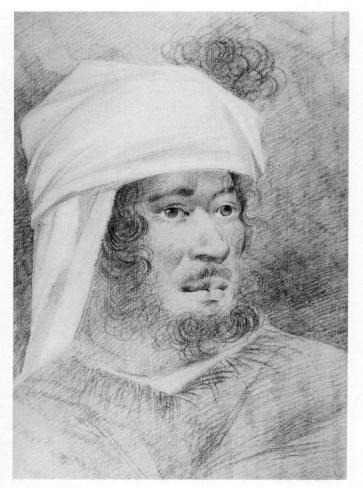

Fig. 62. Portrait heads of Tahitians, by Hodges

them a pig and a dog and with the Customary ceremony presented them to me together with some young plantain trees by way of making and ratifying the Peace,[1] after this we continued our march to the landing place where we imbarqued and went on board, soon after the chief follow'd, with a quantity of fruit, and set down with us to dinner, we had scarce dined before more fruit and two Hogs were brought off to the Ship, so that we were likely to get more by this excursion than by all the presents we had made them; it certainly gave them some Alarm to see so strong a party march into the Country and probably gave them a better opinion of our fire Arms, for I had caused the people on our return to the beach to fire several vollies to let the Natives see we could keep up a constant fire for I believe they had but an indifferent or rather contemptable Idea of Musquets in general, having never seen any fired but at birds &c[a] by such of our people as used to stragling about the Country, the most of them but indifferent sportsmen and Miss'd generally two Shott out of three, this together with their pieces missing fire, being Slow in charging and before the Natives, all this they no doubt took great Notice of and concluded[2] that Musquets were not such terrible things as they had been tought to believe.

SUNDAY *22nd.* I intended to have Saild this Morning had not the Chief assured me last night that if I would stay one day longer we should have a large supply of Provisions, he was in part as good as his word for we got more Bread fruit and Cocoa nutts than we could dispence with, but Pigs which we most wanted came far short of our expectations. Going on Shore in the afternoon I found the Chief just seting down to dinner, I cannot say what was the occasion of his dining so late, several people were imploy'd chewing the peper root about a pint of which juice without any other mixture was the first dish and which was dispatch'd in an instant, a Cup of it was offered to me, but the Brewing alone was sufficient,[3] after this the chief washed his Mouth with Coco-nut Water and eat of Ripe Plantain and Mahee[4] of each not a little and lastly finished his repast by eating or rather drinking about three pints Popoie[5] which is made of Bread fruit, Plantans Mahee &c[a] and deluted with Water till it is about the consistance of custard.

[1] ... another brought a very large hog which he followed us with to the Ship.—f. 218v.

[2] ... as well they might

[3] ... Odiddy was not so nice and took what I refused ...—f. 219.

[4] *mahi*, baked fermented breadfruit.

[5] *popoe*.

MONDAY 23*rd*. Winds Easterly, as it has been ever sence we have been here.[1] The Ship being unmoor'd and every thing in readiness to Sail, at 8 am wieghed and put to Sea, the good old Chief was the last of the Natives who went out of the Ship, when he took leave I told him we should see each other no more at which he wept saying than let your sons come we will treat them well. Oree is a good Man to the utmost sence of the word, but many of the people are far from being of that disposision and seem to take advantage of his old age.[2] The gentle treatment they have ever met with from me and the careless and imprudent manner many of our people have rambled about in their country from a Vain opinion that fire Arms rendred them invincible hath incouraged some of these people to commit acts of Violence no man at Otaheite ever dar'd attempt.

During our stay at this isle we got bread fruit, Cocoa nuts &c[a] more than we could well consume, but Hogs not by far sufficient for our daily expence and yet they did not appear to be scarce in the isle, it must however be Allowed that the number we took away when last here must have thin'd them much and at the same time Stock'd the Natives with our articles, besides we now wanted a proper assortment of Trade our Stock being nearly exhausted and the few Red feathers we had left was here of little Value when compared to what they bore at Otaheite, this obliged me to set the Smiths to work to make different sorts of Iron tools, Nails &c[a], in order to inable me to procure refreshments at the other isles and to support my Credit and influance among them.

MONDAY 23*rd*. As Soon as we were clear of Hauheine we made Sail and steer'd over for the South end of Ulietea, one of the Natives of the first isle took a Passage with us as some others had done from Otaheite.[3] Having but little wind all the afternoon it was dark by such time as we reached the West side of the isle where we spent the night. The same light and variable winds continued till 10 o'Clock y[e] next morning when the Trade wind at East prevail'd and we ventured to ply up to the Harbour, first sending a boat to ly in Anchorage; after makeing a few trips, anchor'd in 20 fathom water, between the two points of the reef which form the entrance on which the Sea broke with Such height and Violence as was frightfull to

[1] *have been here:* left Otahiete.

[2] . . . and Teraderre his grandson and heir is yet but a youth.—f. 219. 'Teraderre' is probably a formal title, Te arii rere or Terii-rere; Terii-rere of Papara, the son of Amo and Purea, had his name so rendered in English.

[3] *one . . . Otaheite:* Orre took the opertunnity to send a man with a message to Opoony.—f. 220.

look at;[1] having all our Boats and Warpes in readiness we presently carried them out and Warped the Ship in to safety where we droped an Anchor for the night. While we were warping into the harbour my old friend Oreo the Chief and Several more came off to see us. The Chief came not empty handed.

WEDNESDAY 25*th*. Rainy Weather, AM Warp'd the Ship up into the Cove which froonts the entrance of the Harbour and higher up than we had ever anchor'd before and there moor'd her, in this situation we commanded the Shores all round us. Whilest this was doing I went on Shore accompanied by Mr F. &c^a^ to make the Chief the Customary present. At our first entering his house we were met by 4 or 5 old Women, Weeping and lamenting, as it were, most bitterly and at the same time cuting their heads with Instruments made of Sharks teeth so that the blood ran p[l]entifully down their faces and on their Shoulders, and what was still worse we were obliged to submit to the Embraces of these old Hags and by that means got all besmear'd with Blood: this ceremony (for it was meerly such) being over, these women went and Washed themselves and immidiately after appear'd as Cheerfull as any of the Company. After I[2] had given my presents to the Chief and his friends he put a Hog and some fruit into my Boat and came on board with us to dinner. In the after-noon we had a vast number of Canoes and people about us from different parts of the isle, they all took up their quarters in our neighbourhood where they remain'd feasting for two or three days. We understood the most of them were Arioe's.

THURSDAY 26*th*. Afforded nothing remarkable except Mr F.[3] seeing a burying place for Dogs, which they call'd *Marai no te oore*,[4] but I think we ought not to look upon this as one of their customs because few Dogs die a natural death, being generally kill'd and eat, besides I see no reason why a Ladies favourate dog should not have as decent a burial here as in England or any other Country in Europe:

[1] . . . After makeing a few trips got before the Channell and with all our sails set and the head way the Ship had acquired, shutt [shot] her in as far as she would go, then droped the anchor and tooke in the sails; this is the method of geting into most of the Harbours, which are on the lee side of these isles, for the channells in general are too narrow to ply in. We were now anchored between the two points of the reef which form the entrance each not more than two thirds the length of a cable from us, and on which the Sea broke with such height and Violence as was frightfull to behold; the sight to people less acquainted with the place would have been terible.—f. 220. The ship had gone through the Rautoanui passage; Cook's anchorage was Haamanino inside.

[2] *After I:* After some little stay and I . . .—f. 220v.

[3] . . . in his botanical excursion

[4] *marae no te uri.*

this certainly may be done without its being a general custom of the Nation.[1]

FRIDAY 27*th.* In the Morning Oreo, his Wife, Son and Daughters and several more of his friends came aboard and brought with them a supply of refreshments.[2] After dinner we went on Shore and were entertained with a Play which ended with the representation of a Woman in Labour, who at last brought forth a thumping Boy near six feet high who ran about the stage draging what was to represent the [3] after him. I had an oppertunity to see this acted afterward, and observed that as soon as they got hold of the fellow who represented the child they f[l]atned his nose or press'd it to his face which may be a Custom a Mong them and be the reason why they have all in general flat, or what we call pug noses.[4]

SATURDAY 28*th.* Mr F. and his party out Botanizing. Spent the day with the Chief and his friends much the same as yesterday.[5]

SUNDAY 29*th.* In the Morning found Several Articles had been Stolen in the night out of our boats lying at the Buoy about 60 or 80 yards from the Ship, went my self to the Chief to complain who immidiately went[6] with me in my boat in pursute of the thief for he was presently inform'd which way they were gone, after we had proceed a good way a long shore to the Southward, we at last land according

[1] *being . . . Nation:* being generally if not allways killed and eat, or else given as an offering to the gods; probably this might be a Marai or Altar were this sort of offering was made, or it might have been the whim of some person to have buried his favourate dog in this manner; but be how it will I cannot think it is a general custom in the Nation, for my own part I neither saw nor heard of such a thing before.—f. 220v.

[2] . . . it is but little we as yet get from any body else.

[3] Afterbirth, presumably; compare following note. The children of nature liked their farce broad.

[4] *which ended . . . noses:* called Mydiddy Harramy, which signifies the Child is Coming which concluded with the representation of a Woman in labour acted by a set of great brawny fellows one of which at last brought forth a Straping Boy about 6 feet high who ran about the stage draging after him a large wisp of Straw which hung by a string from his middle. I had an oppertunity to see this acted another time when I observed, that the moment they got hold of the fellow, who represented the Child they flatened or pressed his Nose; from this I judged that they do so by their Children when born, which may be the reason why all in general have flat noses. This part of the play, what from the newness of the thing and the ludicrous manner it was acted gave us, the first time we saw it, some entertainment and caused a loud laugh, which might be the reason why they acted it so often afterwards; but this like all their other pieces could entertain no more than once, especially us who could gather little from them for want of knowing more of their language.—ff. 220v.–1. 'Mydiddy Harramy': *maititi haere mai*, 'welcome to the child', *lit.* 'child come hither'.—J. R. Forster, *Observations*, pp. 471–2, analyzes the plot of this drama at greater length; see also Wales, pp. 842–3 below.

[5] . . . viz. in entertaining my friends and they me.—f. 221.—Cooper has the entry for 27 May, possibly Cook's 28th, 'Punish'd Chas Williams Coopers Mate for losing his Tools 1 doz^n lashes'.

[6] *who . . . went:* but I found that he not only knew they were gone, but where and by whom and went immediately . . .—f. 221.

to the Chief's directions,[1] and soon after all the articles were produced except the Pinnace's Iron Tiller which I was told was still farther to the Southward, but when I wanted to proceed farther I found the Chief unwilling and actually gave me the Slip and retired into the Country and the people I saw were Alarmed,[2] without him I knew I could do nothing, I therefore sent a man (one of the Natives) after him to desire him to return, he return'd accordingly and we set down and had some thing brought us to eat and drink and in the mean time[3] two Hogs were produced which they intreated me to except which I accordingly did, this satisfied every one, their fears were dissipated and I thought my self not ill of in geting two Hogs for a thing that was already out of my reach, besides I had brought me some articles I did not know we had lost. Every thing be[ing] settld we return'd on board and had the Company of the Chief and his son to dinner. After dinner we all went a Shore where a play was acted for the entertainment of such as would spend their time in looking at it. Besides the Plays which the Chief now and then caused to be acted for our entertainment there were a Set of stroling Players in the Neghbourhood who acted every day, but they were all so much of a piece that we soon grew tired of them, especially, for want of throughly knowing their Language, no intristing circumstance could be collected from them; we well know they can add to or diminish their plays at pleasure; we, our Ship and our Country they have frequently brought on the Stage, but on what account I know not. I make no doubt but it was intended as a Compliment and not interduced but when some of us were present. I generally appear'd at Oreo's Theatre towards the latter end of the Play and twice at the other in order to give my mite to the actors, the only actress[4] was Oreo's Daughter, a pretty brown girl at whose Shrine, on these occasions, many pretty things were offered by her numerous Votarists and I believe was one great inducement why her father gave us these entertainments so often.

MONDAY 30*th*. Early in the Morning, I set out with two boats accompanied by Mess[rs] F., Odiddy, the Chief, his Wife, Son and Daughter for an Estate which Odidde call'd his, situated at the North end of the Island, here I was promised to have Hogs and fruit in a bundance, but when we arrived I found poor Odidde

[1] ... near some houses

[2] ... when they saw I was for going farther, by which I concluded that the tiller was out of their reach also

[3] *some . . . time:* some Victuals set before us, thinking perhaps, that as I had not breakfasted I must be hungry and not in a good humour, thus I was amused till ...—f. 221.

[4] ... at Oreo's theatre

could not command one single thing whatever right he might have to the Whennooa[1] which was now in possession of his Brother, by whom were presented to me with the usual ceremony two small Hogs, in return I made him presents of three times their Value,[2] One of the Hogs I order'd to be immidiately Kill'd and dress'd for dinner, and attended my self to the whole opperation which I shall discribe; the first thing was to Strangle the Hog which was the work of 3 men, the Hog being placed upon his back two of them laid a pretty strong Stick a cross his throat and press'd on each end with their whole weight, the third Man held his hind legs kept him on his back and plug'd up his backside with grass,[3] in this Manner they held him for at least 10 minutes before he was quite dead and in the mean time some hands were Employ'd makeing a fire to heat the oven, which was close by; as soon as the Hog was quite dead they laid it on the fire and Burnt or singed the hair so that it came off with allmost the same ease as if it had been scalded, as they got the hair off one part a nother was applied to the fire &c[a] till the whole was done, but not so clean but that another operation was necessary, which was to carry it to the Water side and scrub it well [with] Sand and Sandy stones, this took off the Scurf &c[a] which this Operation at the fire wou'd not; as soon as this was done and all the Sand and dirt wash'd clean off in the Water it was brought again to the first place and their laid on Clean green leaves in order to be opened; they first riped up the skin of the belly only and seperated the skin from the fatt which lies between it and the inside flesh which they took out, that is that fatt which covers the belly and is in general as soft as the lard, this was laid on a clean leafe, they than riped open the belly and took out the Entrails which were put into a basket and carried away so that I know not what became of them, but am certain they were not thrown away. The Blood was now all taken out and put into a large leafe, then the Lard which was put to the other fat, the Hog was now washed clean both inside and out with fresh Water, Several Hot stones were put into his belly which was afterwards cram'd full with clean green leaves;[4] by this time, or perhaps before, the Oven was sufficently heated, what fire remain'd was taken away, together with some of the Hot stones, the rest were left[5] in the bottom of the hole or Oven which was now covered with

[1] *fenua* here seems to mean 'estate'.

[2] *in return . . . value:* I made him a very ha[n]dsome present in return and Odiddy gave him every thing he had left of what he had collected the time he was with us.—f. 221v.

[3] . . . I suppose this was done to prevent any air from passing or repassing that way,

[4] *which . . . leaves:* which were shaken in under the breast and green leaves cram'd in upon them; . . . f. 222.

[5] *were left:* made a kind of pavement

green leaves on which the hog was laid on his belly, the lard and fatt, after undergoing some washings with fresh Water was put in a Vessel made just then of the bark of Plantain tree, two or three hot stones being put in along with the fat, it was tied up and put in the Oven by the hog as was the blood also prepared in the same manner, round the whole were laid to Bake Plantains, Bread fruit &c[a] then the whole covered with green leaves on which were placed the remainder of the Hot stones and over them more leaves and then any sort of rubbage they could lay their hands upon and lastly finishd the operation by well covering the whole with earth, here it laid two hours and Ten Minutes, then the Oven was opened, the Hog as well as all the other victuals were taken out and laid on green leaves already spread for the purpose on the floor at the one end of a large boat house, such of the Natives who dined with us set down by themselves and we by our selves, that is they were at the one end of the Table and we at the other; the Hog was plac'd before us and the fat and blood before them, which they chiefly if not wholy dined off and said it was Mona-mona ta, that is very good[1] and we not only said but realy thought the same by the Pork. The Hog wieghed about fifty pound, some parts about the Ribs I thought rather over done, but the more thicker parts were excellent, and the Skin which by our way of drissing is generally either hard or tough[2] had by this method a flavour superior to any thing I ever tasted. I have now only to add that during the whole process nothing could be done with more cleanlyness. I have been the more particular in this account because I do not recollect that any one of us ever saw the whol process before nor can I recolect what is said on this Subject in the Journal of my former Voyage.

Soon[3] after we had dined we set out for the Ship with the other Pig and a few races of Plantans which proved the sum total of our great expectations. Poor Odiddy had drank a little too freely either of the juice of peper or our Grog or both and was brought into the boat dead drunk. In our return to the Ship we put a Shore at a place where in a House we Saw four wooden Images standing upon a shelf each about 2 feet in length, they had Turbands about their heads[4] in which were stuck some long feathers. A person in the house

[1] *Mona-mona ta . . . good:* ma-mity, very good victuals . . .—f. 222v. *Monamona ta*, very sweet fresh food. Ma-mity = *maa maitai*, good food.

[2] *is . . . tough:* can hardly ever be eat

[3] *soon:* While dinner was preparing, I took a view of this Whenooa of Odiddies, it was small but a pleasant spot, and the houses were so disposed as to form a very pretty village which is very rarely the case at these isles. Soon . . .—f. 222v.

[4] *they . . . heads:* each had a piece of cloth round the middle, and a kind of Turband on the head . . .—f. 223.

told us they were Eatua's no te Tou tou,[1] that is the gods of the Common people, but this is by no means Sufficient to conclude that they worship them as such or that the Servants or Slaves are not allow'd the same Gods as those of a more elevated rank. I never heard that Tupia made any such distinction,[2] besides these were the first wooden gods we had seen in any of the isles and all the authority we had of their being such was the bare word of, perhaps, a Superstitious person.[3] The people of this isle are in general far more superstitious than at Otaheite or any of the other isles. The first Visit I made the chief after our arrival, he desired I would not suffer any of my people to Shoot the Heron's[4] and Wood Pickers,[5] Birds as Sacred to them as Robin Red-breasts, Swallows, &c[a] &c[a] are to many old women in England. Tupia who was a Priest, and seem'd well accquaint[ed] with their Religion, Traditions, Customs &c[a] paid little or no regard to these Birds. I mention thise things because some among us were inclinable to beleive that they look'd upon these two Birds as Eatua's or Gods.[6] We fell into this opinion when I was here in the Endeavour and some others Still more Obsurd which undoubtedly we should have adopted if Tupia had not undeceived us, a Man of his knowlidge[7] we have not sence met with, concequently have added nothing to his account of their Religion but superstitious Notions.

TUESDAY 31*st*. The Natives being informed that we should sail in a few days began to bring us on board fruit more than usual, amonghest those who came on board was a young man who measured Six feet four Inches and Six-tenths, His Sister, younger than himself, measured five feet ten Inches and a half.

[JUNE 1774]

WEDNESDAY, June 1*st*. A brisk Trade for Hogs and Fruit, Nothing else remarkable.

[1] *atua no te teuteu. Teuteu*, hereditary retainers of a chief.

[2] or that they worshiped any visible thing whatever; . . .—f. 223. These images were probably 'vehicles' for the god, certainly not objects of worship. The god would 'speak' through them if approached with the proper ritual, as he might speak through some living thing. Cf. n. 6 below.

[3] . . . which we were likewise liable to misunderstand.

[4] The Reef Heron, *Demigretta sacra* (Gm.).

[5] There are no woodpeckers in Polynesia. Cook may have meant a kingfisher, *Halcyon venerata* Gm.

[6] These birds were not *atua* or gods, but like many other birds were regarded as 'shadows' or 'reflections' of the gods—i.e. *ata*, the visible representation of gods, one of whom might at some particular time use a particular bird as his 'vehicle'. Different gods used different sorts of birds. Hence the 'sacredness'.

[7] . . . and understanding

THURSDAY *2nd.* In the afternoon had Intillegence that three days before two Ships had arrived at Huaheine, (viz) Captain Furneaux and Mr Banks, the fellow who brought the intelligence described the Persons of Mr Banks and Captain Furneaux so well that I had not the least doubt of the truth and was considering wheather or no I should send over a boat that very night, when a man, a friend of Mr F. said that the whole was a lie, the man who brought the information was now gone a Shore so that the two could not be confronted. I however laid aside all thoughts of sending away a boat till I had more certain information. This Evening we entertained the Natives with fire Works.

FRIDAY *3rd.* I had fixed on this Day for sailing but the intilligence received last night put a Stop to it, but were not sufficient to induce me to send a boat over to Huahine for the more we inquired into it the more reason we had to disbelieve it and at last all our inquiries tended jointly to prove that the whole was a false report.

SATURDAY *4th.* Early in the Morn got every thing in readiness to Sail. Oreo the Chief and his whole family came to take their last leave, accompanied by Oo oorou the Aree de hi[1] and Boba the Aree de hi of Otaha, none of them came empty handed, but Oo oorou brought a pretty large present as this was his first and only Viset, my present in return was suteable to his title, I say title because I believe he posess'd very little more. I made all the others presents sutable to their rank and the service they had done me after which they took a very affectionate leave, Oreo's last request was for me to return and when he found I would not make him the Promise, he asked the name of my *Marai* (burial place)[2] a strange quiston to ask a Seaman, however I hesitated not one moment to tell him Stepney the Parish in which I lived when in London. I was made to repeated it several times over till they could well pronounce it, then Stepney Marai no Tootee was echoed through a hundred mouths at once. I afterwards found that the same question was put to Mr F. by a Person a Shore but he gave a different and indeed more proper Answer by saying no man who used the Sea could tell were he would

[1] *arii rahi*, 'high chief'; cf. p. 233, n. 1.

[2] It is not very likely that the *marae* as burial place had any particular importance in this question, but rather the *marae* as an essential part of a man's social existence and his relationship to the gods: the question was really, What place are you particularly identified with when you are home? Cook's answer, 'Stepney', was therefore quite apposite; because the parish church in Stepney, whether he was buried in its churchyard or not, would be for him the centre of ordinary religious observance; it would have a seat for him, and an altar, its *ahu*; and when he wished to communicate with his god, it would be there. But, unlike the *marae*, it was not a family belonging.

be buried. It is the Custom here as well as in most other Nations for all the great families to have burial places of their own were their bones are entarr'd, these go with the estate to the next heir, as for instance at Otaheite when Toutaha held the sceptre the Marai at Oparre was Marai no Toutaha, but now they say Marai no Otoo. What greater proof could we have of these people Esteeming and loving us as friends whom they wishd to remember, they had been repeatedly told we should see them no more, they then wanted to know the name of the place were our bodies were to return to dust.

As I could not promise or even Suppose that any more English Ships would be sent out to the isles our Companion Odiddee chose to remain in his Native Country, but he left us with great regret, he was a youth of good parts, of a Gentle and Humane disposision but quite ignorant of all their Traditions and Policy both in Religion and goverment, consequently no material knowlidge could have been got from him had I brought him away with us. Just as he was going out of the Ship he ask'd me to Tattaow some Parou[1] for him in order to Shew to any other Europeans who might touch here, I readily complied with his request by giving him a Certificate of his good behavour, the time and were he had been with us and recommended him to the Notice of those who might come to these isles after me.

It was 11 o'Clock before we could get clear of our friends, when we weigh'd and put to Sea, but Odiddee did not leave us till we were almost out of the Harbour,[2] in order that he might have an oppertunity to fire some of the guns, for being his Majestys Birth Day we gave them the Salute at going away. I believe I should have spent the Day with them had not my stock of Trade been wholy expended, they were continually asking for things which I had not to give them, which to me was exceeding disagreeable and made me very desireous of geting away.

When I first came to these isles I had some thoughts of Viseting the famous Island of Bola bola, but having now got all the necessary repairs of the Ship done and got a plentifull Supply of all manner of

[1] *tatau* some *parau*. The meaning is obvious: mark some speech or words—write him a testimonial, in fact.

[2] 'Our Young friend and companion O-Hedidee staying behind, which he was induced to do in consequence of Captn Cook not being able to promise him that a ship should bring him back again But it was not without the deepest distress that he left us; they promis'd him a Handsom young Wife, as one inducement to stay: He was a sensible, well disposed young Man, and had learn't, all our different distinctions in the Ship—Many words &c and been very happy with us, for 7 Months.'—Elliott *Mem.*, ff. 28v–29. Hitihiti had made his own impression: 'At 10 Weigh'd & sail'd out of the harbour, at which time our friend O Diddy left us, universally belov'd by us all.'—Cooper.

refreshments I thought it would be answering no end going there and therefore laid it a side and directed my Course to the West and took our final leave of these happy isles and the good People in them.

*THURSDAY *2nd.* In the after-noon got intillengence that three days before two Ships had arrived at Huaheine. The same report said the one was commanded by Mr Banks and the other by Captain Furneaux, the man who brought the account, said he was made drunk on board the one of them and described the persons of Mr Banks and Captain Furneaux so will that I had not the least doubt of the truth and began to consider about sending a boat over that very evening with orders to Captain Furneaux when a man, a friend of Mr F., happened to come aboard and denied the whole, sa[y]ing it was wāwarre,[1] a lie, the man who brought the information was now gone, so that I could not confront them, and there were none else present who knew any thing about it but by report so that I laid a side sending over a boat till I had better inf[o]rmation. This Evening we entertained the people with fire works on one of the little isles near the entrance of the harbour.

FRIDAY *3rd.* I had fixed on this day for sailing, but the intillegence received last night put a stop to it. The chief had promised to bring the Man on board who first brought the account, but he was either not to be found or would not be found, in the morning the people were divided in their opinions, but in the after-noon all said it was a false report. I had sent Mr Clerke in the Morning to the farther part of the island to make enquir[i]es there, he returned without learning any thing satisfactory: in short whether the report proves true or false it appeared now too ill founded to authorize me to send a boat over or to wait any longer here and therefore on

SATURDAY *4th* early in the Morning got every thing in readiness to sail; Oreo the Chief and his whole family came on board to take their last fare well, accompanied by O ooroo the Aree de hi and Boba the Aree of Otaha and several of their friends. None of them came empty, but Oo ooroo brought a pretty large present, this being his first and only Visit. I distributed amongst them almost every thing I had left, the very hospitable manner I had ever been received by these people, had indeared them to me and given them a just title to every thing in my power to grant. I questioned them again about the Ships at Huaheine and they all to a man deni'd that any was there.

[1] *ha'avare.*

During the time these people remained on board they were continually importuning me to return. The Chief, his Wife and Daughter but especially the two latter, hardly ever seaced weeping, I will not pretend to say whether it was real or feigned greif they shewed on this occasion, perhaps it was a mixture of both, but was I to abide by my own opinion only I should believe it was real. At last when we were about to weigh, they took a most affectionate leave. . . .

As I could not promise or even suppose that more English Ships would be sent to these isles, our faithfull Companion Odiddy choose to remain in his Native Country; but he left us with great regret and nothing but the fear of never returning would have torn him from us.[1] When the Chief Teased me so much about returning, I sometimes gave such Answers as left them some hopes, Odiddy would instantly catch at it, take me on one side and ask me over again. In short I have not words to describe the anguish which appeared in this young mans breast when he went away, he looked up at the ship, burst into Tears and then sunk down into the Canoe. The Maxim that a Prophet has no honour in [h]is own Country was never more fully verified than in this youth. At Otaheite he might have had any thing that was in their power to bestow, whereas here he was not the least noticed. He was a youth of good parts, and like most of his countrymen, of a Docile, Gentle and humane disposition, but in a manner wholy ignorant of their Religion, Goverment, Manners, Customs and Traditions, consequently no material knowlidge could have been gathered from him, had I brought him away: Indeed he would have been [a] better Specimen of the Nation in every respect than the one on board the Adventure[2]. . . .

When I first came to these islands I had some thoughts of visiting the famous Island of Bolabola, but as I had now got on board a plentifull supply of all manner of refreshments, and the rout I had in view Allowing me no time to spare, I laid it a side and directed my Course to the West and took our final leave of these happy isles on which Benevolent Nature, with a bountifull and lavishing hand hath bestowed every blessing man can wish. The Natives, possess'd of the same Benevolent disposition, contribute willingly, cheerfully and

[1] and nothing . . . us *substituted for* the least prospect in the world of his returning would have fixed him with us.—f. 224.

[2] *Indeed . . . Adventure:* G Indeed he would have been a good specimen of the Nation in every respect which the man on board the Adventure is not, he is dark, ugly and a downright blackguard.—The last eight words were apparently included in B, but are there heavily deleted. Cook did not mean that poor Omai was a member of the criminal class, but that his social position was low. Johnson defines 'blackguard' as 'A cant word amongst the vulgar; by which is implied a dirty fellow, of the meanest kind'. Possibly, therefore, Cook was surprised later on by the tremendous success Omai had in England, in circles far removed from those of the blackguard.

with a full hand to the wants of the Navigator. During the Six Weeks we have been at these isles we have had fresh Pork and all the fruits that were in Season in the utmost Profusion, besides fish at Otaheite and Fowls at the other isles; all these arti[c]les we got in exchange for Axes, Hatchets, Nails, Chisels, Cloth, Red feathers, Beads, Knives, Sisers, looking glasses &c[a]; articles which will ever be valuable here. I ought not to have omitted Shirts as very necessary articles in making presents, especially with such who have any connections with the fair sex a shirt here is full as necessary as a piece of gold in England. The Ladies of Otaheite after they had pretty well cleared their lovers of shirts found a method of cloathing them selves with their own cloth. It was their custom to go on shore every morning and to return on board in the evening generally clad in rags which admitted of an excuse to importune the lover for better Clothes and when he had no more of his own, he was to clothe them with new Cloth of the Country which they allways left ashore and appeared again in rags and must again be cloathed so that the same suit might pass through twenty different hands, and be as often, sold, bought and given away.

Before I quit these isles it is necessary to mention all I know concerning the goverment of Ulietea and Otaha.[1] Oreo, so often mentioned is a Native of Bola bola, but is possessed of Whenooa's or Lands at Ulietea, which I suppose he as well as many of his Country got at the conquest. He resides here as Opoonies Lieutenant, and seems to be vested with regal authority and to be the supreme Magistrate in the island, Oo-ooroo who is the Aree by hereditary right seems to have little more left him than the bare title and his own Whenooa or district in which I think he is sovereign. I have always seen Oreo pay him the respect due to his rank and was pleased when he saw me distinguish him from others. Otaha, so far as I can find is upon the very same footing, Boba and Ota are the two Chiefs, the latter I have not seen; Boba is a Stout well made young man and we are told is, after Opoone's death, to Marry his Daughter, by which Mariage he will become Vested with the same regal authority as Opoony has now, by which it should seem that tho a Woman may be vested with regal dignity she cannot have regal power.[2] I cannot find that Opoony has got any thing to himself by the conquest of these isles any farther than providing for his Nobles who have siezed on best part of the lands; he seems to have no demand

[1] Tahaa, the island to the north of Raiatea, within the same reef.

[2] It was really the other way round: the exercise of 'regal power' was a matter of force of personality—e.g. as with Purea. But what Cook means precisely by 'vested with regal dignity' I do not know.

on them for any of the many articles they have had from us. Odiddy has several times enumerated to me all the Axes, Nails &c[a] Opoony is possessed of which hardly amounts to so many as he had from me when I saw him in 1769. Old as this famous man is he seems not to spend his last days in indolence, when we first arrived here he was at Mauraua,[1] soon after he returned to Bolabola and we are now told he is gone to Tubi.[2]

I shall conclude this account of these Islands with some observations on the Watch which M[r] Wales hath communicated to me. At our arrival in Matavai Bay in Otaheite, the Longitude pointed out by the Watch was 2°8′38½″ too far to the West, that is she had lost sence our leaving Queen Charlottes Sound, of her then rate of going 8′34½″; this was in about five Months or some thing more, during which time she had passed through the extremes of both Cold and heat. It was judged that half this Error arose after we left Easter Island by which it appeared that she went better in the Cold than in the hot climates.*—ff. 223v–5v.

SUNDAY 5*th. Winds East. Course S* 67°30′ *W. Dist. Sailed* 69 *Miles. Lat. in South* 16°48′. *Long. made from Ulietea West* 1°12′. Gentle breezes and fine Weather. I have before taken notice of after leaving Ulietea I directed my Course to the West: this was with a View of carrying into execution the resolution I had taken of viseting Quiros's discoveries. At 5 o'Clock in the PM the boddy of Mauroua bore NWBW Bola-bola NE and Ulietea East distant 8 Leagues.[3] At 6 brought to for the night, at day break made Sail. After Sunrise found the Variation 7°7′ East, A Swell from the South.

MONDAY 6*th. Winds East to NE. Course West, Southerly. Dist. Sailed* 79 *Miles. Lat. in South* 16°50′. *Longd. in West* 154°13′. *Long. made from Ulietea* 2°34′. Gentle Gales and Cloudy weather. In the evening shortned Sail and brought to for the night, at the approach of day made Sail. At 11 AM Saw How[e] Island discovered by Captain Wallis which at Noon extended from west to NW distant one League, it is one of those low reef isle's of about [4] Leagues in circuit, the Most land lies on the NE part, the reef extends a good way to the SW and West and hath upon it some little islots. I think Captain Wallis found on the NW side a Channell in within the reef, but whether of a depth sufficient for Shiping or no I know not. The Inhabitants of Ulietea speak of an

[1] Maurua, now called Maupiti; it is a small mountainous island lying about 24 miles west of Borabora.

[2] Tupai or Motu Iti; an atoll about 7 miles NNW of Borabora.

[3] 'The Captain releas'd John Marra Gunners Mate out of Confinement & ordered him to his Duty again.'—Cooper.

uninhabited Isle which they call Mopeha lying to the west[1] to which they go at certain Seasons for Turtle, perhaps this may be the Very Same.[2] Captain Wallis saw upon it Smoaks, signs of inhabitants or people we saw none. Lat 16°48′, Longitude 154°18′ West.[3]

TUESDAY *7th. Winds NE to North. Course S* 74° *West. Dist. Sailed* 81 *Miles. Lat. in South* 17°12′. *Longd. in West* 155°34′. *Long. made from Ulietea West* 3°53′. PM Frish breezes and Cloudy, AM Squally unsettled wea[r] attended with heavy Showers of rain. Lay-to as usual during the night. Swell from the South.

WEDNESDAY *8th. Winds Varble. Course S* 55° *W. Dist. Sailed* 35 *Miles Lat. in South* 17°32′. *Longd. in West* 156°1′. *Long. made from Ulietea West* 4°22′. Most part Variable unsittled weather with heavy Showers of rain. Towards Noon the wind fix'd at NE and the Weather became fair. A very great swell from SSW indicates no land in that direction.

THURSDAY *9th. Winds NE. Course S* 68° *W. Dist. Sailed* 44 *Miles. Long. in West Reck.g.* 156°43′. *Long. in Ulietea* 5°4′. *Lat. in South* 17°48′. Light breezes and Cloudy weather. Swell as yesterday. Men of War and Tropick Birds Daily seen.

FRIDAY *10th. Winds Varible. Course West. Dist. Sailed* 44 *Miles. Long. in West Reck.g.* 157°27′. *Long. in Ulietea* 5°48′. *Lat. in South* 17°48′. *Variation* 8°7′, 8°40′. PM Same Weather, remainder very variable unsettled Weather with rain and a great erregular swell, Mostly from the South.

SATURDAY *11th. Winds East & SE. Course West Northerly. Dist. Sailed* 42 *Miles. Long. in West Reck.g.* 158°9′. *Long. in Ulietea* 6°30′. *Lat. in South* 17°46′. Some times gentle breezes, other times Calm with Showers of rain. Southerly swell still continues.

SUNDAY *12th. Winds SE. Course S* 72°30′ *W. Dist. Sailed* 81 *Miles. Long. in West Reck.g.* 159°29′. *Long. in Ulietea* 7°50′. *Lat. in South* 18°10′. Squally rainy unsettled weather till towards Noon when it became fair. Spent the night Plying under our Top-sails.

MONDAY *13th. Winds SE to East. Course S* 73° *W. Dist. Sailed* 120 *Miles. Long. in West Reck.g.* 161°29′. *Long. in Ulietea* 9°50′. *Lat. in South* 18°45′. Fresh Trade and Cloudy weather. Saw some Men of War Birds.

[1] *lying ... west:* about this situation ...—f. 226.

[2] It was. The atoll Mopihaa or Mopélia lies about 100 miles WSW of Maupiti; Wallis called it Lord Howe Island.

[3] ... From this day to Thursday 16th we met with nothing remarkable.... We general[ly] brought to or stood upon a wind during night and in the day made all the sail we could.

TUESDAY 14*th. Winds Easterly, SW. Course N* 82° *W. Dist.* 74 *Miles. Long. in West Reck.g.* 162°45′. *Long. in Ulietea* 11°6′. *Lat. in South* 18°35′. First part fresh gales, remainder little wind. Reeved Several new ropes, the old decay'd.

WEDNESDAY 15*th. Winds SW, Calm, SW quarter. Course NW. Dist. Sailed* 12 *Miles Long. in West Reck.g.* 162°53′. *Long. in Ulietea* 11°14′. *Lat. in South* 18°27′. PM Calm, remainder light Airs, Saw several Men of War and Tropic Birds.[1]

THURSDAY 16*th. Winds South & SBE. Course N* 50° *W. Dist. Sailed* 25 *Miles. Longde. in West Reck.g.* 163°13′. *Longitude in Ulietea* 11°34′. *Lat. in South* 18°11′. Light breezes and clear weather. At 7 AM saw land from the Mast head bearing NNE, bore down to it.[2] At Noon saw it was a low reef Island or rather a number of small Islots connected together by sand banks & breakers,[3] the extremes bore from NNE to NEBE distant from the Shore six or eight Miles.

FRIDAY 17*th. Winds Southerly. Courses N* 84° *W. Dist. Sailed* 72 *Miles. Longde. in West Reck.g.* 164°28′. *Longitude in Ulietea* 12°49′. *Lat. in South* 18°3′. Gentle breeze and pleasent weather. PM ranged the West and NW sides, so near the Shore that at one time we saw the rocks under us.[4] We saw no inhabitants or signs of any except Birds of which there were a good many and of different sorts and the Coast seem'd to abound with fish. After runing down from its Southern to its Northern extremity which is 2 Leagues without finding anchorage or a Convenient landing place we at 4 o'Clock resumed our Course to the westward. This Isle which I named Palmerston is situated in Lat 18°4′ s, Longitude 163°10′ West, it is composed of six small Islots connected together by Sand banks and breakers and incloseth a Lake which seemed to have a good depth, but we saw no Channell into it. The little Islots were covered with Wood.[5]

[1] 'Served Bread: All our Bread-Fruit & Plantains bring done; a circumstance which would be regretted at any time, much more so now, as the bread is grown very bad.'—Wales.

[2] 'Early in the Morning many Men of War Birds about the Ship, a great Number of Fish of various kinds, Dolphins, Bonetas, Albecores &c &c—none of which however cou'd we get hold of excepting 2 confounded hungry Sharks—the fish & Birds became exceeding numerous as we drew in with the Land.'—Clerke 8952.

[3] . . . inclosing a Lake into which we could see no entrance.

[4] 'Contrary to most of those [islands] we have seen before, the Water seemed very shallow within the reef, and a long Shoal runs off from its S° West Point which we crossed in very shallow Water, and the Ship raised several hundreds of small Sharks, which lay at ye Bottom.'—Wales.

[5] . . . The Situation of this Isle is not very distant from that assigned by Mr Dalrymple for La Sagitaria discovered by Quiros, but by the discription the discoverer has given of it, it cannot be the same, [*deleted* besides I am not satisfied that Quiros took the rout Mr Dalrymple has traced out on his chart.] For this reason I looked upon it to be a new dis-

SATURDAY 18*th*. *Winds SE. Course W¾S. Dist. Sailed* 77 *Miles. Lat. in South* 18°14′. *Longde. in West Reck.g.* 165°58′. *Longde. made Ulietea* 14°19′. Gentle breezes and Clowdy Weather.

SUNDAY 19*th*. *Winds Easterly. Course W¾S. Dist. Sailed* 80 *Miles. Lat. in South* 18°25′. *Longde. in West Reck.g.* 167°11′. *Longde. made Ulietea* 15°32′. *Varn.* 10°36′, 10°9′. Gentle breezes and Clear pleasent weather. Nothing seen remarkable.

MONDAY 20*th*. *Winds East. Course S* 75°30′ *W. Dist. Sailed* 99 *Miles. Lat. in South* 18°50′. *Longde. in West Reck.g.* 168°52′. *Longde. made Ulietea* 17°13′. D° gales which freshned towards Noon at which time thought we Saw Land to the SSW and accordingly hauled up for it.

TUESDAY 21*st*. *Winds East to NE. Course S* 81° *W. Dist. Sailed* 47 *Miles. Lat. in South* 19°23′. *Longde. in West Reck.g.* 170°20′. *Longde. made Ulietea* 18°41′. Gentle breezes and fair Weather. At 2 PM found what we took for land was only Clouds, reassumed our WBS Course, and an hour after saw land from the Mast head in the same direction, as we drew near found it to be an Island the body of which at 5 bore due West distant five Leagues, Shortned Sail and spent the night Plying under Top-sails. At Day break bore up for the Nother point of the Isle and ran along the West Shore at the distance of one Mile from it. A little before Noon preceiveing Some People runing along the Shore and Seeing landing was Practical, Brought-to, hoisted out and Man'd two Boats in one of which I went my self and Mr Pickersgill in the other. Mr F. and his party and Mr H. accompanied us.

WEDNESDAY 22*nd*. As we came near the Shore some People who were on the rocks retired to the woods, as we supposed to meet us and we afterwards found our conjectures right. We landed with ease and took Post on a high rock to prevent a Surprise as the whole Coast was all over run with woods, Shrubery &ca and began to Collect plants &ca under the protection of the Party under Arms, but the approach of the Indians soon made it necessary for us to join which was no sooner done than they appeared in the Skirts of the woods not a Stones throw from us, one of two men who were ad-

covery and named it Palmerston Island, in honour of my Lord Palmerston one of the Lords of the Admiralty.—f. 226.—La Sagitaria was probably Makatea, lat. 15°50′ s, long. 148°14′ w; Palmerston is lat. 18°02′ s, long. 163°12′ w. The two are about 870 miles apart. —Henry Temple, 2nd Viscount Palmerston (1739–1802), a Lord of the Admiralty 1766–77, and of the Treasury 1777–82; his distinction was in social life rather than in politics. He was a member of the Literary Club, and was a pall-bearer at the funerals of both Garrick and Reynolds. For his island, see Chart XXXIV*a* and Fig. 44, p. 240 above.

vanced before the rest threw a Stone which Struck Mr Sparman on the Arm, upon this two Musquets were fired without order[1] which made them all retire under cover of the woods and we saw them no more. Seeing nothing was to be done here we imbarqued and proceeded down a long shore, in hopes of meeting with better Success in a nother place. We proceeded several miles down the Coast without seeing any human being or convenient landing place, at length coming before a small Beach on which lay four Canoes, here we landed by means of a small creek in the rocks, just to take a View of

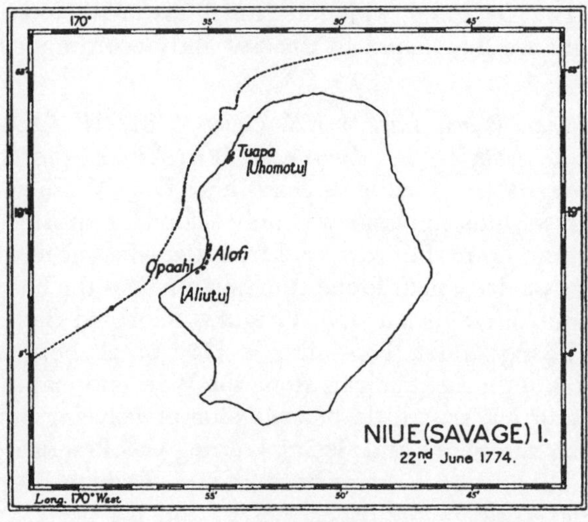

FIG. 63

the Boats and to leave in them some trifles to induce the Natives to believe we intended them no harm. I left a party on the rocks under Arms to keep a good lookout while some of us went to the Canoes where we were but a few minutes before the Indians rushed out of the woods upon us, it was to no effect our endeavouring to bring them to a parly, one of them with the ferocity of a wild Boar advanced a head of the others and threw a dart at us, two or three Musquets discharged in the air did not hinder him from advanceing still farther and throwing a nother, at this instant the party on the rocks

[1] 'One of them threw a large lump of coral at me with his left hand, and hit my left forearm. Lieutenant Pickersgill, who was standing immediately behind me, and came near to receiving this stone on his forehead, carried no musket, and therefore insisted that I should shoot, which I did. Although the small-shot only whistled about the ears of our spiteful enemies (a few may have pierced the skin) it frightened them away. The Captain, however, perhaps with justification, was displeased at this shooting, for he believed that, with more patience, some reconciliation could have been reached.'—Sparrman, p. 129.

began to fire at others who appeared on the hieghts over us, this abated the Ardour of the party we were engaged with and gave us time to retire and then I caused the fireing to cease, the last discharge sent them into the woods from whence they did nor return, we had reason to beleive none were hurt. Seeing no good was to be got of these people or at the isle we return'd on board hoisted in the Boats and made sail to wsw.[1] The Conduct and aspect of these Islanders occasioned my giving it the Name of *Savage Island*,[2] it lies in the Latitude of 19°1′, Longitud 169°37′ West, is about 11 Leagues in circuit, of a tolerable hieght and seemingly covered with wood amongest which were some Cocoa-nutt trees. These Islanders were Naked except their Natural parts, some were painted black. The Canoes were like those of Amsterdam and full as neatly made.

*As we drew near the shore, some people who were on the rocks retired to the Woods, as we supposed to meet us and we afterwards found our conjectures right. We landed with ease in a small creek[3] and took post on a high rock to prevent a Surprise: Here we desplayed our Colours and Mr F. and his party began to Collect Plants &ca; the Coast was so over run with woods, shruberry, Plants, Stones &ca that we could not see forty yards round us. I took two men and with them entered a kind of Chasm which opened a way into the woods; we had not gone far before we heard the Indians approaching upon which I called to Mr F. to retire to the party which I did likewise: we had no sooner joined than the Natives appeared at the entrance of the Chasm not a stones throw from us. We began to speak and make all the friendly signs we could think of to them, which they answered by menaces and one of two men who were

[1] 'return'd on board and Quited this Inhospital and Savage Isle. . . .'—Log. Wales had too much to do on board to go ashore, to his regret, but he makes a comment or two. 'We now learn that they had been attacked twice by the Natives. The first time they landed they took possession of the Island in form, errecting the English Colours as is usual on these Occasions; but whether the Natives took Umbrage at this or not is uncertain; certain it is they attacked them in the very Act & pelted them with stones, and w[h]ether Our people drove away the Natives or the Natives them is a little doubtful. . . . This is the substance of what I had from Mr Hodges whose inteligence I have made use of before when I was not present my self & dare say it is pretty Just.'

[2] It was Niue. Chart XXXIV*b*, Figs. 63, 64.

[3] The Niuean landing-places are not altogether easy to identify, even on the spot, and none of them is good, even though Cook says he landed here 'with ease'. The high upraised coral cliffs are broken only by narrow precipitous gulleys, at the bottom of which are masses of rock and a few minute changing bits of sand (they can hardly be called beach) bare at low tide. An occasional canoe is perched among the rocks. Native tradition about Cook is quite unreliable, because it has confused his landings with those of missionaries and other later-comers, and fantastically embroidered as well. This first landing seems to have been at a place called Tuapa; near by was the chief village of the island, Uhomotu, the residence of the kings of Niue, so that anybody who had known that Cook was on the point of ceremonially annexing the island in the name of his own monarch could have been duly affronted.

advanced before the rist, threw a stone which struck Mr Sparman on the arm; upon this two muskets were fired, without orders, which made them all retire under cover of the Woods, and we saw them no more. After waiting some little time[1] and till we were satisfied nothing was to be done here, the Country being so over run with Shrubery that it was hardly possible to come to parly with [the] Natives, we imbarqued and proceeded down a long shore in hopes of meeting with better success in a nother place. After rangeing the Coast for some miles, without seeing a living soul, or any convenient landing place we at length came before a small beach on which lay four Canoes;[2] here we land[ed] by means of a little Creek formed by the flat rocks before it, with a View of just looking at the Canoes and to leave some Medals, Nails &ca in them, for not a soul was to be seen. The situation of this place was to us worse than the former; a flat rock lay next the Sea, behind it a narrow stone beach, this was bounded by a perpindicular rocky cleft of unequal height whose top was covered with Shrubery, two deep and narrow chasms in the cleft seem'd to open a Communication into the Country, in or before one of these laid the four Canoes which we were going to look at, but in the doing of this I saw we should be exposed to be attacked by the Natives, if there were any, without our being able to defend our selves. To prevent this as much as could be and to secure a retreat in case of an Attack, I orderd the Men to be drawn up on the rock from whence they had a view of the hieghts and only my self and four of the gentlemen[3] went up to the boats, where we had been but a very few Minutes before the Natives, I cannot say how many, rushed down the Chasm out of the wood upon us; the endeavours we made to bring them to a parly was to no purpose, they came with the ferocity of wild Boars and threw thier darts, two or three Muskets discharged in the air did not hinder one of them from advancing still farther and throwing a nother dart or rather a Spear which pass'd close over my Shoulder;[4] his Courage would have cost

[1] During which they performed 'the idle ceremony of taking possession'.—Forster, II, p. 165.

[2] This was most likely Opaahi, a little south-west of what may be regarded as the present island 'capital', Alofi. But we must allow for certain changes in the appearance of these spots in the course of almost two centuries. There was a large village a mile or so inland called Aliutu, now disappeared; so that Cook had perforce picked on another centre of potentially hostile population for his activities.

[3] The Forsters, Sparrman and Hodges. Hodges proceeded to make a drawing of the canoes, till interrupted.

[4] '... one of the Natives rushing suddenly upon him with a Spear, and Cooks piece Missing fire, the Man threw his Spear which pas'd close over Cooks shoulder; and at this moment young Mr Forster made his appearance, and fir'd, wounding the Man, who now retir'd, and join'd his friends with whom they had some skirmishing before; but had it not been for this providentail circumstance, Cooks life would have been in most eminent

him his life had not my musket missed fire, for I was not five paces from him when he threw his spear and had resolved to shoot him to save my self, but I was glad afterwards that it happened otherwise. At this instant the party on the rock began to fire at others who appeared on the heights,[1] this abated the ardour of the party we were engaged with and gave us time to join our people when I caused the fireing to cease, the last discharge sent all the Indians to the woods from whence they did not return so long as we remained, we did not know that any were hurt. It was remarkable that when I joined our party I tried my musket in the air and it went off as well as a peice could do. Seeing no good was to be got of these people or at the isle, as having no Port, we imbarqued and returned on board, hoisted in the boats and made sail to wsw. I had forgot to mention in its proper order, that we put a shore, a little before we came to this last place, where three or four of us went upon the clifts,[2] where we found the Country as before, nothing but Coral rocks all overrun with Shrubery so that it was hardly possible to penetrate into it and we embarked again with intent to return directly aboard, till we saw the Canoes above mentiond, being directed to the place by the opinion of some of us who thought they heard people.

The Conduct and aspect of these Islanders occasioned my nameing it *Savage Island*,[3] it is situated in the Latitude 19°1′ s, Longitude

danger.'—Elliott *Mem.*, f. 29v. This is too dramatic. George Forster was there all the time, and was nearly hit by another spear, which 'slid along my thigh, marking my clothes with the black colour with which it was daubed'. According to Forster, all the party tried to fire, but their muskets missed fire till at last his, loaded with small shot, went off. Hodges then fired with ball, but hit no one.

[1] They were 'coming down by a different path to cut us off', says Forster.

[2] This could only have been at Alofi, about the middle of the west coast of the island. Between Tuapa and Alofi the coast consists of nothing but sheer cliffs; there is one possible landing place, but only through a long cave in the cliffs. This may have been one of the 'curious Caverns' which Cook remarks on later; but its nature he could not have guessed.

[3] The modern Niueans, cheerful industrious people, give a rather pained consideration to the name which Cook bestowed upon their island, and explain the whole matter as one of mistaken intentions. Nothing was farther from the minds of their forebears, they argue, than to attack the visitors; the man who advanced 'with the ferocity of a wild Boar' and threw a dart, and those who did likewise later, were displaying friendship and not enmity—they were merely going through the ritual of the 'challenge', an essential though alarming part of any ceremony of welcome. (The Maoris of New Zealand have a similar ceremony; but it pales into insignificance before the fury and vehemence of the Niuean version.) In addition to this, the challengers had adorned their lips with a scarlet dye, the juice of the *hulahula* banana, and Cook flew to the conclusion that they were cannibals, dripping with the blood of their victims. This tradition, one feels, is rather too obviously made-up. The last part of it is of course a bit of native mythology, 'rationalization', to make the story more persuasive; nor does it explain the first stone-throwing which so alarmed Sparrman and Pickersgill. The daubing black and the feathers of some of the men, on the other hand, might seem to give it some colour; but these were also the panoply of war. Assuming that the Niueans were as savage as Cook thought, they were

169°37′ West. It is about 11 Leagues in Circuit of a round form and good height and hath deep water close to its shores. All the Sea Coast and as far in land as we could see is wholy covered with Trees Shrubery &c[a] amongst which were some few Cocoanut trees, but what the interior parts may produce we know not. To judge of the whole Garment by the skirts it cannot produce much, for so much as we saw of it consisted wholy of Coral rocks all overrun with trees Shrubs &c[a], not a bit of soil was to be seen, the rocks alone supplied the trees with humidity.[1] If these Coral rocks were first formed in the Sea by animals, how came they thrown up, to such a height? has this Island be[en] raised by an Earth quake or has the Sea receeded from it? Some Philosophers have attempted to account for the formation of low isles such as are in this Sea, but I do not know if any thing has been said of high Islands or such as I have been speaking of. In this island not only the loose rocks which cover the Surface but the Clifts which bound the Shore are of Coral stone, which the continual beating of the Sea has in many places formed into a Variety of curious Caverns, some of them very large; the roof or rock over them supported by Pillars which the foaming waves hath formed into a variety of shapes and made more curious than the Cavern it self. In one we saw light was admited through a hole at the top; in a nother place we observed that the whole Roof of one of these Caverns had sunk in and formed a kind of Valley which laid considerably below the circumjacent Rocks.

I can say but little of the Inhabitants which, I believe, are not numerous, they seemed to be stout well made men and were naked except their Natural parts: some of them had their faces, breast and thig[h]s pai[n]ted black. The Canoes were precisely like those of Amsterdam with the addition of a little rising like a gunnel on each side the open part, and had some carving about them which shewed that these people are full as ingenious. Both these islanders and thier Canoes agree very well with the discription M. Bougainvill has

not the only Pacific islanders who looked on newcomers with a jaundiced eye—as other seafarers' journals witness. Cook had had some experience of stone-throwing and spears himself, though not at quite such close quarters. It may be noticed that on this occasion not even Forster embarks on a denunciation of the brutality and inhumanity of 'civilized' men—perhaps because he nearly received a spear himself. His account, II, pp. 163–7, is detailed and interesting. I am indebted to Mr J. M. McEwen, lately Resident Commissioner of Niue, for the story told in the island, as given here. A longer version, with much freely contributed circumstantial detail, is printed in Edwin M. Loeb, *History and Traditions of Niue* (B. P. Bishop Mus. Bull. 32, Honolulu 1926), p. 30. Certainly none of the islanders was hurt.

[1] This is in fact a very accurate description of the appearance of a great deal of the interior—'the whole Garment'—which surprises the modern visitor as much as it did Cook at the skirts. There is no lack of vegetation, and vegetation of large size, growing from what the soil surveyor calls repeatedly 'rocky', 'complex rocky', or 'very rocky loam'.

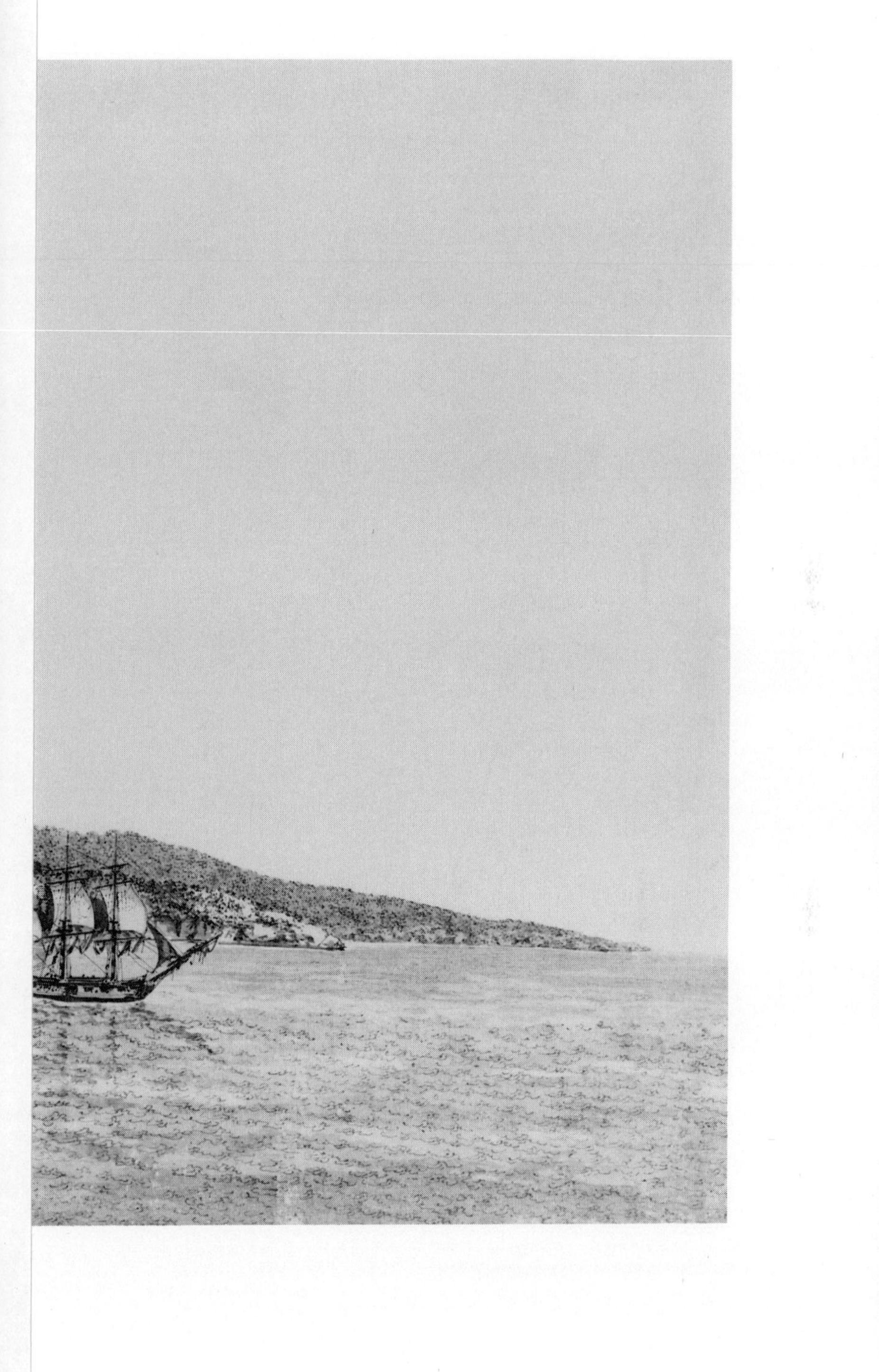

give[n] of those he saw off the isles of Navigators which lie nearly under the same Meridian.*—ff. 226v–8.

THURSDAY 23*rd. Winds ESE & E. Course WSW. Dist. Sailed* 89 *Miles. Lat. in South* 19°49′. *Longde in West Reck.g* 171°50′. *Longde. Ulietea* 20°11′. *Vari.* 10°48′ *E.* Gentle breezes and pleasent Weather.[1]

FRIDAY 24*th. Winds ESE to ENE. Course S* 71°30′ *W. Dist. Sailed* 107 *Miles. Lat. in South* 20°24′. *Longde. in West Reck.g* 173°52′. *Longde. Ulietea* 22°13′. *Vari.* 11°45′. D° Weather. Nothing remarkable.

SATURDAY 25*th. Winds ENE, Calm, Northerly.* Little Clowdy and Hazey at times. In the Evening judgeing our Selves not far from Roterdam shortned Sail and spent the night under our Top-sails. At 6 AM bore away West, at Day light Saw land (Islands) extending from SSW to NNW; the Wind being at NE hauled to the NW with a view of discovering more distinctly the isles in that Quarter but presently after a reef of rocks were seen lying a thwart our Course extending on each Bow farther than we could see, it therefore became necessary to Tack and bear up to the South in search of a Passage that way. At Noon the most Southermost Isle bore SW distant about 4 Miles, near and to the North of this isle were 3 others and Several more to the west: the first four were joined to one a nother by a reef of rocks, we were not certain if this Reef did not join to the one Seen in the Morning as we saw breakers in the intermidiate space.[2]

SUNDAY 26*th. Winds NE, Southerly.* At 3 PM seeing more breakers ahead[3] and having but little wind and a great Easterly Swell, hauled off SE. In the evening the Southern isle bore WNW distant 5 miles and the Breakers last seen SSW½W; here we spent the night for it presently after fell Calm[4] and continued so till 4 AM when we got breeze

[1] 'Caulkers Emp^d Caulking the Main Deck and inside work of the great Cabbin.'—Log.

[2] Cook was coming in towards Tonga from the east, as in 1773, but about a degree of latitude farther north than then. The islands he saw at dawn were those of the Haapai, Kotu and Nomuka groups. The reef that made it necessary to change course was that east of the Kotu group. The 'most Southermost Isle' seen at noon was Telekitonga, the southernmost of four, fifty to seventy feet high, and wooded, that lie north and south on the same sunken reef—the 'Otu Tolu group, or rather a sub-group of the Nomuka group, some others of which Cook could see behind them; though he adds in B f. 228v, 'but Roterdam [Nomuka] was not yet in sight (Lat. 20°23′, Longitude 174°6′ W)'. Between the 'Otu Tolu reef and the one further north, off which he had sheered in the morning, was a deep passage about two miles wide; but looking in that direction from his noon position he would certainly see monitory breakers, even though they were not 'in the intermidiate space'. See Fig. 45, p. 244 above.

[3] There is an irregular narrow shoal stretching to the south from Telekitonga, in one part of which the sea breaks heavily.

[4] . . . and left us to the Mercy of a great Easterly swell which however happened to have no great effect upon the Ship . . . f. 228v.

at South. At Day-light preceiving a likelyhood of a clear Passage between the Isle and the Breakers we stretched to the West and soon after saw more isles a head and on each Bow,[1] but the Passage seem'd open; at length we found soundings in 45 & 40 fathom a clear bottom, this circumstance greatly lessned the danger sence we now had it in our power to Anchor.[2] Towards Noon some people came off in Canoes from one of the isles[3] bring[ing] with them some Cocoa nutts and Shaddocks which they exchanged for Nails, they shewed us Annamocka or Rotterdam[4] which at Noon bore distant Miles, they like wise gave us the names of some of the other Isles and wanted us much to go to theirs.[5] The breeze freshning we soon left them a Stern.

MONDAY 27*th.* Gentle breezes and pleasent Weather. In the PM meeting with nothing to obstruct us, at 5 o'Clock Anchored on the North side of Annamocka about ¾ of a mile from the Shore in 20 fathom water, the bottom Coral Sand, the extremes of the isle extending from S 88° E to SW and a Cove with a Sandy beach S 50° East. As soon as we approached the South end of the isle Several of the Natives came off in their Canoes[6] one of which asked for me by name, a proof that these people have a communication with Amsterdam; as soon as we had Anchored they came a long side with yams and Shaddocks which they exchanged for Small Nails and old rags.[7]

Early in the Morn the Master and I went a Shore to look for fresh

[1] *a head . . . Bow:* both to the SW and NW

[2] *Anchor:* Anchor in case of a Calm or to spend the night if we found no passage.

[3] . . . there were two or three people in each who came boldly a long side

[4] . . . such are the advantages in knowing the proper names to isles. . . . f. 228v. Cook had picked up the name Annamocka (Nomuka) from Tasman, and possibly heard it also when on his previous visit. It was called Rotterdam by Tasman, who was anchored there from 25 January to 1 February 1643, and noted the Tongan name on his chart.

[5] . . . which they called *Comango.* [Mango, 5 miles south-eastward of Nomuka.]

[6] *Several . . . Canoes:* we were met by a number of canoes, laden with fruit and roots, but as I did not shorten sail we had but little traffick with them:—f. 228v.

[7] *as soon . . . rags:* These people importuned us much to go towards their Coast, leting us know, as well as we could understand them, that we might anchor there: this was on the SW side of the island where the Coast seemed to be sheltered from South and SE winds but as the day was far spent I could not attempt to go in there, as it would have been necessary to have sent first a boat in to examine it. I therefore stood for the North side of the Island. . . . Before we had well got to an Anchor, the Natives came off from all parts in canoes, bring[ing] with them yams & Shaddocks, which they exchanged for Small Nails and old rags. One man took a vast likeing to our lead and line, got hold of it and in spite of all the t[h]reats I could make cut the line with a stone, but a discharge of small Shot made him return it and the others less trickish.—ff. 228v–9. It may be pointed out that there is in this paragraph of the text confusion in Cook's writing, which he cleared up in B. The passage 'As soon as we approached the South end of the isle . . . Amsterdam' should logically precede the sentence which goes before: i.e. he (1) approaches the south end (but does not anchor); (2) goes on to anchor on the north side; (3) after he has anchored the natives come alongside to trade.

water, we were received with great Courtesy by the Natives and conducted[1] to a Pond of Brackish Water, the same I suppose as Tasman Water at.[2] In the mean time those in the Boat had loaded her with fruit and roots which the Natives brought down and exchanged for Nails and Beads and on our return to the Ship found the same Traffick carrying there. After breakfast I went a Shore with two Boats to Traffick with the People and ordered the Launch to follow to take in Water. The Natives assisted us to roll the Casks to and from the Pond which was about ⅓ of a Mile, the expence of their labour was a bead or a small Nail. Fruit and roots[3] were brought down in such plenty that the other two Boats were Laden in a trice, sent of cleared and load a second time by Noon at which time the Launch was Laden also and the Botanizing and Shooting parties all come in except the Surgeon for whom we could not wait as the Water was Ebing fast out of the Cove.

TUESDAY 28*th*. In the PM the Launch could not go for Water as there was no geting into the Cove[4] where we landed before and where we took it off, but without the Cove[5] is a very good landing place at all times of the Tide, here some of the Officers landed after dinner, where they found the Surgeon strip'd of his Gun, he having come to the landing place some time after the boats were gone, got a Canoe to bring him on board but he had no sooner got into her than a fellow snatched hold of the gun and ran of with it, as soon as I heard this I hasten'd ashore for fear our people should take such steps to recover the gun as I might not approve. I took two boats with me and landed at the place above mentioned,[6] the few people

[1] *and conducted:* after I had distributed some presents amongst them I asked for water and was conducted . . .—f. 229.—'The Captain & Master went on shore in search of water & were rec'd by the Natives in a very friendly manner, these Islanders are very courteous yet very light fingerd, tho' in other respects without any ill intention. . . .'—Harvey.

[2] This must have been so, though Tasman says the water was fresh, and his estimates of distance are considerably greater than Cook's. The island has no really fresh water, apart from rain water; but only this pond, another not far from the south coast, and the 'Salt Water Lake' or lagoon to which Cook refers below (pp. 448–9). The pond water seeps in from the sea, as in all Tongan ponds (so that digging for water is useless). There are no people living in the vicinity of Cook's pond now: it is surrounded by the usual island undergrowth, and coconuts, taro, yams, manioc and bananas all gone wild.

[3] . . . especially Shaddocks and yams.

[4] . . . with a boat from between half Ebb to half Flood

[5] . . . near the Southern point

[6] *as soon as . . . mentioned:* [*deleted* he followed him but it was to no purpose. As soon as I was informed of this and heard that the officers had taken some of the Arms out of the boat with them I hastened on Shore least they should take any step to recover the gun I might not approve of.] after which no one would put him on board, but would have striped him as he imagined, had he not presented a Tooth-pick case which they no doubt thought was a little gun. As soon as I heard of this I landed at the place above mentioned . . .—f. 229v.

that were there fled at my approach; here I left the Boats and went in Search of our people whom I found down near the beach in the Cove where we had been in the Morning with a good many of the Natives about them, they had taken no step to recover the gun nor did I think proper to take any because I was displeased with the occasion of its being lost, but in this I was wrong and only added one fault to a nother; my Lenity in this affair[1] and the easy manner they had obtained this gun which they thought secure in their possession incourag'd them to commit acts of greater Violence[2] as will soon appear. When the Natives saw no one Molested them on account of the robery they carried their fruit &c[a] to the Boats, so that by the evening they were pretty well Laden and we all return'd on board.

Early in the AM Lieut[t] Clerke and the Master with 14 or 15 men went in the Launch for Water, I did intend to have followed immidiately in a nother boat, but rather unluckily refered it till after breakfast. The Launch was no sooner landed than some of the Natives gather about her, behaving in so rude a manner that the Officers were in some doubt if they should attempt to fill Water, but as they expected me a Shore they got the Casks out of the Boat and with a great deal of difficulty got them fill'd and into the Boat again, in the doing of which the Lieut[t] had his gun snatched from him and carried off. Several of the people were strip'd of one thing or another and some of the Coopers tools were taken away, Our people only fireing one or two Musquets which did no execution, all the time being unwilling to kill any of them if it could be avoided: I landed just as the Launch was ready to put of when M[r] Clerke made me acquainted with the above circumstance.[3] I quickly came to a resolution to oblige the Natives to make restitution and for that purpose ordered all the Marines to be sent on shore[4] and in the mean time remained with one boat, many of the Natives remained about me and behaved with their usual Courtesy, but I made them so sencible of my intention that M[r] Clerk's Musqet was presently brought me, but they

[1] *because . . . affair:* [*deleted* because I was displeased with the occasion of its being lost,] but in this I was wrong [*deleted* and only added one fault to a nother; my Lenity in this affair] . . .—f. 229v. Cook's deletions here, as well as those specified in the previous note, seem to be designed to protect his officers from any possible blame.

[2] *commit . . . Violence:* proceed in these tricks

[3] *Our people . . . circumstance:* and all this was done as it were by stealth, for they laid hold of nothing by main force. I landed just as the Launch was ready to put off; The Natives who were pretty numerous on the beach, as soon as they saw me, began to fly, so that I suspected something happened; I however prevailed on many to stay and M[r] Clerke came and informed me of all the preceding circumstances.—f. 230.

[4] *to be . . . shore:* to be armed and sent on shore. M[r] F. and his party being gone out into the country I order'd two or 3 Guns to be fired from the Ship in order to alarm him, not knowing how the Natives might act on this occasion . . .—f. 230.

made use of many excuses to devert me from insisting on the other. At length the Marines arrived which gave them some alarm in so much that some fled but I prevailed on the greatest part to stay; the first Step I took was to seize on two Large double Sailing Canoes which were in the Cove, one fellow making some resistance I fired at him with Small Shott which sent him limping off, the Natives now convinced I was in earnest fled to a man but on my calling to them several returned and presently after the other Musqet was brought[1] and that moment I ordered the Canoes to be restored to Shew the Natives it was on that account only they were detained, the other things we had lost being of little or no Value.[2] By this time the Launch was a Shore for a nother load of Water and we were permited to fill the Casks without one Man daring to come near.[3] I ordered her to be hoisted in as soon as she was clear as the water we got was not worth the trouble it gave us. Returning from the Watering place we found some of the Natives collected together near the beach from whom we understood that the Man I had fired at was Matte (dead). I treated the Story as improbable and demanded of one of them, a man who seemed of some concequence, the return of a adze which had been taken from us in the morning and told him to send for it, accordingly two men were dispatched, but I soon found that we had quite misunderstood each other for instead of the Adze the wound'd man was brought on a board and laid down at my feet to appearence dead, but we soon found our mistake[4] and that tho he was wounded both in the hand and thigh neither the one nor the other were dangerous. I however sent[5] for the Surgeon a Shore to dress his wounds, in the Mean time I addressed my self to several people to have the Adze return'd,[6] especially to an elderly woman who had always a great deal to say to me from my first landing, but upon this occasion she gave her Tongue free liberty, not one word in fifty I understood, all I could learn from her Arguments was that it was mean in me to insist on the return of so trifling an article, but when she found I was determined She and 3 or 4 more Women went away and soon after the Adze was brought me, but I saw her no more which I was sorry for as I wanted to make her a present on account of the part she seem'd to take in all our transactions, private as well as publick, for I was no sooner return'd from the Pond the

[1] ... and laid down at my feet

[2] ... I was the more indifferent about them

[3] ... except one Man who had befriended us during the whole affair and seemed to disaprove of the conduct of his countrymen.—f. 230–ov.

[4] *but ... mistake:* I was much moved at the Sight, but I soon saw my mistake ...—f. 230v.

[5] *I however sent:* I therefore desired he might be carried out of the Sun and sent

[6] ... for as I had now nothing else to do, I resolved to have it.

first time I landed than this woman and a man presented to me a young woman and gave me to understand she was at my service. Miss, who probably had received her instructions, I found wanted by way of Handsel,[1] a Shirt or a Nail, neither the one nor the other I had to give without giving her the Shirt on my back which I was not in a humour to do. I soon made them sencible of my Poverty and thought by that means to have come of with flying Colours but I was misstaken, for I was made to understand I might retire with her on credit, this not suteing me niether the old Lady began first to argue with me and when that fail'd she abused me, I understood very little of what she said, but her actions were expressive enough and shew'd that her words were to this effect, Sneering in my face and saying, what sort of a man are you thus to refuse the embraces of so fine a young Woman, for the girl certainly did not [want] beauty[2] which I could however withstand, but the abuse of the old Woman I could not and therefore hastned into the Boat, they then would needs have me take the girl on board with me, but this could not be done as I had come to a Resolution not to suffer a Woman to come on board the Ship on any pretence what ever and had given strict orders to the officers to that purpose for reasons which I shall mention in a nother place.

When the Surgeon arrived he dress'd the mans wounds and let him blood and was of opinion he was in no sort of danger as the shott had done little more than penetrate the Skin. In the operation some poultice was wanting, the Surgeon ask'd for ripe Plantains but they brought Sugar Cane and Chewed it to a poulp and gave him it to apply to the wounds, this being more of a Balsamick than the other shews that these people understand Simples.[3] After the mans wounds were dress'd I gave him a Spike Nail and a Knife which to them was of great value, his Master or at least the man who seem'd to own the Canoe took them, most probably to himself. It was rather unlucky this man did not belong to the Isle, but had lately come in one of the two Sailing Canoes from a nother isle in the Nighbourhood. Matters being once more put in order we all return'd on board to dinner.

*I now was informed of a circumstance which was observed on board: several Canoes being a long side when the great guns were

[1] *by way of Handsel:* as a preliminary article

[2] 'It has always been suppos'd that Cook himself, never had any connection with any of our fair friends; I have often seen them jeer and laugh at him, calling him Old, and good for nothing.'—Elliott *Mem.*, f. 29.

[3] Dr John Martin, who did the writing of Mariner's *Tonga*, devoted an appendix to Tongan medical practice, but it has more about surgery than 'simples'.

fired in the morning they all retired but one man who was bailing the Water out of his canoe which laid a long side directly under the guns, when the first gun was fired he just looked up and then quite unconcerned continued his work, nor had the second gun any other effect upon him, he did not stir till the Water was all out of his Canoe and then paddled leasuerly off. This Man had Several times been observed to take fruit and roots out of other Canoes and sell them to us, if the owners did not willingly part with them he took them by force, by which he obtained the appelation of Custom house officer. One time after he had been collecting tribute he happened to be lying along side of a sailing canoe which was aboard, one of her people seeing him looking a nother way or attentively imployed about something or another, took the oppertunity to lighten the Canoe of part of her burthen and then put off and set their sail, but the man preceiving the trick they had played him, darted after them and soon got on board, beat the man who had taken his things which he not only now brought a way but many more which he took from the people in the Canoe. This man had likewise been seen makeing collections on shore at the trading place. I remember to have seen him there and on account of his gathering tribute, took him to be a man of consequence and was going to make him a present, but some of the people present would not let me, saying he was no Areeke, that is Chief. He had his hair allways powdered with some kind of white powder.[1]

Both Mr Cooper and my self being on shore at Noon, Mr Wales could not wind up the Watch at the usual time and as we did not come on board till late in the after noon it was forgot till it was down. This circumstance was of no consequence as Mr Wales had had several al[t]itudes of the sun at this place before it went down and also got some after.*—f. 231–IV.

WEDNESDAY 29*th*. Having got on board a plentifull Supply of roots and some fruits I resolved to sail as soon as we got any Wind for at present it was Calm. In the evining I went a Shore in Company with Mr F. and some of the officers, they made a little excursion into the isle but I did not quit the landing place, the Natives were every were very submissive[2] and obligeing so that had we made a longer stay its probable we should [have] had no more reason to complain of their conduct; while I was now on Shore I got the names of Twenty Islands which lay between the NW and NE, some of them in Sight.

[1] The lime of powdered coral: *lahei*, to lime the hair if you were a commoner, but *penepena* if you were a chief.

[2] *submissive:* courteous

Two which laid most to the West were remarkable on account of their great hight, in the most westermost we judged was a Vulcano by the Continual Column of Smoak we saw assend from the center of the isle, to clear up this point it was necessary we should approach them nearer, accordingly at day-light in the Morning got under Sail with a light breeze at West and Stood to the Northward for these isles, but the wind scanting carried us among the low Islots and Shoals which lie north of Annamocka so that we had to ply to windward. At Noon the middle of Annamocka bore S¼E distant 9 Miles and was at the same time close to one of the islots, those we had in Sight extended from N½W to SEBE½E, and were Sixteen or 18 in Number, the two high Islands bore from NW to NNW½W. Lat Ob^d 20°6′ S. A great Number of Canoes kept about us all the forenoon; the people in them brought for Traffick Various sorts of Curiosities, some roots, fruits and fowls but of these not many; they took in exchange small Nails and Pieces of any kind of Cloth. I believe before they went away they striped the most of our people of the few Clothes the Otaheite Ladies had left them for the Passion for Curiosities was as great as ever.

THURSDAY 30*th*. The Wind being contrary and but little of it the after noon and night was spent in plying with the precaution necessary to such navigation. In the Morning Stretched out for the high Islands having the Advantage of a gentle breeze at WSW. Day no sooner dawned than we saw Canoes coming from all parts, their Traffick was much the same as yesterday or rather better, for out of one Canoe I got two Pigs which were Scarce Articles with them.[1]

[JULY 1774]

FRIDAY 1*st*. Gentle breezes and Clowdy Weather. At 4 o'Clock in the PM we reached the two high Islands, the Southermost and the one on which the Vulcano is or is supposed to be is called by the Natives Amattafoa[2] and the other which is round high and Peaked

[1] 'All this Morning a great many Canoes from the various Low Isles in the Neighbourhood trading and bartering for any trifle in the World—it is fairly the trifling Market—Our People give them old rags in exchange for small Doves—Bows—Arrows &c. &c which are absolutely as worthless as the Rags themselves.'—Clerke.

[2] Tofua. Forster got the name exactly, 'Tofooa'. 'Amattafoa' is a puzzle, and modern Tongans can cast no light on it. J. R. Forster (*Observations*, p. 525) says Cook got it from Tasman (Dalrymple's *Collection*, II); but then where did Tasman get it from? Wales and Gilbert both use the form 'Mattafoa', which suggests they had heard the name independently, and that the Cook-Tasman initial A was the nominative prefix. The Tongan word most similar is *hamatefua*, for a single sailing canoe with outrigger—a word which would most probably have been heard, both in 1643 and 1774; but confusion seems unlikely. The possibility that the island once had the same name as the canoe breaks down

Oghao.[1] We pass'd between the two, the Channell being two Miles wide, safe and without soundings; both are inhabited but neither of them appeared firtile, they lay from Annamocka NNW¼W Distant 11 or 12 Leagues. Amattafoa which is the largest of the two is about 5 Leagues in Circuit. Unfortunately the Summit of this isle during the whole day was covered with heavy clouds, so that we were not able to veryfy whether or no the Smoak we had seen was occasioned by a Vulcano or the burning of the Country, for we could see that great part of the Brow of the Hill had been consumed by fire, this divided our opinions and nothing determined.[2] While we were in the Passage between the two Isles we had little wind, which gave time for a large Sailing Canoe which had been chasing us all day to get up with us as well as several others with Padles which had been thrown a Stern when the breeze was fresh, several of these people came on board the Ship, these as also the others along side continued to exchange articles as usual. I had now an opertunity to verify a fact which before I was in doubt about which was whether or no their great sailing Vessels put about in changeing Tacks or only shifted the sail and so proceeded with either end foremost, the one now by us worked in this Manner, the Sail is Latteen, extended to a Latteen yard above and the foot to a Boom, the yard is slung nearly in the Middle or upon equipoise, so that when they want to change Tacks have only to[3] ease of the sheet and bring the heel or Tack end of the yard to the other end of the Boat and the sheet in like manner: there are notches or sockets at each end of the Canoe in which the end of the yard fixes, in short they work just as the Vessels at the Ladrone Islands described by Lord Anson; when they want to sail large or before the wind the yard is taken out of the Socket and Squared. But all thier Sailing Vessels are not rigged to Sail in this manner, some and those of the largest size are rigged so as to be obliged to Tack. They have a very Short[4] Mast which steps on a kind

before the Wales-Gilbert rendering. Taking a very long shot, one may suggest that the volcanic island had an earlier, or alternative, name, made up of the addition of *maa*—burnt, scorched—to Tofua (though the Polynesian adjective normally follows, not precedes, the noun). The name Tasman got for Kao, it may be noted, was 'Kaybay'.

[1] Kao. It rises to 3,380 feet, in a very beautiful cone frequently obscured by cloud—the sign, according to the local experts, of a northerly wind; it is clear for a southerly. Cook seems to have had a good view.

[2] *veryfy . . . determined:* determine with certainty whether there was a Vulcano or no, but every thing we could see concur'd to make us believe there was.—f. 232a.—Tofua is an active volcano, 1,660 feet at its highest—not particularly 'remarkable on account of' its 'great height' (entry of 29 June) except in comparison with the flat islands to the east; the crater is in the middle of the island, and contains a fresh water lake.

[3] *when . . . to:* when they change tacks, they throw the Vessel up in the Wind . . .—f. 232.

[4] *a very short:* a short, but pretty stout

of roller (fixed on the Fore part of the Platfrom or Deck) in order to raise it with the more ease, the Masts lean very much forward, the head is forked on the two points of which the yard rists at about ⅓ its length from the Tack, as on two Pivots,[1] at about one third its length from the Tack or heel, which when under Sail is confined down between the heads of the two boats by 2 Strong Ropes, one to each Canoe,[2] for all this sort of Sailing Canoe are Double; here the Tack is fixed so that in changing Tacks they must put about, the Sail and boom on the one Tack will lay against the Mast, but on the other it will be clear, just as a whole Mizon which with a boom the whole length of the foot would be no bad representation of one of these sails; however I am not sure if when plying to wind ward they do not unlace that part of the Sail from the yard which is between the Tack and the Mast head and in Tacking shift it and the Boom to leeward, a drawing made of them by Mr H. seems to favour this suposission. The out riggers[3] to these Canoes necessary to support the Mast and yard are of a size sufficient to heave down a Vessel of two or three hundred Tons and were Secured with equal Strength, and the ropes used for shrouds, guies &c^a^ are 4 Inches at least, indeed the Sail, yard and Boom are altogether of such an ennormous weight that strength is required to support them. Mr H. has made several drawings of these Vessels which will not only illustrate but in a manner make the descriptions I have given of them unnecessary.[4] We were hardly through the Passage before we got a fresh breeze from the South, that moment the Natives made haste to be gone and we steer'd to the west all sails set. I had some thoughts of touching at Amsterdam as it lay not much out of the way, but as the Wind was now we could not fetch it and was the occasion of my laying a side going there at all.

Before I proceed with the Sloop to the west it will be necessary to turn back to Annamocka. This Island which is situated in the Latitude of 20°15′, Long^de^ 174°30′ w was first discovered by Captain Tasman and by him Named Rotterdam. It is of a Triangler form each side where of is about three miles and a half or four miles, a Salt-Water Lake which is in it occupies not a sm^l^ part of its Surface

[1] . . . by means of two strong cleats of Wood secured to each side of the yard,

[2] *one . . . Canoe:* one to and passing through a hole at the head of each Canoe . . .—f. 232v.

[3] He does not here give the word 'Outriggers' its usual significance with island canoes—i.e. the arrangement of spars which gives stability to the single canoe—but uses it in its European nautical sense of timbers built to take a strain and projecting beyond the body of the vessel.

[4] See Fig. 47 in this volume; and, for a general collection of Tongan marine craft *Voyage*, II, pl. XLII.

and in a manner cuts off the SE angle.[1] Round the isle, that is from the NW to the South, round by the North and East lies scatered a number of Islots, Sand banks and breakers,[2] we could see no end to their extent to the North and its very probable they reach as far to the South as Amsterdam which together with Middleburg and Pylstaerts make one group of Isles, containing about three degrees in Latitude and two of Longitude: this groupe I have named the Friendly Archipelago as a lasting friendship seems to subsist among the Inhabitants and their Courtesy to Strangers intitles them to that Name.[3] Tasman seems to have seen the northern extremity in about 19°. The Inhabitants of Boscawen and Keppels Isles, discovered by Captain Wallis in 15°53′ and nearly under the same Meridian as this Archipelago, seem, from the little account I have had of them, to be the same Sort of friendly people as these. The Latitude and discriptions of these two isles point them out to be the same as Cocos and Traitors discovered by Lemaire and Schouten, but if they are the same Mr Dalrymple has placed them above 8° too far to the west in his Chart.[4]

The Inhabitants, Productions, &ca of Rotterdam or Annamocka and the Neighbouring isles are much the Same as at Amsterdam. Hoggs and Fowles indeed are scarce, of the former we got but Six

[1] '... In the Heart of the Isle are three large Lakes 2 of salt and 1 of brackish water they all abound in the largest and best wild Ducks I ever saw or tasted ...'—Clerke 8952, 1 July.

[2] All features of the Ha'apai group. Among the names picked up were Nomuka Iki; Mango and Mango Iki; 'Tonamai' (Tonumea); 'Tellefageo' (Kelefesia); these and other islets, reefs and shoals were charted. See Chart XXXV. Cook's 'Tellefageo', Forster's 'Terefetchea', and the modern Kelefesia are together interesting: the two first illustrate the ambiguity of the Polynesian sound rendered both *l* and *r*; while the third shows the mutation of *t* to *k*, and of soft *g* to *s* (cf. the rendering of the English proper name George by Tongan *Seosi*: Mariner wrote this sound as *ch*, the English Methodist missionaries as *j*, the French Catholics as *s*).

[3] The words 'Friendly Archipelago ... Name' are written into a blank space in pencil, after being drafted on a scrap of paper, f. 239. The Log, 29 June, has an addition to it made later, after Add. MS 27887 was copied: 'This Group of Isles, that is Annamocka, Tongatabu, or Amsterdam; Eoowe or Middleburg, Pylstart and the Neighbouring isles; I named the friendly isles, or Archipelago, from the extraordinary courteous and friendly disposition of their inhabitants. Under this appellation we might extend this group of isles much farther to the North, even down to Boscawen and Keppels isles ...' In B we get a combination of this and the pencil addition to the text: 'Friendly Isles or Archipelago, as a firm Alliance and friendship seems to subsist among their Inhabitants, and their Courteous behavour to strangers intitles them to that appellation, under which, we might perhaps extend' etc.

[4] This is a good deduction, though Cook excluded the sentence from B. The strikingly high islet of Tafahi (2000 feet) was discovered by Le Maire and Schouten in 1616, and named Cocos; and by Wallis in 1767, and named Boscawen. Niuatoputapu, about four miles to the south, was named Verraders or Traitors island by Le Maire and Schouten, and Keppel's by Wallis. They lie, roughly, in latitude 15°55′ S, long. 173°50′ W, about 170 miles north and a little east of Tonga—too far north to be reckoned as geographically part of the same group, but always historically connected and now administratively included in it, and often jointly referred to as 'the Keppels'.

and not very many of the latter, yams and Shaddocks were what we got the most of, other fruits being scarcer and not in such great perfection.[1] Not half the isle is laid out in inclosed Plantations as at Amsterdam but the other parts are not less fertile or less cultivated, here is however far more waste land on this isle in proportion to its Size than upon Amsterdam and the People seem much poorer, I mean in respect to Cloth, Matting, Ornaments &c[a] which constitute a great part of the Riches of these people. The people of this isle seem to be more affected with the Leprous or some other Scrofulous disease than any I have yet seen, it breaks out in the face more than in any other parts of the Body. I have seen several who had quite lost their Noses by it.[2] In one of my excursions I happen'd to peep into a house where one or more of these people were, one Man only appeared at the Door or Hole by which I was to enter and he began to Shut me out by drawing a Cord a Cross, but the intolerable Stench which came from his Putrified face was alone sufficient to keep me from entering,[3] his Nose was quite gone and his face ruin'd being wholy covered with ulcers, or rather wholy covered with one ulcer so that the very sight of him was shocking. As our People had not quite got clear of the disease communicated to them by the women of Otaheite I took all immaginable care to prevent its being communicated to these people, and I may venture to assert[4] that my endeavours succeeded. Having just mentiond a House it may not be a Miss to observe that some here differ from those we have seen at the other isles being wall'd round with reeds leaving only a hole like a Port Hole to creep in and Out by,[5] their form is an oblong square, the floor or foundation both narrower and Shorter than at the eve,[6] some thing like one of our Corn Stacks, by this means the water is thrown off from the wall which other wise would decay and rot them. We

[1] '. . . the quantities of Shaddocks and Yams (both excellent in their kind) which this Island produces is almost incredible I'm sure we might have loaded the ship with them had we set about it, we were also pretty plentifully suppli'd with Cocoa Nuts and Bunanoes got some fowls and Fish together with 5 or 6 small Hogs . . .'—Clerke 8952, 1 July.

[2] *who . . . it:* whose faces were ruined by it and Nose quite gone.—f. 233v. This disease seems to have been yaws.—Mariner, Appendix II, pp. cv–vii.

[3] . . . had the entrance been ever so wide,

[4] *may . . . assert:* have reason to believe . . .—f. 233v. Cf. Forster, II, pp. 171–2, on the first landing at Nomuka: 'The hospitality of the natives was exercised in its utmost extent, and one of the handsomest ladies of the island complimented the captain with an offer, which was not accepted. Having examined the watering-place, he returned on board to breakfast, and gave strict orders, that no persons infected with or lately cured of venereal complaints should be suffered to go on shore, and that no woman should be admitted in the ship.'

[5] *being wall'd . . . by:* these being inclosed or Wall'd on every side with reeds neatly put together but not close, the entrance is by a square hole about 2½ feet each way.—f. 233v.

[6] . . . which is about 4 feet from the ground.

were not able to distinguish any King or other Leading Chief amongest them or any person who seem'd to take upon him any thing like that authority. The Woman I have before mentioned and a man which I took to be her husband on some occasions rather distinguished themselves from the rest; this man endeavoured to persuade the people from commiting those acts of Violence at the watering place, he stuck by us during the whole squable and as a reward for his fidillity I gave him a young Dog and a Bitch animals they have not and which they are very fond of.

*... the Man and Woman, before mentioned, which I took to be man and Wife, intrested themselves on several occasion[s] in our affairs, but it was easy to see that they had no great authority. Amongst other things which I gave them as a reward for their service, was a young Dog and Bitch, animals which they have not but are very fond of and know very well by name. Some of the same sort of earthen pots were seen here as were seen at Amsterdam, I am of opinion they are of their own Manufactury or that of some neighbouring isle.

The Road, as I have already mentioned, is on the North side of the isle, just to the Southward of the Southermost Cove,[1] for there are two on this side; the bank is of some extent and the bottom free from rocks, there is 25 and 20 fathoms Water 1 or 2 miles from the shore: Fire wood is very convenient to be got at and easy to be Shiped off; but the Water is so brackish that it is not worth the trouble to fetch it on board, unless one is in great distress for want of that article and can get no better, there is however better, not only on this isle, but others in the neighbourhood, for the people some times brought of some in Cocoanut Shells, which was as good as need be, but probably the springs may be too trifling to Water a Ship.

I have already observed that the SW side of the Island is covered by a reef, or reefs of Rocks and small Isles, if there is a sufficieant depth of Water between them and the island, as there appeared to be, and a good bottom this would be a much securer place for a Ship to Anchor in than the place where we Anchor'd.[2] The Tides

[1] This is not very intelligible: just to the 'southward' of the southernmost cove would bring the ship on shore. Probably 'southward' is a slip for 'northward'. This north coast runs east to west very slightly south; so that although 'southernmost' may be a good word reckoning from the ship's position, on shore 'westernmost' might seem more logical. Hence one should probably read, 'just to the northward of the westernmost cove'.

[2] This is the modern anchorage, between Nomuka and Nomuka Iki, and off the village on Nomuka. It is well protected by the islands and reefs, and is so much the only good Nomukan anchorage (it is even officially called a harbour) that local tradition holds that Cook anchored there, close to Nomuka Iki, and will point to the pond where he watered—for, as it happens, there is a pond near the village something like the one on the north side where he did water.

rises and falls upon a perpendicular about 4 feet and a SE Moon makes high water. The Variation of the Compass was observed to be 11°00′ East.*—f. 234.

FRIDAY *1st.* Mention has already been made of our leaving the Land in the PM of this Day and steering to the West inclining to the South with the Wind at SSE. During night we ran under the three Top-sails only, keeping the Wind on the beam which put it in our power to return back on the opposite Course in case we had met with any dangers. At Day-light made all Sail and Steer'd WBS, at the same time saw Amattafoa bearing EBN.[1] At Noon Latitude in 20°, Long^{de} 176°6′ and Longitude made from Annamocka 1°36′ West.

SATURDAY *2nd.* Winds at SEBS and SSE a gentle gale. At Noon saw Land from the Mast head bearing WNW by Compass which we steer'd for. Our Latitude at this time was 20°3′ Longitude 178°2′ West.

SUNDAY *3rd.* Winds at SEBS gentle breezes and fair Weather. At 4 o'Clock in the PM we discovered the Land to be a small Island, bearing from NW½W to NWBN. At the same time breakers were seen from the mast head extending from SW to West. The Day being already too far spent to make farther discoveries, at 5 o'Clock Shortned Sail, hauled the wind and spent the night making short boards to windward of the Island. At Day-light found our selves farther off than we expected, bore up for it under all the Sail we could set. At 11 o'Clock we reached the NW or Lee side of the isle at a place where Anchorage seem'd probable, but in order to be certain we brought-to hoisted out a boat and sent the Master to sound.[2] At this time 4 or 5 people appeared on the reef which stretch off from the isle and about three times that number on the Shore, as the Boat advanced those on the reef retired to the others and we observed that when the Boat land they all retired to the Woods. At Noon the Boat return'd when the Master informed me that there was no soundings without the reef, through which was a Channel of no more than Six feet water, entering by this Channel he pull'd in for the Shore thinking to speak with the people not more than 20 in number who were Arm'd with Clubs and Spears, but the moment he set his foot on Shore they retired, he left ashore some Medals, Nails and a Knife which they undoubtedly would get as some of them some time after appeared again on the Shore near the place. Near the Reef were seen

[1] ... distant 20 Leagues.—f. 235.

[2] ... and in the mean time we stood on and off with the Ship.

several Turtle which occasioned my giving that name to the Isle.[1] It is situated in the Latitude of 19°48 S, Long^de^ 178°2′ west. It is covered with wood amongest which are Cocoa-nut trees, but it is too small to contain many inhabitants,[2] being not quite a League in length NE & SW and not half that in breadth and is Surrounded by a reef of Coral rocks, which in some places extends two Miles from the isle; some circumstances shew'd the Natives to be a Docile people and that an intercourse might soon have been opened with them, but at this time seeing from the Mast head more breakers to the SSW, which I was willing to explore before night rather than to spend the remainder of the Day about an Island of so little consequence, especially as it afforded no Anchorage in case we should be becalm'd near its Shores,[3] we therefore hoisted in the Boats and stood for the Breakers.

MONDAY *4th*. Winds Easterly pleasent Weather. At 2 o'Clock in the PM we were the length of the Breakers and found they were occasioned by a Coral bank of a bout 4 or 5 Leagues in circuit, by the bearings we had taken we found this to be the same Shoal as we had seen last night.[4] It lies SW from the isle,[5] the Channel between the reef of the latter and it is 3 miles wide: Seeing no more breakers either to the Southward or Westward, and judging there might be Turtils on this Shoal, we equiped two Boats and sent them to look for some but they presently return'd without having seen one, after hoisting them in made Sail to the SW, and as soon as we were clear of the Shoal found a large Swell from SSW which indicated no land near us in that direction.[6] The Variation of the Compass was here 11°46′ E. In the evening Shortned Sail and spent the night makeing Short boards, at daybreak reasumed our former Course all sails set, having but little wind at ENE. At Noon Latitude observed 20°2′, Longitude 178°19′ W.

[1] This sentence Cook added in a blank space in pencil.

[2] . . . probably the few which we saw may have come from some isle in the neighbourhood to fish for Turtle . . .—f. 235–5v.

[3] The islet was Vatoa, a south-eastern islet of the Fiji group, and the only one of that group seen by Cook; it is surrounded by deep water. Chart XXXVI*b*.

[4] . . . Hardly any part of this bank or Reef is above Water, at the reflux of the Waves, the heads of some rocks are to be seen near the edge of the reef where it is the Shoaldest, for in the Middle is deep Water; in short this bank wants only a few little Islots to make it exactly like one of the half drown'd Isles so often mentioned.—f. 235v. This detached reef is called Vuata Vatoa—lat. 19°49′ S, long. 178°13′ W. Chart XXXVI*b*.

[5] . . . about 5 or Six miles

[6] . . . As we pass'd the Isle we observed on the reef some very large Coral rocks, which could not be less than 12 or 15 [feet] high, with small bases in proportion to their size, but spreading or branching out above, so as to form a large round top on which were growing some sort of green plants. I have seen of these sort of Coral rocks under water, but I never saw any like them so high above Water before.—f. 235v. These rocks are called the Three Sisters.

TUESDAY 5*th.* Moderate breezes and fine pleasent Weather. In the evening being in the Latitude 20°8′ S, Long^de 178°34′ the Variation was by an Az^th 12°27′ and by the Amplitude 12°29′ E. At Dark Shortned Sail and hauled up SWBS with the wind on the beam. At Day break made Sail and Steer'd WBS and at Noon found our selves in Latitude 20°37′, Long^de 179°20′ West.

WEDNESDAY 6*th.* Gentle breezes and Dark gloomy weather. Spent the night makeing Short boards. AM Saw a Bird like a gannet.[1] At Noon Latitude observ^d 20°56′, Long^de in 179°30′ E. Steered west. I now reckon my Longit. East from Greenwich.

THURSDAY 7*th.* Gentle gales Easterly and Clowdy weather. In the evening Shortned Sail and spent the night as last. AM saw one of the same sort of Birds as yester and some Tropic birds. Struck and unrigg'd the Fore Top-mast to fix New Trestle trees and Quarter backstays. At Noon Latitude in 20°50′ S, Longitude 178°30′ East.

FRIDAY 8*th.* PM Gentle gales at East, Course WBN. Rigg'd and got up the Fore-Top-mast. At 6 Shortned Sail and at 10 hauled the wind under the Top-sails and spent the night as usual. At Day-break reassumed our proper Course under all Sails set having a fresh gale at NE. At Noon Latitude observ^d 20°42′ Longitude in 177°18′ East.

SATURDAY 9*th.* PM Fresh gales at NE and dark clowdy weather. At 8 hauled the Wind to the Northward under the 3 Top-sails and foresail, thus we spent the night in which the wind veer'd to NW, remained unsettled and was attended with Squals and rain till 8 o'Clock when it began to clear up and became more Settled; found the Variation to be 13°8′ E. Saw a nother of those birds like gannets. At Noon Lat. ob. 20°24′. Long. in 176°15′ East.

SUNDAY 10*th.* PM Little wind at NW, about 4 a Shower of rain brought it round to WSW when we Tack'd and Stood NW, the wind veer'd round by the South to SEBS and increased to a fresh gale, the night was spent makeing short boards and the AM in Steering NW under all Sails. At Noon Lat. in 19°53′, Long^de 175°35′ East.

MONDAY 11*th.* Fresh Trade and pleasent Weather and following Sea. At 6 PM Shortned Sail to Single reef'd Top-sails and brought the Main Top-sail to the Mast; at day-break bore away NWBN and at Noon Steer'd NW[2] being at this time in Latitude 18°26′, Longitude 175°00′ East.

[1] *like a gannet:* of the Pelican kind, white, wings tiped with black and something larger than a Booby.—f. 236. This was probably a Masked Gannet, *Sula cyanops*.

[2] . . . in order to get into the Latitude of Quiros's Isles,

TUESDAY 12*th*. Winds at SE a fresh Trade and Cloudy weather. At 6 PM Shortned Sail and Spent the night as last, day-break reassumed our NW Course all Sails set.[1] At Noon Men of War and Tropick Birds seen. Latitude 17°18′, Long^{de} 173°35′.

WEDNESDAY 13*th*. PM fresh Trade at SE and fair weather. Spent the night laying-to, her head to the Northward as was done for two nights past. AM Little wind and fine weather. At 7 Latitude 16°10′, Long^{de} 173°47′. Variation p^{r} Azth 10°57′ E. At Noon Latitude Observed 16°25′. Longitude 173°31′ E. Tropic birds &c^{a} seen every day.

THURSDAY 14*th*. Gentle Breezes and pleasent Weather. Towards Noon some birds and a piece of Sea weed seen. Course made good NW distance 79 Miles. Lat. in 15°39′, Long^{de} 172°35′.

FRIDAY 15*th*. Winds at ESE, first part gentle breezes latter fresh gales. Steer'd NWBW till 10 pm, then hauled the wind and Spent the remainder of the night making short Boards, at day-break bore away WBN all Sails Set. Variation E. At Noon Lat. in 15°9′, Long^{de} 171°16′ East. Being now in the Latitude of Quiros's land, Steer'd west.

SATURDAY 16*th*. Fresh gales at SE and clear weather. At 4 o'Clock in the PM Mr W. and the Master had Several Lunar observations, as they also had on the two preceeding days, their results reduced to this day at Noon gives 170°56′ East Longitude which differs only 4′ from my reckoning.[2] At day break reassumed our west Course with a very fresh gale at SEBS which blew in Squalls attended with rain and thick hazey weather,[3] at Noon we reckoned we were in Lat. 15°8′ S, Long. 169°18′ East.

SUNDAY 17*th*. Continued to Steer to the West till 3 o'Clock in the PM when we saw land bearing SW upon which we took in the Small Sails, reef'd the Top-sails and hauled up for it having a very Strong gale at SE thick hazey weather. At half past 5 the land bore from SSW to NWBN½W but we were not certain that we saw the whole extent either way. At half past 7 Tack'd judging our selves at this time about two leagues from the land. We stood off till between 1

[1] . . . During Day time we ran under all the Sail we could set, but the nights were spent either laying to or in plying under the Topsails, least we should pass any land in the dark.—f. 236.

[2] B f. 236v *deletes* 'which . . . reckoning'; and the figures 170°56′ have 169°18′ superimposed on them in a blacker ink.

[3] . . . When such Weather happens in this Ocean within the Tropicks it generaly indicates the Vicinity of some high lands—f. 236v.

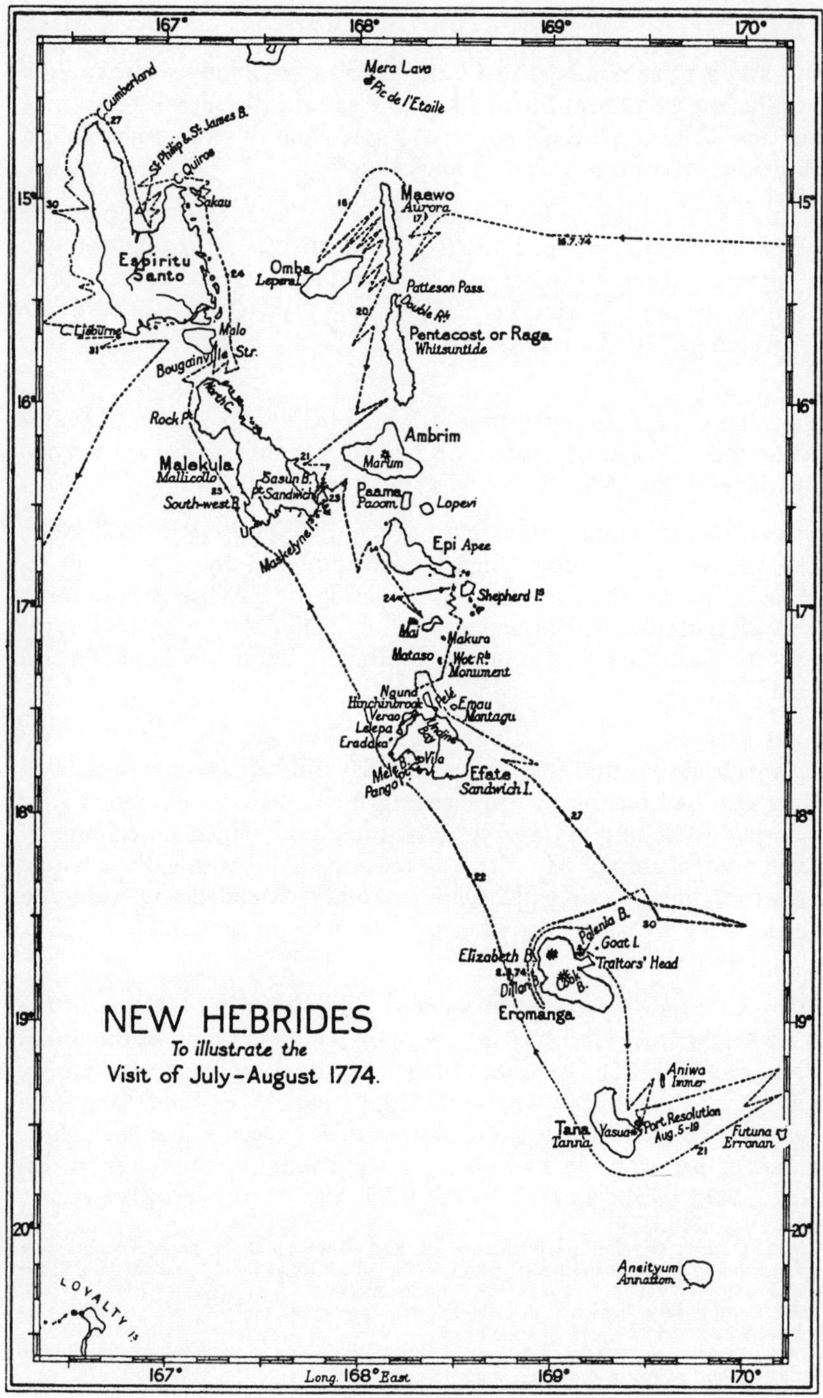
NEW HEBRIDES
To illustrate the
Visit of July–August 1774.
167°
168°
169°
170°
15°
16°
17°
18°
19°
20°
Long. 168° East
Mera Lava
Pic de l'Etoile
Cumberland
St Philip & St James B.
Quiros
Sakau
Espiritu Santo
Maewo
Aurora
Omba
Leper
Patteson Pass
Pentecost or Raga
Whitsuntide
C. Lisburne
Malo
Bougainville Str.
North C.
Rock P.
Ambrim
Marum
Malekula
Mallicollo
Sasun B.
Sandwich
South-west B.
Paama
Paoom
Lopevi
Epi Apee
Maskelyne Is
Shepherd Is
Mai
Makura
Mataso
Wot Rk
Monument
Nguna
Hinchinbrook
Emau
Montagu
Verao
Lelepa
Eradaka
Vila
Mele B.
Pango Pt
Efate
Sandwich I.
Polenia B.
Goat I.
Traitors' Head
Elizabeth B.
Dillon's B.
Cook B.
Eromanga
Aniwa
Immer
Tana
Tanna
Yasua
Port Resolution
Aug. 5-19
Futuna
Erronan
Aneityum
Annattom
LOYALTY Is
16.7.74

Fig. 66

and 2 in the AM then Stood in again. It was no wonder to find we had lost ground in the night for it blew exceeding hard at times and there went a great Sea from the SE, besides several of our Sails were Split and torn to pieces in the night, particularly a Fore Top-sail which was rendred quite useless as a Sail.[1] Being desireous of geting round the Southern ends of the lands or at least so far to the South as to be able to judge of their extent in that direction, for I made no doubt but this was the Australia Del Espiritu Santo of Quiros or what M. D. Bougainville calls the Great Cyclades, and the coast we were now upon the East side of Aurora Island[2] whose Longitude by the Observations we have lately had is 17 ° ′ E.[3]

MONDAY 18*th*. At 3 o'Clock in the PM being about 3 miles from the Shore of Aurora we wore the Ship and Stood off under close reefd Top-sails and Courses, but the gale increasing brought us at last under the latter only. At 2 in the AM wore and Stood in for the Shore which we reached by 7 at which time the North end of Aurora bore WNW distant about two leagues; seeing we lost ground a pace I gave up the design of Plying to the Southward without the isles; bore up, set the Top-sails double reef'd and hauled round the North end of Aurora, in going round the point of this isle we sounded but found no ground with 50 fath of line ¾ of a Mile from the Shore. After geting round the Point hauled up SSW close upon a wind. We had now a Smooth Sea[4] but the wind and weather as stormy as ever. At Noon the North end of Aurora bore NE½N four leagues distant and a high land on the Isle of Lepers[5] which at inter[v]als appeared in Sight bore SBE, our Latitude found by Dble Altitudes and reduced to this time was 15°1½′ S, Longitude 16 ° ′ East.[6]

TUESDAY 19*th*. Very fresh gales at SE attended with heavy Squalls. Continued to Ply to windward all this day between the Isle ot Aurora and Lepers under close reef'd Top-sails and Courses with a view of geting to the South to explore the lands which lies there. At 2 o'Clock in the PM we Tacked about two Miles from the Shore of

[1] 'At ½ past 1 AM Tack'd and Stood in for the land, soon after the Fore Top-sail Split so as to be ever after useless, it having been already worn to the very utmost this was followed by the Spliting of more Sails and the breaking of several ropes.'—Log.

[2] Bougainville's name (1768) for Maewo. It is the north-easternmost of the New Hebrides.—Figs. 65, 66.

[3] 168°30′ East.—f. 236v.

[4] ... having the isle of Aurora to windward.

[5] Bougainville's name; Omba, Oba, or Aoba. Leprosy seems to have been extremely rare, even if it was known at all, on the island; the French may have taken leucodermia, which did exist, for it—or, it has been suggested, the form of ringworm called 'bukwa'.

[6] 168°14′ East.—f. 236v. These figures, to judge from the ink, are the result of later re-calculation.

ye Isle of Lepers and abreast of the Middle of the Isle, at this distance from Shore had no Soundings with a line of 70 fathom. Here we preceived people on the Shore and many beautifull Cascades of Water coming from the adjacent Hills. On the same side of this Isle about 7 miles to the NW of the SE point, at half a mile from Shore we found 30 f^m^ and no ground with 70 fathom a Mile off, here two Canoes came off to us, in the one were 3 men and in the other but one, they came not[1] nearer than a Stones throw, made a Short Stay and then retired a Shore where a good many people were seen Arm'd with Bows and Arrows.[2] On the Side of Aurora we could find no Sounding, ¾ of a Mile from Shore. At Noon the North end of this Isle bore North distant 20[3] Miles and the South end s 24° East. Lat p^r^ Ob^n^ 15°11′, by this Observation as well as the preceeding one I find M.D. Bougainville's discoveries are laid down about 20 Miles too far North, in the Charts which are bound up with the English Translation. As this error is nearly equal and the same way as the one at Otaheite its probable this error runs through the whole Chart of this Sea.[4]

WEDNESDAY 20*th*. Winds at SE, first part very fresh gales and Squally the remainder more moderate. In the evening we fetched up with the South end of Aurora on the NW side of which[5] seems to be a fine bay in which we made some trips to try for Anchorage, but could find no Soundings proper for Anchorage at ⅓ or ½ a Mile from Shore, at this distance had 80 f^m^ dark Sandy bottom, nevertheless I am of opinion there is good Anchorage[6] here nearer the Shore and farther in the beight, and here is no want of Wood or Water, the whole Island from the Sea Shore to the Summits of the hills is covered with the former and every Vally hath a fine Stream of the latter. It is Inhabited, we not only saw people but Smokes rising out of the Woods in many parts.[7] It extends NBW and SBE and is Leagues long in that direction, but its Breadth is inconsiderable, the North end lies in Latitude [8]

[1] *they came not:* all the signs of friendship we could make did not bring them . . .—f. 237.

[2] . . . These people are of a very dark colour and excepting some ornaments at their breast and arms seemed to be intirely naked.—f. 237, *red ink in margin.*

[3] 12 or 15

[4] ABG *note*: 'The Charts bound up with the French Edition must be examined before this error can be laid to M. de Bougainville.' In B marked 'omit.

[5] i.e. on the NW side of the south end.

[6] *good Anchorage:* much less water and secure riding . . .—f. 237. There is a bay, but it is not known as an anchorage; the known anchorages on this coast are farther north.

[7] *It is . . . parts:* We saw people on the shore and some Canoes on the Coast but none came off to us.

[8] B omits this sentence; the island is about 36 miles long and 4 miles across but rises to 2000 feet; the latitude of its northern point is about 14°50′ s.

Leaving the Bay just mentioned at 10 o'Clock in the AM we stretched a Cross the Channel which divides Aurora from Whitsuntide Island which is 1½ League broad,[1] off the North end of the latter Island lies a rock above water not far from the Shore,[2] the rest of the Channel seem'd quite clear. At Noon we were by a good Observation in Lat. 15°   ′, the Island of Whitsuntide extending from ENE to South, the Isle of Lepers from SBW½W to WSW[3] and Aurora from North to NE½E. The SE point of Lepers Island lies from the Channel which divides Aurora and Whitsuntide distant two Leagues, this Island is about   Leagues long in its longest direction which is   and about   in breadth, it rises high in the Middle but its Shores are rather low except some places on the NW side.[4]

THURSDAY 21*st*. Winds at SE a fresh breeze and fine Weather. In the PM we discovered the Seperation between the SW land and Whitsuntide Isla'd.[5] In the Morning we had the whole Channell open, it is two Leagues over and seem'd to be Clear of danger. Whitsuntide Island lies under the same Meridian as Aurora, it extends North and South and is 11 Leagues long in that direction, its breadth is not very considerable. It is of a tolerable height and cloathed with wood except Such parts as seem'd to be Cultivated. Several Smokes were seen riseing out of the woods in all parts of the Island.[6] The SW land at this time extended from SBE to the westward farther than the eye could reach,[7] and we were not sure if the part nearest to us was not

[1] Patteson Passage. Cook uses the name Whitsuntide, after Forster, for Bougainville's Pentecôte; it is now generally Pentecost in English, but the native name is Raga.

[2] Double Rock.

[3] NBW½W to West.—S in the text is a slip for N; cf. the slip when the ship was outside Port Nicholson, p. 285 above.

[4] B omits this sentence, as if Cook had never had time to make the necessary observations. Omba is about 20 miles north-east and south-west, and 9 or 10 miles across its widest part; it rises to 4000 feet.

[5] *In the PM . . . Island:* Whitsun-tide isle appeared joined to the land to the South and SW of it, but in stretching to SW we discovered the separation, this was about 4 o'Clock in the p.m. when the wind veering more to the East made it necessary to resume our Course to the South. We saw people on the shore. . . .—f. 237v.

[6] 'The Shores of Whitsuntide Island are bold, without Inlets . . . the Land high and Mountainous; but exhibits the most beautiful Prospect I ever saw, being cultivated up to the very summit, and divided into rectangular Fields by Fences which appear like Hedges from y[e] Ship, so that one could scarce help imagining one's self in sight of England, with an extensive View of enclosed Fields before one.'—Wales, 19 July. There really seems to be a little overstatement here. The island rises to over 3000 feet, and is densely wooded and well-watered; but Wales must surely have taken natural for cultivated fertility, unless there has been a vast change since. On the other hand, cultivation is inland, and in the bush. No villages would be seen from the sea.

[7] . . . On the part nearest to us, which is of a considerable height, we observed two very large columns of smoak, which I judge assended from Volcanos.—f. 237v. The volcanoes were probably Mounts Marum and Benbow. Volcanic eruptions have altered considerably the western coast of Ambrim that Cook saw.

a seperate Isle, this was verified at 10 o'Clock when in Stretching to SSW the passage opened at SBW½W, this Isle is called by the Natives Ambrrym. Soon after an Elevated land appeared open of the South end of Ambrrym and after that a nother still higher on which is a very high Peaked Mountain, we judged these lands to be two Seperate isles, the first came in Sight at SE and the other at EBS, they appeared to be [10] Leagues distant.[1] Still continuing our Course to SSW for the land a head which at Noon we were about 5 Mile from, it extending from SSE to NWBW round by the SW and appeared to be one continued land, the Isles to the East extended from NEBE to SEBE. Our Latitude by Observation was 16°17′ S.

FRIDAY 22*nd*. Wind at SE a gentle breeze and pleasent Weather. In Standing in for the land we preceived a creek which had the appearence of a good harbour, formed by a point of land or Peninsula projecting out to the North,[2] we just fetched this place at 1 o'Clock PM when we tack'd and stood off till half past 2 in order to gain room and time to hoist the Boats out to examine it. Several people appeared on the Point of the Peninsula and seem'd to invite us a Shore, but[3] the most of them had Bows and Arrows in their hands. In stretching in Shore, by the help of a Tide or Current which we had not before precived, we fetched two Leagues to windward of this place, and by that means discovered a nother opening[4] which I sent Lieut[t] Pickersgill and the Master in two Arm'd boats to Sound and look for Anchorage; Upon their makeing the Sign[1] for the latter, we saild in and anchored in 11 fathom Water Sandy bottom, some thing more than a Cables length from the South Shore and a Mile within the entrance.

Some of the Natives came off to us in their Canoes,[5] two of them were induced to come on board where they made a very Short stay as the Sun was already set; the kind reception these met with induced others to come off by moon light, but I would permit none to enter the Ship or even to come along-side, by this means we got rid of them for the night.[6] They exchanged for pieces of Cloth some few

[1] The first was the two closely neighbouring islands for which Cook got the name Paoom—Paama, Pa Uma or Pau uma and Lopevi; the second Epi, which rises to a sharp peak at 2,770 feet.

[2] Paunomu point, lat. 16°20′ S, on the eastern side of Malekula; the 'creek' was Sasun Bay, a good anchorage in a SE wind.

[3] *but:* probably with no good intent, as

[4] *In stretching . . . opening:* In order to gain room and time to hoist out and arm our boats to reconnoitre the place, we tacked and made a trip off, which occasioned the discovery of a nother port about a League more to the South . . .—ff. 237v–8.

[5] . . . they were very cautious at first, but at last ventured along side . . .—f. 238.

[6] 'Several Canoes came about the Ship so great was their Curiosity that they did not leave the Ship till past 10 at Night, holding up Torches to look at us by. . . .'—Hood.

Arrows, some of which were pointed with bone and diped in Poison or some green gummy substance that could Answer no other end.[1]

In the Morning a good many came round us, some came in Canoes and others swam off. I soon prevaild on one to come on board which he had no sooner done than he was followed by more than we desired:[2] four I took into the Cabbin and made them various presents which they Shew'd to those in the Canoes, thus a friendly intercourse between us and them was in a fair way of being opened when[3] an accident happened which put all in confution but in the end I believe turn'd out to our advantage. A fellow in a Canoe having been refused admittance into one of our boats a long-side was going[4] to Shoot one of the Poisoned Arrows at the Boat-keeper, some[5] interfeering prevented him from doing it that Moment,[6] the instant I was acquainted with this I ran on deck and saw a nother man strugling with him, one of those as I was told who were in the Cabbin and had jump'd out of the window for that purpose, but the fellow got the better of him and directed his Bow again to the boat keeper, but upon my calling to him he directed it to me and was just going to let fly when I gave him a peppering of Small Shott, this Staggered him for a Moment but did not hinder him from holding his bow in the Attitude of Shooting, another discharge of the same Nature made him drop it and the others in the Canoes to Paddle off as fast as they could. Some began to Shoot Arrows from the other side, a Musquet discharged in the air and a four pounder over their heads sent them all off in the utmost confusion; those in the Cabbin leaped out of the Windows, other that were in the ship and on different parts of the Rigging all leaped over board and many quited their Canoes and swam a shore. After this we took no further notice of them, but suffered them to come and pick up their Canoes, and some were soon after prevailed upon to come alongside.[7] We now got every thing in readiness to land in order to try to get some refreshments, for nothing of this kind had been seen in any of thier boats, and to Cut some Wood of which we were in want of.

[1] See p. 465, n. 5 below.

[2] . . . so that not only our decks but rigging was presently filled with them . . .—f. 238, *red ink*.—'. . . repeating the word Tomarr or Tomarro continually, which seemed to be an expression equivalent to the Taheitian Tayo (friend).'—Forster, II, p.205. It may have been the Malekulan *damar*, 'peace', but was more probably *temar*, 'ancestor'; cf. p. 484, n. 4 below.

[3] *thus . . . when:* and seemed very well pleas'd with the reception they met with. While I was thus makeing friends with those in the Cabbin, *red ink*.

[4] *was going:* bent his bow

[5] *some:* some of his Countrymen

[6] . . . and gave time to accquaint me with it

[7] . . . Immediately after the great gun was fired, we heard beating of Drums on Shore, this was probably the Signal for the Country to assemble in arms.—f. 238v.

About 9 o'Clock we landed in the face of about 4 or 500 Men who were assembled on the Shore, arm'd with Bows and Arrows, Clubs and Spears, but they made not the least opposission, on the contrary one Man gave his Arms to a nother and Met us[1] in the water with a green branch in his hand, which [he] exchanged for the one I held in my hand, took me by the other hand and led me up to the crowd to whom I distributed Medals, Pieces of Cloth &c[a]. After M[r] Edgcomb had drawn his Marines up on the beach in such a manner as to Protect the workmen in cutting down wood I made Signs[2] to the Natives that we wanted some to take on board, to which they willingly consented. A small Pigg was now brought down and presented to me for which I gave the bearer a Piece of Cloth,[3] this gave us hopes that a trade would soon be opened for refreshments but we were misstaken, this Pig came on some other account probable as a peace offering, for all that we could say or do did not prevail upon them to bring us above half a Dozen small Cocoanutts and a small quantity of fresh water. They set no sort of Value upon Nails[4] nor did they seem much to esteem any thing we had, they would now and then give an arrow for a Piece of Cloth but constantly refused to part with their bows, they were unwilling we should go into the Country and very desireous for us to go on board, we understood not a word they said, they are quite different to all we have yet seen and Speak a different language, they are almost black or rather a dark Chocolate Colour, Slenderly made, not tall, have Monkey faces and Woolly hair.[5] About Noon after sending what wood we had cut on board we all embarqued and went of after which they all retired some one way and some a nother.

SATURDAY 23*rd*. Having now got on board a small quantity of Wood for present consumption and intending to put to Sea the next Morning in order to take advantage of the moonlight nights which now happened[6] we employ'd this after-noon in seting up our lower & Top-mast Rigging which they stood in need of. Some time last night the Natives had taken away the Buoy from the Kedge Anchor we lay moor'd by, which I now saw a fellow bringing along the Strand to the landing place. I therefore took a boat and went for it accom-

[1] *on the contrary ... us:* on the contrary seeing me advance alone with nothing but a green branch in my hand one man who seemed to be a chief gave his bow and arrows to a nother and met me ...—f. 238.

[2] ... (for we understood not a word of thier language)

[3] ... with which he seem'd well pleased;

[4] ... or any sort of Iron tools

[5] Cook of course had passed from the Polynesian to the Melanesian area of the ocean, and was noticing Melanesian characteristics. See also p. 465, n. 3 below.

[6] *Having ... happened:* Before we had dined the after-noon was too far spent to do any thing on shore ...—f. 239.

panied by some of the Gentlemen; the moment we landed the Buoy was put into our boat by a man who walked of again without Speaking one word; it ought to be observed that this was the only thing they even so much as attempted to take from us by any means whatever and that they seem'd to Observe Strict honisty in all their dealings. Having landed near some of their houses and Plantations which were just within the Skirts of the Woods, I prevaild on one man to let me see them, they Suffered Mr F. to go with me but were unwilling any more should follow. Their houses are low[1] and covered with thick Palm thatch, their form is oblong and some are boarded at the ends where the entrance is by a Square Port hole which at this time was Shut up;[2] they did not chouse we should enter any of them and we attempted nothing against their inclinations; here were about half a Dozen houses, some small Plantations which were fenced round with reeds,[3] about Twenty Piggs and a few Fowles runing about loose, and a good many fine yams lying piled up upon Sticks or kind of Platforms; here were Bread fruit Trees, Cocoa-nutt and Plantain Trees on which were little or no fruit, we afterwards saw an Orange on the beach, proof sufficient that they have of these fruit.[4] We next proceed to the Point[5] of the harbour where we[6] could see the three distant Isles already mentioned the names of which we now obtained as well as the land on which we were which they call *Mallecollo*,[7] a name which we find mentioned by Quiros or at least one so like it that there is not room for a Doubt but that they both mean the same land.[8] After this we proceed to the other side of the Harbour and there landed by invitation[9] but we had not

[1] *Their . . . low:* These houses were something like those at the other isles, rather low

[2] . . . and which they were unwilling to open for us to look in.

[3] . . . as at the Friendly Isles

[4] Proof sufficient? B is more cautious, and reads, 'Here we found on the beach a fruit like an orange called by them   but whether it is fit for eating or no, J cannot say, as this was decayed'. Cook afterwards picked up the name 'Barreeco' for the fruit. 'The ideas of the natural riches of the island of Mallicollo', says Forster (II, p. 223) 'were considerably raised after this confirmation of Quiros's reports'. But oranges did not grow in the New Hebrides. What was found on the beach was probably the bitter and inedible fruit of the wild *Citrus macroptera*, which is fairly common in Melanesian forests.

[5] *Point:* S.E. Point.—It is called Lamap point.

[6] *where we:* where we again landed and Walked along the beach till we

[7] Malekula. But there was no native name for the island as a whole.

[8] The name which Quiros picked up, in April 1606, at Taumako in the Duff islands of the Santa Cruz group, about three hundred miles to the north, was 'Manicolo'. The present editor has fallen into the same error as Cook (I, p. xlviii), in identifying it with Malekula; it was probably Vanikoro, the most southerly of the Santa Cruz group.—B f. 239v. omits the words 'a name . . . land', and substitutes, 'the island which first appeared over the South end of Ambrrijm is called *Apee* [Epi] and the other with the hill on it Paoom.

[9] *by invitation:* at the invitation of some people who came down to the shore . . .—f. 239v.

been a Shore five Minutes before they wanted us to be gone, we complied, put off and proceeded up the Harbour in order to Sound and take a view of it and to search for a stream of fresh Water, for as yet we had seen none but the very little the Natives brought us,[1] nor did we meet with any better success now, but is no reason but there may be some, the day was too far Spent to make a narrow Search and night brought us on board when I understood that not a Canoe had been of to the Ship the whole after noon, so soon was the Curiosity of these people satisfied.[2]

At[3] 7 o'Clock AM weighed and with some variable light Airs of Wind and the Assistance of our Boat towing got out of the Harbour the South point of which at Noon WSW distant two or three Miles, Lat. Ob^{d} 16°24′30″. We now got a gentle breeze at ESE [with] which we stretchd off NE with a view of geting to windward in order to explore the Isles which layd there. While we were geting out of the Harbour we had some little intercourse with the Natives who came off in their Canoes and sold us a few Bows and Arrows,[4] but I think the Most we had along side at one time was only Eight Canoes in each of which might be four or five people. It being low-water when we came out, Vast numbers of people were out on the reefs along the Coast, most probably picking up Shell and other fish which might be there.

The people of this country are in general the most Ugly and ill-proportioned of any I ever saw, to what hath been allready said of them I have only to add that they have thick lips flat noses and. . . .[5]

Their Beards as well as most of their Woolly heads are of a Colour between brown and black, the former is much brighter than the latter and is rather more of hair than wool, short and curly. The Men go naked, it can hardly be said they cover thier Natural parts, the Testicles are quite exposed, but they wrap a piece of cloth or leafe round the yard which they tye up to the belly to a cord or bandage which they wear round the waist just under the Short Ribbs and over the belly and so tight that it was a wonder to us how they could endure it. They have curious bracelets which they wear on the Arm just above the Elbow, these are work'd with threed or Cord and studed with Shells and are four or five inches broad,

[1] . . . which we knew not where they got

[2] . . . As we were coming on board, we heard the Sound of a Drum and I think some other instrument and saw people dancing, but as soon as they heard the noise of the oars and saw us, all was silent.

[3] *At:* Being unwilling to lose the benefit of the Moon light nights, which now happened, at

[4] . . . for pieces of cloth and papers

[5] The sentence is unfinished.

they never would part with one, they also wear round the wrist Hoggs Tusks and rings made of large Shells; the bridge of the Nose is pierced in which they wear an ornament of this form,[1] it is made of a stone which is not unlike alabaster,[2] they likewise wear small ear Rings made of Tortise shell. We saw but few Women and they were full as disagreeable as the Men, their head face and Shoulders were painted with a Red Colour,[3] they wear a piece of Cloth wraped round their Middle and some thing over their Shoulders in which they carry their Children.

Their Arms are Bows and Arrows, Clubs and Spears made of hard or Iron wood,[4] the Arrows are reeds and some are arm'd with a long sharp point made of the Iron wood, others are armed with a very sharp point of bone and covered with a green gummy substance which we took to be poison and the Natives conform'd our Su[pposition] by makeing signs to us not to touch the point.[5] I have seen some Arm'd with two or three of these points with little prekles on the edges to prevent the Arrows being drawn out of the wound.

*. . . only eight Canoes and in each of them four or five people: these Canoes were imployed making several trips, bringing off some new faces every time. I beleive we did not see twenty Canoes in the whole neighbourhood and these were single with out riggers, mostly made out of the trunks of trees, without any ornament and ill built. At the time we came out of the harbour, the Sea was ebbing and vast

[1] The MS leaves a space for a drawing, which, however, was not made; see below, p. 466.

[2] This 'stone' must have been Tridacna shell, rubbed down.

[3] The red colour was, according to Forster, II, p. 231, 'the yellow colour of turmerick'. —'. . . the Women are very ugly & wear a short grass apron round their Waist which reaches to the knees & have more the appearance of the Monkey race than human beings.'—Cooper. This insistence on the likeness to monkeys, which none of the extant drawings of Hodges bears out, is explained by the elder Forster, *Observations*, p. 267: 'In Mallicollo, we observed that the greater part of the skulls of the inhabitants, had a very singular conformation; for the forehead from the beginning of the nose, together with the rest of the head, was much depressed and inclining backward: which causes an appearance in the looks and countenances of the natives, similar to those of monkies.' The bridgeless nose, and possibly the wrinkling of the face in some people, which can be seen in modern photographs, added to the effect. George Forster, II, p. 229, was more appreciative: 'The features of these people, though remarkably irregular and ugly, yet are full of great sprightliness, and express a quick comprehension'.

[4] The *Casuarina equisetifolia* found in the Polynesian islands, and much used for weapons there.

[5] A great deal has been made since of these 'poisoned arrows'. The heads were of human bone, and they were subjected to magic charms, steeped in the juice of certain herbs, smeared with fancied sorts of dirt, and so on. In the ordinary European sense of the word they were not poisoned, but might bring tetanus, and certainly could prove fatal to the native, with his preconditioned and very suggestible mind. The really deadly thing was the charmed human bone. When one of these arrows was later tried on a dog, it suffered no ill effects, being psychologically unprepared—i.e. it did not know it was going to die, and therefore did not die. R. H. Codrington, *The Melanesians* (Oxford 1891), pp. 306–13, has an interesting discussion.

numbers of people were out on the shoals along the Coast, looking as we supposed for Shell and other fish; thus our being on their Coast and in one of their ports, did not hinder them from following thier necessary imployment, by this time they might be satisfied that we intended them no harm, so that had we made a longer stay, it is more than probable we should have been upon a good footing with this Apish Nation, for take them in gener[a]l they are the most ugly and ill proportioned people I ever saw and in every respect different from any we had yet seen in this sea. They are rather a Diminutive Race and almost as dark as Negros, which they in some degree resemble in thier countenances, but they have not such fine features. Thier hair is short and curled, but not so soft and wooly as a Negros, they have flat faces and long heads,[1] they weare a Cord or belt round their waist, just under the short ribs, and over the Middle of the belly, this is tied so tight, that they look as if they had two bellies, the one above and the other below the belt. The men are naked, it can hardly be said that they cover their natural parts, the Testicles are quite exposed, but the Penis is wraped round with a piece of cloth or a leafe, the lower end of which is tied up to the belt. Thier Beards as well as most of their woolly heads are of a Colour between brown and black, the former is much brighter than the latter and is more of hair than wool, but very crisp and curly. Their ornaments are Ear rings mad[e] of Tortise Shell, and Bracelets, a curious one of the latter they wear just above the elbow, it is about 4 or 5 inches broad worked with thred or Cord and studed with shells; round the right wrist they wear Hogs tusks bent circular[2] and Rings made of Shells: and round their left a round piece of Wood, this we jud[g]ed was to ward of the recoiling of the Bow string. The bridge of the nose is pierced in which they wear a piece of white stone about an inch and a half long and of this shape:[3]

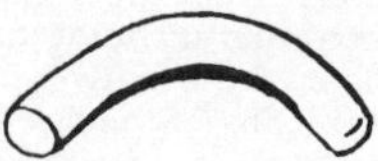

Thier signs of Friendship is a green branch and sprinkling water with the hand over the head.

[1] They are rather . . . heads *substituted for* They are of a very dark colour, inclining to black; little and slender, they have thick lips and flat noses; flat and monkey faces and long and woolly hair, and what adds to these infirmities . . .—f. 240.

[2] Not bent: the top tusk of the hog was knocked out when it was young, so that the bottom tusk grew without interference into a much admired and valued double circular form. Cook was on the edge of the great pig-cult of the New Hebrides, on which a good deal has been written.

[3] The shape here drawn is different from that of another nose ornament reported by Forster, II, p. 221: 'An old woman parted with two semi-transparent bits of selenites, cut

Their Arms are Clubs, Spears and Bows and Arrows the two former are made of hard, or a kind of Iron wood. Their Bows are about 4 feet long and made of a stick split down the middle, they are not circular but in this form.[1] The arrows are made of a sort of reeds, some are armed with a long and Sharp point, made of the hard wood, others are armed with a very sharp point made of bone; the points of these were all covered with a substance which we took for poison, indeed the people themselves confirmed our suspicions by makeing signs to us not to touch the point and giving us to understand that if we were pricked by them we should die, they are very carefull of them themselves, and keep them allways wraped up in a quiver; some of these arrows are Armed with two or three points, each with little prickles on the edges to prevent the arrows being drawn out of the wound. . . .

The Mallicollocans are quite a different Nation to any we have yet met with, and speak a different Language; of about Eighty Words which Mr F. collected[2] hardly one bears any affinity to the language spoke at any other island or place I had ever been at.[3] The letter R is used in many of their words, and frequently two or three together, such words we found difficult to pronounce. I observed that they could pronounce most of our words with great ease.[4] When they express their admiration of any thing they hiss like a goose.

To judge of the Country from the little we saw of it it must be Fertile, but I beleive their fruits are not so good as at the Society and Friendly Isles, their Cocoanutts I am certain are not and their Bread fruit and Plantains did not look to be much better. But their Yams seemed to be very good. We saw no other Animals than those I have already mentioned; they have not so much as a name for a Dog,

into a conical shape, and connected at the pointed ends, by means of a ribbon made of leaves. The diameter of the broad end was about half an inch, and the length of each bit three quarters of an inch. She took it out of the hole in the cartilage of her nose, which was very broad, ugly, and smeared with black paint'. It may have been this example which is shown in *Voyage*, II, pl. XVIII. The semi-transparency mentioned by Forster persuades one that this too was of Tridacna shell, the more usual material of the 'nose-sticks' or other ornaments of the Big Nambas of north-west Malekula. But Speiser, *Ethnographische Materialien aus den Neuen Hebriden und den Banks-Inseln* (Berlin 1923), p. 176, describes a 'quartz-stone' ornament, worn by chiefly persons, like Forster's; and his illustration is like that in the *Voyage*.

[1] The MS has no drawing: that here reproduced is from *Voyage*, II, p. 35. See also *Voyage*, II, pl. XVIII, for a bow of the conventional shape.

[2] The natives, says Forster (II, p. 213), 'with great goodwill sat down on the stump of a tree to teach us their language'.

[3] spoke . . . been at *substituted for* of the more Eastern islands no more than it does to the New Hollanders.

[4] Even the Russian *shtch*, says Forster. The Polynesians, except in Tonga and Samoa, had great difficulty with the sibilant, and generally substituted *h*.

consequently can have none, for which reason we left them a Dog and a Bitch;[1] there is no doubt but they will be taken care of and they were very fond of them.

After we had got to Sea, we tried what effect one of the poisoned arrows would have on a dog, indeed we had try'd it in the harbour the very first night, but we thought the operation had been too Slight as it had no effect. The Surgeon now made a deep incision in the dogs thigh into which he laid a large portion of the poison just as it was scraped from the arrows, and then bound up the wound with a bandage. For several days after we thought the dog was not so well as he had been before but whether this was realy so, or only suggested by imagination I know not; he afterwards was as well as if nothing had been done to him and lived to be brought home to England. I however have no doubt but this stuff is of a poisonous nature, indeed I could see no other purpose it could answer. The people seemed not unacquainted with the art of poisoning for when they brought us Water when we were on shore, they first tasted it and then gave us to understand we might safely drink it.[2] This Harbour, which is situated on the NE side of Mallicollo not far from the SE end in Latitude 16°25′20″ S, Longitude 167°57′23″ East, I named *Port Sandwich*, it lies in SWBS about one league and is one third of a league broad; a reef of Rocks extends out a little way from each point, but the channel is of a good breadth and hath in it from 40 to 24 fathom water; the depth of water in the Port is from 20 to four fathom and so Sheltered that no winds can disturb a Ship at Anchor in it and a nother great advantage is you can lie so near the shore as to cover your people who may be at work upon it.[3]*—ff. 240–1.

SUNDAY 24*th*. Gentle breezes and fair Weather. After stretching to the NE till 3 o'Clock we Tacked and Stood to the South in doing of which we discovered at least three small isles[4] laying off the SE point

[1] From the Society Islands, says Forster, and they were 'sold'.—II, p. 226.

[2] This was nothing to do with poison, but probably simply to guarantee that the water was good.

[3] Cook's luck did not always hold with harbours, but Port Sandwich is said to be the best one in the New Hebrides.

[4] *three small isles*: three or four small Islands which before appeared to be connected.—f. 241v. These were the Maskelyne islands, small and low, five of them in all; they lie on extensive coral reefs, and there is only one good anchorage among them. The name must have been conferred by Wales: for Cook seems to have had something of a distaste for the Astronomer Royal. At the end of the introduction to *Astronomical Observations*, p. lv, Wales writes, 'I cannot conclude, without observing that I have once, in the course of this work, stepped out of my province, and taken a liberty which I would wish not to be censured for. I had been at some pains to determine the situations of a group of small islands, to which I cannot find that any name has been assigned by Capt. Cook: I have therefore ventured to call them by the name of a person to whom I owe very much indeed; one who took me by the hand when I was friendless, and never forsook me when I had occa-

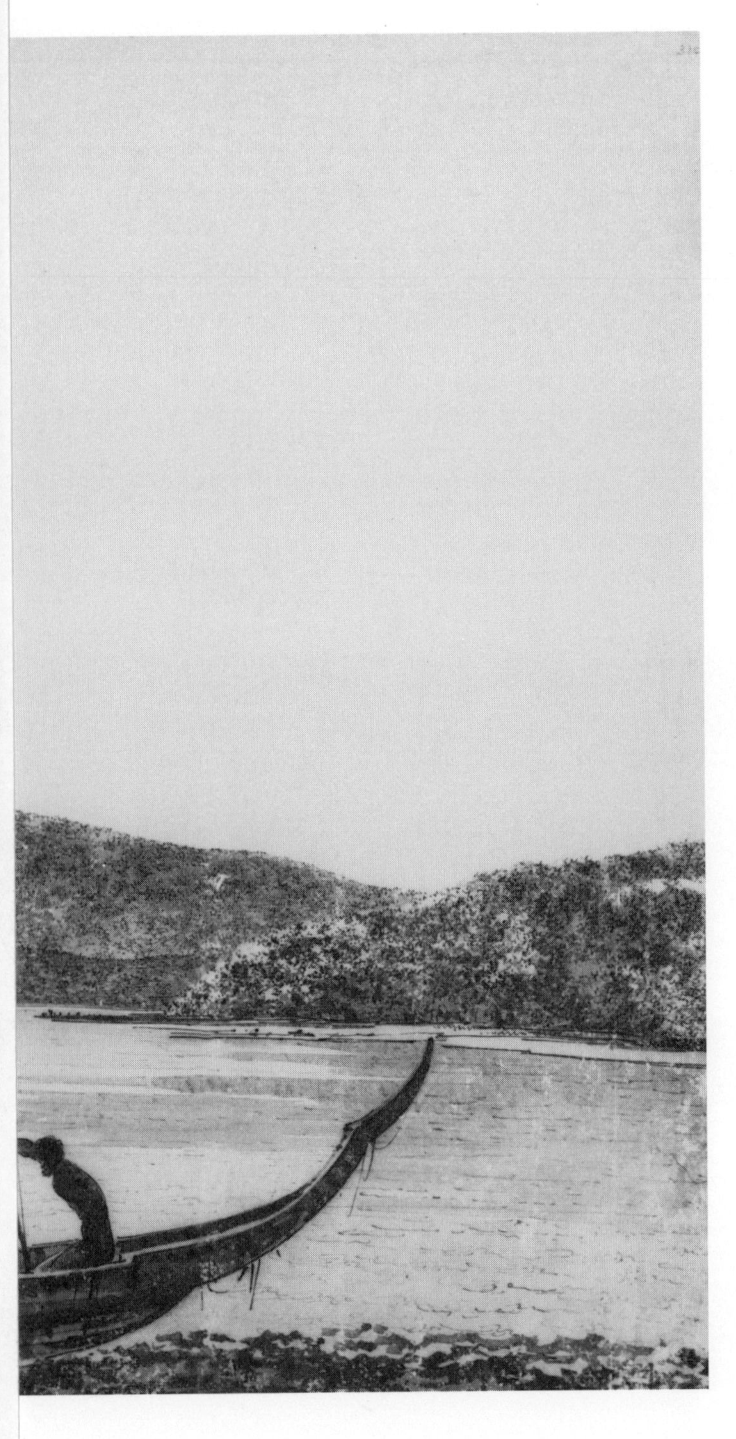

of Mallicollo, within which seem'd to be a good Bay or Harbour. At Sun-set this point bore S 77° West distant [3] Leagues from which the Coast seem'd to trend to the West at the same time we could clearly distinguish the Separation of the three to the East; the Isle of Ambrrym which lies between Whitsuntide Island and Mallecolla bore from N 3° East to N 65° E. The Isle of *Paoom* which lies next to it from N 76° E to S 88° E and the Isle *Apee* which is the Most Southermost extended from S 83 to S 43° East. The Wind Veering to E by N we fetched in with the West side of this last isle by Midnight where we made Short boards till day-break when we made sail to the SE close hauled. At Sun-rise we discovered Several isles in the space between EBS and SEBS the nearest of which we reached at 10 o'Clock, not being able to weather it we Tacked in 14 fathom water a Mile from the Shore. Three high round hills which are on this Island occasioned our calling it Island three hills,[1] it is about four Leagues in circuit and lies   from the South end of Mallicolla distant   Leagues and from the Isle of Apee   .[2]

West half a League from the west point lies a reef of Rocks level with the Sea.[3] At Noon the Island 3 hills bore SEBE distant 3 Leagues and the Isle of Apee from N 20° West to N 60° East. We could see several of what we took for Isles lying off the SE point of the last mentioned Isle and several others to the Southward of the former, in Short we were not Able to distinguish the number of isles a round us. Lat. by Reckoning [16°57′ S][4] Long[de] made from. . . .

The Night before we came out of Port two Red fish about the Size of large Bream[5] and not unlike them were caught with hook and line of which Most of the officers and Some of the Petty officers dined the next day. In the Evening every one who had eat of these fish were seiz'd with Violant pains in the head and Limbs, so as to be

sion for his help; and who, I hope, will not be offended at this public acknowledgement of his favours.' On p. 258, one of the bearings given for the observations of 23 July 1774 is 'Maskelyne's Isles'. This seems to be the first appearance of the name. It must have been through Maskelyne's good offices that Wales went to Hudson's Bay, as well as on this voyage; and he had worked on the *Nautical Almanac*. See Wales's chart, Fig. 65.

[1] Mai or Emae. The three hills rise from 1500 to 2170 feet.

[2] Mai lies roughly SEBE from Malekula about 48 miles; and about 15 miles south of Epi.

[3] The dangerous atoll called Pula Iwa, more exactly 2½ miles WNW of the western point of Mai.

[4] This figure is from Log 887—it is left blank in Log 956: 'the Sky was clouded so that we had no Observation, by our reckoning we were in lat. 16°57′ s'.

[5] The Forsters made no scientific record of this fish at the time; and unfortunately, when two more were caught at Tana, they were being prepared for the pot before anything could be done (George Forster, II, p. 311; J. R. Forster, *Descr. An.*, p. 249), and there is no drawing or detailed description of them. George Forster refers to them as 'red sea breams (*sparus erythrinus*)'; but this fish is confined to the Atlantic. G. P. Whitley, *Poisonous and Harmful Fishes* (Commonwealth of Australia C.S.I.R. Bull. 159, 1943, pp. 12–13), thinks they may have been the Chinaman Fish, *Paradicithys veneratus* Whitley, or Red Bass, *Lutjanus coatesi* Whitley.

unable to stand, together with a kind of Scorching heat all over the Skin,[1] there remained no doubt but that it was occasioned by the fish being of a Poisoness nature and communicated its bad effects to every one who had the ill luck to eat of it even to the Dogs and Hogs, one of the latter died in about Sixteen hours after and a young dog soon after shared the same fate.[2] These must be the same sort of fish as Quiros mentions under the name of *Pargos*, which Poisoned the Crews of his Ships,[3] so that it was some time before they recovered. We had reason to be thankfull in not having caught more of them for if we had we should have been in the Same Situation.

MONDAY 25*th*. In the PM the Wind veer'd to North with which we Stood for the group of Small Isles which lies off the SE Point of Apee, we reached them by 4 o'Clock and thought to have pass'd through one of the Channels but these being narrow and seeing broken water in the one we were steering for, I judged it more Safe to bear up to the South and go without them, but before this could be accomplished it fell Calm, thus we were left to the Mercy of the Currants[4] and Close to the Islands where we could find no Soundings with a line of 180 fathoms.[5] At 8 o'Clock we were relieved by a breeze from SE and we spent the night makeing Short boards. At day-break made Sail and Stretched to the East till after sun-rise when seeing no more land in that direction, and had reson to think there was none near

[1] . . . and numness in the joints . . .—f. 242.

[2] AB *note*, 'It was a Week or ten days before all the gentlemen recover'd'.—There are other witnesses: 'This Evening many of the Officers & people were seized with violent Reachings & excruciating pains from eating the fish (called Groopers) caught last night, also a Pig & sev[l] Dogs who had eat Some part of them were effected, notwithstanding we Boiled a Spoon with them which did not appear at all discoloured.—I remember a similar accident happen'd when I was in the P[ts] Louisa at Tobago in the West Indies with Adm[l] Tyrrell by eating the same kind of Fish that was supposed to have fed on a Copperas Bank whereby many of the Officers & people were seized in like manner. . . . This forenoon the Pig that was seized by eating the above Fish died in great agony, also a Parroquet; upon open[ing] the Pig we found the Lights all turn'd black round the edges.'—Cooper.—Elliott had been the fisherman: 'I caught, in the Night Watch a very fine Fish, which prov'd Poisonous, and by which Myself and three of my Mess Mates were Poison'd and were dangerously Ill, for several days and did not shake off the Effects of it for some time (the Hogs died Mad that eat of the Interals) and it caus'd an interuption to my Survey of *Tanna*, which never got finish'd to this day.'—Elliott *Mem.*, f. 33–3v. But it seems odd that his survey of Tana, which had not yet been seen, should have been interrupted—he must have had some lapse of memory. Forster gives a detailed account of the sickness, II, pp. 237–8, 243–5; on 27 July, he says (p. 244), 'We had not one lieutenant able to do duty; and as one of the mates, and several of the midshipmen were likewise ill, the watches were commanded by the gunner and the other mates'. Elliott had generously presented one of his fish to the lieutenants.

[3] At the Bay of St Philip and St James, Espiritu Santo, in May 1606.

[4] *thus* . . . *Currants:* when our Situation was none of the best, . . .—Log.

[5] . . . We had now land or Islands in every direction and were not able to count the number which laid round us; the Mountain on Paoom was seen over the East end of Apee bearing NNW.—ff. 241v–42.

from the Easterly Swell which we had we Tack'd and Stood for the land, which we had seen to the South having a gentle breeze at SE. In the PM we clearly distinguished the Eastern extremity of the Isle of *Apee* which terminates in a round hillock which at Sun-set bore N 24° W distant , over which appeared the high Mountain on the Isle *Paoom*. The Isles above mentioned which lies off the SE Point of Apee [I called Shepherds Isles, in honour of my Worthy friend D[r] Shepherd Plumian Prof[r] of Astronomy at Cambridge.][1]

The Isles Ambrrym, Paoom and Apee ly nearly in the direction of SSE and NNW of each other; the first is 20 Leagues in Circuit, its Shores are low and the land rises with a gentle assent and forms a tolerable high Mountain in the Middle of the isle, from which assended great Columns of Smoak, but we were not able to determine with any degree of certainty whether it was occasioned by a Volcano or no.[2] We Judged the isle to be well Inhabited from the Vast numbers of Smoaks we saw rising out of the woods in such parts of the isle as came within the Compass of our sight, nor did it appear less fertile. The Isle Paoom we only saw at a distance so that little can be said of it, it is of a considerable hieght but can hardly exceed Eight leagues in circuit, it is remarkable by a high Peaked Mountain near its East end, indeed we were not certain if this Mountain did not belong to a nother isle. Appearences seem'd to favour such a supposission.[3]

The Isle of Apee is not less than 20 Leagues in circuit, its greatest extent is nearly SE and NW in which direction it is not less than 8 or 9 leagues, its breadth is uncertain as we did not see its NE side, but cannot exceed 5 Leagues, it is of an unequal height, covered with wood and inhabited.

In stretching to the South we past to the East of three hills[4] and between a remarkable Peaked Rock, like a sugar loafe and of a con-

[1] I supply the words in square brackets, which Cook obviously forgot to supply himself, from a footnote in A 168, incorporated in the text of B in Cook's last red revision.—There are seven islands and a number of islets and rocks in the group. Antony Shepherd (1721–96), fellow of Christ's College 1747–83, held his chair from 1760; F.R.S. 1763. He held also a long succession of livings. His published works were confined to a preface to an astronomical table, 1772, and a syllabus of a course of lectures on experimental philosophy, 1776. Fanny Burney thought he was 'dullness itself'.

[2] It was.

[3] This was a good guess. Three miles east of Paama is the small island, or volcanic cone, called Lopevi. Paama rises to 1800 feet, but Lopevi to 4,775 feet, and it must have been this peak that Cook saw. Gilbert in his Chart XXXVII*a* shows two islands; the engraved chart (*Voyage*, II, pl. III) shows two only conjecturally.

[4] . . . and like wise of a low isle, which lies on the SE side of it . . .—f. 242. This can only be Makura; but Makura rises to 979 feet, which is hardly low, though it is certainly much lower than Mai.

siderable height, and a small Island, the Channel between them is one Mile broad and 24 fathoms deep, the former, which received the name of Moniment,[1] at Noon bore N 16° East and the Latter which hath on it two high and Peaked hills [Two Hills][2] Lat Ob^d 17°18′30″ s. Longitude made from [Port Sandwich] 45′ East. The Islands to the South extending from s 16°30′ E to 42° west.[3]

TUESDAY 26*th*. At 5 o'Clock in the PM we drew near the Southern land, which, from what we now saw of it, consisted of one large Island, whose Southern and western extremities extended beyond our sight and three or four Small Islands laying along its North side, the two outermost have[4] a good hieght and lay in the direction EBS and WBN from each other distant near 3 Leagues.[5] The light breeze which we had now left us and was Succeeded by a dead Calm which continued till 7 am in which time we had been carried by the Currents 4 Leagues towards the NW. We now saw the western end of the large Island and a Small Islot lying off it.[6] We now got a breeze from the westward and Steer'd SE in order to go between the two Isles above

[1] It is now on the Admiralty chart as Monument Rock; in the *Pacific Islands Pilot* it is called Wot. It is 397 feet high, and inaccessible: 'It is a resort for sea-birds, and, having little or no vegetation, its steep sides, whitened by guano, often give it the appearance of a sail in the distance, particularly on moonlight nights'.—*Pacific Islands Pilot*, II, p. 166.

[2] . . . disjoined by a low and narrow isthmus.—f. 242. This island is Mataso. The northern hill is 1643 feet high, the southern one 465 feet.

[3] *The Islands . . . west:* In this Situation the Moniment bore N 16° East distant 2 miles; Two hills bore N 25° West distant 2 Miles and in a line with the SW part of Three hills and the islands to the South extended from s 16°30′ E to s 42° West.—f. 242v.—There are times when one must read Cook with the closest attention to the chart, and this is one of them. If we regard the New Hebrides as a long screen stretching from north to south, we may say that what had happened so far was this: he had come from the east, round the north-east point of the screen, into the middle of its northern part; in the last twenty-four hours he had sailed through it again out to the east through a cluster of small islands, and then turned round as if he were coming back on to the western side, a little farther south. But, as we shall see in his next entry, he did not complete this movement: he reverted again to the eastern side of the screen, and sailed south. See Figs. 65, 66.

[4] *have:* are much the largest and have

[5] *near 3 Leagues:* 2 Leagues. I named the one *Montagu* and the other *Hinchinbrook* and the large Island *Sandwich*, in honour of my Noble Patron the Earl of Sandwich.—f. 242v. A168 has a note at 'Montague': 'In the Chart the names to these two Isles are misplaced'—i.e. reversed; this is so of the engraved chart (*Voyage*, II, pl. III). Gilbert, Chart XXXVII*a*, has the 'correct' attributions. But cf. p. 509, n. 7. Sandwich Island was Efate; Montagu Mau or Emau; Hinchinbrook Nguna. Montagu was of course Sandwich's family name, and Hinchinbrooke the name of his seat in Huntingdonshire.

[6] *4 Leagues . . . off it:* and a SE swell 4 Leagues to the WNW and passed Hinchinbrooke isle and saw the Wes[t]ern extremity of Sandwich island bearing SSW about 5 Leagues distant, at the same time, discovered a small isle to the west of this direction.—f. 242v. From where Cook was, he could not distinguish Verao and Lelepa, islands close to the west shore of Efate, from Efate itself. The 'western extremity of Sandwich island' was, therefore, probably the western extremity of Lelepa. Close by, on the reef to the west, is Knapp islet, but as this is only 40 feet high it is doubtful whether Cook would distinguish it. The small isle or 'islot' must have been Eradaka, 345 feet high, lying a little south, two miles out from Baffling Point, on the Efate coast.

mentioned.[1] At Noon we were in the Channel which divides the Eastermost from the large Island, the distance from the one land to the other is 1½ league or two leagues but the Channel is not more than a league, being contracted by breakers, the depth to us was unfathomable.[2] At this time our Lat. was 17°31′, Longit. made from [Port Sandwich] East. We could trace the large Island as far as SSE½E but could not see the end of it. The sides of this Isle opposed to us exhibited a most delightfull View, its Shores are low, the land rises with a gentle assent to the hills,[3] it is every where Spotted with Woods and Launds[4] and has the appearance of great fertillity but there is no approaching the Coast in this part, on account of rocks and breakers, but on the west side of the Small Isles above mentioned[5] there seem'd to run in a Bay, which if examined may be found to afford good Anchorage,[6] but this was not so much an object with me as [to] get to the South in order to find the Southern extremity of the Archipeloga. As we pass'd the Eastern Isle several people came down to the strand and by Signs seem'd to invite us on shore.[7] It ought to be remark'd that we have not yet seen a Isle on which we have not either seen people or signs of people, except the Moniment which is only accessable to Birds and by them Inhabit'd.

WEDNESDAY 27*th*. In the PM had[8] variable light airs next to Calm, so that we were apprehensive of being carried back by the Carrents, or rather that we should be obliged to return back through the Channell in order to avoide driving on the Shoals. Soundings we could find none with a line of 160 fathoms. At length we were relieved from our anxiety by a breeze at SW with which we stretchd to SE. At Sun-set the Moniment bore N 14°30′ West and the Eastern Isle

[1] *two . . . mentioned:* Montagu isle and the North side of Sandwich island, above mentioned.—f. 242v. But this is not what Cook first meant. The 'two Isles above mentioned' were 'the two outermost'—i.e. Hinchinbrooke or Nguna, and Montagu or Mau. He did sail between these, a course which also brought him between Montagu and Sandwich (see his next sentence).

[2] . . . with a line of 40 fathoms.—f. 243.

[3] . . . which are of a moderate height

[4] i.e. lawns, open grassy spaces. Cf. Cook on the New South Wales coast: 'The Mountains or Hills are Chequered with woods and Lawns' (I, p. 393); and again, pp. 510, 512 below. Laund was the original form of the word.

[5] *but on . . . mentioned:* but more to the West beyond Hinchinbrook isle,

[6] Undine Bay, formed by the northern coasts of Moso or Verao and Efate, with Nguna and the islands south-east of it, Pele and Kakula—which Cook saw, charted, but did not name (they were the others of the group 'the two outermost' of which he called Hinchinbrooke and Montagu). There is anchorage in the bay, but it is not particularly good.

[7] 'In Passing the S. Eastermost of the Small Isles [Montagu isle] we saw several people on the Shores who seem'd to invite us to them by waving a white Cloth and green branches.'—Log.

[8] *In . . . had:* We had but just got through the Passage, before the West wind left us, to . . .—f. 243.

above mentioned N 28° W dist. [3 Leagues]. The SE end of the large Island seem'd to terminate in a point which bore S 1° East. We continued to Stand to the SE till 4 o'Clock AM when we tack'd and stood to the West. At Sun-rise a new land was discovered bearing South, it appeared in three Hills,[1] seemingly so many Isles, but in order to determine this it was necessary to Tack and Stand towards it. At this time the Eastern Isle[2] bore N 52° West distant [13] Leagues. At Noon we judg'd it to have nearly the same bearing, the New land bore from S½E to SBW[3] distant Leagues. Lat ob^d^ 18°1' S. Longit. made from [Port Sandwich 1°23' East].[4]

THURSDAY 29*th*.[5] Gentle breezes and pleasent Weather. In the Evening found the Variation to be 9°3' East, the Southern land extending from S 31° west to S 61° W. And at Sun-rise from S 35° W to S 71° W[6] and appeared without any Separation,[7] we now made a trip to the west, having the wind at South but so little of it that we drifted faster to leeward than we went ahead. At Noon Lat O^b^ 18°25', Longitude in [169°49'] East;[8] the extremes of the land....

FRIDAY 30*th*. Light Airs next to a Calm all this 24 hours, Stood to the westward till 10 PM then Tack'd and Stood to the SE and East. Soon after Sun-rise the Variation by the Mean of Several Azim^ths^ taken with three Compases was 9°16' East. A little before 8 o'Clock we observed Several distances of the ☉ and ☽, the mean result of those made by me gave the Longitude [170°8'7½"] East and those made by Mr Wales [170°8'15"]. The Watch at the same time gave [169°20'00"] East,[9] the Latitude of the Place of observation was

[1] *it . . . Hills:* makeing in three Hommocs . . .—The land was Eromanga; it has a number of high hills, from 2500 to 3000 feet, and it is not easy to say precisely what Cook saw—possibly Mount Williams (3000 feet) in the north, Mount Robertson (3000 feet) rather more than half way down it, and the three hills, seen as one, of Traitors' Head (2700 feet).

[2] *the Eastern Isle:* Montagu isle

[3] . . . and the three hummoccs seemed to be connected.

[4] The sentence is left unfinished in the MS, f. 262, with a large blank space at the bottom of the page, apparently designed for later completion.

[5] This date and the two following ones are wrong, and what should have been Sunday 31st has disappeared altogether. B, which is very much abbreviated, does not help; nor do the other MSS. Four days of tacking may well have exasperated Cook into missing one of them.

[6] . . . distant about 10 or 12 leagues . . .—f. 243v.

[7] . . . the Three Hummocks mentioned above we now saw belonged to one Island, . . .—f. 243v, *red ink*.

[8] This figure is from Log 956.

[9] The figures in square brackets in this entry are from Log 887. I have worked out the means from Cook's figures: he himself merely gives a mean of the whole—which is, curiously enough, wrong. The full sum is 'Self 1st set 169°59'30", 2nd set 170°16'45"; Mr Wales 1st set 170°03'00", 2nd set 170°13'30"; Mean 170°08'06"'. The correct mean is surely 170°08'11¼". Log 956 does not supply the figures—as Log 887 in its turn has a blank for the longitude the previous day; B and the other MSS omit almost the whole entry.

18°26′ s. A high head or point on the North side of the Island bore s 61° West distant [14] Leagues and at noon it bore s 71° West. Lat Ob^d^ 18°30′ s. Tack'd and Stood to the West with a light breeze at South.

SATURDAY 31*st*. Light breezes between the sw and SE. At Sun-set we saw a new land bearing South[1] and SBW and lying nearly
from the Island we have had in sight the two preceeding days which at this time extended from s 38° w to s 79° w. At Sun rise we again saw the new land, bearing South, but at Noon it was sunk in the horizon, the other Island which we began to despair of reaching was nearly as far distant as yesterday at Noon, notwithstanding we took every advantage of the little wind we had. Obser^d^ Lat 18°35′ s.

[AUGUST 1774]

MONDAY 1*st*. Winds in the SE quarter light breezes, so that we gain'd nothing to windward. At 8 AM the breezes freshning at East s East, we stood South for the North end of the Island which at Noon bore South 23° East, distant Miles. Lat Ob^d^ 18°31′.[2]

TUESDAY 2*nd*. After geting round the Nothern point we rainged the West coast of the Isle at one Mile from Shore, the Natives appeared on several parts of the Coast and seem'd by Signs to invite us on Shore, at length we came to a Bay made by a small bend in the Coast about Miles from the NW point of the isle,[3] at the South part of this bay we found 30 and 22 fathom water near a Mile from Shore; I had some thoughts of anchoring but the Wind which had been at NE Veer'd presently round to NW which was partly on shore, besides I was unwilling to loose the oppertunity we had been so long waiting for to get up to the land we had discovered farther South, therefore continued to rainge along the Coast[4] about the same distance from shore but we soon got out of Soundings. Leagues south[5] of this last Bay, which hath about [2] Miles extent, we saw another rather more extensive,[6] the sun was set before we got the

[1] Cook got the name of this island later as Tanna; the native name was and is Ipari, but it is Tana on the modern chart. Cf. p. 489, n. 4 below.

[2] In the Log Cook gives an entry for 1 August on the variation. 'N.B. Sence we have been a Mongest these Islands, we have found it difficult to determine the Variation with accuracy Our Compasses have given from 8 to 12° the same Compass would vary so much on different days and even between the morning and evening of the same day, when the Ship's change of Situation has been but very little.' He had been using both Gregory's and Knight's compasses.

[3] Elizabeth Bay.

[4] . . . to the South

[5] *Leagues south:* about a league to the south

[6] Dillon Bay.

length of it and [the] wind began to abate.[1] At 8 o'Clock as we were Steering SSE we saw a light a head seemingly a good distance without the land. We had no idea of its being on the isle we had seen to the South for which we were now Steering, but supposed it to be on some low Island or Key which might be dangerous to approach in the Night, for this reason we hauled the wind and spent the night makeing short boards or rather driving to and fro for we had but very little wind. At Day light we could see nothing,[2] but found we had been carried by the Currants considerably to the Northward and attempted to little purpose to regain what we had lost. At Noon the Isl^d[3] Extend^d from S to NNE. Lat Ob^d 18°46′.

WEDNESDAY *3rd.* Finding the Ship not only to drive to the Northward but in Shore also and as we were yet to the Southward of the Bay we had pass'd yesterday, I had thoughts of geting to anchor while we had it in our power to make choise of a Place; for this purpose hoisted out two boats one of which was sent a head to tow and in the other the Master went to Sound for Anchorage and soon after the other boat was sent to assist him: On the South part of the Bay where it was most convenient for us to Anchor no bottom was to be found till close to the beach, and before the other parts could be examined the Ship drived past and made it necessary to call the Boat aboard to two her off from the Northern point, but this service was perform'd by a breeze of wind which very luckily sprung at SW and we hoisted them in and then bore up for the north side of the isle, intending to try once more to get round that way.[4] Mr Gilbert told me he just landed at the South part of the Bay[5] to taste of a Small Stream of Water he Saw there and which he found Salt, so that it must have come from a Pond behind the beach which must have some communicasion with the Sea; he saw some people without Arms but they came not near him.[6] At Sun rise in the Morning we found ourselves a breast of the head[7] and 3 Leagues from it, having had but little wind all night mostly from the South. Being in want of wood I sent two Boats under the Command of Lieut^t Clerk to

[1] . . . I intended not to stop here but to stand to the South under an easy sail all night, but . . .—f. 243v. This evening, narrates Forster, one of the marines fell overboard while drawing water to wash down the decks; the ship was brought to, and he was dragged out and revived with rum. It was William Wedgeborough.—Forster, II, pp. 249–50, 507.

[2] *could see nothing:* saw no more land than the Coast we were upon . . .—f. 244.

[3] *the Isl^d*: we were about a League from the shore of the coast which

[4] *that way:* by the East

[5] *he just . . . Bay:* that at the South part of the bay [i.e. Elizabeth Bay] he found no Soundings till close to a steep stone beach on which he landed

[6] . . . farther down the Coast, that is to the north, he found 20, 24 & 30 fathoms, ¾ of a mile or a mile from shore, the bottom a fine dark Sand.—f. 244.

[7] *the head:* a lofty promontory on the NE side of the island

a Small Island lying off the head to endeavour to cut some, seeing there could be no people to disturb them.[1] At Noon they return'd Empty having not been able to land by reason of a great Surf; there were no people on the Islot, at least they saw none or any thing remarkable. They saw a large batt and caught a Water Snake.[2] The wind veering round to ESE and East so that we could ly up for the head.

THURSDAY 4*th*. At 6 o'Clock in the PM we got in under the NW side of the head where we Anchored in 17 fathom Water half a Mile from the Shore, the bottom black sand. The Point of the head bore N 81° East distant   Miles,[3] the little Islot before mentioned NEBE½E and the NW point of land N 32° west. The Shore here forms a wide and tolerable deep Bay which lies open to ten points of the Compass (viz) from NWBN to East by North.[4] We had reason to form a favourable Idea of the Natives as several attempted to swim off to us as we were Standing in but retired when the boat went a head to Sound.

At day-break I went with two boats to view the coast and to look for a proper landing place, wood and Water. Several people appeared on the Shore and by signs invited us to go to them, I with some difficulty[5] on account of the rocks which every where lined the Coast, put a Shore[6] at one place where a few men came to us to whom I gave pieces of cloth, medals &c[a], for this treatment they offered to haul the boat over some breakers to a Sandy beach, I thought this a friendly offer, but afterwards had reason to think otherwise. When they saw I was determind to proceed to some other place, they ran along the Shore keeping always abreast of the boats and at last directed us to a place, a Sandy beach, where I

[1] . . . in the mean time we continued to ply up with the Ship, but what we got by our sails we lost by the current; at len[g]th, towards noon, we got a breeze at ESE and East with which we could lay up for the head.—f. 244v.

[2] This sea snake is referred to by Forster (II, p. 251) as *Coluber laticaudatus* Linn., and is figured in his drawings, pl. 170. Linnaeus' *Coluber laticaudatus* was a composite of two species, *Laticauda laticaudata* and *Laticauda colubrina* (Schneider); the specimen figured by Forster was the latter. Cf. p. 558, n. 7.

[3] *Miles:* half a league

[4] This was Polenia Bay, the extremes of which are 'the head' to which Cook has referred more than once—Traitors' Head, lat. 18°41′ S, long. 169°11′ E—and the north-east point of Eromanga, eight miles to the north-west. Traitors' Head is a high bluff, rising a little inwards to 2700 feet. The position where Cook was anchored is often called, in error, Port Narevin. There is no port, the name being derived from the native Pot-narivin—*pot*, place; *narivin*, sandy. The 'little Islot' is now called Goat islet; it is precipitous and rocky, five miles north-east of the head.

[5] *I with some difficulty:* I went first to a small beach which is towards the head, here I found no good landing

[6] *put a Shore:* I however put the boats bow to the shore

could step out of the boat without weting a foot.[1] I landed in the face of a great Multitude with nothing but a green branch in my hand I had got from of them,[2] I was received very courteously and upon their pressing near the boat, retired upon my makeing Signs to keep off, one Man who seem'd to [be] a Chief a Mongest them at once comprehending what I meant, made them form a kind of Semicircle round the bow of the boat and beat any one who broke through this order. After distributing a few trinckets a Mongest them[3] I ask'd by signs for fresh water in hopes of seeing where they got it, the Chief immidiately sent a Man for some, he ran to one of their houses and presently return'd with a little in a Bamboo so that I gained but little information by this. I next ask'd by the same means for some thing to eat and they as readily brought me a Yam and a few Cocoa nutts; in short I was charmed with thier behavour, the only thing which could give the least Suspicion was the most of them being Arm'd with Clubs, Darts, stones and bows and Arrows. The Chief made Signs to me to haul the Boat up upon the Shore but I gave him to understand that I must first go on board and then I would return and do as he disired and so step'd into the boat[4] and order her to be put of, but they were not for parting with us to soon and now attempted by force to accomplish what they could not obtain by more gentler means, the gang-board having been put out for me to come in some seized hold of it while others snatched hold of the Oars,[5] upon my pointing a musquet at them they in some measure desisted, but return'd again in an instant

[1] *When they . . . foot:* When they found I would not do as they desired they made signs for us to go down into the bay, which we accordingly did, and they ran along shore abreast of us and their number increased prodigiously; I put in to the shore in two or three places, not likeing the situation did not land: By this time I beleive the Natives conceived what I wanted, as they directed me round a rocky point where on a fine sandy beach I steped out of the boat without weting a foot . . .—ff. 244v–5.

[2] . . . I took only one man out of the boat with me and ordered the other boat to lie at a little dist[ce] off. . . .—f. 245.

[3] *After distributing . . . them:* This man I loaded with presents and gave like wise to others

[4] *The Chief . . . into the boat:* for this reason I kept my eye continualy upon the Chief and watched his looks as well as actions, he made many signs to me to haul the boat up upon the shore and at last sliped into the crowd where I observed him speak to several people and then return to me and made again signs to haul the boat up, and hesitated a good deal before he would receive some Spike Nails I then offered him. This made me suspect something was intended and immidiately steped into the boat . . .—f. 245.

[5] *the gang-board . . . Oars:* The gang board happened unluckily to be laid out for me to come into the boat; I say unluckily, for if it had not been out and the crew had been a little quicker in puting the boat off, the natives might not have had time to have put in execution their design and what followed would not have happened. As we were puting off the boat they laid hold of the gang board and by some means unhooked it off the boats stern; but as they did not take it away, I thought it had been done by accident and ordered the boat in again to take it up, when they themselves hooked [it] over the boats stern and attempted to haul her ashore; some at the same time snatched the oars out of the peoples hands . . .—f. 245v.

seemingly ditermined to haul the boat up upon Shore; at the head of this party was the Chief, and the others who had not room to come at the boat stood ready with their darts and bows and arrows in hand to support them: our own safety became now the only consideration and yet I was very loath to fire upon such a Multitude and resolved to make the chief a lone fall a Victim to his own treachery, but my Musquet at this critical Moment refused to perform its part and made it absolutely necessary for me to give orders to fire as they now began to Shoot their Arrows and throw darts and Stones at us, the first discharge threw them into confusion[1] but a nother discharge was hardly sufficient to drive them of the beach and after all they continued to throw Stones from behind the trees and bushes and one woud peep out now and then and throw a dart, four laid to all appearence dead on the shore, but two of them after wards cript into the bushes, happy for many of these poor people not half our Musquets would go of otherwise many more must have fallen. We had one man wounded in the Cheek with a Dart[2] the point of which was as thick as ones finger and yet it entered above two Inches which shews the force with which it must have been thrown.[3] An arrow struck Mr Gilberts naked breast but hardly[4] penetrated the skin, he was in the Cutter about 30 yards from the shore.[5] After all was over we return'd on board and I orderd the Anchor to be hove up in order to anchoring nearer the landing place, while this was doing several of the Islanders assembled on a low rocky point and there displayed two Oars we had lost in the Scuffle. I looked upon this as a Sign of Submission.[6] I was nevertheless prevailed upon to fire a four pound Shott at them to let them see the effect of our great guns, the ball fell short but frightned them so much that not one afterwards appeared,[7] the Oars they left standing up against the Bushes.

[1] The main endeavour was to get the boat off; 'but more was done to effect this, by a very fine young fellow of a Bowman, than half the Musquets, for he instantly spring into the midst of them, near the Bow of the Boat (his post) and stab'd and hook'd away at so desperate a rate, that he contributed much to the liberation of the Boat . . .'—Elliott *Mem.*, f. 30v.

[2] 'Soln Reardon on the upper lip with a Spear'.—Cooper.

[3] *the force . . . thrown:* that it must have come with great force indeed we were very near them.—f. 246.

[4] *but hardly:* but it probably had struck some thing before for it hardly.

[5] . . . The Arrows were pointed with hard wood.

[6] . . . and that they wanted to give us the Oars,

[7] '. . . one or two of the Guns being fired from the Ship tho they could not be got to bear ('till we hoisted one on the Forecastle) seemed to alarm them much'.—Mitchel.—Of this unhappy clash there exists at Eromanga a very circumstantial tradition. According to this the natives first saw the boats rowing off from Goat Island. Now nobody had ever landed on that island but ghosts, whose habitation it was; and therefore nobody could come from the island but ghosts, and ghosts could do nothing but harm. The panic-

The[1] Anchor was no sooner at the Bows than a breeze of wind sprung up at North which blew right into the Bay which with the best of winds was but an indifferent road and did not seem Capable of supplying all our wants,[2] I therefore resolved to leave it, set our Sails and plyed out accordingly but this was not accomplished at Noon when we observed in Latitude [18°43′ S]. These Islanders are a different race of people to those on Mallecollo and seem'd to speake a quite different language; they are of the Middle Size, have a good Shape and tolerable features, they are of a dark Chocolate Colour and paint their faces with a sort of black or Red Pigment,[3] their hair is very curly and crisp and some what Woolly: I saw some few Women which I thought ugly, they wore a kind of Petticoat made of Palm leaves or some plant like to them. The Men like those of Mallecollo have no other covering than the Case to the Penis which they tie up to a belt or string which they wear round the waist.[4]

FRIDAY 5*th*. About 2 o'Clock in the PM we were clear of the Bay bore up round the head and steered SSE for the South end of the

stricken Eromangans were determined to get rid of them as soon as possible, by any means. If ghosts would have departed at the price of water, well and good, but there was only one small stream at Potnarivin Bay, and that was nearly dry. So force had to be attempted. The chief's name was Narom: he was killed, but no others; and 'the Erromangans saw the ship vanish into air'. I owe this account to Evelyn Cheesman's charming small book, *Camping Adventures on Cannibal Islands* (London 1949), pp. 146–9. It does not explain some parts of Cook's story—why the natives attempted to swim off to the ship, or why they tried to pull the boat on shore—but it bears the marks of good folk-lore. There is a rather different account in the missionary H. A. Robertson's *Erromanga, the Martyr Isle* (1902), pp. 18–20, according to which the visitors were white *nobu* or gods, who had a wonderful fire and lived in a huge floating *lo* or kingdom. This account agrees that only Narom was killed.

[1] *The:* It was now Calm but the

[2] . . . with that conveniency I wished to have, besides I Allways had it in my power to return back to this place in case I found none more convenient farther to the South.—f. 246.

[3] There was a special black earth on Eromanga used for this purpose; the red pigment was a clay from the peak of Nilpon-u-moap—'place of red clay'—near Cook Bay. Both these desirable articles, wherever found, had their place in inter-island trade.

[4] B has here a curious but ethnologically important alteration. For the words 'which they tie . . . the waist' Cook first writes, 'which they tied up to the belt in the same manner'. He then has the red ink alteration, 'which was not tied up to the belt which they wore about their waist'. It is difficult to explain this contradiction from any other source; and the first statement is confirmed by Hodges, *Voyage*, II, pl. XLII—for what that assemblage of classical poses is worth. But it is wrong. The printed page, with some delicacy, hedges: 'the men, like those of Mallicolo, were in a manner naked; having only the belt about the waist, and the piece of cloth, or leaf, used as a wrapper'.—*Voyage*, p. 49, with a reference to p. 34, which does not tell us much more. On this point C. B. Humphreys, without the benefit of Cook's MSS, writes, 'One can only suppose that, in his haste, his usual accuracy in observation deserted him and that his recollection became mixed with that of Malekula, for the *yelau* [penis case] of Eromanga has never been worn inserted in the belt'.—*The Southern New Hebrides* (Cambridge 1926), pp. 134–5. B adds, 'I saw no Canoes with these people, nor had we seen any anywhere about the island, they live in houses covered with thatch and their plantations are laid out by line and fenced round'. Cf. Clerke 8952: 'We saw nothing like a Canoe or Boat among them—whoever of them are desirous of a little party upon the water I believe must conduct themselves upon their own Oars'.

Island having the Advantage of a fresh gale at NW. On the SW side of the head runs in a Deep Bay,[1] seemingly behind the one on the NW side, its Shores are low and the adjacent lands had greatly the appearences of fertility, it is exposed to the SE wind, therefore untill it is better known, the NW Bay must be prefered, in case any Ship should be under the Necessity of touching at this Isle.[2] The high Promontary or Peninsula which disjoins these two Bays I called Traitors head from the treacherous behavour of its inhabetants, but the Island is called by them Erramango of which Traitors-head is the NE point[3] and lies in Latitude 18°43′, Longitude [169°28′] East.[4] As we advanced to the South the New Island we had before seen began to appear in one with the SE end of Erromango bearing S½E distant from each other 10 or 11 leagues. At half past 6 o'Clock in the evening the South point of the last mentioned isle bore due west, by our reckoning from Noon we were in Lat and had now made the circuit of the isle which is . The Middle is situated in Latitude 18° ′ Long[d] 16 ° ′ East[5] and ; its Shores are in places low but there are hills in the Middle[6] which may be seen as also Traitors head 15 Leagues: we had reason to form a favourable Idea of the Soil, as few parts appeared barren and Plantations were every were seen, laid out by line and fenced round, like those we had seen before. After leaving this Island we shaped our Course for the East end of the one to the South, being guided by a great fire we saw upon it. At 1 o'Clock[7] we came near the Shore and made it necessary to shorten Sail and spend the remainder of the night making Short boards. At day break we discovere'd a high table land[8] bearing EBS and a smal low isle bearing NNE which we had passed in the night,[9] Traitors head was still in sight bearing N 20° west and the Island to the Southward extending from S 7° W to S 87° W distant about one League, we now found that what we had taken for a common fire in the Night was a Volcano which threw up vast quantaties of fire and smoak and made a rumbling

[1] Cook Bay.

[2] *in case . . . Isle:* because it is sheltered from the reigning winds; the Winds it is open to, viz. from NWbN to EbN, seldom blow strong.—f. 246v.

[3] Strictly speaking, this is not true; the north-east point of the island is about eight miles further up the coast. Traitors' Head has the native name Wakwi.

[4] . . . It terminates in a Saddle Hill which is of a height sufficient to be seen 16 or 18 leagues.—f. 246v.

[5] Cook seems to have omitted to work out these figures, which are, roughly, lat. 18°48′ S, long. 169°5′ E.

[6] See p. 474, n. 1 above.

[7] . . . in the Morning

[8] . . . (an island) . . .—f. 247. It was Futuna.

[9] . . . without seeing it.—This was Aniwa.

noise which was heard at a good distance.[1] Soon after we had made Sail for the East end of the island we discovered an Inlet which had the appearence of a harbour, as soon as we drew near I sent two Arm'd Boats under the command of Lieut[t] Cooper and the Master to examine and Sound it while we stood on and off with the Ship to be ready to follow or give them any assistance they might want. On the East point were a great number of People Hutts and Canoes, some of the latter they put into the Water and followed our boats but came not near them. It was not long before our boats made the Signal for Anchorage and we stood in accordingly: the Wind being at West, we borrowed close to the west point and pass'd over some Sunken Rocks which would been have avoided by keeping a little more to the East. The wind left us as soon as we were within the entrance and obliged us to drop an anchor in 4 fathom water when the boats were sent again to Sound and in the mean time the Launch was hoisted out and as soon as we were acquainted with the Channel, laid out warps and warped farther in. While this work was going forward Vast numbers of the Natives had collected together on the Shores[2] and a great many came off in Canoes and some even Swam off, but came not nearer than a stones throw and those in the Canoes had their Arms in constant readiness; insensibly they became bolder and bolder and at last came under our Stern and exchanged some Cocoa nutts for pieces of Cloth &c[a]; some more daring than the others were for carrying off every thing they could lay their hands upon[3] and made several attempts to knock the rings of[f] the rudder, the greatest trouble they gave us was to look after the Buoys of our anchors which were no soon let go from the Ship or thrown out of the boats than they lay hold of them, a few Musquets fired without any design to hit had no effect, but a four pounder threw them into great confusion, made them quit their Canoes and take to the water but seeing none were hurt they presently recoverd their fright and returned to their Canoes[4] and once more attempted to take away the buoys, this put us to the necessity of firing a few Musketoon shot over them which had the desired effect and altho none were hurt

[1] 'Saw a very large fire on the shore which at daylight we found to be a Volcano from which issued prodigious clouds of smoke, succeeded by very loud bellowings equal to loud claps of Thunder.'—Cooper.

[2] . . . all armed with Bows Spears &c[a] . . .—f. 247v.

[3] *exchanged . . . hands upon:* made some exchanges. The people in one of the first Canoes, after coming as near as they durst, threw towards us some Cocoa nuts, I went into a boat and picked them up and gave them in return some Cloth & other things; this induced others to come under the Stern and a long side where their behavour was insole[n]t and daring; their was nothing within their reach they were not for carrying off, they got hold of the fly of the Ensign and wanted to tear it from the Staff; . . .

[4] . . . gave us some holloas, florished their weapons

they were afterwards afraid to come near them and at last retired to the Shore and we were suffered to set down to dinner undisturbed. During these transactions a friendly old man in a small Canoe made several trips between us and the shore, bringing with him 2 or 3 Cocoa nutts or a yam each time and took in exchange what ever we gave him: another was on the gang way when the great gun was fired, but he was not to be prevailed upon to stay long after.

SATURDAY *6th.* Wind at South a fresh breeze and fair weather. In the PM after the Ship was moor'd I landed with a strong party of Men at the head of the harbour[1] without any opposition being made by a great number of the islanders assembled in two parties the one on our right and the other on our left, all arm'd with darts, clubs, slings, bows and arrows: after our men were drawn up upon the beach I distributed to the old people presents of pieces of Cloth, Medals &c[a] and ordered two Casks of Water to be fill'd out of a Pond which we found conveniently situated behind the beach,[2] giving the Natives to understand it was what we wanted. We got from them a few Cocoa-nuts which seem'd to be in plenty on the trees, but they would not on any account part with any of their Arms which they held in constant readiness and press'd so much upon us that[3] little was wanting to make them attack us, however no attempt was made, our early embarqueing probably disconcerted their scheme and after that they all retired.[4]

I now found it was practical to lay the Ship nearer to the landing place, and as we wanted to take in a large quantity of both wood and Water it would greatly facilitate that work as well as over-awe the Natives and be more ready to assist our people on Shore in case of an attack, we therefore in the morning went to work to transport her: while this was doing we observed the Natives assembling from all parts to the landing or Watering place where they form'd themselves into two parties one on each side the landing place, we judged there were not less than a thousand people[5] arm'd in the same manner as in the evening. A Canoe conducted some times by one and at other times by 2 or 3 Men would now and then come off

[1] . . . in the SE cornner . . .—f. 248.

[2] 'here we found a Pool of excellent Water not above Twinty yards from the shore and wood for fuel equally as convenient . . .—Log.

[3] *and press'd . . . that:* and in the proper attitude for using them, so that . . .

[4] . . . The friendly old man before mentioned was in one of these parties and we judge from his conduct that his disposition was pac[i]fick.—f. 248. Cf. Clerke 8952: '. . . their behaviour upon this our first Visit was not the most friendly I've ever experienc'd among Indians—they did not insult us tis true but they did by no means seem reconcil'd to the liberty we took in landing upon their Coasts . . .'

[5] *we judged . . . people:* to the amount of some Thousands, . . .—f. 248v.

from them, invite us to go a Shore and bring us a few Cocoa-nuts or Plantains which they gave without asking for any thing in return but I took care they always had some thing. One of those who came off was the old man whose beheavour had attracted our attention yesterday. I gave him to understand by Signs (for we could not understand one another) that they were to lay a side their Arms, took those which were in his Canoe and threw them over board,[1] there was no doubt but he understood me and I believe made it known to his country men on shore for as soon as he landed he went first to the one party and then to the other, and as to himself he was never after seen with any thing like a weapon in his hand. Three fellows coming under the Stern in a Canoe offered a Club[2] for a String of beads and some other trifles all of which I sent down to them, but the Moment they were in their possession they padled off in all haste without makeing any return, this was what I expected and what I was not sorry for as I wanted a pretence to shew the Multitude on shore the effect of our fire arms without materially hurting any of them, having a Musquet[3] ready load[ed] with Small Shott, (N° 3) I gave one of the fellows the Contents into the bargin and when they were above Musquet shott off, order'd 3 or 4 Musketoons or Wall pieces to be fired at them which made them quit the Canoe and keep under her off side and swim with her to the shore, this transaction seem'd to have little or no effect on the two divisions on shore, on the contrary they seem'd to think it sport.

After mooring the Ship by four anchors with her broad side to the landing place, from which she was hardly Musquet Shott, and placeing our Artillery in such a manner as to command the whole harbour, we embarked the Marines and a party of Seamen in three boats and rowed in for the Shore; I have already observed that the two divisions of the Natives were drawn up on each side the landing place, the space between was 30 or 40 yards, here were laid to the most advantage a few bunches of plantains, a yam and two Tara roots, between them and the shore were stuck in the sand four small reeds about 2 feet from each other in a line at right angles to the sea shore, for what purpose they were put there I never could learn;[4]

[1] . . . and made him a present of a large piece of cloth.

[2] *offered a Club:* one of them brandishing a Club, with which he struck the Ship side and commited other acts of defiance, but at last offered to exchang it . . .—f. 248v.

[3] *Musket:* fowling piece

[4] *for what . . . learn:* ABG *note* These reeds remained sticking in the Sand for two or three days after, but I never could learn their meaning.—Mr G. S. Parsonson, of the University of Otago, who has given much study to the New Hebrides, on this passage makes the following comment: 'I think the explanation is simple enough. They were placed to indicate that the food was *tapu*. This was the normal method of indicating that coconut

the old man before mentioned and two more stood by these things and by Signs invited us a Shore, but we were not in a hurry to land, I had not forgot the trap I had like to have been caught in at the last isle and this looked some thing like it; we answered the old men by makeing signs that the two divisions must retire farther back and give us more room, the old men seem'd to desire them so to do but as little regard was paid to them as us. More were continually joining them, and except the 3 old men, not one was without arms: In short every thing conspired to make us believe they intended to attack us as soon as we were on shore. The consequence of such a step was easily seen, many of them must have been kill'd and wounded and we should hardly have escaped unhurt.[1] Sence therefore they would not give us the room we required I thought it was best to frighten them away rather than oblige them by the deadly effect of our fire Arms and accordingly order a Musquet to be fired over the heads of the party on our right for this was by far the Strongest body, the alarm it gave them was only momentary, in an instant they recovered themselves and began to display their weapons, one fellow shewed us his back side in such a manner that it was not necessary to have an interpreter to explain his meaning;[2] after this I ordered three or four more to be fired, this was the Signal for the Ship to fire a few four pound Shott over them which presently dispersed them and then we landed and marked out the limits on the right and [left] by a line. Our old friend stood his ground all the time, tho' diserted by his two companions, the moment we landed I made him a present of Cloth and other things I had taken with me for the purpose.[3] In-

trees, for example, were not to be touched. Moreover, the natives clearly looked upon Cook as a returned ancestor. Hence the very small quantity of food. The offerings to the ancestors were always very small and their quality poor. And they were tapu. I think it significant that the natives showed so little surprise at Cook's arrival. There was excitement, it is true. But they soon showed the greatest familiarity. Cook's colour must have afforded them further proof that he had returned from the dead. He was white. I have a notion, too, that the line of reeds was also designed to discover whose ancestor Cook was—whether that of the party to the left or that to the right'. There seem to have been two different clans present.

[1] . . . two things I equally wished, by every possible means to prevent.—ff. 249–9v.

[2] '. . . one of them turned his backside to us and beat it, like a monkey. For this contemptuous challenge he was sufficiently rewarded, for the Lieutenant of Marines told me he could not restrain himself from aiming a charge of shot at the proffered target.'—Sparrman, p. 145.—This sort of mild obscenity might have been the prelude to worse, and was typical of the gestures with which New Hebrideans, often hot-tempered people, would provoke battle. As Cook rightly judged, there was a very even balance between peace and war. One did not necessarily welcome one's ancestors, who must be 'ghosts'. There had been no hesitation over what to do about ghosts at Eromanga.

[3] Our first care was to draw up the marines in two lines, to guard the waterers. Stakes were driven into the ground on both sides, and ropes fastened to them, leaving a space of fifty or sixty yards clear, for our people to pass and repass unmolested.'—Forster, II, p. 273.

sencibly the Natives came to us seemingly in a more friendly manner, some even came without arms, but by far the greatest part brought them and when we made signs to them to lay them down, they told us to lay down ours first; they climed the Cocoa trees and threw us down the Nutts, without requiring any thing for their trouble, but we took care they were always paid. After filling half a doz^{n} Small Casks with Water and obtaining leave of the old man whose name was [Paowang][1] to cut wood for fireing, just to let the people see what we wanted we return'd on board to dinner after which they to a man retired.[2] I never learnt that any one of them was hurt by our Shott.[3]

SUNDAY *7th.* Wind at SW a fresh gale. In the PM landed again, laded the launch with Water and made three hauls with the Sein in which we caught upwards of 300 lb^{s} of Mullet and other fish. We had been on shore some time before any of the Natives appeared and not above 20 or 30 came to us at last the most of them without arms, our trusty friend [Paowang] made us a present of a small Pig.[4] We were now in hopes they would give us no farther trouble. In the night the Volcano[5] threw up vast quantities of fire and Smoak, the flames were seen to ascend above the hill between us and it, the night before it did the same and made a noise[6] like that [of] thunder or the blowing up of mines at every eruption which happened every four or five Minutes; a heavy shower of rain which fell at this time seem'd to increase it: the wind blew from that quarter and brought such vast quantities of fine Sand or ashes that every thing was

[1] In B Cook begins with 'Paowang', slips into 'Taowang', and then reverts to 'Paowang' without further change. Forster 'Pawyangom'.

[2] *they told us . . . retired:* gave us to understand that we must lie [*sic, altered from* lay *in red*] down ours first; thus all parties stood with their arms in hand. The presents I made to the old people and to such as seemed to be of consequence, had little effect on their conduct. They indeed climed the Cocoa nutt trees and threw us down the Nutts without requiring any thing for them, but I took care, they allways had something in return, I observed [*deleted* that they gave us these with a sparing hand] there were many who were afraid to touch any thing which belonged to us & they seemed to have no notion of exchanging one thing for another. I took the old man, (whose Name we now found to be Paowang) to the Woods and made him understand, I wanted to cut down such and such trees to take on board the Ship, cuting some down at the same time, which we put into one of our boats together with a few small casks of water with a view of leting the people see what it was we chiefly wanted. Paowang very readily gave his consent to cut wood, nor was there one who made the least objections, he only desired that the Coco nutt trees might not be cut down. Matters being thus settle[d] we imbarked and return'd aboard to dinner and immidiately after they went away to a man.'—ff. 249v–50.

[3] *footnote* either on this or the preceding day which was a very happy circumstance . . .—f. 250.

[4] *footnote* which was the only one we got at the isle, or that was offered us. AG this was the only Pig . . .

[5] . . . (which was about 4 miles to the West of us) . . .—f. 250. The volcano is called Mount Yasur or Yasua. It is still in constant activity. See the view, Chart XXXVII*b*.

[6] *a noise:* a long rumbling noise

covered with it,[1] and was also exceeding troublesom to the eyes. In the Morning the Natives again Assembled about the watering place Arm'd as usual, but not in such numbers as at the first. After breakfast we landed in order to cut wood and fill Water, we found many of the Natives inclinable to Peace, especially the old men, while many of the younger sort were very daring and insolent and obliged us to stand with our Arms in hand. After every thing was properly disposed on Shore,[2] I return'd on board and left the party under the Command of Lieut^ts Clerk and Edgcomb, when they came on board to dinner they inform'd [me] the Natives continued to behave in that inconsistant manner they had done in the morning and one man carried his insolence so far that Mr Edgcomb was obliged to fire upon him and believed he was wounded with a Slug shott.[3] While we were at dinner an old man came on board, look'd at some parts of the Ship and then return'd a Shore.

MONDAY 8*th*. In the PM most of the Natives retired as usual, a few who lived in the neighbourhood only remained with whom we were upon a tolerable footing. One of our people having lift an Ax in the woods, it was picked up by one of the Natives and return'd us by our friend.[4]

In the Morning sent the Launch[5] to the other side of the harbour to take in ballast which we were in want of, this work was performed before breakfast after which she was sent for Wood and Water, and in her the people who were employed on this service under the protection of a Serjt^s guard which was now thought sufficient as the Natives seem'd more complaisant than ever, they even, as I was told, invited some of our people to go home with them, on condition they would strip naked as they were.[6]

TUESDAY 9*th*. Wind at SE fair weather. In the AM sent the Launch again to the west side of the harbour for more ballast, the guard and Wooders to the usual place, with the latter I went my self. A good

[1] ... it was a kind of fine sand or like stones ground or burnt to powder,

[2] *After* ... *Shore:* I stayed till I saw no disturbance was like to happen and then

[3] ... after that the others behaved with a little more discrition and as soon as our people came on board they all retired.—f. 250v.

[4] ... some other articles were also returned us which they either had stolen or had been lost through the carelessness of our own people, so carefull were they now not to offend us in this respect.—The point here rather is that the New Hebridean in general did not want any people's property (though cf. 5 and 6 August). It was too dangerous—it would put the thief (or even the quite well-intentioned appropriator) in the owner's power. But the coming of new needs and the breaking down of ancient tabus made these same islanders by the middle of the nineteenth century the worst thieves in the Pacific.

[5] ... under the protection of a party of Marines

[6] ... this shews that they had no design to robb them what ever other they might have. —f. 251.

many of the Natives were collected together as usual whose beheavour tho Arm'd was very pacific[1] as gave us as much room as we desired, so that it was no longer necessary to mark out the ground by a line, they strictly observed the limits without.[2] When I return'd on board to dinner I prevailed on a young man whose name was Wha-agou[3] to accompany me, as we had nothing to eat but salt beef and pork he did but just taste the latter, but eat pretty heartily of yam and drank a glass of Wine.

WEDNESDAY 10*th*. After dinner[4] I shew'd Whaagou all parts of the Ship, I did not observe that any thing fixed his attention a moment or caused in him the least surprise, he had not the least knowlidge of a Goat, Dog or Catt, he called them all Hogs (Bōōga or Bōōgas)[5] he shewed a great desire for a Dog and I accordingly gave him both a Dog and a Bitch, a hatchet and a piece of cloth and then conducted him a Shore, while he was on board some of his friends brought me off a little Sug[r] Cane, a few Cocoa-nutts & a Cock.[6] As soon as we landed the youth and some of his friends took me by the hand in order to conduct me to thier habitations, at least so I understood. We had not gone far before some of the company, for what reason I know not, was unwilling I should proceed in consequence of which the whole company stoped, and if I did not mistake them some were detatched for some fruit &c[a] for me, for I was desired to sit down and wait which I accordingly did, during which time several of our Gentlemen pass'd us, at which they shewed great uneasiness and importuned me so much to order them back that I was at last obliged to comply, they were jealous at our making the least excursions inland or even along the shore of the harbour.

While I was waiting here Paowang came with a present of fruit and roots, brought by about 20 men, in order, as I supposed to make it appear the larger, one carried a small bunch of plantans, a nother a yam, a third a Tara root &c[a] but [two] men might with ease have

[1] *pacific:* Courtious and obliging

[2] . . . As it was necessary for Mr Wales's instruments to remain on shore all the middle of the day, the guard did not come off to dinner as they had done before till releived by others.—f. 251.

[3] Forster 'Fannòkko'.

[4] *After dinner:* Before we sat down to dinner.—f. 251. This is a minor change, but one is curious to know what slip of memory or principle of literary composition prompted it. In any case (to be fussily pedantic) Forster says 'After dinner'.

[5] An obviously Polynesian word; cf. Tahitian and Marquesan *puaa*, Tongan and Rarotongan *puaka*.

[6] *while . . . a Cock:* Soon after he came on board some of his friends came off in a canoe and enquired for him, probably they were doubtfull of his safety, he looked out of the quarter gallery and spoke to them and then they went ashore and soon after return'd with a Cock, a little sugar cane and a few cocoanutts, as a present to me.—f. 251.

carried the whole with ease.[1] This present was in return for some things I had given him in the Morning, I however did not now on that account send him and his train away empty handed.[2] After despatching these people I return'd to Wha-a-gou and his party who were still for detaining me and seem'd to wait with impatience for some thing or a nother,[3] but as night was approaching I press'd them to be gone and so we parted.

Yesterday Mr Forster obtained from these people the Name of the Island (Tanna) and to day I got from them the names of those in the nieghbourhood.[4] They gave us to understand in such a manner which admited of no doubt that they eat human flesh, they began the subject themselves by asking us if we did:[5] they like wise gave us to understand that Circumcision was practised amongest them. While the Launch was taking in ballast on the West side of the harbour, one man employed on this work scalded his fingers in takeing up a stone out of some water, this circumstance produced the discovery of several hot springs at the foot of the clift rather below high-water mark.[6] In the AM Mr F. and his party made an excursion

[1] The gift was no doubt symbolical—another application, it seems, of the ancestor theory of Cook's visit.

[2] *I however . . . empty handed:* however I thought the least I could do now was to pay the porters.—f. 251v.

[3] . . . and were unwilling and seemed to be a shamed to take away the two Dogs without makeing me some return, or at least so I thought;

[4] . . . the one we touched a[t] last is called *Erromango*, the small Isle we discovered the morning we anchored here *Immer*, the table island to the East discovered at the same time, *Erronan* or *Footoona* and an island which lies to the SE *Annattam*: all these islands are to be seen from Tanna.—f. 252. In modern versions and orthography, Eromanga; Aniwa, Immer, or Niua; Futuna; Aneityum; Tana. Forster's information was, in fact, wrong. Cf. Humphreys, p. xv: 'The native of an insular region of moderate size seems never to have a name for his own homeland until he has been a journey away from it. For instance, the proper native name for the island of Tanna is Ipari, which is given it by the natives of the other islands of the sub-group, all of which are in sight of it, when they point to it or mention it in any connection. The word *tanna* means 'ground' or 'earth' in the Waisisi dialect, and Captain Cook's [i.e. Forster's] mistake in thinking, when he pointed to the ground, that the native would give him the name of the island, and not of the object at which his finger pointed, was perfectly understandable from his point of view, but took no note of the workings of the native mind. . . . Curiously enough, the name given by Cook has survived to this day, and there has never been any question of calling this island by the native name given it by its neighbours, or any other. . . . The native name for Eromanga is, reciprocally, that given it by the Tannese when they speak of it or point to it'. The inhabitants of Futuna call Tana *Ekiamo*; but the tendency nowadays is for everybody to use the names used by Europeans.

[5] . . . otherwise we should never have asked them such a question. I have heard people argue that no Nation would be cannibals, if they had of other flesh to eat, or did not want victuals, and so lay the Custom to necessity; the people of this island can be under no such necessity, they have fine Pork and Fowls and plenty of roots and fruit; but sence we have not actually seen them eat human flesh, it will admit of some doubt that they are Cannibals.—f. 252. Forster, however, got pretty explicit information, II, p. 300; and the Tanese and other New Hebrideans were, and enjoyed being, cannibals.

[6] 'Found the water which discharged it self from the Rocks under the Volcano extremely warm, in which we dipped two Men (for some disorder) tho, not without its first cooling'.—Mitchel, description of Tana.

into the country, he met with civil treatment from the Natives and saw several fine Plantations of Plantains, Sugar Cane, roots &c[a]. The people now, especially those in our neighbourhood are so well reconciled to us that they take no notice of our going a Shooting in the woods.

THURSDAY 11*th*. Wind at South with some heavy showers of rain in the night. In the pm two or three boy's got behind some thickets and threw 2 or 3 stones at our people, who were cuting wood, for which they were fired at by the petty officers present. I was much displeased at such an abuse of our fire Arms[1] and took measures to prevent it for the future. During the night and all the next day the Volcano made[2] a terrible noise throwing up prodigeous colums of Smoak and fire at every erruption;[3] at one time great stones were seen high in the air. In the AM beside the necessary work of Wooding and Watering, we struck the main-top-mast in order to fix new Tristle-trees and a pair of new back stays. M[r] F. made a little excursion up the hill on the west side the harbour where he found three places from whence assended Smoak or Steam of a Sulpherous smell,[4] they seem'd to keep pace with the Volcano, for at every erruption the quantity of smoak or steam was greatly increased and forced out of the ground[5] in such quantities as to be seen at a great distance which we had before taken for the smoak of common fire; it is at the foot of this hill the hot springs before mentioned are.

FRIDAY 12*th*. In the After-noon M[r] F. carried his botanical excursions to the other side of the harbour and fell in with Paowang's house where he saw most of the articles I had given him hanging on the adjoining bushes, probably they were in his eyes of so little Value as not to be worth house room.[6] Some of the gentlemen accompanied

[1] *I was . . . Arms:* I who was on shore at the time, was alarmed at hearing the report of the Muskets and saw two or three boys run out of the wood, but when I knew the cause I was much displeased at such a Wanton use being made of our fire arms . . .—f. 252v.

[2] *made:* was exceeding troublesome and made

[3] . . .which happened every 3 or 4 Minutes . . .—The trouble with this volcano was that an evil spirit called Iaramus lived in the vent playing with fire and red-hot stones. The spirits of the dead also congregated there. 'The crater', writes Mr Parsonson, 'is about 1200 feet deep and about three quarters of a mile across. The peak is about 600 feet high, rising in a cone above a bare plain. On the landward side there is a lake. The scene is most desolate and awe-inspiring'. There is another interesting description in Miss Cheesman's *Things Worth While* (1957), pp. 189–91.

[4] . . . from cracks or Fissures in the Earth the ground about them was exceeding hot and pearched or burnt;

[5] . . . so as to rise in small Columns

[6] George Forster, who was on the expedition, gives a different explanation, and does not fail to draw a moral. 'Little bits of their cloth, which they wear as sashes or belts, were suspended on the bushes which surrounded the green; and the presents which Paw-

Mr F. to the hot places he was at yesterday. [A thermometer] placed in a little hole made in one of them rose from 80[1] to 170. Several other parts of the hill emited Smoak or Steam all the day, the Volcano was unusally furious and filled all the circumjacent air with its ashes so that the drops of rain which fell was mixed with its ashes, it mattered not which way the wind blew we were sure to be troubled with them.[2] The Natives gave us now very little trouble and we made little excursions inland with safety, they would however have been better pleased if we had confined our selves to the Shore, as a proof of this, some of them undertook to conduct the gentlemen to a place where they might see the mouth of the Volcano, they very readily embraced the offer and were conducted down to the harbour before they preceived the cheat.

SATURDAY 13*th*. Wind at NE gloomy weather. The only thing remarkable to day was old Paowang dining with us on board. I took the oppertunity to shew him several parts of the Ship and various articles all of which he looked upon with the greatest indifferency.[3]

SUNDAY 14*th*. Wind northerly, weather as yesterday. After breakfast we made up a party consisting of 9 or 10 and set out in order to see if we could not have a nearer and better View of the Volcano, we first went to one of those burning or hot places before mentioned, having a Thermometer[4] with us we made a hole in the ground where the greatest heat seem'd to be into which we put it; in the open air the mercury stood at   but here it presently rose to and stood at 110[5] which is only two below boiling Water.[6] The Earth in this place was a kind of Pipe clay or whitish marl which had a sulpherous smell and was soft and wet, the upper surface only excepted which was crusted over with a thin dry crust, on which

yangom had received, among which was a laced hat, were placed in the same manner like so many trophies. This was a convincing proof to me of the general honesty of the people towards each other'.—II, p. 304.

1 . . . which it stood at in the open air . . .—f. 253.

2 *so that . . . them:* The rain which fell at this time was a compound of Water, Sand and Earth, so that it might very properly be called showers of mire. Let the wind blow which way it would, we were sure to be plagued with its ashes unless it blew very strong indeed from the opposite direction.—f. 253.

3 *all of which . . . indifferency:* in hopes of finding out some thing which they might value and be induced to exchange refreshments for, for what we got of this kind was trifling, but he looked upon every thing that was shewed him with the greatest indifferency; nay he hardly took notice of any one thing except a wooden Sand box which he seem'd to admire and turned it two or three times over in his hand.—f. 253. The sand was of course for drying ink.

4 . . . of Fahrenheits construction . . .—f. 253v.   5 An error for 210?

6 . . . It remained in the hole two minutes and a half without either rising or falling.

was Sulpher and a Vitriolick substance which tasted like Alumn: the whole space was no more than eight or ten yards square, near to which were some fig-trees who spread their branches over a part of it.[1] This extraordinary heat seem'd to us to be caused by the Steams of boiling liquid, most probably Water impregnated with Sulpher. I was told that some of the other places were larger than this, but we did not wait to look at them but proceeded up the hill through a Country covered with Trees, Plants, Shrubs, &c^{a}. The Bread fruit and Cocoa-nutt trees which seem'd to be Planted here by Nature were in a manner choked with Shrubery, creeping vines, &c^{a}. Every now and then we met with a house, some few people and Plantations, we found of the latter in different states, some of long standing, others lately cleared and clearing and before any thing had been planted; the clearing a piece of ground for a plantation seem'd to be a work of much labour, especially when we consider the tools they have to do it with which are of the same kind as at the other isles, but much inferiour, with these they cut or lop of the branches of the trees,[2] dig under the roots and there burn the branches and the small Shrubs and plants which they root up; thus they distroy both root and branch. The Soil, at least the upper surface,[3] seemed to be chiefly composed of decayed leaves and plants and the Sand or ashes which the Volcano sends forth over all its neighbourhood. Happening to turn out of the common path we came into a plantation where there was a Man at work, he either out of good Nature or to get us the sooner out of his territories, undertook to be our guide, we had not gone with him far before we met a nother fellow standing at the junction of two roads with a Sling and a Stone in his hand, both of which he thought proper to lay aside when a Musquet was pointed at him, the Attitude we found him in and the ferosity which appear'd in his looks and his beheavour after, led us to think he meant to defend the path he stood in; he pointed to the other along which he and our guide led us, he counted us several times over and kept calling for assistance[4] and was presently joined by two or three more one of which was a young Woman with a Club in her hand; they presently conducted us to the brow of a hill and pointed to a road which led down to the harbour and wanted

[1] . . . and seemed to like their situation.

[2] *with these . . . trees:* G Their methods is however judicious and as expeditious as it can well be. They top off the small branches of the trees

[3] *at least . . . surface:* G in some parts is a rich black mould

[4] *he pointed . . . assistance:* G he in some measure gain'd his point, our guide took the other road and we follow'd, but not without suspecting he was leading us wrong; the other man went with us likewise, he counted us several times over and hollowing, as we judged for assistance

us to go that way, we refused to comply and returned to the one we had left which we pursued alone our guide refusing to go with us; after assending a nother ridge as closely covered with Wood as those we had come over, we saw still other hills between us and the Volcano which discouraged us from proceeding farther especially as we could get no one to be our guide and therefore came to a resolution to return, we had but just put this into execution when we met twenty or thirty of the Natives collicted together and were close at our heels, we judged their design was[1] to oppose our advancing into the Country but now they saw us returning they suffered us to pass unmolested and some of them put us into the right road and accompanied us down the hill, made us to stop in one place where they brought us Cocoa nutts, Plantains and Sugar Canes and [what] we did not eat on the spot, brought down the hill for us; thus we found these people Civil[2] and good Natured when not prompted by jealousy to a contrary conduct, a conduct one cannot blame them for when one considers the light in which they must look upon us in, its impossible for them to know our real design, we enter their Ports without their daring to make opposition, we attempt to land in a peaceable manner, if this succeeds its well, if not we land nevertheless and mentain the footing we thus got by the Superiority of our fire arms, in what other light can they than at first look upon us but as invaders of their Country; time and some acquaintance with us can only convince them of their mistake.[3]

MONDAY 15*th*. In the PM I made an excursion in company with Mr Wales on the other side of the harbour, where we met from the Natives very different treatment [from what] we had done in the

[1] *collected . . . was:* G which the fellow before mentioned had got collected together with a design, as we judged,

[2] *Civil:* G hospit[ab]le, civil

[3] *in what . . . mistake:* G under such circumstances what opinion are they to form of us; is it not as reasonable for them to think that we come to invade their Country as to pay them a friendly visit; time & some acquaintance with us, can only convince them of the latter; these people are yet in a rude state, and if we can judge from circumstances & appearences, are frequently at War not only with their Neighbours, but amongst themselves, consequently must be jealous of every new face. I will allow, that there are many exceptions to this rule to be found in this Sea, but there are few Nations who will willingly suffer you to make excursions far into their country.—The Log adds, 'PM nearly compleated wooding and Watering AM Cleaned the Ship inside and out. Several people on shore on liberty trucking with the Natives, some few for fruits, but the greatest part for Curosities Such as Bows, arrows, Darts and such like trifles'.—Cook's observation was very just, and he might well have regarded his expedition, comparatively speaking, as a great success. The New Hebrideans were extremely sensitive about visitors going beyond the beach. Natives from other islands always carried on their business on the beach. John Williams the missionary was killed in 1839 only when he persisted in going beyond the the beach. On the other hand, the Log makes it clear that trading on the beach could be perfectly amicable. Compare the entry for 12 August above.

morning, these people, in whose neighbourhood lived our friend Paowang, being better acquainted with us than those we had seen in the morning, shewed a readiness to oblige us in every thing in their power: here was a little Stragling Village consisting of a few house which need no other discription than to compare them to the roof of a thatched house taken of the walls and placed on the ground, the figure was oblong and open at both ends, some indeed had a little fence or wall of reeds at each end about 3 feet high, some seem'd to be intended for more families than one as they had a fire place near each end,[1] there [were] other mean and small hovels which I understood were only to Sleep in, in one of these which with some others stood in a Plantation but separated from them by a fence, I understood was a dead Corps, they made Signs that he slipt or was dead, circumstances sufficiently pointed out the latter. Curious however to see all I could I prevailed on an elderly man to go with me within the fence which surrounded it, one end of the hut was closed up the same as the sides the other end had been open but now shut up with Matts which he would not suffer me to remove,[2] he also seem'd unwilling I should look into a Matted bag or basket which hung to the end of the hutt, in which was a piece of roasted yam and some kind of leaves all quite fresh: thus I was led to believe that these people dispose of the dead some thing in the same manner as at Otahiete. The Man had about his neck fastned to a String two or three locks of human hair and a Woman present had several; I offered some thing in exchange for them but they gave me to understand this could not be done as they belonged to the person who laid in the hutt. A similar custom to this is observed by the New Zealanders.[3] Near most of their larger houses are placed upright in the ground in a square position about 3 feet from each other the Stems of four Cocoa-nut trees, some of our gentlemen who first saw these seem'd to think they had a Religious tendancy, but I was now fully

[1] *the figure . . . end:* G some are open at both ends and others are partly closed with reeds and all are covered with Palm thatch; some are 30 or 40 feet long and 14 or 16 broad.—The reeds were probably those of the plant called *ning* or *nuing*, 'wild cane' or cane-grass, *Miscanthus japonicus*, generally used for that purpose; the roof and the outer walls were thatched with dried wild sugar cane, very thick.

[2] *within . . . remove:* G to the hutt, which was seperated from the others by a reeded fence, built quite round it at the distance of 4 or 5 feet from it, the entrance was by a space in the fence made so low as to admit one to step over. The two sides and one end of the hut was closed or built up in the same manner and with the same materials as the roof, but the other end had been opened but was now well closed up with Matts, which I could not prevail on the man to remove or suffer me;

[3] *A similar . . . Zealanders:* G a similar custom to wearing the hair is observ'd by the people of [Otaheite] and likewise by the New Zeelanders; the former make Tamau of the hair of their deceas'd friends, and the latter make Ear-rings and Necklaces of their teeth . . .—For 'Tamau' (*taamu*) see the description in I, p. 126.

satisfied they were to hang cocoa upon to dry.[1] Thier houses are generally built in an open Area where the air has a free circulation, in some are a large tree or two whose spreading branches afford an agreeable shade and retreat from the Scorching Sun.

This part of the Isle was well cultivated open and airy, the Plantations were laid out by line and Planted with Plantains, Sugar Canes, yams and other roots and well stocked with Bread, Cocoa-nutt and other fruit trees. In our walk we met with old Paowang who with some others accompaned us to the landing place and brought down with them a few Cocoa-nutts and a yam which they gave to me, and then we parted they returning home and we on board. In the AM having compleated our wood and Water, a few hands were only employed ashore Cuting stuff for brooms, the rest were imployed on board seting up the rigging and puting the Ship in a Condition for Sea. Mr F. in his excursion to day Shot a Pigeon[2] and in the Craw found a fruit which was either a wild Nutmeg or very much like one.[3]

TUESDAY 16*th*. Winds northerly fair Weather. In the PM Mr F. and I[4] took a Walk to the Eastern Sea shore in order to have a sight of an Island to the SE which these People called Annattom; the high table Island we discovered the Morning we anchored here is called Irromang or Foottoona and the flat isle lying off the harbour Immer.[5] I observed that in their Sugar Plantations were dug holes or Pitts about 4 feet deep and 5 or six in diameter, we were made to understand that these Pitts were to catch Ratts which when once in they could not get out and so were easy killed, these animals which are distructive to the Canes are here in plenty.[6] In the Morning after having got every thing in readiness to put to Sea and waited for nothing but a wind we found the Tiler sprung and other ways deffective in the Rudder head and by some strange neglect we had

[1] G for when I asked, as well as I could, the use of them, a man took me to one loaded with Cocoanutts from the bottom to the top; no words could have informed me better.—'Some of our gentlemen' seems to point to J. R. Forster, but George Forster gives a clear account (II, pp. 303–4) of the use of these coconut stems as poles across which were fastened the sticks to which the nuts were hung.

[2] The Pacific Pigeon. Cf. p. 262.

[3] . . . he took some pains to find the tree, but his endeavours were not attended with success.—f. 254. There are several species of wild nutmegs in the New Hebrides: *Myristica guillauminiana*, *M. inutilis*, *etc.*

[4] *Mr F. and I:* a party of us. . . .—The party was Cook, the two Forsters Cooper, Pickersgill, Patten, Hodges and Sparrman—so we learn from Forster, II, p. 333.

[5] *in order . . . Immer:* in order to take the bearing of Annatam and Erronan or Footoona but the horizon proved so hazey that I could see neither but one of the natives gave me as I afterwards found the true direction of them.—f. 254.

[6] . . . the canes I observed were planted as thick as possible round the edges of these Pitts, so that the ratts in coming at them are the more liable to tumble in.

never a spare one on board and this was not known till now we wanted it. While the Carpenter was unshiping the old tiler I went ashore to cut down a tree to make a new one, but as we knew but of one fit for the purpose which stood near the watering place and this Paowang had disired might not be cut down and I had promised it should not proper application was therefore necessary in order not to give umbrage to the Natives. Therefore as soon as I landed I sent for old Paowang and as soon as he came made him a present of a Dog and a large piece of Cloth and then made known to him that our great steering Paddle was broke and that I wanted that tree to make a new one, he presently gave his consent as well as several others present and we set people to work to cut it down. It was easy to see that this Method which I took to Obtain the tree was very agreeable to all the people present.[1] After this I returned on board with Paowang who stayed dinner. After the tiler was unshiped we found that by scarfing a piece to the inner end and liting it farther into the rudder head it would still perform its office and the Carpenters and smiths were set about this work. When the gentlemen who had been on Shore returned on board to dinner I learnt from them that an old man whose name was   and as they understood King or Chief of the Island, was then at the landing place.

WEDNESDAY 17*th*. After dinner I went a Shore with Paowang, saw the old Chief and made him a present with which he retired; his name was [Geogy] he seem'd to be very old[2] and had with him a Son near

[1] *I went ashore . . . present:* sent the Carpenter a shore to look at it and an officer with a party of Men to cut it down provide[d] he could obtain leave of the Natives, if not to send to acquaint me with it; He understood that no one had any objection and set the people to work to cut it down, but as the tree was large this was a work of some time and before it was down word was brought me that our friend Poawang, was not pleased with it and I gave orders to desist, as we found that by Scarfing a piece to the inner end of the tiller and leting it farther into the Rudder head, it would still perform its office; but as it was necessary to have a spare one on board, I went on shore, sent for Paowang, made him a present of a Dog and a piece of Cloth and than made him understand that our great steering paddle was broke and that I wanted that tree to make a new one; it was easy to see how well pleased every one present was with the means I took to obtain it and with one Voice gave their consent so that Paowang gave his consent also which he, perhaps, could not have done without the others for I do not know that he had either more property or authority than the rest.—f. 254v.—The tree, says Forster, was a casuarina, 'highly valued at Tanna, and so very scarce, that they are obliged to go to Irromanga, where it grows more plentifully, in order to supply themselves with clubs'.—II, p. 339.

[2] *saw the old chief . . . very old:* to pay a Visit to an old Chief who was said to be king of the island; but this was a doubt with me, Poawang took little or no notice of him, I made him a present after which he immidiately went away, as if he had got all he came for; his Name was Geogy and they gave him the Title of Areekee, he was very old but had a merry open countenance. He wore round his waste a broad red and white chequered belt, the materials and Manufacture of which seemed the same as those of Otaheite cloth but this was hardly a mark of distinction.—ff. 254v–5. Forster gives the old man's name as Yogài, and his son's as Yatta.

fifty years of Age. A great number of people were at this time at the landing place and some few were a little troublesome, daring and insolent[1] whilest the others behaved with courtesy and friendship.

In the Morning sent the Guard a Shore as usual, about 10 o'Clock I went a Shore and found in the crowd Old Yeoki[2] and his son, he soon made me understand that he wanted to dine with me on board, accordingly I brought him, his son and two more on board, they all called themselves Kings or cheifs,[3] but I did not believe any one of them had any pretentions to that title over the whole island.[4] I shewed them all over the Ship which they viewed with surprise and uncommon attention. We happened to have for their entertainment a kind of a Pye or Pudding made of Plantains and some sort of greens which we had got from the Natives, of this and yams they made a hearty dinner.[5] After makeing each of them a present of a Hatchet, a Spike Nail, and piece of cloth and some Medals they were conducted a Shore and immidiately retired.[6]

THURSDAY 18*th*. In the PM M[r] F. and I went to the west side of the Harbour to try the degree of heat of the hot Springs, in one of which the mercury in the Thermometer rose to 191 from 78 which it stood at in the open air. At this time it was high-water and within two or three feet of the spring which we judged might be in some degree cooled by it but the next morning we found just the contrary for repeting the experiment when the tide was out the Mercury rose no higher than 187, but at a nother Spring which bubbles out in large quantities from under a steep rock at the SW corner of the harbour, the Mercury rose to 202½ which is only 9½ below boiling water; I have already said that these Springs are at the foot of the same hill on the side of which we saw the hot places and Smokes ascend before mentioned: this hill belongs to the Same Ridge in which the Volcano is: the Ridge is of no great height[7] nor is the Volcano at the

[1] . . . which I thought proper to put up with as our stay was nearly at an end.

[2] Geogy

[3] *Kings or Cheifs:* Areekes (Kings)

[4] . . . it had been remarked that one of these Kings had not authority enough to order one of the people up into [a] cocoa nutt tree to bring him down some nutts, altho he spoke to several, and was at last obliged to go himself; and by way of revenge as it was thought, left not a nutt on the tree, took what he wanted himself and gave the rest to some of our people.—f. 255. —Cook was perfectly correct in his disbelief that there was any king of the whole island. The mark of New Hebridean social organization was indeed the great number of clans and chiefs on the same island—too many for social cohesion.

[5] . . . for as to Salt Beef and Pork they would hardly taste it.

[6] 'Punish'd W[m] Tow Marine 1 dozen for trading with the natives when on guard on shore'.—Cooper.

[7] *I have already . . . height:* The hot places before mentioned are from about three to four hundred feet perpendicular above these Springs and on the Slope of the same ridge as the Volcano, that is there is no vally between them but such as are formed in the ridge it self.—f. 255v.

highest part of it but on the SE side and contrary to the Opinion of Philosophers, which is that all Volcanos must be at the summits of the highest hills, here are hills in this island more than double the height of the ridge I have been speaking of. Nor was the Volcano on the isle of Ambrrym (which I now have not the least doubt of there being one if not two) on the highest part of the Island but seem'd to us to be in a Vally between the hills:[1] to these remarks must be added [a] nother which is that during wet or moist weather the Volcano was most vehement. Here seems to be [a] feild open for some Philosophical reasoning on these extraordinary Phenomenon's of nature, but as I have no tallant that way I must content my self with stateing facts as I found and leave the causes to men of more abilities.

FRIDAY 19*th.* Winds northerly a gentle gale. In [the PM] the Tiller was finished and Shiped, so that we only waited for a fair Wind to put to sea. In the AM as the wind would not admit of our geting to sea I sent the guard on [shore] with Mr Wales as usual and at the same time a party to cut up and bring off the remainder of the tree we had cut a spare tiller of. A good many of the Natives were, as usual, assembled near the landing place and unfortunately one of them was Shott by one of our Centinals, I who was present and on the Spot saw not the least cause for the commiting of such an outrage and was astonished beyond Measure at the inhumanity of the act, the rascal who perpetrated this crime pretended that one of the Natives laid his arrow across his bow and held it in the Attitude of Shooting so that he apprehen[d]ed himself in danger, but this was no more than what was done hourly and I beleive with no other View than to let us see they were Armed as well as us: what made this affair the more unfortunate it not appearing to be the man who bent the Bow but a nother who was near him. After this unhappy affair most of the Natives fled and when we imbarked to go on board they retired to a man and only a few appeared in the afternoon[2] amongest whom was Wha-a-you who I had not seen sence the day he dined on board. During the night the Wind Veered round to SE. At 4 AM began to unmoor and at 8 got under sail and Stood out to Sea, leaving the Launch behind to take up a Kedge Anchor and hawser we had out to cast by and was obliged to Slip. As soon as were clear of the harbour we brought-to to wait for the Launch and to hoist her and the other boats in which was employment till Noon, when we

[1] Ambrim is a centre of considerable volcanic activity: ranges rise from all its shores to form a circle round a tremendous crater, in which are separate cones. The highest peak on the island is Mount Marum, 4,380 feet; so that Cook's observation was not inaccurate.

[2] i.e. the afternoon of Saturday 20th, ship time.

made Sail and Stretched to the Eastward with our Starboard tacks on board in order to take a nearer View of the Island of Erronan the same as we discover'd in the morning of the 5th.

*As I had nothing to do I went on shore with them and found a good number of the Natives collected about the landing place as usual, to whom I distributed all the presents I had about me and then went on board for more. In less than an hour returned, just as our people were geting some large logs into the boat; At the same time four or five of the Natives steped forward to see what we were about, and as we did not allow them to come within certain limmits unless it was to pass along the beach, the sentery ordered them back, which they readily complied with. At this time I had my eyes fixed on them and observed the sentery present his piece (as I thought at the men) and was just going to reprove him for it, because I had observed that when ever this was done, some or another of the Natives would hold up their arms, to let us see they were as ready as us, but I was astonished beyond measure when the sentry fired for I saw not the least cause. At this outrage, most of the people fled, it was only a few I could prevail upon to remain; as they ran off I observed one man to fall and was immidiately taken up by two others who led him into the water, washed his wound and then led him off. Presently after some came and described to us the nature of his wound, which I now sent for the surgeon to dress, as I found the man was not carried far. As soon as the Surgeon came I went with him to the man, which we found expiring; the ball had struck his left arm, which was much shattered, and then entered his body by the short ribs, one of which was broke. The rascal who perpetrated this crime, pretended that a Man had laid an arrow a Cross his bow and was going to shoot it at him, so that he apprehended himself in danger, but this was no more than what they had always done, and I believe with no other view than to shew they were armed as well as us, at least I have reason to think so, as they never went further. What made this affair the more unfortunate, it not appearing to be the man who bent the bow, that was shott, but another who stood by him.[1] This unhappy affair threw the Natives into the utmost con-

[1] The sentry concerned was the marine William Wedgeborough, a not very attractive person; but it is not easy to give a satisfactory last word on this incident. There were others who took the matter more easily than Cook did, for instance Cooper; and others who thought Cook was quite wrong. To Cooper, it seems, the life of an 'insolent' native was of no particular value: 'This forenoon a Centinel on shore fired at one of the natives for attempting to fire an arrow at him, which shatter'd the Elbow of his left Arm & enter'd his side, he was immediately taken to a small distance & expired in a quarter of an hour, this act of hostillity has been often offered to our Centinels before unnoticed which has totally rendered them disregarded by the natives to a great degree of insolence: the rest

sternation the few that were prevailed on to stay ran to the plantations and brought Cocoa nutts &c[a] and laid [them] down at our feet, so soon were these daring people humbled.

When I went on board to dinner they retired to a man and only a few appeared in the after-noon amongst whom were Paowang and Whā ā-gou, this young man I had not seen sence the day he dined on board, both he and Pā-o-wang promised to bring me fruit &c[a] the next morning but our early departure put it out of their power.

SATURDAY 20*th*. During the night the wind had veered round to SE; as this was favourab[l]e for geting out of the harbour, we at 4 a.m. began to unmoor and at 8 wieghed our last anchor and put to Sea. As soon as we were clear of the land, I brought-to to wait for the Lau[n]ch which was left behind to take up a Kedge Anchor &

of the natives on the Beach quite passive & undisturbed.'—Elliott's account (*Mem.*, ff. 32v–33) is possibly coloured by reminiscence, and he may have been unconsciously arguing a case: 'In this state of things with respect to the Natives, Tho I have several times said that Capt[n] Cook was a Most Brave, Just, Humane, and good Man, and the fittest of all others for such a Voyage; yet I must think, that here, and upon another occasion (which I shall notice, in its proper place) He lost sight, of both justice, and Humanity. The circumstance was this; Capt[n] Cook, told the officer of Mariens, that his Men were not to fire, until fir'd upon. And he repeated the orders to the *Sentrys*; one day the Natives appear'd particularly Insolent, and one of them came repeatedly within a Sentry's lines, the Soldier told him to keep back, which only made him more insolent, He then shew'd the Man his Musquet, and push'd him by, upon this the Man took an Arrow, laid [it] across his Bow, and drew it, but looking at it, he took it from the Bow, and replac'd it with one that he lik'd better, and drew it to the last stretch; in this situation, not 5 Yards distance stood the Sentry; Now the question was, whether the sentry was to recieve a Poison'd Arrow into him (for he was sure to be hit) or he to save himself, was to shoot the Man; the sentry choose the latter, and he instantly level'd his Musquet and Shot the Man; for which Capt[n] Cook order'd him on board, and had him brought to the gangway to be flogged, but was induc'd through the per[s]wasions of all the officers, to forego the flogging, but kep't him in Irons a considerable time'. Neither Cooper nor Elliott was an eyewitness, and certainly Forster, who gives a circumstantial account (II, pp. 350–3) was not. According to him, Edgcumbe, the lieutenant of marines, had deliberately given the sentries orders directly contrary to Cook's—which reads like nonsense; and equally nonsense seems the remark, 'the officer's right to dispose of the lives of the natives remained uncontroverted'. Sparrman (p. 151), a less biased writer, says that Edgcumbe and the naval lieutenants defended Wedgeborough, arguing that he was 'entitled to believe he was not posted there simply to provide a target for arrows'.—Wales sided with Wedgeborough, and calls Forster's account 'one of the most malignant pieces of misrepresentation and abuse in his whole book'. One attempt to shoot a sentry had already been made, and was only prevented by another native who was standing by; and Edgecumbe's orders to the sentries were simply, if there was no alternative to shooting, to shoot in time. The only 'person of moment' who saw the whole transaction, he says, was Whitehouse, one of the master's mates. He concludes, 'I have already proved from the testimony of the only person who saw the whole, for Captain Cook saw only a small part of it, that the centinel did strictly obey Captain Cook's orders as long as he could, and, in consequence thereof, was obliged to shoot him in his own defence. Mr. Whitehouse has assured me, that he is absolutely certain Captain Cook is, himself, mistaken in saying, that there was room to suppose it was not the man who drew the arrow that was shot. I never heard that there was the least reason for such a supposition,'—Wales, *Remarks*, pp. 83–8. Forster gives his last word on the subject thus: 'So much I know, that the matter was discussed in my hearing, with much warmth, between the officers and Captain Cook, who by no means approved of their conduct at that time.'—*Reply*, p. 9. This is interesting but proves nothing on the main point.

hawser we had out to cast by. About day break a noise was heard in the Woods nearly abreast of us on the East side of the harbour, it was not unlike singing of Psalms; I was told that the same had been heard about the same time on other mornings, but it never came to my knowlidge till now when it was too late to known the occasion of it. Some were[1] of opinion that at the East point of the harbour (where we observed in coming in, some houses boats &c[a]) were some thing or a nother, sacred to Religion, because some of our People [who] had attempted to go to this point were prevented by the Natives. I thought and do still think, it was only owing to a desire they on every occasion shew'd of fixing bounds to our excursions, so far as we had once been we might go again, but not fa[r]ther with their consent, but by encroaching a little every time our excursions were insensibly extended without giving the least umbrage, besides these morning ceremonies, whether Religious or not, were not performed down at that point, but in a part where some of our people were daily.[2] I cannot say what might be the true cause of these people shewing such a dislike to our makeing little excursions into their Country; it might be owing to a natural jealous disposition, or perhaps to their being accustomed to hostile visits from their neighbours or quarrels amongst themselves, circumstances seemed to shew that such must frequently happen; we observed that they are very expert and well accustomed to Arms and seldom or never travel without them. It is possible all this might be on our account, but I can hardly think it, we never gave them the least molestation, nor did we touch any part of their property, not even Wood and Water without first having obtained their consent. The very Cocoa-nutts hanging over the heads of the Workmen were as safe as those in the middle of the isle. It happened rather luckey that there were many Cocoa-nut trees near the skirts of the harbour, which seemed not to be private property, so that we could generally prevail on some or other to bring us some of these nutts when nothing would induce them to bring any out of the

[1] Some were *substituted for* M[r] F. was now

[2] There is conflict of testimony here. 'Every morning, at day-break, we heard a slow solemn song or dirge sung on this point, which lasted more than a quarter of an hour. It seemed to be a religious act, and gave us great reason to suspect that some place of worship was concealed in these groves. . . .'—Forster, II, pp. 300–1. Forster even reports 'signs that we should be killed and eaten' if they went beyond the point.—p. 300. This seems to display a rather romantic imagination, which had fed on Druids and certain ingredients of the forested Teutonic past. The natives were most probably practising for some great feast, or for celebrating a new season with new music— the Tanese spent a great deal of time 'singing heathen songs' (to use the missionary phrase), but they were not songs of religion. New Hebridean 'religion' is a ticklish subject, and need not be gone into. Possibly the second remark from Forster indicates some warning against less friendly clans, or even some local magician, 'disease-maker', living apart, with death at his disposal—though in Tana these people generally inhabited a spot close to the volcano.

Country. We were by no means wholy without refreshments, for besides the fish which our seine now and then provided us with, we got daily some fruits or roots from the Natives, tho' but little in comparison to what we could consume; The reason why we got no more might be our having nothing to give them in exchange which they thought a valuable consideration; they had not the least knowlidge of Iron consequently Nails and Iron tools Beeds &c[a] which had had so great a run at the more Eastern isles were of no value here and Cloth can be of no use to people who go naked.[1] The Produce of this island are Bread fruit, Plantains Cocoa nuts, The fruit like a Nectrine,[2] Yams, Tarra, a sort of Potato,[3] Sugar Cane Wild figs, a fruit like an orange which is not eatable and some other fruits & nuts whose names I have not and I have no doubt but the Nutmegs before mentioned were the produce of this Island.[4] The Island not only produceth all the fruits and roots that are to be found at Otaheite but some others.[5] The bread fruit Cocoa nutts and Plantains are neither so plenty nor so good as at Otaheite, on the other hand Sugar Canes and yams are not only in greater plenty but superior in qualitey and vastly larger, we got one of the latter which wieghed 56 pounds every Ounce of which was good. Hogs did not seem to be scarce but Fowles we saw but few. These were all the domestick animals they have. Land Birds are not more numerous than at Otaheite and the other Islands, but here are[6] some small Birds with very beautiful plumage which we had nowere seen before. Here are as greater[7] variety of Trees and Plants as at any isle we have touched at that our botanist[s] have had time to examine. I believe these people live chiefly on the produce of the land and that the Sea contributes but little towards their subsistance; whether it is because the Coast does not abound with fish or that they are bad fishers I know

[1] *Deleted* and secondly something may be attributed to the excessive passion which prevailed amongst our selves for curiosities of every kind, sence the natives could obtain more for a bow and an arrow, or even a dart than for a whole load of fruit, it was but Natural for them to bring that to a Market which was the easiest carriage and perhaps of least Value.

[2] By this Cook probably means the Tahitian *vi*, or 'vi-apple', to give one of its numerous European names, *Spondias dulcis*.

[3] The local variety of sweet potato or *kumara*.

[4] This sentence is a red ink addition, on a separate slip, numbered f. 257.

[5] A *note* 'Besides several sorts of Figs, here are Oranges or a fruit exactly like them, which they call Barreeco; it is Sour and bitter and not to be eat, nor do I know that the Natives make any use whatever of it. This Isle produceth none of that fruit which we call Apples and are so plenty at Otahiete.' B and G *note*, 'There are no apples at this isle that we have seen, but there are 5 or 6 sorts of Figs and some very good'. Apples here probably means the Jambo (rose-apple, mountain apple, Malay apple), *Eugenia malaccensis*.

[6] Land Birds ... here are *substituted for* Here are most of the sorts of land birds which are at the other isles together with

[7] *Sic*, the sentence being imperfectly altered from 'Here are likewise a greater variety of Trees and Plants than at ...'.

not, perhaps both, I never saw any sort of fishing tackle amongst them or any one out fishing except it was on the shoals or along the shores of the harbour, watching to strike with a dart such fish as came within their reach, and in this they were expert, they seemed much to admire our catching fish with the Seine and I believe were not well pleased with it at last. I make no doubt but they have other methods of catching fish beside striking them. We understood that the little isle of Immer was chiefly inhabited by fishers and that the Canoes we frequently saw pass to and from that isle and the East point of the harbour were fishing Canoes. These Canoes were of unequal sizes, some are 30 f^{t} long, 2 broad & 3 deep, they are composed of several pieces of Wood sewed together with bandage[s] in a very clumsy manner, the joints are covered on the out side by a thin battan champhered off at the edges over which the bandages pass.[1] They are Navigated by either Paddles or sails, the sail is latteen, extended to a yard and boom and hoisted to a short mast; some of the large Canoes have two sails and all of them have outriggers.

At first we thought the People of this isla^{d} as well as those of Erromango were a race between the Natives of the Friendly Islands and those of Mallicollo, but a little acquaintance with them convinced us that they had little or no affinity to either except it be in their hair which is a good deal like what the people of the latter Island have. The general colours are Black and brown, it grows to a tolerable length and is very crisp and curly; the[y] separate it into small locks and wold or cue them round with the rind of a slender plant down to about an Inch of the ends, and as the hair grows, the wolding is continued. Each of these cues or locks are something thicker than common whip Cord and looks like a parcel of small strings, hanging down from the crown of their heads.[2] Their Beards, which is strong and bushy, are in general short. The Women do not wear their hair so but croped, nor do the boys till they approach man-

[1] The joints . . . pass *substituted for* so that they are by no means a master piece of workmanship *deleted.* Add. MS 27889, f. 79, has a note, 'Tanna Boats deformed as if they broke thier Backs'. The ocean-going canoes were seaworthy vessels, however.

[2] they had little . . . their heads: *substituted for deleted passage* they had no affinity to the latter except in their hair, which altho it is not quite so woolly is very near it and may be disputed whether it be wool or hair, be it the one or the other, it is very crisp and Curly and grows to a tolerable good length if we have not been deceived by their method of wearing it, which is thus; the whole head of hair is divided into a vast number of small locks, each lock cue'd with the fine fibers of some plant, from the root to the end, as the hair grows the cue is lengthened, till in some they hang down over their shoulders, but some of our gentlemen observed them lengthen these cues by other hair, which may be the case with all that are long. Each of these cues are something thicker than common whip cord. The reason of their dressing their hair in this manner may be to prevent it from intangling together; but I rather think the fashion is from Custom.—f. 259. This style no longer exists on Tana.

hood; some few men, women and Children were seen who had hair like ours; it was easy to see that these were of a nother nation and I think we understood they came from Arronan; It is to this isld they ascribe one of the two languages which they speak and is nearly if not exactly the same as that spoke at the friendly islands, it is therefore, more than probable that Erronan is peopled from that Nation and by long intercourse with Tanna and the other islands each have learnt the others language, which they now speak indiscriminately. The other language which the people of Tanna speake, and as we understood, those of Erromanga and Annattom, is properly speaking their own, and is different to any we had before met with. It bears no affinity to that spoke in Mallicollo hence it should seem that the people of these islands are a distinct Nation of themselves.[1] Mallicollo, Apee &c[a] were names intirely unknown to them, they even knew nothing of Sandwich island which is much the nearer; I took no little pains to know how far their geographical knowlidge extended and did not find that it exceeded the limmits of their horizon. These people are of the middle size, rather slender than otherwise, many are little, but few can be called tall or stout;[2] the most of them have good features and agreeable countinances, are like all the Tropical Race, active and nimble, but these seem to excell in the use of Arms, but do not seem to be fond of labour, they never would put a hand to assist in any work we were carr[y]ing forward, which the people of the other islands would take a delight in, but what I judge most from, is their makeing the Women do the most laborious work, of them they make pack-horses, I have seen a woman carrying a large bundle on her back, or a Child on her back and a bundle

[1] One can comment on the foregoing, without entering into a lengthy dissertation, only in generalities about as broad as Cook's own. He was right in seeing similarities to the people of the Friendly Islands. The New Hebrideans are mostly Melanesian in type, but with some mixture of Polynesian blood, particularly in the east and south. In Tana, though not in Malekula, this mixture is very evident: stature and hair are Melanesian, but facial features and head form are much nearer Polynesian. The colour, even, of the Tanese may be the Polynesian brown. Among the great number of New Hebridean languages and dialects there are certain broad divisions as one moves from north to south. In the south the languages of Futuna and Aniwa and a few other islands are basically Polynesian; they are most closely related to those of Tonga, Samoa, and other western Polynesian islands. The languages of Tana, Aneityum and Eromanga are in general distinct from this group; but there was going and coming, and Cook could easily have heard something like Tongan on Tana. Malekula and the other northern islands on the other hand spoke Melanesian tongues, related to those of Fiji to the east and New Caledonia to the west—with, on the whole, a common grammatical structure but much difference in vocabulary. Cook may certainly be forgiven for the paucity of his linguistic observations.

[2] 'People are in general well made, in many parts of their bodys cutt in shape of Lizards . . .'—Mitchel. Cf. Forster: 'They cut the flesh with a bamboo, or sharp shell, and apply a particular plant, which forms an elevated scar on the surface of the skin, after it is healed. These scars are formed to represent flowers, and other fancied figures, which are deemed a great beauty by the natives.' Only one man was observed with any tattooing.—II, pp. 277–8. For Hodges's drawings, see Fig. 72.

under her arm and a fellow struting before her with nothing but a club, or a spear or some such like thing in his hand;[1] we have frequently seen little troops of women pass to and fro a long the beach, laden with fruit and roots escorted, as it were, by a party of men under arms; now and then we have seen men carry a burdthen at the same time but not often, I know not on what account this was done or that an armed troop was necessary, when we first saw it we thought they were moving out of the neighbourhood with their effects but we afterwards saw them both carry out and bring in allmost every day. I cannot say the women are beauties but I think them handsome enough for the men and too handsome for the use that is made of them. Both sex are of a Very dark Colour but not black, nor have they the least character[i]stic of the Negro abo[t] them; they make themselves blacker than they really are by painting their faces with a Pigment of the Colour of black lead, they also use a nother sort which is red and a third sort brown, or a Colour between red and black, all these, but especially the first they lay on with a liberal hand, not only on the face but on the neck shoulders and breast.[2] The Men wear nothing but a belt and a case to the Penis, which is tied up to the belt; this case is some times of Cloth, but more generally of the leaves and small branches of a certain plant.[3] The Women wear a kind of Peticoat which is made of the filaments of the Plantain tree, Flags or some such like thing which reaches below the knee. Both sex wear ornaments, such as braclets, Earings, necklaces and Amulets; the braclets are chiefly worn by the men and made some of Sea Shells and others of Cocoa nut shells, Amulets is a nother Ornament worn by the Men, those of most Value are made of a greenish stone;[4] the green stone of New zeland was valued by them for this purpose. Necklaces were chiefly worn by the women and made mostly of shells; Ear Rings were worn in common, those Valued most were made of Tortoise shell, some of our people got of this shell at the Friendly isla[n]ds and brought it here

[1] This, though the fruit of personal observation, is not quite just. Men carried burdens, and heavy ones; but not on the back or under the arm, like a woman. They needed a pole, with a man at each end—or with a man in the middle, and a load at each end. There was an etiquette about these things.

[2] 'The paints are reserved for the face; they are red ochre, white lime, and a colour shining like black lead; all these they mix with coco-nut oil, and lay on the face in oblique bars, two or three inches broad. The white colour is seldom employed, but the red and black is more frequent, and sometimes each covers one half the face.'—Forster, II, p. 277. The 'black lead' pigment was from the burnt oily fruit of the candlenut *Aleurites moluccana*. The red colour was an ochre from Aneityum; the white was lime.

[3] a plant like ginger'—Forster, II, p. 277. Perhaps *Zingiber zerumbet*; but the leaves generally used were those of the banana, *Hibiscus tiliaceus*, or *Coleus* spp.

[4] Probably this was some sort of serpentine, though ornaments of this stone are more characteristic of the islands to the north-east—e.g. Woodlark and the Trobriands.

to a good market it being of more value to these people than any thing we had besides; from this I conclude that they catch but few Turtle, we however saw one in the harbour just as we were geting under sail. I observed that towards the latter end of our stay they began to ask for hatchets and large nails; it is likely they had found out that they made better tools than Stone, bone or shells, of which all their tools I have seen are made. Their stone hatchets at least all those I saw, were not made like adzes as at the other islands but more like an ax—in this form 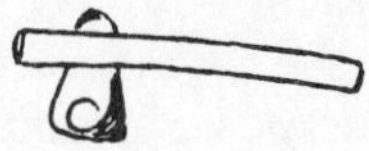 ; in the helve, which is pretty thick, is made a hole into which the stone is fixed. These people seem to have as few Arts as most I have seen, besides knowing how to cultivate the ground they have few others worth mentioning; they know how to make a Course kind of Matting and a Course sort of cloth of the bark of a tree which is used chiefly for belts.[1] The workmanship of their Canoes I have before observed are very rude and their arms, with which they take the most pains, in point of neatness come far short of some others we have seen.

Their Arms are Clubs, spears or Darts, Bows and Arrows and Stones; the Clubs are of three or four kinds and from 3 to 6 feet long.[2] They seem to place the greatest dependence on the Darts, which are poi[nted] with three bearded edges, in throwing the dart, they make use of a becket, that is a piece of stiff platted Cord about six inches long, with an eye in on[e] end and a knot at the other, the eye is fixed on the fore finger of the right hand and the other end is hitched round the dart where it is nearly on an equipoise. They hold the dart between the thum and remaining fingers, which serve only to give it direction, the Vilocity or force being communicated to it by the becket & finger, the former flies off from the dart the Instant there is no more occasion for [i]t, Viz. when the Velocity of the dart becomes great[er] than that of the hand, but it remains on the finger ready for another dart. With Darts they kill both birds and fish and are sure of hitting a mark the compass of the crown of a hat at the distance of 8 or 10 yards, but at double this distance its a chance if the[y] hit a mark the Size of a mans body,[3] although they

[1] Matting was woven of pandanus and coconut leaves: coconut generally made the coarser kind. The Tanese belts seem simply to have been strips of the bark of some large tree—e.g. the banyan—not bark converted into tapa.

[2] *Deleted* The spear seems not to be a common weapon it is made of hard wood and is about 10 feet long and pointed at one end.

[3] But cf. Elliott: '. . . with their Bows they could shoot a Bird in the bush; and I have seen 6 of them, placed in a line, at 20 yards distance and they have fix'd every Spear, ina soft Coconut'.—*Mem.*, f. 32. See also Forster, II, pp. 278–9.

will throw one 60 or 70 yards. They always throw with all their might let the distance be what it will. Darts Bows and arrows are to them as Muskets are to us, the arrows are made of reeds and pointed with hard wood, some are bearded and some not; those for shooting birds have two, three and some four points. The stones they make use of are for the most part the branches of Coral Rocks, from 8 to 14 inches long and from an inch to an inch and a half in diameter.[1] I know not if they use them as missive weapons. Allmost every one carries a Club and besides it, either darts or a Bow and Arrows, but never both; those who had stones kept them generaly in their belts. I cannot conclude this account of their arms without adding an intire passage out of Mr Wales's Journal.[2] As this gentleman was continually a shore among them he had a better oppertunity to see the feats which they performed than any of us; this passage is as follows:

'I must confess I have been often lead to think the Feats which Homer represents his heros as performing with their Spears a little too much of the marvelous to be admitted into a Heroic Poem, I mean when confined within the straight stays of Aristotle; nay even so great an Advocate for him as Mr Pope, acknowlidges them to be *surprising*. But sence I have seen what these people can do with their wooden ones; and them badly pointed and not of a very hard nature either, I have not the least exception to any one passage in that Great Poet on this account. But if I can see fewer exceptions I can find infinite number more beauties in him as he has, I think scarce an action, circumstance or discription of any kind whatever relateing to a spear, which I have not seen & recognised amongst the People, as their whirling motion and whistling noise as they fly. Their quivering motion as they stick in the ground when they fall. Their medi[t]ating their aim when they are going to throw and their shaking them in their hand as they go along &ca &ca.'

We know nothing of the Religion of these people and but very little of their Goverment. They seem to[3] have Chiefs amongst them, at least such have been pointed out to us by that Title, but these, as I have already observed, seemed to have very little authority over the rest of the people.[4] Old Geogy was the only one the people were

[1] Forster, who gives a good account of those terrifying weapons the New Hebrides clubs (II, pp. 279–80), treats this as a club—'a piece of coral rock, about eighteen inches long, and two in diameter, rudely shaped into a cylinder. Sometimes this is likewise made use of as a missile weapon'.

[2] This sentence and the following one, and the extract from Wales, form no part of the original journal, but are added as a separate slip, f. 261.

[3] They seem to *substituted for* it is certain that they

[4] *Deleted after* 'people': indeed we are not to suppose one Chief can have any authority in the district of a nother.—Chiefs did in fact have the power of life and death over members of their own clans.

ever seen to take the least notice of, whether this was owing to high rank or old age I cannot say on several occasions I have seen the old men respected and obeyed. Our friend Paowang, who I never heard called a Chief, seemed to be much respected in our neighbourhood and yet I have many reason[s] to beleive that he had not, by right, any more authority than many of his neighbours, and that few if any were bound to obey him or any other person in our neighbourhood, for if there had been such a one, we certainly should some how or a nother have known it.

I named the Harbour, Port Resolution after the Ship as she was the first who ever entered it. It is situated on the North side of the Most Eastern point of the Island and about ENE from the Volcano; in the Latitude of 19°32′25½″ S and in the Longitude of 169°44′35″ East. It is no more than a little creek runing in SBW½W three quarters of a Mile and is about half that in breadth. A shoal of Sand and Rocks lying along the East side makes it still narrower. The depth of Water in the harbour is from 6 to 3 fathoms and the bottom is sand and mud.[1] No place can be more convenient for takeing in Wood and Water, for both are close to the shore. The Water Stunk a little after it had been a few days on board but afterwards turned sweet, and even when it was at the worst the Tin Machine would in a few hours sweeten a whole Cask. This is an excellent contrivance for sweetning Water at sea and is very will known in the Navy.[2] Mr Wales (from whom I had the Latitude and Longitude) found the Variation of the needle to be 7°14⅕′ East and the Dip of its South end 45°02⅓′.*—ff. 256–62v.

SUNDAY 21*st*. Fresh gales at SE and fair weather. Continued to stretch to the East[3] till Middnight when having pass'd the Isle of Erronan tacked and spent the remainder of the night in makeing two boards and at sunrise as no new land was to be seen, we Stretched to SW in order to get to the Southward of Tanna and to have a nearer View of the Island Annattom,[4] which at Noon extended from S½E to S½W distant about 10 Leagues, the Harbour of Tanna bore N 86° west and the Island from S 88° west to N 64° west, Traytors head N 58° West and the Isle of Erronan N 86° East distant [5] Leagues.[5] This last isle is by some call'd Footoona, it is the most

[1] Chart XXXVII*b*. Cook would find his port unusable now; thirty years ago it was silted up, and the bottom seems likely to have been raised by seismic action.

[2] See p. 10, n. 1 above.

[3] . . . in order to have a nearer view of Erronan . . .—f. 263.

[4] . . . to see if any more land laid in that direction, for an extraordinary clear morning had produced the discovery of none to the East.

[5] . . . At Noon observed in Latitude 20°33′30″, the situation of the lands around us were as follows: Port Resolution bore N 86° West distant 6½ leagues, the isld of Tanna

Eastern in this Archipeloga situated in Lat 19°[31]′ Long^{de} [170°21′] East, it did not appear to be above [5] Leagues in Circuit, but is of a considerable height and flat at top. At the NE side appeared a little Peak seemingly disjoined from the isle but we believed it was connected by low-land. Annattom, which is situated [9] Leagues from Tanna in Latitude 20°[3]′ S Longitude [170°04′] East, seem'd to be only a small Island of a moderate height and hilly surface. I had almost forgot to mention the little Isle of Immer which lies NBE½E distant [4 Leagues] from the Port of Tanna, it is low and flat and as we have been informed, inhabited chiefly by fishers.[1]

MONDAY *22nd*. Wind at SE and ESE a fresh breeze. At half past 2 pm[2] bore up round the SE end of Tanna and ran a long the South side at the distance of one league from Shore, it seemed to be a bold Coast without the guard of any Rocks and the Country appeared to be full as fruitfull as in the neighbourhood of the Harbour.[3] At 6 o'Clock the high land on Erromanga appeared over the West end of Tanna bearing N 16° west, At 8 we were past the isle and Steer'd NNW for the one we left on ye 27th of last month, in order to finish the Survey[4] of it and the other Isles to the NW. At Noon we observed in Latitude 18°18′30″, Traytors head bore S 54° East distant Leagues.

TUESDAY *23rd*. Wind at ESE a fresh gale and fair weather. At 4 PM we began to draw near the Island we were steering for which at this time extended from N 42° E to NW.[5] As we were not like to have any intercourse with the Inhabitants of this fine isle by which we might obtain its true name, I called it *Sandwich Island*[6] in honour of My Noble Patron the Earl of Sandwich, the Northwestermost of the two Isles which lie on the NE side I name Muntagu and the Southeastermost [Hinchinbrook].[7] Sandwich Island (Lat [17°22′ S] Long^{de}

extended from S 88° west to N 64° W, Traytors head N 58° W distant 20 leagues, the island of Erronan N 86° E distant 5 Leagues and Annattom from S½E to S½West distant 10 Leagues.—f. 263.

[1] The figures given in square brackets in the four preceding sentences are from the Log. These sentences are omitted from B, which substitutes the passage printed in the previous note. In the last sentence I have, following the Log, substituted 'Leagues' for 'Miles'—as I have done elsewhere more than once.

[2] . . . when seeing no more land to the South

[3] . . . and made a fine appearence

[4] ABGH *note*: The word Survey, is not to be understood here, in its literal sence. Surveying a place, according to my Idea, is takeing a Geometrical Plan of it, in which every place is to have its true situation, which cannot be done in a work of this kind.

[5] *we began . . . NW:* we drew near the SE end and ranged the South coast, which we found to trend in the direction of W and WNW for about nine leagues . . .

[6] It was Efate.

[7] Cf. p. 472, n. 5. This present occasion must be that of naming Montagu Island, which Cook has mentioned already in B under the date 26 July—almost a month earlier than this. But even here he has not yet named Hinchinbrook—Nguna according to the earlier entry, Mau according to this one; for it must be noted that 'the Chart' does not 'misplace'

[167°40′ E]) lies NW and SE and is   Leagues long in that direction and about [24] in circuit,[1] from its Shores which are low the land rises with a gentle Slope to the hills which are in the middle of the isle whose summits are covered with Wood; a Luxuriant Vegetation, beautifully diversified between Woods, Launds and Plantations seem'd to spread it self over the whole island;[2] near the middle of the SW side and close to the Shore lay three or four small Islands within which seem'd to be safe Anchorage.[3] We continued to range the Coast of this isle to its NW extremity off which lies a small Island[4] which we pass'd at 8 o'Clock and then Steer'd NNW for the SE end of Mallicollo which at half an hour past Six AM bore N 14° E distant 7 or 8 Leagues and the Island three hills S 82° East. Soon after we saw the Islands Apee Paoom and Ambrrym; the land comprehended under the name of Paoom appeared to us now to be two Islands, some thing like a Seperation was seen between the Hill and the land to the West.[5] We approached the SW side of Mallicollo to within half a league and ranged the coast at that distance. From the SE end it trends west a little southerly[6] to a pretty high point or head land[7] which obtained the name of S.W. Cape, between which and the SE end the Coast seem'd to form several projecting points, or else they[8] were so many small isles lying under the shore, we were certain of one about a League and a half short of the Cape. Close to the NW point of the Cape is a round rock or Islot, connected to the Cape by breakers which helps to shelter a fine bay, formed by an elbow in the coast,

the names now given. It was Cook himself who misplaced them in revising his journal. The two passages give some indication of the time lag between the composition of the two versions. B omits most of this sentence and the following one.

[1] The figures given in square brackets in this sentence are from the Log.

[2] 'In short so far as may be Judged from what we have seen from the Ship this is one of the most beautiful & desirable Islands we have yet seen in the South Seas.'—Wales.

[3] The coastal outline on the chart is not good here. The islets of Eratapu, Erakor, Fila, and Mele have been suggested; but Cook may have mistaken other features of the coast for islets—including the low wooded peninsula which ends in Pango point, at the entrance to Mele Bay. Behind this peninsula, on the eastern side of Mele Bay, is indeed safe anchorage—the harbour of Vila, now the port of entry for the New Hebrides, and the seat of two Resident Commissioners, British and French. But Cook had not that gift of prophecy which would have been necessary to foresee the Condominium.

[4] This passage, in conjunction with the chart, which follows it quite literally, is extremely baffling till one notes that in B, f. 263v, 'NW' is altered to 'western'. The geography then becomes intelligible; for there is no island off the north-western point of Efate, except Moso (or Verao), which was comparatively large, and to Cook was part of 'Sandwich Island' itself. Cook seems to mean the islet called Hat Island or Eradaka, which lies about two miles westward of the coastal feature called, not unsuitably, Baffling Point.

[5] The 'Hill' was Lopevi, the 'land to the West' was Paama. Cf. p. 460, n. 1 above.

[6] . . . for 6 or 7 leagues and then NWbW 3 leagues . . .—f. 263v.

[7] . . . situated in Latitude 16°29′ and

[8] *between which . . . else they:* The coast, which is low, seemed to be indented into Creeks and projecting points, or else these points

from the reigning winds.[1] Numbers of People appeared on all parts of the Coast and some attempted to come of to us in Canoes, but as I would not wait their attempt was fruitless. From the S. W. Cape the Coast trends NBW but the most advanced land bears from it NWBN and seem'd to terminate in a point.[2] We followed the direction of the Coast which we were two miles from at Noon and by Observation in Latitude 16°22′30″ S which is nearly in the parallell with [Port Sandwich] and [26] miles west of it[3] which limits the breadth of Mallicollo; the S. W. Cape bore S 26° East distant [7] Miles and the Most advanced land NWBN.

WEDNESDAY *24th.* Gentle gales at SE and fine weather. In the PM steer'd for the most advanced point of land which we reached at half past 3 o'Clock and then found the Coast turn more and more to the North. We followed it to its northern extremity which we got length off by 7 o'Clock at which time we were so near the shore as to hear the people who were assembled round a fire they had made on the beach; the night being dark we tacked in 20 fathom water, sandy bottom,[4] and made a trip to the South till the Moon appeared after which resumed our Course to the North, hauld round the point and spent the night in Bougainville's Passage. We were well enough assured of our situation at Sunset by seeing the land on the North side of the Passage extending as far as NW½W.

At Sun-rise found our selves nearly in the middle of the Passage, the NW end of Mallicollo extending from S 30° E′ to South 58° west, the land to the North from N 70° W′ to N 4° E and the isle of Lepers N 30° E distant [11 or 12] Leagues. Variation of the Compass 10°31′ E.

[1] To follow the foregoing description with any success a large-scale chart is really imperative, and one must bear in mind that the western side of Malekula has not been properly surveyed even yet. Cook's 'pretty high point or head land' is on the *west* coast (see p. 510 above), and, to judge from his text, he seems to have given the name 'S.W. Cape', which has not been perpetuated, to a comparatively large piece of coast, which has attained only the status of a broken line on the present-day chart. This broken line comes to a slight projection about half way up—i.e. a short distance north-west of the more certainly charted Caroline bay, itself about 1½ miles NNW of the island of Ur or Toman, at the south-west point of Malekula. This is the 'small isle' Cook was certain of, 'about a League and a half short [B East] of the Cape'. The cape, or point, or head land, seemed high to Cook because of a hill, 1030 feet, at the northern end of a short range, a little in from the shore; and it is further marked by a rock close to the shore, now known as Sugarloaf rock. The northern end of the broken line runs on to West point, where the chart becomes more certain again: this is 'the NW point of the Cape'. The 'round rock or Islot' off it is Ten Stick islet, on a reef which runs north from the point; and the 'fine bay' is South-west bay, where there is good anchorage and shelter from winds from the west and round by the south to north-east.

[2] Rock Point.

[3] *and* [*26*] . . . *of it:* and our never failing guide the Watch shewed that we were 26′ west of it, . . .—f. 264.

[4] . . . on edging off from the shoar we presently got out of Sounding[s]

Made sail and bore up for the East coast of the northern land, along which lie several low woody isles[1] of small extent except the Southermost which[2] is 6 or 7 leagues in circuit and forms the north east point of Bougainville's passage; continued to range the coast of these Isles at half a league from shore and at noon were by Observation in ye Latitude of 15°23′, the Isle of Lepers extending from EBN to EBS distant 7 or 8 Leagues, a bluf head where the Coast we were upon seem'd to terminate bore NNW½W distant 10 or 11 Leagues and an Island East of it, seen from the Mast-head, bearing NBW½W.[3]

We will now return to Mallicollo and finish the account of that Island which lies nearly NW and SE and is [18½] Leagues long in that direction extending from the Lat of 16° ′ to 15°4′, its greatest breadth is [8 leagues][4] and lies at the SE end from whence it grows narrower and narrower to two thirds of its length where it is but 7 or 8 miles broad and is occasioned by a wide open bay on the SW side.[5] The Country about the SE end as far as the SW Cape is luxuriantly cloathed with wood[6] from the Sea Shore to the Summits of the hills, to the NW of that Cape it is spoted with Launds,[7] some of which seem'd to be cultivated, and the Summits of the hills are barren. As you advance to the North the land falls insencibly lower and lower and is less and less covered with wood, I believe it is well inhabited[8] as we saw smokes by day and fires in the night in all parts of the Country.

THURSDAY 25*th*. PM wind at SE a gentle gale. As we advanced to the NNW along a fine Coast covered with trees, we preceived low-land stretching out from the bluf head before mentioned towards the isle but did not seem to join it. We were not sure if the low-land joined to the head or was it self an island; we had already pass'd several projecting points[9] of unequal heights which we were not able to deter-

[1] *and bore up . . . isles:* and steer'd NBE and after wards north along the East Coast of the Northern land, with a fine breeze at SE. We found this Coast, which at first sight appeard to be continued, to be composed of several small low woody isles . . .—f. 264–4v.

[2] . . . on account of the day I named St Bartholomew it . . .—f. 264v. This was Malo.

[3] The 'bluff head' was Cape Quiros; the island Sakau.

[4] I have substituted this figure from the Log for the original MS text ' miles'. The figure 18½ for the length is from the Log also; which gives the direction of the island as NW½N and SE½S.

[5] Cook is here referring to the distance between the eastern shore of this unnamed bay and the coast below Port Sandwich.

[6] . . . and other productions of Nature

[7] *it is . . . Launds:* the Country is less wooded but is agreeably chequered with Lawns . . . —f. 264.

[8] *it . . . inhabited:* it is a very fertile island and well inhabited

[9] *we were . . . points:* I intended to have gone through this channell, but the approach of night made me lay it aside and steer without the island. During the after-noon we pass'd some small isles, lying under the shore and had observed some projecting points . . . —f. 264v.

mine whether they were realy such or Islands, be they either the one or the other they seem'd to form some good bays or harbours, behind these was a ridge of Mountains which terminated at the bluf point. Some white places were seen in the clifts which we judged to be chalk.[1]

At ten o'Clock we were the length of the Northern isle[2] where we spent the night makeing short boards. At Sun-rise the bluf-head which obtained the name of Cape [Quiros] bore west, for which we steered Passing to the North of the isle[3] and a long the low land before mentioned which we found to join to the Cape: At this time an elevated Coast appeared in sight extending from N west to the Southward behind the Cape and was a bout Leagues beyond it.[4] After doubling the Cape we found the Coast trend away to the South[5] and to form a very large and deep bay of which the land above mentioned was its western boundaries. Every thing Conspired to make us beleive this was the Bay of St Philip and St James discovered by Quiros in 1606. To determine this point it was necessary to search it to the very bottom for at this time we could see no end to it, for this purpose hauled the wind on the Larboard tack, having a gentle breeze at South which at Noon began to veer towards East and being well over to the Western shore, tacked and stood to NE.[6] Latitude 14°55′30″, Longde 167°3′ East, the Mouth of the Bay extending from N 64° W to S 86° East.[7]

FRIDAY 26*th*. After Standing an hour and a half to the NE, tacked and stood again up the bay with a gentle breeze at ESE. A NE Swell hurtled us over to the West shore so that at half past 4 PM we had to tack again 2 miles from the Shore in 120 fathom water, a Muddy bottom: we were no sooner about than it fell Calm[8] and we were apprehensive we should be obliged to Anchor in a great depth upon a lee shore, at last a breeze sprung up at ESE and put an end to our apprehensions. During the Calm we observed Numbers of the Na-

[1] In this description 'ridge of Mountains' rather overdoes the height of the land. The 'white places . . . in the clifts' were not chalk, but apparently patches of old coral rock on the face of Table Peak, 'which show out from among the foliage to a great distance, when the sun shines on them' (*Pacific Islands Pilot*, II, p. 211). Table Peak is only 1200 feet high, and from this height the land descends to the cape. But the land is higher to the west.

[2] *Northern isle:* island which lies off the head,

[3] . . . (which is of a moderate height and 3 leagues in circuit)

[4] *from N . . . beyond it:* to the north as far as NWBW.—f. 265.

[5] . . . a little Easterly

[6] *for this . . . to NE:* The Wind being at South we had to ply up and first stretched over for the West shore, which we were three miles from at Noon . . .

[7] . . . this last deriction was the bluf head distant 3 Leagues.

[8] *we were . . . Calm:* The bluf head or East point of the Bay bore N 53° East. We were no sooner Tacked than it fell calm and left us to the mercy of the swell, which continued to hurtle us towards the shore . . .

tives assembled on the Shore in sever[l] different places and some came of in two Canoes, but all the Signs of Friendship we could make did not induce them to come a long side or near enough to receive any thing from us, at last they took fright at some thing and suddenly retired a shore. None of tham had any other covering than a little long grass like flags fastned to a belt and hanging down nearly as low as the knee before and behind;[1] their colour was very dark and their hair was either woolly or croped short which made it appear so. The Canoes were single with outriggers.[2]

The night was spent in plying to no purpose for at day-break we found we had advanced nothing, after this our tacks were more advantageous, but the wind which was at South left us to a Calm at 10 o'Clock. At Noon we observed in 15°5′ s and was about 7 or 8 Miles from the head or bottom of the bay, which terminated in a low beach behind which is an extensive flat covered with wood, bounded on each side by a ridge of Mountains.

SATURDAY 27*th*. At 1 PM the Calm was succeeded by a gentle breeze at NBW with which we stood up the bay till 3 when being but about two Miles from the shore, I sent away M[r] Cooper and the Master[3] to sound and reconnoitre the Coast and in the mean time we stood off and on with the Ship, this gave time for three sailing Canoes who had been following us some time to come up with us; there were 5 or 6 Men in each; they came near enough to take hold of such things as were thrown them fastned to a rope but would not come along side.[4] They were the same sort of people as we saw last night[5] and had some resemblance to those of Mallicollo but seemed to be stouter and better shaped, and so far as we could judge spoke a different language which made us believe they were of a nother Nation: probably the

[1] Cf. Wales, 27 August: 'The Dress of the Natives who came off to the Ship consisted only of a String which was tied very tight round the Waist, and a long narrow strip of Cloth, which, I think, passes between their legs and under their Girdle from whence the two ends hang down before and behind, almost as low as their knees. To this may be added a sort of Coronet of Cocks feathers which they wear on their head'.

[2] . . . The Calm continued till near 8 oClock in which time we had drove into 85 fathom water and so near the shore that I expected we should be obliged to Anchor; a breeze of wind sprung up at ESE and first took us on the wrong side but contrary to all our expectations and when we had hardly room to veer, the Ship came about and we filled on the starboard tack and stood off NE thus we were relieved from the apprehensions of being forced to an anchor in a great depth on a lee shore and in a dark and obscure night.—ff. 265v–6.

[3] . . . in two boats . . .—f. 265v.

[4] 'While we were lying too for the Boats 3 Canoes with 5 or 6 of the Natives came off to us, and with much coaxing approached near enough to take some Medalls, Nails & pieces of Otahitee Cloth which were lowered down to them by a string, They began to gather Courage & would I believe soon have ventured on board had they not seen our boats Coming off . . .—Wales.

[5] . . . indeed we thought they came from the same place . . .

same as Annamoka and the neighbouring isles, as one of them, on some occasion, mentioned the Numerals as far as five or Six in that language, some other circumstance increased the Probabillity such as giving us the Names of such parts of the Country as we pointed to, but we could not obtain from them the Name of the Island.[1] Some had hair short and crisp which looked like wool,[2] others had it tyed up[3] on the crown of the head and Ornamented with feathers like the New Zealanders, their other Ornaments were Braclets and Necklaces and one wore some thing like a white shell on his fore-head.[4] Some were painted with a kind of black Pigment. It did not appear to me that they had any other weapons with them than darts and fish gigs intended only for strieking of fish. The Canoes which were by no means a master piece of workman Ship, were fitted with outriggers.[5] The Sail was trianglar, extended between two sticks one of which was the Mast and the other the Yard or boom, at least so they appeared to us who only saw them under Sail at some distance off. They remained by us till they saw our boats returning and then they Paddled in for the Shore.[6] When the boats got on board M[r] Cooper informed me that they had landed on the beach at the head of the bay near a fine River which fell into the bay, by a narrow but strong stream over the beach; it being near low-tide the Water was perfectly sweet and fresh, but at high-water the tide was supposed to flow into it;[7] they found 3 fathom water close to the beach and 50 & 55 f[ms] two Cables length off.[8] Some people were seen on the beach both to the right and left, but our people did not attempt an interview the others seem'd desirous to avoid but imbarked after leaving some Medals and other things on the beach.

Before the boats got on board we had got the wind at SSE which blew

[1] It does not seem that Espiritu Santo as a whole ever had a native name, though the south-eastern portion is now referred to as Marina. There are, as we have seen, other islands for which the same observation holds. Cf. Wales, 27 August: 'If I interpreted their Signs right they seemed to be very friendly inclined, and endeavoured to understand and answer such Questions as we put to them: and amongst others told us the Land which forms y[e] West side of the Bay is called *Tafonia*; but they gave us three or four different Names for as many different Parts of it'.

[2] *such as giving . . . wool:* they understood us when we asked the names of the adjacent lands in that language; some indeed had black short frizled hair like the Mallicoleans, . . . —f. 265v.

[3] *tyed up:* long and tyed up

[4] Several species of white univalve shells were worn on the forehead as ornaments.

[5] *The Canoes . . . outriggers:* Their Canoes were much like those of Tanna and Navigated in the same manner or nearly so.—f. 266.

[6] . . . notwithstanding all we could say or do to detain them.

[7] *a fine . . .into it:* a fine river or stream of fresh Water, so large and deep that they judged boats might enter it at high water, . . .—f. 266.—This was Quiros's River Jordan (native Eora or Yora); its accessibility for large boats varies.

[8] . . . without which they did not sound, and where we were with the ship we had no soundings with a line of 170 fathoms.

directly down the bay, in which we had already spent two days and it was probable we should spind a nother before we could get to an Anchor, we were in want of little we could expect to find here and had no time to spend in amusements. On these considerations I ordered the boats to be hoisted in and to make sail and steer down the bay. During the fore part of the night the Country was prettily illuminated with fires from the Sea shore to the Summits of the hills,[1] we judged they were occasioned by the Natives burning the roots of trees, underwood &c[a] on the places they clear for new Plantations as we had seen done at Tanna.[2] All the AM we had but little wind so that we advanced but little. At Noon Observed in Lat 14°39½′, [the SE point] bore S 48° East and the NW point of the Bay N 82° west distant [5] miles, in this Situation the west shore of the Bay was about miles from us.[3]

It was not unanimously concluded that this was the bay of S[t] Philip and S[t] James, as the Port of *Vara Cruz* was not to be found,[4]

[1] ... but this was only on the West side of the bay.

[2] ... At day-break found ourselves two thirds down the bay, and as we had but little wind it was noon before we were the length of the NW point, ...—f. 266.

[3] This sentence provides another example of those which are less informative than the Log, though it is possible that the blank represents an hiatus due to a slip in copying the Log. Log 956 reads, 'Hoisted in the Boats and made Sail down the bay the NW point of which at Noon bore N 82° West distant 6 Miles, and the SE point S 48° East distant 8 Leag[s] Lat. 14°39′30″ Longitude 165°58′ East. I called the former Cape Cumberland and the latter Cape Quirios [*sic*]. This is undoubtedly the Bay of S[t] Philip and S[t] Iago discovered by Quiros, in [1606] and the anchorage at the head of it is what is called the Port of *Vera Cruz*.'

[4] Forster, II, pp. 372–3: 'it is still somewhat doubtful....' Wales was sceptical to start off with, but was converted: '[26 August] Towards the Eastern Corner is a pretty large Brook runing with great rapidity into the sea & at some Distance a small stream or two of Water Ousing through the beach: but these can never surely be the Rivers Quiros writes of, if they are he must have far exceeded the *Poetica Licentia* and I fear much that even the Priviledges of a Traveller, extensive as they are generally said to be will scarce bear him out. However this may be it is certain we saw not the least appearance of his Port of *Vera Cruz* which would Contain a thousand sail of Ships, and were even unfortunate enough not to find Anchorage for a single Ship at any prudent distance from the Shore. It is possible this may not be y[e] Bay of S[t] Phil. & James; but the first he mentions, & if so, we shall find it round y[e] North-west point of this Bay.' [27 August] 'I here take the Opportunity to conclude what I have to say concerning the Bay of S[t] Phillip & James, and by the bye, it is now clear that that we have just left is what was called so by Quiros, seeing that we have not the least appearance of any more land either to the southward, Westward, or Northward'. 'The first he mentions': this is not altogether clear, but I think Wales is referring to a passage in Torquemada's account of the voyage of Quiros, printed in Dalrymple's *Collection*, II, p. 136, ' The captain and pilot hearing the description of this port, and that to leeward of it there was the appearance of another large bay, they ordered to bear away....' This other large bay would then be the portion of the coast between Sakau Island and Sugmar Point, at the bottom of which is Hog Harbour. The port of Vera Cruz, which could contain a thousand ships, lay, wrote Torquemada, between the two rivers Jordan and Salvador. By 1774 the Salvador seems to have dried up. Clerke accepted the bay but could not otherwise accept Quiros: 'On the N°ermost part of this Isle is the Bay of S[t] Phillip and S[t] James where Quiros staid 36 days with his 3 Vessels. He has given a most pompous description of this Country in his Memorials to the King of Spain wherein he solicits the settlement of these Isles; however I firmly believe M[r] Quiros's Zeal and warmth for his own favourite projects has carried him too far in the

for my own part I had no doubt about it, I found general points to agree very well with Quiros's discription, and as to what he calls the Port of Vara Cruz is undoubtedly the Anchorage at the head of the bay which in some places may extend farther off than where our boats sounded:[1] it was but natural for them to give a name to a place, independant of so large a bay, where they laid so long at Anchor. Port is a vague term, like many others used in geography, and is very often applied to a much less sheltred place than the head of this bay. The Officers observed that there is seldom any surf on the beach, as grass and other plants grew close to high-water mark which is a sure sign of Pacifick anchorage; they judged that the tides rose about 4 feet and that boats might enter the River[2] at high-water, so that it is very prob[ab]le it is one of those mentioned by Quiros and appearence inclined us to believe we saw the other. The beach at the head of the bay [is]   miles extent and where our boats landed it is about   yards broad. The Bay hath [20] Leagues Sea Coast, [Six] on the East side which lies in the direction of [S½W and N½E, two] at the head and [Twelve] on the west side which lies in the direction of [SBE and NBW from the head down to two thirds of its length and then NWBN to the NW Point].[3] The two Capes which form the entrance lie in the direction of N 53° west and S 53° East distant [Ten] Leagues from each other. The bay is every were free from danger and unfathomable, except near the shores which are for the Most part low and have Sounding a little way off; this low shore is no more than a little[4] strip of low-land between the sea and the foot of the hills.

I have already said that the bay as well as the flat land above it is bounded on each side by a ridge of hills, the one to the west is very high[5] and double and extends the whole length of the Island. An extraordinary luxuriant vegetation is every where to be seen from the Sea Shore to the summits of the highest hills, of all the productions of Nature this Country was adorn'd with the Cocoa-nut tree were the most conspicuous. The sides of the Mountains were

qualities he has attributed to this Country; for fine and fertile as it certainly is, I'm afraid he's there given it too prolific a Soil and luxuriant a Clime; at least if we may be allow'd to judge, from what we cou'd observe of this Country and the productions of the Neighbouring Isles. . . .'—'Account of the Great Cyclades', following 31 August. Clerke refers to Quiros's eighth memorial, printed by Dalrymple, II, pp. 162–74.

[1] *sounded:* landed. There is nothing in Quiros's account of the Port which contridicts but rather confirms this supposition;

[2] . . . which seemed to be pretty deep and broad within, . . .—f. 266v.

[3] This last sentence again is given more fully in the Log than here. The portion in square brackets must have been added to the Log after Add. MS 27886 was written up, and then have been copied only into B.

[4] *little:* very narrow

[5] The volcanic ridges here rise to 4000 feet.

checkered with Plantations[1] in which were seen Plantans &c[a], these together with the many fires we have seen by night and Smokes by day make it highly probable the country is well inhabited.[2]

SUNDAY 28*th.* In the PM with a light breeze at East doubled [Cape Cumberland] from which the Coast trends S 48° west for about miles and then gradually round to South, SSE and SEBS. During night and most part of the Morning it was calm so that at Noon [Cape Cumberland] bore N 47° E dist[t] only Leagues.[3] Lat Ob[d] 14°50′30″.

MONDAY 29*th.* Light airs next to a Calm all these 24 hours. PM Variation p[r] Az[th] 9°40′ East. Noon observed Latitude 14°59′ the Land extending from NNE½E to SSE½E.

TUESDAY 30*th.* In the AM the Calm was succeeded by a breeze from SE and SSE, tho' right in our teeth it was better than none as it inabled us to ply up the coast, which at Noon extended from NNE to SE½E distant from the nearest shore 4 Leagues, Lat Ob[d] 15°20′.[4]

WEDNESDAY 31*st.* Fresh breeze at SSE and fair weather. At 3 PM Tacked in 75 fathom water one Mile from the Shore before a low sandy flatt where several of the Natives made their appearence. After this we continued to make boards of two and three hours as was most advantageous. At Noon the South end of the Island bore N 62° East miles,[5] this is what forms the NW point of Bougainvill's Passage: the South side of the Isle which forms the NE point bore N 85° East and the NW end of Mallicollo from S 72° E to S 54° East. Latitude Observed 15°45′ S.

[SEPTEMBER 1774]

THURSDAY 1*st.* Moderate breezes at SE and ESE fair Weather. In the PM without makeing any more board[s] we doubled the South point of the Island, to the East of which the Coast is and seem'd to form little bays or creeks, with some low isles lying of it toward the SE end behind [St. Bartholomew's Island] so that SE as well as most of the East Coast of [Espiritu Santo] is covered with small Islands which without answering any other end cannot fail makeing some good harbours. After stretching to the East N East till 5 o'Clock the bore from to S 75° E, the SW end N 82° west, and the Island

[1] . . . and every Vally watered by a stream of Water . . .—f. 267.

[2] . . . and very fertile

[3] *at Noon . . . Leagues:* Log 'At Noon . . . the NW Point of the Bay in a line with the first Point to the South of it N 37° East distant 7 Leagues'.

[4] 'We've made but a poor hand of it these 3 days past; these light Airs and Calms detain us most confoundedly, and now begin to grow very tedious'.—Clerke.

[5] *miles:* distant 4 Leagues . . .—f. 267v.—'dist[t] 10 or 11 Miles'.—Log.

of Mallicollo from S 31° E to S 53° E, and haveing made the Circuit of [the isle] and with it finished the Survey of the whole Archipelago so that I had no more business there, besides the Season of the year made it necessary I should think of returning to the South. With this View we tacked and hauled to SSW with our Larboard tacks aboard.[1] At Sun-rise the next morning we saw no more land. At Noon we were in Lat 16°34′ S, Long^{d} 16 ° E. [Longitude made 0°45′ W.][2]

*[27th] The East point of this Bay, I name *Cape Quiros*, in memory of the first discoverer, it is situated in Latitude 14°56′00″ S, Longitude 167°13′ East. The NW point I named *Cape Cumberland* in honour of His Roy^{l} Highness the Duke,[3] it lies in the Latitude of 14°38′45″ S, Longitude 166°49½′ East and is the NW extremity of this Archipelago, for after doubling it, we found the Coast to trend gradually round to the South and SSE. The 28th and 29th we had light airs and Calms, so that we advanced but little; in this time we took every oppertunity when the horizon was clearer than Common to look out for more land, but none was seen; by Quiros's track to the North, after leaving the bay above mentioned, it seems probable that there is none nearer than Queen Charlottes Island, discovered by Captain Carteret which lies about 90 leagues NNW from Cape Cumberland and which I take to be the same with *St^{a} Cruz*.[4]

TUESDAY 30*th*. The Calm was succeeded by a fresh breeze at S.S.E. which inabled us to ply up the Coast. At noon observed in 15°20′, afterwards stretched in East to within a mile of the Shore and then tacked in 75 fathom, before a sandy flat on which several of the natives made their appearence. We observed on the sides of the hills several plantations that were laid out by line and fenced round.

WEDNESDAY 31*st*. At Noon the South or SW point of the island

[1] Rather than fill in all Cook's gaps at length in this paragraph I print the following passage from the Log: 'In standing to the East ward, weathered the South end of the Island and stood into Bougainvilles passage till 5 oClock, when having made the circuit of the isle, tacked stood out again and hauled to the Southward, Mallicollo extending from S 31° E to S 53° E, the South point of the Island which forms the NE point of the Passage S 75° E and the NW point of the Passage N 82° West distant 10 miles from this point which is in Latitude 15°40′ Long. 166° 59 East I take my departure.'

[2] This longitude and those by account and watch given in square brackets, 2–4 September, are from the Log; the others from B.

[3] Henry Frederick, Duke of Cumberland (1745–90), brother of George III; a man on whom it is impossible to lavish any particular encomium, unless it is an encomium to say with the *Dictionary of National Biography* that, though coarse and brutal in everyday life, he was not without taste. He certainly subscribed to Burney's *History of Music*.

[4] The Banks group is nearer than the Santa Cruz group, although a little to the east. Cook's last remark is almost, but not quite, correct. Carteret discovered, or rediscovered, the Santa Cruz group, which he called Queen Charlotte's Islands, on 12 August 1767. Mendaña's Santa Cruz, as a particular island, was Ndeni. Carteret, who lost four men here, in a brush with the natives caused by his master's stupidity and disobedience, called it Egmont.

bore N 62° E distant 4 Leagues, this point forms the NW point of what I call Bougainvill's Passage,[1] the NE point at this time bore N 85° East and the NW end of Mallicollo from S 54° East to S 72° East, Lat. Ob[d] 15°45′ S. In the afternoon, in stretching to the East, weathered the SW point of the island from which the coast tren[d]ed East Northerly. It is low and seemed to form some Creeks or Coves and as we got farther into the Passage we preceived some small low isles lying along it, which seemed to extend behind S[t] Bartholomew island.[2] Having now finished the Survey of the Whole Archipelago and the Season of the year makeing it necessary I should return to the South, while I had yet some time left to explore any lands I might meet with between this and New Zeland, where I intended to touch to refresh my people and recrute our stock of wood and Water, for another Southern Cruse:[3] with this view, at 5 PM we Tacked and hauled to the Southward with a fresh gale at SE at this time the NW point of the passage or the SW point of the Island *Tierra Del Espiritu Santo*, the only remains of Quiros's Continent, bore N 82° West distant 3 Leagues I named it *Cape Lisburne*,[4] its situation is in Latitude 15°40′, Long[de] 165°59″ E: In the foregoing account of these Islands I have neither been particular enough in situation nor discription. I thought by treating these subjects by themselves, would, together with the annexed Chart,[5] convey to the reader a better idea of them than if this had been done in order as they were explored.

The Northern islands of this Archipelago were first discovered by that great Navigator Quiros in 1606, and not without reason supposed to be a part of the Southern Continent, which at that time and

[1] Now called Bougainville Strait, between Malekula and Espiritu Santo (including Malo).

[2] Malo. I give the identifications of these islands again, for the reader's convenience, as part of Cook's summary.

[3] Cf. pp. 325–8 above. Cook was now once more modifying his plan of action somewhat, owing to 'the Season of the year' and the necessity of recruitment. He had not let the Forsters into the secret—which accounts for George Forster's rather silly passage dated 1 September: 'We proceeded at present to the southward, and prepared to cross the South Sea in its greatest breadth towards the extremity of America; and though our crew were much weakened by living entirely upon salt meat in a hot climate, yet it was intended not to touch at any place by the way; a project, which if it had been put in execution, would doubtless have proved fatal to some of them, whose bad constitution would not prompt them to support such an abstinence. Fortunately, after standing on the same course for three days, we fell in with a large land, which had never been visited by any European navigator before, and which entirely altered the plan of our proceedings for the remaining part of our stay in the South Seas'.—II, p. 376. Wales comments furiously on this, *Remarks*, p. 89.

[4] The Hon. Wilmot Vaughan (1728–1800), 4th Viscount Lisburne 1766, Earl of Lisburne 1776; a politician of some prominence, a member of the Board of Trade 1768–70, and a Lord of the Admiralty 1770–82. He was one of the men who signed Cook's instructions for this voyage.

[5] This particular chart is no longer extant. Presumably it was the basis for the one in the printed *Voyage*, II, pl. III. See Fig. 66, and Wales's chart, Fig. 65.

untill very lately was supposed to exist. They were next visited by M. de Bougainville in 1768, who, besides landing on the isle of Lepers, did no more than discover that it was not a connected land, but composed of islands which he called the great Cyclades; but as we, not only, ascertained the extent and situation of these islands, but added to them several new ones which were not known before and explored the whole, I think we have obtained a right to name them and shall for the future distinguish them under the name of the *New Hebrides.*[1] They are Situated between the Latitude of 14°29′ and 20°4′ South and between 166°41′ and 170°21′ East Longitude and extend 125 Leagues in the direction of NNW½W and SSE½E.

The most Norther[n] island is that called by M. de Bougainville *Peake of the Etoile*,[2] it is situated according to his account in Latitude 14°29′, Longitude 168°09′ and NBW 8 leagues from Aurora. The next island which lies farthest North is that of *Tierra Del Espiritu Santo.* It is the most Westermost and largest of all the Hebrides being 22 leagues long in the direction of NNW½W and SSE½E, 12 in breadth and 60 in circuit, we have obtained the true figure of this island very accurately. The land of this Island especially the West side is exceeding high and Mountainous and in many places the hills rise directly from the Sea. Except the Clifts and beaches every other part is covered with wood or laid out in Plantations. Besides the Bay of St Philip and St Iago, the isles which lie a long the South and East Coast, cannot, in my opinion, fail of forming some good Bays or Harbours.[3]

The next considerable island is that of *Mallicollo*,[4] to the SE; it extends NW and SE and is 18 Leagues long in that direction, its greatest breadth which is at the SE end, is 8 leagues, the NW end

[1] Why this particular name? one may ask. Why should Cook pick on the Hebrides to make new? Nothing could be more violently unlike the Hebrides than this dispersed group of islands, with their heavy covering of tropical rain-forest and their volcanoes. I can only suggest that he named the New Hebrides and New Caledonia in conjunction, and that their contiguity gave him the solution for two problems in nomenclature at once: just as the Hebrides lay off the coast of Scotland, so did the New Hebrides lie off the coast (or at least near enough to it not to make the analogy absurd) of New Scotland. In any case we get a pleasant name for islands which have had, since Cook's day, a rather unpleasant history.

[2] *Pic de l'Etoile* (named after Bougainville's ship), Star Peak, or Mera Lava. Quiros had called it San Marcos. Bougainville's position is not far out. Geographically, it is rather the most southern member of the Banks group, though that group administratively is reckoned in with the New Hebrides. Cook did not see it himself, though, says Forster (II, p. 199), 'My father had a momentaneous glimpse of it . . . but the clouds which moved with great velocity soon involved it.'

[3] There are a number of good anchorages, but only one place that attains the dignity of the name of harbour—Hog Harbour, on the east coast. In the Bay of St Philip and St James (locally known as Big Bay), 'the area of depths suitable for anchorage is very restricted and terminates abruptly'.—*Pacific Islands Pilot,* II, p. 212. Quiros found this

[4] Malekula. See Fig. 67.

is 2 thirds this breadth and near the middle one third, this contraction is occasioned by a wide and pretty deep bay on the SW side. To judge of this island from what we saw of it, it must be very fertile and well inhabited; The land on the Sea Coast is rather low and lies with a gentle Slope from the hills, which are in the Middle of the island. Two thirds of the NE Coast was only seen at a great distance, therefore the delineation of it on the Chart can have no pretentions to accuracy; but the other parts I apprehend are without any material error. *St Bartholomew*[1] lies between the SE end of Tierra del Espiritu Santo and the North end of Mallicollo, the distance between it and the latter is Eight miles; this is the Passage through which M. de Bougainville went[2] the middle of which is in latitude 15°48′.

The *Isle of Lepers*[3] lies between Spiritu Santo and Aurora Island, 8 leagues from the former and 3 from the latter, in latitude 15°22′ and nearly under the same Meridian as the SE end of Mallicollo; It is of an Egg like[4] figure, very high and 18 or 20 leagues in circuit; the limmits of this isle was determined by several bearings, but the lines of the shore was traced out by guess, except the NE part, where there is Anchorage half a mile from Shore.

Aurora, *Whitsuntide*, *Ambrym*, *Paoom* and its neighbour, *Apee*, *Three Hills* and *Sandwich* islands, lie all nearly under the Meridian of 167°26′ or 30′ East, extending from the Latitude of 14°51′30″ to 17°53′30″. The Island of *Aurora*[5] lies NBW and SBE and is 11 leagues long in that direction, but I believe it hardly any where exceeds 2 or 2½ in breadth, it hath a good height and hilly surface and every were covered with wood, except where the Natives have their dwellings and Plantations. *Whitsuntide Isle*[6] lies 1½ leagues to the South of Aurora and is of the same length and lies in the direction of North and South, but it is something broader than Aurora I^d^, it is of a good hieght and cloathed with Wood, except such parts as seemed to be cultivated which were pretty numerous. From the South end of Whitsuntide Island to the North side of Ambrrym[7] is 2½ leagues; this island is about 17 Leagues in circuit, its shores are rather low, but the land rises with an unequal ascent to a tolerable high mountain in the middle of the island from which ascended great columns of Smoak, but we were not able to determine whether this was occa-

[1] Malo.
[2] *Deleted* he calls it 5 leagues broad which shews him a bad guesser of distance.—In H the words 'which shews . . . distance' are heavily deleted. The strait is 7½ miles wide.
[3] Omba or Aoba.
[4] A rather angular egg, to be sure.
[5] Maewo.
[6] Pentecost or Raga.
[7] Ambrim or Ambrym.

sioned by a Volcano or not:[1] The island seemed to be fertile and will Inhabited by the great [n]umber of Smoaks we saw rise out of the Woods, in such parts of the island as came within the compass of our sight, for it must be observed that we did not see the whole of it, and we saw still much less of *Paoom*[2] and its neighbour,[3] I can say no more of this island than that it towers up to a Great height in the form of a round hay stack, its extent, as also the one by it (if there are two) cannot exceed 3 or 4 leagues in any direction, for the distance between Ambrrym and Apee is hardly 5 and they lie in this space and East from Port Sandwich distant about 7 or 8 leagues. The Island of *Apee*[4] is not less than 20 Leagues in circuit, its longest direction is about 8 leagues NW and SE, it is of a considerable height and hath a hilly surface, diversified with woods and Lawns, the West and South parts especially, for as to the others we did not see. *Shepherds Isles* are a group of small Isles of unequal extent, extending off from the SE point of Apee, about 5 leagues in the direction of SE. The Island *Three Hills*[5] lies South 4 leagues from the Coast of Apee, and SE½S distant 17 leagues from Port Sandwich. To this and what hath been already said of it I shall only add, that WBN 5 miles from the west point is a Reef of Rocks on which the Sea Continualy breaks.

Nine leagues in the direction of South from Three Hills, lies *Sand-[w]ich Island. Two hills*, the *Monument* and *Montagu* islands[6] lies to the east of this line and *Hinchinbrook*[7] to the West as also two or three small isles which lie between it and Sandwich Island to which they are connected by breakers. *Sandwich Island* is 25 Leagues in Circuit, its greatest extent is 10 leagues and lies in the direction of NW by W and SE by E. The NW Coast of this island we only Viewed at a distance, therefore the Chart in this part may be faulty, so far as it regards the line of the Coast but no farther. The distance from the SE end of Mallicollo to the NW end of Sandwich island is 22 leagues in the direction of SSE½E. In the same direction lies *Erromango*, *Tanna* and *Annattom*.[8] The first is 18 leagues from Sandwich island and is 24 or 25 leagues in Circuit; the middle of it lies in the Latitude of 18°54′, Longitude 169°19′ E and is of a good hieght as may be gathered from the distance we were off when we first saw it.

Tanna lies 6 leagues from the South side of *Erromango*, it extends SEBS and NWBN and is about 8 leagues long in that direction and every were about 3 or 4 leagues broad.[9] The Harbour is situated

[1] Cf. p. 459, n. 7 above.
[2] Paama.
[3] Lopevi.
[4] Epi.
[5] Emae or Mai.
[6] Mataso, Wot, and Emau or Mau.
[7] Nguna.
[8] Eromanga, Tana, Aneityum.
[9] *Deleted* consequently it must be 22 in circuit.

on the north side of the most eastern point of the isle about ENE from the Volcano in Latitude 19°33′, Longitude 169°44′35″, it is no more than a little Creek runing in SBW½W three quarters of a Mile and about half that in breadth; a shoal of Sand and rocks lying along the East side makes it still narrower, in the harbour is from 6 to 3 fathom water a bottom of Sand and Mud and room to moor with half a Cable each way. No place can be more convenient for Wooding and Watering, the Water stunk a little after it had been a few days on board, but after wards turnd sweet, and even when it was at the worst the Tin Machine would in an hours time sweeten a whole Cask; this is a most excellent contrivance for sweetning water. It is high-water in this harbour at the full and Change of the Moon [about 5^h45^m][1] and the tides rises and falls upon a perpendicular [three feet]. I named this Harbour *Port Resolution* after the Ship as she was the first who ever entered it. The isle of *Immer*[2] lies in the direction of NBE½E four leagues from Port Resolution in Tanna and the Island of *Erronan* or *Footoona*,[3] East distant 11 leagues: This is the most easte[r]n island of all the Hebrides, it did not seem to be above 5 leagues in circuit, but it is of a considerable height and flat at top: on the NE side is a little Peak, seemingly disjoined from the isle, but we thought it was connected by low land.[4] *Annattom* which is the Southermost Island is situated in the Latitude of 20°3′, Longitude 170°4′ and S 30° East 11 or 12 leagues from Port Resolution: it is of a good height and hilly Surface and more I must not say of it. Here follows the Lunar observation made by Mr Wales for assertaining the Longitude of these islands reduced by the Watch to Port Sandwich in Mallicollo and Port Resolution in Tanna—

Port Sandwich	Mean of 10 Sets of Obser^ns before —	167°56′33¾″	East Longitude
	——— 2 D^o ——— at ———	168 02 37½	
	——— 20 D^o ——— after ———	167 52 57	
	Mean of these means ———	167 57 22¾	
Port Resolution	Mean of 20 Sets of Obser^ns before —	169°37′35″	East Longitude
	——— 5 D^o ——— at ———	169 48 48	
	——— 20 D^o ——— after ———	169 47 22½	
	Mean of these means ———	169 44 35	

It is necessary to observe, that each set of observations, consists, of between Six and ten observed distances of the Sun and Moon or

[1] Figure omitted and supplied from *Voyage*, II, p. 84.
[2] Aniwa.
[3] Futuna.
[4] It is so connected.

Moon and Stars, so that the whole number amounts to several hundreds and these have been reduced by means of the Watch to all the islands, so that the Longitude of each is as well assertained as the two Ports above mentioned, as a proof of this I shall only observe that the difference of Longitude between the two Ports pointed out by the Watch, and by the observations did not differ from each other two miles. This also shews to what degree of accuracy these observations are capable of, when multiplyed to a considerable number, made with different Instruments and with the Sun and Stars on both sides of the Moon; by the last method, the errors which may be either in the Instruments or Lunar Tables, destroy one another and likewise those which may arise from the observer himself, for some men may observe closer than others. If we consider the number of observations that may be obtained in the course of a Month (if the weather is favourable) we shall, perhaps, find this method of finding the Longitude of place[s] as accurate as most others, at least it is the most easiest to put in practice and attended with the least expence to the observer; every ship that goes to foreign parts is, or may be, supplied with a sufficient number of Quadrants at a small expence, I mean good ones, proper for makeing these observations, for the difference of the price between a good and bad one I apprehend can never be an object with an officer.[1] The most expensive article, and what is in some measure necessary in order to come at the utmost accuracy, is a good watch; but for common use and where the utmost accuracy is not required, one may do without. I have some were before in this Jour[n]al observed that this method of finding the Longitude is not so difficult, but that any man with proper applycation and a little practice may soon learn to make these observations as well as the astronomers themselves. I have seldom[2] found any material difference between the observations made by Mr Wales and those made by the officers at the same time.[3] In finding the variation of the Magnetick Needle, we found, as usual, our Compases differ among themselves, some times near 2°; the same compass too would sometimes make nearly this difference in the Variation on different days and even between the morning and evening of the same day when our change of situation has been but very little. By the mean of the observations which I made about Erromango and

[1] At any rate, if the officer was Cook; but he perhaps put too high a valuation on a number of his fellows.

[2] seldom *substituted for* never.

[3] *Deleted* as may be seen at large in my Logg book.—It is obvious that Cook's officers were improving with practice. Cf. the pains Green took to train the junior men in observation on the first voyage—e.g. I, p. 9, n. 2; p. 225, n. 2.

the SE part of these islands the Variation of the Compass was 10°5′48″ East and the mean of those made about Tierra del Espiritu Santo gave 10°5′30″ E.[1] Having occasionally mentioned the Currents, I shall now observe that we allways found them set towards the NW and were most sinsibly felt on the North side of Sandwich island and about the shores of Erromango, but this might be owing to the Calms which we had there, which made us observe their effects more than could have been done with a fresh breeze of wind. Indeed if it had not been for these Calms, I question if we had discovered there were any attall, especially at any distance from Shore. A modern circumnavigator observed that while the Sun is in the Northern hemisphere the Currents set to the West, and when in the Southern to the East.[2] I have now crossed a part of this ocean within the Tropicks three times when the Sun was in the Northern hemisphere and have not been able to discover that there is any current atall seting either East or West, clear of the lands. My opinion is not supported by my rickoning alone, but those of the other officers also, and likewise by some Journals, kept on board the Dolphin by men on whose judgement I know I can depend. So many concuring testimonies is certainly of more weight than M. de Bougainvilles Journal alone.*—ff. 267–71.

FRIDAY *2nd*. Moderate breezes at SE and ESE, Clowdy but fair weather. Course made good to Noon S 24° West, distance 101 Miles. Lat Observ[d] 18°6′. [Long. Acco: 165°38′.]

SATURDAY *3rd*. First part gentle breeze and fair Weather, remainder Clowdy and hazey with Showers of rain and light airs next to a Calm. At 5 PM Lat 18°22′ Longitude [165°26′] the Variation was 10°50′ East. Lat p[r] Acco[t] at Noon 19°00′. [Long Acco: 165°13′.] Longitude made sence yesterday 20′ west.

SUNDAY *4th*. Light breezes at East and ESE. At 5 PM the sky cleard up and we found the Variation to be 10°51′ E. Lat 19°15′ Longitude 16 ° ′ E. In the AM when the Lat was [19°49′, Longitude 164°53′]

[1] *Note by Cook, marked marginally* 'omit': This is considerably more than M[r] Wales [made] it to be at Tanna; I cannot say what might occasion this difference in the variation between the Sea and on shore, unless it was influanced by the land, for I have no doubt but the variation found at Sea is nearest the truth.

[2] The 'modern circumnavigator' was Bougainville. He writes that on several dates he found himself by ship's reckoning to the east of the longitudes fixed by observation by Verron, his astronomer. 'All these differences shew, that from the isle of Taiti, the currents had carried us much to the westward. . . . I must however observe, that whilst the sun was in the southern hemisphere, our reckoning has been to the westward of the observations; and that, after he passed to the other side of the line, our differences have changed.'—*Voyage* (English ed.), pp. 299–300.

the Amp'd gave 10°21′ and the Azth 10°7′ East. At 8 o'Clock as we were Steering to the South we discovered land bearing SSW distant 8 or 10 Leagues. At Noon it extended from SSE to WBS without our being able to see the termination of it; the nearest part was distant from us about Six Leagues. It appeared high with hills. Latitude Observed 20°00′, Long^{d} in 16 ° ′ East. [Acco: 164°43′ Watch 164°02′.]

MONDAY *5th*. Continued to Stand to the South with a light breeze at East till 6 PM[1] when we were three leagues from the land the extremes of which bore from SEBS to WBN. Some openings appeared in the coast to the West so that we could not tell if it was continued;[2] the extremes to the SE seem'd to terminate in an elevated point (at least we could see no land beyond it) which I named *Cape* [*Colnett*] after one of my Midshipmen who first saw this land.[3] We saw breakers betwixt us and the Shore, but could not tell if they were connected to it, some time before sunset two or three Canoes were seen under sail coming off to us as we supposed, but if that was their design they soon gave it up.

After a few hours Calm we got a gentle breeze at SE and spent the night standing off and on. At Sun-rise the horizon being clear we could see the land extending from SE[4] round by the SW to NWBW. The openings to the West still appeared and a reef or breakers seem'd to extend all along the Coast at some distance off.[5] It was to us a matter of no great moment whether we plyed up the Coast to the East or bore down to the west.[6] I chose the latter and after runing two leagues down the out side of the Reef (for such it proved) we came to an opening or a place free of breakers which had the appearence of a good Channel[7] and which I sent two Arm'd boats to Sound and in the mean time we stood on and off with the Ship. It was necessary to arm the boats as Ten or Twelve Sailing Canoes were near us, we had observed them coming off from the Shore all the Morning from different parts, and some were laying on the reef fishing; as soon as they were got together they came down to us in a body and some of

[1] *6 PM:* 5 in the Evening when we were stoped by a Calm.—f. 272.

[2] *continued:* one connected land or a group of islands,

[3] Cape Colnett is in lat. 20°30′ S, long. 164°46′ E. It may be here noted that Chart XXXVIII transfers the name to what is pretty clearly Cape Baye, a prominent point about 20°57′ S. James Colnett had an interesting career, and was one of the pioneers of the fur-trade on the north-west coast of America. See p. 876 below.

[4] *from SE:* to the SE of Cape Colnett and

[5] *at . . . off:* connected with those we discovered last night.

[6] *East . . . west:* SE . . . NW

[7] . . . through which we might get in for the land, where I wanted to go, not only to visit it but also to have an oppertunity to observe an Eclips of the Sun which was soon to happen.—f. 272v.

them were within hail when we began to hoist out our boats which probably gave them some allarm as they retired again to the reef, but we afterwards saw our boats go along-side one or two. As soon as the boats made the Signal for a Channel we stood in and took them

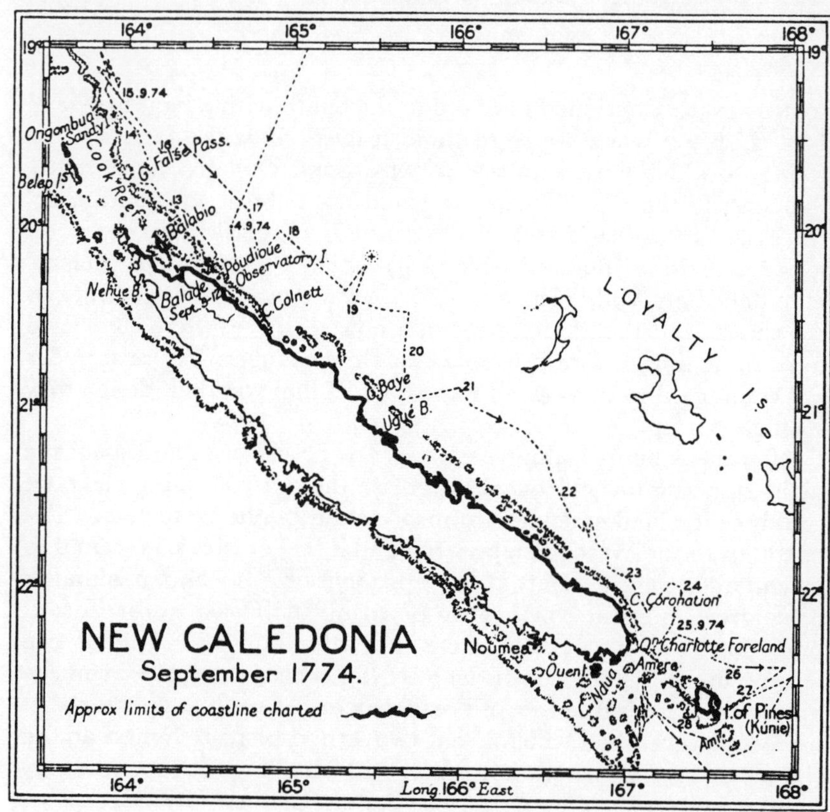

FIG. 68

aboard as they were coming off:[1] the officer informed [me] there was Soundings just within the Channel of 16 & 14 fathom bottom fine sand, also said he had put a long side two Canoes, the people [in] them gave him some fish,[2] in one was a robust young man whom he under-

[1] *As soon . . . coming off:* We now saw that what we had taken for openings in the Coast was low land and that it was all connected excepted [*sic*] the western extremity which was an Island known by the name of Balabea as we afterwards learnt. As soon as the Boats made the Signal for a Channell and one of them placed on the point of the Reef on the weather side of the Channel, we stood in with the Ship and took up the other boat in our way.

[2] *the people . . . fish:* and found the people very obligeing and civil, they gave him some fish, & in return he presented them with medals &c^{a}.

stood was a Prince or Chief. After sending a boat to lay upon the Weather East point of the Channel we stood in and then hauld up S½E for a Small sandy isle we saw lying near the shore,[1] Soundings from 15 to 12 f^m^ a fine Sandy bottom, these soundings continued for about three[2] miles, after which it shoalned to 6, 5 & 4 f^m^. This was on the tail of a Shoal which lay to the East a little without the sandy isles.[3] Being over this we found 7 & 8 fathom which gradually shoalned to 3 f^m^, this last was near the shore. At length after makeing a trip we Anchored in 5 fathom the bottom fine sand mixed with mud, the Sandy isle EBS distant ¾ of a Mile and one or some thing more from the shore of the Main which extended from SEBE to ,[4] an Island which the Natives called *Balabea*[5] and the Channel through which we came nearly north 4 miles distant. The little sandy isle and its shoals and the one without effectually shelters this anchoring place from the reigning winds. We were accompaned to this anchorage by all the Boats we had seen in the morning, which were joined by some others from the Shore so that we had hardly Anchored before we were surrounded by a Vast number of People,[6] the most of them without Arms; at first they were a little Shy, but it was not long before we prevail'd on the people in one Canoe to come near enough to receive some presents we lowered down to them by a line to which they tyed in return two fish which stunk intollerable as did those they gave us in the Morning, these mutual exchanges soon brought on a kind of Confidence so that two ventured aboard[7] and presently after the Ship was full of them and we had the Company of several at dinner in the Cabbin. Our dinner was Pease Soup, Salt Beef and Pork which they had no curiosity to taste, but they eat some yam which they call *Oobee*, which is not much unlike Oofee the

[1] . . . and was followed by all the Canoes.

[2] *three:* 2

[3] *sandy isles:* small isle to the NE.—f. 273.

[4] *to* : round by the South to WNW

[5] . . . bore NWbW . . .—This addition is essential to the meaning of the passage, and Cook can only have omitted it from the MS by a slip. 'Balabea' = Balabio. It appears that Cook made his way inside the long and dangerous barrier reef through the Amoss passage, between the western end of Balade reef on the south-east and the south-east end of Cook reef on the north-west; and then turned south ('hauld up S½E') to anchor inside the 'little sandy isle' he later called Observatory Isle, now known as Pudiu or Poudioué. It was called by the natives 'Pordúa', says Clerke, 6–7 September. Forster renders it 'Poozooe'. Chart XXXIX*a* gives a view of the harbour.

[6] . . . in Sixteen or eighteen canoes,

[7] '. . . great No of Indians came onboard swiming from ye shore, bring with them their weapons of War, & sold them for Nails & old peices of Cloth, which they seem very fond of, Their Weapons of War are Spears made of very hard black wood about 12 or 14 feet in length, which they thro' with a small sling upon ye fore finger, they use Slings to Thro' stones having a bag tied before them with stones in it made on purpose, & they have short Clubs about 3 or 4 feet long & carv'd curiously at ye big end, they have also fish gigs which have 3 or 4 prongs & are jagged.'—Harvey.

name they are called by at all the isles we have been at except Mallicollo.[1] Nevertheless we found these people spoke a language quite new to us and like all those we have lately seen had no other[2] covering than a little case to the Penis which was suffered to hang down. They were curious to look into every cornner of the Ship which they viewed with some attention; they had not the least knowlidge of Goats, Hogs, Dogs or Catts, they had not so much as a name for one of them; they seem'd fond of Iron, large spike Nails especially, and pieces of red cloth or indeed any other colour, but red was their favourite.

TUESDAY *6th.* Wind Easter, Clear weather. In the PM I embarked with two armed boats in order to land, having with us one of the Natives who had attatched himself to me. We landed on a Sandy beach before a great number of people who crowded together with [no] other intent than to see us, for many of them had not so much as a stick in their hands, consequently we were received with great courtesy.[3] I made presents to all those my friend pointed out to me which I observed were either old men or other of some note at least so they appeared to me; he took not the least notice of some Women who stood behind.[4] Here we met with the same Chief Mr Pickersgill had seen in the boats in the Morning;[5] after we had been some little time a shore he called for Silence was instantly obeyed and then made [a] short Speach, a little while after a nother chief did the same, it was extraordinary to see with what attention they were heard and the profound silence which was observed, only two or three old men answered to every sentance[6] by noding their heads and giving a kind of grunt, signifying as I thought their approbation. It was not possible for us to know what was said in these Speaches, we had reason to conclude they were favourable to us on whose account they were undoubtedly made, I kept my eyes fixed on the people all the time and saw nothing to induce me to think otherwise. Whilest we were with them we enquired by signs for Fresh water, some pointed along shore to the East others to the west, my friend offered to conduct us

[1] This generalization is rather too wide, though of course basically correct. The New Zealand, Tahitian, Marquesan and Easter Island word was *uhi*; the Tongan and Tanese *ufi*; the New Caledonian *ubi*; the Malekulan word is given in *Voyage*, II, 'Table' following p. 364, as *Nanram.*

[2] *had no other:* I may say quite naked, having hardly any other . . .—f. 273.

[3] . . . and the surprise natural for people to express at seeing people and things so new to them as we must be. . . .—f. 273v.

[4] . . . and held my hand when I was going to give them some beads and medals.

[5] . . . whose name we now understood was Teabooma: . . .—Cf. p. 544, n. 3 below.

[6] *only . . . sentance:* their speaches were composed of short sentances, to each of which two or three old men answered . . .

to some and embarked with us for that purpose, we rowed about two miles along shore to the East where the Coast was mostly covered with Mangoroves,[1] entering amongest them by a narrow creek or River we were brought to a little stragling Village where we landed, indeed this was necessary for we could proceed no farther in the boat. This was above all the Mangroves where the Country on one side the River was finely Cultivated and laid out in Plantations of Sugar,[2] yams and other roots and Watered by little rills, conducted by art from the main stream whose Source was in the hills. Here we were given to understand we might Water, it was excellent but far for us to fetch and troublesome to get at, here were some Cocoa-nutts which did not seem to be over loaded with fruit, we heard the Crowing of Cocks but saw none or any thing else to enduce us to believe they had any thing to spare us but good Nature and Courtious treatment. We saw on a fire an earthen Jarr (in which were roots bakeing) which did not hold less than six or eight gallons,[3] no one can doubt of these being of their own Manufactury. As we proceeded up this creek or river Mr F. shott a duck flying[4] which was the first use these people saw made of fire arms, my friend beged it of me and when we landed he told his Countrymen in what manner it was killed. The day being far spent and the tide not permiting a longer stay we tooke leave of these people and returned on board a little after sun-set.[5]

In the Morning we were viseted by some hundreds of the Natives, some came off in Canoes, others swam off so that before 10 o'Clock our decks[6] were quite full, my friend was one of the number who brought me a few roots, but all the others came empty in respect to refreshments, but brought with them some arms such as Clubs, darts, &ca which they exchanged away, indeed these things gener-

[1] The mention of mangroves argues that the boat went at least as far as Point Bailly, which is low and covered with these trees; but there are a number of streams flowing down to the sea on this part of the coast, and precise identification of the place is probably impossible.

[2] ... Plantains

[3] '... a round earthen pot, which could hold four or five gallons. It was very clumsily shaped, had a large belly, and consisted of a reddish substance, which was totally covered with soot both without and within.'—Forster, II, p. 389. These pots were made only in the northern part of the country, by the women, who were secretive about the process; but it seems to have been by the coil technique.

[4] It was George Forster who shot the duck, according to his own account (II, p. 386)—probably one of the only common duck in New Caledonia, the Australian Grey Duck, *Anas superciliosa pelewensis* Hartl. and Finsch.

[5] ... From this little excursion, I found that we were to expect nothing from these people but the privilege of visiting their country undisturbed for it was easy to see that they had little else but good Nature to spare us. In this they exceeded all the nation[s] we had yet met with, and although it did not fill our bellies it left our minds at ease.—f. 274.

[6] ... and all other parts of the ship

ally found the best Market with us, such was the prevailing Passion for curiosities, or what appeared new. As I have had occasion to make this remark more than once before, the reader will think the Ship must be full of such articles by this time, he will be misstaken, for nothing is more Common than to give away what has been collected at one Island for any thing new at a Nother, even if it is less curious, this together with what is distroyed on board after the owners are tired with looking at them, prevents any considerable increase.

After breakfast I sent Lieutenant Pickersgill with two armed boats to look for fresh water, Mr Wales and Lieutenant Clerk went to the sandy isle to make preparations for observing an Eclips of the [sun] which was to happen in the after noon. Mr Pickersgill soon return'd having found nearly a breast of the Ship a stream of Water far more convenient than the one we were at before. After ordering the Launch to be hoisted out to compleat our Water, I went to the Island to assist in the observation.

WEDNESDAY *7th*. About one PM the Eclips came on, Clouds interposed and we lost the first contact. We were more fortunate in the end, which was observed[1]

	Apr^t^ time h ′ ″
By Mr Wales with Dollonds 3½ f^t^ Achromatic Refractor at	3 28 49¼
—Mr Clerke with Birds 2 f^t^ Reflector at	3 28 52¼
and by me with an 18 Inch Reflector made by Watkins	3 28 53¼
Latitude of the isle or place of Observation	20°17′39″ South
Longitude p^r^ Dist^ce^ of the ☉ & ☽ and ☽ and ☆^s^ 48 sets	164° 41′ 21″ East
D^o^ p^r^ Watch - - - - - -	163 58 0
D^o^ p^r^ Eclips	

Mr Wales measured the quantity eclipsed by a Hadlies Quad^t^ a method I believe never before thought of, I am of opinion it answers the purpose of a Micrometer to a great degree of accuracy and that it is a valuable discovery and will be a great addition to the use of that most usefull instrument.

After all was over we returned on board where I found Teabooma

[1] There are so many hiatuses in the following seven lines of the MS that it seems preferable to delete them altogether and substitute the full passagef rom B, f. 274v. The figure for the longitude by eclipse is not given.

the Cheif, the same as made the first speach yesterday. Soon after I got aboard he sliped out of the Ship without my knowlidge and by that means miss'd the Present I intended him. Towards the evening I went a shore to the Watering place. The Water was taken up at a fine stream about $\frac{1}{3}$ of a mile from the sea Shore where it ran into a little creek and mixed with the Salt Water, it was necessary to have a small boat in the Creek to float the Casks down to the beach over which they were rolled and then taken into the Launch. A small boat could only enter this Creek at high-water.[1] Notwithstanding the great number of the Natives that were aboard the Ship there was not a few at the watering place, but no people could behave with more civility than they did.[2] This eveng departed this life Simon Monk, Ships Butcher,[3] occasioned by a fall down the fore hatch-way last night.

In the AM the Watering party went aShore under the protection of a Guard as before. Some time after a party of us went to take a View of the Country having two of the Natives to be our guides who conducted us up the hills by a tollerable good path way, meeting in our rout several people most of whom followed us so that at last our train was numerous, some indeed wanted us to return back, but we paid no regard to their Signs and they seem'd not uneasy when we proceeded. At length we reached the Summit of one of the hills from whence we saw the Sea[4] between some Advanced hills at a considerable distance on the opposite[5] side of the Island.[6] Between those advanced hills and the ridge we were upon is a large Vally through which ran a Serpentine river which added no little beauty to the prospect.[7] The plains along the Coast on the side we lay appeared

[1] . . . excellent wood for fuel was here far more convenient than water, but this was an article we did not want.—f. 274v.

[2] 'This Afternoon 2 or 300 of the Natives onboard the Ship many came off in Canoes but great numbers swimming off in various large parties—they all behav'd exceedingly well except one who was detected in stealing a Bayonet—he was immediately turn'd out of the Ship and was seemingly much blam'd by his own Countrymen.'—Clerke 8953.

[3] . . . a man much esteemed in the ship . . .—f. 275. 'He was a laborious man, indefatigable in his employment, though he seemed to be near sixty years old'.—Forster, II, p. 395. —'. . . beloved alike by both his comrades and superiors (which is rare enough).'—Sparrman, p. 175.

[4] . . . in two places

[5] . . . or SW

[6] . . . This was a usefull discovery, by which we were able to judge of the breadth of the land which in this part did not exceed leagues.—f. 275. *Voyage*, II, p. 110, gives the figure as 10.

[7] *which added . . . prospect:* on the banks of which were several plantations and some villages, whose inhabitants we had met on the road and found more on the top of the hill gazing at the Ship as might be supposed.—f. 275, *red ink*. The party had climbed the north-eastern of the two ranges that enclose the valley of the Diahot river, the largest river in New Caledonia, and saw the sea on the other side of the island between the peaks of the south-western range—to judge from the engraved chart, it was the sea of and about Nehue Bay.

from the hills to great advantage, the winding Streams which ran through them which had their direction from Nature, the lesser streames conveyed by art through the different plantations, the little Stragling Villages, the Variaty in the Woods, the Shoals on the Coast so variegated the Scene that the whole might afford a Picture for romance. Indeed if it was not for the Fertility of the Planes and some few spotts in the Mountains the Country would be called a D[r]eary waste, the Mountains and other high places are for the Most part incapable of Cultivation, consisting chiefly of solid Rocks,[1] the little soil which is upon them is scorchd and dryed up with the Sun, it is never the less coated with a kind of Coarse grass and other plants and here and there are trees and Shrubs. The Country in several respects bore a great affinity to some parts of New Holland under the same Parallel; here were the same sort of white barked trees[2] and I believe severl other Plants, the Woods free from under wood; Alternately, Sandy and Mangrove shores and here and there a rocky point[3] and several other similarities which struck every one who had seen both Countries. We could see from the hills, the reef extending all along the North Coast and towards the NW, that is off Balabea it extended out to Sea till it was lost in the horizon. After having made the observations[4] we decended the mountains by a different road which brought us down to their Plantations in the Planes, which I observed were laid out with great judgement and cultivated by much labour: I observed several old plantations laying in fallow, some seemingly but lately laid down and others of a longer date, some pieces of which they were again begining to dig up, the first thing they do is to set fire to the grass &c[a] which had over run its Surface.[5] Our excursion was finished by noon when we return'd a board to dinner, bring[ing] one of our guides with us, the other having left us, the fidelity of the one which remaind was rewarded at a small expence to us but valuable to him.

THURSDAY 8*th*. In the PM we made a little excursion along the Coast to the Westward, but met with nothing remarkable, the Natives every where behaving with all the civility imaginable.[6] A Fish was

[1] . . . many of which are full of Mundick,

[2] Eucalypti, as Forster's description (II, p. 391) makes plain.

[3] *alternately . . . point:* the reefs on the Coast . . .—f. 275v.

[4] . . . and our guides not chusing to go farther

[5] . . . Recruiting the land, by leting it lay some years untouched is observed by all the Nations in this Sea, they seem to have no notion of manuring the lands, at least I have no where seen it done.

[6] *but met . . . imaginable:* in company with M[r] Wales. Besides makeing observations of such things as came we got the names of several places, which I then thought were islands but upon farther enquiry, found they were districts on this same land.—f. 275v.

procured from the Natives by my Clerk[1] and given to me after my return a board, it was of a new genius, something like a sun fish,[2] without the least suspicion of its being of a poisonous quality we had ordered it for supper,[3] but luckaly for us the opperation of describeing and drawing took up so much time till it was too late so that only the Liver and Roe was dressed of which the two Mr Forsters and my self did but just taste. About 3 or 4 o'Clock in the Morning we were siezed with an extraordinary weakness in all our limbs attended with a numness or Sensation like to that caused by exposeing ones hands or feet to a fire after having been pinched much by frost, I had almost lost the sence of feeling nor could I distinguish between light and heavy bodies,[4] a quart pot full of Water and a feather was the same in my hand. We each of us took a Vomet and after that a sweat which gave great relief. In [the morning] one of the Pigs which had eat the entrails was found dead, the Dogs got the start of the Servants of what went from our table, so that they escaped, it soon made the dogs sick and they t[h]rew it all up again and were not much effected by it. In the Morning when the Natives came on board and saw the fish hanging up, they immidiately gave us to understand it was by no means to be eat, expressing the utmost abhorrance of it, and yet no one was observed to do this when it was to be sold or even after it was bought.

The guard and Watering party was sent a Shore with the last of our empty Casks to fill with water and also some people to Cut shrubery for Brooms.

FRIDAY 9*th*. Fresh gales at East and fair Weather. In the PM I received a Message from the officer on duty a shore that Teabooma the Chief was come down with a present, consisting of a few yams and sugr Canes. I sent him in return amongest several other things a Dog and a Bitch,[5] the former was red and white, the latter all red or the Colour of an English fox.[6] When the officer came aboard in the even-

[1] *A fish . . . Clerk:* In the afternoon a fish was struck by one of the natives near the Watering place, which my Clerk purchased

[2] . . . with a large ugly head . . .—f. 275v. It was a Toadfish, *Lagocephalus sceleratus* (Gm.).

[3] Forster's account is slightly different. 'It was of the genus, by Linnaeus named *tetraodon*, of which several species are reckoned poisonous. We hinted this circumstance to captain Cook, especially as the ugly shape, and large head of the fish, were greatly in its disfavour; but he told us he had eaten this identical sort of fish on the coast of New Holland, during his former voyage, without the least bad consequences. It was accordingly preserved for the next day, and we sat down very chearful, in expectation of a fresh meal'.—II, p. 403. It seems true that Cook was stubborn about food.

[4] . . . that is such as I had strength to move

[5] . . . both young, but nearly full grown . . .—f. 276.

[6] . . . I mention this because they may prove the Adam and Eve of their species in this Country.

ing, he inform'd me that Teabooma came attended by about twenty Men so that it looked like a Visit of cerimony, it was some time before he was satisfied the Dog and Bitch was intended,[1] but as soon as he was convinc'd he could hardly contain himself for joy.[2] Early in the AM I sent Lieutenant Pickersgill and the Master[3] to explore the Coast to the West and to see whether it was continued or only Isles, judging this would be better effected in the boats than in the Ship as the reefs would oblige the latter several leagues from land.

After breakfast sent a party a shore brooming, my self and the two M^r F^s confined aboard, but much better, a good sweat last night had a good effect.

SATURDAY 10*th*. Wind Easterly a very fresh gale. In the PM a man was seen a shore and a long side the Ship said to be as white as a European, from the accounts I had of this man (for I did not see him my self) his whiteness was not from hereditary descent but from some disease.[4]

AM a party a shore as usual, Mr F. and his party Botanizing. Many of the Natives on board.

SUNDAY 11*th*. Wind and Weather as yesterday. Nothing remarkable.

MONDAY 12*th*. Wind continues to blow fresh at East. In the evening the Boats returned when the officers reported that from an elevated point they reached the morning they set out, they took a view of the Coast, Mr Gilbert was of opinion he saw the termination of it to the west but Mr Pickersgill thought it extend beyond their sight, from this place they proceeded to the Island of Balabea,[5] they agree'd in one thing which was that there was no passage for ye ship but as it was dark before they reached it and left it again in the morning before day-break, this proved a fruitless expedition. The other two days were spent in recovering the Ship. As they went down to the Island they saw abundance of Turtle, the Violence of the wind and sea rendered it impractical to stricke any. The Cutter was very near foundering by suddinly springing a leek and filling with Water, they

[1] *intended:* intended him

[2] . . . and sent them away immediately

[3] . . . with the Launch and Cutter . . .—f. 276v.

[4] . . . such have been seen at the Society isles. A fresh Easterly wind, and the Ship laying a mile from the shore, did not hinder these good natured people from swiming off to us in shoals of 20 or 30, and returning the same way.—f. 276v. Cf. Clerke for a note on this albinoism: '. . . this Afternoon I saw a man onshore as white as Europeans in general are with light colour'd Hair, nothing inclining to the Woolly order which is the general case here with the head furniture; it had a most singular and striking appearance to see a white fellow naked running about among these dark colour'd Gentry, it really appear's to me highly unnatural and disgusting'.

[5] . . . (accompanied by two of the Natives)

were obliged to heave several things overboard before they could free her & stop the leek. From a fishing boat they met coming in from the reef they purchased as much fish as gave all the people a good Meal, and they were received by Teabi the Chief of Balabea and his people with great Curtesy who came in crowds to see them, this made it necessary for our people to draw a line on the ground within which the Natives were given to understand they were not to come; one of them happened[1] to have a few Cocoa-nutts which one of our people wanted to purchas, but as the other was unwilling to part with them he ran off but when he saw he was followed by the man who wanted to make the purchas, he sat down on the Sand and made a Circile round him, as he had seen our people do, and signified none were to come within it which was accordingly observed: as this story was well attested I thought it not unworthy a place in this Journal.

As I was willing to have the Cutter repaired before we put to sea to incounter with shoals the Carpenters were set to work upon her in the Morning and the Launch was employed to replace the water which had been expended the three preceeding days. Mention hath been made of my puting a Dog and a Bitch a shore, I also wanted to lay a foundation for stocking the Country with Hogs having kept some alive for such purpose's. As Teabooma the Chief had not been seen sence the day he got the Dogs, I took a young Boar and a Sow with me in the boat and went up the Mangrove creek to look for my friend [2] but when we came there we were told he lived at some distance off but they would send for him, but whether they did or no I cannot say, in short he did not come, and as the tide would not permit us to stay much longer, I resolved to give them to any man I could find of some note; our guide we had to the hills happened to be here, I made him understand I wanted to leave the two pigs a Shore, which I had now ordered out of the boat; several people present made signs to me to take them away one of which was a grave elderly man, him I made understand that it was my intention they should remain there, at which he shook his head and repeated his signs to take them away; but when they saw I did not do it they seemed to consult what was to be done, and at last our guide told me to carry them to the *Alekee* (Chief),[3] accordingly I ordered them

[1] *one . . . happened:* a restriction which they observed and which one of them soon after turned to his own advantage, for happening . . .—f. 277.

[2] The MS has a space left here, presumably for a name; B reads 'friend in order to give them to him'.

[3] Cf. Forster, II, p. 381: 'Their language, if we except the word areekee and one or two more, had no affinity with any one of the various languages which we had heard in the South Sea before'.

to be taken up by my people, for none of the others would come near them; our guide conducted us to a house wherein were seated in a circle eight or ten middle aged men to whom I and my Pigs were interduced and with great courtesy I was desired to sit down, when I began to expatiate on the merits of the two Pigs, shewing them the distinction of their sex, telling them how many young ones the female would have at a time, in short I multiplyed them to some hundreds in a trice, my only view was to enhance the Value of the present that they might take the more care of them, and I had reason to think I in some measure succeeded. In the mean time two men had left the Company, it was not long before they returned again with six yams which were presented to me and then I took leave and returned aboard. Here was a pretty large scatering Village and a good deal of Cultivated land, regularly laid out in plantations, mostly planted with Tarro or Eddy roots, some yams, Sug^r Cane & Plantains: the Tarro Plantations were prettily Watered by little rills, continually supplyed from the main Channel where the Water was conducted by art from a River at the foot of the mountains. They have two methods in Planting and raising these Roots, some are planted in square or oblong Plantations which lay perfectly horizontal and sunk below the common level of the adjacent lands, so that they can let in as much water upon them as is necessary. I have generally seen them wholy covered 2 or 3 inches deep, but I do not know if this is always necessary; others are planted in ridges about 4 feet Broad and 2½ in height, on the midle or top of the ridge is a narrow gutter along which is conveyed a small stream of Water which Waters the roots planted on each side, the plantations are so judiciously laid out that the same stream will Water several. These ridges are some times the divisions to the horizontal plantations, where this method is used[1] not an Inch of ground is lost. Perhaps there may be some diffirence in the roots which may make these two methods of raising them necessary.[2] I cannot say I have observed it, some are better tasted than others and they are not all of one Colour, be this as it will they are a very wholsome root and the tops make excellent greens and are eat as such by the planters. On these plantations men women and Children were at work.

[1] . . . which is for the most part observed, when a Pathway or something of that sort is not necessary, . . .—f. 278.

[2] There may have been some difference, but both methods are characteristic of the cultivation of the 'wet' taro—at which, as Cook noticed, the New Caledonians were extremely expert. Some of their 'canals', bringing water to terraced plantations, were five or six miles long. There are other varieties of taro, of the 'dry' sort, which do not require this refinement of cultivation but are generally a coarser and less-favoured food.

TUESDAY 13*th*. PM fresh gales at East. All our Water Casks being filled and got on board, I order the Kedge Anchor to be taken up and the Launch to be hoisted in. In the mean time I went a shore and by Vertue of our being the first discoverers of this Country took posession of it in his Majestys name and as a farther testimony had an Inscription engraved on a large tree close to the Shore near the Watering place, seting forth the Ships Name date &c[a] &c[a].[1] This being done we return'd aboard and then hoisted in all the Boats in order to be ready to put to sea in the morning.[2]

*I shall conclude our transactions at this place with some acco[t] of the Country and its Inhabitants. The latter are a strong robust active well made people, Courteous and friendly and not in the least addicted to pelfering, which is more than can be said of any other nation in this Sea. They are nearly of the same colour as the people of Tanna, but these have better features, more agreeable countenances and are a much stouter race, some were seen who measured Six feet four inches.[3] I have seen some who had thick lips, flat noses and full cheeks and in some degree the features and countenance of a Negro. Two things contributed to the forming of such an Idea, first their ruff mop heads and secondly their besmearing their faces with black pigment. Their hair and Beards in general black, the former is very much frizzled so that at first sight it looks like that of a negro, but it is nevertheless very different and is both Coarser and stronger than ours; some who wear it long tye it up on the Crown of the head, some suffer only a large lock to grow on each side the head, which they tye up in a club, others again and these not a few, and likewise all the women, wear it croped short. These rough heads most probably want frequent scratching, for this purpose they have a most excellent instrument, which is a kind of Comb made of Sticks of hard wood, from 7 to 9 or 10 Inches long and about the thickness of Kniting Needles, a number of these, seldom exceeding 20, but generally fewer, are fastened together at one end parallel to, and near a tenth part of an inch from, each other, the other ends, which are a little pointed, will spread out or open like the Sticks of a fan,

[1] . . . as I had done at all others we had touched at, where this cerimony was necessary. —f. 278. But B does not say specifically that he took possession of the country.

[2] From this point the MS has 7½ pp. blank before resuming—no doubt left for a description of the country, which is here supplied from B, ff. 278–82.

[3] The New Caledonians are Melanesian, their closest relatives racially being the people of the northern New Hebrides, though they themselves were in some respects more primitive. Their language was Melanesian—if one may use the singular language where there were so many distinct dialects (sixteen major groups alone, it is said) some quite incomprehensible to the speakers of others. At the same time they had a common, neolithic, culture, the source of which is doubtful. Cook's further meditations on the 'origin of this Nation' should be read in the context of these remarks.

by which means they can beat up the quarters of a hundred lice at a time. These combs or scratchers, for I believe they serve the purpose of both, they allways wear in their hair on the one side or other of the head; an Instrument of this kind the people of Tanna used for the same purpose, theres were forked and never I think exceeded 3 or 4 prongs and some times only a small pointed Stick. Their Beards, which are of the same crisp nature as their hair, they, for the most part wear short. Swelled and ulcerated legs and feet are very common amongst the Men; swelled Testicles are likewise very Common, I know not whether this is occasioned by a disease or by tying the Coat or covering of the Penis too teight; this like the people of Tanna and Mallicollo is allmost their only covering and is made generally of the bark of a tree and some of leaves: all small pieces of cloth, paper &c[a] that they got from us was generally applied to this use. They do not tye it up to the belt as at Tanna, but suffer it to hang down, nor do they untie it when they want to make water, but piss through all, and when done shake off what drops may hang to the coat. We have seen Coarse Garments amongst them made of a sort of Matting[1] but I never saw them worn, except when out in their Canoes and unemployed. Some have a kind of Concave cylindrical stiff black caps,[2] these seemed to be a great ornament a mong them, and we thought only worn by men of note or Wariors, a large sheet of our strong paper, when ever they got one, was generally applied to this use, so that these men only ornamented or cloathed the head and tail. The Womens dress is a short Petticoat made of the small filaments of the Plantain tree, laid over a cord to which they are fastned and tyed round the waist; the Petticoat is made at least Six or eight inches thick, but not one inch longer than necessary for the use they seemed to be designed for. The outer filaments are dyed black and as an additional ornament the most of them have a few Pearl Oyster shells fixed to the right side. The generall Ornaments of both sex, Are Ear rings of Tortoise shells, necklaces or amulets made of both shells and stones and Braclets made of large Shells which they wear above the elbow. They have punctures or marks on the skin on several parts of the body,[3] but none I think are black as at the eastern island[s]. I know not if they have any other design than ornament; the people of Tanna are marked much in the same

[1] The 'matting' of the New Caledonians, used for these coarse garments, sails, and anything else for which a rough textile was required, was generally woven of pandanus. Their bark cloth was beaten from the banyan (*Ficus prolixa*), *Hibiscus tiliaceus*, or paper mulberry (*Broussonetia papyrifera*).

[2] These were most often woven of the threads of coconut leaves.

[3] Tattooing was not very important in New Caledonia, though used; and curiously enough, women were more tattooed than men.

manner. Was I to judge of the Origin of this Nation, I should take them to be a race between the people of Tanna and the Friendly isles or between Tanna and the New Zealanders or all three; their language in some respects is a mixture of all. In their desposition they are like the Natives of the friendly isles, in affability and honesty they rather exceed them.[1] Notwithstanding their pacific desposition they must some times have wars, as they are well provided with offensive weapons, such as Clubs, Spears, Darts and Slings for throwing stones. The Clubs are about two feet and a half long and variously formed, some are like a Cyth others like a pick ax, others have a head like a Hawk and some have round heads and all are neatly made; many of their Darts and Spears are no less neat and ornamented with Carvings; the Slings are as simple as possible, but the stones they use they take some pains with, to form them into a proper shape, which is some thing like an egg, supposeing both ends to be alike, that is like the small end. They use a becket in the same manner as at Tanna in throwing the dart which I believe is much used in striking fish &c[a] at which they seem very dextrious, indeed I do not know that they have any other methods of catching large fish, I neither saw hooks nor lines a mongst them. It is needless to mention their working tools as they are made of the same Materials and nearly in the same manner as at the other islands, their axes indeed are a little different, some at least, which may be owing to fancy as much as custom.[2] Thier Houses or at least the most of them are circular, something like Behives and full as close and warm, the entrance is by a small door or long square hole just big enough to admit a man to enter double. The side walls are about 4½ feet high, but the roof is high and peaked to a point at the top above which is a post or stick of wood which is generally ornamented with either carving or shells or both. The framing is of small spars reeds &c[a]

[1] '... we always found the inhabitants Friendly wherever we landed conducting us to the most convenient places for our boats and repose at night and in that cordial manner which gave us pleasure in accepting of their good offices. These people are of a black complexion and in general have woolly hair their Features regular and pleasing in our Rambles both up into the country and along shore found them well disposed offering us their little services with the greatest pleasure imaginable. The women wear a long fring about 6 inches deep folded many times round their waist, the end secured and fastened to an handsom shell of the pearl kind which is all the Ladies dress its made of a silky colourd grass and sometimes dyed Black it looks decent and becoming. The men treat them with more respect then I have seen the generallity of the Islanders. In return we have no reason to believe them unfaithfull. The men crow[d]'ed on board in great numbers, The Ladies always paid their visits alongside not one could ever be preswaded to come on board.'—Gilbert, 29 September.

[2] A number of these artifacts, with a cylindrical cap and a comb, are presented from Hodges's drawings in *Voyage*, II, pl. XX. For the cap, see also Fig. 73*b* in this volume.

and both sides and roof is[1] thick and close covered with thatch made of coarse long grass. In the inside of the house are set up posts to which cross spars are fastned & platforms made for the conveniency of laying any thing upon: some houses have two floors one above the other. The floor is laid with dry grass and here and there matts are spread,[2] for the principal people to sleep or sit on. In the most of them were two fire places and most commonly a fire burning, and as there was no vent for the smoak but by the door, the whole house was not only smoaky but hot too, in so much that we, who were not used to such smoaky holes, could hardly indure to be in them a moment. This may be the reason why we find these people so chilly when in the open air and have no exercize; we have frequently seen them make little fires any where, and hurtle[3] round them with no other View than to warm them selves. Smoaky houses too may be necessary to keep out the Moskitoes which are pretty numerous here. In some shape their houses are neat, besides the ornaments at top, I have seen some with carved door post[s]. Upon the whole their houses are better calculated for a Cold than a hot climate & As there are no partitions in them they can have little privacy. Houshold Utentials are confined to very few articles, the Earthen Jarrs before mentioned is the only article worth noting, every family has at least one of them, in which they bake their roots and perhaps Fish &c[a]. The fire by which they Cook their victuals is on the out side of the house in the open air: at each are three or five pointed stones fixed in the ground, their pointed ends being about six inches above the surface, in this form those of three stones are only for one Jarr and those of five for two; The Jarrs do not stand on their bottoms but lie inclined on their bilge or side: the reason of these stones is obviously to keep the Jars from risting on the fire in order that it may burn the better. Their chief subsistance must be in roots and fish and the bark of a tree (which I am told grows in the West Indias) which they roast and are almost continually chewing, it has a sweetish & insipid tas[t]e and was liked by some of our people.[4] Cocoanuts, bread fruit, Plantains and Sugar Cane are by no means plenty. Bread fruit are very scarce and Cocoa nutt trees are small and but thinly planted and neither the one nor the other seem to yeild much increase. To judge

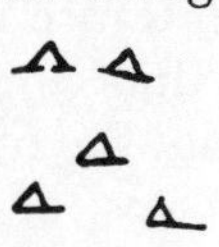

[1] and both . . . is *substituted for* over it is laid bark of trees and then the whole is . . .—The thick cork-like bark of the tree called Niaouli, *Melaleuca viridiflora,* was much used for this purpose.

[2] *deleted* as I supposed

[3] 'Hurtle' had an old sense of 'jostle'.

[4] This was the *Hibiscus tiliaceus*, says Forster, 'insipid, nauseous, and affording little nutriment'.—II, pp. 407–8. Sparrman, p. 168, mentions *Hibiscus esculentus* or okra, and three or four other foods, including cooked spiders, 'a food they eat quite readily'.

of the Inhabitants by the number we saw every day one must think them numerous, but I believe it is not so, but that at this time they were Collected from all parts to see us; Mr Pickersgill observed, that down the coast to the West, he had seen but few people and we know they came daily from the other side of the land over the mountains to see us. But although[1] the Inhabitants may not be numerous the Country upon the whole is not thinly peopeled, especially on the Sea Coast and in the plains and Vallies where it is cultivatable. It seems not to be a Country able to support many inhabitants; Nature has been less bountifull to it than any other Tropical island we know in this Sea. The greatest part of its surface or at least what we have seen of it consists of barren rocky Mountains, the grass &ca which grow on them is of no use to people who have no cattle to eat it. The sterility of the Country will apologize for the Natives not contributing to the wants of the Navigator. The Sea perhaps may in some measure make up for the difficiency of the land, a Coast surrounded by reefs and shoals as this is cannot fail of being stored with fish. I have before observed that the Country has a great resemblance to new south Wales in New Holland and some of its natural productions are the same particular[ly] the tree which is covered with a soft white and ragged bark that is easily picked off, and is, as I have been told, the same that in the East Indies is used for caulking of ships. The wood is very hard, the leaves are long and narrow and of a pale-deadish green and a fine aromatic,[2] so that it[3] may properly be said, to belong to that Continent; nevertheless here are several plants &ca which are common to the Eastern and nothern islands and even a species of the Passion flower, which I am told has never before be[en] known to grow wild any where but in America.[4] Our Botanists did not complain for want of employment while we lay here, every day brought in some thing new, either in Botany or Natural history; land Birds indeed are not numerous, but several are new, one of which is a kind of Crow, or at least so we called it, for it is not half so big and its feathers are tinged with blue,[5] some very

[1] But although *substituted for* I have observed, that we met many the day we went to the hills, those were not all, several companies were assembled on the hills, from the other side of the land in order to see the Ship, as might be supposed, amongst these were several Women and even some children. However though

[2] It was the commonest New Caledonian tree, Niaouli, *Melaleuca leucadendron*.

[3] 'it' refers to the country and not to the tree; i.e. the country might be said to belong to the continent of New Holland. The words 'and some of its natural productions ... aromatic' are inserted in the original text, f. 280v; this syntactical confusion causes the printed version, *Voyage*, II, p. 124, to go wrong.

[4] *Passiflora aurantia* Forster f. See Fig. 53.

[5] This was probably the New Caledonian Cuckoo-shrike, *Graucalus caledonicus* (Gm.), of which a drawing by George Forster exists, as well as three others by an artist unknown.

beautifull turtle Doves[1] and other small birds, such as I never saw before.

All our endeavours to get the name of the whole Island proved enefectual, probably, it is too large for them to know by one name;[2] when ever we made this enquiry they allways gave us the Name of some district or place which we pointed to; I, as hath been before observed, got the names of several with the Name of the King or Cheif of each; hence I conclude that the Country is divided into several districts, each governed by a Cheif, but we know nothing of the extent of his power. *Balade* was the Name of the district we were at and *Tiā Booma* the Chief, he lived on the other side the ridge of hills, so that we had but little of his Company and therefore could see but little of his power. *Tea* seems to be a title which is prefixed to the Names of all or most of their Chiefs or great men, my friend honoured me with this title calling me Tiācook.[3]

Their dead they entarr in the ground, I saw none of their burrying places my self, but several of the gentlemen did, in one, they were informed, laid the remains [of] a Chief who had been killed in battle, his grave, which had some resemblance to a large Mole hill, was decorated with Spears, Darts, Paddles &c[a] all stuck upright in the ground round about it.

The Canoes which these people make use of, are in some shape like unto those of the Friendly isles, but the most heavy clumsy Vessels I ever saw: they are what I call double Canoes, made out of two large trees hollowed out, and with a raised gunel about ten inches high, and closed at each end with a kind of bulk head of the same height, so that the whole is like a long square trough about 3 feet shorter than the body of the Canoe, that is a foot and a half at each end; two Canoes thus fitted are secured together about three feet asunder, by means of cross spars, which project about a foot over each side, over these spars is laid a deck or very heavy platform made of planks and small round spars on which they have a fire hearth & generally a fire burning & they carry a Pot or Jarr to dress

It somewhat resembles a small crow and its dark feathers have the blueish tinge mentioned by Cook. Latham (*General Synopsis of Birds*, 1781, p. 377) calls it the New Caledonian Crow.

[1] The country has half-a-dozen doves and pigeons, and a specific identification could not be risked here.

[2] This was so.

[3] Sparrman, p. 158: 'Ti Buma, which means the Chief Buma'; and '*Eriki*, as the word for chief, was sometimes used, but mostly *ti*'. Forster, II, p. 380: 'shewed him one of their number whom they named *Teà-booma*, and stiled their *arèekee*, or king'. Sparrman has certainly omitted a syllable. It appears that Cook was received by the tribe of Pouma, though Pouma may also have been the chief's personal name—cf. 'Teabi' above. Père Lambert, however, says that a high chief was called 'Téama'; that 'Téa' was the title of the eldest son of a high chief.—*Moeurs et Superstitions des Néo-Calédoniens* (Noumea 1900), p. 79.

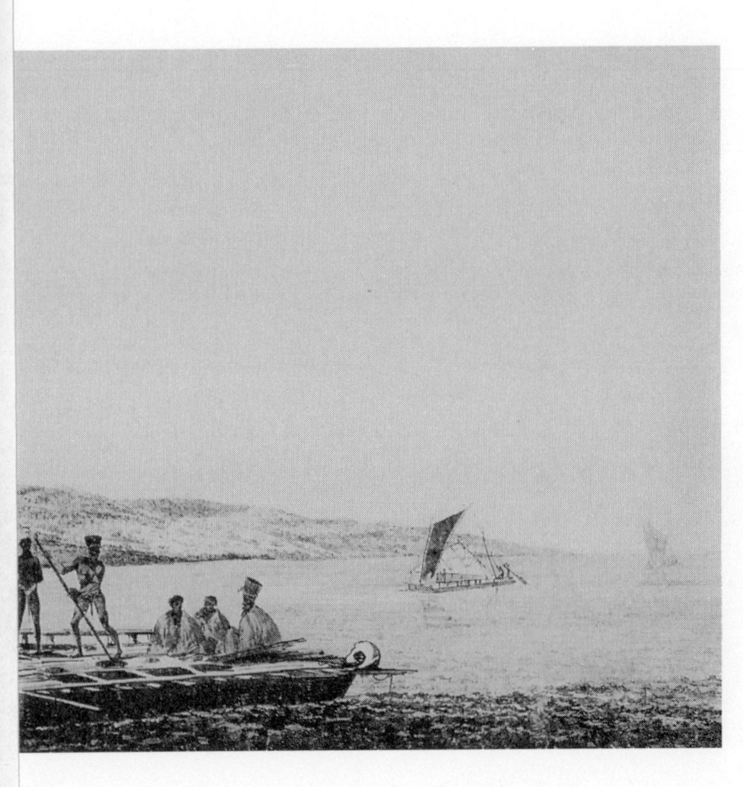

their victuals. The space between the two Canoes is laid with plank and the rest with spars: on one side of the deck and close to the edge is fixed a row of knees, pretty close to each other; the use of which are, to keep the masts yards &c[a] from rolling over board. They are Navigated by one or two Latteen sails, extended to a small latteen yard, the end of which fixes in a notch or hole in the deck, the foot of the sail is extended to a small boom: the sail is composed of pieces of matting and the ropes are made of the coarse filiments of the plantain tree, twisted into cords of the thickness of a finger; three, four or more such cords marled together serve them for Shrouds guies &c[a].[1] I thought they sailed very well,[2] but they are not attall calculated for rowing nor padling; their method of proceeding when they cannot sail is by sculling, for which purpose there are holes in the boarded deck or platform through which they put the Sculls, which are of such a length that when the blade is in the water the loom[3] or handle is 4 or 5 feet above the deck; the man who workes it, stands behind it and with both his ha[n]ds sculls the vessel forward. This method of proceeding is very slow for which reason I think them but ill calculated for fishing, especially for striking of Turtle, which I think can hardly ever be done in them. Their fishing Implements, such as I have seen, are Turtle netts, made, I believe, of the filaments of the plantain tree twisted; small hand netts with very small Meshes, made of fine twine, and fish gigs; I believe their general way of fishing is to lie on the reefs in shoal Water and strike the fish that may come in their way. They may however have other methods of fishing, which we had no opertunity to see as no boat went out while we were here,[4] all their time and attention was taken up with us. Their Canoes are about 30 feet long and the deck or platform about 24 in length and 10 in breadth; we had not at this time seen any timber in the country so large as the hulls of these Canoes were made on.[5] It was observed that the holes made in the several parts in order to sew them together were burnt through but with what Instrument we never learnt, most probable with an instrument of stone;[6] this may be the reason why they were so fond of large spikes, seeing at once that they would answer this purpose; I was

[1] The larger ropes were twisted from coconut husk.

[2] In spite of the cumbrous look of these double dug-outs, they are said to have been very seaworthy, and could carry as many as twenty men.

[3] The 'loom' was the shaft of an oar.

[4] They did: by hook and line, traps, and the use of some vegetable drug in the Polynesian manner.

[5] The trunks of the pine called *Araucaria columnaris*, which caused such excitement and argument later, were used.

[6] A good guess: heated stones were applied to the wood till it was burnt through.

convinced they were not wholy designed for edge tools, because every one shewed a desire to have the Iron belaying-pins which were fixed in the Quarter-deck rail, and seemed to value them far more than a spike nail, altho' it might be twice as big. These pins (being round) was perhaps the very shape of the tool they wanted to make of the nails. I did not find that a hatchet was quite so Valuable as a large spike, small nails was of little or no value and Beads, looking glasses &c[a] they did not admire. The Women of this Country and likewise those of Tanna, are, so far as we can judge, far more Chaste than those of the Eastern islands. I never heard that one of our people obtained the least favour from any one of them; I have been told that the Ladies here would frequently devert themselves by going a little aside with our gentlemen as if they meant to grant them the last favour and then run away laughing at them. Whether this was Chastity or Coquetry I shall not pretend to determine, nor is it material sence the Consequences were the same.*—ff. 278–82.

At Sun-rise on the Morning of the 13th we got under sail with a fine gale at EBS and steered for the same Channel we came in by, indeed we were not sure we could get to sea by any other. At half past 7 we were in the middle of it, Observatory isle bore S 5° East distant four miles and the East end of Balabea WBN½N, this was the Northermost land we had in sight and lies within the same reef as guards the Coast of Ballade. As soon as we were clear of the reef we hauld the Wind on the Starboard tack with an intent to ply round the SE end of the land; but M[r] Gilbert the Master, on whose judgement I had a good opinion, being of opinion that he had seen the Western extremity of the land and that it would be easier to get round by the NW I gave over Plying and bore up along the out side of the Reef, steering NNW, NW and NWBW as it trended. At Noon the Isle of Balabea bore from S½W to SBW½W distant [13] miles. What we judged to be the west end of the other land[1] bore SW½S and the direction of the reef was NWBW. Latitude observed 19°53′20″, Longitude from Observatory isle 14′ west.

WEDNESDAY 14*th*. Fresh gales easterly and fair weather. PM continued to range a long the reef till half past 3 before we came to any seperation or Channel leading within it, here we thought was one from the strong tide or current seting out, it lies with the Isle of Balabea bearing [SBE½E][2] from this place the reef turn'd away north for 3 or 4 Leagues and then inclined to NW. We followed its

[1] *other land:* great land . . .—f. 283; i.e. the main island. Cook was now outside the Cook reef, a barrier which runs north-west from Amoss passage for nearly a hundred miles.

[2] This was Great False passage, practicable only for boats.

directions till 5 o'Clock, passing what appeared to us to be two other openings,[1] we also raised more land, but at a great distance, which seemed to be connected with the other so that Mr Gilbert was miss-taken when he judged he saw the Western extremity.[2] At this time the land bore WBN½N[3] and the reef seem'd to extend NWBN. Hauled the wind on the Starboard tack and spent the night plying. At Sun-rise the Island of Balabea bore S 6° East and the land seen last night west, the direction of the reef NW. Ranged along it, but having but little [wind] made no great progress, indeed I was affraid to come near for fear of a Calm in a place where there was not a possibility of anchoring. At Noon observed in Latitude 19°28′ S, Longitude made from Observatory isle 27′ west. We had now lost sight of the isle of Balabea and could only see the land to the West of it which bore WBS½S, we were not sure if it was continued or isles, some partitions appeared in the coast which made some parts of it look like the latter; a multitude of shoals rendred a nearer approach to it exceeding dangerous, if not impractical.

THURSDAY 15*th*. PM a gentle breeze at ESE with which we steered NWBW, NWBN and NNE along the out side of the reef, following its direction. At 3 o'Clock we past a low sandy isle lying near the outer edge.[4] At 6 o'Clock we were a breast of a point of the reef from which it turned away WNW½W and seemed to terminate in a point which was seen from the Mast head: the Northerly direction it had lately taken had carried us almost out of sight of land, what we now saw of it bore SWBS distant about 10 Leagues. In ranging along the reef we preceived some places where the sea did not break, among other there was a large space on the SE of the sandy isle which we judged to be a Channell, but within it were extensive shoals. The night was spent makeing short boards with the wind at NEBE & ENE.[5] At Sun-rise made sail and steer'd NWBW, at this time saw neither land nor breakers. Two hours after saw the latter extending NW farther than the eye could reach, but no land was to be seen, so that

[1] Not practicable as passages.

[2] The land now seen was the Belep islands, the northernmost part of New Caledonia, some twenty miles north-west of the main mass.

[3] . . . distant 20 Miles, . . .—f. 283.

[4] . . . in Latitude 19°25′.—f. 283v. Ongombua, a low sandy island in the middle of the Ongombua passage, to which Cook refers a few lines further on.

[5] . . . At Sunset we could but just see the land which bore SW by S about 10 leagues distant. A clear horizon produced the descovery of no land to the westward of this direction; the reef too trended away WBN½N and seemed to terminate in a point which was seen from the Mast head, thus every thing conspired to make us beleive that we should soon get round these Shoals and with these flatering expectations we hauled the wind, which was at ENE and spent the night makeing short boards.—f. 283v.

we had all the reason in the world to believe that we had seen its termination to the NW. We were already carried far out of sight of land and there was no knowing how much farther we might be carrid before we found the ends of the shoals, the exploreing of them must, and was now attended with great risk, a gale of wind or a Calm, both of which we had often enough experienced, might have been attended with fatal consequences.[1] Sence we had seen the termination of the land to the NW and from the hills of Ballade its extent to the SW it became now a necessary object to know its SE Extremity,[2] rather than to spend time in exploreing shoals, which when done would have answered little end. It is sufficient to know that they cannot extend farther North than M. Bougainvills track in Latitude 15°00′ S but I think it not attall improbable but that they may extend to the west as far as the Coast of New South Wales, the Eastern extent of the isles and shoals off that Coast between the Latitude of 15° & 23° were not known and M. Bougainville meeting with the Shoal of Diana above 60 Leagues from the Coast, together with the signs he had of land to the SE (Page 303) all conspire to increase the Probability. The semilarity of the two Countries might also be advanced as a nother argument. I must confess it is carrying conjectures a little too far to pretend to say what may lay in a space of 200 leagues, it is however in some degree necessary if it was only to put some future Navigator (if any should come into these parts) on his guard.[3]

When I found that the Shoals did not terminate with the land, I determined to follow their direction no longer but to ply back to the

[1] *the exploring . . . consequences:* These considerations together with the risk we must run in exploreing a sea strewed with shoals and where no anchorage without them is to be found, induced me to abandon the design of proceeding round by the NW and to ply up to the SE in which direction I knew there was a clear Sea.—f. 284. It was the work of D'Entrecasteaux, in 1792, to explore and chart the side of the island that Cook was thus forced to leave unseen.

[2] *its SE extremity:* how far it extended to the East, or SE while it was in our power to recover the coast, for by follo[w]ing the direction of the Shoals we might be carried so far to leeward as not to be able to beat back without considerable loss of time.—f. 284.

[3] The foregoing sentences from 'It is sufficient' Cook neither included nor adapted in B (in which his entries for the 15th and 16th are very much re-arranged)—perhaps because he thought better of his reasoning. In H he adds the note, 'By Captain Survilles track, communicated to me by C. Crozet it appears that Caledonia & its shoals, cannot extend much farther West & makes it probable we saw the whole'. See p. 657 below. To the north of the New Caledonian dangers there were the D'Entrecasteaux reefs, but beyond these (lat. 17°50′) there was clear sea for over 400 miles directly north, as far as the south-eastern end of the Solomons: so far he was right. To the west, as far as the Great Barrier off the coast of Queensland, there were isolated reefs, but no great reef-system. No one, however, knowing Cook's experience in these latitudes, would blame him for carrying his conjectures a good distance. The passage in Bougainville, p. 303, to which he refers, runs, 'For twenty-four hours past, several pieces of wood, and some fruits which we did not know, came by the ship floating; the sea too was entirely falling, notwithstanding the very fresh S.E. wind that blew, and these circumstances together gave me room to believe that we had land pretty near us to the S.E.'

SE. We therefore Tack'd and stood close hauled on the Larboard Tack with the Wind at NEBE, we were at this time in the Latitude of [19°7'] Longde [163°57' E]. We did but just weather the point of the reef we had past the preceeding evening, and what rendred our situation still more dangerous, the breeze began to fail us. At Noon the low sandy Isle (before mentioned) seen from the Mast head in one with the westermost land bearing S 44° West. The Variation of the Compass was found in the morning to be from 10°8' to 10°11' E.

FRIDAY 16*th*. At 3 PM it fell Calm and we were left to the Mercy of a great swell which set directly upon the reef which was hardly one league from us, we Sounded but could find no ground with a line of 200 fathoms.[1] I ordered the Pinnace and Cutter to be hoisted out and sent a head to tow, but they were of little use against so large a swell. At 7 a light breeze sprung up at NNE, it lasted no longer than middnight:[2] from that time the boats were kept a head till day-light when we found our selves out of sight of the reef, so contrary to our expectation that we could not account for it. The Variation by the mean of three Compasses was found to be 10°24' East.

After breakfast some of the gentlemen went in one of the boats to shoot birds, about 11 o'Clock a breeze sprung up at SSW when we call'd them aboard by signal, hoisted in the boat and made sail to ESE; they kill'd but three or 4 birds, one of which was a booby of a new kind.[3] At Noon we observed in Lat 19°35' which was considerably more to the South than we expected[4] and very well accounted for our geting off from the Reef in the night, a favourable circumstance which happened very oppertuneately.

SATURDAY 17*th*. At 2 PM the breeze left us to a Calm which continued till 9 when it was succeeded by light airs from ENE and East with which we advanced slowly to the SE. At Sun-set the Island of Balabea was seen bearing S 7° west and the westermost land S 77° west. At Noon the Island bore S 68° west distant 10½ Leagues. Latitude observed 19°54' S.

SUNDAY 18*th*. Light Airs Easterly, that is between the NEBE &

[1] There almost seems here an echo from the first voyage; I, pp. 377–9. Possibly there was some danger of becoming 'embayed' where the reef turns east from the Ongombua passage.

[2] *a light . . . midnight:* a light air at NNE kept her head to the Sea; it lasted no longer than midnight, when it was succeeded by a dead Calm.—f. 284.

[3] 'At 11 hoisted in the Boats & made all sail—a vast Number of fish about, but a tantalizing sight is ye only share we can attain of them—We've seen neither reef nor Land today.'—Clerke 8953. The booby was the Australian Brown Booby, *Sula leucogaster plotus* Forster.

[4] . . . and shewed that a Current or tide had been in our favour all night . . .—f. 284v.

SEBE. Kept Plying on the most advantageous tacks. At Sun-set the Isle of Balabea bore S 78° west. At Sun-rise the horizon being hazey we could see no land, at 10 it was more clear and we saw land which we judged to be Ballade. At Noon Observed Lat 20°4′ South.

MONDAY 19*th*. Gentle breezes between ENE and SSE dark gloomy weather with some rain. Plying as before.

TUESDAY 20*th*. PM little wind at SE and hazey till sunset when the sky cleared up and we saw the land bearing SBE about Leagues distant. Continued to stretch to the East with a gentle gale at SBE till Sun-rise, when the wind Veering more to the East we stood in for the land which at Noon extended from Cape Colnet, which bore N 78° W distant [6] Leagues, round by the South to the East beyond our sight.[1] Latitude observed 20°41′, Longit made from Observatory isle [1°8′] East.[2]

WEDNESDAY 21*st*. Light breezes Easterly and Clear weather. At 5 PM the Var^{n} was 10°35′30″ East and at 7 in the preceeding AM it was 10°27½′ East. Continued to stand in shore till Sun-set at which time we were between two and three leagues off, the Coast extended from S 42½° East to N 59° west round by the South. Two small isles were without the last direction distant from us about 5 miles,[3] on one of them was an elevation like a Tower.

Several more appeared on different parts of the Coast to the west and so numerous that they looked not unlike the Masts of a fleet of Ships, I must susspend my judgement upon them for the present.[4] The two small isles above mentioned as well as some others more to the East, laid upon a reef which extended a long the Coast not less than 4 or 5 miles off, several openings appeared in the reef, which probably opened a way into good Harbours. The Country was mountainous and had much the same asspect as about Ballade. We now Tacked and stood off all night with a light breeze at SE which at Sun-rise was succeeded by a Calm which confined us to the place we were then in. At Noon we were about [Six] Leagues from the coast which extended from N 74°30′ west to S 30° East, Lat Ob^{d} 20°55′30″, Long^{de} made [1°28′][5] East.

[1] . . . and the Country appeared with many hills and Vallies.

[2] 'Long. 165°49′ E'.—Log.

[3] These islets are difficult to identify; but comparison of Chart XXXVIII and the engraved chart, together with Cook's not very satisfactory description, suggests that they were the Harcourt isles, about 10 miles down the coast from Cape Baye, and two or three miles north of Ugué bay.

[4] . . . as we shall most likely know what they are before we leave the coast.—f. 284v.—'. . . much resemblance to the Masts of a fleet of Ships lying at Anchor—not that any one thought they were such'.—Log.

[5] Figure supplied from Log.

THURSDAY 22*nd*. Light airs and Calm till 10 PM when we got a faint land breeze at SW, it continued till 10 AM when it was succeeded by the Sea breeze at EBS, with the former we steered up along shore and with the latter in for it. At sun-rise it was cloudy over the land, as soon as they cleared away we found we had made a good advance in the night. At Noon we were about [5] Leagues from the Coast which extend from N 78° west to S 26° East.[1] In this last direction the land seem'd to terminate (or trend more to the South) in a lofty Promontary which I named *Cape Coronation* it being the day that ceremony was performed on His present Majesty: it is situated in Latitude [22°02′] Longitude [167°7½′] East. The NE side of this land from its NW extremity up to this Cape deviates but very little from the direction of

FRIDAY 23*rd*. Variable light breezes and Calms; stood in shore so long as the sea breeze lasted which [was] till sun-set, at which time we were between 3 and 4 Leagues from the land, Cape Coronation bore S 31½° East and some breakers lying off the Coast SW.[2] After some hours calm we got a light land breeze which carried us two leagues to SE when it was succeeded by Calms and Variable light airs from the East. At Day-break an elevated point appeared in sight beyond and just open of Cape Coronation, bearing S 23° East, it proved to be the SE extremity of the Coast situated in Latitude [22°16′ S] Longitude [167°14′] East and obtained the name of [*Queen Charlottes Foreland*].[3] At Noon it bore S 12° E and Cape Coronation SBW distant 8 miles. Lat. Ob^{d} 21°53½′ S.

SATURDAY 24*th*. PM as we stood in SE & SSE for the land with a light breeze at NE & ENE we saw in a Vally on the South side of Cape Coronation a vast cluster of those elevated objects before mentioned and some low-land under [the Foreland] was wholy covered with them, various were the opinions and conjectures about them and occasioned the laying of several trifling Wagers. Smoak was seen at the first place all the day,[4] we also saw Smokes daly on several parts of

[1] . . . Lat. ob. 21°25′30″ Longit. made from Observatory isle 2°4′ East,—f. 285.

[2] . . . probably they were connected to those we had seen before.

[3] It is now called Cape Queen Charlotte.

[4] *various were . . . day:* we could not agree in our opinions what they were, I had no doubt but what they were a singular sort of trees, being too numerous to be any thing else; a great deal of smoak kept rising all the day from amo[ng]st those near the Cape.—f. 285v. A195 and G have a footnote at this point as follows: 'Mr F. was positive that this smoak was caus'd by some Internal and Perpetual fire; my representing to him that there was no smoak here in the morning, would have had no effect, had not this Eternal fire of his, gone out before night, and no more smoak was seen after. He was still more positive, that the elevations or Trees, were all stone Pillars, produced by nature, something like the Giants Causeway in Ireland.' B begins with this footnote; but in his later red ink revision Cook deleted it as a note and included it in his text, substituting 'Our Philo-

the Coast, a sure sign of the whole being inhabited. We had observed on several parts of the Coast, especially a little to the NW of Cape Coronation, the appearence of bays or inlets but when near the shore we found they were large Vallies or Planes covered with wood and were so far from what they appeared to be that they terminated at the sea in projecting points. There is likewise great reason to beleive that the whole NE Coast is covered by a reef, as we never came near the land that we did not see it. I judge that it extends nearly in a Parallel direction with the Coast and about 4 or 5 miles from it; some breakers were seen about this distance off the above mentioned Cape.[1] At sun-set the wind veering round to the South we tacked and stood to SE all night it not being safe to stand any nearer the land in the dark. At day break we found that the Currents had carried us far to the North of our reckoning, whereas on the NE Coast they generally set us to the SE of our reckoning. We now stood in again S & SW for the land with a very faint breeze varying between ESE and SSE. At Noon Observed in Lat 21°59′30″. Cape Coronation bore west

sophers' for 'Mr F' and 'Pillars of Bizaltes' for 'stone Pillars'. It appears that Forster grew very dogmatic, and Wales (23 September) could not resist a little private fun. 'The Appearance of the Land hereabouts is materially different from what it was near the Place where we Anchored. Here the Trees & Verdure are of a fine bright Green and seem chiefly to grow on the higher parts of the Land; but the greater part, even here, is almost entirely destitute of this lovely Cloathing, and seems to [be] a redish Clay or Rock. The Shores, in most places, and all the low Land spoken of above exhibits a most extraordinary appearance, and seems as if it was full of exceeding high, upright, ragged Pillars of Wood or Stone; but which nevertheless I take to be Trees of a singular Nature: they are, if trees they be, certainly such as we have not seen before. One Gentleman in the True Spirit of the *Ancient* Philosophy Asserts & swears to it also that they are Pillars of Bizaltes such as compose the Giants' Cawsway in Ireland & that he can see with his Glasses the Joints very distinctly. I have often been struck with Surprise at the Excellency of this Gentlemans Eyes & Glasses or the Imperfection of My own. He has seen Oranges & Lemons Growing on y[e] trees at 3 Miles Distance & sworn positively to a Bird flying at upwards of one. I think it ought to be mentioned to the honour of M[r] Ramsden that the Glass these feats have been done with was made by him, & is a common 2 feet Achromatic spy-Glass.'—To this may be added Clerke, 25 September: 'We have seen for some days past on various parts of this Land, something growing which has been a matter of dispute among us: the Naturalist is very certain they are the Bisaltics or Giants causeway; some believe them one thing, and some another, for my own part, I believe they are Trees from their being so plentifully interspers'd about the Country and indeed from their appearance in general; but must own, if they are, they are of a most extraordinary and peculiar Growth. We see them in very thick clusters, probably 2 or 300 of them together, very high, streight, and of a Pyramidical form, they very much resemble a large body of Rocks with spiral Tops very thick upon them. Hope tomorrow or next day will satisfy our curiosity and determine this matter.' Forster II, pp. 434–6, gives a very mild version of the affair. The phenomena were those very peculiar conifers known as *Araucaria columnaris* or *Araucaria cooki* (R. Br.), Cookpine or *pin colonnaire*, which grow to upwards of 100 feet high, their branches rarely longer that 6 feet, and shortest on the biggest trees.

[1] The sentences 'We had observed . . . Cape' are omitted in B, as if Cook thought he had gone too far in statement. But he is quite right about the reef: indeed New Caledonia is practically surrounded by a barrier, in some places below the level of the sea, generally level with it, and distant from the north-east coast one to fifteen miles. Inside are further reefs and shoals. On the whole, Cook was fortunate not to get too close; and when he did go inside, to find a tolerable passage.

southerly distant 7 Leagues and [the Foreland] s 38° west. For several days past a kind of Water Moss, such as is found in stagnated places, has been seen floating on the Sea in great quantities.[1]

SUNDAY 25*th.* Winds faint and variable so that we advanced but slowly as it was necessary to proceed with caution, for[2] at Sun-set we saw a low Island lying off [the Foreland] some distance from the land,[3] it was of that sort which are generally surrounded with shoals; at the same time a new land[4] was discovered bearing s 24° East, 12 Leagues distant. At Sun-rise it bore SSE½E the farthest point of land on the Main beyond [the Foreland] bore s 43° w and Cape Coronation N 70° west. At Noon the said Cape bore N 67° west distant 6½ Leagues, Lat in p^r Ob^n 22°10′ s.

MONDAY 26*th.* As we advanced to SSW with a light breeze at ESE in expectation of geting round the end of the land, we raised by little and little more low Isles beyond the one already mentioned and at last we saw they were connected by Sand banks and reefs,[5] which seem'd to extend home to the Main and shut up the Passage a long shore. We stood on till half an hour past 3 pm when we preceived from the deck rocks level with[6] the surface of the Sea on a Shoal which spited out from the little Isle towards the Main but we could not be sure that it joined, the Wind was too faint and unsittled to look for a Passage in the Ship and the day was too far spent to send away the boat as it would have been dark before they got back.[7] I prefer'd hauling to the SSE to see if we could get round the small Isles, we had a fine breeze at East, but it continued no longer than 5 o'Clock when it was succeeded by a dead Calm; our situation was now worse than ever,[8] we were but a little way from the Shoals, which instead of turning to sw as we expected, they took a SE direction towards the SE land and seem'd wholy to shut up the Passage between the two.[9] At

[1] Probably either *Diplanthera uninervis* (Forsk.) Aschers or *Najas graminea* Delile.

[2] *for:* As we advanced to SSW the coast beyond the Foreland began to appear in sight, and . . .—f. 285v.

[3] *off . . . land:* SSE about 7 Miles from the Foreland. . . .—This corresponds with the position of the wooded islet called Nuare, inside the reefs between New Caledonia and the Isle of Pines.

[4] *new land:* round hill

[5] *Sand . . . reefs:* breakers or seemed to be; . . .—f. 286.

[6] *level with:* just peeping above

[7] *a Shoal . . . back:* the Shoal above mentioned, it was now time to alter the Course, the day was too far spent to look for a passage near the shore, as we could find no bottom to anchor to spend the night.

[8] *our situation . . . ever:* we sounded but a line of 170 fathoms did not reach the bottom;

[9] *SE land . . . two:* hill we had seen the preceding evening and seemed to point out to us that it was necessary to go round that land.

this time the most advanced point of land on the SW side of the Main bore S 68° west distant 9 or 10 Leagues: beyond this point we judged the SW Coast would take the same direction as the NE, indeed this was necessary in order to join that part of it we had seen from the hills of Ballade. At 7 o'Clock a faint breeze from the North inabled us to steer out East and to spend the night with less anxiety than otherwise we should have done. During the Calm we sounded but found no ground with a line of 150 f^m^. On these low Isles were many of those elevations already spoke of, every one were now satisfied they were trees, except our Philosophers who still maintained they were Stone Pillars. About day break the wind shifting to SSW we stretched to the SE for the isle in that direction in order to try to get round it, for we saw no likelyhood of a passage any other way. At Noon observed in Latitude 22°16′, Longitude made from Observatory isle 2°53′45″ East, the Main or the land we had left extended from N 68° W to S 78° west and the SE Isle from S 7° west to S 15° East, a hill near the middle, remarkable because the only one in the isle, bore S 4°30′ E.

TUESDAY 27*th*. In the PM the wind veered to SSE and increased to a fresh gale. Continued to stretch to East and NE till 2 AM when we tacked and stood SW with a very fresh gale at SE; we had some hopes of weathering the isle, but we fell a few miles short of our expectation, for at 10 o'Clock we had to tack, being about one mile from the East shore of the isle, the Hill bearing west, the extremes from NWBN to SW and some low isles lying off the SE point SBW, these seem'd to be connected to the large isle by breakers. Had no soundings with 80 fathoms of line. The Skirts of this isle is wholy covered with the trees so often mention[ed][1] on which account it obtained the name of *Isle of Pines*.[2] We stood off under single reef'd Top-sails till Noon when we made another attempt to weather the isle. Lat 22°32′20″, Long^de^ made 3°12′45″ East. The Mercury in the Thermometer stood at Noon at 68¾ which is lower than it has been sence the 27th of last February.

[1] 'I am now perfectly convinced that those same extraordinary Appearances are Trees as we were very near some of them but nothing of the sort ever sure had so singular a form. They must be also amazing large as every other thing on the Isle appeared but as so many bunches of Reeds when compared to them.'—Wales, 27 September.

[2] . . . They had much the appearance of tall pines the round hill, before mentioned, is on the SW side and is of such a height as to be seen 14 or 16 leagues. The island is about miles in circuit and situated in Lat. 22°38′, Longit. 167°40′ E.—f. 286v. The Isle of Pines has the alternative name of Kunie; it is 29 miles ESE of Cape Ndua, the southernmost point of New Caledonia. The hill, Pic Nga, is 872 feet high. The trees Cook saw near the coast have all gone. Though very close this day, he was too far north to notice the opening of the narrow passage between Kunie and the lesser island of Kutomo. The 'low isles lying off the SE point' which he mentions above are the South East Islets, Ami and Ana. For the general appearance of the island, see Chart XXXIX*a*.

WEDNESDAY 28*th*. Fresh gales at SE and ESE. Two attempts we made to weather the isle before Sun-set proveing fruitless, I determined[1] to stretch off till middnight and than stretch in, assisted by the winds and Currents we found our selves at day-break several leagues to windward of the isle of Pines and bore away large round the SE end and was soon after able to determine the figure and extent of the Island which is Situated in the Latitude of [22° 38′] Longitude [167°40′] East and Leagues distant from . It hath nearly a round form and is about Leagues in circuit, the elevated hill in the middle makes it conspicuous. It is inhabited. The Coast from the SE to west round by the South is covered with small isles, Sand banks and breakers, and excepting those which lie off the SE side, seem to be unconnected: most of the low isles are covered with the same sort of lofty trees as ornament the borders of the great isle. We continued to range along the outside of the small isles and reefs at ¾ of a league distance and as we pass'd one we raised others, so that they seem'd to form a chain extending to the low isles lying off the Main.[2] At Noon observed in Latitude 22°44′36″, the hill on the isle of Pines bore NEBE and the extremes from N 19½° E to N 79° East, and Cape Coronation N 32½° W distant 17 Leagues.

THURSDAY 29*th*. Very fresh gales Easterly. Continued to range the Coast of the isles as above mentioned, steering NWBW with a View of falling in with the Main a little to the SW of [the Foreland]. At 2 pm two low isles were seen four points on our Larboard bow,[3] they were connected by breaks which seem'd to join those on our Starboard; this made it necessary to haul off SW in order to go without them, the impractibility of which appeared at 3, when a continued reef was seen extending from the two isles to the SE.[4] This discovery made us get our tacks on board and haul out close to the wind. After sailing an hour and a half in this manner we were brought close to the Reef and obliged to tack, from the Mast-head the breakers were seen to

[1] Cook writes 'tertimed', which I cannot see as other than an extraordinary slip.

[2] *Main:* Foreland

[3] *four . . . bow:* bearing SWBS

[4] To understand what was now happening see Chart XXXVIII, Fig. 68, or even better a modern chart with the reefs and shoals clearly marked. Cook was sailing into a large bay, a sort of isosceles triangle, of which the sides were formed by the reefs and shoals which run south-east and south from the southern end of New Caledonia, and of which the base was a line from South Reef on the west to South East islets. There were numerous islets on his port or larboard side, and what the two were that he has mentioned it is difficult or impossible to say with confidence. He got over to the western side of this bay, and as the afternoon wore on and the easterly gale increased in strength, of course found himself very uncomfortably on a lee shore. Next day, instead of tacking out to the south as quickly as possible, he pushed north into the apex of the triangle. Such was scientific passion.

extend as far as ESE, the smoothness of the Water made it probable they extend to the North of East and that we were in a manner surrounded by them. At this time the hill on the Isle of Pines bore N 71°30′ E, [the Foreland] N¼W, and the farthest point of land in sight NW distant 15 or 16 Leagues: this direction of the SW Coast which was rather with the Parallel of the NE assured us that it extended no farther to the SW than what we now saw. After a short trip to the NNE we stood again to the south in order to have a nearer and better View of the shoals at[1] Sun-set, we gained nothing by this but the Melancholy prospect of a sea strewed with Shoals: we were now about one mile from the reef to leward of us and contrary to expectation had soundings in   fathoms,[2] the bottom fine sand, but Anchoring in a strong gale with a Chain of breakers to leeward was the last resource, it was thought safer to spend the night makeing short boards over that space we had in some measure made our selves acquainted with in the day. Proper persons we stationed to look out and each man held the rope in his hand he was to manage, to this we perhaps owe our safety,[3] for as we were standing to the Northward the People on the Fore Castle and lee gang-way saw breakers under the lee-bow which we escaped by the expeditious manner the Ship was tack'd. Thus we spent the night under the terrible apprehensions of every moment falling on some of the many dangers which surrounded us. Day-light shewed that our fears were not ilfounded and that we had spent the night in the most eminent danger hav[g] had shoals and breakers continually under our lee at a very little distance from us.[4] We found by the bearings and situations of the lands a round us that we had gained nothing to wind-

[1] *at:* before

[2] *we were . . . fathoms:* and no way to clear them but by returning by the same way we came in. We tacked nearly in the same place we had tacked before and on sounding found   fathoms . . .—f. 287.

[3] *Proper persons . . . tack'd:* we perhaps ow our safety to a good lookout and the very brisk manner the Ship was managed . . .—f. 287; and so G. But Cook thought better of this, and in his London revision deleted 'perhaps' and added some key words in red, so that his final version reads, 'we ow our safety to the Interposition of Providence a good look-out' &c. It is evident that Providence, so scandalously treated by Hawkesworth on an earlier occasion (see I, p. ccl), this time was to receive proper justice.

[4] 'We passed the Night standing too & from amongst these terrible Reefs expecting the ship to be brought up by some or other of them every Minute: to mend the Matter, it turned out exceeding dark, and I realy think our situation was to be envyed by very few except the Thief who has got the Halter about his Neck.'—Wales. 'In sailing round the Isle of Pines, in the Evening, we found ourselves, in a most dangerous situation, for the Men at the Mast Heads, call'd out *Breakers ahead,* we hauld up several Points, still *Breakers ahead*; in fact we found that we had been Running into a Net of Breakers (or reefs) and no way out, but as we had come in; which was now right in the Winds Eye: The Winds increas'd, as Night came on, and every way we stood for an Hour, the Roaring of Breakers was heard, so that was a most anxious, and perilous Night, at last Daylight appear'd . . . —Elliott *Mem.*, f. 34.

ward during the night. I was now almost tired of a Coast I could no longer explore but at the risk of loosing the ship and ruining the whole Voyage, but I was determined not to leave it till I was satisfied what sort of trees those were which had been the subject of our speculation.[1] With this view[2] we stood to the north in hopes of finding anchorage under some of the isles on which they grow, we however kept the wind till[3] stoped by the shoals which lie extended between the Isle of Pines and [Queen Charlottes Foreland]. We found soundings of them in 55, 40 & 36 fathoms, bottom fine sand: the nearer we approached to these Shoals the more we saw of them so that we were as far of as ever from knowing if there was any passage between these two lands.

But a little to leeward were those low isles discovered on the 25 and 26th on which were many of the trees we had in view; we edged down to the nearest and as we drew near saw it was unconnected with the neighbouring reefs and that it was probable we should find anchorage on the lee or west side.[4] After hauling round the point of the reef which lay round it we attempted to ply to windward in order to get more under shelter of the isle, a Reef to the North confind us to a narrow Channell thro' which ran a Tide[5] against us, which rendered this attempt fruitless and we were obliged to Anchor in 39 fathom the bottom fine Coral sand, the isle WBN one Mile distant. This was no sooner done than I ordered a boat to be hoisted out and went ashore accompaned by the Botanists to take a view of those trees and to see what else the isle produced; we found the trees to be a kind of spruce pine, very proper for Spars which we were in need of; after makeing this discovery I hastened aboard in order to have more time after dinner.

FRIDAY 30*th*. After dinner I landed again with two boats accompaned by several of the officers and gentlemen, takeing with me the Carpenter and some of his crew to cut down such trees as we wanted; while this was doing I took the bearings of the distant lands: the hill on the isle of Pines bore S 59°30′ E, the low point [of Queen Charlottes Foreland] N 14°30′ west and the high land over it[6] N 20° west and the most advanced point of land to the SW, W half South distant [6 or 7] Leagues: we had from several bearings deter-

[1] . . . especially as they appeared to be of a sort usefull to shiping and had not been seen any where but in the Southern part of this land.—f. 287v.

[2] . . . after makeing a trip to the South to weather the Shoals under our lee,

[3] . . . about 8 o'Clock

[4] . . . we therefore stood on, being conducted by an officer at the mast head,

[5] *Tide:* Current

[6] . . . seen over two low isles . . .—f. 288.

mined the true posission of the Coast from [the Foreland] to this point which [I shall distinguish by the name of Prince of Wales Foreland, it is situated in the latitude of 22°29′ S, Longit. 166°57′ E. It is of a considerable height and when it first appears above the horizon looks like an island].[1]

From this [Cape] the Coast trend[ed] NW nearly, this is rather too northerly a direction to join that part of the Coast we saw from the hills of Ballade, but as it was very high land which opened of the [Cape] in this direction it is probable lower land which we could not see might have opened sooner, or else the Coast afterwards takes a more westerly direction,[2] be this as it may we pretty well know the extent of the Land by having it confin'd within certain points.[3] On this little isle which was a mere sand bank not exceeding half[4] a mile in circuit were, besides the Pines, a variety[5] of other trees, Shrubs and Plants which gave sufficient employment to our botanists the time we stayed upon it, which occasioned it to be called [Botany Isle].[6] Here were several Water Snakes,[7] some Pigeons[8] and Doves,[9] seemingly different to any we had seen. One of the

[1] There is an unusually large hiatus in the MS here. The name 'Prince of Wales Foreland' in B is a red ink substitution for a deleted 'S.W. Cape' (as in G). The 'true position' of the coast is not in fact very well defined, and Cook's figures are sufficiently out to cause some confusion. His Prince of Wales Foreland is indeed an island, Wen or Ouen, separated from the main island by the rather narrow Woodin channel. In its northern part it rises to 925 feet. The position of this high point is about lat. 22°25′ S, long. 166°49′ E, so that Cook was not far out.

[2] I do not, I must confess, follow this line of argument. The coast inside Wen does take a more westerly direction as far as Noumea. It then turns north-westerly again, running roughly parallel with the north-eastern side of the island; but before it joins 'that part of the Coast we saw from the hills of Ballade', it inclines more to the north again. For 'afterwards' B reads 'more to the north west in the same manner as the NE coast'; so it is possible that Cook thought the northern side of the island inclined more to the west than it does.

[3] ... I however still entertain'd hopes of seeing more of it, but in this I was disapointed. —f. 288. The words 'but ... disapointed' are in red ink.

[4] *half:* $\frac{1}{2}$

[5] *Pines, a variety:* Pines the Etoo tree of Otaheite and a variety ...—f. 288. The additional words are interlinear in red.

[6] The small islets scattered over the line of reefs between Cape Queen Charlotte and the Isle of Pines were in the nineteenth century known collectively as the Botany Isles. This particular one was Améré, lying on its own little reef, lat. 21°27′ S, long. 167°6′ E.

[7] Forster (II, p. 438) identified this snake as *Anguis platura* but J. R. Forster subsequently (*Descr. An.*, p. 257) called it *Anguis laticauda*; this appears to be a deliberate emendation, for another undoubted *platura* identification of the elder Forster (pl. 171 from Tahiti) is not changed in the later work (1844, p. 229). The Linnean name *Anguis laticauda* has never been satisfactorily assigned, but it is likely that J. R. Forster in 1844 was following Latreille's comprehensive reptilian treatise of 1802, where *laticauda* was used for a 'species' of *Hydrophis*. Latreille himself had two species confounded. See also p. 560, n. 2 below.

[8] Forster (II, p. 438) says, 'We saw several large beautiful pigeons which we could not shoot'. These were very likely the Giant Pigeon of New Caledonia, *Ducula goliath* Gray, which owing to steady persecution is now largely restricted to mountain forests and remote localities.

[9] Two predominantly green fruit doves and a small ground dove occur in New Caledonia, but none was recorded here by the Forsters.

officers shott a Hawke[1] of the very same sort as our English fishing hawkes, this and a small bird[2] was all the land birds we got. People had been there but lately, by the number of fire places, Branches and leaves of trees near them hardly in the least decayed: probably they had been here Turtling as the remains of some were seen. The hull of a Canoe laid wrecked in the sand, it was precisely of the same sort as we had seen at Ballade, we are now no longer at a loss to know of what trees they make their Canoes, they can be no other than the Pines. On this little isle were some which measured twenty inches diameter and between Sixty and Seventy feet in length and would have done very well for a Fore-mast for the Resolution if one had been wanting. Sence trees of this size are to be found on so small a spot is it not reasonable to expect to find some vastly larger on the Main and on the larger isles; if appearences have not deceived us we can assert it. If I except New Zealand, I know of no Island in the South Pacifick Ocean where a Ship could supply herself with a Mast or a Yard, was she ever so much distress'd for want of one; nay you cannot even get a Studing-sail boom of Wood attall fit for the purpose much less a lower mast or yard; thus far the discovery may be both usefull and Valuable. My Carpenter who is a Mast-maker as well as a Ship-wright, two professions he learnt in Deptford yard, concequently acquainted with all the various sorts of Timber and their uses in Shiping, is of opinion that these trees would make exceeding good Masts. The Wood is White, closer grained than fir and seemingly tougher.[3] Turpentine had exuded out of most of the trees which the Sun had inspissated in to a Rosin, which was found sticking to the trees and laying about the roots. These trees shoot out their brance in the same manner as all the Pine kind, with this difference that these are vastly smaller & shorter, so that the knots become nothing when the tree is worked for use, and what is most extraordinary in them is, the larger this tree the shorter and smaller are the branches,[4] this was what lead our Philosophers into the extravagant notion of them being Natural Pillars of Stone.

The Seed is produced in cones but we could find one that had any in it, or that was in a proper state for a botanical examination. Besides these there was a nother tree or shrub of the spruce or fir kind

[1] The Osprey, a cosmopolitan bird-of-prey. The form found here is *Pandion haliaetus microhaliaetus* Brasil.

[2] A flycatcher, *Petroeca* sp.

[3] *closer . . . tougher:* close grained tough and light . . .—f. 288v.

[4] *and what . . . branches:* I took notice that the largest trees had the smallest and shortest branches, and were crowned as it were, at the top by a spreading branch like a bush; . . . —f. 289.

but it was very small.[1] Having got half a score small spars to make Studding-sail booms, Boats Masts &c[a] and night approaching we returned with them aboard.[2]

At low-water Mr Gilbert had from the Mast-head reconoitred the Sea around us and found the whole strewed[3] with small Islots, Sand banks and breakers,[4] some connected and others not, so that it was very probable a Passage might be found a Mongest them quite into the Main and even all along the SW Coast, but when I considered the little Advantages that could accrue by exploreing this Coast, as its extent was already pretty well determined, the great risk we must run,[5] and the time it would require on account of the dangers attend ing it I determined not to risk the Ship down to leeward amongest these shoals, where we might be so hemed in as to find it difficult to return.[6] Now it was that I wished to have had the little Vessel set up, the frame of which we had on board, with her the Coast might have been explored with little risk, but it was too late, the Season of the year was too far advanced to spare time to set her up and afterward make use of her in these parts, and to the South she was not wanting.[7] After such an explanation few (I believe) will blame me for put[ting] again to sea at day-light in the morning with a gentle breeze at EBN. We had to make some tacks before we could clear the

[1] This was not another sort of tree, but simply the young stage of *Araucaria columnaris*, which has a more pyramidal, symmetrical and spruce-like shape than the older tree.

[2] . . . We also found on the isle a sort of Scurvy grass and a Pla[n]t which we called Lambs quarters, which when boiled eats like spinage.—f. 289. The scurvy grass might have been either *Sesuvium portulacastrum* or *Tetragonia expansa*; the lambs' quarters was probably *Atriplex jubata*—though possibly, again, *Tetragonia expansa*, the 'New Zealand spinach'; all three plants are common on sandy beaches and coral sand islets about New Caledonia like the one now visited. Wales went on shore with the boats, saw a number of birds—which flew away on being fired at—and an abundance of very large water-snakes, ringed black and white, 'a very torpid sort of Reptile'. This description points to the Hydrophid *Laticauda colubrina* (Schneider), often found in large numbers on coral islets: it is not exactly a torpid reptile, but likes to lie warming itself in the sun, or after sunset upon rocks which still retain the heat, and it will be attracted by any fire lit on the beach at night. Wales adds, 'After getting on board we had a rich repast indeed of our Greens & a Piece of salt Pork. The fear of being affected by eating [vegetables] after so long an Abstinence from them induced me to eat rather spareingly, and accordingly I felt no bad effects from them; but some of those who ate very plentifully suffered very severe gripings attended with a loosness.'

[3] *whole strewed:* whole to the west to be strewed

[4] . . . to the utmost extent of our horizon.

[5] *we must run:* attending a more accurate Survey.

[6] . . . and by that means loose the proper season for returning to the South.

[7] *Now it was . . . wanting:* It was now that I wished to have had the little Vessel set up, the frame of which we had on board: I had considered about seting her up when we were last at Otaheite this I found it could not be done without neglecting the Calking and other necessary repairs of the Ship or staying longer there than the rout I had in view would admit; it was now too late to think of seting her up and to use her in exploreing this coast afterwards, and to the South she could be of no use. These reasons induced me to try to get without the Shoals, that is to the Southward of them.—f. 289–9v.

breakers to leeward, the wind too began to fail us, so that [at] Noon we had not advanced above 3 Leagues from our last anchoring place.[1]

[October 1774]

SATURDAY 1*st*. Continued to advance slowly to SSE with a faint breeze at ENE till 3 PM when it fell Calm, The swell assisted by the Currents set us fast to SW to the breakers which were yet in sight in that direction,[2] thus we continued till 10 o'Clock when a light breeze sprung up at NNW and we steer'd ESE[3] not daring to steer to the South round the Shoals till day-light. At 3 AM the wind veered to SW, blew hard and in squals attended with rain, so that we were obliged to proceed with our Courses in the brales and Top-sails on the Cap[4] till day-break when the Hill on the Isle of Pines bore North, and distance from the shore in that direction was about four Leagues.

We had now a hard gale at SSW and a great sea, and had reason to rejoice of having got clear of the shoals before this gale overtook us, which we could now make no other use of but to stretch to ESE with our starboard tacks aboard and where we might hope to find a Clear sea. At Noon we were out of sight of land and in Latitude [22°41′] S, Longitude made from the Isle of Pines [0°38′ East].[5]

When this gale came on every thing conspired to make me think it was the Westerly Monsoon, nevertheless I cannot believe it can properly be comprehended under that name for two reasons, first, it is near a Month too soon for these winds to blow, and secondly we do not know that these winds reach this place attall;[6] be this as it may the wind seemed to be now fixed in the SW quarter and made it impossible for us to return to the Coast we had left, and when I

[1] '. . . at 6 AM wieghed and Stood out to Sea with a gentle breeze at ENE which afterwards veer'd to East & EbS and fell by little and little, nevertheless it together with the help of the Currents which were in our favour, carried us some miles from the dangers we most dreaded, and then it fell Calm & the Currant ceased to act any longer in our favour. This Current is no more than a Tide which sets Six hours one way and Six hours the other, but its direction was not easy determined where there was so many different Channels for it to pass through. We availed our selves of the clearness of the day and Observed a great many distances of the Sun and Moon which reduced to Noon when the Lat. was 22°34′30″ gave 167°24′ East.'—Log.

[2] 'We saild again on the 30th—And in going out, had it not been for the intervention of providence, a good lookout and quick working, we must still have been lost, for the Breakers were seen close under our Bows when the Ship was thrown Instantly about, and by that means saved, and proceeded to sea.'—Elliott *Mem.*, f. 34.

[3] . . . the contrary course we had come in

[4] That is, he had all his sails closely furled.

[5] Figure from Log, 'Acco: cor[rected]'.

[6] *for two . . . attall:* for several reasons; it is near a month too soon for these Winds; we know not that they reach this place atall and lastly it is very common for Westerly winds to blow within the Tropicks; however I never found them to blow so hard before, or so far Southerly . . .—f. 289v.

considered that summer was at hand, the Sea which was yet to explore to the South which could only be done in summer, the state and condition of the Ship already in want of some necessary stores and the vast distance we were from any European Port where we could get supplies in case we should be detained by any accident in this Sea [a]nother year, I did not think it adviseable to loose time even in attempting to regain the Coast, and thus I was constrained as it were by necessity to leave it sooner than otherwise I should have done. I called the land we had lately discovered *New Caledonia*.[1] If we except New Zeeland it is perhaps the largest Island in the whole South Pacifick Ocean; it is situated between [19°37′] and [22°30′] south Latitude and [163°37′] and [167°14′] East longitude extending [NW½W] and [SE½E about 87] Leagues, its breadth is not very considerable, no where (I believe) exceeding [10 leagues]. It is a Country full of Hills and Vallies of various extent both for height and depth. To judge of the whole by the parts we were upon, from these hills spring vast number of rivulets which greatly contribute to fertilize the planes and supply all the wants of the Inhabitants in the manner I have already observed. The Summits of most of the hills seemed to be barren, some few are Cloathed with Wood as are all the planes and Vallies.

*By reason of these hills, many parts of the Coast, when at a distance from it, appeared to be indented, or to have great inlets between the hills, but when we came near the shore we always found such places to be shut up with low land, and also observed low-land to lie a long the Coast between the Sea Shore at the foot of the hills, that is in all such parts as we came near enough to see, it is therefore reasonable to suppose that the whole Coast is so, I am like wise of opinion that the whole or greatest part is guarded by reefs or shoals, which renders the access to it very dangerous, but at the same time they guard the Coast from the Violence of the wind and Sea, make it abound with fish, secure an easy and safe Navigation along the Coast for Canoes &c[a] and most likely form some good harbours for Shipping. Most, if not every part of the Coast is inhabited, the Isle of

[1] For this name cf. New Hebrides, p. 521, n. 1 above. It has been said that Cook gave the name because the country reminded him of Scotland; but so far as we know he had never seen Scotland, though no doubt he knew it was a hilly country. Certainly he knew that not so far to the north were a New Britain and New Ireland; and to the south-west he had himself added a New South Wales to the map; so why not round out the United Kingdom with a New Scotland? True, there was a Nova Scotia already in existence; but that was in a different hemisphere, and the fact could anyhow be side-stepped by using a different name for Scotland, even if another Latin one; and New Caledonia certainly tripped more easily off the tongue than Nova Caledonia, and perhaps sounded better than New Scotland. Anyhow it completed the circle well enough. And it helped with the island group he had so recently come from.

Pines not excepted, we saw either smoaks by day or fires by night where ever we came. In the extent which I have give to this land is included the broken or rather unconnected lands to the NW as they are deliniated in the Chart, as they may be connected as well as not, we were however of opinion that they were isles and that *New Caledonia* terminated more to the SE but this at most can only be called a well founded conjecture, be these lands either the one or the other, it is by no means certain that we saw their termination to the west. I think not, as the Shoals did not terminate with the land we saw, but kept their NW direction; . . . Mr Wales determined the Longitude of that part of *New Caledonia* we explored by 96 sets of Observations, which were reduced to one another by our trusty guide the watch. I found the Variation of the Compass to be 10°24′ E; this is the mean variation given by the three Azimuth Compasses which we had on board, which would differ from each other a degree and a half and some times more; I did not find the least difference in the Variation between the NW and SE parts of this land, except it was at anch^r before Balade, where it was found to be less than 10° but this I did not regard as I found such a uniformity out at Sea, and it is there where Navigators want to know the variation. While we were on the NE Coast I thought the Currents set to SE and to west or NW on the other side, but they are by no means considerable and may as probably be channels of Tides as regular currents. In the narrow Channels which divide the shoals and those which communicate with the Sea, the tides run strong, but their rise and fall are inconsiderable, not exceeding 4 feet and the times of high and low-water are not regular.*—ff. 289v–91.

SUNDAY *2nd.* Very fresh gales at SSW and South with which we continued to stretch to the East having a very high Sea from the same direction as the wind. In the AM the gale abated so as to bear all the reefs out and Top g^t sails set. At Noon observed in La^t 23°18′, Longitude made in [169°49′] East and [1°54′] East from the Isle of Pines.[1]

MONDAY *3rd.* PM Little Wind Southerly and a great swell from the same direction. Boobies, Tropick and Men of War birds seen. 11 o'Clock being nearly in the same Lat as the preceeding noon and 15′ more east, we got the wind westerly, it fixed at SWBW and blew a strong gale, by squals attended with rain. This banished all thoughts of returning to the Coast of Caledonia and we stretched to the SSE keeping about a point from the wind. The Southerly swell was suc-

[1] . . . and about 42 leagues South of the *Hebrides*.—f. 290.

ceeded by one from SW as high as the former. At Noon had fair Weather, observed in Lat 24°4′ S, Longitude in [170°11′ E Acco:] and from I. Pines [2°31′ Acco: cor] East.[1]

TUESDAY 4*th.* Fresh gales as above and fair weather. PM Lat 24°, Long 1 ° ′ the variation p[r] Az[th] and Amp[d] was , AM squally with showers of rain. At Noon Lat [25°26′] Lon[g] [Acco 171°03′] and from I. Pines [3°23′ Acco: cor].

WEDNESDAY 5*th.* PM Wind WSW squally with showers of rain. Lat [26°51′] Long [Acco: 171° 37′ Watch 170°50′30″] Variation 10°24′ East. AM fresh gales at West fair Weather. Saw an Albatross, the first we have seen sence we have been with[in] the Tropick. Noon Lat. 26°51′, Long 1 ° ′ and from I. Pines [3°57′ E].

THURSDAY 6*th.* Fresh gales and very squally. Reefed the Top-sails. AM the Wind abated, at 6 it veering to south, Tacked and stood to the West and soon after it fell calm. Noon Lat 27°52′, Long [171°43′ E]. Caulkers at work caulking the Dicks.[2] Had a boat in the Water to shoot birds for the pot, no sport.

FRIDAY 7*th.* Calm all this 24 hours. PM shott two Albatrosses which were geese to us. Variation 9°53′, AM 11°14′ East.

SATURDAY 8*th.* At 1 PM a breeze sprung up at South, soon after it veered to and fixed at SEBS and blew a gentle gale attended with pleasent weather. Stretched to WSW. AM Var 12°14′ E. Noon Lat 28°25′. Long[de] [170°26′ E] and from I. Pines [2°46′ E].

SUNDAY 9*th.* Gentle breezes at SE and clear weather. In the evening M[r] Cooper struck a Porpoise with a Harpoon, it was necessary to have two boats in the Water before we could kill him and get him on board. It was six feet long, a female of that sort which Naturalists call Dolphin of the Ancients, they differ from the other sort in the head and jaws, which in these are long and pointed: this one had [88] teeth in each jaw.[3] The Harslet and lean flesh was to us a feast, the latter eat a little liverish but had not the least taste of fish. We eat it[4] broiled and fryed first soaking it in warm water; in-

[1] Most of the figures supplied in the text from this point to Monday 17th, p. 569 below, are from the Log. Cooper adds a note for the present date, 1 a.m., 'About this time we Cross'd the Tropic of Capricorn the 5th time'.

[2] *sic.*—We had neither Pitch Tar nor Rosin left to pay the seams, this was done with Varnish of Pine and afterwards covered with Coral Sand, it made a cement which far exceeded my expectation.—f. 291v.

[3] The Common Dolphin, *Delphinus delphis* Linn., described in detail by J. R. Forster (*Descr. An.*, p. 280) and painted by his son.

[4] . . . Roasted

deed little art was required to make any kind of fresh meat sute our taste who had been living so long on salt.[1]

At Noon Lat Observed 28°54′30″, Longitude [169°21′ Acco:] and [1°41′ E] from I. Pines.

MONDAY 10*th*. Gentle breezes between S and SW and pleasent weather. PM observed several Distances of the Sun & Moon, the mean result gave 169°30′ E Longitude. The Variation of the Compass being the Mean of several Az[ths] taken by three compasses was [13°9′20″] East, Lat 28°58′ S. At Day-break as we were standing to the West, an Island was discovered bearing SWBS. Soon after we sounded and had 22 fathom water, the bottom Coral Sand, our distance from the Isle was about 3 Leagues. In Plying up to the isle we found not less than 22 nor more than 24 f[m], the same sort of bottom, some times mixed with broken shells. At Noon the isle extended from S 37° E to S 20° W. A Hill nearly in the middle of the Isle bore south 3 miles distant. Lat observed 29°57′ S,[2] Long[d] made from I. Pines [28 Miles E Long Acco: 168°06′ Watch 167°21′.]

TUESDAY 11*th*. Gentle gales at SE and ESE. After dinner hoisted out two boats in which my self, some of the officers and gentlemen went to take a view of the Island and its produce, we found no difficulty in landing behind some rocks which lined part of the coast[3] and defended it from the Surf. We found the Island uninhabited and near a kin to New Zealand, the Flax plant, many other Plants and Trees common to that country was found here but the chief produce of the isle is Spruce Pines which grow here in vast abundance and to a vast size, from two to three feet diameter and upwards, it is of a different sort to those in New Caledonia and also to those in New Zealand and for Masts, Yards &c[a] superior to both. We cut down one of the Smallest trees we could find and Cut a length of the uper

[1] 'PM at 6 many Porpoises being about the Bows, one was struck with the Harpoon, but found we were in danger of loosing him, by not being able to give him the necessary play in the Ship, so hoisted out the 2 small Boats, One of which he tow'd right in the wind's eye at an incredible rate to a great distance—however they at last shot him, and brought Him onboard at 7. We then hoisted in the Boats and made sail again. This Porpoise we cut up and eat; I've often heard it averr'd that the Haslet of a Porpoise is little inferior to that of a Hog. I readily agree, that it is very little inferior to a Hogs Haslet, but in my Opinion the flesh of Him is vastly superior to any Haslet whatever [8953 vastly superior to the Haslet of any Animal or fish on the Earth beneath or in the Waters under the Earth]. I really think myself that it is exceeding good, and I'm sure it had the universal approbation of every Man onboard here, that was fortunate enough to get a slice of Him'. —Clerke. Mitchel less eloquently says, 'The porpoise was divided to the sick &c &c which was devoured eagerly—it exceeds the flesh of Seal & in short is a very dainty & good fresh Meat'.

[2] This figure is clearly a slip for 28°57′ S, as in the Log.

[3] . . . on the NE side . . .—f. 292.

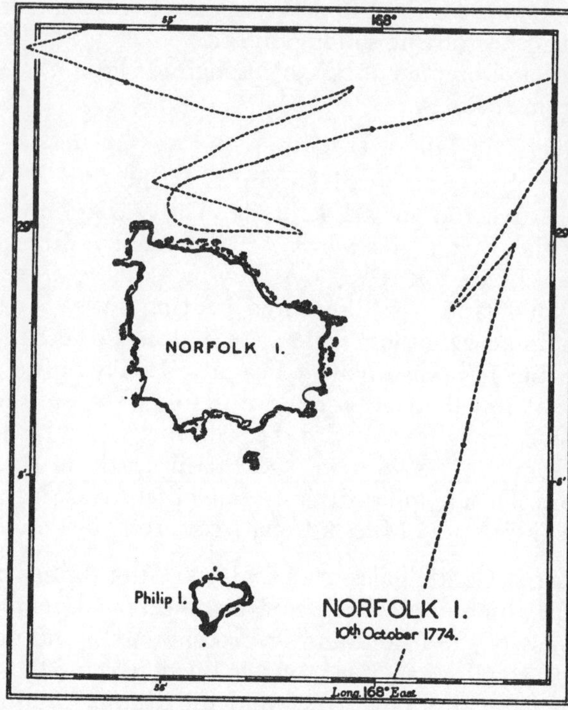

FIG. 70

end to make a Topg[t] Mast or Yard. My Carpenter tells me that the wood is exactly of the same nature as the Quebeck Pines.[1] Here then is a nother Isle where Masts for the largest Ships may be had. Here are the same sort of Pigions,[2] Parrots[3] and Parrokeets[4] as in New Zea-

[1] . . . We found it uninhabited and were undoubtedly the first who ever sit foot upon it. We found many trees and plants Common to New Zealand and in particular the flax plant which is rather more luxurient than in any part of that Country but the chief produce is a sort of Spruce Pine, which grows here in great abundance and to a large size Ma[n]y trees were as thick breast high as two men could fathom and exceeding straight and tall, it is of a sort between that which grows in New-Zeeland and that in New Caledonia and the foliage is some thing different from both. The wood is not so heavy as the former nor so light and close grained as the latter and is a good deal like the Quebec pine For about two hundred yards from the shore, the ground is covered so thick with Shrubs & Plan[t]s as hardly to be penetrated. Farther inland the Woods were perfectly clear and free from under wood & the soil seemed to be rich and deep.—ff. 292, 293 (the last two sentences are written on f. 293, a separate slip, in red ink). The tree was the Norfolk Island Pine, *Araucaria excelsa*.

[2] *Hemiphaga novaeseelandiae spadicea* (Latham) now extinct.

[3] The Long-billed Parrot *Nestor productus* Gould, now extinct. It was never found in New Zealand.

[4] The Norfolk Island Parrot *Cyanoramphus novaezelandiae cookii* (G. R. Gray). Another form occurs in New Zealand.

land, Rails and some small birds.[1] The Sea fowl are White Boobies,[2] guls, Tern &c[a] which breed undisturbed on the Rocks and in the Clifts. The Coast is not distitute of Fish, our people caught some which were excellent while in the boats a long-side the rocks. I took posission of this Isle as I had done of all the others we had discovered, and named it *Norfolk Isle*, in honour of that noble family.[3] It is situated in the Latitude of 29°00′ S, Longit of [168°16′] East,[4] it is about [5 leagues] in circuit of a good height and its shores are steep and rocky. Here is good Soundings and Anchorage about this isle, a bank of Coral Sand mixed with Shells on which we found from [19] to [35 or 40] fathom Water, surrounds it, and extends, especially to the South, [7] Leagues off and perhaps as far or farther every other way only we had no oppertunity to determine it, on the NW & North side is 20 & 19 fathom, one quarter of a mile from the shore and very good anchorage. I had almost forgot to mention that the isle is supplied with fresh Water and produceth a bundance of small Cabbage Palms, we cut down and brought off as many as the little time we had would admit.[5] Upon the whole here

[1] The Forsters obtained a flycatcher known as the Scarlet-breasted Robin, *Petroeca multicolor* (Gm.).

[2] The Masked or Blue-faced Booby, *Sula dactylatra personata* Gould.—There are several different species of the other birds here mentioned by Cook: see 'The Birds of Lord Howe and Norfolk Islands', by A. F. Bassett Hull in *Proc. Linn. Soc. N.S.W.*, 1910–11, pp. 34–5.

[3] *that . . . family:* the Noble family of Howards.—f. 291v. Gilbert and Wales are more selective—'after the Dutchess of Norfolk'. I do not know why Cook felt that family particularly deserving of commemoration in the Pacific. Chart XXXIX*b*.

[4] . . . the latter was determined by Lunar observations made on this, the preceeding and following days and the Latitude was determined by a good Observation at Noon.—ff. 291v–2. But there are a number of minor differences over these and other figures in the various MSS, not particularly significant except that they mark the thirst for accuracy. The latitude is given in the Log, as here, as 29°; in B as 29°01′, subsequently altered in red ink to 29°02′30″. The longitude is 168°06′ in the Log—perhaps a slip. The Log gives the circuit as 16 miles, B as 5 leagues; the maximum sounding on the bank is 32 fathoms in the Log, 35 or 40 in B.

[5] . . . On the isle is fresh Water and abundance of Cabbage Palms, Wood Sorril, Sow-Thistle and Samphire, with which the Shores in some places abound. We brought on board as much of each sort as the time we had to gather them would admit. The Cabbage trees or palms were not thicker than a mans leg & from 10 to 20 feet high, they are of the same Genus with the Cocoanut trees, with large pinnated leaves like them and are the same as the second sort found in the Northern parts of New [Holland *deleted*] South Wales (Vide Hawkesworth Voyage Vol. 3, p. 624). The Cabbage is properly speaking the Bud of the tree. Each tree produceth but one Cabbage, which is situated at the Crown where the leaves spring out and is inclosed in the Stem. The cuting off the Cabbage effectually distroys the tree, so that no more than one can be had from the same stem. The Cocoanut tre[e] and some others of the Palm kind produce cabbage as well as these. This Vegetable is not only wholesome but exceeding palatable and proved the most agreeable repast we had had for some time.—f. 292. This is a very late addition (as the reference to Hawkesworth alone would show), almost all in red ink; the sentences describing the cabbage tree are marginal. It is in fact a curious amalgam of Wales (who contributed most of it, see p. 869 below), Banks-Hawkesworth ('with large pinnated leaves . . . New South Wales', and the sentence on other trees of the palm kind producing cabbage), and Cook himself,

are many good refreshments to be got but we had no time to spare to benefit by them. Whilest I was a shore I observed that an East and West Moon must make high-Water or nearly so, and that the Tides must rise six or eight feet perpendicular. The Variation of the Compass was 11°9′ East.[1]

The approach of night brought us all on board, when we hoisted in the Boats and stretched to the ENE with the Wind at SE. At midd-night Tack'd, stood to the South and weathered the Island on the south side of which lay some high Islots or rocks, which serve as roosting and breeding places for birds.[2] Being clear of the isle we stretched to the South[3] with a fresh breeze at ESE. My design was to touch at Queen Charlottes Sound in New Zealand, there to refresh my people and put the Ship in a condition to cross this great ocean in a high Latitude once more. At Noon Norfolk Isle bore NBE distant 7 Leag[s] Lat Ob[d] 29°21′ S. Depth of Water [from 19 to 32] fathom.

WEDNESDAY 12*th*. Fresh breezes and Clear Weather. Sounded at 1 and at 2 o'Clock but had no ground, the first time with 44 fathoms and the Second with 70, so that Judged we were on the verge of the bank at Noon. During the night the Wind came more favourable and inabled us to proceed to the South with very little deviation to the west. At Noon Lat 31°1′ S, Longit [Acco: 167°47′ Watch 167°2½′] East.

THURSDAY 13*th*. Gentle gale at EBN & NEBE pleasent Weather. PM Lat 31°31′, Longit same as at the preceeding Noon, the Variation was 9°35′ E. AM Lat 32°33′, It was 9°45′ East. Noon Lat 34°3′[4], Longit [Acco: 168°20′ Watch 167°35′] East.

on the destruction of the tree. The cabbage tree is here the palm called Nikau in New Zealand, *Rhopalostylis sapida* (Solander's *Areca sapida*). Forster (*De Plantis Esculentis*, pp. 66–7) writes, 'Reperitur spontanea in Nova zeelandia usque ad aestuarium Charlottae reginae et frequens in Norfolciae insula deserta. Huius praecipue Cor sive Caput in deliciis est apud nautas Europaeos, et cum oleo et aceto parari solet'. The information that it was eaten with oil and vinegar is interesting—evidently it was treated as a salad vegetable and not vulgarly boiled. What is called today the cabbage tree (*Cordyline australis*) branches freely; the Nikau only most exceptionally. For other annotation see the relevant page of Wales's journal, p. 869 below.

[1] *The Variation . . . East:* The morning we discovered the I[d] the Variation was found to be 13°9′ E but I think this observation gave too much as others which we had both before and after gave near 2° less.—f. 292v (final revised version).

[2] . . . On this as also on the SE side is a sandy beach, whereas most of the other shores are bounded by rocky clifts which have 20 and 18 fathom water close to them at least so we found it on the NE side, and with good anchorage; . . .—f. 292–2v. Cook had a better experience of landing on Norfolk Island than many who came after him.

[3] . . . inclining a little to the West . . .—f. 292v.

[4] The MS reads here 34°3′, which seems like an accidental transference from the following entry. The Log gives the figure 32°55′.

FRIDAY 14*th*. Wind at NEBN fine pleasent Weather. Steer'd SE.[1] PM Lat 33°9', Longit [168°43⅔'] E. Var 9°54' E. Noon Lat. 34°3'. Long [Acco: 169°26'] E.

SATURDAY 15*th*. PM Moderate gales & Clear Weather. At 6 Lat [34°24'] Longit 169°53' Variation 10°10' East. AM Fresh gales and Clowdy. Saw some Diving Petrels (small Divers).[2] Noon Lat Ob[d] 35°32'30". Longitude [170°50' Watch 170°11'] East and [2°50' E] of Norfolk isle.

SUNDAY 16*th*. Fresh breeze at NNE and pleasent Weather. At PM altered Course to SEBS. Many Little divers or Diving Petrels about the Ship, such as are common on the Coast of N. Zealand. Noon Lat Observed 37°32'. Long[de] in [Acco: 172°41' Watch 171°56'] East and from Isle of Norfolk [4°35' E].

MONDAY 17*th*. PM Fresh gales Northerly and Cloudy weather. At 4 Sound[d] no ground with a line of 140 fathoms. Middnight heavy Squalls[3] with rain, Thunder and Lightning. Wind shifted to SW, remain'd unsetled: Split the Jibb to pieces, lost great part of it, remains good for little, being much worn. Day-break saw Mount Egmont (covered with everlasting snow) bearing SE½E; sounded 70 fathoms, muddy bottom, distance off shore 3 Leagues. Wind Westerly a fresh gale, Steer'd SSE for Queen Charlottes Sound. Noon Cape Egmont ENE distant 3½ or 4 leagues, the Mount hid in the Clouds, judged it to be in one with the Cape. Lat Ob[d] 39°24' Long[de] in [Watch 173°1'].

TUESDAY 18*th*. Very strong gales at Westerly and Cloudy. Steered SSE for Queen Charlottes Sound. At 7 Close reefed the Fore & Main Top-sails and handed the Mizen Top-sail, got down Top g[t] yards and hauled the wind close. At 11 Stephens's Isle SEBE. At middnight Tacked and made a trip to the North till 3 AM then bore up for the Sound under double reef'd Top-sails and Courses. At 9 hauled round point Jackson through a Sea which looked Terrible, occasioned by the Tide, Wind[4] & Sea, but as we knew the Cause it did not alarm us; At 11 Anchored before Ship Cove the strong fluries from the land not permiting us to get in.

WEDNESDAY 19*th*. PM As we could not move the Ship I went into the Cove to try to catch some fish with the Sein. As soon as I landed I looked for the bottle I had left behind in which was the Memd[m] it

[1] . . . all sails set, the Variation increased but slowly
[2] The New Zealand Diving Petrel, *Pelecanoides urinatrix* (Gm.).
[3] . . . from the North
[4] *the Tide, Wind:* a rapid tide a high wind . . .—f. 294.

was gone, but by whom it did not appear. Two hauls with the Sein procured us only four small fish, after shooting a few[1] old Shags and robing the Nests of some young ones we returned aboard. AM being little wind, weighed and Warped into the Cove and there moored a Cable each way, Intending to wait here to refresh the Crew, refit the Ship in the best manner we could and compleat her with Wood and Water. We unbent the Sails to repair several having been much damage'd in the late gale, the Main and Fore Course, already worn to the utmost, was condemned as useless. Struck and unriged the Fore and Main Topmasts to fix moveable Cheeks[2] to them for want of which the Trestle trees were Continually breaking. Set up the Forge to make bolts for the above use and repair what was wanting in the Iron way. Set up the Astronomers Observatory on shore in the bottom of the Cove and Tents for the reception of a Guard, Sail-makers, Coopers &c[a]. Ordered Vegetable, of which here were plenty, to be boiled with Oatmeal & Portable Soup every Morning for breakfast and with Pease and Portable Soup every day to dinner for all hands.[3] We now found that some Ship had been here sence we last left it not only by the bottle being gone as mentioned above, but by several trees having been Cut down with Saws and Axes which were standing when we sailed. This Ship could be no other than the Adventure Captain Furneaux.[4]

THURSDAY 20*th*. PM Fresh gales at NW and fair weather. Sent all the Sails wanting repairs a Shore to the Tent and in the AM several empty Casks. Carpenters employed fixing Cheeks to the Top-masts, Caulkers caulking the sides and Seamen overhauling the rigging.[5] Winds Southerly Hazey Cloudy weather.

FRIDAY 21*st*. Wind Southerly with continual rain.[6]

SATURDAY 22*nd*. First part D[o] Weather, remainder Clear pleasent weather, which admited us to go on with our works and for my self and the Botanists to viset several parts of the Sound and a mongest

[1] *after . . . few:* we in some measure made up for this difficiency by shooting several birds which the flowers in the garden had drawen thither, some . . .

[2] *cheeks:* chocks or knees

[3] . . . over and above their usual allowance of salt meat.—f. 294v.

[4] *We now . . . Furneaux:* In the after-noon as M[r] Wales was seting up his observatory, he discover'd that several trees had been cut down with saws and axes, which were Standing when we last left this place, and a few days after the spot where an Observatory, clock &c[a] had been set up was also found in a place different to that where M[r] Wales had his; it was therefore now no longer to be doubted but that the Adventure had been here after we left it.

[5] *Carpenters . . . rigging:* Every body went to work on their respective employments, one of which was to Calk the Ship sides, a thing much wanting . . .

[6] *with . . . rain:* 'a Strong gale with continual Rain, so that no work could go forward'. —Log.

others our gardens on Motouara which we found allmost in a state of Nature and had been wholy neglected by the Inhabitants, nevertheless many Articles were in a florishing state.[1] None of the Natives having as yet made their appearence we made a fire on the isle, judgeing the smoke would draw their attention towards us.

SUNDAY 23*rd*. Variable light airs and pleasent weather. Every one[2] who chused were at liberty to go a shore.

MONDAY 24*th*. Pleasent weather. AM went on with the various works in hand. Two Canoes were seen coming down the Sound but retired behind a point on the west side upon discovering us as was supposed. After breakfast I went in a Boat to look for them accompani'd by the Botanists. As we proceeded a long shore we shott sever[l] birds, the report of our guns gave notice of our approach and the Natives discovered them selves[3] by hollaing to us but when we came before their habitations only two men appeared on a rising ground,[4] the rest had taken to the Woods and hills, but the moment we landed they knew us again, joy took place of fear, they hurried out of the woods, embraced us over and over and skiped about like Mad men.[5] I made them presents of Hatchets, Knives, Cloth & Medals and in return they gave us a quantity of fish. There were only one or two amongest them whose faces we could well recolect, the account they gave us of our other friends whom we inquir'd after by name were variously understood concequently ended in nothing.[6] After a short Stay we took leave and returned aboard, they promiseing to come to the Ship in the Morning and bring with them fish which was all I wished for by the intercourse.

TUESDAY 25*th*. Winds SW pleasent Weather. Early in the Morning our friends paid us a Viset and brought with them a quantity of fish which they exchanged for Otaheite cloth &c[a] [7] and then returned to their habitations.

[1] . . . and shewed how well they liked the Soil in which they were planted.

[2] *Every one:* 'PM all hands at Work. AM after washing the decks and Scrubing betwixt wind and Water, all . . .'—Log.

[3] . . . in Shag Cove [i.e. the present Resolution Bay.]—f. 295.

[4] . . . with their arms in hand

[5] . . . but I observed that they would not suffer some women who made their appearence to come near us.—f. 295, *red ink*.

[6] *There were . . . nothing:* 'There were only a few amongst them whose faces we could recognise and on our enquiring why they were afraid of us and for some of our old acquentances by name, they talked a great deal about killing which was so variously understood by us that we could gather not[h]ing from it, so that after a short stay we took leave and returned aboard.'—f. 295.

[7] '. . . a plentifull Cargoe of Fish, the Market at the old stand, a little piece of Otahite Cloath purchases an excellent dish of them.'—Clerke. Cooper, 26 October, also mentions 'Mouldy Bisquit' as a return for fish.

WEDNESDAY 26*th.* PM fresh gales Southerly with rain. AM Variable light Airs and fair Weather. The Carpenters had no sooner finished the Cheeks to the Top-masts than we found one of the fore Cross-trees broke, set them to work to make a new one out of the Spare Anchor Stock. Got into the after hold four Launch Load of Shingle ballast and struck down Six guns from off the Deck, keeping no more than Six Mounted. Our good friends the Natives stick by us and supply us plentifully with fish.

THURSDAY 27*th.* Variable gentle breezes and pleasent weather, favourable for the carrying on of our works which increase upon us the more we examine and look into things.

FRIDAY 28*th.* PM Wind and Weather as before. AM fresh gale Westerly fair weather. Rigged and fidded the Topg[t] Masts. Went on a Shooting party to the west bay, Viseted the place where I left the Hogs and fowls, saw no vestige's of them or of any people being there sence. Viseted some of the Natives who gave us some fish in return for some trifles I gave them. Soon after we left them M[r] F. thought he heard the squeaking of a Pig in the woods hard by their habitations, probably they may yet have those they had when we were last here. Returned on board[1] with about a Doz[n] and a half of Wild fowl, Shaggs and Sea Pies.[2] Sence the Natives have been with us a report has risen said to come first from them, that a ship has lately been lost, some where in the Strait, and all the crew Killed by them, when I examined them on this head they not only denied it but seem'd wholy ignorant of the matter.

*... [a ship] had been lately lost in the Straits, that some of the people got on shore and that the Natives stole their Cloathes &c for which several where shot: but afterwards when they could fire no longer the Natives got the better and killed them with their Patapatoos and eat them. But that they had no hand in the affair, which they said happend at Vanua Aroa[3] near Teerawhitte which is on the other side of the Strait. One man said it was two Moons ago; but another contradicted him and counted on his fingers about 20 or 30 days. They discribed by actions how the Ship was beat to pieces by going up and down against the Rocks till at last it was all scattered abroad.

[1] The MS reads 'Returned about', but unless Cook meant to give a time, he seems to have made a verbal slip. He may have intended 'Returned aboard'. All the other MSS read 'In the evening returned on board with about a dozen' etc.

[2] ... The sportsmen who had been out in the woods near the Ship were more successfull among the small birds.—f. 295v.

[3] I know of no place name corresponding to this: *whenua aroha* or *aroa* is presumably the Maori equivalent. Wales, to whom the story was first told, gives the name as Venua Arow.

The next day some others told the same story or one nearly to the same purport and pointed over the[1] East Bay, which is on the East side of the Sound for the place where it happened. These stories made me very uneasy about the Adventure and I desired Mr Wales and those on Shore to let me know if any of the Natives should mention it again or to send them to me for I had not heard any thing from them my self. When Mr Wales came on board to dinner, he found the very people on board who had told him the story on shore and pointed them out to me. I enquired about the affair and endeavoured to come at the truth by every method I could think on, All I could get from them was Caurey[2] (No) and not only denied every Syllable of what they had said when on shore but seemed wholy ignorant of the matter—so that I began to think our people had Misunderstood them and that the story refered to some of their own people and boats.*—f. 296.

SATURDAY 29*th*. Wind variable with much rain which did not hinder our friends from bringing us a supply of fish.[3]

SUNDAY 30*th*. Wind Southerly a fresh gale with showers of rain. Natives a board most of the day tradeing with green talk, hatchets &ca. One of the officers found in the Woods not far from our tents a fresh hens egg, a proof that the Poultry that we left here are living, the Natives tell us that they lost those I gave them in the Woods.

MONDAY 31*st*. AM Wind at NE fine pleasent weather. Our Botanists went to Long Island where some of the party saw a Hog, a boar as they judged,[4] so wild that it took to the woods as soon as it saw them. It is probably one of those Captain Furneaux left behind and brought to this isle by the Natives. Sence the Natives did not distroy these Hogs when in their posession, we cannot suppose they will attempt it now, so that there is little fear but that this Country will soon be stocked with these Animals, both in a wild and domistick state. I am in doubt that the goats I put ashore are killed, for if they killed the goats why should they not the hogs also.[5]

[1] *sic;* perhaps 'to' was intended. [2] *Kaore or kahore.*

[3] 'Cleaned the Ship betwixt decks.'—Log.

[4] *Hog . . . judged:* a large black boar as it was described to me

[5] 'AM wind Northerly Pleasent Weather. Employ'd Wooding, Watering, repairing Casks, Sails, makeing bolts to secure the Tops, Calking the Sides and overhauling the rigging. Took the New Driver and the Jibb belonging to the boat in frame to make a Jibb for the Ship and to repair small Sails having no thin Canvas left.'—Log.—'The Carpenter has found many of the planks in our upper works drawn off the Timbers at least a quarter of an Inch which took a number of Ragg'd Bolts & Nails to secure it to again.'—Cooper. Obviously the ship had come to her repair base none too soon. Rag-bolts—'those which are jagged or barbed, to prevent working in their holes' (Smyth, *Sailor's Word-Book*).

[NOVEMBER 1774]

TUESDAY *1st.* Very strong gales Westerly. Fidded the Fore Topmast and Set up the fore rigging. Cast off the Main Shrouds for the Caulkers to come at the seams in and under the Chains. A Number of Strangers viseted us to day and brought with them some fish, but their principle article of trade was green talk and other trifles,[1] our old friends left us on Sunday evening and have not been with us sence.

WEDNESDAY *2nd.* First and Middle parts strong gales at SW with rain. Latter fine pleasent Weather which inabled us to resume of our Works the bad Weather had put a stop to. My self accompanied by the Botanist viseted the East side of the Sound, shott a few Pigions and other birds and returned aboard in the evening without meeting with any thing remarkable. I now learnt that a number of the Inhabitants had been on board Most of the day tradeing with their usual Articles.

THURSDAY *3rd.* Variable light breezes and pleasent weather. Fided the Main Top-mast and set up the Main & Top-mast rigging. Compleated the Ship with Wood and Water and nearly finished all our other works except Caulking which goes on slowly, as having only two Caulkers and a great deal to do and which must absolutely be done before we can put to sea.[2]

[1] *A number . . . trifles:* we were visited by A Number of strangers; they came from up the Sound; and brought with them but little fish, the chief articles of their trade was Women and green stones or talk are two articles which seldom came to a bad market. Some of the largest pieces of green talk were got to day I had ever seen.—ff. 295v–7 (f. 296 is a separate slip). This was a first version, which was altered to omit the mention of women, so as to read 'was green stone or Talk are articles which never came to a bad market. . .'—the syntax still being alarming.

[2] In the Log this entry, or the substance of it, comes under 4 November. B, f. 297, has a shortened version of it for the 3rd, which is deleted and the following substituted, in red ink: 'M[r] Pickersgill met with some of the Natives who related to him the circumstances of a Ship being lost and the people killed; but added with great earnestness that it was not them who did it'. In the Log for 3 November we come once again upon the name of Marra: 'Punished Jn[o] Marra with a Doz[n] Lashes for Drunkenness and going out of the Ship without leave'.—'. . . for attempting to secrete himself in one of the Natives Canoe with intention of getting on shore', says Clerke; or, in 8953, 'with intention of deserting from the Ship'. Whether this time Marra wanted to desert is doubtful, and Cook in his Log entry does not make that the charge. Marra in his own account (p. 305) adverts to 'seven or eight young red painted blue-lip'd cannibal ladies' of Queen Charlotte Sound, and says, 'The gunner's mate, who had been confined in irons for endeavouring to leave the ship at Ottaheite, was here punished with twelve lashes for going ashore without leave in pursuit of one of those beauties'. There is a further reference: 'The same Gunner, attempted to leave us here that did at Otaheite, and Cook declar'd that if he was not well assurd that the fellow would be killd and Eat before morn[g] he would have let him go'.—Elliott *Mem.*, f. 35.

FRIDAY 4*th*. Fine pleasent Weather. Most of the Natives retired up the Sound to their habitations there.[1] Went over to Long Island to look for the Hog which had been seen there, found it to be one of the Sows Captain Furneaux left behind the same as was in the posession of the Natives when we were last here. From a Supposion of its being a boar I had carri'd over a Sow to leave with him but brought her back when I found the Contrary.[2]

SATURDAY 5*th*. Light breeze Westerly and pleasent Weather. Early in the morning our old friend[s] paid us a second Viset and brought us a supply of fish. At 8 o'Clock went in the Pinnace up the Sound accompanied by Mr F. and his party. I had some thoughts of finding the termination of it or to see if it communicated with the sea,[3] in our way we met with several people out fishing of whom we made the necessary enquiries, they all agree'd that there was no passage to Sea by the head of the Sound. After proceeding five Leagues up, which was farther than I had ever been before, we met a Canoe conducted by four or five men who confirm'd what the others had told us; we then enquired if their was any passage to the East and understood them there was, this was what I suspected for from the Hill I first discovered the Strait I saw a Bason into which the tide had access & recess, but I did not know whether it was an Arm of the Sound or an inlet of the Sea;[4] to determine this point I laid aside the scheme of proceeding to the head of the Sound and went to this Inlet, which is on the SE side of the Sound four or five leagues above Ship Cove, here we found a large settlement of the Natives who received us with great courtesy; our stay with them was short as we found incouragement to persue the object we had in view and accordingly proceeded ENE down the Inlet which we at last found to open into the Sea by a Channell about a mile wide in which ran a very strong tide. It was four o'Clock in the after noon before we had made this discovery which opens a new passage into the Sound and as we came to a resolution[5] to return aboard that same evening we were obliged to

[1] *to their . . . there:* indeed I had taken every gentle method to obliged [*sic*] them to be gone, for sence these new comers had been with us, our old friends had disapeared and we had been without fish.—f. 297.

[2] as the leaving her there would have answered no end.

[3] *or to . . . sea:* or rather to see if I could find any passage out to Sea by the SE as I suspected from some discoveries I had made when first in this Sound.

[4] *this was . . . Sea:* in the very place where I expected to find one . . .—f. 297v.

[5] *here we found . . . resolution:* A little within the entrance on the SE side, at a place called Kohèghe-nooee [Ko Heke-nui], we found a large Settlement of the Natives, the Cheif whose name was Tringo-boohee [? Te Ringapuhi or Te Ringaopuhi] and his people, which we found to be some of those who had lately been on board the Ship, recieved us with great courtesy; they seemed to be pretty numberous here and in the neighbourhood; our stay with them was short, as the information they gave us incouraged us to prosue

defer viseting a large Hippa or strong hold built on a rising ground on the North side a little within the entrance whose inhabitants seem'd to invite us to them and without makeing any stop proceeded for the Ship which [we reached] by 10 o'Clock bring[ing] with us some fish we had got from the Natives and a few birds we had shott, amongest which were some of the same sort of Ducks we got in Duskey Bay and we have reason to think they are all to be found here as the Inhabitants of this place have[1] a particular [name] to each.[2]

SUNDAY 6*th*. Wind NE, Gloomy weather with some rain. Had a present from one of the Natives whose name was *Pedero*[3] of a Staff of honour,[4] in return I dress'd him in an old suit of Clothes with which he was not a little proud: having got him and a nother in a communicative mood we began to enquire of them if the Adventure had been here and they gave us to understand in a manner which admited of no doubt that soon after we were gone she arrived and Stayed here about   Days,[5] and farther asserted that neither her or any other Ship had been Stranded on the Coast as had been reported. After breakfast I took a number of men over to Long Island to endeavour to catch the Sow but we returned without being able to see her. [Pedero] dined with us, eat of every thing at table and drank more Wine than any of us.[6]

the object we had in view. Accordingly we proceeded down the Arm, ENE and EbN leaving several fine Coves on both sides and at last found it to open out into the Strait by a Channell about a mile wide in which ran out a Strong tide, we had also observed one seting down the Arm all the time we had been in it, it was now about 4 oClock in the After-noon and in less than an hour after this tide ceased and was succeeded by the flood which came in with equal Strength. The out let lies SEbE and NWbE and nearly in the direction of ESE and WNW from Cape Terawhittee. We found 13 fathoms water a little within the entrance clear ground: It seemed to me that a leading Wind was necessary to go in and out of this passage on account of the Rapidity of the tides, I however had but little time to make observations of this nature as night was at hand and I had resolved . . . —f. 297v. This was Tory Channel, which got its name from the New Zealand Company's brig *Tory* in 1839. Its Cook Strait entrance is in fact less than half a mile wide. See Fig. 32.

[1] *have:* knew them all by the drawings—and had . . .—f. 298.

[2] '. . . the Utmost sociallity subsists between us and the Natives—numbers of Visits are paid and repaid Upon various Occasions . . .'—Clerke 8953.

[3] ? Pitirau.

[4] No doubt a *taiaha*.

[5] 'We made two pieces of paper, to represent the two ships, and drew the figure of the Sound on a larger piece; then drawing the two ships into the Sound, and out of it again, as often as they had touched at and left it, including our last departure, we stopped a while, and at last proceeded to bring our ship in again; but the natives interrupted us, and taking up the paper which represented the Adventure, they brought it into the harbour, and drew it out again, counting on their fingers how many moons she had been gone.'—Forster, II, pp. 456–7.

[6] 'Punish'd Jn° Keplin with a dozen lashes for leaving the Boat when on duty and declareing he would go with the Indians He thought proper to come back of himself'.—Gilbert.

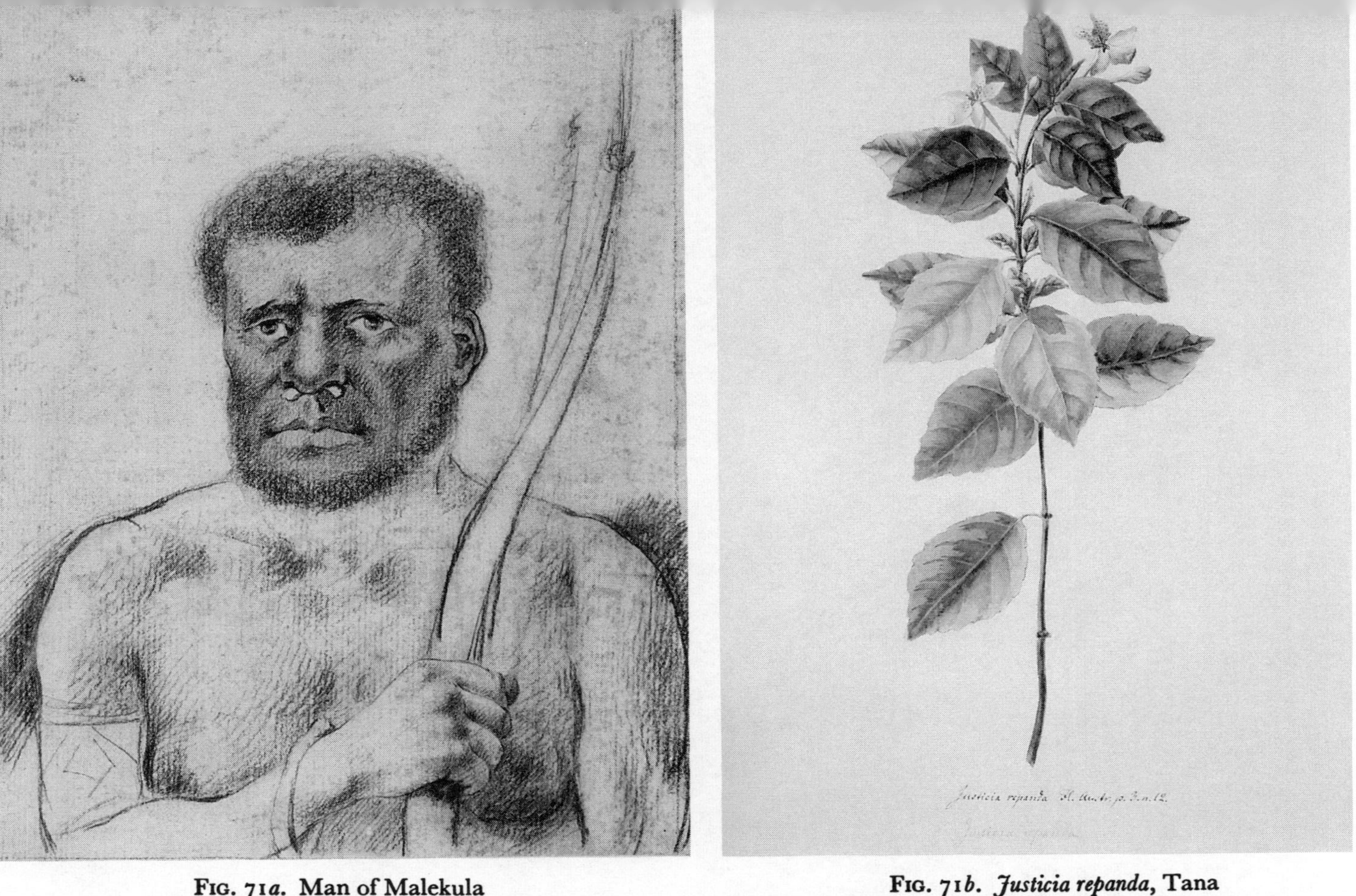

FIG. 71*a*. Man of Malekula

By Hodges.—B.M., Dept. of Prints and Drawings

FIG. 71*b*. *Justicia repanda*, Tana

B.M. (N.H.), George Forster, 'Botanical Drawings', I, pl. 7

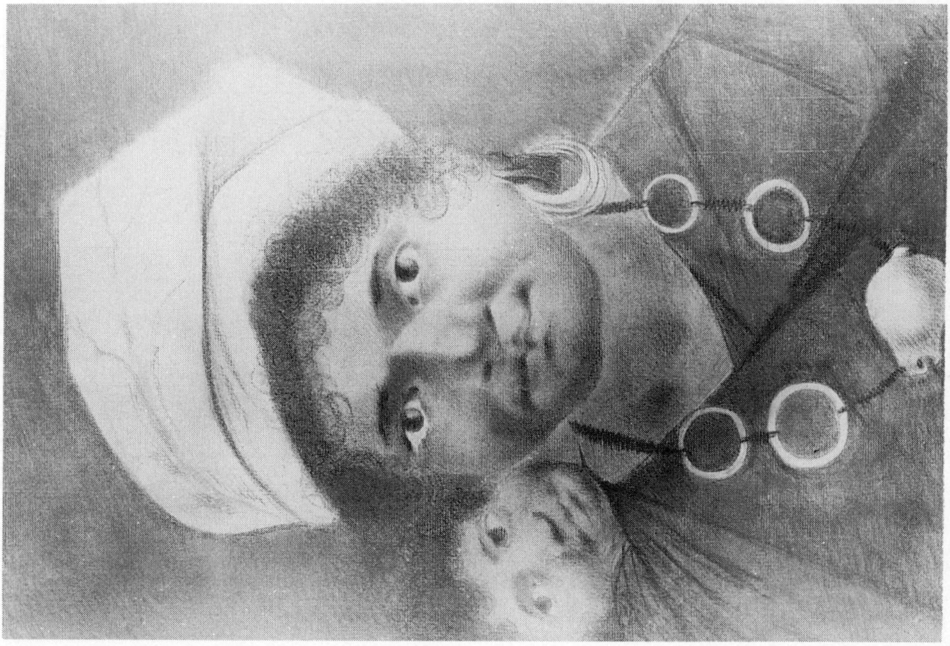

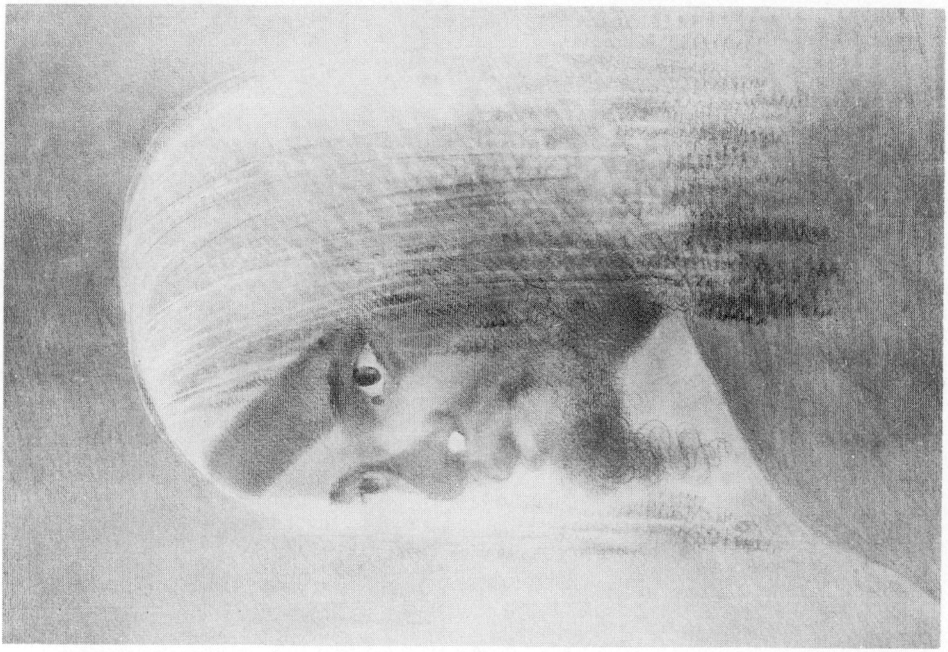

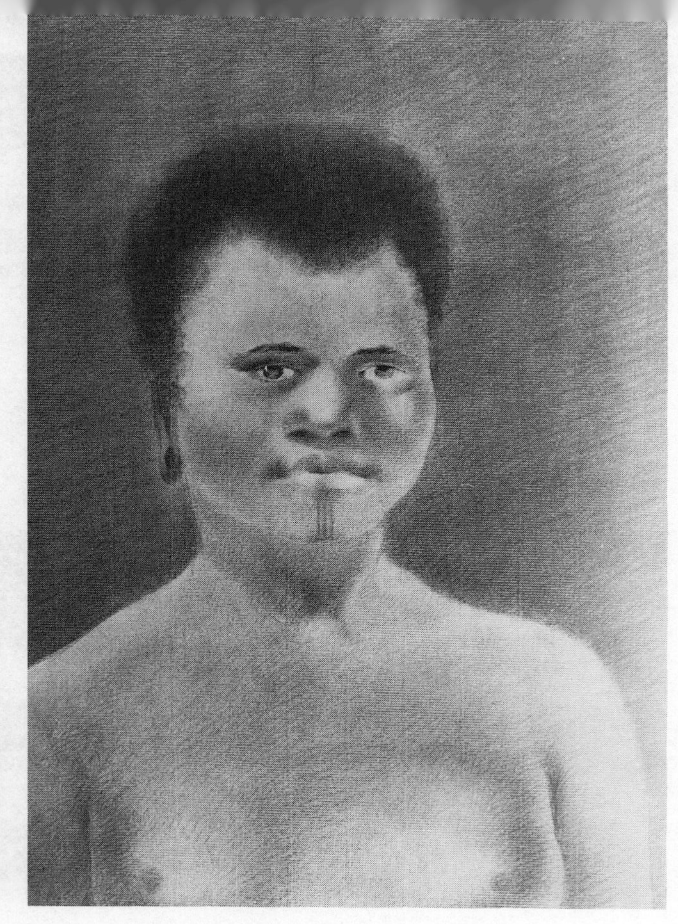

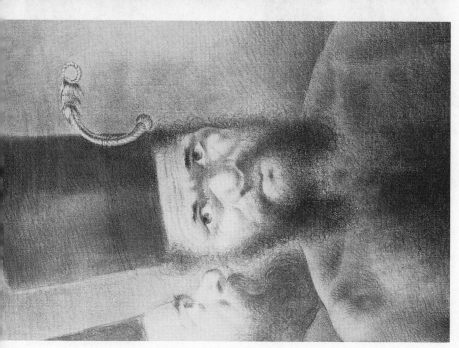

Fig. 73. Portrait heads of natives of New Caledonia

(*left*) Man; (*right*) Woman. Crayon drawings by Hodges.—Commonwealth National Library

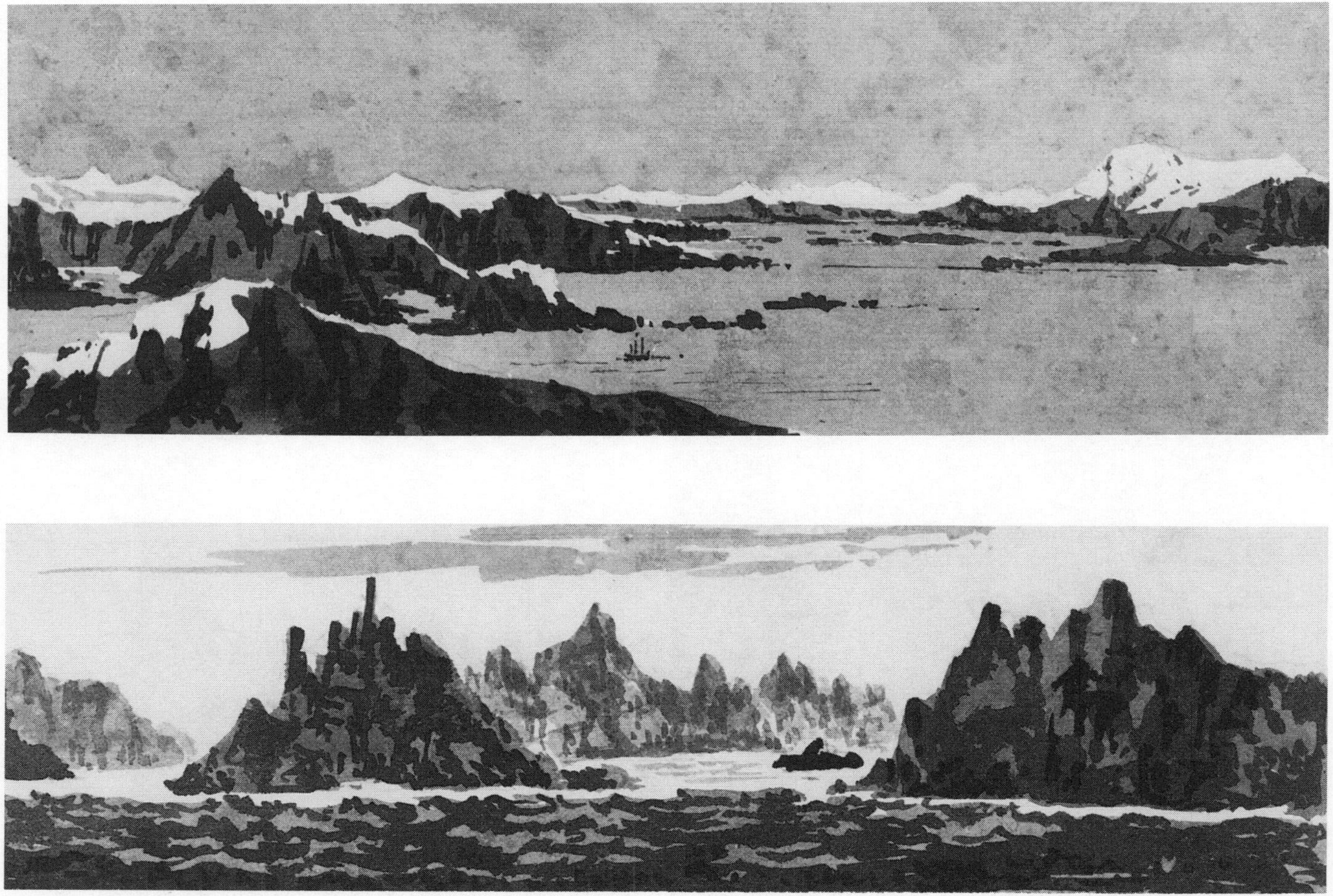

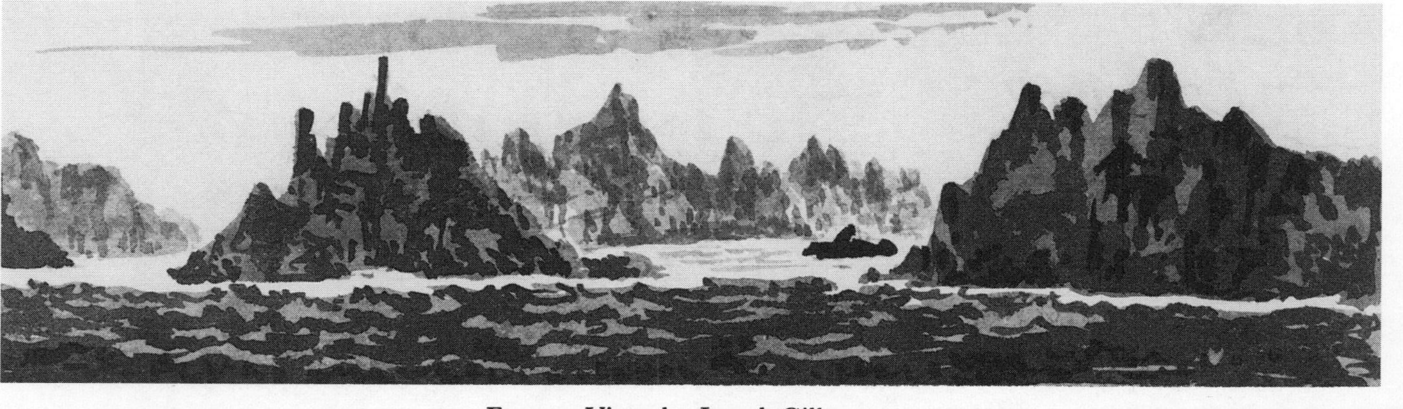

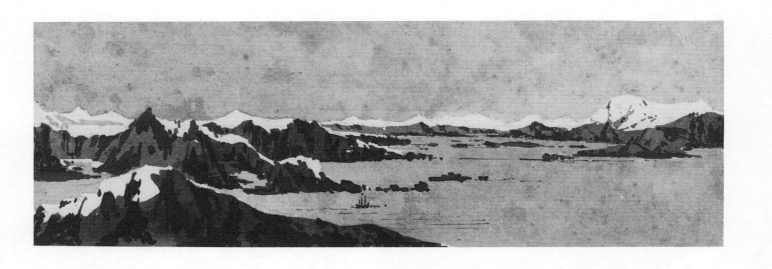

FIG. 74. Views by Joseph Gilbert

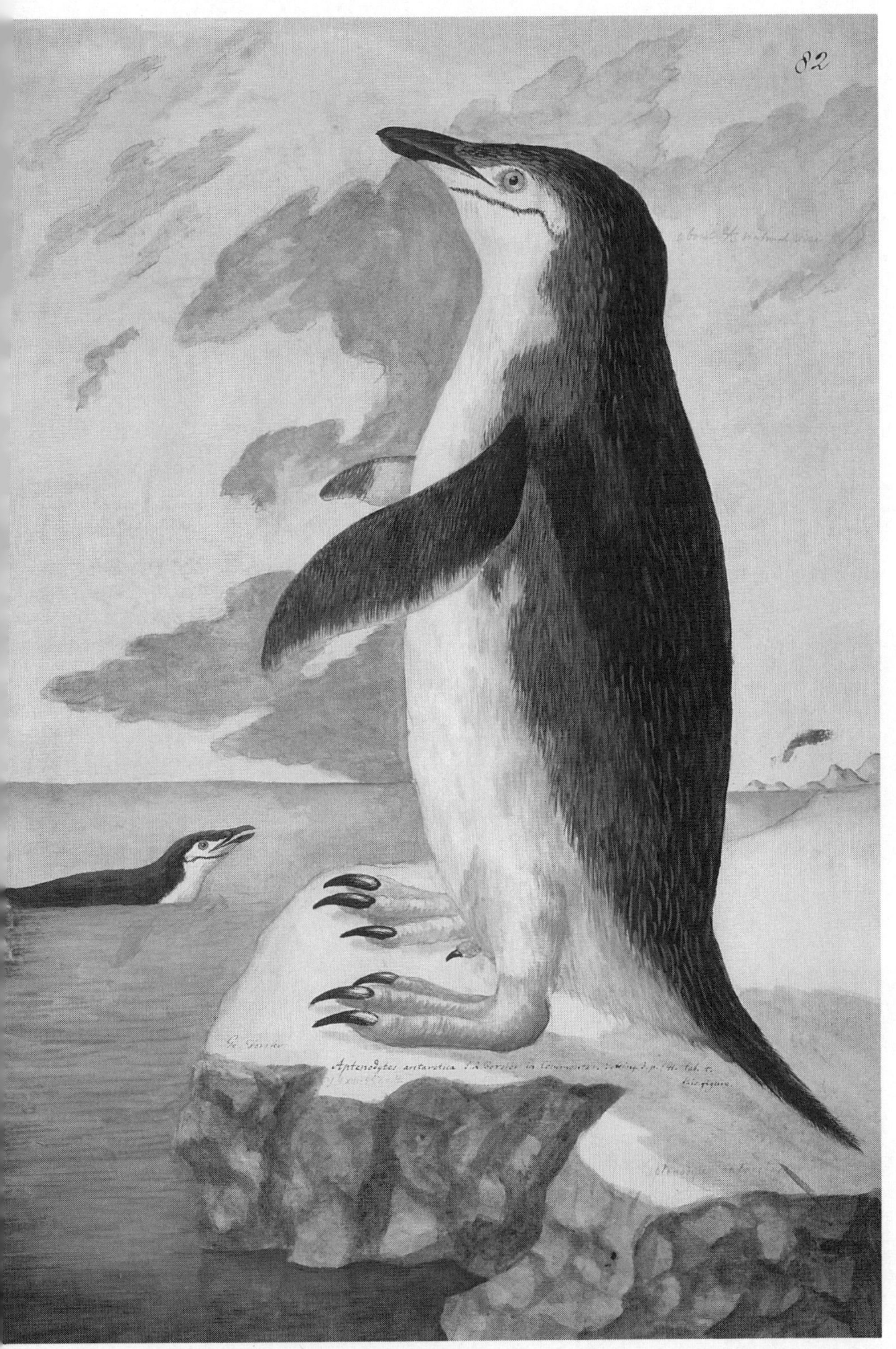

FIG. 75. Bearded Penguin on an ice floe

Pygoscelis antarctica (Forster). Drawing by George Forster in B.M. (N.H.)—'Birds', pl. 82

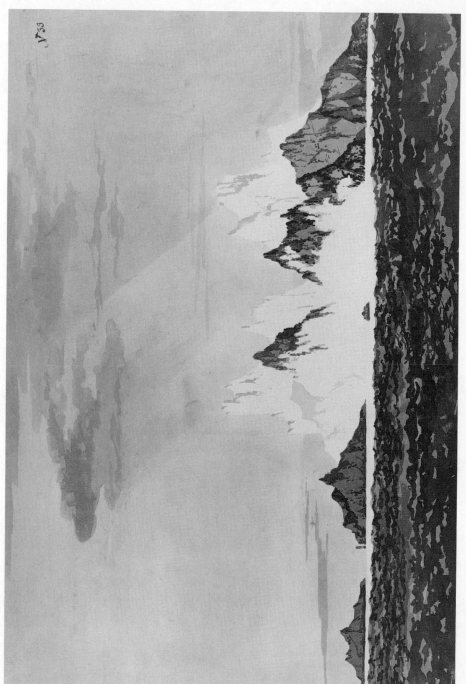

Fig. 76. View of South Georgia, [illegible] January [illegible]

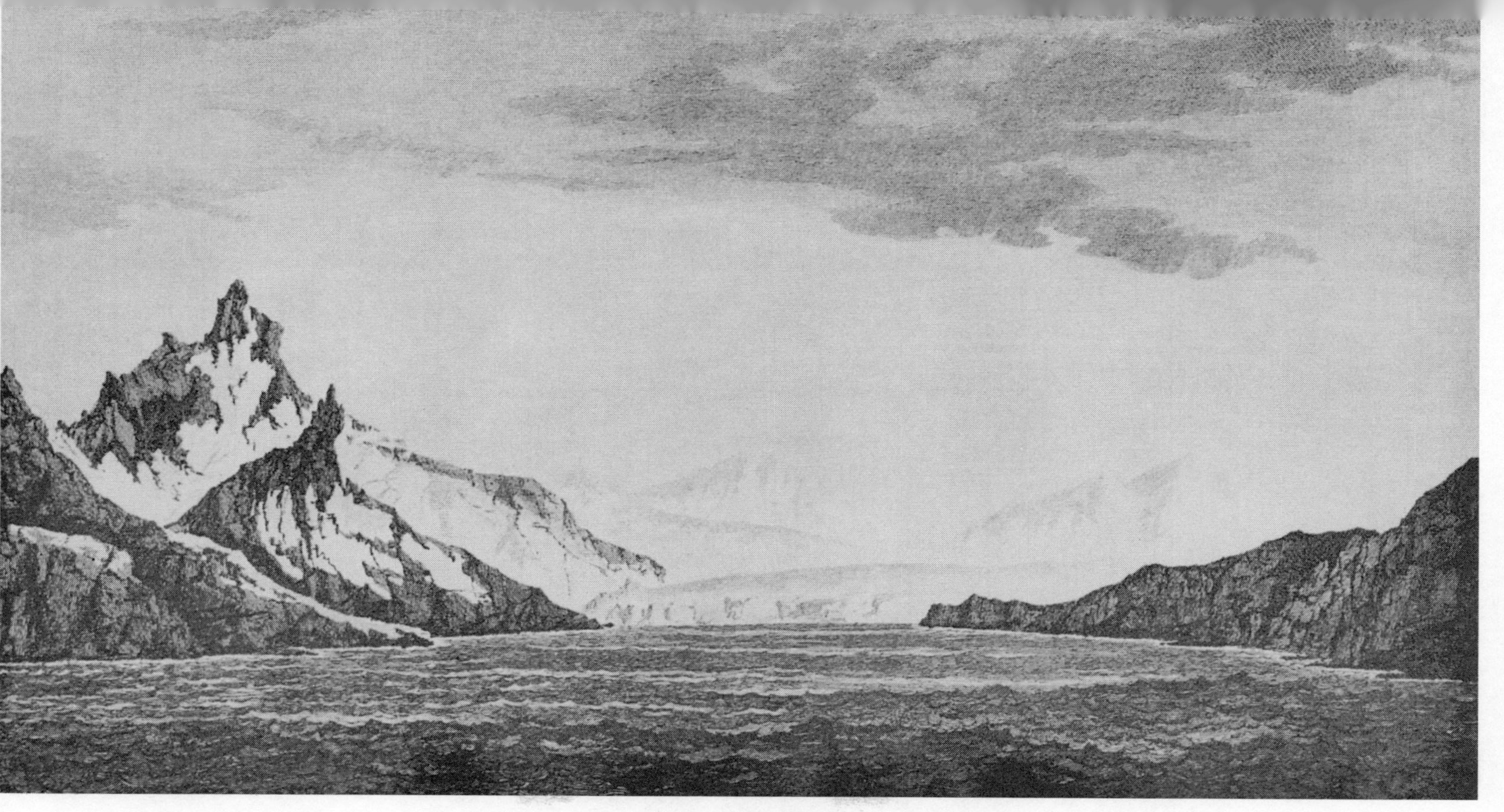

FIG. 77. View of Possession Bay, South Georgia

Engraved by S. Smith after Hodges

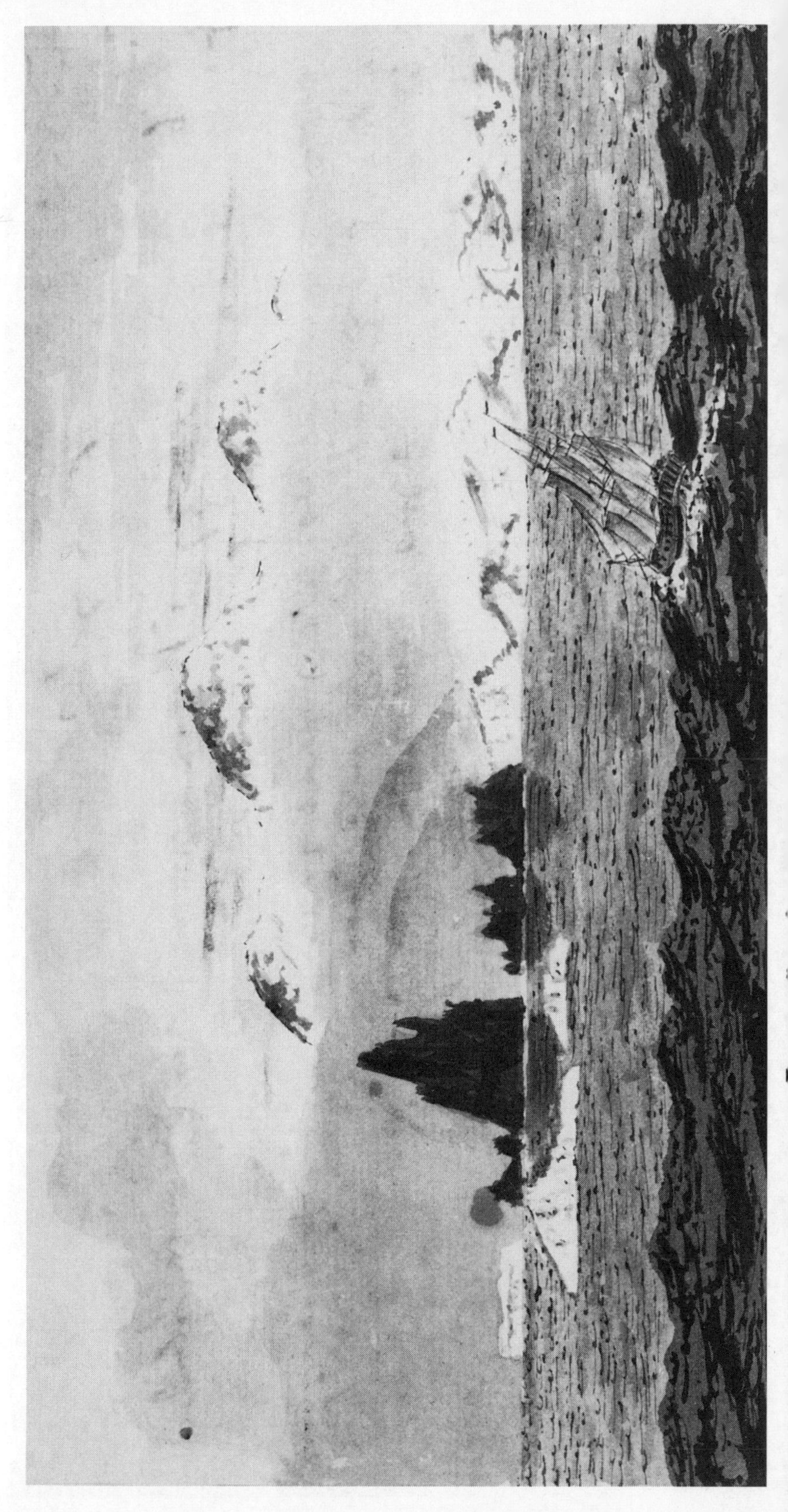

*SUNDAY 6*th*. Wind at NE Gloomy weather with rain. Our old friends having taken up their aboad near us, one of them whose name was Pedero, (a man of some note,) made me a present of a Staff of honour, or such as the cheifs generally carry; in return I dressed him in an old suit of cloathes with which he was not a little proud, he had a fine person and a good presence and nothing but his Colour distinguished him from a European. Having got him and a nother into a communicative mood, we began to enquire of them if the Adventure had been there during my absance and they gave us to understand in such a manner as admited of no doubt, that soon after we were gone, she arrived, that she stayed between ten and twenty days and had been gone ten Months. They likewise asserted that neither she or any other Ship had been stranded on the Coast as had been reported. This assertion and the manner they related to us the coming and going of the Adventure made me easy about her, but did not wholy set aside our doubts of some disaster having happened to some other strangers. Besides what has been already related, we have been told that a ship had lately been here and was gone to a place called Terato which is on the North side of the Strait. Whether this story relates to the former or no I can not say, when I have questioned the Natives about this matter they have always dinied all knowledge of it and of late have avoided mentioning it. It is but a few days ago that one man receiv'd a box on the ear for naming it to some of our people.

After breakfast I took a number of hands over to long island in order to catch the Sow, to put her to the boar and remove her to some other place, but we returned without seeing her; some of the Natives had been there not long before us, as their fires were yet burning; they undoubtedly had taken her a way. Pedero dined with us, eat of every thing at table and drank more Wine than any one of us without being in the least affected by it.[1]*—f. 298.

MONDAY 7*th*. A fresh gale at NE attended with rain which put a stop to Calking.

TUESDAY 8*th*. First part rain remainder fair weather which enabled us to go on with Calking, the Seams we are obliged to pay with a kind of putty made of Cooks fat and Chalk,[2] for as to Pitch and Tarr

[1] The previous four sentences are a very late addition to the text, in red ink, and run into the margins of ff. 298, 300v. They include a footnote, here omitted, on the report of a ship that went to Terato.

[2] . . . the gunner happening to have a quantity of the latter on board.—f. 294v. Cook ordered John Ramsay to supply the boatswain with 400 lb of fat 'for the necessary uses' of the ship as early as 1 September.—p. 951 below. Chalk must have had many uses on board (for making marks, whitening, lubricating, etc.); why it was among the gunner's stores is not clear.

we have had none for some Monthes Past and a Cask of Varnish of Pine which served as a substitute for all purposses is now expended. Put two Piggs, a Boar and a sow a Shore in the Cove next without Cannibal Cove, its hardly possible for all the methods I have taken to stock this Country with these animals to fail.[1]

WEDNESDAY *9th.* Winds Westerly or NW, Squally with rain, got every thing off from the Shore, unmoor'd and hove short on the best bower, waiting for the Calkers to finish their work. Our friends the Natives brought us a seasonable and large supply of fish. I made my friend [Pedero] a present of an Oyle Jarr which made him as happy as a prince.

*Our friends brought us a large and very Seasonable supply of fish; I made my friend Pedero a present of an empty Oyle Jarr which made him as happy as a prince; soon after he and his party left the Cove and retired to their proper place of a boad with all the treasure they had got from us. I beleive they must give away many of the things they have at different times got from us, to their friends and Neighbours, or else purchass Peace with them of their more powerfull Enemies; for we never see any of them after they are once in their posession and every time we have visited them, they have been as much in want of Hatchets, Nails &c[a] to all appearence as if they never had had any amongst them. I am satisfied that the people in this Sound, which are upon the whole pretty numerous, are under no regular form of Goverment, or so united as to form one body politick; the head of each Tribe or family seems to be respected and that respect may on some occasions command obedience, but I doubt if they either have a right or power to inforce it. The other day when we were with Tringo-boohee, the people came from all parts to see us, which he endeavoured to prevent, he even went so far as to throw stones at some, but I observed that very few paid any regard to either his words or actions, and yet this man was spoke of as a Chief of some note. I have before made some remarks on the evils attending these people for want of a Union among themselves and the more I am acquented with them the more I find it to be so. Notwithstanding they are *Cannibals*, they are naturaly of a good disposission and have not a little share of humanity.*—ff. 298v–300.

THURSDAY *10th.* Fresh gales at NW and fair weather. PM hove up the anchor and drop'd out of the Cove and then anchored in a clear

[1] . . . We also [have] reason to believe the [*sic*] some of the Cocks and Hens which I left here still exist although we have not seen any of them, as a Hens Egg was some days ago found in the woods, almost new laid.—f. 298v, *red ink in margin.*

place for the more readier geting under-sail in the morning. After this a party of us spent the afternoon a shore, we land where were two families of the Natives, variously employed, some sleeping, others makeing Matts, dressing Victuals &c^{a}.[1] One little girl I observed was heating stones at a fire, curious to know what they were for I remained by her, for I thought they were to dress some sort of Victuals but I was misstaken for as soon as the stones were made hot, the girl took them hout of the fire and gave them to an hold Women who was siting in the hut, she put them in [a] heap and then laid over them a large handfull of green Sellery, over it a coarse Mat and then squated herself down upon her heels over all, thus she made what one may call a Dutch Warming-Pan on which she sit as close as a hare to her seat.

I should hardly have mentioned this circumstance if I had thought it had been done with no other view than to warm the old Womans back-side, I rather think it was done with a view of curing some disorder she might have upon her, which the Steams ariseing from the green Celery might be specifick, I was lead to think so by there being hardly any Celery in the place (we having gathered it long before) and grass of which here was plenty would have kept the stones from bur[n]ing the Mat just as well, if that was all it was intended for, besides the woman looked to me to be sickly and not in a good state [of] health.—f. 300.

At Daylight AM weighed and stood out of the Sound with a gentle breeze at WNW. At 8 hauled round the two brothers and steered for Cape Campbel which is at the SE entrance of the Strait.[2]

Mr Wales having from time to time communicated to me the observations he had made in this Sound, for determining the Longitude, the mean results of which gives 174°25′07½″ East for the bottom of Ship Cove where the observations were made the Latitude of which is 41°5′56½″ South. In my Chart constructed in my former Voyage this place is laid down in 184°54′30″ W equal to 175°5′30″ East, the error of the Chart is therefore 0°40′ and nearly equal to what was found at Duskey Bay; by which it appears that the whole of *Tavaipoenammoo*, is laid down 40′ too far East in the said Chart, as well as in the Journal of the Voyage; but the error in *Eahei-no-mauwe* is not more than half a degree or 30′ because the distance between Queen Charlottes Sound and Cape Palliser has been found to be greater by

[1] *dressing Victuals &c^{a}:* roasting fish and fir[n]-roots . . .f. 300.

[2] Add. MS 27886 ends at this point. B *adds* at 4 in the after-noon passed Cape Campbel at the distance of 4 or 5 leagues and then steered SSE½E, with the Wind at NW a gentle gale and Cloudy weather.—f. 300.

10′ of Longitude than it is laid down in the Chart. I mention these errors not from a supposition that they will much effect either Navigation or Geography, but because I have no doubt of their existance, for from the multitude of observations which Mr Wales took the situation of few parts of the world are better assertained than that of Queen Charlottes Sound. Indeed I might with equal truth say the same of all the other places where we have made any stay at. For Mr Wales, whose abilities is equal to his assiduity, lost no one observation that could possibly be obtained.[1] Even the situation of such Islands as we past without touching at are by means of Mr Kendalls Watch determined with almost equal accuracy. The Error of the Watch from Otaheite to this place was only 43′39¼″ in Longitude, reckoning at the rate it was found to go at at that Island and at *Tanna*. But by reckoning at the rate it was going when last at this place and from the time of our leaving it to our return to it again which was near a year the error was 19′31″,25 in time, or 4°52′48¾″ in Longitude. This error can not be thought great if we consider the length of time and that we had gone over a space equal to upwards of three quarters of the Equatorial Circumference of the Earth and through all the Climates and Latitudes from 9° to 71°. Mr Wales found its true rate of going here to be that of gaining 12″,576 on mean time per day. The Mean Result of all the observations which he made for assertaining the Variation of the Compass and the dip of the south end of the Needle the three several times we have been here gave 14°09⅕′ East for the former and 64°36⅜′ for the latter.

FRIDAY 11*th*. In the morning the wind veered round by the west to South and forced us more to the East than I intended. At 7 o'Clock in the evening the Snowey Mountains bore WBS and Cape Palliser North ½ west dist^t^ 16 or 17 leagues. From this Cape I shall, for the third time, take my departure. After a few hours calm a breeze sprung up at North with which we steered SBE all sails Set, with a view of geting into the Latitude of 54° or 55°. My intention was to

[1] The preceding two sentences are a red ink revision of the following, which almost conveys the impression that Cook thought Wales was going a little too far in accuracy; but that as he had done so, his efforts must be mentioned. 'As Mr Wales had made so many observations in the Sound for determining the Longitude, I thought it was proper to say what the results were, otherwise I should hardly have mentioned these errors; from a supposition that few will think them of such consequence as either to effect Navigation or Geography. In justice to Mr Wales I must say that he was quite indefatigable and lost no one observation that could possibly be obtained.'—f. 300v. Perhaps the wording in the text represents the final resolution of Cook's little mortification over the correction of the first voyage figures for Queen Charlotte Sound and the charting of New Zealand: cf. p. 174, n. 2 above.

cross this vast Ocean nearly in these Parallels, and so as to pass over those parts which were left unexplored last summer.[1]

SATURDAY 12*th*. In the morning the wind increased to a fine gale. At Noon observed in Latitude 43°13′30″, Longitude in 176°41′ E. An extraordinary fish of the Whale kind was seen, some called it a Sea Monster.[2] I did not see it myself. In the after-noon our old companions the Pintado Peterels began to make their appearences.

SUNDAY 13*th*. In Morning the wind veered to WSW. At 7 saw the appearence of land to the SW, hauled up towards it and soon found it to be a Fog bank, after wards steered SEBS and soon after saw a Seal. At noon Latitude in by account 44°25′, Longitude 177°31′ E. Foggy weather which continued all the afternoon. At 6 in the evening the wind veered to NEBN, increased to a fresh gale attended with thick hazey weather. Course steered SE½S.

MONDAY 14*th*. AM saw a nother Seal. At noon Latitude in 45°54′, Longitude 179°29′ E.[3]

TUESDAY 15*th*. In the AM the wind veered to the westward, the Fogg cleared away but the weather continued Cloudy. At Noon Latitude 47°30′, Longitude 178°19′ West, for having passed the Meridion of 180° East I reckon my Longitude West of the first Meridian viz Greenwich. In the evening heard Penguins and the next morning

WEDNESDAY 16*th*. Saw some pieces of Sea or Rock weed. At Noon a fresh gale from the West and fine Weather. Latitude Observed 49°33′. Longitude in 175°31′ West.

THURSDAY 17*th*. Morning fresh gales and hazy weather. Saw a Seal and several pieces of weed. At noon Latitude in 51°12′, Longitude

[1] 'Carpenters Employed repairing the Chain Pumps, spoiled for want of use, no signs of a leaky Ship.'—Log. Cook has now gone over to civil time; this entry is for 11 November a.m.

[2] 'We saw a whale on the 12th, about twelve yards long, with an oblong blunt head, on which were two longitudinal furrows, and as many upright ridges. It had small eyes, two semilunar apertures, from whence it occasionally spouted the water, and was mottled all over with white spots. It had two large fins behind the head, but none on the back. This extraordinary creature seems to have been intirely unknown before.'—Forster, II, p. 482. This description, if taken literally, cancels itself out as a verisimilitudinous description of a whale. The large fins 'behind' the head must have been also below it; and the 'semilunar apertures' were probably the features enclosing the blow hole. Dr R. A. Falla writes, 'There is certainly something queer about the whale, an abnormal specimen, probably a sperm whale. White blotches occur on these otherwise black mammals when they have been gripped by the suckers of large squids. Perhaps in this case the head had been disfigured by squid attacks and the grooves might well have been caused by a wound healing'. If this conjecture fails, the 'Monster' must be let go unidentified.

[3] 'PM this Afternoon the Carpenter came aft and reported that the Ship made a considerable quantity of Water forward. Upon examining we found the defect above ye water line considerably and that she only leak'd when plunging—we suppos'd it nothing more than the Caulking having rotted and wash'd out, but must wait fair Wea^{r} to examine more distinctly into it.'—Clerke 8953, 15 November.

173°17′ West. The Wind veered to the North and NEBN, blew a strong gale by squals which expended an old Main Topg^t sail and obliged us to double reef the Top-sails, but in the evening the wind moderated and veered to WNW and we loosed a reef out of each Top-sail.[1] Found the Var^n of the Compass to be 9°52′ E being then in the Latitude 51′47″, Longitude 172°21′ W and the next morning

FRIDAY 18*th* in the Latitude of 52°25′, Longitude 170°45′ East[2] it was 10°26′ E. Towards Noon had moderate and Cloudy weather and a great swell from the West. Some Penguins and pieces of Sea weed seen.

SATURDAY 19*th*. Steered ESE with a very fresh gale at North, hazy dirty Weather. At Noon Latitude in 53°43′, Longitude 166°15′ W.

SUNDAY 20*th*. Steered EBS with a moderate breeze at North attended with thick hazy weather. At Noon Latitude 54°8′, Longitude 162°18′ W.

MONDAY 21*st*. Winds mostly from the NE a fresh gale attend with thick hazy dirty weather. Course SEBS. Latitude at Noon 55°31′, Long 160°29′. Abundance of Blue Peterels and some Penguins seen.

TUESDAY 22*nd*. Fresh gales at NWBN and NBW and hazy till towards Noon when the weather cleared up and we observed in Lat 55°48′. Long in 156°56′ W. In the after-noon had a few hours Calm after which the wind came at SSE and SEBS a light breeze with which steered East northerly. In the night the Aurora Australis visible, but very faint and noways remarkable.

WEDNESDAY 23*rd*. In the Latitude of 55°46′, Longitude 156°13′ W the Variation was 9°42′ East. We had a Calm from 10 o'Clock in the Morning till Six in the evening when a breeze sprung up at West, at first it blew a gentle gale but afterwards freshned.[3] Our Course was now E½N.

THURSDAY 24*th*. A fresh breeze at NWBW and NBW,[4] Noon Latitude in 55°38′, Longitude 153°37′ West. Foggy in the night, but on

[1] '. . . in takeing in the small sails the fore topg^t sail (being much worn) split to pieces and the most of it blew overboard. At 6 out reefs and set main Topg^t sail and bent another fore Topg^t sail. A heavy swell from the Northward.'—Log.

[2] 'East' is a slip for 'West'.

[3] '. . . a very heavy swell going, and the weather being perfectly calm, it rowls us about most confoundedly.'—Clerke. For this date (his 24th) Clerke records seeing piebald porpoises, penguins, albatrosses, black shearwaters, and small blue petrels.

[4] 'Hauled up the Small Bower Cable to get plank to repair the gunners Store room doors.'—Log.

FRIDAY 25*th.* Had a fine gale at NW attended with clear pleasent weather. Course steer'd EBN.[1] In the evening being in the Latitude of 55°8′, Longitude 148°10′ W the Variation by the Mean of two Compasses was 6°35½′ E.

SATURDAY 26*th* and SUNDAY 27*th.* Had a steady fresh gale at NNW with which Steered East and at Noon on the latter we were in the Latitude of 55°6′, Longitude 138°56′ west.[2] I now gave up all hopes of finding any more land in this Ocean and came to a Resolution to steer directly for the West entrance of the Straits of Magelhanes, with a View of coasting the out, or South side of Terra del Fuego round Cape Horn to Strait La Maire. As the world has but a very imperfect knowlidge of this Coast, I thought the Coasting it would be of more advantage to both Navigation and Geography than any thing I could expect to find in a higher latitude. In the after-noon of this day the Wind blew in squalls and occasioned the Main Topg^{t} mast to be carried away.

MONDAY 28*th.* A very strong gale Northerly, hazy rainy weather which obliged us to double reef the Fore and Main Top-sails, hand the Mizen Top-sail and get down the Fore Top-g^{t} yard. In the morn^{g} the bolt rope of the Main Top-sail broke and occasioned the Sail to be split.[3] I have observed that the ropes to all our sails, the Square Sails especially, are not of a Size and strength sufficient to wear out the canvas. At Noon Latitude in 55°20′, Longitude 134°16′ west. A great swell from NW. Albatrosses and Blue Peterels seen.

TUESDAY 29*th.* Towards noon the Wind abated and we loosed all the reefs out of the Top-sails, rigged a nother Topg^{t} mast and got the Yards a cross. AM little wind and hazy weather. At midnight calm which continued till noon the next day, when a breeze sprung up at East, with which we stretched to the northward. At this time we were in the Latitude 55°32′, Longitude 128°45′ West. Some Albatrosses and Peterels seen. At 8 PM the Wind veered to NE, & we Tacked and stood to ESE.

[1] 'Sailmakers repairing Sails to which use converted some of the Boat sails having no new Canvas sutable.'—Log.

[2] 'We've had a fine steady Gale and following Sea these 24 Hours, and run the greatest distance we've ever reach'd in this ship.'—Clerke. The distance run was 183 miles. From 25 to 29 November the ship did nobly, her daily distances in miles being 140, 168, 183, 160, 152.

[3] '. . . split the Sail to pieces and the most of it b[l]ew away'.—Log.—'[8 a.m.] Carried away the Tiller rope . . .'—Log.

[DECEMBER 1774]

THURSDAY December 1*st*. Thick hazy foggy weather with drizling rain and a moderate breeze of Wind which at 3 o'Clock in the after noon fell to a Calm, at this time we were in the Latitude of 55°41′, Longitude 127°5′ W. After four hours Calm the Fog cleared away and we got a Wind at SE with which stood NE.

FRIDAY 2*nd*. Fresh breeze at SE and hazy fogy weather except a few hours in the morning when we found the Variation to be 1°28′ East. Latitude 55°17′, Longitude 125°41′ W. The Variation after this was supposed to increase for on

SUNDAY 4*th* in the morning, being in Latitude 53°21′, Longit. 121°31′ W it was 3°16′ East and in the evening in Latitude 53°13′, Longit. 119°46′ West it was 3°28′ East.

MONDAY 5*th* at 6 o'Clock in the Evening in Latitude 53°8′, Longitude 115°58′ West it was 4°1′ East. For more than 24 hours past we have had a fine gale at South which enabled us to steer East with very little deviation to the North and now it veered to SW and blew a steady fresh gale and we continued to steer East, inclining a little to the South.

TUESDAY 6*th* had some Snow Showers. In the evening being in the Latitude 53°13′, Longitude 111°12′ the Variation was 4°58′ E and the next morning

WEDNESDAY 7*th*. Being in the Latitude 53°16′, Longitude 109°33′ it was 5°01′ East. The Wind was now at West a fine pleasent gale with now and then showers of rain. Nothing remarkable till

FRIDAY 9*th* at Noon when being in the Latitude of 53°37′, Longitude 103°44′ W the Wind veered to NE and after wards came insencibly round to the South, by the East and SE attended with cloudy hazy weather and some showers of rain.

SATURDAY 10*th* At Noon Latitude in 54°00′, Longitude 102°7′ West, a little before pass'd a small bed of Sea weed. In the after-noon the wind veered to SW blew a fresh gale attended with dark cloudy weather. We steered East half a point North and the next day

SUNDAY 11*th* at Six in the evening, being in the Latitude of 53°35′, Longitude 95°52′ W the Variation was 9°58′ E. Many and various sorts of Albatross about the Ship.

MONDAY 12*th*. The Wind veered to the West, NW and in the evening to North and at last left us to a Calm which continued till Midd-night when we got a breeze at South, which soon after veered to and fixed at West, with which steered East and on

WEDNESDAY 14*th*. In the morning found the Variation to be 13°25′ East, Latitude 53°25′, Longitude 87°53′ West, and in the Afternoon,[1] being in the same Latitude and the Longitude of 86°2′ W it was 15°3′ East and increased in such a manner that on

THURSDAY 15*th* in the Latitude of 53°30′, Longitude 82°23′ West it was 17°00′ East and the next evening

FRIDAY 16*th*. In the Latitude of 53°25′, Longitude 78°40′ it was 17°38′ East. About this time saw a Penguin and a piece of weed and the next morn a Seal and some diving Peterels.[2] For the three pre-ceeding days the wind has been at west a steady fresh gale, attended now and then with showers of rain or hail.

SATURDAY 17*th*. At 6 o'Clock in the Morning, being nearly in the same latitude as above and in the Longitude of 77°10′ W the Varia-tion was 18°33′ E, and in the after-noon it was 21°38′, Latitude in at that time 53°16′ S, Longitude 75°9′ West. In the Morning as well as in the after-noon I took some observations to determine the Longi-tude by the Watch, the results reduced to noon gave 76°18′30″ West Longitude: at the same time the Longitude by my reckoning was 76°17′ W, but I have reason to think that we were about half a degree more to the West than either the one or the other:[3] our Latitude at the same time was 53°21′ S. We steered EBN and E½N all this day under all the sail we could carry with a fine fresh gale at NWBW in expectation of seeing the land before night but not making it before 10 o'Clock we took in the Studding sails, Topg[t] Sails, and a reef in each Top-sail and steered ENE in order to make sure of falling in with Cape Deseado.[4] Two hours after made the land, extending from NEBN to EBS about 6 Leagues dist[t]. Upon this discovery we wore and brought to with the ships head to the South and then sounded and

[1] 'Albatrosses and blue Petrels daily seen.'—Log.

[2] Possibly the Magellanic Diving Petrel, *Pelecanoides magellani* Mathews.

[3] The MS has here a deleted footnote: 'but this so inconsiderable, in this Lat. as not to be worth correction'. Cook may have deleted it because he concluded that error was always worth correction. G also has it. A has a slightly different form of words for text and note.

[4] Cape Deseado is the north-west extreme of Desolation Island, behind which is the Pacific entrance to the Strait of Magellan. It is a low cape, surrounded with rocks; see Chart XL. Magellan's Cabo Deseado, the northern point of the island, is now called Cape Pillar.

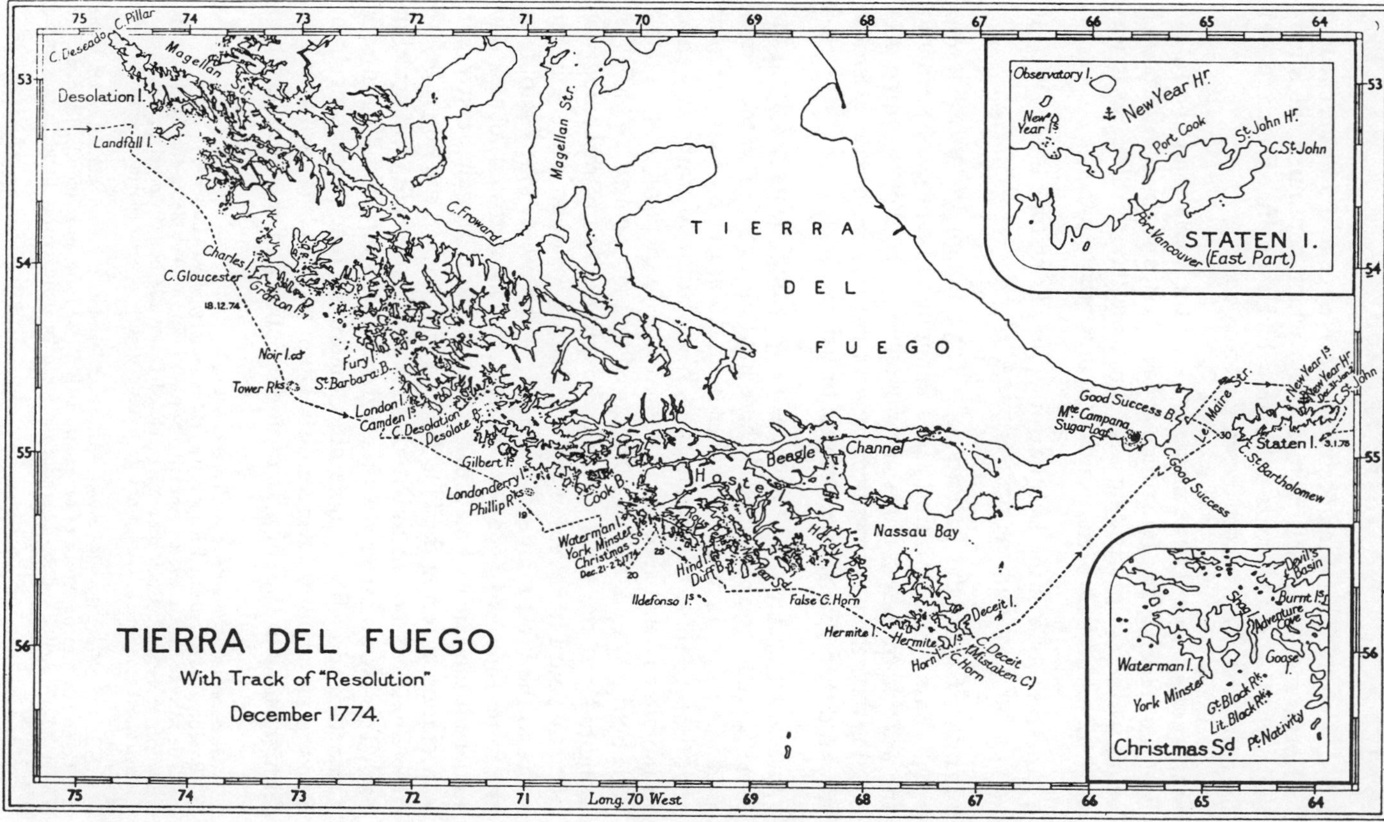
TIERRA DEL FUEGO
With Track of "Resolution"
December 1774.
TIERRA
DEL
FUEGO
STATEN I.
(East Part)
Observatory I.
New Year Is.
New Year Hr.
Port Cook
St. John Hr.
C. St. John
Port Vancouver
Christmas Sd.
Waterman I.
York Minster
Gt. Black Rk.
Lit. Black Rks.
Pt. Nativity
Devil's Basin
Burnt Is.
Adventure Cove
Goose I.
Shag I.
C. Deseado
C. Pillar
Magellan Str.
Desolation I.
Landfall I.
C. Froward
Magellan Str.
Charles I.
C. Gloucester
Grafton Is.
18.12.74
Noir I.
Fury I.
St. Barbara B.
Tower Rks.
London I.
Camden Is.
C. Desolation
Desolate B.
Gilbert Is.
Londonderry I.
Phillip Rks.
Cook B.
Waterman I.
York Minster
Christmas S.
Dec. 21-27.1774
Ildefonso Is.
Hind I.
Duff B.
Hoste
Hardy
Beagle
Channel
Nassau Bay
False C. Horn
Hermite I.
Hermite Is.
Horn I.
C. Horn
C. Deceit
(Mistaken C)
Deceit I.
Good Success B.
Mte. Campana
Sugarloaf
C. Good Success
Le Maire Str.
Staten I.
3.1.75
C. St. Bartholomew
New Year Is.
New Year Hr.
C. St. John
Long. 70 West
75
74
73
72
71
70
69
68
67
66
65
64
53
54
55
56

Fig. 79

found 75 fathoms water, the bottom stones and shells. The land now before us can be no other than the west Coast of Terra del Fuego and near the West entrance to the Straits of Magelhanes. As this was the first run that had been made directly a Cross this ocean in a high Sothern Latitude[1] I have been a little particular in noteing every circumstance that appeared attall Intresting and after all I must observe that I never was makeing a passage any where of such length, or even much shorter, where so few intresting circumstance[s] occrued, for if I except the Variation of the Compass I know of nothing else worth notice. The weather has neither been unusually Stormy nor cold, before we arrived in the Latitude of 50° the Mercury in the Thermometer fell gradually from 60 to 50 and after we arrived in the Latitude of 55° it was generally between 47 and 45, once or twice it fell to 43°; these observations were made at Noon. I have now done with the SOUTHERN PACIFIC OCEAN, and flatter my self that no one will think[2] that I have left it unexplor'd, or that more could have been done in one voyage towards obtaining that end than has been done in this.

Soon after we left New Zealand, Mr Wales contrived and fixed up an Instrument which very accurately measured the Angle the Ship rolled when sailing large & in a great sea and lay down when sailing upon a wind. The greatest Angle he observed her to Roll was 38°, this was on the 6th Inst. when the Sea was not unusually high, so that it cannot be reckoned the greatest Roll she had made. The most he observed her to heel or lay down when sailing upon a wind was 18°, this was under Double reef'd Topsails & Courses.[3]

SUNDAY 18*th*. At 3 o'Clock in the morning we sounded again and found 110 fath the same bottom as before. We now made sail with a fresh gale at NW and steered SEBE along the coast which extended from *Cape Deseado* which bore N 7° E to ESE. A pretty high ragged

[1] AG and at first B have here a footnote by Cook: 'It is not to be suppos'd that I can know what the Adventure may have done'. In B this is altered to 'It is not to be supposed that I could know at that time that the Adventure had made the Passage before me'.

[2] *and flatter . . . think:* A I hope those who honoured me with this employ will not think . . .—The passage originally ran thus in B, in which Cook, making the alteration, failed to delete the words 'I hope those who honoured me'; for simplicity I delete them now, as does *Voyage*, II, p. 170. H reads, 'I have now done with the South Pacific Ocean, will any one say that I have left it unexplored', etc.

[3] The foregoing paragraph is added to the MS as a separate slip of paper, f. 304. Wales describes his apparatus in his log, 13 November 1774. 'It having been frequently disputed what the greatest Angle is that a Ship lies down to when going on a wind, & that she will roll to in a high sea & calm weather, to try that on board the Resolution I fixed up, while at New Zealand, a graduated Arch of a Circle to one of the Cross Beams of the Ship that passed through my Cabbin'; pivoting upon this was a long slender rod weighted at the bottom, the upper end being an index to point out the degrees of movement. Wales notes many observations after this date.

isle, which lies near a league from the Main and S 18° E Six leagues from Cape Deseado, bore N 49° E distant 4 Leagues, it obtained the name of *Land-fall.*[1] At 4 o'Clock we were North and South of the high land of Cape Deseado[2] distant about 9 Leagues, so that we saw none of the low rocks said to lie off it. The Latitude of this Cape is about 53°00′ S[3] Longitude 74°40′ West. Continued to range the Coast at about two leagues distance and at a 11 o'Clock past a projecting point which I called *Cape Gloucester*; it shows a round surface of considerable height and has much the appearence of being an Island,[4] it lies SSE½E distant 17 leag[s] from the Isle of Landfall. The Coast between them forms two bays, strewed with rocky Islots, Rocks and Breakers. The Coast appeared very broken, with many inlets, or rather it seemed to be composed of a number of Islands,[5] the Land is very mountainous, rocky and barren, spoted here and there with tufts of wood and patches of snow. At Noon C. Gloucester bore North distant 8 miles and the most advanced point of land to the SE which we judged[6] to be *Cape Noir*, bore SEBS distant 7 or 8 leagues. Latitude Ob[d] 54°13′ S, Longitude made from Cape Deseado 54′ East. From C. Gloucester, off which lies a small rocky Island, the direction of the Coast is nearly SE but to Cape Noir, for which we steered, the Course is SSE distant about 10 Leagues. At 3 o'Clock we past Cape Noir which is a steep rock of considerable hieght, and the SW point of a large Island which seemed to lie detatched a league or a league and a half from the main.[7] The land of the Cape, when at a distance from it, appear'd to be an island disjoined from the other, but upon a nearer approach found it to be connected by a low neck of land. At the point of the Cape are two rocks, the one is peaked

[1] There are two islands of unequal size; lat. 53°19′ S, long. 74°11′ W. The name persists.

[2] The high land *behind* Cape Deseado, no doubt. Cape Pillar, the northernmost point of Desolation Island, reaches a height of 2779 feet.

[3] D *note* In the Chart of the Straits of Magelhanes, bound up with the English Voyages, the Latitude of this Cape is said to be 52°52′S, and I make no doubt but this is its true Latitude, but the Longitude is erronious. . . —The 'English Voyages' is Hawkesworth, and the chart, 'in which are Inserted the Observations and Discoveries of Capt[n] Byron, Capt[n] Wallis and Captain Carteret', is in vol. I. The longitude there noted is 76°45′W. The true position is now given as 52°44′S, 74°45′W.

[4] Cape Gloucester is the western extremity of Charles island, the largest of the Grafton islands.

[5] Tierra del Fuego hereabouts, says the *South America Pilot*, 'consists of islands, islets and rocks almost innumerable'; an observation which holds for the whole of the, at times, dangerous shore off which Cook was now sailing. Fortunately for him this was merely an incidental part of his voyage, and did not call for close investigation. Indeed some of the coast has not been closely investigated even yet, and the Admiralty charts of south-western Tierra del Fuego still depend, in the main, on the *Beagle's* surveys in 1830–4.

[6] *we judged:* D proved

[7] The island is Noir Island. The cape is an unmistakable steeple shape. Cook's 'league or a league and a half' is an underestimate. The island is 15 miles WSW of Kempe island, part of 'the main'.

like a Sugar Loafe, the other is not so high and shews a rounder suffarce, and SBE two leagues from the Cape are two other rocky Islets.[1] This Cape is situated in the Latitude of 54°30′ S, Longitude 73°33′ West. After passing the two Islots[2] we steered ESE, crossing the great Bay of *St Barbara,* we could but just see the land in the bottom of it which could not be less than 7 or 8 leagues from us. There was a space which lies in the direction of ENE from Cape Noir, where no land was to be seen; this may be the Channell of St Barbara which opens into the Straits of Magelhanes, as mentioned by Frezier; we found the Cape to agree very well with his discription, which shews that he laid down this Channell from good memoires.[3] At 10 o'Clock, drawing near the SE point of the Bay, which lies nearly in the diriction of S 60° E from Cape Noir, 18[4] leagues distant, we shortned sail and spent the night standing on and off.

MONDAY 19*th*. At 2 o'Clock in the morning made sail and steered SEBE along the coast and soon passed the SE point of the bay of St Barbara which I called *Cape Desolation,*[5] because near it commenced the most desolate and barren Country I ever saw, it is situated in the Latitude of 54°55′ S, Longitude 72°12′ West. About 4 leagues to the East of this Cape is a deep Inlet, at the entrance of which lies a prety

[1] The Tower Rocks.

[2] *the two Islots*: D the rocks above mentioned

[3] *which shews... memoires:* D which, at least, shews that he had good authority for laying down this Channel, notwithstand[ing] subsequent Navigators have not found it.—Cf. Clerke 8953.—'This Cape Noir forms the N°thern part of the Western Mouth of the passage of St Barbe [a very liberal interpretation, considering the position of the island]; this passage was found by accident in a French Tartane call'd the St Barbara in May 1713. Monsieur Frezier gives a very clear account of this incident in the Course of his Voyage which was translated into English in 1717 and the Coast hereabouts agrees very well with the Chart he has there given of it.'—Frézier was a French engineer officer, who in 1712–14 made a survey of the Pacific side of South America for Louis XIV. His 'Voyage' in its English dress was *A Voyage to the South Sea, and along the Coasts of Chili and Peru*... (London 1717). The chart in this book to which Clerke refers was pl. XXXII, 'in which may be seen two new Discoveries. The one is a Passage into *Tierra del Fuego,* through which chance carry'd the Tartane S. *Barbara,* commanded by *Marcanil,* out of the Streights of *Magallon* into the *South-Sea,* on the 15th of May, 1713...'—p. 285. 'This Streight is perhaps the same as that of *Jelouchte* [=Jelouzel: see p. 590, n. 1 below], which Monsieur *de Lisle* has laid down in his last Map of *Chili*; but as the *English* Memoirs, which he has been pleas'd to shew me, seem to place it South of Cape *Frouvart* [i.e. Cape Froward, in Magellan Strait], it may be suppos'd that they are two different streights.'—p. 287. I do not know what these 'English memoirs' were. The 'great Bay of St Barbara' was the broad opening, 11½ miles wide, between Fury island and London island (one of the Camden group), which leads to two channels into Magellan Strait, the Barbara channel running north, and the Cockburn channel running east and then north.

[4] 18 is corrected from '15 or 17'.

[5] The rugged, many-peaked Cape Desolation is the southern point of Basket island, and is the northern entrance point to Bahia Desolada or Desolate Bay. One would hardly judge from Chart XL that it is the south-east point of 'the bay of St Barbara': there is intervening land marked, quite properly—the Camden islands. One can only assume that Cook took these to be islands actually in the bay. Even then the chart shows the cape as much more prominent, in the general run of the coast, than it really is.

large Island and some others of less note.[1] At 10 o'Clock, being about a league and a half from the land, we sounded and found 60 fathom water a bottom of small stones and shells. The wind which had been fresh at NBW began to abate and at Noon it fell Calm, at which time we observed in Latitude 55°20′ s, Longitude made from Cape Deseado 3°24′ East, in this situation we were about 3 leagues from the nearest shore which was that of an island which I named *Gilbert Isle* after my Master.[2] It is near of equal height with the rest of the Coast and shews a surface composed of several peaked rocks of unequal height. A little to the SE of it were some smaller Islands and without them breakers.[3] I have before observed that this is the most desolate coast I ever saw, it seems to be intirely composed of Rocky Mountains without the least appearence of Vegetation, these Mountains terminate in horroable precipices whose craggy summits spire up to a vast hieght, so that hardly any thing in nature can appear with a more barren and savage aspect than the whole of this coast. The inland mountains were covered with Snow but those on the Sea Coast were not; we judged the former to belong to the Main of Terra del Fuego and the latter to be islands so ranged as apparently to form a Coast. After 3 hours Calm we got a breeze at SEBE and after makeing a short trip to the South, stood in for the land, the most advanced point of which we had in sight bore East, distant 10 leagues; this is a lofty Promontory lying ESE 10 leag[s] from Gilbert isle and situated in Latitude 55°26′ s, Longitude 70°25′ west. From the situation we now saw it, it terminated in two high towers and within them a hill shaped like a Sugar Loafe. This Wild rock obtained the name of *York Minster*.[4] Two leagues to the westward of this Head, appeared a large

[1] The 'deep Inlet' must be the large tract of water that includes Desolate Bay, which runs northward for about twelve miles. By the 'prety large Island' Cook perhaps means Stewart island. At this point he has a note, 'Nearly in this situation some Charts place a Channel leading into the Straits of Magelhanes, under the name of Straits of Jelouzel'; which was a guess that might have been right, but was wrong. Desolate Bay does lead into the Beagle Channel, and so into the Atlantic in about 55°10′ s. Cook probably got the name 'Straits of Jelouzel' from Robert de Vaugondy's map of Magellan Strait in de Brosses, *Histoire des Navigations aux Terres Australes*, II, pl. III. 'Jelouzel' is a corruption of Jelouchet̩é, a name that must have been conferred by Beauchesne-Gouin's expedition of 1699–1701 to the coasts of Chile and Peru (see de Brosses, II, pp. 113–25; E. W. Dahlgren, *Voyages français à destination de la Mer du Sud avant Bougainville, 1695–1749*, Paris 1907). The first map to show the strait is that of G. Delisle, referred to by Frézier, p. 589, n. 3 above: 'Carte de Paraguay, du Chili, du Détroit de Magellan &c.', 1703—where we have the legend 'Détroit nomme Jelouchet̩é par ceux du pays'. Delisle cites Brouwer, Narborough, and Beauchesne as his authorities: the name is not in the first two, and he gives other Beauchesne names on the map.

[2] The name remains, but there are two islands, certainly not distinguishable as two from Cook's position.

[3] The outer islands of the Londonderry group, and the sea breaking on the Phillip Rocks, a few miles south-west of them.

[4] It is the southernmost high point of Waterman island. Its peaks succeeded in reminding Cook—a Yorkshireman, we must not forget—of that edifice. The next man to de-

Inlet,[1] the west point of which we fetched in with by 9 o'Clock when we Tacked in 41 fathom Water half a league from the Shore; to the westward of this inlet was a nother with several Islands lying in the entrance.[2]

TUESDAY *20th.* During the preceding night had little wind Easterly which in the morning Veered to NE and NNE but it was too faint to be of use and at 10 we had a Calm, when we observed the ship to drive from off the shore out to sea and we had made the same obser^{n} the day before; this must have been occasioned by a current, the melting of the Snow must increase the inland Waters and cause a stream to run out of most of these inlets. At Noon observed in Latitude 55°39′30″ S. York Minster bore N 15° E distant 5 Leagues and a round hill just peeping above the horizon, which we judged to belong to the Isles of St Ildefonso, bore E 25° S 10 or 11 leagues distant. At 1 o'Clock a breeze sprung up at EBS. I took the oppertunity to stand in for the land with a view to going into one of the many Ports which seemed open to receive us, in order to take a view of the Country and recrute our stock of Wood and Water. In standing in for an opening which appeared on the East side of York Minster we had 40, 37, 50 and 60 f^{ms} Water a bottom of small stones and shells; when we had the last Soundings we were nearly in the middle between the two points which forms the entrance to the Inlet, which we observed to branch in to two Arms, both of them lying in nearly north and disjoined by a high rocky point. We stood for the Eastern branch as being clear of islots, and after passing a black rocky islot, lying without the point just mentioned, we sounded and found no bottom with a line of 170 fathoms.[3] This was altogether unexpected and a circumstance that would not have been regarded if the breeze had continued, but at this time it fell Calm, so that it was not possible to extricate our selves from this disagreeable situation.[4] Two Boats were

scribe it was FitzRoy of the *Beagle*, who was in Christmas Sound in 1830. 'The promontory of York Minster is a black irregularly-shaped rocky cliff, eight hundred feet in height, rising almost perpendicularly from the sea. It is nearly the loftiest as well as the most projecting point of the land about Christmas Sound . . .'; and again, 'I fancied that the high part of the Minster must have crumbled away since he [Cook] saw it, as it no longer resembled "two towers", but had a ragged, notched summit, when seen from the westward.'—*Narrative of the Surveying Voyages of . . . Adventure and Beagle* (1839), I, pp. 407, 411.

[1] Cook Bay.

[2] This other inlet seems to have been the inward curve of the large Londonderry island, with the islets of the group lying before and within it.

[3] For this and the ensuing pages see Chart XL, inset of Christmas Sound, which Cook drew pretty accurately, and where all his names remain. FitzRoy remarked that Cook's 'sketch of the sound, and description of York Minster, are very good, and quite enough to guide a ship to the anchoring place'.—*Narrative*, I, p. 407. See also Fig. 79, inset.

[4] *This was . . . situation:* D this was a circumstance we did neither foresee nor expect, nor would it have been regarded, if the breeze had not now left us to a great swell which rolled in from Sea and broke in a dreadfull Surf on all the shores around us.

hoisted out and sent a head to tow, they would have availed but little if a breeze of wind had not, about 8 o'clock, sprung up at SW which put it in my power either to stand out to Sea, or up the inlet, prudence seemed to point out the former, but the desire of finding a good Port and learning something of the Country got the better of every other consideration and I resolved to stand in, but as night was approaching our safety depended on geting to an Anchor. With this view we continued to Sound but always in an unfathomable depth. Hauling up under the East side of the land which divided the two Arms and seeing a small Cove a head I sent a boat to Sound for anchorage and we kept as near the shore as the flurries from the land would admit in order to be able to get into this place if there was anchorage.[1] The Boat soon returned and informed us that there was 30 and 25 fathom Water a full Cables length from the shore, here we Anchored in 30 fathom (the bottom Sand and broken shells) and carried out a Kedge[2] and hawser to steady the Ship for the night.

WEDNESDAY 21*st*. Calm and pleasent Morning; after breakfast I set out[3] with two boats to look for a more secure anchoring place. We no sooner got round or above the point under which we were anchored than we found a Cove in which was Anchorage in 30, 20 and 15 f^ms^ the bottom stones and sand.[4] In the bottom of the Cove is a small stoney beach, a small Vally covered with wood and a small streamlet of fresh Water so that here was every thing we could expect to find in such a place, or rather more for we shot three geese out of four which we saw and caught some young ones which we after wards let go.[5] After discovering and sounding this Cove, I sent Lieut^t^ Clerke who commanded the other boat, on board with orders to remove the Ship into this place, while I proceeded farther up the Inlet. I presently found that the land we were under, which disjoined the two Arms as mentioned before, was an Island at the northern end of which the two Channels united.[6] After this I hasted on board and found every thing in readiness to wiegh, which was accordingly done

[1] *but as night . . . anchorage:* D but as our safety depended on geting to an Anchor before dark, I sent away a boat to sound for anchorage under the west shore and we kept as near to it with the Ship and [i.e. as] the flurries of wind from off it would permit in order to be ready to push into any Corner the boat might find. . . .

[2] *Kedge:* A D Kedge Anchor.

[3] *after breakfast . . . out:* D In the morning I sent the Master to search the Cove, in which we lay, for fresh Water, he soon returned without finding any. Besides the want of Water this place was not sheltered from the Sea winds, I therefore set out

[4] Adventure Cove, near the northern end of what proved to be an island; it is small, but was large enough for the *Resolution.*

[5] Probably the Kelp Goose, *Chloëphaga hybrida* (Molina), painted by George Forster, who wrote 'Terra del Fuego 1774' on the plate.

[6] Shag Island.

and all the Boats sent a head to tow the ship round the point, but at this moment a light breeze came in from Sea, too scant to fill our sails so that we were obliged to drop the Anchor again for fearing of falling upon the point and carry out a Kedge to windward: which being done, hove up the Anchor, warped up to and wieghed the Kedge and proceeded round the point under our staysails and there anchored with the best-bower in 20 fathom and moored with the other bower, which laid to the North in 13 fathom. Thus moored we were shut in from the Sea by the point above mentioned, which was in one with the East point of the Inlet; some islots off the next point above us, covered us from the NW from which quarter the wind had the greatest fetch; our distance from the shore was about one third of a mile. Thus situated we went to work to clear a place to fill Water, cut wood and set up a Tent for the reception of a guard, which was thought necessary as[1] we had already discovered that barren as this country is it was not without people, altho' we had as yet seen none.[2] Mr Wales also got his observatory and Instruments on shore, but it was with the greatest difficulty he could find a place of sufficient stability and clear of the Mountains which every were surrounded us, to set them up in, and at last was obliged to content himself with the top of a rock, not more than 9 feet over.[3]

THURSDAY *22nd.* Sent Lieutenants Clerke and Pickersgill, accompanied by some of the other officers, to examine and draw a sketch of the Channel on the other side of the island[4] and I went my self in a nother boat accompanied by the Botanists, to survey the Northern parts of the Sound. In my way I landed on the point of a low isle which was covered with herbage, part of which had been lately burnt, we likewise saw a hut, signs sufficient that people were in the neighbourhood. After I had taken the necessary bearings, we proceeded round the East end of Burnt Island and over to what we judged to be the Main of Terra del Fuego,[5] where we found a very fine harbour, incompassed by steep rocks of vast height down which ran many limpid streams of Water. At the foot of the rock are some tufts of trees fit for little else but fuel. This Harbour, which I shall distinguish by the [name of] *Devil's Bason*, is divided as it were into

[1] *which . . . as:* A this last was necessary as Mr Wales proposed to set up his Observatory and have his Instruments ashore and

[2] *altho' . . . none:* D as appeared by some fire places we had seen.

[3] This sentence is written on a separate slip, f. 309.

[4] *Sent Lieutenants . . . island:* D Early in the morning sent Lieutenant Pickersgill, who I frequently employed on these occasions, to Examine and draw a sketch of the Channell on the other side of the isle, he was accompanied by some of the other officers, whose business was to shoot what game they met with for this was become a necessary object to be attended to:

[5] It was in fact the 'main' of the large island called Hoste Island.

two, an inner and outer one, the communication between them is by a narrow channell of 5 fathoms deep. In the outer Bason I found 13 and 17 fathom water and in the inner 17 & 23 fathom. This last is the most secure place that can be, but nothing can be more gloomy than it is, the vast hieght of the Savage rocks which incompass it deprived a great part of it, even on this day, of the meridion Sun; the outer harbour is not quite free of this illconveniency, but far less so than the other and is rather more commodious and equally safe. It lies in the direction of North 1½ miles dist[t] from the East end of Burnt island, I likewise found a good anchoring place a little to the West of this harbour, before a stream of Water which comes out of a lake or large reservoir which is continually supplied by a Cascade falling into it. Leaving this place we proceeded a long the shore to the Westward and found other harbours which I had no time to look into. In all of them is fresh Water and wood for fuel, but except these little tufts of Shrubery, the whole Country was a barren Rock, doomed by Nature[1] to everlasting sterility. The low islands and even some of the higher which lie scatered up and down the Sound are indeed mostly covered with shrubs & Herbage; the Soil a black rotten Turf evidently composed by length of time of decayed Vegetables.[2] I had an oppertunity to verify what we had observed at Sea, viz. that the Sea Coast is composed of a number of large and small Islands and that the numerous inlets are formed by the junction of several channels, at least so it is here. On one of the low islands we found several huts which had lately been inhabited, near them was a good deal of celery[3] with which we loaded our boat and returned on board at 7 o'Clock in the evening. In this expedition we met with little game, one duck, three or four shags and about the same number of Rails or Sea Pies[4] was all we got. The other boat had been aboard some hours before; they had found two Harbours on the West side of the other Channel, the one large and the other small, but both safe and commodious, but by the sketch which M[r] Pickersgill had taken the access to them appeared rather intricate.[5] I was now told of a Melancholy circumstance

[1] A has here a footnote, 'Drawing N° 60 will prove this assertion'. But where, alas! is Drawing N° 60?

[2] *Vegetables:* A Plants &c[a].

[3] *Apium graveolens.* Cook used it on the first voyage, and Wales now says, 'nothing could be more awful to outward appearance than the Place we are now in; but when we came to land on it we found Plenty of good Wood; besides great quantities of the best wild Cellery I ever tasted, and I think but little inferior to the Garden Cellery in England'.—20 December.

[4] Quoy's Black Oyster Catcher, *Haematopus ater* Vieillot and Oudart.

[5] These harbours are on the east side of Waterman Island. The larger one is March Harbour, so named by FitzRoy, who anchored there on 1 March 1830 and stayed three weeks. Cook called the other Port Clerke. See below, 23 December.

which had happened to one of our Marines, he had not been seen sence 11 or 12 o'Clock the preceding night, it was supposed that he had fallen over board out of the head where he was last seen and was drownded.[1]

*FRIDAY 23*d*. Fine pleas[t] weather. Sent Lieu[t] Pickersgill in the Cutter to explore the East side of the Inlet, my self[2] went in the Pinnace to the West, with an intent to go round the isle we were at Anchor under, which I shall distinguish by the name of *Shag Island*—in order to view the Passage leading to the harbour M[r] Pickersgill discover'd yesterday, on which I made the following observations. In coming from Sea leave all the rocks and Islots lying off and within York Minster on your larboard side and the black rock which lies off the South end of Shag Island on your Starboard, and when abreast of the South end of that Island, haul over for y[e] W[t] shore, taking care to avoide the beds of weed you will see before you, as they allways grow on rocks, some of which I have founde 12 fathoms under water; but it is allways best to keep clear of them. The entrance to the large Harbour or *Port Clerke* lies just to the North of some low Rocks, lying off a point on Shag Island, the harbour lies in WBS a mile & a half and hath in it from 12 to 24 fathom Water, Wood and fresh Water. About a mile without this harbour is or seem'd to be another, which we did not examine, it is form'd by a large isle which covers it from the South and East winds; without this Isle, that is between it and York Minster, the Sea seem'd to be strew'd with islots, rocks and breakers. In the proceeding round the South end of Shag Island, we observ'd the Shags to breed in vast numbers in the Clifts of the Rocks, some of the old ones we shott, but we could not come at the Young ones, which are by far the best eating. On the East side of the isle we saw some Geese, with some difficulty we landed and got three which at this time was thought [a] valuable acquisition. About 7 o'clock in the evening we got aboard; M[r] Pickersgill who had got aboard just before, inform'd me that the land opposite to us was an Island, which he had been round: on another isle more to the north he found many[3] Terns eggs and that without the great isle, between it and the East head, he found a Cove in which were many geese, one only of which he got besides

[1] D . . . this was the more probable as when he was last seen he was going to the head and appeared to be a little in liquor. This was the same Marine who shot the man at Tanna. —'PM Found Will[m] Wedgeborough Marine missing who we imagine fell over board last night as he was seen very much in Liquor at 12 O'Clock & was drown'd'.—Cooper.

[2] D . . . accompaned by the two M[r] Forsters and M[r] Sparman

[3] *many:* D some hundreds of.

some young goslings. This information of Mr Pickersgills induced me on

SATURDAY 24*th* to make up two Shooting parties; Mr Pickersgill and his assoceates went in the Cutter and my self and the botanists in the Pinnace. Mr Pickersgill went to the NE side of the large Island opposite us, which obtain'd the name of *Goose Island*; and I went by the SW side. As soon as we got under the Isle, we found plenty of Shags in the Clifts, but without waiting to spend our time and shott in shooting, we proceeded on, and presently found sport enough; for on the South side of the isle were abundance of[1] Geese; it happen'd to be the Moulting season and the most of them were ashore for this purpose and could not fly. There being a great surf on the Shore, we found great difficulty in landing and very bad climing over the rocks when [we] were landed, so that hundreds escaped us, some into the Sea and others into the isle; we however, by one method and another, got Sixty two with which we return'd aboard in the evening, all heartily tired; but the acquisition of so many geese over ballanced every other consideration, and we sit down with a good appetite to supper on part of what the preceeding days had produced. Mr Pickersgill and his associates got aboard some time before us with 14 Geese; so that I was able to make a distribution to the whole Crew, which was the more exceptable on account of the approaching festival.[2] I now learnt that a number of the Natives, in 9 Canoes, had been along-side the Ship, and some on board; little address was necessary to persuade them to either the one or the other; they seem'd to be well enough acquainted with Europeans, and had amongst them some of their Knives. ye next morning

SUNDAY 25*th* they made us another visit; I found them to be of the same Nation as I had formerly seen in Success Bay,[3] and the same[4]

[1] *were abundance of:* D the Rocks were covered with

[2] 'The Captain serv'd out to the ships Company a Goose to ev'ry 3 men for a Xtmass Dinner.'—Cooper.—'Our sailors well pleased to see their ship safe at anchor, had already begun their holiday the evening before, and continued to carouse during two days without intermission, till captain Cook ordered the greatest part of them to be packed into a boat, and put ashore, to recover from their drunkenness in the fresh air.'—Forster, II, p. 506.

[3] They were a different 'nation': those Cook had seen in Success Bay were Onas, who did not use canoes; these were probably a sub-tribe of Yahgans, who spent a great deal of time in their canoes. They 'seemed to be good natured inoffensive people'.—Log. The best commentary on Cook's description of them is E. Lucas Bridges, *Uttermost Part of the Earth* (1948), chap. 3 and *passim.*

[4] *and the same:* DH they also seemed to be the same sort of People as are frequently seen in the Straits of Magelhanes

which M. de Bougainville distinguishes by the name of Pecheras[1]—a word which these had on every occasion in their mouths. They are a little ugly half starved beardless Race; I saw not a tall person amongst them. They were almost Naked; their cloathing was a Seal skin; some had two or three sew'd together, so as to make a cloak which reach'd to the knee, but the most of them had only one skin hardly large enough to cover their shoulders, and all their lower parts were quite naked. The Women, I was told, cover their privities with a flap of Seal skin, but in other respects were cloathed as the Men; they as well as the Children remain'd in the Canoes. I saw two young Children at the breast, as naked as they were born; thus they are inured from their infancy to Cold and hardships. They had with them bows & Arrows & darts, or rather harpoons made of bone and fitted to a staff. I suppose they were intended to kill Seals and fish; they may also kill Whales with them in the same manner as the Esquimaux's do; I know not if they are so fond of train Oyle but they and every thing they have about them smell most intolerable of it. I order'd them some Bisket; but I did not observe that they were so fond of it as I have heard said;[2] they were much better pleas'd when I gave them some Medals, Knives &c[a]. The Women & Children, as I have before observ'd, remain'd in the Canoes, which were made of Bark, and in each was a fire, over which the poor Creatures huddled themselves; I cannot suppose that they carry a fire in their Canoes for this purpose only, but rather that it may be allways ready to remove a shore wherever they land; for let their method of obtaining fire be what it will, they cannot be allways sure of finding dry fuel that will take fire from a spark. They likewise carry in their Canoes large Seal hides, which I judged was to shelter them when in the Canoes and to serve as covering to their hutts ashore, and may occa-

[1] 'After dinner we proceeded by rowing along the coast of Terra del Fuego . . . we distinguished some savages upon the low point of a bay, where I intended to touch. We went immediately to their fires, and I knew again the same troop of savages which I had already seen on my first voyage in the straits. We then called them *Pécherais*, because that was the first word they pronounced when they came to us, and which they repeated to us incessantly, as the Patagonians did their *shawa*.'—Bougainville, pp. 163–4. Whether Cook's people were in fact the same as Bougainville, and later FitzRoy, met in Magellan Strait, is perhaps a little doubtful, though the word 'Pecheray' certainly links them. FitzRoy (*Narrative*, II, p. 132) refers to 'a small and very miserable horde, whose name I do not know', and whose usual exclamation was 'Pecheray'. He did not regard them as Yahgans. The word is a problem. Dr Thomas Bridges, in his MS Yahgan dictionaries (B.M. Add. MSS 46177–80) has nothing like it. The *Beagle* narrative devotes some interesting pages to it (I, pp. 313–15), concluding, 'there evidently is something of a superstitious nature connected with the word; but our frequent attempts to find out its precise meaning, were unsuccessful'. On the other hand, FitzRoy (II, p. 358), though speaking of different people—he mentions 'the Huilliche or Araucanian language'—says it was 'always uttered in a begging, or whining tone', and obviously sees no 'superstitious' connection.

[2] DH but this might be owing to the badness of it, but be this as it will,

sionally serve them for Sails. They all retir'd before dinner and did not wait to pertake of our Christmas Cheer, indeed I beleive no one invited them, and for good reasons, for their dirty persons and the stench they carried about them was enough to spoil any mans appetite, and that would have been a real disapointment, for we had not experienced such fare for some time, Roast and boiled Geese, Goose pies &c[a] was victuals little known to us, and we had yet some Madeira Wine left, which was the only Article of our provisions that was mended by keeping; so that our friends in England did not perhaps, celebrate Christmas more cheerfully than we did.

MONDAY 26*th*. Little wind next to a Calm and fair weather, except in the morning when we had some showers of rain. In the evening the natives made us another viset; it was a Cold evening and distressing to see them stand trembling and naked on the deck and I could do no less than give them some Baize and old Canvas[1] to cover themselves.[2]

TUESDAY 27*th*. Fine pleas[t] weather. Having already compleated our water, I order'd the Wood, Tent and observatory to be got onboard and as this was work for the day, a party of us went away in two boats to shoot Geese. We proceeded round by the South side of Goose Island and pick'd up in all thirty one. On the East[3] side of Goose island, to the North of the East point, is good Anchorage in 17 fathom water, where it is intirely land-lock'd. This is a good place for Ships to lay in who are bound to the West; on the North side of this isle I observ'd three fine Coves, in which were both wood and Water, but it being near night I had no time to sound them, but I have no doubt but there is Anchorage; the way to come at them is by the West end of the isle. When I got aboard I found every thing was got off from the shore, the launch in, so that we now only waited for a Wind to put to Sea. The Festival which we celebrated at this place occasion'd my giving it the name of *Christmas Sound.**—A 209–11.

The entrance which is 3 leag[s] wide is Situated in the Latitude of 55°27′, Longitude 70°16′[4] West[5] and in the direction of N 37° West from S[t] Ildefonso Isles distant ten leagues. These isles are the best land mark for finding the Sound. *York Minster* which is the only remark-

[1] '. . . . gave each a knife, and a piece of old Canvas . . .'—Log.

[2] *to cover themselves:* DH which they received with greater satisfaction than any thing I had given them before, and would have given me in return any thing they had.

[3] *East:* D North East

[4] 16′ corrected from 08′; A 8′.

[5] *in the Latitude . . . West:* D on the East side of York Minister,

able land about it will hardly be known by a stranger, by any discription which can be given of it, because it alters its appearences according to the different situations it is Viewed from. Besides the black rock which lies off the South end of *Shag* island, there is a nother about midway between this and the East shore. A[1] Copious discription of this Sound is unnecessary, as few would be benefited by it, the Sketch which accompanies this Journal[2] will be a sufficient guide for such Ships as Chance may bring here; Anchorage, Tufts of wood and fresh Water will be found in all the Harbours and Coves. I whould advise no one to Anchor very near the Shore for the sake of anchoring in a moderate depth of Water, because near the Shore I generally found a rocky bottom. The refreshments to be got here are precarious, as it consists chiefly in wild fowl and may probably never be got in such plenty as to supply the Crew of a Ship, and fish, so far as we can judge, are scarce, indeed the plenty of Wild Fowl made us pay less attention to fishing; here are however plenty of Muscles, they are not very large but well tasted,[3] and very good. Celery is to be found on several of the low islots and where the Natives have their habitations. The Wild Fowl are Geese, Ducks, Sea Pies, Shags, and that sort of Gull so often mentioned in this Journal under the name of Port Egmont Hen. Here is a kind of Duck which our people called Race-horses on accountof the great swiftness theyruns upon the Water for they cannot fly, the wings being too short to support the body in the air.[4] This Bird is at the Falkland isles, as appears by Pernety's Journal,[5] page 244. The Geese too are there[6] and seem to be very well described under the Name of Bustards, page 213. They are much smaller than our English tame geese and eat as well as any I ever tasted.[7] They have short black Bills and yellow feet, the Gander is all white, the female is spoted black and White or grey, with a large white spot on each wing.[8] Besides the birds above mentioned, here are several other aquatick and some land birds, but of the latter not

[1] *A:* D as there is no danger that I know of, but what is visible, a

[2] Chart XL must be the 'sketch' which Cook refers to—or at least a copy of it.

[3] *they are . . . tasted:* D H they are not large but exceeding well tasted and we felt no ill effects by eating them

[4] The Magellanic Steamer Duck, *Tachyeres pteneres* (Forster.)

[5] Antoine Joseph Pernety (1716–1801), a Benedictine, went to the Falklands with Bougainville as chaplain in 1763. He later left his order and became librarian to Frederick the Great until 1783. He accumulated an odd set of beliefs and wrote an odd variety of books: the one Cook refers to is his *Journal historique du voyage fait aux îles Malouines et au détroit de Magellan* (Berlin 1769, Paris 1770), of which an English translation appeared in 1771.

[6] *there:* A there the same . . .

[7] *They are . . . tasted:* D H In size, they are between a Duck and a Goose, and make a noise some thing like the former,

[8] They were the Kelp Goose, *Chloëphaga hybrida.*

many.[1] From the knowlidge which the Inhabitants seem to have of Europeans, we cannot suppose that they live here continually but retire to the North during the Winter. I have often wondered that these people do not cloath them selves better, sence nature hath certainly provided materials; they might line their Seal skin cloaks with the skins and feathers of Aquatick birds; they might make their cloakes larger and might make of the same skins other sort of cloathing, for I cannot suppose they are scarce with them, they were ready enough to part with those they had to our people, a thing they hardly would have done if they had not known where to have gone and got more. In short of all the Nations I have seen the Pecheras are certainly the most wretched.[2] They are doomed to live in one of the most inhospitable climates in the world, without having sagacity enough to provide themselves with such necessaries as may render life convenient. As barren as this Country is it produceth a number of unknown plants and gave sufficient employment to Mr Forster and his party. The tree which produceth the Winters bark[3] is found here in the woods, the holly-leaved berbery[4] and some other sorts which I know not, but I believe are common in the Streights of Magalhaens.[5] We found a berry, which we called cran berries, because they are nearly of the same Colour, size and shape; they grow on a bushy plant which is pretty plenty near the shores, these berries have a bitterish taste rather insipid but may be eat either raw or in tarts and are eat by the natives.[6]

WEDNESDAY 28*th*. At 4 o'Clock in the Morning began to unmoor and at 8 weighed and stood out to Sea with a light breeze at NW which

[1] D H As barren as this Country is, it afforded Mr Forster a number of unknown plants and gave sufficient employment for him and his people all the time we were here.

[2] *I have often . . . wretched:* D H The Hutts which we saw were rather different to those I had formerly seen in Success bay, but not a bit better addapted for Winter habitations: their food is seal flesh, fish, Shells and birds, or what ever comes in their way, they do not seem to be more nicer in their food than in their persons, in short one sees nothing about them that is not disgusting in the highest degree. It seems extraordinary that these people do not clothe themselves better, sence Nature has certainly provided materials and they seem'd most sencibly to feel the want of better: they might make their cloaks much larger and of the same sort of skins make other and more warmer cloathing, the Skins and feathers of Aquatick birds might be appli'd to the same use, which they now only use in making a kind of Cap or bonnet, which is more for ornament than use, in short of all the Nations I have seen the Pecheras are the most wretched and are the most deserving our compassion.—Cf. Darwin, *Naturalist's Voyage* (ed. 1888), p. 216: 'There is no reason to believe that the Fuegians decrease in number; therefore we must suppose that they enjoy a sufficient share of happiness, of whatever kind it may be, to render life worth having'. Nevertheless since Darwin they have decreased in number.

[3] *Drimys winteri;* cf. I, p. 51.

[4] *Berberis ilicifolia* Forster.

[5] *but I believe . . . Magalhaens:* D but as I have already observed, there is hardly a tree fit for any other use but firing.

[6] *Pernettya mucronata.*

afterwards freshned and was attended with rain. At Noon the East point of the Sound (*Point Nativity*) bore N½W distant one league and a half and St Ildefonso Isles SE½S distant seven leagues; the Coast seemed to trend in the direction of EBS but the weather being very hazy nothing appeared distinct. We continued to steer SEBE and ESE with a fresh breeze at WNW till 4 PM when we hauled to the South in order to have a nearer view of St Ildefonso Isles. At this time we were a breast of an Inlet which lies ESE about 7 Leagues from the Sound, but it must be observed that there are some isles without this direction.[1] At the West point of this inlet are two high peaked hills,[2] and below them to the East two round hills or isles which lie in the direction of NE & SW of each other.[3] An Island or what appeared to be an Island laid in the entrance.[4] Another but smaller inlet appeared to the west of this,[5] indeed the Coast appeared indented and broken as usual. At half past 5 o'Clock the Weather clearing up gave us a good sight of St Ildefonso Isles; they are a group of Islands and rocks above Water,[6] situated about Six leagues from the Main and in the Latitude of 55°53′ S, Longitude 69°41′ West.

We now resumed our Course to the East and at Sun-set the most advanced land bore SEBE¾E and a point which I judged[7] to be the West point of Nassau Bay, discovered by the Dutch Fleet under the Command of Admiral Hermite in 1624,[8] bore N 80° East Six leagues distant. In some Charts this point is called False Cape Horn,[9] as being the Southern point of Terra del Fuego, It is situated in Latitude 55°39′ S. From the Inlet above mentioned to this false Cape the derection of the Coast is nearly East half a point South distant 14 or 15 leagues. At 10 o'Clock shortned sail and spent the night makeing short boards under the Top-sails.[10]

THURSDAY 29*th*. At 3 o'Clock in the Morning made sail and steered SEBS with a fresh breeze at WSW the Weather some what hazy. At this

[1] The inlet was Duff Bay: the 'isles without this direction' I think Morton and Henderson islands.

[2] The double peaks of Leading Hill, on Hind Island, visible for eighteen or twenty miles; they are a good mark for the entrance to Duff Bay.

[3] To identify here with any confidence, one needs to take up Cook's position. But one may conjecture that the 'round hills or isles' were Mount Jane, at the eastern tip of Rous peninsula, and the hill facing it across the entrance of New Year Sound, on Hardy peninsula.

[4] Hind Island.

[5] Rous Sound.

[6] D . . . fit only for the habitations of Birds:

[7] *I judged:* D proved

[8] Cf. I, p. 52, n. 4.

[9] It still is. Cook's judgment was right. False Cape Horn rather resembles the real cape; it is the southernmost point of the Hardy peninsula, lat. 55°43′ S, long. 68°03′ W.

[10] *shortned sail . . . Top-sails:* D shortned sail to the three Top-sails and spent the night standing on and off, because I would not miss seeing the whole of the Coast quite to Cape Horn.

time the West entrance to Nassau bay extended from NBE to NE½E and the South side of Hermites isles EBS. At 4 Cape Horn, for which we now steered, bore EBS, it is known at a distance by a high round hill over it, a point to the WNW shews a surface not unlike this, but their situations alone will allways distinguish the one from the other. At half past 7 we passed this famous Cape and entered the *Southern Atlantick Ocean*. It is the very same point of land which I took for the Cape when I passed it in 1769, which at that time I was doubtfull of:[1] it is the most Southern point of land on Hermites Islands (a group of Islands of unequal extent lying before Nassau bay) and situated in the Latitude of 55°58′[2] and in the Longitude of 68°13′ W, according to the observations made off it in 1769; by the observations which we had in Christmas Sound and reduced to the Cape by the Watch and others which we had afterwards and reduced back to it by the same means places it in 67°19′. It is most probable that a mean between the two, viz. 67°46′, will be nearest the truth.[3] On the NW side of the Cape are two peaked Rocks like Sugar loaves, they lie NWBN & SEBS by compass of each other, some other stragling low rocks lie west of the Cape and one South of it but they are all near the Shore.

From Christmas Sound to Cape Horn the Course is ESE½E distant 31 leagues. In the direction of ENE three leagues from Cape Horn is a rocky point which I called *Misstaken* Cape: it is the southern point of the Eastermost of Hermites isles.[4] Between these two Capes there seemed to be a passage directly into Nassau bay, some small Isles were seen in the passage and the Coast on the West side seemed to form some good bays or Harbours.[5] In some Charts Cape Horn is laid down as belonging to a small island, this was neither verified nor contridicted by us,[6] several breaks appeared in the Coast both to the East and West of it and the hazy weather rendered every object indistinct. The summits of some of the hills were rocky, the sides and Vallies seemed to be covered with a green Turf and Wooded in tufts. From Cape Horn we steered EBN½N which direction carried us without the Rocks which lie off Misstaken Cape; these rocks were White with the Dung of Fowls, and vast numbers were seen about

[1] I, p. 49.

[2] A or 59′ South...—The now accepted latitude is 55°59′.

[3] This is a bad assumption. The longitude is 67°16′ W, so that the observations and the watch together brought Cook, with 67°19′, very close to the truth. Perhaps the sentence is another minute example of his affection for the observations made on the first voyage.

[4] Cape Deceit; the easternmost of the Hermite group is Deceit Island, and the cape is its south-east point. Cook's name has disappeared.

[5] This is so; the isles are Maxwell, Saddle and Jerdan; and there are two harbours, St Martin's Cove and Port Maxwell, on the east side of Hermite Island.

[6] It is the south extreme of Horn Island, itself the southernmost of the Hermite group.

them. After passing these Rocks, steered NE½E and NE for Strait La Maire with a view of looking into Success bay to see if there were any traces of the Adventure having been there. At 8 o'Clock in the Evening drawing near the Strait, we shortned sail and hauled the Wind. At this time the Sugar loafe[1] on Terra del Fuego bore N 33° West, the point of Success bay just open of the Cape of the same name bearing N 20° E and Staten land extending from N 53° E to 67° East.

Soon after the wind died away and we had light airs & Calms by turns, till near Noon the next day, during which time we were driven by the Current over to Staten Land. The calm was succeeded by a light breeze at NNW with which we stood over for Success bay assisted by the Currents which set to the North. Before this we had hoisted our Colours and fired two guns[2] and soon after saw a Smoake rise out of the Woods above the South point of the Bay which I judge was made by the Natives, as it was at the place where they resided when I was here in 1769. As soon as we got off the Bay I sent Lieutenant Pickersgill to see if any traces remained of a Ship having been there lately and in the mean time we stood on and off with the Ship. At 2 o'Clock the current turned and set to the South, and Mr Pickersgill informed me when he returned on board that it was falling Water ashore; this is contrary to what I had observed when I was here before, for I thought then that the flood came from the North. Mr Pickersgill saw not the least signs of any Ship having been there lately. I had in[s]cribed the Ships name on a Card, which he nailed to a tree, at the place where the Endeavour Watered. This was done with a view of giving Captain Furneaux some information in case he was behind us and should put in here. On Mr Pickersgills landing he was courtesly received by several of the Natives who were cloathed in Guianaco and Seal skins and had on their Arms braclets, made of Silver Wire and worked some thing like the hilt of a sword and were no doubt the manufactury of some Europeans. They were the same sort of People as we had seen in Christmas Sound and like them repeated the word Pechera on every occasion. One man spoke a good deal to Mr Pickersgill, pointing first to the Ship and then to the bay as if he wanted her to come in. Mr Pickersgill said the Bay was full of Whales and Seals, we had observed the same in the Strait especially on the Terra del fuego side where the Whales in particular were

[1] Monte Campana.

[2] 'All the Fore Noon working to windward in the Straits, about 10 fir'd 2 Guns as a signal to the Adventure supposing her to be in Success Bay, which Captain Cook has some idea of.'—Clerke.—A '. . . but now we saw this could answer no end, as no Ship was in the bay; . . .'

exceeding numerous.[1] As soon as the boat was hoisted in which was not till near Six o'Clock we made sail to the East with a fine breeze at North, for sence we had explored the South Coast of Terra del Fuego I resolved to do the same by Staten land, which I believe to have been as little known as the former. At 9 o'Clock the Wind freshned and veered to NW, we tacked and stood to SW in order to spend the night which proved none of the best, being stormy and hazey with rain.

SATURDAY 31*st*. At 3 o'Clock bore up for the East end of Staten land, which at half past 4 bore S 60° E, the West end S 2° E and the land of Terra del Fuego S 40° West. Soon after I had taken these bearings the land was again obscured in a thick haze and we were obliged to make way as it were in the dark, for it was but now and then we got a sight of the land. As we advanced to the East we preceived several islands[2] of unequal extent lying off the land, there seemed to be a clear passage between the Eastermost and the one next to it to the west, I would gladly have gone through this Passage and anchored under one of the islands[3] to have waited for better weather (for on sounding we found only 29 fathom water) but when I considered that this was runing to leeward in the dark I chose to keep without the islands and accordingly hauled off to the north. At 8 o'Clock we were abreast of the most Eastern isle[4] distant from it about 2 miles and had the same depth of Water as before. I now shortned sail to the three top-sails, to wait for clear weather for the fog was so thick that we could see no other land than this island. After waiting an hour and the Weather not clearing up, we bore up and hauled round the East end of the island for the sake of smooth Water and anchorage if I found this necessary. In hauling round the end of the island we found a strong race of a Current like unto broken Water, but we had no less than 19 fathoms, we also saw on the island abundance of Seals and Birds, This was a temptation too great for people in our situation to withstand, to whom fresh Provisions of any kind was acceptable; this determined me to anchor in order to have an oppertunity to taste of what we now only saw at a distance. At length after

[1] '. . . there are a greater abundance of Whales & Seals rowling about these Straits, than I suppos'd were to be met with in any part of the World: a fair Account of them wou'd appear incredible—the Whales are blowing on every point of the Compass and frequently taint the whole Atmosphere about us with the most disagreeable effluvia that can be conciev'd.'—Clerke.

[2] The New Year Islands—Cook's name, Chart XL. There are five of them. Also Fig. 79.

[3] One wonders why here and so often later Cook altered his original 'isle[s]' or 'islot[s]' (as in A) to 'island[s]'. He may have thought it 'sounded better': there is no accounting for authors.

[4] Observatory Island.

makeing a few boards, fishing as it were for the best ground, we anchored in 21 fathom water a stony bottom about a mile from the island which extended from N 18° E to N 58½° West and soon after the Weather cleared up and we saw Cape St John, or the East end of Staten land bearing S 75° E distant 4 leagues; we were sheltered from the South Wind by Staten land and from the north wind by the island, the other isles laid to the West and secured us from this wind, but beside being open to the NE and East we also laid exposed to the WNW winds which might have been avoided by anchoring more to the west, but I made choice of this situation for two reasons, first to be near the Island we intended to land upon and secondly to be able to get to sea with any wind.

After dinner hoisted out three boats and landed with a large party of men, some to kill seals, others to catch or kill birds fish or what came in our way. To find of the former it mattered not where we landed for the whole shore was covered with them and by the noise they made one would have thought that the island was stocked with Cows and Calves. On landing we found they were a different Animal to Seals, but in shape and motion exactly resemble them, we called them Lions on account of the great resemblance the Male has to a land Lion.[1] Here were also the same sort of Seals which we found in New Zealand generally known by the name of Sea Bears, at least so we called them:[2] They were all so tame, or rather so stupid as to suffer us to come so near as to knock them down with a stick but the large ones we shot as it was rather dangerous to go so near them. We also found on the island abundance of Penguins and Shaggs, the latter had young ones almost fledged and just to our taste; here were geese and Ducks but not many; Birds of prey and a few small birds. In the evening we returned on board with our boats well Laden with one thing or a nother.[3]

[JANUARY 1775]

SUNDAY Janry *1st* 1775. Finding that nothing was wanting but a good harbour to make this a tolerable place for Ships to refresh at, whom Chance or design might bring here, I sent Mr Gilbert with

[1] They were *Otaria byronia* Blainville, the Southern Sea Lion.

[2] *Arctocephalus australis* Zimmermann, the Southern Fur Seal.

[3] 'Observ'd the small Island covered with Seals, Sea Lions & Birds of different kinds, hoisted out the Boats & sent them on shore with several of the Officers & ships Company to kill Sea Lyons & Seals to make Oil for the use of the Ship. At 8 the Boats return'd on board loaded with Sea Lions, Seals, Geese, Shags & Penguins, the shores of the Island being entirely covered with them, some of the Lions weighing nearly 1000 lbs Weight. AM Hoisted the Launch out & sent her with the other Boats to bring off those imazing animals whilst hands are employ'd on board taking off the Skins & blubber.'—Cooper.

the Cutter over to Staten land to look for one, appearences promised success in a place opposite to the Ship. I also sent two other boats for the Lions &c^a^ we had killed the preceeding evening and soon after I went my self[1] and observed the Suns Meridion altitude at the North East end of the island which gave the Latitude 54°40′05″ s. After shooting a few geese and some other birds and lading the Boat with young Shags, we returned on board to dinner and soon after the other boats came on board laden with Sea Lions, Sea Bears &c^a^. The old Lions and Bears were killed cheifly for the sake of their Blubber or fat to make oil of for except their Harselets which were tollerable the flesh was too rank to be eat with any tolerable relish. But the young Cubs we found very Palatable[2] and even the flesh of some of the old Lionesses were not much a miss, but that of the Old Lions was abominable. In the after noon I sent some people on shore to skin and cut off the fat of those who yet remained dead a shore, for we had already got more carcases on board than necessary, and I went my self in a nother boat to collect birds. About 10 o'Clock Mr Gilbert returned from Staten land where he had found a good Port situated 3 leagues to the westward of Cape St John and in ye direction of North a little Easterly from the NE end of the Eastern island. It may be known by some small Islands lying in the entrance, the channel, which is on the East side of these Islands, is half a mile broad. The Course in is SWBS, turning gradually to WBS and west, the harbour lies nearly in this last direction and is near two miles in depth and in some places near a mile broad and hath in it from 50 to 10 fathoms Water, a bottom of Mudd and sand. Its shores are covered with Wood fit for fuel and there are in it several Streams of fresh Water. On the Islands were Sea Lyons &c^a^, such an innumerable quantity of Gulls as to darken the air when disturbed and almost suffocated our people with their dung, which they seemed to void by way of defence and it stunk worse than Assafettida or as it is commonly called Devil's dung. They also saw several Geese, Ducks and Race Horses which is also a kind of duck.[3] The day on which this port was descovered occasioned my calling it *New Years Harbour*, it would have been more convenient for Ships bound to the West or round Cape Horn, had it been so situated that they could have put to sea with an

[1] A (accompanied by Mr F.)

[2] *The old . . . Palatable:* A on whose flesh all hands dined to day and found it good eating, the young ones especially. . .—Cooper, 2 January, writes, 'Today boil'd Shags & Penguins in the Coppers for the Ships Company's Dinner'; so at least fresh food did not lack in quantity.

[3] *Such an . . . duck:* A and some Aquatick birds.—The passage in B is in red ink, and mainly on a separate slip. These odorous islands were called the Gull Isles (Chart XL, inset of New Year's Harbour).

easterly and northerly wind.[1] The ill conveniency is of little consequence sence these winds are never known to be of long duration. The Southerly and Westerly are the prevailing winds, so that a Ship can never be detained long in this port.

MONDAY *2nd.* As we could not sail in the morning for want of Wind, I sent a party of men on shore to the Island on the same duty as yesterday. Towards noon we got a fresh breeze of Wind at west but it came too late and I resolved to wait till the next morning.[2]

TUESDAY *3rd.* At 4 o'Clock when we weighed with a fresh breeze at NWBW and stood for Cape St John which at half past 6 bore NBE distant about 4 or 5 miles. Sence this Cape is the Eastern point of Staten land, a description of it is unnecessary. It may however not be amiss to say that it is a rock of considerable height and situated in the Latitude of 54°46′ S Longitude 64°07′ W with a rocky islot lying close under the north part of it. To the Westward of the Cape about five or six miles is an Inlet which seemed to divide the land, that is to communicate with the Sea to the South; between this inlet and the Cape was a Bay but I cannot say of what depth.[3] In sailing round the Cape we met with a very strong current from the South, it made a race which looked like breakers and it was as much as we could do with a strong gale to made head against it. After geting round the Cape I hauled up along the South Coast and as soon as we had brought the wind to blow off the land it came upon us in such heavy squals as to oblige us to double reef our Top-sails: it afterwards fell by little and little and at Noon ended in a Calm. At this time Cape St John bore N 20° E distant 3½ leagues, Cape St Bartholomew or the SW point of Staten land S 83° W, two high detatched rocks N 80° West and the place where the land seemed to be divided, which had the same appearence on this side, bore N 15° West 3 leagues distant. Latitude observed 54°56′. In this situation we sounded but had no

[1] A which cannot be done without turning out, and this cannot always be done in a Channell bounded on each side by high lands as this is.—This passage is deleted from the text of B.

[2] 'Hoisted in the Launch having got from the sea Lyons pun[cheon]s of bluber and 4 Boat loads of penguins and shaggs which are exceeding good eating in those seas only.'—Gilbert.—Or possibly only in those seas did Gilbert and his fellows, after all they had been through, feel that penguins and shaggs were exceeding good eating.—Cf. Wales, 3 January: 'It [Staten Land] affords good Plenty of Ducks & Geese like those we met with in Christmas Sound, and as to Sea Fowl such as Pengwins Shags Gulls &c they are innumerable of which most of our People eat and thought very good: I must confess I did not much relish them but the Ducks & Geese are as good as any I ever tasted . . .'. See also p. 615, n. 2 below.

[3] The inlet is Port Cook, which does not divide the land, but is separated only by a low isthmus from Port Vancouver, running in on the south side. The bay is St John Harbour.

bottom with a line of 120 fathoms. The Calm was of very short duration, a breeze presently sprung up at NW but it was too faint to make head against the Current and we drove with it back to the NNE. At 4 o'Clock the Wind veered at once to SBE and blew in squals attended with rain. Two hours after, the squals and rain subsided and the Wind return'd back to the west and blew a gentle gale. All this time the Current set us to the North, so that at 8 o'Clock Cape S[t] John bore WNW dist[t] about 7 Leagues. I now gave over plying and steered SE with a resolution to leave the land, judgeing it to be sufficiently explored to answer the most general purposes of Navigation and Geography. The annexed Chart[1] will very accurately shew the direction extent and position of the Coast along which I have sailed either on this or my former Voyage and no more is to be expected from it. The Latitudes have been determined by the Suns Meridion altitude which we were so fortunate as to obtain every day except the one we sailed from Christmas Sound, which was of no consequence sence its latitude was known before. The Longitudes have been settled by Lunar observations as hath been already mentioned. I have taken 67°46′ for the Longitude of Cape Horn from this meridion, the Longitude of all the other parts are deduced by the watch by which the extent of the whole must be determined to a few miles and whatever error there may be in Longitude it must be general, but I think it highly probably that the Longitude is determined to within a quarter of a degree. Thus the extent of Terra dell Fuego from East to West and consequently that of the Straits of Magalhaens will be found less than most Navigators have made it.[2]

In order to illustrate this and to shew the situations of the neighbouring lands and by this means make the annexed Chart of more general use, I have extended it down to 47° of Latitude.[3] But I am

[1] i.e., when he first wrote, Chart XL.

[2] At this point in A, but not elsewhere, Cook has the following footnote: 'The reason of my not laying down the Straits of Magelhanes in this Chart, was, my not having such good memoirs, as must be in the Admiralty; when I can have recourse to them, it shall be done; I shall only observe that Cape Pillar at the West end of the Strait must lie in the longitude of 74°. The Author of Lord Ansons Voyage says, they made 2½° of Longitude between Cape Virgin Mary and Strait Le Maire, Feuillee says he made 3°25′ between the said Cape and Cape S[t] Johns on Staten Land. Therefore, according to the former, Cape Virgen Mary, at the East end of the Strait, must lie in the Longitude of 68°00′ West, and according to the latter in 67°32 West.'

[3] The 'annexed Chart' is now a new one, not that referred to in A (n. 2 above). It is engraved in the *Voyage*, II, pl. II. From this sentence of the text to the end of the following paragraph Cook has redrafted considerably in red ink, taking up and expanding the short discussion in his footnote in A (n. 2 above). There are two of these red ink drafts, B ff. 314 (portion only) and 315–5v. I print from f. 315–5v. The *Voyage*, II, pp. 198–9, has a shortened version, which makes no reference to the figures which Cook here leaves blank, except for the longitude of Cape Virgin Mary (the north point of the eastern entrance of Magellan Strait, now Cape Virgins), which is given as 67°52′. The accepted figure at the present day is 68°21′ W.

only answerable for the inaccuracy of such parts as I have explored my self. In laying down the rest I had recourse to the following authorities:

The Longitude of Cape Virgin Mary, which is the most essential point as it determines the length of the Straits of Magalhaens, is deduced from Father Feuillee[1] and Commodore Anson. The former made 3°25′ difference of Longitude between it and Cape S[t] John and the latter between it and Straits La Maire. Now as Cape S[t] John lies in 64°07′ Cape Virgin Mary by Father Feuillee must be in 67°32′; and as Straits La Maire is in 6 ° ′ Cape Virgin Mary by Commodore Anson must lie in the mean of the two is which is the Longitude I have made use of and which I have reason to think cannot be far from the truth. The Straights of Magalhaens and the East Coast of Patigonia is laid down from the observations made by the late English and French Navigators. The West Coast of America from Cape Victory to the Latitude of is from the discoveries of Sarmienta a Spanish Navigator,[2] communicated to me by M[r] Stuart F.R.S.[3] Falkland Islands are Copied from a sketch take[n] by Captain M'Bride who Circumnavigated them in His Majestys Ship Jason in 176[6][4] and their distance from the main is agreeable to the run of the Dolphin under the Command of Commodore Byron, from Cape Virgin Mary to Port Egmont and from Port Egmont to Port Desire. Each of which

[1] Louis Feuillet (1660–1732), sometimes called in error Feuillée, a Franciscan, a French scientific traveller of great distinction, particularly in astronomy and botany. Among other important travels was his voyage round the Horn to Chile and Peru, 1707–11, of which he published an account in 1725; in this he had some rather bitter differences with Frézier.

[2] Pedro Sarmiento de Gamboa, a distinguished Galician sailor who went on Mendaña's voyage to the Solomons, and later, as a result of Drake's irruption into the Pacific, was sent to survey the Strait of Magellan. He discovered the Sarmiento Channel south through the Chilean islands in 1579, and made a valuable survey—'a voyage down the western coast, and through the Strait of Magalhaens, that has never been surpassed', said Captain P. P. King, who could speak with authority (*Narrative of the Surveying Voyages*, I, p. 565). In 1581 he was despatched by Philip II to found a colony in the Strait to bar it against intruders. On his way to Spain in 1586 to secure supplies he was captured by a privateer belonging to Sir Walter Raleigh, and his settlers perished of starvation. He wrote a history of the Incas. 'This Sarmiento hath caried the name to be the best Navigator in all Spaine, and that hee hath sayled the furthest of all others.'—Lopez Vaz in Hakluyt (MacLehose ed.), XI, p. 273.

[3] The only Stuart who seems to fit is, surprisingly, James Stuart (1713–88) the architect and painter—'Athenian Stuart', so called because of his and Nicholas Revett's celebrated *Antiquities of Athens* (1762); he was elected F.R.S. in 1768. He had possibly got hold of a copy of the edition of Sarmiento, *Viage al estrecho de Magallanes . . . 1579 y 1580*, published in Madrid in 1768, and sent Cook the book or material from it—Cook could not read Spanish but he could read a map. Presumably, like other gentlemen of the Royal Society, he met Cook in the period between the first and second voyages. See also p. xli above.

[4] Captain John McBride commanded the *Jason* frigate which took out marines to garrison Port Egmont, in the Falkland Islands, in 1766; it was he who, in December of that year, discovered Bougainville's settlement at Port Louis. See I, pp. lxxxix–xc.

runs were made in a few Days, consequently no material error could well happen.

The SW Coast of Terra del Fuego, with respect to Inlets, islands &c[a] may be compaired to the Coast of Norway, for I doubt if there is an extent of three leagues on the whole coast where there is not an inlet or harbour which will receive and shelter the largest shiping. The worst is, that untill they are better known, one is, as it were obliged to fish for anchorage. There are several lurking rocks upon the Coast but happily none of them lie far from the land, the approach to which may be known by sounding, supposeing the weather to be so obscure that you cannot see the land; for to judge of the whole by the parts we have sounded it is more than probable that there is Soundings all along the Coast, and for several leagues out to sea: upon the whole this is by no means that dangerous Coast it has been represented.

Staten land lies nearly EBN and WBS and is 10 leagues long in that direction and is no where above 3 or 4 leagues broad, the coast is rocky, much indented and seemed to form several bays or inlets. It shews a surface of Craggy Hills which spire up to a vast height, especially near the west end.[1] Except the Cragy summits of these hills, the greatest part was covered with trees and shrubs or some sort of Herbage and there was little or no snow up[on] it.[2] The Currents between Cape Deseado and Cape Horn set from West to East, that is in the same direction as the Coast, but they are by no means considerable. To the East of the Cape their strength is much increased and their direction is NE to wards Staten Land, they are rapid in Strait Le Maire and a long the South Coast of Staten land and set like a Turrent round Cape S[t] John and then takes a NW direction and continue to run very strong both within and without New Years Isles. While we lay at anchor within these Islands I observed that the Current was strongest during the flood and that on the Ebb its strength would be so much impared that the Ship would some times Ride head to wind when it was at West & NWN. This is only to be understood where the Ship laid at anchor, for at the very time that we had a strong current seting to the Westward, M[r] Gilbert found one of equal strength near the Coast of Staten

[1] A the other parts being neither so high nor so rocky.

[2] Cf. Wales, 3 January: 'At 8 oClock bore away and left Staten Land in a sort of Pet; but as I bear it no ill-will I shall take the liberty of stopping a little to give a short account of it. It did not appear to me by far so frightfull as it seems to have done to the relator of Lord Anson's Voyage, and I think appears to advantage after being conversant with the black bare Rocks on the s.w. side of *Terra del Fuego*'. He remarks on the trees and the luxuriant grass.

Land, seting to the Eastward. Probably this was an Eddy Current or Tide.[1]

If the tides are regulated by the Moon it is high Water by the Shore at this place, on the days of the new and full moon about 4 o'Clock. The perpendicular rise and fall is very inconsiderable, not exceeding four feet at most. In Christmas Sound it is high Water at half an hour past two o'Clock on the days of the full and Change and Mr Wales observed it to rise and fall upon a perpendicular 3 feet Six inches, but this was during the Neap Tides, consequently the Spring Tides must rise higher. To give such an account of the Tides and Currents on these Coasts as Navigators might depend on would require a multitude of observations and in different places, the makeing of which would require some time. I confess my self unprovided with meterials for such a task and believe that the less I say on this subject the fewer Misstakes I shall make, but I think I have been able to observe, that in Strait La Maire the Southerly Tide or Current (be it flood or ebb) begins to act on the days of the New and full Moon about 4 o'Clock; this remark may be of use to Ships who pass the Strait. Was I bound round Cape Horn to the West and not in Want of wood or Water or any other thing that might make it necessary for to put into port, I would not come near the land attall, for by keeping out at Sea you avoide the Currents, for I am satisfied that they loose their force at 10 or 20 leagues from land and at a greater distance there is none.[2] During the time we were upon the Coast we had more Calms then storms and the Winds so variable that I question if a passage might not have been made from East to West in as short a time as from West to East, nor did we experience any cold Weather. The mercury in the Thermometer at noon was never below 46 and while we laid in Christmas Sound it was generally above Temperate. At this place the Var. was 23°20′ East. A few leagues to the sw of Straits Le Maire it was 24°, and at Anchor within New years Isles it was 24°20′ East. These isles, especially the one we landed upon, is so unlike Staten land that it deserves a particular description. It shews a surface of equal height and elevated about 30 or 40 feet above the Sea, from which it is defended by a rocky Coast, the inner part of the isle is covered with a kind of Sword grass, which is very green and grows to a great length, it grows in large tufts and

[1] The last two sentences are in red ink on a separate slip, f. 316. There are red ink revisions in the first part of the paragraph also.

[2] Cf. Cook's discussion of the Horn route, I, pp. 58–9. It is true that the Cape Horn current is strongest near the land. The reader who wishes to check Cook against more recent experience will find a succinct discussion in the *South America Pilot*, Part II (1928) pp. 9–10.

on little hillocks of two or three feet in diameter and as many or more in height; they seem to be composed of the roots of the plant matted together.[1] Among these hillocks are a vast number of Paths made by Sea Bears and Penguins by which they retire into the very center of the isle, it is nevertheless exceeding bad traveling for these paths are so dirty that one is some times up to the knees in mire.

Besides this plant there were some other grases, a kind of heath[2] and some Celery. The whole surface was moist and wet and on the Coast were several small streams of Water. The sword-grass, as I call it, seems to be the same as grows in Falkland isles, which M. de Bougainville calls gladiolus or gramen, page 51 and Pernety, Corn-flags. The Animals which Inhabit this little spot are Sea Lyons, Sea Bears, a variety of aquatick and some land birds. The Sea Lion is pretty well described by Pernety, but these have not such fore feet or fins as the one he has given a plate of, but such fins as the one he calls a Sea wolf, nor did we see any so large as he speaks of, the largest were not more than 12 or 14 feet in length and perhaps 8 or 10 in circumference. They are not of that sort described under the same name by Lord Anson, but for aught I know these are more like a lion of the Wood, the long hair with which the back of the head, the neck and shoulders are covered gives them greatly the air and appearences of one. The other part of the body is covered with a short hair little longer than that of a cow or a horse and the whole is a dark brown. The female is not half so big as the male, it is covered with a short hair of an ash or light dun Colour. They live as it were in herds, upon the rocks and near the Sea shore.[3] As this was the time for ingendering as well as bringing forth thier young, we have seen a Male with 20 or 30 females about him and was always very attentive to keep them all to himself by beating off every other male who attempted to come into his flock; others again have a less number and some no more than one or two, and here and there we have seen one lying growling in a retired place by himself and would neither suffer males nor females to come near him, we judged these were old and superannuated. The Sea bears[4] are not by far so large as the Lions but rather larger than a Common Seal; they have none of that long hair which distinguishes the lion, it is all of an equal length and finer than that of the lion, something like an otters and the general Colour

[1] (*Dactylis caespitosa* Forst. f.) *Poa flabellata* Hook. f.

[2] Possibly *Pernettya mucronata* Linn. f., which was described from specimens collected by Forster, in Baeck's herbarium; though this was a shrub Cook had met with more than once before, remarking on its berries.

[3] They were the Southern Sea Lion.

[4] The Southern Fur Seal.

is a kind of Iron grey. This is the sort which the French call Sea Wolfs and the English Seals; they are however defferent from the Seals we have in Europe and in North America. The Lions may too, without any great impropriety, be calld over grown Seals for they are all of the same Species. It was not attall dangerous to go among them,[1] they either fled or laid Still, the only danger was in going between them and the Sea for if they took fright at any thing they would come down in such numbers that if you could not get out of their way you would be run over. Sometimes when we came suddenly upon them or Waked them out of their sleep (for they are slugish sleeping animals) they would raise up their heads, snort and snarl and look as fearce as if they meant to devour one in a moment, but by retorting it upon them I observed that they allways run away, so that they were down right bullies. The Penguin is an amphibious bird so well known to most people that I shall only observe that they are here in prodigious numbers and we could knock down as many as we pleased with a stick.[2] I cannot say they are good eating, I have indeed made several good meals of them but it was for want of beter victuals. They either do not breed here, or else this was not the Season, for we saw neither egs nor young ones. Shags breed here in vast numbers and we took on board not a few, as they are very good eating. They take certain spots to themselves and build their nests near the edge of the clifts on little hillocks which are either those of the sword grass or else they are made by the Shags building on them from year to year.[3] There is a nother sort rather smaller than these which breed in the clefts of rocks.[4] The geese are of the same sort as we found in Chrismas Sound,[5] there were but few and some had young ones. Mr Forster shott a Goose which was different from these, it was larger with a grey plumage and black feet.[6] The other sort make a noise exactly like a duck. Here were some ducks[7] but not many and

[1] A not one of our people was attack'd by them,

[2] The Magellanic Penguin, *Spheniscus magellanicus* (Forst.). 'They were of the size of small geese, and of that species which is the most common in the neighbourhood of the Straits of Magelhaens. The English at the Falkland Islands have named them jumping-jacks. They sleep very sound, for Dr. Sparrman met one of them, which he kicked several yards by accidentally stumbling over it, without breaking its sleep, till by repeatedly shaking the bird, it awoke. When the whole flock was beset, they all became very bold at once, and ran violently at us, biting our legs, or any part of our clothes. They are excessively hard-lived, for having left a great number of them, seemingly dead on the field of battle, and going in the pursuit of the rest, they all at once got up, and walked off with great gravity.'—Forster, II, p. 519.

[3] Probably the Imperial Cormorant, *Phalacrocorax atriceps atriceps* King: in South Georgia it frequently nests on top of hummocks of tussock grass.

[4] This may have been the Magellanic Shag, *Phalacrocorax magellanicus* (Gm.).

[5] The Kelp Goose.

[6] The Upland Goose, *Chloëphaga leucoptera* (Gm.).

[7] The Crested Duck, *Anas specularioides* King, was taken here.

several of that sort which we called race horses,[1] we shot some and found them to weigh 29 or 30 pound, those who eat of them said they were very good. The Oceanic[2] birds were Guls, Terns,[3] Port Egmont hens[4] and a large brown bird the size of an Albatross, and which Pernetty calls Quebrantahuessas, we called them Mother caries Geese and found them pretty good eating.[5] The land birds were Eagles or Hawkes,[6] Bald headed Vultures[7] or what our seamen called Turkey Buzzards, Thrushes[8] and a few other small birds.[9] Our Naturalists found two new spicies of birds, the one is about the size of a Pigeon,[10] the Plumage as white as milk, they feed a long shore, probably on shell fish and Carrion, for they have a very disagreeable smell. When we first saw these Birds we thought they were the Snow Peterel, but the moment they were in our possession the misstake was discovered, for they resemble them in nothing but size and Colour. These are not web-footed. The other sort was a Species of Curlews, nearly as big as a heron, it has a variegated plumage, the principle colours whereof are light grey, and a long crooked bill.[11] I had almost forgot to mention that here are Sea-Pies,[12] or what we called when in New Zealand, Curlews, but we only saw a few stragling pairs. It may not be a miss to observe that the Shags are the same bird which M. Bougainville calls saw-bills but he is misstaken in saying that the Quebrantahuessos are their enemies, for this bird is of the Peterel tribe and feeds wholy on fish[13] and is to be found in all the high Southern Latitudes. It is wonderfull to see how the defferent Animals which inhabited this little spot are reconciled to each other, they seem to have entered into a league not to disturb each others tranquillity. The Sea lions occupy most of the Sea Coast, the Sea bears take up thier aboad in the isle; the Shags take post on the highest clifts, the Penguins fix their

[1] The Magellanic Steamer Duck, *Tachyeres pteneres*.

[2] *Oceanic:* A other Aquatick

[3] Several kinds of gulls and terns occur in the south of South America.

[4] Probably the Chilean Skua, *Catharacta skua chilensis* (Bonaparte), which breeds in Tierra del Fuego and on the outlying islands.

[5] The Giant Petrel. *Quebrante huesos*, 'the bone-breakers'; the English common names are Nellie or Stinker. Cook has met them before.

[6] Both the Southern Caracara, *Polyborus plancus* (J. F. Miller) and Forster's Caracara, *Phalcoboenus australis* (Gm.), were taken and sketched by George Forster here.

[7] This was no doubt the Chilean Turkey Vulture, *Cathartes aura jota* (Molina).

[8] *Turdus magellanicus* King, the Magellanic Thrush.

[9] Other small birds taken included the Magellanic Babbler, *Scytalopus magellanicus* (Gm.); the Thorn-tailed Creeper, *Aphrastura spinicauda* (Gm.); and the Patagonian Cinclodes, *Cinclodes patagonicus* (Gm.).

[10] The Sheath-bill, *Chionis alba* (Gm.)

[11] The Black-faced Ibis, *Theristicus caudatus melanopis* (Gm.).

[12] Quoy's Black Oyster Catcher.

[13] Actually Bougainville was right: the Giant Petrel catches fish, is a predator and also a scavenger.

quarters where there is the most easiest communication to and from the sea and the other birds chuse more retired places. We have seen all these animals mix together like domesticated Cattle and Poultry in a farm yard, without the one attempting to disturb or molest the other; Nay I have often seen the Eagles and Vultures seting on the hillocks among the Shags, without the latter either young or old being desturbed by it. It may be asked how these birds of prey live, I suppose on the carcases of Seals and birds which die by various causes and probably not a few where they are so numerous. This very imperfect account is written more with a view to assist my own memory than to give information to others; I am neither a botanist nor a Naturalist and have not words to describe the productions of Nature either in the one Science or the other.

WEDNESDAY *4th.* Having left the land the preceeding evening as already mentioned we saw it again this morning at 3 o'Clock bearing West. Wind continued to blow a steady fresh breeze till 6 in the PM when it shifted in a heavy squal to SW; it came so suddenly upon us that we had not time to take in the Sails and was the occasion of carrying away a topg^t mast, a Studding sail boom and the loss of a Fore studding sail. The Squall ended in a heavy shower of rain, but the wind remained at SW; our Course was SE with a view of discovering that extensive coast which Mr Dalrymple lies down in his Chart in which is the Gulph of St Sebastian.[1] I designed to make the Western point of that Gulph in order to have all the other parts before me. Indeed I had some doubts about the existence of such a Coast and this appeared to me to be the best rout to clear it up and to explore the Southern part of this ocean.[2]

[1] Forster adverts to Dalrymple in a footnote (II, p. 523) to a passage on the 'latest charts published in England and France': 'See Mr. Dalrymple's Memoir of a Chart of the Southern Ocean, and the Chart itself, which bear an indisputable testimony of the laudable enthusiasm with which that gentleman has prosecuted his enquiries on this subject'. But the enthusiasm with which the gentleman prosecuted his enquiries was so untempered by scepticism that one with difficulty regards it as quite laudable. Dalrymple's 'Chart of the Ocean between South America and Africa. With the Tracks of Dr Edmund Halley in 1700 and Monsr Lozier Bouvet in 1738' was published in April 1769, and the accompanying *Memoir* in May 1769. The *Memoir*, p. 5, runs, 'The extensive tract of land to the eastward of America was taken from Ortelius's map, 1586; he calls the gulph St. Sebastiano: this map places the N.W. point in the same position La Roche does in 1675, and the Lion in 1756'. 'Ortelius's map' is not, as one might think it would be, the world-map reproduced in I, fig. 3; it is apparently his map of the New World (1587, not 1586), with its Golfo de Sebastiano; this is reproduced in R. A. Skelton's *Decorative Printed Maps* (London 1952), pl. 15. The large gulf penetrating Terra Australis in this longitude appeared (without a name) as early as 1531, in the world map of Oronce Finé. The world chart of 1569 by Mercator, who here follows Finé, first gives this gulf the appellation Golfo di San Sebastiano, apparently transferred from the harbour on the Brazilian coast similarly named by Vespucci on his southward voyage of 1501–2. Ortelius copied Mercator. See the detail of Dalrymple's chart, Fig. 80 overleaf.

[2] 'The people tired of eating Penguins and Young Shags, they prefer Salt Beef and

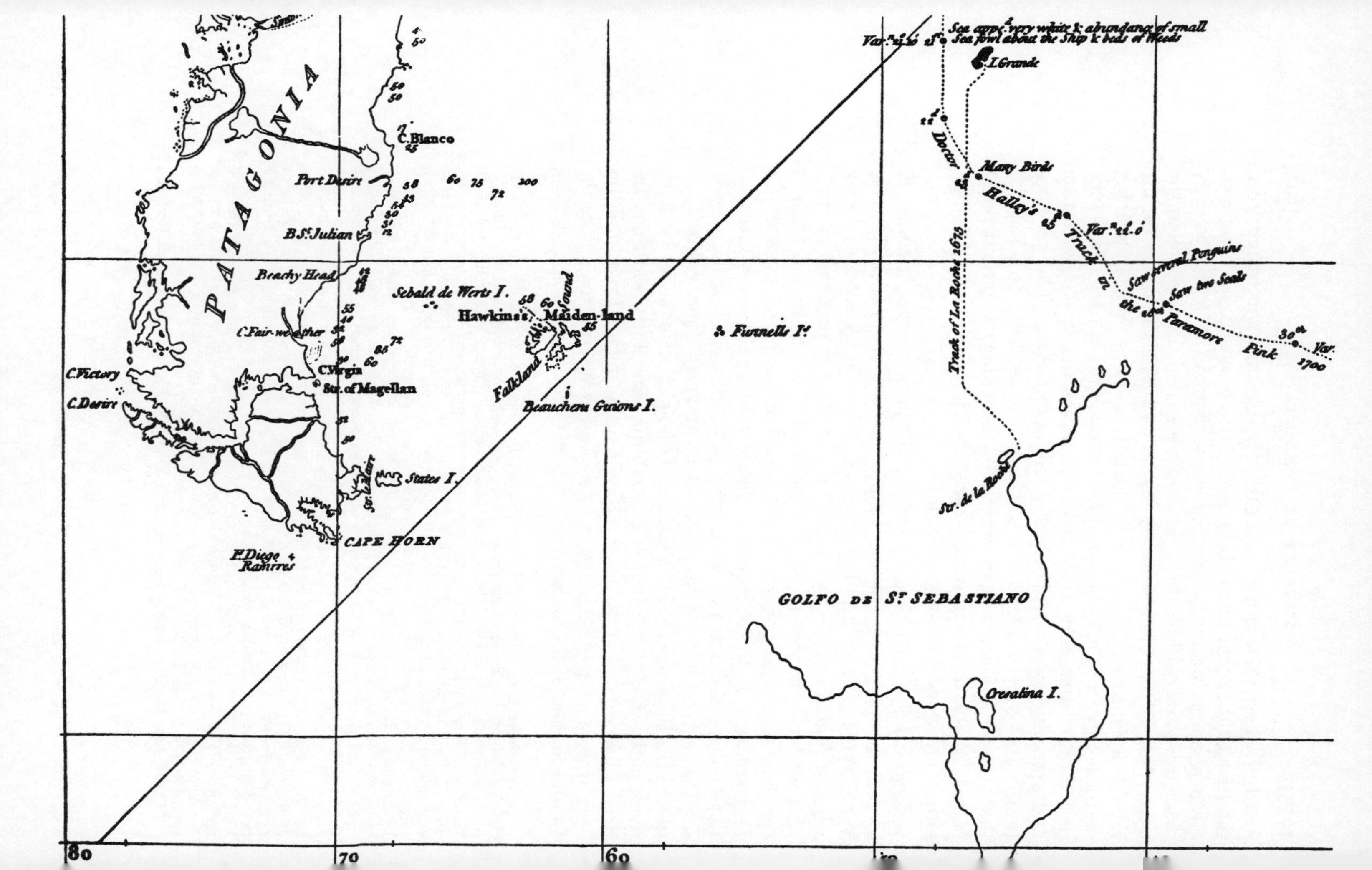

PATAGONIA
C. Blanco
Port Desire
B. St. Julian
Beachy Head
C. Fair-weather
C. Virgin
Str. of Magellan
C. Victory
C. Desire
States I.
CAPE HORN
F. Diego Ramirez
Sebald de Werts I.
Hawkins's Maiden-land
Falkland Sound
Beauchene Guions I.
Furnells Is.
Sea appd very white & abundance of small Sea fowl about the Ship & beds of Weeds
Var. 21.30
I. Grande
Doctor
Many Birds
Halley's Track
Var. 22.0
Track of La Roche 1675
Saw several Penguins
Saw two Seals
the Paramore Pink
Var. 1700
Str. de la Roche
GOLFO DE St. SEBASTIANO
Oresalina I.
80
70
60

THURSDAY 5*th*. Fresh gales at West and Cloudy weather. At Noon observed in 57°09′, Longitude made from Cape St John 5°2′ East. At 6 o'Clock in the PM being in the Latitude 57°21′ and in the Longitude of 57°45′ W the Variation was 21°28′ East.[1]

FRIDAY 6*th*. At 8 o'Clock in the evening, being then in the Latitude of 58°9′ S, Longitude 53°14′ West, we close reefed our Top-sails and hauled to the North with a very strong gale at West attended with a thick haze and sleet. The situation just mentioned is nearly the same as Mr Dalrymple assigns for the SW point of the Gulph of St Sebastian, but as we saw neither land nor signs of any, I was the more doubtfull of its existence and was fearfull that by keeping to the South I might miss the land said to be discovered by La Roch in 1675 and by the Ship Lion in 1756,[2] which Mr Dalrymple places in 54°30′ Latitude and 45° of Longitude; but on looking over D'anvill's Chart I found it laid down 9° or 10° more to the West,[3] this difference of situation was to me a Sign of the uncertainty of both and determined me to get into the Parallel as soon as possible and this was the reason of my hauling to the north at this time.

Pork to either.'—Log, 4 January.—'About 11 this fore Noon there was the most extraordinary Halo about the Sun I ever saw—it measur'd somewhat more than 22° from the Suns nearest Limb—it was in many places very thick and dark between the Limbs of it and the Sun and the Colours of the edges of the Halo a good deal resembled those of a rainbow'. —Clerke. There must have been a veil of cirrus cloud, though Clerke does not mention it, to produce this effect, which presaged bad weather: within two days it duly came.

[1] 'The Carpenters at work upon a spar we got at Norfolk Island forming it into a Main Top Gallant Mast.'—Clerke, 5 January; and 6 January (ship time): 'Carpenters converting the Mast of ye Sloop we have in store into a Main Top Gallant Mast—the Norfolk Island spar proving but indifferent.'—It was full of knots and too heavy, says Cooper.

[2] Antoine de la Roche, a London merchant of French parentage, in 1674 went on a trading voyage to Peru. It was his intention to return through the Strait of Le Maire, but high winds and currents carried him, in April 1675, to the east, where he discovered land; he anchored in a bay and remained for fourteen days in tempestuous weather, in sight of snow-covered mountains; when the weather cleared he saw further high land covered with snow to the south-east and south. He then departed for Brazil, and in 45° S discovered 'a very large and pleasant island', with a good port, but no people. Post-Cook writers conjectured that the first discovery was South Georgia; though the large and pleasant island had never been seen since. Burney thought it not improbable that La Roche had first sighted the southern part of the Falklands, and that the 'island' was Cape Santa Elena, a large projecting headland on the coast of Patagonia in lat. 45°.—Burney, III, pp. 395–403. The *León* was a Spanish merchant ship which on her homeward passage from Valparaiso round the Horn in mid-1756 was also carried east, the snow frozen on her rigging. On 29 June she sighted a small island, and then 'a Continent of land . . . full of sharp and craggy mountains of frightful aspect'; she was in sight of this land, in lat. 54°50′, for three days. The Frenchman Ducloz Guyot, who was on board, showed his journal to the geographer d'Après de Mannevillette, who communicated an abstract to Dalrymple; the latter published it, as well as accounts of La Roche, Halley and Bouvet, in his *Collection of Voyages, chiefly in the Southern Atlantick Ocean* (1775). This land must have been South Georgia.—Burney, V, pp. 136–42.

[3] Jean-Baptiste Bourguignon d'Anville (1697–1782), one of the most celebrated of French geographers, who left behind him 211 maps and plans and 78 memoirs. He was remarkable both for his learning and his caution. The 'chart' Cook refers to is his hemispheric world map of 1761, which places the 'I. de S. Pierre découv.? en 1756' in long. 36°–37° W of Ferro; i.e. 54° or 55° W of Greenwich, as against Dalrymple's 45°.

SATURDAY *7th.* Towards the Morning the gale abated and the Weather cleared up and the wind veered to WSW where it continued till middnight, after which it veered to NW; we were at this time in the Latitude of 56°4′ S, Longitude 53°36′ West, we sounded but found no bottom with a line of 130 fathoms. I still kept the Wind on the Larboard tack, having a gentle breeze and pleasent Weather. On

SUNDAY *8th* at Noon a bed of Sea weed past the Ship. In the afternoon in the Latitude of 55°4′, Longitude 51°45′ W the Variation was 20°4′ East.

MONDAY *9th.* Wind at NE attended with thick hazy weather. Saw a Seal and a piece of Sea weed. At Noon Latitude in 55°12′ S, Longitude 50°15′ West. The Wind and Weather continuing the same till towards middnight when the latter cleared up and the former Veered to West and blew a gentle gale. We continued to ply till 2 o'Clock the next morning

TUESDAY *10th* when we bore away East and at 8 ENE. At Noon observed in Latitude 54°35′ S, Longitude in 47°56′ West. A great many Albatroses and Blue Peterels about the Ship. I now steered East and the next morning

WEDNESDAY *11th* in the Latitude of 54°38′, Longitude 45°10′ West the Variation was 19°25′ East. In the after-noon saw several Penguins and some pieces of weed. Spent the night lying to & on

THURSDAY *12th* at day-break bore away and steered East northerly with a fine fresh breeze at WSW. At Noon Observed in Latitude 54°28′ S, Longitude in 42°08′ West, which is near 3° E of the Situation in which M[r] Dalrymple places the NE point of the Gulph of S[t] Sebastian, but we had no other signs of land than seeing a Seal and a few Penguins; on the Contrary we had a Swell from ESE, which could hardly have been if any extensive tract of land laid in that direction. In the evening the gale abated and at Middnight it fell Calm.

FRIDAY *13th.* The Calm attended by a thick Fogg continued till 6 o'Clock in the Morning, when we got a Wind at East but the Fogg still continued. We stood to the South till noon when being in the Latitude of 55°07′ Tacked and stretched to the North with a fresh breeze at EBS and ESE. Cloudy wea[r]. Saw several Penguins and a Snow Peterel which we looked upon to be signs of the vicinity of ice, the air too was much colder than we had felt it sence we left New Zealand. In the afternoon the Wind veered to SE and in the night to SSE and blew fresh with which we stood to the NE.

At 9 o'Clock the next morning saw[1] an Island of ice, as we then thought, but at noon we were doubtfull whether it was ice or land; at this time it bore E¾S distant 13 Leagues, our Latitude was 53°56½', Longitude 39°24' West. Several Penguins, small divers, a snow Peterel and a vast number of blue Peterels about the Ship. We had but little wind all the morning and at 2 PM it fell Calm. It was now no longer doubted but that it was land and not ice which we had in sight: it was however in a manner wholy covered with snow. We were farther confirmed of its being land by finding Soundings at 175 fathoms, a muddy bottom, the land at this time bore EBS about 12 leagues distant. At 6 o'Clock the Calm was succeeded by a breeze at NE with which we stood to SE. At first it blew a gentle gale, but afterwards increased, so as to bring us under double reefed Top-sails and was attended with Snow and Sleet.

SUNDAY 15*th*. We continued to stand to the SE till 7 in the morn^{g} when the Wind veering to the SE tacked and stood to the North. A little before we tacked we saw the land bearing EBN. At Noon the mercury in the Thermometer was at 35½°. The Wind blew in Squals attended with Snow and Sleet and we had a great sea to encounter. At a Lee Lurch which the ship took Mr Wales observed her to lay down 42°. At half an hour past 4 PM we took in the Top-sails, got down topg^{t} yards, wore the Ship and stood to the SW under two Courses. At Middnight the storm abated so that we could carry the Top-sails double reefed.

MONDAY 16*th*. At 4 in the Morning wore and stood to the East with the Wind at SSE a moderate breeze and fair. At 8 o'Clock saw the land extending from EBN to NEBN. Loosed a reef out of each Top-sail, got Topg^{t} yards across and set the Sails. At Noon observed in Latitude 54°25½', Longitude in 38°18' West, the land extending from N½W to East Six or eight leagues distant. It appeared to be very mountainous and rocky and was allmost wholy covered with Snow.[2] In this Situation we had 110 fathom water. The Northern extreme was the land which we first saw and proved to be an Island which obtained the name of *Willis's Island* after the person who first saw it.[3]

[1] *blew fresh . . . saw: MS before revision* blew a fresh gale with which the cold increased, notwithstanding we kept standing to the North. The mercury in the Thermometer at 6 oClock in the morning Saturday 14th stood at 35° and at Noon it stood at 37½°. At oClock saw . . .—f. 323; and similarly A.

[2] 'The Land which we are now off is exceeding high Steep and Cliffy and covered in most Places with Snow which gives it so much the appearance of Ice Islands at a distance that I now think it possible that which we saw in the Latit. of 67 in ye Year 73 and that in ye Lat of 71 in ye year 74 might possibly be land also.'—Wales, log, 16 January.

[3] Thomas Willis, the 'Wild & drinking' midshipman. There are more than one island,

At this time we had a swell from the South which made it probable no land was near us in that direction: but the Cold air which we felt and the vast quantity of Snow on the land in sight induced us to think that it was extensive and I chose to begin with exploring the Northern Coast. With this view we bore up for Willis's Island all sails set, having a fine gale at SSW. As we advanced to the North we preceived a nother isle lying East of Willis's island and between it and the Main. Seeing that there was a clear passage between the two isles,[1]

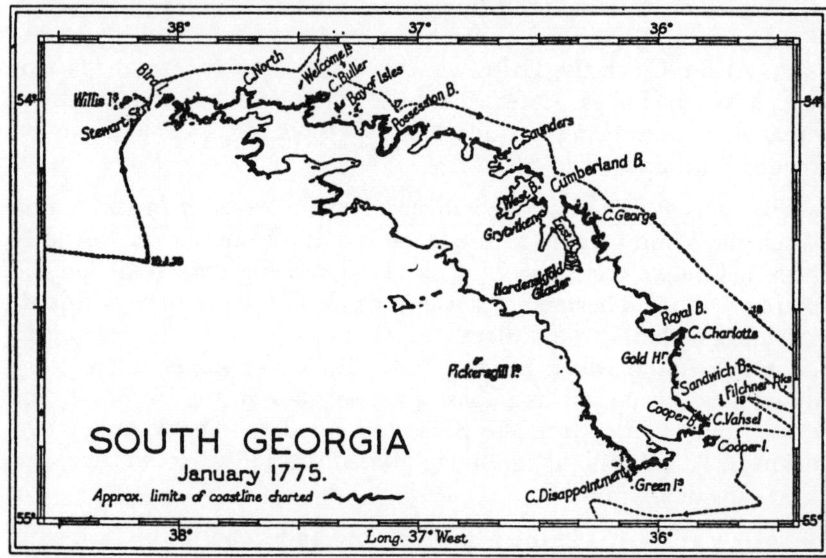

FIG. 81

we steered for it and at 5 o'Clock we were in the Middle of it and found it to be about two miles broad. Willis's isle is a high rock of no great extent, near to which are some rocky islots. It is situated in the Latitude of 54°00′ S, Longitude 38°23′ W. The other isle which obtained the name of *Bird isle,* on accou^t of the vast number that were upon it,[2] is not so high but of greater extent and lies close to the NE[3] point of the Main land which I called *Cape North.* So much as we saw of the SE Coast of this land it lies in the direction of S 50° East and N 50° W, it seemed to form several Bays or inlets and we observed huge masses of snow or ice in the bottoms of them, especially in one which lies 10 miles to the SSE of Bird isle. After geting through the

now separately named, and a number of rocks; the whole group is known as the Willis islands. Main Island, which Willis first saw, rises to 1800 feet.

[1] Stewart Strait. For this, and the next half-dozen pages, see Fig. 81.

[2] This is still true, and the island is a protected area for birds and seals.

[3] This is a slip for NW.

Passage we found the North Coast to trend EBN for about 9 miles and then East and East Southerly to *Cape Buller*[1] which is a 11 miles more. We coasted or ranged the Coast at one league distance till near 10 o'Clock when we brought to for the night and on Sounding found 55 fathoms a muddy bottom.

TUESDAY 17*th*. At 2 o'Clock in the morning made sail in for the land with a fine breeze at SW. At 4 Willis Island bore WBS distant 32 Miles, Cape Buller to the west of which lies some rocky islots,[2] bore SWBW and the most advanced point of land to the East S 63° E. We now steered along shore at the distance of 4 or 5 miles off till 7 o'Clock, when seeing the appearence of an Inlet we hauled in for it and as soon as we drew near the shore, hoisted out a Boat in which I (accompanied by Mr Forster and his party) imbarked with a View of reconoitring the Bay before we ventured in with the Ship. When we put off from the Ship which was about 4 Miles from land we had 40 fathom water. I continued to sound in going in for the shore, but could find no bottom with a line of 34 fathoms, which was the length of the one I had in the boat, and which also proved too short to sound the Bay, so far as I went up it. I found it to lie in SWBS about two leagues and to be about two miles broad and well sheltered from all Winds, and I judged there might be good Anchorage before some sandy beaches which appeared on each side, and likewise near a low flat isle near the head of the Bay.[3] As I had come to a resolution not to bring the Ship in, I did not think it worth my while to go and examine these places where it did not seem probable that any one would ever be benifited by the descovery.

The head of the Bay, as well as two places on each side, was terminated by a huge Mass of Snow and ice of vast extent, it shewed a perpendicular clift of considerable height, just like the side or face of an ice isle; pieces were continually breaking from them and floating out to sea. A great fall happened while we were in the Bay; it made a noise like Cannon. The inner parts of the Country was not less savage

[1] Lat. 53°58′ S, long. 37°22′ W. The cape was named after John Buller (1721–86), M.P. for East Looe 1747–86 and a Lord of the Admiralty 1765–79, Lord of the Treasury 1780–2. The Bullers were a well-known Cornish family, members of which held seats in the county continuously from 1620 to 1832, and did pretty well for themselves out of politics. See Namier, *Structure of Politics*, II, pp. 398–413.

[2] The Welcome islets—a later name.

[3] Cook's judgment on this day, it appears, was not at its best. Possession Bay, where he was, is the windiest place in South Georgia. As for anchorage, the *Antarctic Pilot* (2nd ed., 1948, p. 107) says, 'Assistance bay, which forms the head of Possession bay, affords possible anchorage, in a depth of 13 fathoms (23m8), mud, near the glacier. Westerly and south-westerly winds, however, blow with great force here, and the ice from the glacier, though not large, would be a constant trouble'. We do not know where Cook landed (next paragraph). See Fig. 77.

and horrible: the Wild rocks raised their lofty summits till they were lost in the Clouds and the Vallies laid buried in everlasting Snow. Not a tree or shrub was to be seen, no not even big enough to make a tooth-pick. I landed in three different places, displayed our Colours and took possession of the Country in his Majestys name under a descharge of small Arms. Our Botanists found here only three plants, the one is a coarse strong bladed grass which grows in tufts, Wild Burnet and a Plant like Moss which grows on the rocks.[1] Seals or Sea Bears were pretty numerous,[2] they were smaller than those at Staten land: perhaps the most of those we saw were females for the Shores swarm'd with young cubs. We saw none of that sort which we call Lions, but here were some which Lord Anson describes under that name,[3] at least they appeared to us to be of the same sort and are in my opinion very improperly called Lions; I was not able to see the least grounds for the comparison. Here were several Flocks of Penguins, the largest I ever saw, we brought some on board which weighed from 29 to 38 p^ds^.[4] It appears by M. Bougainvilles account of the Animals of Falkland Islands that this Penguin is there and seems to be very well described under the name of first class of Penguins, P.64.[5] The Oceanic birds were Albatross,[6] Common Gulls[7] and that sort which I call Port Egmont hens,[8] Terns,[9] Shags,[10] Divers,[11] the New White Bird[12] and a small Duck such as are at the Cape of Good Hope and known by the name of Yellow-bills;[13] we shot two and found them most delicate eating. All the Land birds we saw consisted in a few small Larks,[14] nor did we see any Quadrupedes. Mr Forster indeed saw some dung which he judged to have come from a Fox or some animal of that kind.[15] The land or rather rocks bordering on the Sea Coast, was

[1] The grass was the tussock grass *Poa flabellata* Hooker fil.; the Wild Burnet, *Acaena adscendens* Vahl. subsp. *georgiae-australis* Bitter, collected by Forster. The cushiony flowering plant *Colobanthus crassifolius* seems to have been mistaken for a moss.

[2] The Southern Fur Seal.

[3] The Elephant Seal, *Mirounga leonina* (Linn.).

[4] The King Penguin, *Aptenodytes patagonicus* J. F. Miller.

[5] 'The penguin of the first class is fond of solitude and retired places. It has a peculiar noble and magnificent appearance, having an easy gait, a long neck when singing or crying, a longer and more elegant bill than the second sort, the back of a more blueish cast, the belly of a dazzling white, and a kind of palatine or necklace of a bright yellow, which comes down on both sides of the head, as a boundary between the blue and the white, and joins on the belly.' (Forster's translation.)

[6] Various albatrosses occur at South Georgia.

[7] Probably the Southern Black-backed Gull, *Larus dominicanus* Licht.

[8] The Brown Skua.

[9] Probably the Wreathed Tern, *Sterna vittata* Gm.

[10] The South Georgian Blue-eyed Shag, *Phalacrocorax atriceps georgianus* Lönnberg.

[11] The South Georgian Diving Petrel, *Pelecanoides georgica* Murphy and Harper.

[12] A Sheath-bill, *Chionis alba* (Gm.).

[13] The South Georgian Teal, *Anas georgica* (Gm.). It does not occur at the Cape of Good Hope.

[14] The Antarctic Pipit, *Anthus antarcticus* Cab.

[15] No record exists of any native dog or fox from South Georgia.

not covered with snow like the inland parts, but all the Vegetation we could see on the clear places was the grass above mentioned. The rocks seemed to contain Iron. After having made the above observations, we set out for the Ship and got on board a little after 12 o'Clock with a quantity of Seals and Penguins, an exceptable present to the Crew. It must however not be understood that we were in want of Provisions, we had yet plenty of every kind, and sence we had been on this Coast I had ordered, in addition to the common allowance, Wheat to be boiled every morning for breakfast, but any kind of fresh meat was prefered by most on board to Salt; for my own part, I was now, for the first time heartily tired of salt meat of every kind and prefer'd the Penguins, whose flesh eat nearly as well as bullocks liver, it was however fresh and that was sufficient to make it go down. I called the Bay we had been in *Possession Bay*, it is situated in the Latitude of 54°5′ s, Longitude 37°18′ West and a 11 Leagues to the East of Cape North. A few miles to the West of Possession Bay between it and Cape Buller, lies the *Bay of isles*, so named on account of several small isles lying in and before it. As soon as the boat was hoisted in we made sail a long the Coast to the East with a fine breeze at wsw. From Cape Buller the direction of the Coast is s 72°30′ East for the space of a 11 or 12 Leagues, to a projecting point which obtained the name of *Cape Saunders*.[1] Beyond this Cape is a pretty large Bay, which I name *Cumberland Bay*. In several parts in the bottom of Cumberland Bay as also in some others of less extent lying between Cape Saunders and Possession Bay were vast tracts of frozen snow or ice not yet broke loose.[2] At 8 o'Clock, being just past Cumberland Bay and falling little Wind we hauled off the Coast, from which we were distant about 4 Miles and had 100 Fathoms Water.

We had variable light airs & Calms[3] till 6 o'Clock the next Morning, when the wind fixed at North and blew a gentle breeze, but it lasted no longer than 10 o'Clock when it fell allmost to a Calm. At Noon Observed in Latitude 54°30′ s, we were about 2 or 3 leagues from the Coast which extended from N 59° W to s 13° west, the land in this last direction was an isle which seemed to terminate the Coast

[1] Presumably after the distinguished and taciturn Admiral Sir Charles Saunders (1713?–75), under whose command Cook had served in the St Lawrence in 1759. 'Sir Charles Saunders, who loves no dish like a French ship'; 'That brave statue, Sir Charles Saunders'—Horace Walpole, *Letters* (ed. Toynbee), VIII, p. 266; IX, p. 292. It will be recollected that Cook had called a cape in New Zealand after him.—I, p. 257.

[2] Cook here notices the glaciers so much a feature of the South Georgian landscape. Cumberland Bay has two arms, West and East; into East Cumberland Bay falls the Nordenskjöld glacier, the greatest in the country. In this bay also, on the shore of King Edward Cove, is the present-day principal settlement of the island, Grytviken.

[3] *& Calms:* A so that we advanced but little

to the East. The nearest land to us was a projecting point which terminated in a round Hillock, it was, on account of the day, named *Cape Charlotte.*[1] On the West side of Cape Charlotte lies a Bay which obtained the name of *Royal Bay*, the West point of which I named *Cape George*, it is the East point of Cumberland Bay and lies in the direction of SEBE from Cape Sa[u]nders Distant 7 leagues. Cape George and Cape Charlotte lies in the direction of S 37° E and N 37° west[2] distant 6 leag^s from each other. The isle above mentioned was called *Coopers isle*, after my first Lieutenant. It lies in the direction of SBE distant 8 leagues from Cape Charlotte. The Coast between them forms a large Bay which I named *Sandwich.*[3] The Wind was variable all the after-noon, so that we advanced but little, in the night it fixed at South and SSW and blew a gentle gale attended with showers of Snow.

THURSDAY 19*th.* Was wholy spent in plying, the wind continuing at South and SSW, clear pleasent weather but cold. At sun-rise a new land was seen bearing SE½E, it first appeared in a Single hill like a Sugar Loafe; some time after other detatched pieces appeared above the Horizon, near the hill. At Noon observed in Latitude 54°42′30″ S. Cape Charlotte bore N 38° W distant 4 leagues and Coopers Isle South 31° W, in this situation a lurking rock which lies off Sandwich Bay, 5 miles from the land,[4] bore W½N distant 1 mile. Near this rock were several breakers ᵀn the after-noon we had a prospect of a ridge of mountains, behind Sandwich bay, whose lofty and icey summits were elevated high above the Clouds. The Wind continued at SSW till 6 o'Clock when it fell to a Calm. At this time Cape Charlotte bore N 31° west and Coopers Island WSW. In this situation we found the variation by the Az^th to be 11°39′ and by the Amplitude 11°12′ E. At 10 o'Clock a light breeze sprung up at North with which we steered to the South till 10, then brought to for the night.

FRIDAY 20*th.* At 2 o'Clock in the morning made sail to SW round Coopers Island, it is a rock of considerable height about 5 miles in circuit and lies one from the main.[5] At this isle the Coast takes a SW direction for the space of 4 or 5 leagues to a point which I called

[1] 18 January was the Queen's birthday.

[2] The directions are back to front: they should be N 37° W and S 37° E.

[3] This sentence rather misinterprets the relation of Cooper Island to the coast, though perhaps pardonably so from Cook's point of observation. Chart XLI (which compare with Fig. 81), is a better statement. The south-eastern limit of Sandwich Bay is Cape Vahsel; and Cooper Island is, as it were, round the corner formed by the cape. See also Fig. 76.

[4] Probably Filchner rocks, NNE of Cape Vahsel. They seem to be marked on the Cook charts, though unnamed.

[5] A Latitude 54° 51′ South, Longitude 35°54′ W.

Cape Disappointment off which lie three small isles,[1] the Southermost of which is green low and flat & lies one league from the Cape. As we advanced to SW land opened of this point in the direction of N 60° West and 9 leagues beyond it. It proved an Island quite detatched from the Main and obtained the name of *Pickersgill Island* after my third officers. Soon after a point of the main beyond this Island came in sight in the direction of N 55° West which exactly united the Coast at the very point we had seen and set the day we first came in with it and proved to a demonstration that this land which we had taken to be part of a great Continent was no more than an Island of 70 leagues in Circuit.[2] Who would have thought that an Island of no greater extent than this is, situated between the Latitude of 54° and 55°, should in the very height of Summer be in a manner wholy covered many fathoms deep with frozen Snow, but more especially the SW Coast, the very sides and craggy summits of the lofty Mountains were cased with snow and ice, but the quantity which lay in the Vallies is incredable, before all of them the Coast was terminated by a wall of Ice of considerable height. It can hardly be doubted but that a great deal of ice is formed here in the Winter which in the Spring is broke off and dispersed over the Sea:[3] but this isle cannot produce the ten thousand part of what we have seen, either there must be more land or else ice is formed without it. These reflections led me to think that the land we had seen the preceeding day might belong to an extensive tract and I still had hopes of discovering a continent. I must Confess the disapointment I now met with did not affect me much, for to judge of the bulk by the sample it would not be worth the discovery. This land I called the *Isle of Georgia* in honor of H. Majesty.[4] It is situated between the Latitudes

[1] Green Islets—Cook's name on the engraved chart; 'the Southermost is green, low and flat'—A 321. They 'appeared to have some verdure on them'.—Forster, II, p. 525.

[2] Cf. Clerke, 17 January: 'the Captain and Botanical Gentry went on shore to take possession of this new Country (Southern Continent I hope) . . .'—followed by his 'Account of this Isle', 20 January: 'I did flatter myself from the distant soundings and the high Hills about it, we had got hold of the Southern Continent, but alas these pleasing dreams are reduc'd to a small Isle, and that a very poor one too—as to its appearance in general I think it exceeds in wretchedness both Terra del Fuego and Staten Land which places 'till I saw this, I thought might vie with any of the works of Providence in that particular.'

[3] Cf. p. cii above. Although there are many glaciers in South Georgia, the bergs that calve from them generally break up and melt before they can reach the open sea. Cook, however, forms a valid theory of the origin of bergs.

[4] Cook, it is alleged, did not honour His Majesty unprompted. 'As it had been the main object of our voyage to explore the high southern latitude[s], my father suggested to captain Cook, that it would be proper to name this land after the monarch who had set on foot our expedition, solely for the improvement of science, and whose name ought therefore to be celebrated in both hemispheres, [here follows the appropriate quotation from Horace]. It was accordingly honoured with the name of Southern Georgia, which will give it importance, and continue to spread a degree of lustre over it, which it cannot

of 53°57′ and 54°57′ South and between 38°13′ and 35°54′ West Longitude, it extends SEBE and NWBW and is 31 leagues long in that direction and its greatest breadth is about 10 Leagues.[1] It seems to abound in Bays and Harbours, the NE coast especially, but the great quantity of Ice must render them inaccessable the greatest part of the year or at least it must be dangerous lying in them on account of the breaking up of the Ice clifts.[2]

It is remarkable that we did not see a River or stream of fresh Water on the whole coast. I think it highly probable that their are no Perennial Springs in the Country and that the Interiour parts, as being much elevated, never enjoys heat enough to melt the Snow in such quantities as to produce a River or stream of Water. The Coast alone only receives warmth sufficient to melt the snow and this only on the NE side, for the other, which is in a great degree deprived of the Suns rays by the great height of the Mountains[3] and lying exposed to the Cold South Winds, seemed from its aspect to be doomed by Nature to Frigidity the greatest part of the year.[4] It was from a supposition that the Sea Coast of a Land situated in the Latitude of 54° could not in the very height of summer be wholy covered with snow, that I supposed Bouvet['s] discovery to be large Islands of Ice. But after I had seen this land[5] I no longer doubted the existence of Cape Circumcision, and did not doubt but that I should find more land than I should have time to explore. With these Ideas I queted this Coast and directed my Course to the East South East for the land we had seen the preceeding day. The Wind was very variable till noon when it fixed at NNE and blew a gentle gale, but it increased in such a manner that before 3 o'Clock we were reduced to our two Courses and obliged to strike Topg[t] yards. We were certainly very fortunate in geting clear of the land before this gale overtook us; it is hard to say what might have been the consequence had it come on while we were on the North coast. This Storm was of short duration, for at 8 o'Clock it began to abate and at Middnight it was little wind and we took the oppertunity to Sound, but found no bottom with a line of 180 fathoms.

derive from its barrenness and dreary appearance'.—Forster, II, pp. 525–6. Even after this the royal bounty did not extend to J. R. Forster. A minor point is that Forster's name ('Southern') is not Cook's.

[1] South Georgia is about 116 miles long NW and SE, and about 20 miles wide.

[2] *or at least . . . clifts:* A at least it is reasonable to think so: if the Winter could [cold] bear any sort of proportion to that of the Summer. During the time we have been about this land, the Mercury in the Thermometer at Noon has generally been between 39 and 41.

[3] *Mountains:* A savage Mountains

[4] A The Frigid, Gloomy and Savage aspect which nature has given to this Country exceeds every thing that could have been imagined.

[5] A and the manner these ice islands were formed

SATURDAY 21*st*. The Storm was succeeded by a thick Fog attended with rain, the Wind veered to NW and at 5 o'Clock in the Morng it fell Calm, which continued till 8 and then we got a breeze Southerly with which we stood to the East, till 3 in the after noon when the Weather became some what clear, we made Sail and Steered North in search of the land. At half past Six we were again involved in a thick Mist which made it necessary to haul the Wind and spend the night makeing short boards.

SUNDAY 22*nd*. Variable light airs next to a Calm and thick Foggy weather till half past 7 o'Clock in the evening when we got a fine breeze at North and the weather was so clear that we could see two or three leagues round us; we laid hold of the oppertunity and steered to the west, judgeing we were to the East of the land. After runing 10 miles to the west the Weather became again Foggy and we hauled the Wind and spent the night under Top-sails.

MONDAY 23*rd*. At 6 o'Clock in the Morning the fog cleared away so that we could see 3 or 4 miles. I took the oppertunity to Steer again West with the Wind at East a fresh breeze, but two hours after a thick fog obliged us to haul the wind again to the South. At 11 o'Clock a short interval of clear weather gave us a Sight of 3 or 4 rocky Islots extending from SE to ENE two or three miles distant; but we did not see the Sugar Loafe peak before mentioned, indeed two or three miles was the utmost we could see. We were well assured that this was the land we had seen before and which we had now been quite round and therefore could be no more than a few detatched rocks, inhabited by Birds of which we saw vast numbers, especially Shags who gave us notice of the nearness of land before we saw it. These Rocks lie in the Latitude of 55°00′ S and S 75° E distant 12 Leagues from Coopers isle. The interval of clear weather was of very short duration before we had as thick a fog as ever, attend with rain, on this we tacked in 60 fathom Water and stood to the North, and thus we spent our time involved in a continual thick Mist and for aught we knew surrounded by dangerous rocks; the Shags and Soundings were our best Pilots, for after we had stood a few miles to the North we got out of Soundings and saw no more Shags. The day and the succeeding night was spent in makeing short boards and at 8 o'Clock the next morning

TUESDAY 24*th* Judgeing our selves not far from the rocks by some stragling shags which came about us we sounded in 60 fathom Water, the bottom Stones and broken Shells. Soon after saw the rocks bearing SSW½W four miles distant, but still we did not see the peak, it was no doubt beyond our horizon which was limeted to a short distance, indeed we had but a transitory sight of the other rocks before they were again lost in the Fog. With a light air of Wind at North and a great swell from NE we were able to clear the rocks to the West and at 4 in the PM judgeing our selves to be 3 or 4 leagues east and west of them I steered South, being quite tired with cruzing about them in a thick fog. Nor was it worth my while to spend any more time in waiting for clear weather only for the sake of having a good sight of a few stragling rocks. At 7 o'Clock we had at intervals a clear Sky to the West which gave us a sight of the Mountains of the Isle of Georgia bearing WNW about 8 Leagues distant. At 8 o'Clock we steered SEBS and at 10 SEBE with a fresh breeze at North attended with a very thick fog, but we were in some measure acquainted with the Sea we were runing over. The rocks above mentioned obtained the name of *Clerke's Rocks*,[1] after my second officers, he being the first who saw them.

WEDNESDAY 25*th*. Steered ESE with a fresh gale at NNE attended with very Foggy weather, till towards the evining when the sky became clear and we found the Variation to be 9°26′ East, being at this time in the Latitude of 56°16′ S, Longitude 32°9′ W.

THURSDAY 26*th*. Having continued to steer ESE with a fine gale at NNW till day-light this morning, when seeing no land to the East, I gave orders to steer South. At this time we were in the Latitude of 56°33′ S, Longit 31°10′ west. The Weather continued clear and gave us an oppertunity to observe several distances of the Sun and Moon for the correcting our Longitude, which at Noon was 31°04′ west, the Latitude observed 57°38′ S. We continued to steer to the South till

FRIDAY 27*th*[2] At Noon, at which time we were in the Latitude of 59°46′ S and had so thick a fog that we could not see a Ships length. It was therefore no longer safe to sail before the Wind as we were soon to expect to fall in with ice and therefore hauled to the East having a gentle breeze at NNE. Soon after the fog cleared away and we resumed our Course to the South till 4 o'Clock when it returned again as thick as ever and made it necessary for us to haul upon a wind. I now reckoned we were in the Latitude 60° and farther I did

[1] They lie in two groups about 35 to 40 miles ESE of Cooper Island; the highest of the western group rises to 800 feet. For the ship's track round them, see Chart XLI.

[2] '[a.m.] Found the Miz. Topmast sprung, six Inches above the Cap; struck it and made another fid hole to let the Sprung part come into the Cap ...'—Log.

not intend to go, unless I met with some certain signs of soon meeting with land, for it would not have been prudent in me to have spent my time in penetrating to the South when it was, at least as probable, that a large tract of land might be found near Cape Circumcision; besides I was now tired of these high Southern Latitudes where nothing was to be found but ice and thick fogs. We had now a long hollow swell from the West, a strong indication that there was no land in that direction. I think I may now venture to assert that that extensive coast, laid down in Mr Dalrymple's Chart of the Ocean between Africa and America, and the Gulph of St Sebastian does not exist. I too doubt if either Le Roche or the Ship Lion ever saw the Isle of Georgia, but this is a point I will not dispute as I neither know where they were bound or from whence they came, when they made the discovery; if it should be the same, Mr Dalrymple has placed it half a degree of Latitude too far South and 7° of Longitude too far West, and M. D'Anville 15 or 16 degrees, the only two Charts I have seen it inserted in; but be it how it will, I will allow them the merit of leading me to the discovery, for if it had not been on these maps, it is very probable I had passed to the South of it.

At 7 o'Clock in the evening the fog receded from us a little and gave us a sight of an ice island, several Penguins and some Snow Peterels, we sounded but found no ground at 140 f^ms^. The fog soon returned again and we spent the night makeing boards over that space we had in some degree made our selves acquainted with in the day.

SATURDAY 28*th*. At 8 o'Clock in the morning we stood to the East with a gentle gale at North, the weather began to clear up and we found the Sea strewed with large and small ice, several Penguins, Snow Peterels and other birds were seen and some Whales. Soon after we had sun shine, but the air was cold, the mercury in the Thermometer stood generally at 35, but at Noon it was at 37, the Latitude by observation was 60°04′ S, Longitude 29°23′ W. Continued to stand to the East till half an hour past two o'Clock PM, when we fell in all at once with a vast number of large Ice islands, and a Sea strewed with loose ice,[1] the Weather too was become thick and hazy attended with drizling rain and sleet and made it the more dangerous to stand in among the ice, for which reason we tacked and stood back to the West with the Wind at North. The Ice islands, which at this time surrounded us, were nearly all of equal height and shewed a flat even Surface, but they were of various extent, some were two

[1] 'vast quantities of loose Ice which we find floating about on all sides of us . . .'—Clerke.

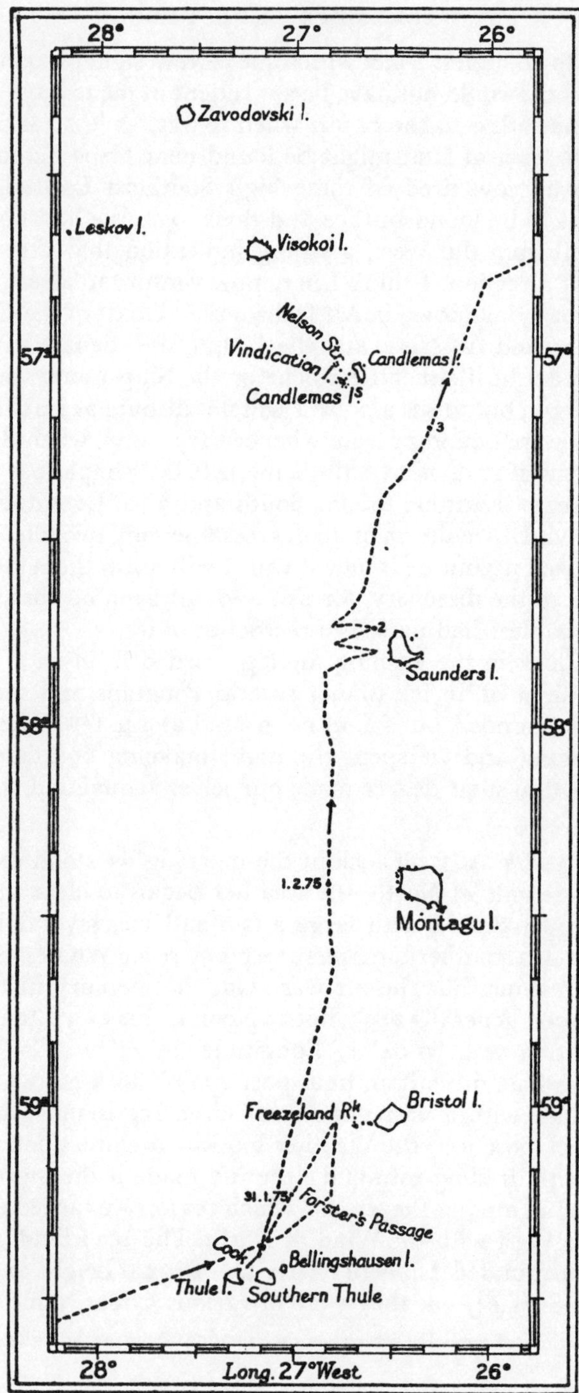

FIG. 82. The South Sandwich Islands

or three miles in circuit.[1] The loose ice was what had broke from thes isles.[2]

SUNDAY 29*th*. In the morning the Wind fell and veered to SW and we steered NE, but this Course was soon interrupted by numerous ice islands, and having but very little Wind we were obliged to steer such Courses as carried us the clearest of them, so that during this 24 hours we hardly made any advance one way or a nother. Abundance of Whales and Penguins were about us all the day. The Weather was fair but dark and gloomy.

MONDAY 30*th*. At Middnight the Wind began to freshen at NNE with which we stood to NW till 6 in the morning, when the wind veered to NNW and we Tacked and stood to NE and soon after sailed through a good deal of loose ice and pass'd two large islands. Except a short interval of clear weather about 9 o'Clock, it was continually foggy with either snow or sleet. At Noon we were by our reckoning in the Latitude of 59°30′ S, Longitude 29°24′ West. We Continued to stand to NE with a fresh breeze at NNW and at 2 o'Clock pass'd one of the largest Ice islands we had seen the Voyage and some time after passed two others, which were much smaller. Weather still Foggy with sleet and the Wind continued at NBW with which we stood to NE over a Sea strewed with ice.

TUESDAY 31*st*. At half an hour past six o'Clock in the Morning, as we were standing NNE with the wind at West, the fog very fortunately cleared away a little and we discovered land ahead 3 or 4 miles distant; on this, we hauled the wind to the North, but finding we could not weather the land on this tack, we soon after tacked in 175 fathom Water three miles from the shore and about half a league from some breakers. Soon after we had tacked, the weather cleared up a little more and gave us a tolerable good sight of the land. That which we had fell in with proved three rocky islots of considerable height, the outer most terminated in a lofty Peak like a Sugar Loaf and obtained the name of *Freezland Peak*, after the Man who first discovered it[3] (Lat 59°00′ S, Longit. 27°00′ W). Behind this Peak, that is to the West[4] of it, appeared an elevated coast, whose lofty and

[1] This is a description of typical tabular bergs.

[2] In spite of this definite statement, it seems probable that this 'loose ice' was the northern edge of the pack; p. ciii above.

[3] Samuel Freezland (perhaps originally Friesland) a Dutch A.B. It is 'a magnificent structure with a towering pillar of rock' 900 feet high and a secondary peak of about 620 feet.—*Antarctic Pilot*, p. 127. The three 'islets' are called 'Freezlands Rocks' on Chart XLII; now Freezeland, Wilson and Grindle Rocks. See Fig. 78.

[4] This is a slip for east, repeated in A and H; it is noted in the margin of A by a later hand, and is corrected in print.

snowey summits were seen above the Clouds, it extended from NBE to ESE. I called it *Cape Bristol*,[1] in honour of the Noble family of *Hervey's*. At the same time a nother elevated Coast appeared in sight, bearing SWBS and at noon it extended from SE to SSW from 4 to 8 Leagues distant, at this time the observed latitude was 59°13′30″ S, Longitude 27°45′ W. I called this land *Southern Thule* because it is the most southern land that have yet been descovered: it shews a surface of vast height and is every where covered with Snow.[2] Some thought they saw land in the space between Thule and Cape Bristol; it is more than probable that these two lands are connected and that this space was a deep Bay which I called *Forsters Bay*.[3] At 1 o'Clock finding that we could not Weather Thule, we Tacked and stood to the North and at 4 Freezland Peak bore East distant 3 or 4 Leagues; soon after it fell little wind and we were left to the mercy of a great Westerly swell which set right upon the shore; we sounded but a line of 200 fathoms found no bottom. At 8 o'Clock the weather, which had been very hazy, cleared up, and we saw Cape Bristol bearing ESE, it terminated in a point to the North beyond which we could see no land; this discovery relieved us from the disagreeable anxiety of being carryed by the swell upon the most horrible Coast in the World[4] and we continued to stand to the North all night with a light breeze at west.

[FEBRUARY 1775]

WEDNESDAY Febry 1*st*. At 4 o'Clock in the Morning we got a faint breeze at SW, at the same time we got sight of a new coast, which at 6 o'Clock bore N 60° East. It proved a high promontary which I named *Cape Montagu*, situated in Latitude 58°27′ S, Longitude 26°44′ W and 7 or 8 leagues to the North of Cape Bristol, we saw land from space to space between them, which made us conclude that the whole was

[1] It was Bristol Island, which rises to 3600 feet, though only five miles long east to west. Cook was experiencing typical South Sandwich weather of the better kind—i.e. it was at least possible to see bits of the islands, not entirely lost in fog, mist and snow.

[2] 'This being the southernmost extremity of the land, my father named it Southern Thule, a name which captain Cook has preserved.'—Forster, II, p. 536. This story at least is not an unlikely one, as Forster would be more in touch with legend than was Cook. There are three islands: the westernmost is Thule; the middle, the largest one, rising to the 3,660 feet of Mount Harmer, is now called Cook; the easternmost is Bellingshausen. See Fig. 82.

[3] Forster's Passage, 27 miles across.

[4] 'What we've hitherto seen of this Land is I believe as wretched a Country as Nature can possibly form—the shores are formed of rocky and Icy Cliffs and precipices—we've not yet seen a Hole we cou'd shove a Boat in, much less the Ship; we here and there see Points of Land which must doubtlessly form Bays &c but the intermediate spaces are quite chok'd up with Ice, which breaks off in perpendicular Cliffs into the Sea as high as the adjacent shores; at some short intervals when the Haze clears a little, we see Mountains of immense bulk and height a distance in Land, but totally cover'd with Snow as is the whole face of the Country throughout.'—Clerke.

connected.[1] I was sorry I could not determine this with greater certainty, but prudence would not permit me to venture near a Coast, subject to thick fogs, on which there was no anchorage, and where every Port was blocked or filled up with ice and the whole Country, from the summits of the Mountains down to the very brink of the clifts which terminate the Coast, was covered many fathoms thick with ever lasting snow. The clifts alone was all which was to be seen like land. Several large Ice islands lay upon the Coast, one of which attracted my notice; it had a flat surface, was of a considerable extent both in height and circuit and had perpendicular sides, on which the Waves of the Sea had made no sort of impression, by which I judged that it had not been long at sea and conjectured that it might have lately come out of some bay on the coast where it had been formed. At Noon we were East and West of the Northern part of Cape Montagu, distant about 5 Leagues and Freezland Peak bore s°16′ East distant 12 leagues, Latitude Obs[d] 58°25′ s. In the Morning the Variation was 10°11′ East.

At 2 o'Clock in the after noon, as we were standing to the north with a light breeze at sw we saw land bearing N 25° East distant 14 leagues, Cape Montagu bore at this time s 66° East. At 8 it bore s 40° E Cape Bristol SBE and the new land extending from N 40° to 52° East, and we thought we saw land more to the East and beyond it. We continued to steer to the north all night and at 6 o'Clock the next morning

THURSDAY *2nd* a new land was seen bearing N 12° E about 10 leagues distant, it appeared in two hummocks just peeping above the horizon and we soon after lost sight of them and got the wind at NNE a fresh breeze with which we stood for the northermost land we had seen yesterday, which at this time bore ESE. We fetched in with it by 10 o'Clock, but could not weather it and was obliged to tack 3 miles from the Coast which extended from EBS to SE, it had much the appearence of being an island of about 8 or 10 leagues circuit, it shews a surface of considerable hieght whose summit was lost in the Clouds and like all the other lands covered with a sheet of snow and Ice, except on a projecting point on the north side and two hills seen over this point which probably might be two islands. These only were

[1] Montagu Island, the largest of the group, 6½ miles across and 4,500 feet high. But of course the 'land from space to space' between it and 'Cape Bristol' was an illusion; the two islands are 31 miles apart. It is possible that in the existing poor weather conditions Cook saw heavy pack ice, which he took for land, between the two islands. Dr Herdman (to whom I owe this suggestion) considers that at this time of year the northern limit of ice may well have extended up to Southern Thule.

clear of snow and seemed to be covered with a green turf.[1] Some large Ice islands laid to the NE and some others to the South. We stood off till Noon and then stood in for the land again, in order to verify whether it was an Island or no. The Weather was now become very hazy, which soon turned to a thick fog, put a stop to discovery and made it not safe to stand for the land, so that after having run the same distance in as we had run off, we tacked and stood to NW for the land we had seen in the Morning, which was yet at a considerable dist^{ce}. Thus we were obliged to leave the other, under the supposition of its being an Island, which I named *Saunders*, after my honourable friend Sr Charles.[2] It is situated in the Latitude of 57°49′ S, Longitude 26°44′ West and North distant 13 Leagues from Cape Montagu. At 6 o'Clock in the evening the Wind shifted to the West and we tacked and stood to the North. At 8 the fog cleared away and gave us a sight of Saunders's Isle extending from SEBS to ESE. We were still in doubt if it was an island, for at this time land was seen bearing EBS which might or might not be connected with it. It might also be the same as we had seen the preceeding evening,[3] but be this which way it will, it was now necessary to take a View of the land to the North before we proceeded any farther to the East.[4] With this view we stood to the north with a light breeze at WBS which at 2 o'clock in the morning of

FRIDAY *3rd* was succeded by a Calm which continued till 8, when we got a breeze at EBS attended with hazy weather. At this time we saw the land we were looking after and which proved to be two isles; the day on which they were discovered was the occasion of calling them *Candlemas Isles* (Latitude 57°11′ S, Longitude 27°06′ W). They are of no great extent, but have a considerable height and were covered with Snow; a small rock was seen between them, perhaps there may lie more, for the Weather was so hazy that we soon lost sight of them and did not see them again till Noon, at which time

[1] A *note:* Some were of opinion that it was nothing but a bare Rock which is rather more probable than its being cover'd with a green turf.—The words 'than its . . . turf' are added to the note in Cook's hand. G has the note as far as 'probable'; B, f. 332 has it, deleted.—Green patches are not unlikely to have been seen—not tussock grass, which does not grow on the South Sandwich islands, but probably some cryptogam, such as favours penguin rookeries; the islands are a great resort for penguins.

[2] Cf. p. 623, n. 1 above.

[3] It probably was—what Cook refers to in the preceding entry in the words 'we thought we saw land more to the East and beyond it'. But it was not land. Chart XLII has a bulge of land in this position, unnamed; in the engraved chart this is reduced to a line with the inscription 'Large Ice Isles'—which were probably what was seen, if the appearance was not merely an effect of heavy cloud.

[4] 'Serv'd double distill'd Spirit for the people's Grog having no more Cape Brandy or Arrack on board, which is mix'd 7 to 1, a very hot disagreeable mixture, tho' weak.'—Cooper.

they bore West distant 3 or 4 leagues.[1] A great swell from the North assured us that there was no large land in that direction, we were however obliged to Stand to the NE as the Wind kept veering to the South in which rout we met with several large ice islands, loose ice and many Penguins, and at Midnight came at once into extraordinary White water, which alarmed the officer of the Watch so much that he tacked the Ship instantly, some thought it was a float of ice, others that it was shallow Water, but as it proved neither the one nor the other, it is probable it was a shoal of fish.[2]

SATURDAY *4th.* We stood to the South till 2 o'Clock in the morning, when we resumed our Course to the East with a faint breeze at SSE which ended in a Calm at six. I took the oppertunity of the Calm to put a boat in the Water to try if there was any current, the tryal proved there was none. Some Whales were playing about us and abundance of Penguins, a few of the latter were shot,[3] they proved to be of the same sort as we had seen among the ice before and different to both those on Staten land and those we got at the Isle of Georgia.

[1] The Candlemas Islands provide a better example of observation on the part of Cook than of some navigators who came later. Bellingshausen, who proved the insular nature of the South Sandwich group in general, thought there were three of them, being probably deceived at a distance by the low snow-free part of the larger of the two, looking as if it were separate. C. A. Larsen, manager of a Norwegian whaling expedition in 1908, reported only one, as did the German South Polar expedition of 1910–12. It was left to the *Discovery II* expedition of 1929–31 to put the matter beyond doubt, and to vindicate Cook by giving separate names to the two islands, Candlemas and Vindication. The strait between them, Nelson Strait, is about two miles wide; a reef extends half-way across from Vindication, on which is the rock that Cook saw, together with others that he thought might exist ('perhaps there may lie more'). The largest is now called Cook Rock. See Fig. 82.

[2] 'Just before 12 this Evening I saw a change in the Colour of the Water that a good deal alarm'd me—it was a large patch as perfectly white as milk of about a 100 Yards diameter; the Weather was Cloudy and very dark and when we first observ'd this extraordinary appearance, it was close under the lee Bow. I immediately put the Helm down for I apprehended danger from it, but what with the large swell and little Winds she miss'd stays and of course fell round off into it. I threw over the Lead but cou'd find no Ground; I took up a bucket of water upon a supposition it might possibly be small Ice, but there was not the least particle of Ice or any other perceptible matter in the water, so what cou'd occasion this strange change in the Colour of it, I'm still at a loss to divine—some are of opinion it might be the spawn of Fish—possibly it might, but for my own part I've frequently seen large quantities of Spawn which in the Night has a very extraordinary show in the Water—but I never had any idea and have very little now of its affecting so very great a change as we last night met with.—A swell from the NW: Many Whales, Penguins, Fulmers &c &c &c about and many Ice Isles around. Observ'd Lat^{de} 56°44′ s.'—Clerke, who was the officer of the watch. This discoloration of the sea-water continues to puzzle modern observers. Dr Herdman writes: 'I have never seen this milky water myself, though I do know that others have—and in recent years. Almost certainly it has nothing to do with the animal life, and it is much more likely to be a physical condition due to melting ice or some sharp temperature change. Any big concentration of 'krill' (whale food) would almost certainly have resulted in the presence of *feeding* whales; and although dense concentrations of fish are known near South Georgia, these attract millions of birds'.

[3] This was no doubt the Antarctic Pengiun, *Pygoscelis antarctica*, which is abundant at the South Sandwich islands.

It is remarkable that we have not seen a Seal sence we left that Coast.[1] At Noon we were in the Latitude of 56°44′ s, Longit 25°33′ w. At this time we got a breeze at East with which we stood to the South with a view of gaining the Coast we had left. But at 8 o'Clock the Wind shifted to the South and made it necessary for to tack and stand to the East, in which Course we met with several ice Islands and some loose ice; the Weather continued hazy with snow and rain.

SUNDAY 5*th*. This day we saw no Penguins, we also observed that the Sea was changed to its usual Colour, whereas all the time we were about the land or rather from our falling in with the Isle of Georgia, to this day it had been of a pale or Milkish colour, the same as Water tinged with milk: this Colour was not caused by the reflection of Clouds, &c[a] as is sometimes the case, because it kept the same Colour after it was taken up out of the Sea, had we been all the time in Soundings I should have thought that had been the Cause of it, but as we were not I confess myself at a loss how to account for it: let what will have been the cause I no where ever saw Sea Water of so pale a Colour before. The Sea resuming its usual colour and the Penguins leaving us, as it were all at once, made us conjecture[2] that we were leaving the land behind us and that we had already seen its northern extremity. At Noon we were in the Latitude of 57°8′ s, Longitude 23°34′ west, which was 3°00′ of Longitude to the East of Saunders isle; it was not possible for us to gain this westing without much time for in the after noon the Wind shifted to that direction; this however enabled us to stretch to the south and to get into the Latitude of the land, that if it took an East direction we might again fall in with it. In the Latitude of 57°15′ s, Longitude 23°00′ w the Variation was 5°18′ East.

MONDAY 6*th*. We continued to steer to the South and SE till noon at which time we were in the Latitude of 58°15′ s, Longitude 21°34′ West and seeing neither land nor signs of any, I concluded that what we had seen, which I named *Sandwich Land*[3] was either a group of

[1] AGH have a footnote here, 'As this is the breeding Season, it is very probable, that this Southern land is too Cold'. B f. 333 has the note, but deleted, with Cook's characteristic 'could' for 'cold'.

[2] The passage 'we also observed . . . made us conjecture' is in the MS, f. 333, marked 'omit' in Cook's hand, but is not deleted; at the beginning he has written, interlineally, 'which made me conjecture'. The other MSS have the passage. Why Cook should wish to omit it (it is not in the printed version) I cannot guess: he is not as a rule averse from admitting ignorance or perplexity.

[3] 'which I named Sandwich land' is an interlinear addition, not in A or G. H has a footnote by Cook, 'I gave this land the Name of *Sandwich* in honor of the Earl of Sandwich'.—'Captain Cook at first gave it the general name of Snowland, but afterwards

Islands or else a point of the Continent, for I firmly beleive that there is a tract of land near the Pole, which is the Source of most of the ice which is spread over this vast Southern Ocean: and I think it also probable that it extends farthest to the North opposite the Southern Atlantick and Indian Oceans, because ice has always been found farther to the north in these Oceans[1] than any where else which, I think, could not be if there was no land to the South, I mean a land of some considerable extent; for if we suppose there is not, and that ice may be formed without, it will follow of Course that the cold ought to be every where nearly equal round the Pole, as far as 70° or 60° of Latitude, or so far as to be out of the influence of any of the known Continents, consequently we ought to see ice every where under the same Parallel or near it, but the Contrary has been found. It is but few ships which have met with ice going round Cape Horn and we saw but little below the sixtieth degree of Latitude in the *Southern Pacifick Ocean.* Whereas in this ocean between the Meridion of 40° West and 50° or 60° East we have found Ice as far north as 51°. Bouvet found some in 48°[2] and others have seen it in a much lower Latitude. It is however true that the greatest part of this Southern Continent (supposeing there is one) must lay within the Polar Circile where the Sea is so pestered with ice, that the land is thereby inacessible. The risk one runs in exploreing a coast in these unknown and Icy Seas, is so very great, that I can be

honoured it with that of Sandwich Land. . . . It remains very doubtful, whether the different projecting points of Thule, Cape Bristol, and Cape Montague, form one connected land, or several distinct islands; and this may probably continue undetermined for ages to come, since an expedition to those inhospitable parts of the world, besides being extremely perilous, does not seem likely to be productive of great advantages to mankind'. —Forster, II, p. 539. Such is the perversity of mankind, however, that the group was visited again in less than fifty years. Bellingshausen with the Russian naval vessels *Vostok* and *Mirny* discovered the three northern islands of the group, unsighted by Cook, Zavodovski, Visokoi and Leskov (which he called collectively the Traverse Islands) on 22–23 December 1819; and then passed south-eastward of the others. He brought back drawings, precisely defined, of Saunders, Montagu, Bristol and Southern Thule.

[1] Southern Atlantick and Indian Oceans . . . these Oceans *altered from* Southern Atlantick Ocean, that is between Africa and America . . . this Ocean.—The other MSS have the earlier form. Evidently Cook thought over his data again after his first version. The most northerly part of the Antarctic continent is the Trinity peninsula of Graham Land, south-eastward of Cape Horn; its northernmost extreme is in lat. 63°09′, long. 56°46′ W. Enderby Land, from lat. 67°10′, long. 45° E to about lat. 66°, long. 55° E, is roughly south of Madagascar. The coast from Kaiser Wilhelm Land to Wilkes Land, lat. 66°30′–66°05′, long. 86°–136° E, is south of the eastern part of the Indian Ocean and the western half of Australia. It appears then that Cook's second thoughts were an improvement on his first —though the continent is some degrees farther south of the Atlantic than in other places. In such thoughts we must of course take account of his reserved judgment over the nature of 'Sandwich Land'. For the movements of ice see Fig. 10; and for the effect of the cold water current from the Weddell Sea, pp. lix, cvi above.

[2] A has a footnote here in Cook's hand, 'M[r] Dalrymple, in his Momoir to the Chart of this Ocean, I think, mentions Ice being seen in Lat[d] 36°–'. The following words in the text, 'and others . . . Latitude', seem to be an adaptation of this.

bold to say, that no man will ever venture farther than I have done and that the lands which may lie to the South will never be explored. Thick fogs, Snow storms, Intense Cold and every other thing that can render Navigation dangerous one has to encounter and these difficulties are greatly heightned by the enexpressable horrid aspect of the Country, a Country doomed by Nature never once to feel the warmth of the Suns rays, but to lie for ever buried under everlasting snow and ice. The Ports which may be[1] on the Coast are in a manner wholy filled up with frozen Snow of a vast thickness, but if any should so far be open as to admit a ship in, it is even dangerous to go in, for she runs a risk of being fixed there for ever, or coming out in an ice island. The islands and floats of ice on the Coast, the great falls from the ice clifts in the Port, or a heavy snow storm attended with a sharp frost, would prove equally fatal. After such an explanation as this the reader must not[2] expect to find me much farther to the South. It is however not for want of inclination but other reasons. It would have been rashness in me to have risked all which had been done in the Voyage, in finding out and exploaring a Coast which when done would have answerd no end whatever, or been of the least use either to Navigation or Geography or indeed any other Science; Bouvets Discovery was yet before us, the existence of which was to be cleared up[3] and lastly we were now not in a condition to undertake great things, nor indeed was there time had we been ever so well provided. These reasons induced me to alter the Course to East, with a very strong gale at North attended with an exceeding heavy fall of Snow, the quantity which fell into our sails was so great that we were obliged every now and then to throw the Ship up in the Wind to shake it out of the Sails, otherways neither them nor the Ship could have supported the wieght. In the evening it ceased to snow, the weather cleared up, the Wind backed to the West and we spent the night makeing two short boards under close reefed Topsails and fore-sail.

TUESDAY *7th.* At Day-break resumed our Course to the East with a very fresh gale at SWBW attend by a high sea from the same direction. In the after noon, being in the Latitude of 58°24′ S, Longitude 16°19′ west, the variation was 1°52′ East. Only 3 Ice islands seen to day. At 8 o'Clock shortned sail and hauled the Wind to the South East for the night, in which we had several showers of snow and sleet.

[1] 'may be' erased in A and 'are' substituted by Cook.
[2] *must not:* A of this Journal will hardly
[3] *the existence . . . cleared up:* A the extent of which we had no knowlidge

WEDNESDAY *8th.* At Day-light resumed our East Course with a gentle breeze and fair weather. After sun-rise being then in the Latitude of 58°30′ s, Longit 15°14′ w the variation by the mean results of two Compasses was 2°43′ E. These observations were more to be depended upon than those made last night, there being much less Sea now than then. In the after-noon pass'd three ice islands. The night was spent as the preceding one.

THURSDAY *9th.* At Six o'Clock in the Morning, being in the Latitude of 58°27′ s, Longit 13°04′ west the Variation was 0°26′ East and in the after-noon, being in the same Latitude and about a quarter of a degree more to the East, it was 0°02′ West. This situation may therefore be taken for the point through which the line passeth where the Compass has no variation. We had a Calm the most part of the day, the Weather fair and clear, excepting now and then a snow shower. The Mercury in the Thermometer at Noon rose to 40, whereas for these several days past it has been no higher than 36 or 38. We had several Ice islands in sight but no one thing that could induce us to think that any land was in our neighbourhood. At 8 o'Clock in the evening a breeze sprung up at SE with which we stood to NE.

FRIDAY *10th.* During the preceding night the Wind freshned and veered to South, which enabled us to steer East. The Wind was attended with Showers of Sleet and Snow till day light when the weather became fair, but piercing cold, so that the Water on deck was frozen and at Noon the mercury in the Thermometer was no higher than 34½. At 6 o'Clock in the morning the variation was 0°23′ west being then in the Latitude of 58°15′ s, Longit 11°41′ west, and at 6 o'Clock in the Evening, being in the same Latitude and in the Longitude of 9°24′ w, it was 1°51′ West. In the evening the Wind abated and during the night it was variable between the South and West. Ice Islands continually in sight.

SATURDAY *11th.* Wind Westerly light airs, attended with heavy Showers of Snow in the Morning, but as the day advanced the Weather became fair cleare and serene. Still continuing to Steer East, at Noon observed in 58°11′ Latitude, Longitude in at the same time 7°55′ w. Thermometer 34⅔. In the after noon we had two hours Calm, after which we had faint breezes between the NE and SE.

SUNDAY *12th.* At 6 o'Clock in the Morning, being in the Latitude of 58°23′ s Longitude 6°54′ West the variation was 3°23′ w. Had variable light airs next to a Calm all this day, and the Weather was fair and clear, till towards the evening when it became Clouded with snow Showers and the air very cold. Ice Islands continually in sight, the most of them small and breaking to Pieces. Not the least signs of land to be seen. Yesterday, Sour Krout, a most necessary and valuable article, was all expended.

MONDAY 13*th*. AM had fresh gales at SSE, and fair Weather. At 6 o'Clock, being in the Latitude of 58°03′, Longitude 5°37′ W the Variation was 4°25′ West. In the after-noon the wind increased, the Sky became Clouded and soon after had a very heavy fall of snow, which continued till 8 or 9 o'Clock in the evening, when the Wind abated and veered to SE, the sky cleared up and we had a fair night, attended with so sharp a frost that the Water in all our Water Vessels on Deck was in the Morning covered with a sheet of ice. The mercury in the Thermometer was as low as 29° which is 3° below freezing, or rather 4 for we generally find the water freeze when the Mercury is at 33°. Continue to see Ice Islands.

TUESDAY 14*th*. Towards noon the Wind veered to the South and increased to a very strong gale and blew in heavy squals attended with snow; at intervals between the squals the weather was fair and clear, but exceeding cold. We continued to steer East inclining a little to the North and in the after-noon cross'd the first Meridion or that of Greenwich in the Latitude of 57°50′ S. At 8 o'Clock in the evening close reefed the Top-sails, took in the Main sail and steered East with a very hard gale at SSW and a high sea from the same direction: but last night we had the Sea from ESE both of which was a sign that no land was near us to the South. Thermometer no higher to day than 32½. Islands of Ice allways in sight.

WEDNESDAY 15*th*. Very strong gale at SW and fair weather. At day break set the Main sail and loosed a reef out of each Top-sail and steered ENE till noon, at which time we were in the Latitude of 56°37′ S, Longitude 4°17′ East, when we steered NE in order to get into the Latitude of Cape Circumcision. Some large ice islands in sight and the air nearly as Cold as yesterday. At 8 o'Clock in the evening shortned sail and at 11 hauled the Wind to the NW, not daring to stand on in the night, for by this time the wind had greatly abated, and we had a prodigeous high sea from the same direction.

THURSDAY 16*th*. During the night the Weather was foggy with snow showers and a smart frost. At day break bore away NE with a light breeze at West which at Noon was succeeded by a calm and fair weather:[1] our Latitude at this time was 55°26′ s, Longitude 5°52′ East. In this situation we had a great swell from the Southward but no ice in sight. At 1 o'Clock in the PM a breeze sprung up at ENE and we stood to SE till Six then tacked and stood to the North under double-reef'd Top-sails and Courses, having a very fresh gale attended with Snow and sleet which fixed to the Masts and rigging as it fell and coated the whole with ice.

FRIDAY 17*th*. The Wind continued veering by little and little to the South till midnight when it fixed at SW being at this time in the Latitude of 54°20′ s, Longitude 6°33′ East. I steered East having a prodigious high sea from the South which assured us no land was near in that direction.

SATURDAY 18*th*. In the Morning it ceased to Snow, the Weather became fair and clear and we found the variation to be 13°44′ West. At Noon we were in the Latitude of 54°25′, Longitude 8°46′ East. I thought this a good Latitude to keep in to look for Cape Circumcision, because if the land had ever so little extent in the direction of North and south we could not miss seeing it, as the northern point is said to lie in 54°.We had got a great swell from the South so that I was now well assured it could only be an island and it was of no consequence which side we fell in with. In the Evening Mr Wales made several observations of the Moon and the Stars Regulus and Spica, the mean results at 4 o'Clock when the observations were made for finding the time by the watch, gave 9°15′20″ East Longitude, the Watch at the same time gave 9°36′45″. Soon after the variation was found to be 13°10′ W. It is nearly in this situation where Mr Bouvet had 1°00′ East; I cannot suppose that the Variation has altered so much sence that time but rather think he had made some misstake in his observations: there can be none in ours, the uniformity for some time past is a proof of this, besides we found 12°08′ west variation nearly under this Meridian in Jan^ry^ 1773. During the Night the Wind veered round by the NW to NNE[2] and blew a fresh gale.

SUNDAY 19*th*. At 8 o'Clock in the Morning we saw the appearence of land in the direction of EBS or that of our Course, it proved a mere fog bank which soon after disapeared. We continued to steer EBS and SE till[3] 7 o'Clock in the evening, when we were in the Latitude of

[1] 'Calm with Open Cloudy W^r^. We're most confoundedly jumbled today not a breath of Wind stirring, and a heavy Sea rowling from ½ the Points of the Compass but principally from the SEward . . . no Ice in sight'.—Clerke 8953.

[2] A with which we continued to steer to the East . . .

[3] *We continued . . . till:* A for we continued this Course near 26 Leagues, after it was first seen, without seeing afterwards either land or signs of any; I should not have men-

54°42′ S, Longitude 13°03′ E and the wind having veered to NE we tacked and stood to NW under close reefed Top-sails and Courses, having a very strong gale attended with snow showers.

MONDAY 20*th*. At 4 o'Clock in the Morning, being in the Latitude of 54°30′ S, Longitude 12°33′ East we tacked and stretched to NE with a fresh gale at NW attended with Snow showers and sleet.[1] At Noon we were in the Latitude of 54°08′ S, Longitude 12°59′ E and steered East with a fresh gale at WBN and tolerable clear weather. At 10 o'Clock we brought to least we might pass the land in the night of which we had however not the least signs.

TUESDAY 21*st*. At Day-break made sail and bore away East and at Noon we observed in Latitude 54°16′ S, Longitude 16°13′ E which was 5° to the East of the Longitude Cape Circumcision was said to lie in, so that we began to think that no such land ever existed. I however continued to steer East inclining a little to the South till 4 o'Clock in the after noon of the next day, when we were in the Latitude of 54°24′ S, Longitude 19°18′ E. We had now run down 13° degrees of Longitude in the very Latitude Bouvets land was said to lie in, I was therefore well assured that what he had taken for land could be nothing but an Island of Ice, for if it was land, it is hardly possible we could have miss'd it, was it ever so small, besides sence we left the Southern lands, we had not met with the least signs of any, but even suppose we had, it would have been no proof of the existence of this land, for I am well assured that neither Seals, Penguins or any of the Oceanic birds are indubitable signs of the Vicinity of land. I will allow that they are found on the Coasts of all these Southern lands, but are they not allso to be found in all parts of this Southern Ocean. There are however some Oceanic or aquatic birds which point out the Vicinity of land, especially shags which seldom go out of sight of it, and Gannets, Boobies and Men of War birds I believe seldom go very far out to Sea. As we were now no more than two degrees of Longitude from our rout to the South after leaving the Cape of Good Hope, it was to no purpose to proceed any farther to the East under this parallel, knowing no land could be there; but as an oppertunity now offered of clearing up some doubts[2]

tioned this att all, had not this been the Situation, where we were to expect to find Cape Circumcision, it also shews how we are deceiv'd by appearences. At length, at

[1] A and a great sea from the North

[2] A which some had . . .—These words seem to argue that some of the officers had been convinced of the existence of land by the conditions in mid-December 1772 (pp. 59, 63 above). Cook goes on in A, 'It must be remembered, that when we first fell in with the field ice, after leaving the Cape of Good Hope; that we thought we saw land in the direction of SWBS but that we had afterwards reason to beleive we were mistaken'. Cf. the extract from Cooper in the following note.

of our having seen land farther to the South, I steered SE to get into the Situation in which it was supposed to lie. We continued this Course till 4 o'Clock the next morning and then SEBE and ESE till eight in the evening, at which time we were in the Latitude of 55°25′ S, Longitude 23°22′ E, both deduced from observations made the same day, for in the Morning the sky was clear at intervals and afforded an oppertunity to observe several distances of the Sun and Moon which we had not been able to do for some time past, having had a constant succession of bad weather. Having now run over the place where the land was supposed to lie without seeing the least signs of any it was no longer to be doubted but that the Ice hills had decieved us as well as Mr Bouvet.[1] The Wind by this time had veered to the North and increased to a perfect storm attended, as usual, with snow and sleet, we handed the Top-sails and hauled up ENE under the Courses. During the night the Wind abated and veered to NW which inabled us to steer more to the North having no business farther South.[2]

I had now made the circuit of the Southern Ocean in a high Latitude and traversed it in such a manner as to leave not the least room for the Possibility of there being a continent, unless near the Pole and out of the reach of Navigation; by twice visiting the Pacific Tropical Sea, I had not only settled the situation of some old discoveries but made there many new ones and left, I conceive, very little more to be done even in that part. Thus I flater my self that the intention of the Voyage has in every respect been fully Answered, the Southern Hemisphere sufficiently explored and a final end put to the searching after a Southern Continent, which has at times ingrossed the attention of some of the Maritime Powers for near two Centuries past and the Geographers of all ages. That there may be a Continent or large tract of land near the Pole, I will not deny, on the contrary I am of opinion there is, and it is probable[3] that we have seen a part of it. The excessive cold, the many islands and vast floats of ice all tend to prove that there must be land to the South and that this Southern land must lie or extend farthest to the North opposite the Southern Atlantick and Indian Oceans, I have already assigned some reasons, to which I may add the greater degree of cold which we have found in these Seas, than in the Southern Pacific Ocean under

[1] 'NB. This day at Noon we suppose the ship nearly in the same Lattitude & Longitude she was in on the 15th of December 1772 where we fell in with a large field of Ice which we stood along for upwards of 30 Leagues, seeing many Penguins & snow Birds & in great expectation of finding land, but now we can see neither Ice, Birds, or the least signs of land whatever.'—Cooper, 22 February.

[2] A as we knew nothing was there.

[3] *am of . . . probable:* A firmly beleive it and its more than probable

the same parallels of Latitude. In this last Ocean the Mercury in the Thermometer seldom fell so low as the freezing point, till we were in Sixty and upwards, whereas in the others it fell frequently as low in the Latitude of fifty four: this was certainly owing to there being a greater quantity of Ice and extending farther to the North in these two Seas than in the other, and if Ice is first formed at or near land, of which I have no doubt, it will follow that the land also extends farther North. The formation or Coagulation of Ice Islands has not, to my knowledge, been throughly investigated: Some have supposed them to be formed by the freezing of the Water at the Mouths of large Rivers or great Cataracts and so accumulate till they are broke of by their own weight.[1] My observations will not allow me to acquiesce in this opinion because we never found any of the Ice which we took up incorporated with Earth or any of its produce which I think it must, had it been coagulated In land waters. It is also a doubt with me that there are any Rivers in these Countries, the interior parts being so much elevated as never to enjoy heat sufficient to melt the snow in any quantity. It is very certain that we saw not a River or stream of Water on all the coast of Georgia, or on any of the Southern lands; nor did we ever see a stream of Water run from any of the Ice Islands. How are we then to suppose that there are large rivers in these Countries, the Vallies are covered many fathoms deep with everlasting snow and at the sea they terminate in Ice clifts of vast heights. It is here where the Ice islands are formed, not from streames of Water, but from Consolidated snow which is allmost continually falling or drifting down from the Mountains, especially in Winter when the frost must be intence. During that Season, these Ice clifts must so accumulate as to fill up all the Bays be they ever so large, this is a fact which cannot be doubted as we have seen it so in summer; also during that season the Snow may fix and consolidate to ice to most of the other coasts and there also form Ice clifts. These clifts accumulate by continual falls of snow and what drifts from the Mountains till they are no longer able to support their own weight and then large pieces break off which we call Ice islands. Such as have a flat even Surface must

[1] A this way of reasoning, in my opinion is very obsurd, for that degree of cold which is necessary to form an Ice Island, at the mouth of a River; would, I should suppose, freeze up the River itself.—In B, f. 338v, Cook at first includes this passage, though rather more politely, and then recasts it as follows in the text. We have here a reference to an older argument for the existence of the southern continent, drawn from the finding of icebergs in high latitudes. It was assumed that sea water did not freeze: where then could ice islands have come from but from some great source of fresh water—i.e. rivers? And rivers obviously presupposed land. Hence, no doubt, the rivers laid down in Terra Australis by sixteenth-century mapmakers; and hence, in more recent and mature shape the hypothesis on the origin of Antarctic ice published by Philippe Buache in 1757.

be of the Ice formed in the bays and before the flat Vallies,[1] the others which have a spired unequal surface must be formed on or under the side of a Coast, composed of spired Rocks and precepices, or some such uneven surface, for we cannot suppose that snow alone, as it falls, can form on a plain surface, such as the Sea, such a variety of high spired peaks and hills as we have seen on many of the Ice isles. It is certainly more reasonable to suppose that they are formed on a Coast whose Surface is something similar to theirs.[2] I have observed that all the Ice islands of any extent, and before they begin to break to pieces, are terminated by perpendicular clifts or sides of clear ice or frozen snow, always on one or more sides, but most generally all round. Many, and those of the largest size, who had a hilly and spired surface, have shewed a perpendicular clift or side from the summit of the highest peak down to its base. This to me was a convincing proof that these, as well as the flat isles, must have broke off from a substance like themselves, that is from some large tract of ice.[3]

When I consider the vast quantity of Ice we have yearly seen and the vicinity of the places to the Pole where it is formed, where the degrees of Longitude are very small, I am lead to believe that these Ice Clifts extends in some parts a good way into the Sea, such parts especially as are sheltered from the Violence of the Winds; it may even be doubted if ever the Wind is violent in the very high Latitudes and that the Sea will freeze over, or the snow which falls upon it, which amounts to the same thing, we have instances in the Northern Hemisphere; the Baltick sea, the Gulf of S[t] Laurence, the Straits of Bell-isle and many other equally large Seas are frequently frozen over in Winter; nor is this attall extraordinary, for we have found the degree of cold at the surface of the sea, even in summer, to be two degrees below the freezing point, consequently nothing kept it from freezing but the Salts it contained and the agitation of its surface; when ever this last ceaseth in Winter, when the frost is set in and there comes a fall of Snow, it will freeze on the Surface as it falls and in a few days or perhaps in one night form such a sheet of ice as will not be easy broke up; thus a foundation will be laid for it to acumu-

[1] This is really a pretty good account of the origin of tabular bergs, though to judge from Cook's wording he had not heard of glaciers.

[2] Cook had not come at the idea of the 'weathering' of icebergs; or rather—for he knew quite well that they decay and disintegrate, as the journal makes abundantly plain—he did not realize that a great many of the inequalities or extraordinary appearances he had seen were due to weathering. His theory is that the berg breaks away directly from the land, carrying the 'impression' of the coast with it. Where he speaks of a 'hilly' surface he is undoubtedly thinking of the characteristic seracs of the glacier berg.

[3] Perhaps he is thinking of glacier bergs, perhaps also of some weathered berg that had split away from another, and would so have a 'perpendicular clift or side'.

late to any thickness by falls of snow, without it being attall necessary for the Sea Water to freeze.[1] It may be by this means that these vast floats of low ice we find in the Spring of the Year are formed and after they break up are carried by the Currents to the North; for from all the observations I have been able to make, the Currents every where in the high Latitudes set to the North or to the NE or NW but we have very seldom found them considerable. If this imperfect account of the formation of these extraordinary floating islands of ice, which is written wholy from my own observation, does not convey some usefull hints to some abler pen, it will however convey some Idea of the Lands where they are formed, Lands doomed by nature to everlasting frigidness and never once to feel the warmth of the Suns rays, whose horrible and savage aspect I have no words to describe; such are the lands we have descovered,[2] what may we expect those to be which lie more to the South, for we may reasonably suppose that we have seen the best as lying most to the North, whoever has resolution and perseverance to clear up this point by proceding farther than I have done, I shall not envy him the honour of the discovery but I will be bold to say that the world will not be benefited by it.

I had at this time some thoughts of revisiting the place where the French discovery was said to lie,[3] but when I considered that if they had realy made this discovery, the end would be as fully answered as if I had done it my self, we know it can only be an island and if we may judge from the degree of cold we found in that Latitude it can-

[1] Cook is struggling with the dogma that sea-water did not freeze: hence his remark that the freezing of snow that falls on the sea 'amounts to the same thing'. The observation that the temperature at the sea's surface was below freezing point (i.e. the freezing point of fresh water) was correct; the reasoning that the salinity of the water and its movement kept it from freezing was correct also; and so was the further reasoning that falls of snow would add thickness to the ice. But Cook had had no opportunity, luckily for the expedition, to watch the sea in comparatively shallow water actually freezing round him, or to trace the process by which, freezing once having started, it spread and consolidated. Hence his theory that the sea might be frozen over without being actually frozen itself.

[2] *some abler pen . . . discovered:* A some abler pen, as intended, it will however convey some Idea of the horribleness of the Country's where they are formed; Country's which I have but barly attempted to describe; Indeed I have no words to paint a Country in more gloomier colours, than the Author of Lord Ansons Voyage, has given to Staten land and yet I do assert, that it is a paradise when compared to these Southern lands.—'The Author of Lord Ansons Voyage' himself makes a comparison (pp. 74–5): 'I cannot but remark, that though Terra del Fuego had an aspect extremely barren and desolate, yet this Island of *Staten-land* far surpasses it in the wildness and horror of its appearance . . . nothing can be imagined more savage and gloomy, than the whole aspect of this coast': and so on to everlasting snow and frightful precipices.

[3] The reference here cannot be to Bouvet's land, which Cook believed he had disposed of, but to Kerguelen's—which lay about 45 degrees east of where he now was, and 5 to 7 degrees north.

not be a fertile one. Besides this would have kept me two Months longer at sea and in a tempestious Latitude which we were not in a condition to support, our sails and rigging were so much worn that some thing was giving way every hour and we had nothing left either to repair or replace them.

We had been a long time without refreshments, our Provisions were in a state of decay and little more nourishment remained in them than just to keep life and Soul together. My people were yet healthy and would cheerfully have gone wherever I had thought proper to lead them, but I dreaded the Scurvy laying hold of them at a time when we had nothing left to remove it. Besides it would have been cruel in me to have continued the Fatigues and hardships they were continually exposed to longer than absolutely necessary, their behavour throughout the whole voyage merited every indulgence which was in my power to give them. Animated by the conduct of the officers, they shewed themselves capable of surmounting every difficulty and danger which came in their way and never once looked upon either the one or the other to be a bit heightned by being seperated from our companion the Adventure. All these considerations induced me to lay a side looking for the French discoveries and to steer for the Cape of Good Hope, with a resolution however of looking for the isles of Denia and Marseveen, which are laid down in Dr Halley's Variation Chart, in the Latitude of [41½] S and about [4] of Longitude to the East of the Meridian of the Cape of Good Hope.[1] With this view I steered NE with a hard gale at NW and thick weather and on

SATURDAY 26*th*[2] at Noon we saw the last Ice island, we were at this time in the Latitude of 52°52′ S, Longitude 26°31′ East. The next day our Latitude at Noon was 50°34′ S, Longitude 28°37′ E, the Mercury

[1] *which are . . . Hope:* A laid down in Dr Halleys and Mr Dalrymples charts.—The figures in square brackets occur in none of the MSS, and are supplied from the printed *Voyage*. These illusory isles seem to have had their origin in icebergs: they first appeared on Dutch charts of the seventeenth century, and maintained their position with some cartographers until the early years of the nineteenth. Dalrymple (*Memoir of a Chart of the Southern Ocean*, p. 6) doubted their existence, referring to Halley's adoption of them thus: 'I suppose he had some authority for doing so, although I have not met with any, except that Van Keulen says, they have been seen by the Dutch company's ships, but he gives no circumstances'. Horsburgh (*Directions for sailing to and from the East Indies*, I (1809), p. 80) plumps for the iceberg theory. Halley, after his voyages in the *Paramour* pink (1698 and 1699–1700), published two isogonic charts, one of the Atlantic (1701) and one of the world (1702). The latter was republished by Mount and Page in 1745, with the isogonic lines redrawn by the mathematician Charles Leadbetter to show the variation in the preceding year; and again in 1757, with still newer variation data up to 1756. It is to the 1745 chart that Cook refers (see p. 671 below).

[2] Saturday was the 25th.

in the Thermometer was no higher than 41.[1] Continued to steer NE till

[MARCH 1775]

WEDNESDAY March 1*st* when the wind abated and veered to the South with which we steered West in order to get farther from Mr Bouvets track which was but a few degrees to the East of us. We were at this time in the Latitude of 46°44′ S, Longitude 33°20′ E and found the Variation to be 23°36′ W.

It is some what remarkable that all the time we have had the late Northerly winds, which have been regular and constant for several days past, the Weather has always been thick and Cloudy, but as soon as they came South of West, it cleared up and was fine pleasent weather. The Barometer began to rise several days before this change happened; but wheather on account of it or our coming Northward cannot be determined.[2] The next day at Noon, being in the Latitude of 46°30′ S, Longitude 31°46′ E the Mercury in the Thermometer stood at 47, which is the same as it stood at the 9th of Febry 1774 in the Latitude of 55½°; on the 17 of the same month and under the same Latitude as we are now, it stood at 55. Such was the difference in the temperature of the air between the Southern Pacific Ocean and this we were now in. The Wind remained not long at South before it veered round by the NE to NW, blew fresh and by squalls attended as before with rain and thick Misty weather. On

FRIDAY the 3*rd* in the PM had some intervals of clear weather and we found the Variation to be 22°26′ W, Latitude in at this time 45°08′ S, Longitude 30°50′ East. The following night was very stormy, the wind blew from SW and in excessive heavy squalls, at short intervals between the squals the wind would fall allmost to a Calm and then come on again in such fury that neither our sails nor rigging could withstand it; several of the Sails were Split and a middle Staysail[3] wholy lost. The next morning the gale abated and we repaired the Damage we had sustained in the best Manner we could.[4] We con-

[1] A Monday 27*th*. Continued to stretch to NE with the wind at NW a very fresh gale and squally, and which increas'd in such a manner, that in the evening, we were reduced to our two low sails. The night was very foggy and obscure and we spent it making short boards. Tuesday 28*th*. At day-light, set the Top-sails double reefed and stretched to the East, Wind at NNW a very hard gale, at Noon we were in the latitude of 47°58′ South, Longitude 31°45′ East. Thermometer at 47°. In the evening, saw two Seals, a Port Egmont Hen and a piece of sea weed; spent the night, which was thick and hazy, making short boards.

[2] This paragraph is written on an additional slip, f. 341.

[3] The words 'already worn to raggs' are here deleted.

[4] *The next morning . . . could:* A In the morning the gale moderated and we set the Top-sails close reefed and shifted such sails as had been torn in the night, that is such as we had any spare ones of; for the number of our sails, as well as every other thing, were by

tinued standing to the North till the Evening when the Wind had veered to NW, we tacked and stood to SW being at this time in the Latitude of 43°20′ S, Longitude 29°50′ W.

MONDAY *6th.* The Wind returning back to the West, obliged us to tack and stretch to the North. Thermometer 44.[1]

TUESDAY *7th.*[2] In the PM had some intervals of Clear weather when Mr Wales, Mr Clerke and Mr Gilbert observed several distances of the Sun and Moon, the result shewed that our reckoning was without any error.[3]

WEDNESDAY *8th* being in the Latitude of 41°30′ S, Longitude 26°51′ E, the Wind having veered to NW we tacked and stood to SW. At Noon the Mercury in the Thermometer rose to 61 and we found it necessary to put on lighter cloathes. The Wind continued invariably fixed between the NW and West and we tooke every advantage to get to the West, by tacking when ever it shifted any thing in our favour, but as we had a great swell against us our tacks were rather disadvantageous. We daily saw Albatrosses, Peterels and other Oceanic birds but not the least signs of land.

FRIDAY *10th.* We used the last of our Raisins which were put on board by the Victualling Office three years ago, and we thought them but little worse by keeping. It is a custom in the Navy for no ships to be supplyed with Flour, Raisins or suet for a longer time than Three Months, from a supposistion that these articles will not keep good longer, but if this is the Reason it is not well founded, for they have been found to keep as well if not better than any other of our Provisions, nothing more is required but to pack them in good and well seasoned Casks and to see that they are good when packed: I have always found Seamen prefer flour and fruit to Salt Beef and I am well assured that the one is more wholesom and nourishing than the other.[4] I do not mean to insinuate that no Salt Beef should be

this time very much reduced. Before Noon we were able to carry single reefed Topsails, the wind had so much abated, but it continued at WSW and West and was attended with a very high Sea from the same direction.

[1] A At Noon Observ'd in Latitude 43°49′. Thermometer 50°. The preceeding night we had thick weather with rain and lightning. In the afternoon the Wind was variable between the North and West; it at last fixed at West and blew a fresh gale, attended with a very high sea.

[2] A At noon observed in Latitude 42°24′ S, Longitude 26°51′ East. Thermometer 52½°. At this time we had a prodegious high sea from the West.

[3] *the result . . . error:* A their results reduced to Noon was very consonant with my reckoning.

[4] *I have . . . the other:* A The flour which we now made use of was put onboard at the same time: I cannot say that it is not the worse for keeping, on the contrary some Casks were a little damaged and so was all our other Provisions, as well they might, after having been three years onboard and pass'd through such a variety of climates. I have ever

served in the Navy, but, only to shew that the want of a longer proportion of flour &c[a] is hurtfull to the Service. I am well convinced that some improvements might be made in the Victualling which would greatly contribute to the health of Seamen and in the end be a saving to the Crown, but this is not a place for the full discussion of this subject.[1]

SATURDAY 11*th*. In the Latitude of 40°40′ S, Longitude 23°47′ E the Variation was 20°48′ W.[2] The Mercury in the Thermometer this day at Noon was no higher then 52. This sudden fall was occasioned by the Wind veering or shifting from NW to SW which caused the Mercury to fall no less than 10°, such was the different state of the air between a notherly and southerly wind. The next day we had a few hours Calm; we put a boat in the water and shot some Albatrosses and Peterels which at this time were highly exceptable.[3] We were now nearly in the Situation where the isles we were in search after are said to lye, we however saw nothing that could give us the least hopes of finding them.

MONDAY 13*th* the Calm continued till 5 o'Clock in the AM when it was succeeded by a breeze at WBS with which we stood to NNW and at Noon observed in Latitude 38°51′ S, which was upwards of 40 Miles more to the North than our Log gave us, and the Watch shewed us that we had been set to the East also. If these differences did not arise from some strong current, I know not how to account for it. Very strong Currents have been found on the Africa Coast, between Madagascar and the Cape of Good Hope, but I never heard of their extending so far from the land, nor is it probable they do, or that this current has any connection with that on the Coast, but some stream which is neither lasting nor regular which we happened to fall into,[4] but these are points which require much time to investigate and must therefore be left to the industry of future Navigators. We were now two degrees to the North of the Parallel in which the isles of

found Seamen prefer Flour and Fruit to Salt Beef; I have often, in the Course of this Voyage left it to their choice and have always found that they never took up above, or hardly, one third of their allowance in the latter article and I have found by my own experience, that the other is more Wholesome and nourishing.

[1] The whole of this entry, though not deleted, is marked marginally by Cook, 'Omit'; and it does not appear in the *Voyage*—presumably to avoid any public criticism, even implied, of naval practice.

[2] These were evening figures, says A, which adds, 'Soon after it fell little wind and veered more to the South and inabled us to haul more to the West, but the Sea ran so high that the Ship hardly made any way against it'.

[3] A Saw a Sun fish . . .—'Hoisted the Boat in, having killed 4 large Albatrosses & 18 diff[t] kinds of small Petrels.'—Cooper.

[4] A we met with nothing of this kind in going to the Southward from the Cape of Good Hope.

Denia and Marseveen are said to lie in, we had seen nothing to incourage us to persevere in looking after them and I found it would take up some time longer to find them or to be satisfied that they did not exist. Every one was impatient to get into Port and for good reasons, as we had had nothing but stale and Salt Provisions to live upon for a long time and for which every one had lost all taste.[1] These reasons induced me to yield to the general wish and to Steer for the Cape of Good Hope with a gentle breeze at SSW which afterwards veered round by the SE to ENE and increased to a strong gale. At the time we bore away we were in the Latitude of 38°38′ S Longitude 23°37′ E.

TUESDAY 14*th.*[2] The observed Latitude at Noon was only 17 Miles to the North of that given by the log, so that we had either got out of the strength of the Current or it had ceased. In the PM in the Latitude of 37°10′, Longitude 21°45′ E the Wind suddenly and in a heavy Squal shifted to NW with which we stood to NE under single reefed Top-sails and Courses.

WEDNESDAY 15*th.* As the day advanced the gale increased and blew in such heavy squals as soon brought us under our Courses, after spliting the Top-sails. The observed Latitude at Noon, together with the watch shewed that we had had a strong current seting to SW, the contrary direction we had found it to set on some of the preceding days as hath been mentioned. In the Evening the gale abated so as to admit us to carry the Top-sails close reefed.

THURSDAY 16*th.* At Day light saw two Sail in the NW quarter, standing to the westward, one of them shewed Dutch Colours. At 10 o'Clock we Tacked and stood to the west also, being at this time in the Latitude of 35°09′ S, Longitude 22°38′ E. I now in persuance to my Instructions demanded from the Officers and Petty officers the Log Books and Journals they had kept, which were delivered to me accordingly and Sealed up for the Inspection of the Admiralty.[3] I

[1] *Every one . . . taste:* A Every one was impatient to get to the Cape and for good reasons, for we had now been above four Months without any manner of refreshments, except the little we got at *Terra del Fuego* and *Staten Land*; our sea Provisions were indeed yet good considering their age; but the time we had been living upon them was enough to tire any one.

[2] A Got the guns out of the hold and Mounted them.—No doubt this was in preparation for ceremonial occasions at the Cape and later.

[3] Officers and gentlemen were on their honour; the men's chests were searched. Charts and drawings were included in the demand: 'so that I can safely say', writes Elliott mournfully, 'that notwi[t]hstanding all the pains I had taken, the next day I had not a figure to shew, any more than if I had never been the Voyage'.—*Mem.*, ff. 39v–40. The confiscatory system, indeed, however necessary from Admiralty points of view, did not encourage the keeping of proper journals by anybody who was not driven by a demon of

also enjoined them and the whole crew not to devulge where we had been till they had their Lordships permission so to do. In the after noon the Wind veered to the west and increased to a hard gale which was of short duration for the next day it fell and at Noon veered to SE.[1] At this time we were in the Latitude of 34°49′ S, Longitude 22°00′ E and on sounding found 56 fathoms water. In the evening Saw the land in the direction of ENE about Six leagues distant and during all the fore part of the night there was a great fire or light upon it.

SATURDAY 18*th*. Day break saw the land again bearing NNW Six or seven Leagues distant, depth of Water 48 f^{ms}. At 9 o'Clock, having little or no wind, hoisted out a boat and sent on board one of the two ships before mentioned, which were about two leagues from us, but we were too impatient after News to regard the distance. Soon after a breeze sprung at West with which we stood to the South and presently three Sail more appeared in sight to windward, one of which shewed English Colours. At 1 PM the boat returned from on board the Bownkerke Polder, Captain Cornelis Bosch, a Dutch Indiaman from Bengal; Captain Bosch very obligingly offered us sugar, Arrack and whatever he had to spare. Our people were told by some English Seamen on board this Ship that the Adventure arrived at the Cape of Good Hope Twelve Months ago and that one of her boats crew had been Murdered and eat by the People of New Zealand, so that the story which we heard in Queen Charlottes Sound was now no longer to be doubted, it was to this effect: that a ship or boat had been dashed to pieces on the Coast, but that the crew got safe on shore; on the Natives who were present stealing some of the strangers clothes, they were fired upon till all their ammunition was spent, or as the Natives express'd, till they could fire no longer, after which the Natives fell upon them, knocked them all on the head and treated them as above mentioned; this was the substance of what our people understood from them; when I examined them about it they denied their knowing any thing about the matter or that any thing of the kind had happened and never after would mention it to any one,

self-expression. It may be doubted if any official person ever read any journal except Cook's—and, in the Board of Longitude, perhaps Wales's; but at least the market was protected from a flood of poor publications.

[1] 'PM confin'd Messieurs Maxwell, Loggie and Coglan for going into the Galley with drawn knives and threatening to stab the Cook . . . [AM] Read the Articles of War to the Crew; the Captain upon examining the Prizoners finding Mr Loggie somewhat less culpable than the other two dismiss'd him from confinement.'—Clerke, 16 March. The young gentlemen were 'confin'd in Irons', says Cooper; who notes, 20 March, that 'The Captain releas'd the two gentlemen out of confinement they having made a concession for their behaviour & promis'd to behave better for the future'.

consequently I thought our people had missunderstood them. I shall make no ref[l]ections on this Melancholy affair untill I hear more about it. I must however observe in favour of the New Zealand[er]s that I have allways found them of a Brave, Noble, Open and benevolent disposition, but they are a people that will never put up with an insult if they have an oppertunity to resent it.[1]

We had light airs next to a calm till 10 o'clock the next Morning when a breeze sprung up at West and the English Ship which was to windward bore down to us, she proved to be the True Briton, Captain Broadly from China. As he did not intend to touch at the Cape, I put a letter on board him for the Secretary of the Admiralty.[2] The account which we had heard of the Adventure was confirmed to us by this ship; we also got from them a parcel of old News papers, which were new to us and gave us some amusement in reading; but these were the least favours which we received from Captain Broadly, he with a Generosity peculiar to the Commanders of the India Companies Ships, sent us fresh provisions, Tea and other articles, which were very acceptable and deserves from me this publick acknowlidgement. In the after noon we parted Company, the True Britton stood out to Sea and we in for the land, having a very fresh gale at West which split our Fore Top sail in such a manner that we were obliged to bring another to the Yard. At 6 o'Clock we tacked within 4 or 5 Miles of the shore and as we judged about 5 or 6 leagues to the East of Cape Auguilas. We stood off till Middnight, when the wind having veered round to the South, we Tacked and stood a long shore to the west. The Wind kept veering more and more in our favour and at last fixed at ESE and blew for some hours a perfect huricane, as soon as the Storm began to subside we made sail and hauled in for the land. On

TUESDAY 21*st* at Noon the Table Mountain over the Cape Town bore NEBE distant 9 or 10 Leagues. By makeing use of this bearing and distance to reduce the Longitude shewn by the watch to the Cape Town, the error was found to be no more than 18′ in Longitude which she was too far to the East, and the greatest difference we have found between it and the Lunar observations sence we left New

[1] The whole of the preceding sixteen lines, 'to be doubted . . . resent it' is, although not deleted, marked marginally by Cook 'omit', and the two words 'a Mystery' substituted. The passage, it is clear, now seemed to him useless repetition; and in his final revision, he was planning to print a chapter supplied by Furneaux, which would include Burney's report on the tragedy.—For the last sentence, 'I must however observe . . .' A reads simply, 'I shall only observe, in favour of these people, that I have found them no wickeder than other Men'.

[2] *I put . . . Admiralty:* I took the oppertunity to write to the Secretary of the Admiralty, just to acquaint him where I was.

Zealand has seldom exceeded half a degree and allways the same way.[1] The next Morning, being with us Wednesday 22nd but with the people here Tuesday 21st [2] we anchored in Table Bay, where we found several Dutch Ships, some French and the Ceres Captain Newte, an English East India Company Ship from China bound directly to England, by whom I sent a Copy of this Journal, Charts and other Drawings to the Admiralty which Captain Newte was so obliging as to take charge of and as he intended to make but a very short stay at St Helena will probably be the first that carries the news of our arrival to England. Before we had well got to an anchor, I dispatched an officer to acquaint the Governor with our arrival and to request the necessary stores and refreshments, which were readily granted. As soon as the officer returned we saluted the Garrison with 13 Guns which Compliment was immediately returned with an equal number. I found here a letter from Captain Furneaux acquainting me with the loss of Ten of his best men together with a boat in Queen Charlottes Sound. This together with a great part of his Bread being damaged was the reason he could not follow me in the rout I had proposed to take. He also informed me that he had sailed over the place where Cape Circumcision was said to lie, so that here is another proof that it must have been Ice and not Land which Bouvet saw.[3]

The next day I went on shore and waited on the Governor Baron Plettenberg and other Principal officers who[4] Received and treated us during our whole stay with the greatest politeness, and contributed all in their power to make it agreeable.[5] And as there are few people who are more obligeing to strangers than the Dutch in general at this place, and no place where refreshments of all kinds are to be got in such abundance we enjoyed some real repose after the fatigues of so long a voyage.

[1] Here follow the last words of A: 'It would not be doing justice to Mr Harrison and Mr Kendal if I did not own that we have received very great assistance from this usefull and valuable time piece as will more fully appear in the course of this Journal'—followed by Cook's signature.

[2] 'Having gained a Day by circumnavigating the Globe by an East course shall now make an allowance for it, by having two days of the same name.'—Log.

[3] The preceding three sentences are supplied on a separate slip, f. 346; they are a rather abbreviated version of a later entry (p. 658 below). Both passages are given, as an illustration of Cook's reshaping of the journal.

[4] *and other . . . who:* H Mr Hemmy the Second Governor, Major Prehn the Commander of the Troops and the Master Attendant or Equipagie. Governor . . .—The word 'Equipagie' is not in Cook's hand, and seems to have been written in for him by a Dutchman. In f. 345v, Cook starts out in this way, but gives up over 'Equipagie', and deletes and alters to produce the text as printed.

[5] 'Went with Capt Cook to the Governour & obtained leave to carry on shore & erect my Observatory & Instruments. Also agreed with the Widow Xieman For the use of the Ground whereon they stood before, and where Messieurs Mason & Dixon Observed.'—Wales.

The good treatment of all kinds which strangers meet with at the Cape of Good Hope and the necessity of breathing a little fresh air, has interduced a custom which is not common any where else, at least I have no where seen it so strictly observed, this is for all the officers which can be spared out of the Ships to reside on shore: we followed this Custom, my self, the two Mr Forsters and Mr Sparman took up our aboad with Mr Brant a gentleman well known to the English by his obligeing readiness to serve them.[1]

My first care after our arrival was to procure fresh baked Bread, fresh Meat, Greens and Wine for those who remained on board and with these articles they were provided every day during our Stay, which soon restored them to their usual strength. We had only three Men on board which were thought necessary to send on Shore for the recovery of their health; these I provided quarters for at the rate of Thirty Stivers, or half a Crown per day, for which they were provided with Victuals, Drink and Lodging.[2]

We now went to work to repair all our defects, for which purpose we, by permission, errected a Tent on shore to which was sent our Casks and Sails to repair. We also struck the Yards and Top-masts in order to repair and overhaul the rigging which we found in so bad a condition that almost every thing except the standing Rigging was obliged to be replaced with New, which was purchased here at a most exorbitant price. In the Article of Naval Stores, the Dutch here, as well as at Batavai, take a shamfull advantage of the distress of Foreigners. That our Rigging, Sails, &c^a^ should be worn out will not be wondered at when it is known that during this circumnavigation of the Globe, that is sence we left this place to our return to it again, we have sailed no less than   a distance I will be bold to say, was never sailed by any Ship in the same space of time before.[3]

[1] *Deleted* he has lately been appointed Port-keeper at False Bay where he resides during the Winter Season.—Cook and Brand (Brant, Brandt) seem to have been by now on the friendliest terms. Christoffel Brand became known as the 'governor' of Simonstown (in False Bay), which he 'governed' for twenty years. He was the forbear of some men very distinguished in South African history.

[2] It is not to be thought that the rest of the ship's company did not get on shore. Elliott *Mem.*, f. 40v, is our informant. 'In the mean time, as it was convenient, Captn Cook gave leave to the Officers, as well as the Men, to go on shore, for pleasure, or refreshment, and it was no uncommon thing in our Rides in the Country, to see three of the Sailors on a Horse, in full sail, and well filld with grog—at other times I have seen them Laying asleep by the roadside, and the Horses standing over them; all this must not be wonderd at, when it is considerd how long they had been confin'd, and I will here do them the justice to say that *No Men* could behave better, under every circumstance than they did....'

[3] The blank in the preceding line is in G also. Cook apparently worked out the sum later: *Voyage*, II, pp. 265–6, reads, 'we had sailed no less than twenty thousand leagues; an extent of voyage, nearly equal to three times the equatorial circumference of the earth, and which, I apprehend, was never sailed by any ship in the same space of time before. And yet, in all this great run, which had been made in all latitudes between 9° and 71°,

One of the French that were at Anchor in the Bay was the Ajax Indiaman bound to Pondicherry, commanded by Captain Crozet, who was Second in Command with Captain Morion,[1] who sailed from this place with two Ships in March 1772 as hath been already mentioned, but instead of going from hence to America as was said, he stood away for New Zealand, where in the Bay of isles he and some of his people were killed by the Inhabitants. Captain Crozet who succeeded to the Command, returned by way of the Philippine isles with the two Ships to the isle of Mauritius. Captain Crozet seemed to be a man possessed of the true spirit of a discoverer and to have abilities equal to his good will;[2] he in a very obligeing manner communicated to me a Chart wherein was delineated not only his own discoveries but that of Captain Kerguelen, which I found laid down in the very situation where we searched for it, so that I can by no means conceive how both us and the Adventure missed it. Besides this land, which Captain Crozet told us was a long but very narrow island extending East and West,[3] Captain Morion in about the Latitude 48° S and from 16° to 30° of Longitude, East of the Cape of Good Hope, discovered Six Islands which were high and barren.[4] These together with some islands lying between the line and the Southern Tropick in the Pacific Ocean,[5] were the principle dis-

we sprung neither low-masts, top-mast, lower nor top-sail yard, nor so much as broke a lower or top-mast shroud; which, with the great care and abilities of my officers, must be owing to the good properties of our ship'. I have not seen the original of this passage.

[1] i.e. Marion du Fresne; see pp. liv–lv, lxix above. Julien Marie Crozet (1728–82) had great experience in the service of the French East India Company, by whom he was properly and highly esteemed. He was Marion's second in command in the *Mascarin*, and a more prudent man, and brought the ship back to Port Louis (Brittany) in November 1773. He later commanded a naval vessel in the American War of Independence. See the interesting paper by H. F. Buffet, *L'Explorateur Port Louisien Julien Crozet* . . . in the Société d'Histoire et d'Archéologie de Bretagne *Mémoires* 23 (1943), pp. 41–66. I have been fortunate in using an offprint with later corrections by M. Buffet.

[2] Crozet in his turn had an abundant admiration for Cook: see I, p. 274, n. 4. Relations with the French were good. Forster, II, p. 554, remarks that 'We became acquainted, in the course of our stay, with M. Crozet, who, attended by all his officers, dined with us, upon captain Cook's invitation, and entertained us with many curious particulars relating to his voyage'. Cook, on the other hand, shunned the Spanish officers at the Cape, though Wales got on well with them and gave them a sextant.

[3] This is hardly an accurate description, though the main island of the Kerguelen group is certainly about 75 miles from north-west to south-east.

[4] The Prince Edward islands (Cook's name on his third voyage) lat. 46°36′ to 46°53′ S, long. 37°45′ to 37°57′ E; and the Crozet islands, lat. 45°55′ to 46°30′ S, long. 50°05′ to 52°15′ E.

[5] After leaving New Zealand the French directed their course to Amsterdam and Rotterdam; they missed these islands of Tasman's but saw, 6 August 1772, a chain of low-lying islands in lat. 20°9′, long. 182° E of Paris. On 12 August at daybreak they saw another island, an arid, steep and mountainous peak, in lat. 16°, long. 182°30′ E of Paris; this they called *Isle du point du jour*—'Daybreak Island'. If these positions were anything like accurate the first chain may have been some of the Lulunga or Kotu group of the Tongan islands, stretching north for about twelve miles from lat. 20°07′, long. 174°42′–46′ W. But in that case one would have thought they would have seen Tofua and Kao as well;

coveries made in this Voyage, which we were told was ready for publication.[1] By this Chart it appeared that a Voyage had been made by the French across the South Pacifick Ocean in 1769, under the Command of one Captain Surville, who on condition of his making discoveries, had obtained leave to make a Trading Voyage to the Coast of Peru. He fited out, and took in a Cargo in some part of the East Indies, proceeded by way of the Philippine isles, passed near new Britain and discovered some land in the Latitude of 10° s, Longitude 158° East to which he gave his own name. From hence he steered to the South, passed but a few degrees to the West of New Caledonia, fell in with New Zealand at its Northern extremity and put into Doubtless Bay, where it seems he was when I passed it on my former Voyage in the Endeavour. From New zealand Captain Surville Steered to the East, between the Latitude of 35 and 41° s untill he arrived on the Coast of America where in the Port of Callao, in attempting to land he was drowned.[2] These Voyages of the French, tho' undertaken by private Adventurers, have been productive of some usefull discoveries, as well as contributing in exploaring the Southern Ocean. That of Captain Surville clears up a Misstake, which I was led into by immagining the Shoals off the West end of New Caledonia to extend to the West as far as New Holland: It proves that there is an open Sea in this space and that we saw the NW extremity of that Country. From the same gentleman we learnt that it was a Ship from New Spain which had been at Otahiete before our first arrival and that in her return she had discovered some isles in the Latitude of 32° s and under the Meridian of 130° West:[3] some other isles, said to

possibly the weather was overcast. 'Daybreak Island' may have been Fonualei, lat. 18°09′, long. 174°11′ W., a sharp and well defined peak of 600 feet, about 40 miles NNW of Vava'u. Niua Fo'ou is another possibility, lat. 15°36′, long. 175°39′ W.; it is 853 feet high and volcanic, but it is well wooded.

[1] But nothing was published before Crozet's account, edited by the Abbé Rochon, *Nouveau Voyage à la Mer du Sud*, in 1783. Alexis Marie Rochon (1741–1817) was a distinguished astronomer and physicist, who sailed on Kerguelen's first voyage.

[2] The voyage of Jean François de Surville (1717–70) has never been adequately documented. He left Pondicherry on 2 June 1769, and sailed by way of the East Indies and the Philippines as a blind to his real purpose, the exploitation of a fancied island which was half Tahiti, half 'David's Land'. Turning south, he passed through the Solomon Islands without connecting them with the sixteenth-century discovery, fought bloodily there with the natives and gave the land he had discovered not his own name, but that of *Terre des Arsacides*—'Land of Assassins'. (The south-eastern extremity of the island of San Cristobal is now called Cape Surville.) Passing to the west of New Caledonia, as Cook says, he fell in with New Zealand not at its northern extremity but just south of Hokianga, on the west coast, when Cook was on the east side of the North Island, almost opposite. He sailed round the north of the country and put into Doubtless Bay, but was not in the bay when Cook passed it. See I, pp. cxvi, 223, n. 3; Corney, *Voyage of Captain Don Felipe Gonzalez . . . to Easter Island* (Hakluyt Society, 1908), pp. lii–lxii; McNab, *Hist. Rec. N.Z.*, II, pp. 230–347; and, for a brief account, my *Exploration of the Pacific*, pp. 291–2, 384–5.

[3] The Spaniards of the *Aguila*, on her two voyages to and from Tahiti, 1772–3 and 1774–5, had sighted and charted 22 islands new to them: of these, seven were altogether

be discovered by the Spaniards, appeared on this Chart, but these discoveries of the spaniards, Captain Crozet seemed to think, were inserted from no good authority. Probably more authentick accounts may be got here after, but it will hardly be necessary to resume the Subject unless all the discoveries, both Ancient and Modern, are laid down in a Chart and then an explanatory Memoir will be necessary and such a Chart I intend to construct when I have time and the necessary materials. We were likewise informed of a later Voyage which had been under taken by the French under the command of Captain Kerguelen which had ended highly to the disgrace of that Commander.[1]

On the 6th of Apl the Royal Charlotte, Captain Clemints from China, put in here and sailed again the 10th. By her I transmitted to the Secretary of the Admiralty two of the officers Journals.[2] I had forgot to mention that on my arrival here, I found a letter from Captain Furneaux wherein was confirmed the loss of Ten of his best Men, together with a boat in Queen Charlottes Sound and that this together with the finding a great part of his Bread damaged was the reason he could not follow me in the rout I had proposed to take. He acquainted me, that after leaving New zealand he got into the Latitude of 60° and kept in that Latitude till he doubled Cape Horn and in his rout to the Cape of Good Hope he ran over, as well as us, the place where Bouvets discovery was said to lye, so that we have another proof that it was ice and not land which he saw.[3]

While we lay in Table Bay several Foreign Ships put in and out, bound to and from India, viz. English, French, Deans, Swedes and three Spanish Frigates, two of them going to and one coming from Manila. It is but very lately that the Spanish Ships have touched here,

new discoveries—Tauere, Haraiki, Tatakoto, Amanu, Hikueru, Tahanea and Raivavae. All except the last were sighted on the outward passages, and are in the Tuamotus—i.e. between lats. 14° and 25° s. and longs. 134° and 149° w. Raivavae in the Australs is in lat. 23°52′ and long. 147°41′; it was discovered on 5 February 1775 and it is questionable whether Crozet would have heard of it. The *Aguila* in any case could not have discovered anything in the position given to Cook, because there was nothing there to discover. La Pérouse was later instructed to look for the reported isles. Corney, II, p. 180, has a long note partly bearing on the point, and suggests that 32 may have been a transposition of 23—Crozet's information then being a confused reference to Easter Island. But there seems no reason why anybody should have been confused over Easter Island by 1775.

[1] Kerguelen's second voyage, of 1773, in which he was disillusioned over the nature of his discovery.

[2] Cook gives in his Log, between 23 March and 27 April, full details on the overhaul and repair of the ship. In the midst of them, for 10 April, he has the entry, 'Strong gales and squally weather. The Cutter sunk along side which occasioned the loss of the Masts, Sails and oars, and the Jolly boat broak adrift, drove out to Sea and was lost'. Ordinarily such an incident would certainly have been mentioned in his Journal; but it is clear that he was not inclined to devote overmuch space to the incidents of a stay in a known port.

[3] The preceding two sentences, though not deleted, are marked in the margin 'omit'. Cf. p. 654 above.

and those were the first that were allowed the same privilidges as other European friendly Nations; those which had put in here before, were not allowed to remain longer than what was absolutely necessary, nor were any of the people suffered to come out of the Ships. This was thought a hardship even by the Governor and Council here, and as they had no express orders in what manner they should be treated, they wrote home for Instructions and received for answer that they were to be treated in the same manner as other nations.[1]

On examining the Rudder, the Pintles were found to be loose and we were obliged to unhang it and have it on shore to repair.[2] We were also delayed for want of Caulkers to Caulk the Ship which was absolutly necessary to be done before we put to Sea. The Dutch Caulkers being employed on their own Ships, so that none could be spared to assist us. At length I obtained two from one of the Dutch Ships and the Dutton English Indiaman coming in from Bengal, Captain Rice obliged me with two more so that by the 26th of April this work was finished; and having got on board all necessary stores and a fresh supply of Provisions and Water, we took leave of the Governor and other principal officers[3] and the next Morning repaired on board, and soon after, the Wind coming fair, we weighed and put to Sea as did also the Spanish Frigate Juno from Manila, a Deanish Indiaman and the Dutton. As soon as we were under sail we saluted the Garrison with thirteen guns which Compliment was immidiately returned; the Spanish Frigate and Deanish Indiaman both saluted us as we passed them and I returned each Salute with an equal number of guns.[4] As soon as we were clear of the Bay the Deanish ship Steered for the East Indies, the Spanish Frigate for

[1] This sentence and the previous one from 'those which had . . .' are marked marginally 'omit'.

[2] The pintles were the metal bolts or elbows attached to the rudder, on which it turned. From the Log we learn that the rudder was unhung and sent on shore on 4 April, and hung again on the 15th.

[3] Forster, II, p. 555: 'After taking leave of all our friends, and particularly of Dr. Sparrman, who had shared the perils and distresses of our voyage, and whose heart had endeared him to all who knew him, we came on board. . . '. Sparrman (p. 201) says, 'I might have joined the *Resolution* on her homeward passage, free of charge and with the greatest comfort, but it was my intention first to explore the unknown interior of the continent. . . . I went on board to take my leave and accompany her past Robben Island, where a very friendly parting took place, as Mr. Forster quotes in Vol. II, p. 555'. This seems to dispose of any great weight in Elliott's remark (*Mem.*, f. 41), 'Here Mr Sparman left us, conceiving himself not handsomly treated, at different times during the Voyage, by the Elder Mr Forster'. But writing twenty-five years after the voyage, Sparrman, a good-tempered man, may quite well have forgotten any Forster unpleasantnesses. He did not arrive home in Sweden till July 1776.

[4] The Spanish and the Danish ships, says Elliott, 'ran out on each side of us, and saluted us, Music playing on board the Dane all the time, & this was done in Compliment to Captn Cook, and had a very pretty effect'.—*Mem.*, f. 41.

Europe and we and the Dutton for St Helena. Depending on the goodness of Mr Kendals Watch, I resolved to try to make the island by a direct course, it did not deceive us and we made it accordingly on the 15th of May at Day-break in the Morning in the direction of WNW about 14 leagues distant.[1] It was 8 o'Clock in the evening before we got the length of the Northern point of the island when I dispatched a boat with an officer to acquaint the Governor who we were, without which no ship is allowed to pass the forts. We were so much delayed by the Calms and the Current which set to NE that it was middnight before we got to an Anchor in the Road before the Town or Chappel Vally which is on the NW side of the island.

At Sun rise the next Morning the Castle and Dutton each Saluted us with 13 guns and on my landing to wait on Governor Skottowe I was saluted by the same number from the Castle, each of these salutes were taken up by the Ship.[2] I received a very pressing invitation, both from Governor Skottowe and his Lady, a very accomplished Woman and a Native of the island, to take up my aboad with them during my stay and also offered me the use of a Horse to ride out whenever I thought proper. We next paid our respects to the Lieutenant Governor Mr a Gentleman highly esteemed by all who have the honour of his acquaintance.[3] In these visits we were accompaned by Captain Rice and several persons of Note who were returning from India on board his Ship, viz. Mr Graham and his Lady, Col Macleane, Mr Lawrel, the Honble Mr Stuart, son to the Earl of Bute, and several others and with them we dined with the Governor, where such an elegant dinner was served up as surprised me, who had never seen more of the island than the barren rocks which compose its borders, and the accounts which I had heard of it had not conveyed to me a better idea. In order therefore to gain some knowlidge of it from my own observations, I took a ride into the Country the next morning in company with Mr Stuart and Mr George Forster. We no sooner got out of the Vally and reached the

[1] Cook at this stage of the voyage was evidently in high spirits, as well he might be. Cf. Elliott again: 'The day before we saw St Helena, the Dutton spoke us, and said they were afraid that we should miss the Island, but Captn Cook laugh'd at them, and told them that he would run their jibboom on the Island if they choose, and on the 15th of May we made the Land . . .'—*Mem.*, f. 41v. This pleasantry may be taken as one of the greatest tributes to John Harrison ever paid.

[2] *Each . . . ship:* H We returned the former with an equal number and the latter with two less.

[3] In spite of Cook's tribute to this gentleman, he does not appear to have picked up his name. It was Daniel Corneille, Esq., lieutenant-governor from 1769. John Skottowe was governor, 1764–82, in which latter year he was succeeded by Corneille.—Brooke, *History of the Island of St Helena* (London 1808), pp. 256, 258–9. Skottowe was a son of Thomas Skottowe, on whose farm at Great Ayton Cook had spent his early years, his father being 'hind'.

Summit of the first hill than I was agreeably surprised with the prospect of a Country finely diversified with hill and vally, Wood and Lawn and all laid out in inclosures. The fences are mostly of stone or a bank of earth planted with Furze, the seeds of which were brought from England about Sixty Six years ago, and have succeeded so well that they are now spread over the whole Island and are of the greatest Utility, not only for fences and fuel, but by planting them on the barren lands, have so increased the Soil in a few years that many Acres of good pasture land have by this means been obtained. Excepting the Kitchen gardens, near the Country houses of the principle Inhabitants, and some plantations of Eddy roots[1] in the Watery Vallies, the whole island is laid out in pasture and better I no where ever saw. Wood is rather scarce, it grows chiefly in groves, the trees are Natives of the island, small, thinly planted and free from under wood. The Hills are steep and the Vallies deep and in general well watered except at a place called long Wood, where I was told there is no Water.

The Second day after our arrival, the whole company was entertained at the Governors Country House which is situated in a vale, with the Sea in front which to people who are confined the greatest part of the year to the Sea shore, can be no great addition to the prospect; the View of the Country is in part cut off by a large heavy wall, so that as you approach the place it looks more like a prison than the Country seat of the first person on the island. The house is small and old, but the garden which is in the front, is large and well stocked with the necessary articles both for use and ornament. Here was a live Oak tree which seemed to like its situation, and some of the finest Peaches I ever tasted.

The next day the two Mr Forsters and my self dined with a party at the Country house of one Mr Masons, at a remote part of the island, which gave me an oppertunity to see the greatest part of it, and I am well convinced that the island in many particulars has been missrepresented. It is no wonder that the account which is given of it in the narrative of my former Voyage should have given offence to all the principle Inhabitents. It was not less mortifying to me when I first read it, which was not till I arrived now at the Cape of Good Hope; for I never had the perusal of the Manuscript nor did I ever hear the whole of it read in the mode it was written, notwithstanding what Dr Hawkesworth has said to the Contrary in the Interduction.[2]

[1] i.e. taro, presumably for the feeding of slaves.

[2] See I, pp. ccxlv–xlix. Cook's, and St Helena's, mortification was due to Hawkesworth's unsuspecting use of the journal of Joseph Banks. 'Dr. Hawkesworth's account of captain Cook's first voyage round the world, in the Endeavour, had reached this island

In the narrative, my Country men at St Helena are charged with exercizing a wanton cruelty over their Slaves, they are also charged with want of ingenuity in not having Wheel Carriages, Wheel Barrow's and Porters Knotts to facilitate the task of the labourer. With respect to the first Charge, I must say, that perhaps, there is not a European settlement in the world where slaves are better treated and better fed than here, out of the many of whom I asked these questons not one had the least shaddow of Complaint.[1] The Second charge, tho of little consequence is however erronious for I have seen every one of the three Articles that are said not to be on the island; they have Carts which are drawn sometimes by men and sometimes by oxen, and Wheel Barrows have been used in the island from the first settlement and some are sent Annually out from England in the store Ship.[2] How these things came to be thus missrepresented, I can not say, as they came not from me, but if they had I should have been equally open to conviction and ready to have contridicted any thing, that upon proof, like this, appeared to be ill-founded, and I am not a little obliged to some people in the isle for the obligeing manner they pointed out these Mistakes. Whoever views St Helena in its present state and can but conceive what it must have been originally will not hastily charge the people with want of Industry, tho' perhaps they might apply it to more advantage, was more land appropriated to planting of Vegetables, Roots, and even Corn, articles that are always wanting to Shipping, and where they would meet with a good market and reward the Planter for his industry. They raise no grain and their Gardens produce little more than what serves the Tables of the Principle Inhabitants, which amount to about four hundred; the Slaves, which are about fourteen hundred, subsist cheifly on Yams, Rice and fish, but the garrison which consist of five or six hundred men, depend wholy on the Mother Country for their daily bread. By the apparent fertility of the island one would immagine,

some time before; it had been eagerly perused, and several articles, relative to this settlement, were now taken notice of with great good humour and pleasant raillery. The total want of wheelbarrows, and the ill-treatment of the slaves, which are spoken of in that account, were reckoned particularly injurious, and captain Cook was called upon to defend himself. Mrs. Skottowe, the sprightliest lady on the island, displayed to advantage her witty and satirical talents, from which there was no other escape left, than to lay the blame on the absent philosophers whose papers had been consulted.'—Forster, II, pp. 560–1. The lady, thought Sparrman (p. 202), 'probably troubled the naval officers more than many an ocean storm, although they were otherwise dauntless enough in their own element'.

[1] The slave code of St Helena, dating from the latter part of the seventeenth century, was certainly stringent enough, but that is an imperfect index to actual conditions a hundred years later. Very much more humane ordinances were introduced by the East India Company in 1791 and 1792.—Brooke, *op. cit.*, pp. 355–62, 378–409.

[2] 'There are many wheelbarrows and several carts on the island, some of which seemed to be studiously placed before captain Cook's lodgings every day.'—Forster, II, p. 560, n.

was it properly managed, it would alone support far more than the whole number of Inhabitants, whereas in its present state, the land does not subsist above one fourth part, exclusive of what is supplied the Shiping, which of late years has not amounted to much, but now they say they can supply all the companies Ships with as much fresh meat as they can want and I have no doubt of the fact, for they had at this time about two thousand five hundred head of Cattle, three thousand Sheep, besides Goats, Hogs and Powltry. And as very little of these articles falls to the share of the soldier or the slave, it is clear they must have a good deal to spare to shipping. The oxen, which are of the English breed, weigh between four and five hundred weight, some more and some less and better beef I no where ever met with: the sheep are also of the English breed, are rather small and the meat well tasted; the Hogs seemed to be of a mixed breed between the English and Chineas and the goats are of a strong hardy race. It appeared that the island would mentain double the number of Cattle that were at this time upon it, for I saw not a pasture where the grass was eat up, but this was owing to the rains they had lately had, which made the pastures so good and as this is not always to be depended on, the island one year with another will not support above five hundred head of Oxen more than what are now upon it.

It sometimes happens, as I was told, that they have no rain for twelve or fifteen Months and then there is a want of grass and if the Catele are numberous they are lost for want of food. The uncertainty of having a Constant Supply of Grass discourages them from increasing the number of Cattle above three thousand, and the uncertainty of wanting it discour[a]ges them from converting the overpluss grass into hay and laying it up for time of scarcity. Thus they are kept between hope and fear from making any sort of improvements in the mode in which the island is now managed and it is not likely to be altered so long as the greatest part of the land remains in the hands of the Company and their servants; without industerous planters this island can never florish and be in a condition to supply shipping with all necessary refreshments.

W[it]hin these three years a new Church has been built, a neat edifice and sufficiently large; some other new buildings were in hand and a commodious landing place for boats has been made, which adds both strength and beauty to the place; an excellent new Road is made up Gallows hill, the rock on the right of the vally and the old Road on the other side repaired, all at the companies expence. No hilly country hath better roads than are in this island, they are so judiciously laid out, that you can assend and desend the steepest hills with ease; every man who keep a slave is obliged to send him or some person for him, five days in the year to repairing the Roads and as there is generally more than sufficient for that purpose, the overplus time is employed in planting furzes and grass on the Commons and barren lands.

The two preceding evenings before we sailed Mr Graham and Mr Laurel gave each of them a ball: it is to these gentlemen we are obliged for a sight of the celebrated beauties of St Helena, and I should not do my Country women at this island justice if I did not confirm the report of common fame; they have fine persons, an easy and genteel deportment and a bloom of Colour unusual in a hot climate.

On SUNDAY *21st* in the evening the whole party took leave of the Governor who attended us to the water side and on my going off was saluted with 13 guns from the garrison, and soon as we got under sail and put to Sea with the Dutton in company, were saluted with a like number, which salutes were returned by the ship. During the time we lay at this isle we finished some repairs of the Ship, painting and scraping, which we had not time to do at the Cape; we also filled all our empty Water Casks and the crew was served with fresh beef which was purchased here at five pence per pound.[1]

I have already mentioned, that after leaving the Cape we steered a direct Course for St Helena. For the first Six days, that is till we got into the Latitude of 27°, Longitude 11½° West of the Cape, the Winds were Southerly and SE, after this we had variable light airs for two days which were succeeded by a wind at SE which continued to the island, except a part of one day when it was at NE. In general the wind blew faint all the Passage which made it longer than Common. On makeing the island the Ship was 1°17′ of Longitude ahead of my reckoning, kept by the Log without any regard paid to the Watch or Lunar Observations, and by some reckonings she was more; near 20′ of this error arose the first day, after which it increased in a pretty equal proportion near 4′ of Longitude per day, an error so trifling that it is not easy to say what might be the cause of it, it is however most probable owing to a Current which set to the west or NW. By a series of Observations made at the Cape Town and at James fort in St Helena, at the former by Messrs Mason and Dixon and at the latter by Mr Maskelyne the present Astronomer Royal, the difference of

[1] In the Log, 16 May, Cook mentions losing a kedge anchor which had been carried out to steady the ship, the hawser breaking. On the 18th, the ship received not merely a supply of fresh beef, but also '8 men discharged from the [East India] Companies Service'; which last, added to a stowaway from the Cape mentioned by Forster (II, pp. 556–7), must have made a very full ship.

Longitude between these two places is [24°12′15″][1] only two miles more than Mr Kendals Watch made. The Lunar observations made by Mr Wales, before we made, and after leaving the island and reduced to it by the Watch, gave [5°51′] for the Longitude of James fort which is only 5 miles more west than by Mr Maskelynes. In like manner the Longitude of the Cape Town was found within 5′ of the truth. I mention this to shew how near the Longitude of places may be found by the Lunar method even at Sea by the assistance of a good Watch.

After leaving St Helena the Dutton was ordered to steer NWBW or NW by Compass, in order to avoide falling in with Ascension at which isle it was said an illicit trade had been carried on between the officers of the Companies Ships and some Vessels from North America, who of late years have frequented the isle on pretence of fishing for Whales or Catching Turtle, when their real design was to wait the coming of India Ships. In order to put a stop to this trade, so pernicious to the Company and commerce in general, the Company sent out orders to St Helena to order all their homeward bound ships to steer the Course above mentioned till they are to the northward of Ascinsion, thinking that this Course would carry them clear of these Smuglers. We kept Company with the Dutton till Wednesday 24th when having put a Packet on board her for the Admiralty containing some of the Officers Journals, we parted company, she continuing her Course to the west and we steered for Ascension, where it was necessary for me to touch to take in Turtle for the refreshment of my people as the salt Provisions they had to eat was what had been in the Ship the voyage.[2] We made this isle on the morning of the 28th and the same evening anchored in Cross Bay on the NW side of the isle in 10 fathom water the bottom a fine Sand and half a mile from the shore. The Cross Hill, so called on account of a Cross or flag-staff errected upon it, bore by Compass S 38° E and the two extreme points of the Bay extended from NE to SW.

We remained here till the evening of the 31st and notwithstanding we had several parties out every night, we got but twenty four Turtle, it being rather too late in the Season; however as they wieghed between four and five hundred pounds each, we thought our selves not ill of. We might have caught fish in any quantity, especi-

[1] This figure and that in square brackets three lines below are supplied from the printed *Voyage*, all the MSS being blank.

[2] While at St Helena Cook, ever an experimenter with any new invention connected with a ship, got from Captain Rice of the *Dutton* what he calls 'one of Foxon's Hydrometers or perpetual Log', and Wales 'Foxon's Hydrometer or patent Log-Reels'. In the Log, 26 May, he says, 'it was set a going this day at Noon, but at 10 in the eveng the

ally of that sort called Old Wives,[1] I no where ever saw such abundance, there were also Cavalies,[2] Congor Eels and various other sorts but the catching of them was not attended to, the object was Turtle. On the island are abundance of Goats and Aquatick birds such as Men of War[3] and Tropick birds,[4] Boobies,[5] &c[a]. The Island of Ascension is about ten miles in length in the direction of NW and SE and about five or six in breadth, it shews a surface composed of barren Hills and Vallies, on the most of which not a shrub or plant is to be found for several miles and where we see nothing but stones and Sand, or rather Slags and Ashes, an indupitable sign that the isle at some remote time has been distroyed by a Volcano, which has thrown up vast heaps of stones and even hills. Between these heaps of stones, we find a smooth even surface, composed of Ashes and sand and very good traveling upon it, but one may as easy walk over broken glass bottles as over the stones, if the foot deceives you you are sure to get cut or lamed as happened to some of our people. A high Mountain at the SE end of the isle seems to be left in its original state and to have escaped the general distruction. The Soil is a kind of white Marl which yet retains its vegetative qualities and produceth Purslain, Spurg and one or two grasses,[6] on which the Goats subsist, and it is at this part of the isle where they are to be found as well as the Land Crabs, which I am told are very good: I was told that about this part of the isle is some very good land on which might be raised many necessary Articles, and some have been at the trouble of sowing Turnips and other usefull vegetables. I was also told that there is a fine spring in a Vally which disjoines two hills, which are on the top of the Mountain above mentioned, besides great quantities

Common Log got foul of the Worm, by which means we lost both the one and the other'. The worm was replaced, and from 7 June the ship's log was discontinued off and on in favour of experiments with the hydrometer, till 26 July, when Cook sums up, 'I think it is neither so convenient nor so accurate as the common log'. Foxon's was one of the two 'perpetual logs' tested by Captain Phipps on his Arctic voyage in 1773—'both constructed upon this principle, that a Spiral, in proceeding its own length in the direction of its axis through a resisting medium, makes one revolution round the axis'; the 'spiral' outboard was connected by worm gearing to a dial in the ship, recording the distance run. Phipps reported favourably on its performance in smooth water.—*Voyage* (1774), p. 97. In spite of Cook's adverse report, the future lay with the perpetual (or patent) log, which provided a cumulative record of the distance sailed.

[1] *Balistes vetula* Linn.

[2] *Caranx* sp.

[3] The Ascension Frigate Bird, *Fregata aquila* Linn.

[4] The White-tailed Tropic Bird, *Phaëton lepturus ascensionis* (Mathews) and the Red-billed Tropic Bird, *P. aethereus* Linn., both breed on Ascension Island.

[5] Probably the Blue-faced or Masked Booby, *Sula dactylatra* Lesson.

[6] The Purslain was *Portulaca oleracea* Linn., which was collected by Sparrman, wide-spread; the spurge, *Euphorbia origanoides* Linn., collected by Forster, endemic in Ascension Island. The 'grasses' were *Aristida adscensionis* Linn., which, collected by Forster, was first described from the island, and (probably) species of *Polypogon*.

of fresh Water in holes in the rocks, which the person who gave me this information believed was collected from rains; but these supplies of Water can only be of use to the traveler or to those who may be so unfortunate as to be ship-wrecked on the island, as seems to have been the fate of some not long ago, as appeared by the remains of a Vessel or wreck we found on the NE side. By what we could judge she seemed to have been a Vessel of about 150 Tons[1] burdthen. Those who saw the wreck conjectured from the manner several parts were burnt, that she had taken fire at Sea and the Crew had run her ashore to save themselves.

While we lay in the road a Sloope of about 70 Tons burdthen came to an Anchor by us, she belonged to new York which place she left in Febry and had been to the coast of Guiney with a Cargo of goods and was come here to take in Turtle to carry to Barbadoes. This was the story the Master, whose name was Greves, was pleased to tell and which may in part be true, but I believe the Chief view of His coming here was the expectation of meeting with some of the India Ships. He had been about the island near a Week and had got on board twenty Turtle. A Sloop belong[ing] to Bermuda who was sailed but a few days, with one hundred and five on board, which was as many as She could take in, but having turned several more on the different sandy beaches, they had rip'd open their bellies, taken out the Eggs and left the Carcasses to putrefy, an act as inhuman as ingerous[2] to those who came after them. Part of the account I have given of the interior parts of this island I received from Captain Greves, who seemed to be a sencible intillegent man and had been all over it: he sailed the Morning of the same day we did. Turtle as I am told are to be found at this isle from the Month of Janry to June; the method of catching them, is to send people on shore to the several sandy bays to watch their coming on shore to lay their Eggs, which is allways in the night, and then to turn them on their backs till there is an oppertunity to take them off the next day. It was recommended to us to send a good many men on shore to each beach, where they were to lay quiet till the Turtle were ashore and then to rise and turn them at once; this method may be the best when the Turtle are numerous, but when there are but few, three or four men are sufficient for the largest beach, who ought to keep Patroling of it close to the wash of the surf during the night, by which method they will see all that comes ashore and cause less noise than if there were more of them. It

[1] H left a space for the burden of the ship, which Cook fills in himself, 'of 120 Tons'.

[2] What Cook meant by this is not quite certain. G 'ingenerous', *Voyage* 'injurious'. The text of H reads 'ingerous', and Cook writes carefully in the margin 'injurious', so this may be what he first intended.

was by this method we caught the most we got,[1] and this is the method by which the Americans take them. Nothing is more certain, than all the Turtle which are found about this island come here for the sole purpose of laying their eggs, for we find none but females and of all those which we caught not one had any food worth mentioning in its Stomach, a sure sign, in my opinion, that they must have been a long time without any and this may be the reason why the flesh of them is not so good as some I have eat on the Coast of New South Wales which were caught on the spot they fed.

The Watch made 8°45′ difference of Longitude between St Helena and Ascension, which added to 5°49′ the Longitude of James fort in St Helena, gives 14°34′ for the Longitude of the Road of Ascension, or 14°30′ for the Middle of the island, the Latitude of which is 8°00′ S. The Lunar observations made by Mr Wales and reduced to the same point of the island by the Watch gave [14°28′30″][2] West Longitude by observation. But as the Watch could hardly deceive us in so short a run and time as from the one isle to the other, the Longitude pointed out by it ought in my opinion to take place of that deduced from observation.[3]

On WEDNESDAY 31*st* of May we left Ascension and steered to the Northward with a fine gale at SEBE. I had a great desire to visit the Island of St Mathew[4] in order to settle its situation, but as I found the winds would not allow me to fetch it, I steered for the Island of Fernando de Norono on the Coast of Brazil, in order to determine its Longitude, as I could not find this had yet been done. Perhaps I should have done a more exceptable service to Navigation if I had gone in search of the Isle of St Paul and those Shoals which are said to lie near the Equator and about the Meridian of [20°][5]

[1] They got twenty-four: 'weighing', says Forster, II, p. 578, 'from three to four hundred pounds each. They lasted us three weeks, one and sometimes two being killed every day, and the ship's company receiving as much as they could eat of this wholesome and palatable food'. Since the flesh was 'wholesome and palatable', they were almost certainly Green Turtles, *Chelonia mydas* (Linn).

[2] Figure from the printed *Voyage*.

[3] by observation . . . from observation *substituted for the following deleted*: which is more by   than it is laid down in Mr Maskelyne's British Mariners guide, where he says, it was settled by Observations of a more delicate nature than those of the Sun and Moon, but till I know what these delicate observations were, the Longitude deduced from them must give place to that given by the Watch, which ha[r]dly deceived us in so short a run and time as from the one isle to the other and no man will doubt but the Situation of St Helena must be well settled.—f. 356.—This is not the only place, as we have seen, where Cook displays some impatience with Maskelyne.

[4] This was a supposititious island, believed by sixteenth-century chroniclers and cartographers to have been discovered by the Portuguese in the later fifteenth century, and laid down on the charts in approximately 2° S and 7° or 8° W. See Barros, printed in Crone's *Voyages of Cadamosto* (Hakluyt Society 1937), p. 112 and n. 1; also Peckham's *A True Report*, in Hakluyt (MacLehose ed.), VIII, p. 127.

[5] Figure printed.

west, as neither their situation nor existance are well known.[1] The truth is I was unwilling to prolong the passage in searching for what I was not sure to find,[2] nor was I willing to give up every object which might tend to the improvement of Navigation and Geography for the sake of geting home a Week or a fortnight sooner. It is but seldom that oppertunities of this kind offer and when they do they are but too often neglected. In our Passage to Fernando de Norono, we had steady fresh gales between the SE and ESE attended with fair and Clear weather, and as we had the advantage of the Moon a day nor night did not pass without making Lunar observations for the determining our Longitude. In this run the Variation of the Compass gradually decreased from 11° ′ W[3] which it was at Ascinsion to 1°00′ W which is what we found it off Fernando de Norono, this was the Mean result of two Compasses one of which gave 1°37′ and the other 0°23′ West.

FRIDAY June 9*th* at Noon, we made the Island of Fernando de Norona bearing SWBW½W distance Six or 7 Leagues as we afterwards found by the Log, it appeared in ditatched and peaked hills, the largest of which looked like a Church Tower or steeple. As we drew near the SE end, or part of the isle, we preceived several detatched sunken rocks, lying near a league from the Shore on which the Sea broke in a great surf. After standing very near these rocks we hoisted our Colours and then bore up round the North end of the isle, or rather a group of little islots, for we could see that the land was divided by narrow Channels. On the one next the Main island is a strong fort, besides several others on this last mentioned island, all of which seem'd to have every advantage that Nature can give them, and so disposed as wholy to command all the Anchoring and landing places about the island. We continued to Steer round the Northern point, till the Sandy beaches (befor which is the Road for Shipping) began to appear and untill all the forts and the Peaked hill were open to the westward of the said point. At this time, and on a gun being fired at one of the forts, the Portuguese Colours were displayed and the example followed by all the other forts. As the purpose for which I made the island was now answered I had no intention to anchor and therefore after firing a gun to leeward we made sail and stood away to the Northward with a fine fresh gale at ESE, the Peaked hill or Church Tower bore S 27° W distant about 4 or 5 miles and from this point of view it leans or over hangs to the East.

[1] Now known as St Paul rocks, a volcanic group, in lat. 0°56′ N, long. 29°22′ W.
[2] Cf. I, p. 66 and n. 3 on that page.
[3] Printed 11° West.

This Hill is nearly in the Middle of the island which no were exceeds two leagues in extent and shews a hilly unequal surface, mostly covered with Wood and Herbage.[1]

Ulloa[2] says, 'this Island hath two Harbours, capable of receiving ships of the greatest burthen, one is on the North side and the other on the NW. The former is in every respect the Principal, both for shelter and Capacity and the goodness of its bottom, but both are exposed to the North and West, though these winds particular the North are periodical and of no long continuance.' He further says, that you anchor in the North harbour, which is no more than what I would call a Road, in 13 fath. water one third of a league from shore, bottom of fine sand; the Peaked hill above mentioned, bearing SW 3° Southerly. This road seems to be very well sheltered from the South and East Winds. One of my Seamen was on board a Dutch India ship who put in at this isle in her way out in 1770. They were very sickly and were in want of Refreshments and Water; the Portuguese Supplyed them with some Buffaloes and Fowls and they Watered behind one of the beaches at a little Pool which was hardly big enough to dip a Bucket in.[3]

By reducing the Observed Latitude at Noon to the Peaked hill, its Latitude will be 3°53′ S, and its Longitude by the Watch, carried on from St Helena is 32°34′ West and by Observations of the Sun and Moon, made before and after we made the isle and reduced to it by the Watch 32°44′30″ W. This was the mean result of my observations, the results of those made by Mr Wales, which were more

[1] 'The Appearance of this Island, usually called Ferdinando de Noronha, is perhaps the most romantic of any in the World, on account of the great Number of very singularly shaped Rocks which are on it, and it is yet farther diversified, by the irregularity of its Surface. It is well covered with Wood in those Parts which are not Cultivated, but appears to have many Plantations on it, & is on ye whole extremely beautiful.'—Wales.

[2] Antonio de Ulloa (1716–95), a Spanish admiral of strong and wide scientific interests, though not himself deep or exact in research; and one of the ornaments of the intellectual renaissance in the Spain of his day. As a young man he was sent out to South America in 1735 to accompany La Condamine and other French scientists in important geodetic work, and was then engaged in the defence of the Pacific coast against Anson's expedition. Captured during his voyage home by an English privateer, he was welcomed in London as a man of eminence, made F.R.S. and allowed to return immediately to Spain (1746). For some years he was virtually ignored by his own government; but on the accession of Charles III his fortunes improved. In command of a squadron sent in 1779 to fall on Florida he displayed the endearing trait of being so sunk in scientific studies that he forgot to read his instructions. At the subsequent court-martial he was honourably acquitted but removed from active service, and devoted the rest of his life to stimulating various applications of science in Spain. Cook seems to be quoting from the English translation of his *Relacion histórica del viage a la América meridional* (1748), editions of which, under the title of *A Voyage to South America*, appeared in 1758, 1760 and 1772.

[3] *Deleted* Captain McBride, I think touched here either in going to or returning from Falkland Islands, he no doubt can give a better account of this isle than I can. My only view for making of [*sic*] it was to determine its Situation, which I have reason to think has been done with such accuracy as to admit of little doubt.—ff. 357v–8.

numerous, gave about a quarter of a degree less. The mean of the two will be pretty near the Watch and probably nearest the truth.[1] By knowing the Longitude of this isle we are able to determine that of the adjacent East Coast of Brazil which according to the Modern Charts lies about [sixty or seventy leagues][2] more to the west. We might very safely have trusted to these Charts, especially the Variation Chart for 1744 and Mr Dalrymples of the Southern Atlantic Ocean.[3]

SUNDAY 11*th* at 3 o'Clock in the after-noon we crossed the Equator in the Longitude of 32°14′ W: we had a fresh gale at ESE which blew in Squals attend by showers of rain which continued at certain intervals till Noon the next day, after which we had 24 hours fair Weather.

TUESDAY 13*th*. At Noon being in the Latitude of 3°49′ North, Longit. 31°47′ West the Wind became Variable between the NE and South, and we had light airs and squalls by turns, attended by hard Showers of rain and for the most part dark gloomy weather, which continued till the evening of

THURSDAY 15*th* where in the Latitude of 5°47′ N, Longitude 31°00′ West we had three Calm days, in which time we did not advance above Ten or Twelve Leagues to the North. We had fair weather and rain by turns and the Sky for the most part obscured and Sometimes by heavy dence Clouds which broke in excessive showers of rain.

SUNDAY 18*th* at 7 o'Clock in the evening the Calm was succeeded by a breeze at East, which the next day increased and veered to and fixed at NE, with which we stretched to NW with our Tacks on board; we made no doubt but that we had now got the NE trade wind, as it was attended with fair weather, excepting now and then some light showers of rain and as we advanced to the North the wind increased and blew a fresh Top gt gale.

WEDNESDAY 21*st*. I ordered the Still to be fitted to the largest Copper, which held about Sixty-four gallons. The fire was lighted at 4 o'Clock in the Morning and at Six the Still began to run, it was continued till Six o'Clock in the evening in which time we obtained 32 gallons of fresh Water, at the expence of one bushel and a half of Coals, which was about three quarters of a bushel more than what

[1] The position of Fernando de Noronha is lat. 3°50′ S, long. 32°25′ W.

[2] Printed.

[3] It is odd that Cook is using the variation chart for 1744, and not that for 1756 (see p. 647, n. 1 above). It rather staggers the system, as Clerke might have said. For Dalrymple's chart see p. 615, n. 1 above.

was necessary to have boiled the Ships Companies Victuals only, but the expence of fuel was no object with me. At this time the Victuals was dressed in the small Copper and the other applyed wholy to the Still and every method made use of to obtain from it the greatest quantity of fresh Water possible, as this was my sole Montive for seting it to work. The Mercury in the Thermometer at Noon was at 84½, and higher it is seldom found at Sea, had it been lower more Water, under the same circumstances, would undoubtedly have been produced, for the colder the air is, the cooler you can keep the still, which will condence the Steam the faster. Upon the whole this is a usefull invention; but I would advise no man to trust wholy to it, for altho' you may, provided you have plenty of fuel and good Coppers, obtain as much water as will support life, you cannot, with all your efforts, obtain Sufficient to support health, in hot climates especially, where it is the most wanting, for I am well convinced that nothing contributes more to the health of Seamen than having plenty of Water.

The Wind now remained invariably fixed at NE and ENE and blew fresh with Squalls attended with Showers of Rain and the Sky for the Most part Clouded.

SUNDAY 25*th*. In the Latitude of 16°12′ N, Longitude 37°20′ W, We saw a Sail to Windward and steering down upon us, we Shortned Sail in order to speak her, but seeing she was Dutch by her Colours we made sail again and left [her] to persue her course which we supposed was to some of the Dutch Settlements in the west Indias. In the Latitude of 20° N, Longitude 39°45′ W the Wind began to Veer to EBN and East, but the weather continued the same, that is we continued to have clear and cloudy weather by turns, light squalls and showers. Our Course was between NWBN and NNW till noon on

WEDNESDAY 28*th* after which our Course made good was NBW being at this time in the Latitude of 21°21′ N, Longitude 40°06′ W. Afterwards the Wind began to blow pretty steady and was attended with fair and clear weather.

FRIDAY 30*th* at 2 o'Clock in the Morning, being in the Latitude of 24°20′ N, Longitude 40°47′ W, a Ship steering to the Westward passed us within hail, we judged her to be English as they Answered us in that Language, but we could not understand what they said and they were presently out of sight.

In the Latitude of 29°30′, Longit. 41°30′ the Wind began to slaken and veer more to the SE. We now began to see of that Sea Plant which is commonly called Gulf Weed,[1] from a supposition that it comes out of the Gulf of Florida, indeed for any thing I know to the contrary it may be a fact, but it seems not necessary as it is certainly a plant which vegetates at sea. We continued to see of it, but allways in small pieces, till we reached the Latitude of 36°00′, Longitude 39° W, beyond this situation we saw none.

WEDNESDAY 5*th* of July. In the Latitude of 32°31′30″ N, Longitude 40°29′ W the Wind veered to the East and blew very faint, the next day it was Calm and the two following days we had Variable light airs and Calms by turns and at length on

SUNDAY 9*th* it fixed at SSW and increased to a fresh gale with which we Steered first NE and then ENE with a View of making some of the Ozores or Western isles.

TUESDAY 11*th*. In the Latitude of 36°45′ N, Longit. 36°45′ W we saw a sail which was steering to the West, the next day we saw three more and on

THURSDAY 13*th* at 5 PM we made land which proved to be the Island of Fayal, the SW point of which at 7 bore N 40° East distant Six leagues, at the same time we saw the isle of Pico, under which we spent the Night making short boards. At day-breake the next Morning, made sail for the Bay of Fayal, where at 8 o'Clock we Anchored in 20 fathom Water, a Sandy bottom and something more than half a Mile from Shore: here we moored NE and SW being directed so to do by the Master of the Port, who came on board before we droped Anchor and directed us where to come to for which he demanded his fee; it was but a trifle and I was sorry I could not pay it as it was demanded as *Port Charges* and not as Pilotage; every Merchant Vessel which Anchors in the Road is obliged to pay a Certain sum, about three Shillings, but if she comes from any part South of the line, she pays considerable more.

After being moored, the SW point of the Bay bore S 16° West, the Church at the NE end of the Town N 38° West, the NE point of the Bay N 33° East, the W point of S[t] Georges Isle N 42° E and the Isle of Pico extending from S 46° E to 74° East, distant about four miles.[2] As my chief design for stoping here was to give M[r] Wales an oppertunity to make some observations to find the Rate of the Watch, the better to enable us to determine with certainty the Longitude of

[1] *Sargassum bacciferum*, a sort of seaweed found in the Gulf Stream, the Sargasso sea and elsewhere.

[2] *Deleted* Note the above bearings are by Compass, the Variation not being allowed, as I was not sure of its quantity.

these Islands, The Moment we had Anchored, I sent an officer accompanied by Mr Wales on shore to wait on the English Consul and to notify our arrival to the Governor and request permission for Mr Wales to make observations on shore for the purpose above mentioned. They were met on the Beach by Mr Dent who acted as Consul in the absence of Mr Gathorne[1] and who not only got leave for Mr Wales [to] land his Instruments but accomodated him with a convenient place in his garden to set them up so that he was enabled to observe equal Altitudes the same day. The ceremony of Saluting was here omited, as the Governor refused to return Gun for Gun. We found riding in the Bay the Pourvoyeur, a large French Frigate, an American Sloop and a Portuguese Brig from the River Amazon laden with Provisions for the Cape Verde isles which she missed and was obliged to steer for this place.

During our stay the Ships Company was Served with fresh beef, and we took on board about fifteen Tons of Water which was brought off in boats belonging to the place at the rate of about three Shillings per Ton. Strangers are not denied the liberty of Watering with their own Boats and People, but the many ilconveniences attending it more than over ballances the expence and has interduced a kind of general Custom the same as at Madeira to hire Shore boats. These come on board, take your empty Casks and return them full, without any further trouble.[2] The Water is tolerable,[3] it is taken out of a Well which is about One hundred yards behind the beach and just within the Walls of the Town.[4] Fresh provisions for present use may also be had at a very reasonable rate, such as fresh beef, Vegetables and fruits and Hogs, Sheep and Poultry for Sea Stock, but I do not know that any Sea Provisions except Wine are to be got. The Bullocks and Hogs are very good, the latter especially, but the Sheep are very small and wretchedly poor.

We were not more obliged to Mr Dent for the readiness he Shewed in procuring us such of these articles as we wanted, than by the very liberal and hospital entertainment we met with at his house which was open to accommodate us both night and day.

The Town is called *D'horta* and is seated in the bottom of the Bay close to the edge of the Sea, it is defended by two Castles, one at each end of the Town or Corner of the Bay and a wall of stone work extending from the one to the other. It makes a fine appearence from

[1] Mr Gathorne, we learn from a later deletion, had 'lat[e]ly gone to London'.
[2] *Deleted* it is not even necessary to send a Man with them.
[3] *Deleted* it is neither the best nor worst,
[4] *Deleted* Wood for fewel may be had here in any quantity, but it also must be purchased.

the Road.[1] But if we except the Jesuites College, the Monasteries and Churches, all the other buildings have nothing to commend them neither on the out side nor in, the Inside walls being only white washed and there is not a glass window in the place except what are in the Churches and in a Country house which belonged to the English Consul, all those belonging to the Portugues were Letticed which makes them look like Prisions. This City[2] is like all others belonging to the Portuguese Crowded with Religious buildings, here are no less than three Monasteries of Men and two of Women and Eight Churches including those belonging to the Monasteries and the one in the Jesuites College. This College is a fine structure and is seated on an elevation in the pleasentest part of the City; sence the expulsion[3] of that order it has been in the hands of the Crown who make no other use of it than for the Courts of Justice to meet in so that very probably it will soon be no better than a heap of ruins.

The Island of Fayal is finely Cultivated, at least what I saw of it, and I was told that it was every where the same. The chief produce is Wheat and Indian Corn, with which they supply Pico and some of the other Islands.[4] Fayal altho' the most noted for Wine, do's not raise sufficient for their own Consumption, this Article is raised on Pico where there is no Road for Shipping so that it is brought to Fayal and from thence sent a broad, cheifly to America, thus it has got the name of Fayal Wine. Many of the principal people in Fayal, especially those of the City of de Horta, have Vineyards in Pico, which produceth little else but fruit and some are brought daily to De Horta for present consumption. The best Wine is said to be made on Pico of all the Ozores or Western isles, which are nine in number and all of them except it raise Corn and Cattle as well as Wine. St Michiels produceth a good deal of Flax which they Manufacture into Coarse Linnen with which they not only supply the other isles and Madeira, but send some yearly to the Brazils. Flax is also raised in Fayal, but I believe not sufficient for its own consumption. St Maries is famous for makeing Coarse earthenware from which all the other isles are supplied, but the entering into the particular productions of each isle is more than I intend, because a better account of these

[1] and a wall . . . Road *substituted for* and a wall of Stone Work between them, which is also continued out to the sw head of the Bay, so that when you first enter it seems a very strong place, but it is quite otherwise these works are much out of repair, without Cannon and garrisoned with only one hundred men. In like manner one is deceived by the City, which makes a grand and fine appearances from the Road, and which is probably heighted by the Country Houses, situated in a Country richly Cultivated, . . . f. 365.

[2] This City *substituted for* This little Town, for it by no means deserves the Name of a City

[3] expulsion *substituted for* abolishing

[4] with which . . . Islands *substituted for* but as it supplyes the Isle of Pico with Provisions they have little to export.

Matters may be had, I prosume, any day in London from the English Merchants who have resided upon them than any I can give, all I intended was to point out the Shelter and Refreshments they afford to Shipping, things which are not well known.

The Island of Fayal is three Leagues in breadth North and South, and as I was told by the Inhabitants eight or nine in length from East to West, but we have great reason to think that not only this isle, but all the others, have not that extent, the Inhabitants believe they have, or as they are represented in our Books of Navigation. The Bay is situated at the South East end of the isle before the City de Horta, and faceing the West end of the isle of Pico, it is 2 Miles broad and ¾ of a Mile deep and is shaped like the segment of a circle; the depth of Water is from 20 to 10 and 6 fathoms, a clean Sandy bottom, except near the Shore, especially that of the SW head off which the ground is Rocky and likewise without the line which joins the two points, so that it is not safe to anchor far out. The bearing taken when at anchor, before mentioned, will direct any one to the best ground. It is by no means a bad road, the only Wind you have to fear is that which blowes from between SSW & SE, the former indeed is not dangerous because with it you can always get to Sea. A Portuguese Captain informed me, that about half a league from the Road in the direction of SE, that is in a line between it and the South side of Pico, lies a Rock about 22 feet under water, on which the Sea breaks in hard gales from the South: the said Captain allso informed me, that of all the Shoals which are laid down in our Charts and Books of Navigation about these isles, not one has any existance but the one between the isle of St Michiel and St Mary called Hormingan.[1] This account may be believed without relying intirely upon it. Two observations of the Suns Meridian Altitude gave the Latitude of the Road to be 28°[2] 31′55″ N and the Longitude was found by Lunar Observations as follows, viz.

	°	′	″
Seven days Observans before we arrived and Reduced to it by the Watch	28	24	30
Four Sets observed at Anchor	28	33	15
Two days observations after leaving it & reduced back as above	28	53	22
Mean	28	27	02

[1] Hormigon, the highest of the northern part of the Formigas rocks, which, together with a bank of the same name, lie between São Miguel and Sta Maria, the two south-eastern isles of the Azores.

[2] A slip for 38°.

	°	′	″
By the Watch (which was found to go nearly as at the Cape)	28	55	45
By Lunar Observations made by Mr Wales	28	24	0

A North and South Moon makes high-water on the Change days and the Tide rises between 4 and 5 feet. There runs a pretty Strong tide between Fayal and Pico both Flood and Ebb: the Flood comes in from SW and Ebb from NE but out at Sea their direction is East and West.

N.B. Bay of Fayal reduced from Plymouth by the watch will be found to lie in the Longitude of 28°48′ W which is probably nearer the truth than that deduc'd from observations.

MONDAY 18*th*[1] about Noon the French Frigate sailed for Madeira for the same purpose as she came here, viz. to take in sweet wine, she was to go next to Tenerif on the same account and then home to Rochelle.[2]

WEDNESDAY 19*th* at 4 in the Morning we left the Bay and steered for the West end of St Georges isle, which we found to lie Leagues in the direction of NE½E from the Road or Bay of Fayal. This isle we found to be about 9 Leagues in length, in the direction of WNW and ESE, its breadth is inconsiderable. After passing the point of this isle, we steered for the Isle of *Tercera*, leaving *Gratiosa* on our Larboard. This isle, which is not above eight or ten Leagues in circuit, lies in the direction of NEBE from the West end of St George distant Eight leagues, and in the Latitude of 29°09′ N nearly, for the Weather being Cloudy and heazy we had no observation at Noon, but our reckoning could not be much out in so short a Run. At 2 o'Clock in the after-noon were not more than a League from the West end of Tercera, when we edged away along the NW Coast, having a fresh gale at SW attended with hazey rainy weather which made me give up the design of steering along the Coast to the Eastern point, in order to assertain its length. At 4 o'Clock the NE point boare S 27° East distant 5 or 6 Leagues, we now stood away from the Isle in the direction of NEBE½E with the wind and weather as before; but about Middnight, in a very heavy shower of rain, the wind Shifted to the North, where it fixed and blew a gentle breeze with fair weather till

[1] *sic*; it should be Monday 17th or Tuesday 18th.

[2] The Log, 19 July (i.e. Tuesday 18th civil time) has the domestic detail, 'The English Consul and the Captain of the Garrison dining on board, they were saluted with 9 Guns on their coming on board and going on Shore'.

SATURDAY 22*nd* when after two hours Calm, in the Latitude of 39°38′ N we got the wind at West, the next day it fixed at WNW and increased to a fresh [gale] with which we Steered directly for the Lizard and on

SATURDAY 29*th* we made the Land about Plymouth; Maker Church, at 5 o'Clock in the after-noon, bore N 10° west distant 7 Leagues, this bearing and distance shew that the error of Mr Kendals Watch in Longitude was only 7′45″, which was too far to the west.[1]

* * *

TUESDAY 11*th*.[2] In the Latitude of 36°45′ N, Longit. 36°45′ W we saw a sail which was steering to the West, the next day we saw three more, and on Thursday the 13th at 5 o'Clock in the Evening we made the Island of Fayal, one of the Ozores, and soon after that of Pico, under which we spent the night making short boards. At Day break the next Morning bore away for the Bay of Fayal or De Horta where at 8 o'Clock we anchored in 20 fathom Water, a clean sandy bottom and some thing more than half a mile from the Shore. Here we moored NE and SW, being directed so to do by the Master of the Port, who came on board before we droped Anchor and directed us where to come to. When moored the SW Point of the Bay bore S 16° W and the NE Point N 33° E; the Church at the NE end of the Town N 38° W, the West point of St George's Island N 42° E and the Isle of Pico extending from N 74° E to S 46° E distant four or five Miles. We found in the Bay the *Pourvoyeur*, a large French Frigate, an America Sloop and a Brig belonging to the place; she came last from the River Amazon, where she took in a Cargo of Provisions for the Cape Verd Islands, but not being able to find them she steered for this place, where she Anchored about half an hour before us.

As my sole design for stoping here was to give Mr Wales an oppertunity to find the Rate of the Watch, the better to enable us to fix with some degree of certainty the Longitude of these Islands, The moment we Anchored I sent an officer to wait on the English Consul, and to Notify our arrival to the Governor and to request permission for Mr Wales to make observations on shore for the purpose above mentioned. Mr Dent, who acted as Consul in the absence of Mr Gathorne, not only procured this Permission, but accomodated M^r^

[1] In H Cook adds to this entry the sentence, 'The next day anchor'd at Spithead', and his signature.

[2] I here give the second version of the closing pages of Add. MS 27888, ff. 359v–63v, as revised by Cook from ff. 364–7v, and printed, in a form further revised, in *Voyage*, II, pp. 282–9. See the Textual Introduction, pp. cxxii–iii.

Wales with a convenient place in his garden to set up his Instruments, so that he was enabled to observe equal Altitudes the same day. We were not more obliged to Mr Dent for the very obliging readiness he shewed in procuring us this and every other thing we wanted, than by the very liberal and hospitable entertainment we met with at his house, which was open to accomodate us both night and day.

During our Stay the Ships Company was served with fresh Beef, and we took on board about 15 Tons of Water, which was brought off in the Country Boats at the rate of about three Shillings per Ton. Ships are allowed to Water with their own Boats, but the many ilconveniences attending it more than over ballances the expence of hiring shore boats which is the most general Custom. Fresh Provisions for present use may be got such as Beef, Vegetables and Fruit, and Hogs, Sheep and Poultry for Sea Stock all at a pretty reasonable price. But I do not know that any Sea Provisions except Wine are to be had. The Bullocks and Hogs are very good, but the Sheep are very small and wretchedly poor.

The chief produce of Fayal is Wheat and Indian Corn with which they supply Pico and some of the other Isles. The Chief Town is called Villa de Horta, it is seated in the bottom of the Bay close to the edge of the sea and is defended by two Castles, one at each end of the Town or bottom of the Bay, and a Wall of stone work, extending along the Sea Shore, from the one to the other. But these works are suffered to go to decay and serve more for Shew than strength. They heighten the Prospect of the City which makes a fine appearence from the Road, but if we except the Jesuites College, the Monasteries and Churches, there is not another building that has any thing to recommend it either on the out side or in. There is not a glass window in the place, except what are in the Churches and a Country house which lately belonged to the English Consul, all the others are Letticed which makes them looke like Prisions to an Englishman. This little City, like all others belonging to the Portuguese is Crowded with Religious Buildings, here are no less than Three Monasteries of Men and two of Women, and Eight Churches, including those belonging to the Monasteries and the one in the Jesuites Collage. This Collage is a fine structure and is seated on an elevation, in the pleasantest part of the City. Sence the expulsion of that order, it has been suffered to go to decay and will, probably, in a few years be no better than a heap of ruins.

Fayal, altho' the most Noted for Wine, does not raise sufficient for their own consumption. This article is raised on Pico, where there is no Road for Shipping, brought to De Horta and from thence Shiped a broad, chiefly to America, thus it has acquired the name of Fayal Wine.[1]

The Bay or Road of Fayal is situated at the East end of the isle, before the Villa de Horta and faceing the West end of Pico. It is two Miles broad and ¾ of a Mile deep and hath a semicircular form; the depth of Water is from 20 to 10 and even 6 fathoms a Sandy bottom, except near the shore, and particular the SW head, off which the bottom is Rocky, also without the line which joins the two Points of the Bay, so that it is not safe to anchor far out. The bearing before mentioned, taken when at Anchor, will direct any one to the best ground. It is by no means a bad Road, the most dangerous Winds are those which blow from between the SSW and SE, the former is not so dangerous as the latter, because with it you can always get to Sea. Besides this Road there is a small Cove round the SW Point, called Porto Pieri, in which I am told a Ship or two may lay in tolerable safety, and in which they some times heave small vessels down.

A Portuguese Captain informed me, that about half a League from the Road, in the direction of SE, that [is] in a line between it and the South side of Pico, lies a sunken Rock, over which is 22 feet water and on which the Sea breaks in hard gales from the South. He also assured me, that of all the Shoals which are laid down in our Charts and Pilot Book[s] about these isles, not one has any existance, but the one between the Island of St Michiel and St Mary called Hormingan. This account may be believed without relying intirely upon it. He further informed me that it is 45 Leagues from Fayal to the Island of Flores, & that there runs a Strong Tide between Fayal and Pico, the Flood seting to the NE and the Ebb to the SW, but that out at Sea the direction is East and West. Mr Wales observed the times of high and low Water by the Shore and concluded that it must be high-water at the Full and Change about 12 o'Clock and that the Water riseth about 4 or 5 feet.

The Distance between Fayal and Flores was confirmed by M. Rebiers, Lieutenant of the French Frigate, who told me that after being by estimation two Leagues due South of Flores, they made 44 leag^s^ on a SEBE Course by Compass to St Catherines point on Fayal.

	°	′	″	
I found the Latitude of the Ship at Anchor in the Bay	38	31	55	N

[1] *Deleted paragraph following this one:* The Ozores, or Western Islands, which are Nine in number, belong to the Crown of Portugal and are Governed by a General, who resides at Tecera, but I believe each Island has a seperate Governor under him residing on it. From the best accounts I can obtain, they are situated between the Latitude of and and between the Longitude of and West.—f. 361–IV.

	° ′ ″
By a mean of 17 sets of Lunar Observations taken before we arrived & and reduced to the Bay by the Watch made the Longitude	28 24 30 W
By a mean of 6 sets after leaving it and reduced back by the Watch	28 53 22
West Longitude by observation	28 38 56½
D° by the Watch	28 55 45
Error of the Watch on our [arrival at Portsmouth	16 26½
True longitude by the watch	28 39 18½][1]

I found the Variation of the Compass, by several Azimuths, taken by different Compasses on board the Ship to be 22°30′ W, which agree'd very well with the like observations made by Mr Wales on Shore and yet the Variation thus found is greater by 5° than we found it to be at Sea, for the Azimuths taken on board the Evening before we came into the Bay gave no more than 16°18′ West Variation, and the evening after we came out 17°33′ West.

I shall now give some account of the Variation as we found it in our run from the Island of Fernando de Norono to Fayal. The least Variation we found was 0°37′ W, this was the day after we left Fernando de Norono and in the Latitude of 0°33′ S Longitude 32°16′ W. The next day, being nearly in the same Longitude and in the Latitude of 1°25′ N, it was 1°23′ W and we did not find it increase till we got into the Latitude of 5°, Longitude 31° W. After this our Compasses gave different Variation, vizt from 3°57′ to 5°11′ West, till we arrived into the Latitude of 26°44′ N, Longitude 41° West, where we found 6°0′ W. After this it increased gradually, so that in the Latitude of 35° N, Longitude 40° West it was 10°24′ W. In the Latitude of 38°12′ N, Longitude 32½° W it was 14°47′ and in sight of Fayal 16°18′ West as mentioned above.

WEDNESDAY 19*th* at 4 o'Clock in the Morning we left the Bay and steered for the West end of St Georges Island, which lies in the direction of NE½E distant about Six Leagues from the NE end of Fayal. St Georges Island is about 9 Leagues in length in the direction of WNW and ESE, its brea[d]th is inconsiderable. After passing the point of

[1] The page ends with the words 'on our'. The words and figures between square brackets are supplied from *Voyage*, II, p. 287.

this Isle we steered for the Island of Tecera, leaving Gratiosa on our Larboard: this Island is about 10 Leagues in Circuit and lies in the direction of NEBE from the West end of St Georges Island, distant Eight Leagues.

At 2 o'Clock in the afternoon we were not more than one League from the West end of Tecera, having run 13 Leagues from the West end of St Georges Island. We now edged away for the North side with a view of rangeing the Coast to the Eastern point, in order to assertain the length of the isle. But the Weather coming on very thick and hazy and night approaching I give up the design and hauled off from the Land in the direction of NEBE½E, with a very fresh gale at SW attended with rain. We have now seen and pretty well determined the situation of five out of the Nine Islands which compose this Archipelago. By which and from the information of M. Rebiers and Mr Gilbert, my Master, I have endeavour'd to settle that of the other four also, as it may be of use to the Navigator, either in verifying or correcting his Longitude. In constructing the following Table I have two observed Latitudes given, viz. the Bay of Fayal and the Road of St Maries; the former observed by us and the latter by Mr Gilbert.[1] From the above Data's, the situation of the Several Islands will be as follows, viz.

	Latitude	Longitude
The Middle of Corvo		
The Middle of Flores		
Bay of Fayal, at the East end of the Id		
Peak on Pico		
Middle of St Georges Island		
Middle of Gratiosa		

After leaving these Islands, I made the best of my [way] for England. On Saturday the 29th we made the land near Plymouth and the next morning anchored at Spit-head. Having been absent from England Three Years and Eighteen Days, in which time I lost but four men and one only of them by sickness.[2]

[1] As Gilbert was one of 'us', Cook, I should guess, meant to write 'Rebiers' here and slipped into the wrong name. If the observation was by Gilbert, it must have been on some former voyage.

[2] The last word may be young Mr Elliott's. 'The same day Captn Cook, with Messrs Forster, Wales Hodges, and my Messmate Grindal set out for London: The latter we now found (and not till now) had Married a very handsome young Lady, and left her, within an hour after, on our leaving England.'—*Mem.*, f. 44v.

APPENDIX I

Cook's Letters and Reports on and about the Voyage

1. To Furneaux

[*Not all of Cook's communications to Furneaux on the voyage are here given, but some only that appear to throw light on his plans or character. The following is printed from P.R.O. Adm 1/1610 (Admiralty In Letters, James Cook, 1772 to 1775), copies enclosed in Cook's letter to the Admiralty Secretary, Philip Stephens, from Spithead, 30 July 1775. These are all certified 'a Copy—J:Cook'. They are entered in the Canberra Letter Book. The directions for rendezvous were enclosed one within another, under the general date 15 July 1772: the first was for Madeira, the second for St Iago.*]

Third Rendezvous, to proceed to the Cape of Good Hope where you are to refresh the sloops Company and take on board such provisions &c as you may stand in need of and may be able to procure, If I do not arrive at or before the Expiration of Six weeks, reckoning from the time of your first arrival, you are then to Open the enclosed Secrete Instructions, and proceed as therein directed.

Given under my hand on board
His Majesty's Sloop Resolution
J: Cook

To
Capt[n] Furneaux

By Capt. James Cook, Comm[r]
of His Majesty's Sloop Resolution

After having waited at the Cape of Good Hope the time limeted by the Rendezvous (Viz[t]) Six Weeks, you are hereby required and directed to put to Sea with the Sloop you Command and carry into Execution, as far as in you lay, the enclosed Instructions, which are an Exact Copy of those I have from their Lordships.

On all such land as you may Discover on your rout to the Southward and can land thereon you are to Erect on the most conspicuous parts of the coast post[s] or Marks at the Feet of which leave letters in Bottles given [*sic*] an Account of your proceedings, time you departed from thence, the rout you intend to take and such other informations as you think Necessary, and also during your stay in any port or place, you are on some hill or other conspicuous place to hoist a S[t] George's Ensign in the day and make fires in the Night & fire Guns, or take such other Method as your Situation will admit to point out to me the place w[h]ere you are in case

I should happen to be upon the coast at that time; But if you should fail of discovering land in your rout to the Southward or Westward, or the land you discover should be in so high a Latitude that you cannot Winter upon it, In either of these cases you are, as soon as the season of the year may render it unsafe for you to continue in high Lattitudes, to make the best of your way to Queen Charlottes Sound in New Zealand, where you are to remain untill the next season approaches for returning to the Southward, taking care before you depart to leave directions in the Manner abovementioned near the watering place in Ship Cove; and if you should put into any port on the Southern parts of New Zealand, either before you arrive at the abovementioned Sound or after you depart from it, you will also make use of the forementioned methods to point out the place were you are. It is recommended to you that while you are upon the Southern parts of New Zealand to Endeavour to procure Speciements of the different Stones you may find in the Country, as an Opinion has lately been started that some of them contain Menerals or Metal. If after all your Endeavours to join me before you leave New Zealand should prove ineffectual you will Neve[r]theless Continue to put in practice the same Methods towards filiciating[1] a meeting as you had done before, all of which I myself will put in Execution in case I shall happen to be before you.

Given under my hand on
board His Majestys Sloop
Resolution at Sea
this 15th of July 1772
J: Cook

To
Captn Tobs Furneaux
Commander of His Majesty's
Sloop Adventure

2. To the Admiralty Secretary

[*Printed from P.R.O. Adm 1/1610; only the signature is in Cook's hand. Endorsed 'Recd 7th Sepr & Read'. Entered, with minor differences, in the Canberra Letter Book.*]

Sir

Please to Acquaint my Lords Commissrs of the Admiralty with the arrival of His Majesty's Sloops Resolution and Adventure at this place late in the Evening of the 28th of last month and that havg taken on board as much wine as they can conveniently Stow I intend to put to sea again this Evening. Least it is thought that the tryal made of the Resolution between Sheerness & Plymouth was not sufficient to form a just judgement of her qualities, and the clamour raised against her not yet subsided; I beg leave, once more, to assert that so far from finding her crank, I find her remarkable stiff and to have as many other good Qualities as can be found

[1] An attempt, no doubt, at 'facilitating'.

in one ship and Captain Furneaux is equally as well Satisfied with the Adventure; In point of sailing they are well Match'd, the Little difference is in favour of the Resolution;

I am Sir
Your most Humble Serv[t]
JAM[s] COOK

Resolution, at Madeira the 1st
of August 1772

Phil. Stephens Esq[r]

3. COOK TO ?

[*Windsor Castle Library, Georgian Papers, no. 1359; holograph. The name of the person addressed nowhere appears: it may have been a personal letter to Stephens, or even to Palliser—though no other letter to Palliser has survived. It has been printed, not quite correctly, in Fortescue,* Correspondence of George III (*1927*), *II, pp. 372–3.*]

Resolution, at Madeira 1st Aug[t] 1772

Sir

I have now the pleasure to acquaint you that the Resolution answers in every respect as well, nay even better than we could expect, she steers works, sails well and is remarkably stiff and seems to promise to be a dry and very easy ship in the Sea; In our passage from Plymouth we were once under our Courses but it was not wind that obliged the Resolution to take in her Topsails tho' it blow'd hard, but because the Adventure could not carry hers, in point of sailing the two Sloops are well match'd what difference there is is in favour of the Resolution. I arrived here late in the evening of the 28th of last month and shall put to Sea again this evening having got on board all our Wine water &c[a].

Three days before we arrived a person left the Island who went by the name of Burnett he had been waiting for M[r] Banks arrival about three months, at first he said he came here for the recovery of his health, but afterwards said his intention was to go out with M[r] Banks, to some he said he was unknown to this Gentleman, to others he said it was by his appointment he came here as he could not be receiv'd on board in England, at last when he heard that M[r] Banks did not go, he took the very first oppertunity to get of the Island, he was about 30 Years of age and rather ordinary than otherwise and employ'd his time in Botanizing &c[a]. Every part of M[r] Burnetts behaviour and every action tended to prove that he was a Woman, I have not met with a person that entertains a doubt of a contrary nature, he brought letters of recomendation to an English House where he was accomodated during his stay, It must be observed that M[rs] Burnett must have left London about the time we were first ready to sail.

I am
JAM[s] COOK

4. To the Admiralty Secretary

[*P.R.O. Adm 1/1610; only the signature is in Cook's hand. Entered in Canberra Letter Book.*]

Sir

In obedience to their Lordships directions signified to me by your Letter of the 2nd of May last I have Caused several trials to be made of the Inspissated juce of Malt by making of it into Beer, by mixing, from Eight parts of Water to one of Juce, to twelve of water to one of Juce, the Beer made by this last proportion had a Strong taste of the Juce but became Sour soon after it was made, owing I think, to the very hot weather it was brew'd in, which caused to[o] great fermentation, indeed all the Experiments were made in hot weather when the Thermometer was at 79° or 80 and for that reason unfavourable to the Juce; the Beer made from it is of a very Deep Colour and has rather a burnt taste, but no ways disagreeable and was very well liked by the people in general; More hops I apprehend is Necessary, for there remained not the least taste of them, only one thing more is wanting to render it a Valuable and usefull Article, that is to hinder it from fermenting, for all the time we were in hot climates, that is when the Thermometer was at 65° and upwards, it was in a Continual State of fermentation in So Much that the Casks were not able to Resist its efforts, and every Method we took to stop it proved inefectual, with some care and a good deal of Trouble we have preserv'd about half of it with which I Shall Make experiments from time to time.

Mr Pelham Secretary to the Commissioners of the Victualing put on board a few Jarrs of Juce Containing about five pints Each, of his own preparing, which promises fair to Answer all that is expected from it.

I am
Sir
Your most Humble Servt
Jams Cook

Resolution at the Cape of Good
Hope 16th of Novr 1772

Phillip Stephens Esqr

5. To the Admiralty Secretary

[*P.R.O. Adm 1/1610; only the signature is in Cook's hand. Entered in Canberra Letter Book, with slight variants as noted.*]

Resolution, Cape of Good Hope 18th Novr 1772.

Sir

Please to acquaint their Lordships that I left Madeira with His Majesty's Sloops Resolution and Adventure the 1st of August, touched at St Iago took on board some refreshments and Departed again in two Days, and on the 30th of last Month arrived at this place without any Material occurences happening. I find the Sloops to Answer as well as Ships can do and the crews were, and Continue healthy; from this last Circumstance I thought to have made my Stay very Short here, waiting for some Articles of Provisions hath kept me longer than I intended; being at length Compleat, as you will see by the inclosed State of the Sloops, shall put to sea without loss of time.

Lieutenant Shank, First of the Adventure, having requested Leave to quit in Order to return home, and the Surgeons having Reported the same to be absolutely Necessary for the Restablishment of his health, I granted it him accordingly, and appointed Mr Kemp to be First Lieutenant of the Adventure and Mr James Burney one of my midshipman to be Second in his room, which I hope will meet with their Lordships approbation; Copies of the Letters and orders on this affair you will herewith receive. I must beg leave to assure their Lordships that Mr Shank has quited the Sloop with the greatest eluctancy,[1] and nothing but his bad State of health would have Obliged him to give up a Voyage on Which he had Set his heart. On My arrival at this place, I learnt, that about Eight months ago two French Ships (La Fortune & Gross Ventre) from the Mauritius Discovered Land in the Meridian of that Island and in about Latitude of 48° a long which they Sail'd Forty Miles till they came to a bay into which they were about to enter when they were drove off the Coast and Seperated by a Gale of wind, the La Fortune Arrived at the Mauritius Soon After and the Captain is Since gorne [*sic*] to France to give an Account of the discovery and touched here about three Months ago in his way; the Gross Ventre is lately arrived at the Mauritius from Batavia with a Cargo of Arrack, this Account we have by a Ship who left the Island two days after the other Arrived [in][2] which time Nothing about the Discovery transpired, Also in March last two French Frigates from the same Island touched here in their way to the South Sea, had on board the Man Bougainvill brought from the Otaheite[3] and who Died before the Ships left this place; they are to touch Some were on the Coast of America before they proceed round Cape Horn the rout they intended to take.

The Paintings which Mr Hodges has made of Madeira Port Praya and this place I have packed up and left here to be forwarded to you by the first Safe Opportunity Vizt One large painting of this place one Small one of part of Funchall and One of port praya all in Oil Colours and Some others in Water Colours of little Note.

I am Sir,
Your most Humble Servt
JAMs COOK

Resolution, Cape of Good Hope
Novemr 18th 1772

Phillip Stephens Esqr

1 *sic;* CLB reluctance.
2 Supplied from CLB.
3 *the Otaheite:* CLB Otaheita.

6. To Banks

[*Mitchell Library MSS. Reproduced in facsimile in* Hist.Rec.N.S.W., *Vol. I, Part 1.*]

Resolution Cape of Good Hope
18th Novr 1772

Dear Sir

Some Cross circumstances which happened at the latter part of the equipment of the Resolution created, I have reason to think, a coolness betwixt you and I, but I can by no means think it was sufficient to me to break of all corrispondance with a Man I am under m[a]ny obligations too

I wish I had some thing intresting to communicate, but our passage here has rather been barren on that head; We touch[ed] at St Iago where we remain'd two days and Mr Forster got some things there new in your way. Mr Brand[1] has got for you a fine Collection as I am told. I depart from hence in a Day or two well Stored with every necessary thing, but I am told the French from the Mauritius have got the start of me: about Eight Months ago two Ships from that Island discovered Land in the Latitude of 48° and about the Meridian of the Mauritius along which they saild 40 Miles till they came to a bay into which they were about to enter when they were seperated and drove off the Coast by a gale of Wind, the one got to the Mauritius soon after and the other is since arrived from Batavia with a Cargo of Arrack as the report goes here. Also in March last two Frigates from the same Island touched here in thier way to the South Sea having on board the man Bougainville brought from Otahiete and who died before the Ships departed from hence a circumstance I am realy sorry for, these Ships were to touch some were on the Coast of America and afterwards to proceed round Cape Horn.

I am in your debt for the Pickled and dryed Salmon which you left on board, which a little time ago was most excellant, but the eight Casks of Pickled salted fish I kept for my self proved so bad that even the Hoggs would not eat it; these hints may be of use to you in providg for your intinded expeditation,[2] in which I wish you all the Success you can wish your self and am with great esteem and respect

Dr Sir

Your most Obliged Humble Servt
JAMS COOK

Joseph Banks Esqr

[1] The agent who acted for Cook at the Cape in the purchase of supplies, with whom Banks had become acquainted on the homeward passage of the *Endeavour* in March–April 1771.

[2] *sic;* Cook probably refers to Banks's projected South Seas expedition; but in fact Banks at this date was on the point of leaving Scotland for London, after his expedition to Iceland —his hopes for an independent voyage to the South Seas already over.

7. To the Admiralty

[*The following 'Extract of a letter' was printed in* The General Evening Post, *London, 19 April 1773. The original document has not been found among the records.*]

Extract of a letter from Captain Cook of his Majesty's sloop Resolution, dated at the Cape of Good Hope the 19th of November, 1772.

I did myself the honour to acquaint your Lordships in my last with my arrival at Madeira in company with the Adventure. I left that island on the 1st of August, touched at St. Jago, filled our water, and departed again in two days, and on the 30th of last month arrived at this place without any thing remarkable happening in our passage. The crews of both sloops are healthy; and I must say your Lordships could not have made choice of two finer vessels in every respect for such a voyage, more especially the Resolution, which has every quality I could wish to find in a ship. I now wait for nothing but a wind to get out of the bay, after which I shall proceed to the Southward without loss of time.

8. To John Walker

[*General Assembly Library, Wellington, New Zealand.*]

Cape of Good Hope 20th Novr 1772

Dear Sir

Having nothing new to communicate I should hardly have troubled you with a letter was it not customary for Men to take leave of their friends before they go out of the World, for I can hardly think my self in it so long as I am deprived from having any Connections with the civilized part of it, and this will soon be my case for two years at least. When I think of the Inhospitable parts I am going to, I think the Voyage dangerous, I however enter upon it with great cheerfullness, providence has been very kind to me on many occasions, and I trust in the continuation of the divine protection; I have two good Ships well provided and well Man'd. You must have heard of the Clamour raised against the Resolution before I left England, I can assure you I never set foot in a finer Ship. Please to make my best respects to all Friends at Whitby and beleive me to be with great regard and esteem

Your Most affectionate Friend
Jams Cook

9. To Furneaux

[*P.R.O. Adm 1/1610, enclosure in Cook to Stephens, 30 July 1775. Signature only in Cook's hand. Entered in Canberra Letter Book.*]

By Capt. James Cook &c

Whereas Several Months must elapse before His Majesty's Sloops Resolution & Adventure, can proceed on Discoverys to the South, my intention therefore is, to employ that time in exploring the unknown parts of the Sea, to the East & North by first proceeding to the East between the Latitude of 41° & 45° South untill I arrive in the Longitude of 140° or 135° West of Greenwich, if in this Rout I discover no Land then to proceed directly to the Island of Otahiete where I intend to take in water & such refreshments as are to be got, afterwards to return back to this place by the shortest Rout, & after taking in wood & water to proceed to the South in order to explore the unknown parts of the Sea between the Meridian of New Zealand & Cape Horn. You are therefore Required & directed to put to sea & proceed with me with His Majesty's Sloop under your command and in case of Seperation, by any unavoidable accident before we reach Otahiete, you are first to look for me in the same place you last Saw me & not meeting me in three days, you are to proceed to Matavai Bay in the Island of Otahiete, where you are to wait untill the 20th of August, if I do not arrive before that time then to put to sea and make the best of your way back to this place, where you are to waite until the 20th of November, not being join'd by me by that time you are to put to Sea and carry into Execution there Lordships Instructions.

Given under my hand on board His
Majesty's Sloop Resolution in
Queen Charlottes Sound New
Zealand the 4th day of June 1773

J Cook

To
Captain Tob[s] Furneaux
Commander of His Majesty's
Sloop Adventure

10. To the Admiralty Secretary

[*P.R.O. Adm 1/1610; holograph. Endorsed 'Recd 27 June 1775 & Read'. It is not in the Canberra Letter Book.*]

Sir

Having this Moment spoke with the True Britain India Man, I take the oppertunity to accquaint you that His Majesty's Sloop Resolution is within two days Sail of the Cape of Good Hope. I lear[n]t from a Dutchman yesterday that Captain Furneaux sailed from the Cape for England, twelve Months ago; you must therefore know the former part of my proceedings and a full account of the latter shall be sent you by the very first oppertunity after my arrival at the Cape. I have the satisfaction to say, that I have met with no one accedent and the Crew, thus far, hath injoyed a good state of health.

I am with great respect

Sir

Your Most Humble Serv[t]

Jam[s] Cook

Resolution at Sea
19th March 1775.

To Philip Stephens Esq[r]

11. To the Admiralty Secretary

[*P.R.O, Adm 1/1610. Only the signature and the date at the head are in Cook's hand. Entered in the Canberra Letter Book.*]

22nd March 1775

Sir

As Captain Furneaux must have inform'd you of my proceedings prior to our final Separation, I shall confine this letter to my Transactions afterwards. The Adventure not arriving in Queen Charlottes Sound before the 26th of November, I put to Sea and after spending two days looking for her on the Coast, I stood away to the South, inclining to the East. I met with little interruption from ice till we got into the Latitude of 66° where the Sea was so covered with it that we could proceed no farther; We then steered to the East inclining to the South, over a Sea strewed with Mountains of Ice; and crossed the Antarctick Circle in the Meridian of 146° West. After this I found it necessary to haul to the North, not only to get clear of the ice Islands, which were very numerous, but to explore a large space of Sea we had left nearly in the middle of the Ocean in that direction. After geting to the Latitude of 48° I edged away to the East and then again to the South, till we arrived in the Latitude of 71° 10′ Longitude 106½° West, farther it was not possible to go, all the Sea to the South being wholy covered with a solid Sheet of ice, in which were Ice Mountains whose lofty summits were lost in the clouds. Hetherto we had not seen the least signs of land, or any one thing to encourage our researches, nevertheless I did not think the Pacific ocean sufficiently explored and as I found we were in a condition to remain in it another year I resolved to do it and accordingly stood away to the North and searched in vain for Juan Fernandes land. I was more successfull with Easter Island, where I made a short stay and next visited the Marquesas, from the Marquesas I proceeded to Otaheite and the Society Isles, where we were received with a hospitality altogether unknown among more civilized Nations; these good people Supplyed all our wants with a liberal and full hand, and I found it necessary to spend six Weeks with them. I left these Isles on the 4th of June, proceeded to the West, touched at Rotterdam, stayed two or three days and then continued our rout for Terra del Espiritu Santo of Quiros which we made the 16th of July. I found this land to be composed of a large group of isles, (many of them never seen by any European before) lying between the Latitude of 14° and 20° and nearly under the Meridian of 168° East. The exploring these isles finished all I had intended to do within the Tropic, accordingly I hauled to the South intending to touch at New Zealand, but on the 4th of September in the Latitude of 20° I fell in with a large Country, which I called New Caledonia. I coasted the N E Coast of this Country and partly determined the extent of the S W. I found the whole so incompass'd with Shoals that the risk we ran in exploring it was very great. We were at last blown off the Coast and as it was now time for us to return to the South, I was obliged to leave it unfinished and to continue our route to Queen

Charlottes Sound, where we arrived on the 6th of October. I remain'd here refiting the Sloop and refreshing my people till the 9th of November, when I put to Sea and proceeded directly for Terra del Fuego, but over such parts of the Sea as I had not visited before; I choose to make the West entrance of the Straits of Magalhanes, that I might have it in my power to explore the S W and South Coast of Terra del Fuego, which was accordingly done, as well as that of Staten land. This last Coast I left on the 3d of Janry last and on the 14th in the Latitude of 54° Longitude 38° West we discovered a Coast which from the imence quantity of Snow upon it and the vast height of its Mountains, we judged to belong to a great Continent, but we found it to be an isle of no more that 70 or 80 leagues in circuit. After leaving this land I steered to S E and in 59° discovered another, exceeding high and Mountainous, and so buried in everlasting snow that it was necessary to be pretty near the Shore to be satisfied that the foundation was not of the same composition. I coasted this land to the North and found it to terminate in isles in that direction. There isles carried us insencibly from the Coast which we could not afterwards regain, so that I was obliged to leave it without being able to determine whether it belonged to a Continent extending to the South or was only a group of isles. Our thus meeting with land gave me reason to believe there was such a land as Cape Circumcision, so that I quited this Horrid Southern Coast with less regret. But our second Search for Cape Circumcision was attended with no better success then the first and served only to assure us that no such land existed. At length after having made the Circuit of the Globe, and nothing more remained to be done, the Season of the year and other circumstances, unnecessary I presume to mention, determined me to steer for the Cape of Good Hope where I arrived on the date hereof and found the Ceres, Captain Newte bound directly for England, by whom I transmit this together with an account of the proceedings of the whole Voyage and such Surveys, Views and other drawings as have been made in it. The Charts are partly constructed from my own observations and partly from Mr Gilbert my Master whose judgment and asseduity, in this as well as every other branch of his profession is exceeded by none. The Views are all by Mr Hodges and are so judiciously chosen and executed in so Masterly a manner as will not only shew the judgment and skill of the artist but will of themselves express their various designs, but these are not all the works of that indefaticable gentleman, there are several other Views, Portraits and some valuable designs in Oyl Colours, which for want of proper Colours, time and conveniences, cannot be finished till after our arrival in England. The other Gentlemen whom Goverment thought proper to send out, have each contributed his share to the success of the Voyage; I have received every assistance I could require from Mr Wales the Astronomer; Mr Kendals Watch has exceeded the expectations of its most Zealous advocate and by being now and then corrected by Lunar observations has been our faithfull guide through all the vicissitudes of climates.

In justice to my Officers and Crew, I must say they have gone through the dangers and fatigues of the Voyage with the utmost constancy and cheerfullness, this together with the great skill, care and attention of Mr Patten the Surgeon, has not a little contributed to that uninterrupted good state of health we have all along enjoyed, for it cannot be said that we have lost one man by sickness sence we left England.

If I have failed in discovering a Continent it is because it does not exist in a Navigable Sea and not for want of looking after, Insurmountable difficulties were the bounds to my researches to the South. Whoever has resolution and paseverence to find one beyond where I have been, I shall not envy him the honour of the discovery, but I will be bold to say, that the world will not be benefited by it. My researches has not been confined to a Continent alone, but to the isles and every other object that could contribute to finish the exploring the Southern Hemisphere, how far I may have succeeded I submit to their Lordships better judgment and am with the greatest respect

Sir
Your most Obedient
Humble Servt
JAM^{S} COOK

Resolution in Table Bay Cape
of Good Hope
March 22nd 1775

Philip Stephens Esqr

12. TO THE ADMIRALTY SECRETARY

[*Canberra Letter Book. No signature, and no day of the month given in the date. The letter does not appear among others from Cook relating to the voyage in the relevant Admiralty records, P.R.O.*]

Resolution Cape of Good Hope
April 1775.

Sir

By the Ceres Captain Newte I had an oppertunity to acquaint you with the Arrival of His Majesty's Sloop under my Command at this place on the 22nd of last Month. At the same time I transmited a Journal of my proceedings during the whole Voyage together with every necessary drawing for the illustration of the said Journal. I am under no doubt but they will arrive safe, but to guard against every accident I thought proper herewith to transmit to you, by the Royal Charlotte Captain Clements, two of the Officers Journals or Log-books, and shall if another oppertunity offers before I leave this place, which will be in twelve or fourteen days, transmit those[1] of the Officers.

I am with great respect
Sir
Your most humble Servant

Philip Stephens Esqr

[1] Possibly this word read originally 'others'.

13. To the Admiralty Secretary

[*P.R.O. Adm 1/1610; only the signature is in Cook's hand. Entered in the Canberra Letter Book.*]

Sir

This is the third Letter I have had the honour to transmit to you sence my Arrival at ye Cape of Good Hope, the first, which was accompanied by a copy of my Journal & various drawings, was forwarded by ye Ceres East Indiaman, the Second together with ye Journals of two of ye Officers, by ye Royall Charlotte, and this comes by the Dutton with whom I saild from ye Cape the 27th of last Month. The probability of this ship being at home before us, as we touch at Assencion and she not, induced me to put on board her Lieutenant Coopers Journal, Some remarks and a chart of Mr Pickersgills, and a Journal kept by one of ye Mates, this Journal is Accompanied by very accurate charts of all the Discoverys we have made, executed by a Young man who has been bred to the Sea under my care and who has been a very great assistant to me in this way, both in this and my former Voyage.[1] I have the Honour to be with great respect

Sir

Your Most Humble Servt

Jam^{s} Cook

Resolution at Sea
May 24th 1775
Lat. 13° S
Long. 10° W^{t}

Philip Stephens Esqr

14. To the Admiralty Secretary

[*Canberra Letter Book; not in Admiralty records, P.R.O. The copy is undated, but presumably the letter was written on 31 July or 1 August, to which latter date belong some important reports.*]

Sir

Please to Acquaint their Lordships with the arrival of His Majestys Sloop Resolution under my Command at Spithead on the 30th Instant where I left her to the Direction of the first Lieutenant and in Obedience to their Lordships Instructions, have repaired to London to lay before them a full Account of my proceedings during ye Whole Voyage which you will here with receive together with charts of Lands I have either discovered or explored and such of Mr Hodges's drawings as were not Transmited to you from the Cape of Good hope but the paintings made by this Gentleman are yet on board the Sloop, For particulars I must beg leave to refer you to my Letter dated at the Cape of Good Hope the 22^{d} of last March a Copy whereof is here enclosed, as also two others, I had an Opportunity to write afterwards, the last was by the Dutton East Indiaman dated the

[1] No doubt this refers to Isaac Smith (see App. VII, p. 875 below).

22nd of May. The same day we parted Company and I steered for y[e] Isle of Ascension in Order to get some Turtle which we found so scarce as to oblige us to waite Three days. From Ascension I steered for and made the Island of Fernando De Noronha in Order to ascertain its Longitude and I made the Western Isles and put in at Fyall for the same purpose, where I remained four days the only Delay this rout has occasioned. It is with pleasure that I acquaint you that my people Continued healt[h]y to the last and that I have only lost four Men since I left England one died of a Consumption, two were drowned and one was killd by a Fall down the Forehatchway The behaviour of my Officers & Crew during y[e] whole Course of y[e] Voyage merits from me the highest recommendations and I Shall be happy if my Conduct meets with their Lordships approbation.

I am &c

J.C.

Phil: Stephens Esqr

15. To Latouche-Tréville

[*Bibliothèque Nationale, Paris, MSS, Nouv.Acq.Fr. 9439. Printed by E. T. Hamy in* Bull. de géographie hist. et descript. *(1904), p. 207; and by J. Forsyth in* Mariner's Mirror, *xlv (1959). Latouche was a young French naval officer ambitious to be a Pacific explorer.*]

Monsieur,

Je n'ai reçu la lettre très obligeante que vous m'avez fait l'honneur de m'écrire que bien après sa datte, ce qui sans doute n'est arrivé que par une erreur fort étrange de la part du maître de poste. Ce qui a encore retardé ma réponse est que, comme je ne suis pas absolument maître de la langue françoise, j'ai été obligé de la mettre aux mains d'un ami pour me la traduire, ce qui m'a privé jusqu'à présent de vous faire mes très humbles remercîmens du grand compliment que vous avez eu la bonté de me faire sur mes deux voyages, aussitôt que j'aurois bien voulu.

Il ne me suffit donc point d'avoir les applaudissemens de ma nation seule, parce que ce n'est pas pour elle que j'ai travaillé en particulier, mais pour toute l'Europe. Et si ma conduite a l'approbation de la nation françoise, je ne dois point m'embarrasser des autres.

Votre nation, Monsieur, n'a pas peu contribué aux découvertes de la mer du Sud. Et nous avons bien raison de regretter que vous en ayez été privé de votre part, parce que ce n'est que par des hommes d'un génie aussi entreprenant que le vôtre que nous devons attendre de grandes choses de ce côté-là. Car je soutiens que celui qui ne fait qu'exécuter des ordres ne fera jamais grandes figures dans les découvertes.

Il y a encore bien des parties dans l'océan Pacifique qui ne sont point découvertes, et il seroit à souhaiter que vous fussiez un jour ou l'autre employé à ce service-là que vous avez tant à cœur. Et si un pareil événement arrivoit, vous pouvez me demander tout ce qui dépend de moi à ce sujet. Et en même temps, s'il y a quelque chose en particulier dont vous ayez envie de vous informer concernant mon dernier voyage, je vous le communiquerai très volontiers, comme il sera exposé au public, aussitôt que les estampes qui doivent l'accompagner seront gravées.

Il faut avant que je conclue que je vous dise que toutes les envies qu'on avoit de trouver un continent dans la Mer du Sud sont toutes évanouies, c'est-à-dire dans une latitude où la mer est navigable, car depuis le 60° et plus la mer du Sud est si parsemée de glaces de toutes espèces qu'on n'y navigue qu'avec beaucoup de danger.

Il ne m'a pas été possible d'aller plus loin que le 71°10. J'ai pourtant trouvé terre au 59° et sous le 27e méridien Ouest de Greenwich ou Londres, mais je n'ai jamais pu déterminer si c'étoit un groupe d'îles ou une partie d'une grande terre s'étendant dans le Sud. Ceci a été la seule terre que j'aie trouvée dans le Sud, excepté celle qui est déjà connue. Je me flatte que vous voudrez bien continuer la correspondance dont vous m'avez honoré et je suis avec toute vérité, Monsieur,

Votre très obligé et fidèle serviteur

JAMES COOK[1]

Mile End,
London,
6th Sept. 1775

16. TO JOHN WALKER

[*Dixson Library MSS, Public Library of New South Wales, Sydney.*]

Mile End London Sepr 14th 1775

Dear Sir

I now sit down to fullfill the promise I made you in my last which was to give you some account of my late Voyage and which I am more at liberty to do, as it will be published as soon as the drawings which are to accompany it can be got engraved. I left the Cape of Good Hope on the 22nd of Novr 1772 and proceeded to the South till I got into the Latitude of 55° where I met with a Vast field of Ice and much fogy weather and large isles or floating Mountains of Ice without Number. After some trouble and not a little danger, I got to the South of this field of ice and after beating about some time for land in a Sea Strewed with Ice, I on the 17th of Janry 1773 Cross'd the Antarctick circle and the same evening I found it unsafe, or rather impossible to stand farther to the South for Ice; we were at this time in the Latd of 67° 15′S, Longitude 40° East of Greenwich. Seeing no signs of meeting with land in these high Latitudes I stood away to the Northward to look for that which as I was informed at the Cape of Good Hope, had lately been discovered by the French, in about the Latitude of 48½° and Longitude 57° or 60°. This land, (if any) I did not find probably owing to hard Westerly gales I met with which might carry me

[1] The formal ending only is in Cook's hand.

somthing to the Ea[s]t of its situation. While I was looking for this land the Adventure was separated from me, this did not hinder me from proceeding again to the South to the Latitude of 61° and 62° which was as far as the Ice and prudence would allow me; I kept between this Latitude and 58° without Seeing any signs of land, till I thought proper to Steer for N. Zealand, where I anchored in Dusky Bay on the 26th of March. This Bay lies on the SW point of N. Zealand and abounds with Fish and Wild Fowl, on which we refreshed for near Seven Weeks and then Sailed to Queen Charlottes Sound where I found the Adventure and who had been here Six Weeks.

I left this Sound on the 7th of June and proceed with the two Ships to the East between the Latitude of 42° and 47 till we got into the Longitude of 136° West. Dispairing of finding land in the high Latitudes I bore up for Otaheite, as it was now necessary for us to get into Port as the Adventures Crew was very sickly. In our run to Otaheite we discovered in Latitude 17° Some low isles and on the 17th of Augt we anchored at Otaheite, but not before we were within an ace of loosing the Resolution. At this Isle we remained 16 days, got plenty of fruit, but very little fresh Pork, the people seemed not to have it to spare. I next Visited Huaheine and Ulietea where the good people of these isles gave us every thing the isles produced with a liberal and full hand and we left them with our dicks [*sic*] crowded with Pigs and Rigging loaded with fruit. I next visited Amsterdam, in Latitude 21° an Island discovered by the Dutch in 1642; it is one of those happy isles on which Nature has been lavishing of her favours and its Inhabitants are a friendly benevolent race and ready [to] supply the wants of the Navigator. From this isle I steered for New Zealand and after having been some days in sight of our Port, the Adventure was again Separated from me, after which I saw her no more. After waiting something more then 3 weeks for her in Queen Charlottes Sound, I put to Sea and stood to the South where I met with nothing but Ice and excessive cold bad Weather. here I spent near four months, beating about between the Latitude of 48° and 68° and once I got as high as 71°10′ and farther it was not possible to go for Ice, which lay as firm as land, here we saw Ice Mountains whose lofty Summits were lost in the Clouds. I was now fully satisfied that there was no southern Continent, I never the less resolved to spend some time longer in these Seas and with this resolution I stood away to the North and on the 14th of March 1774 I found and anchor'd at Easter Island, the only land I had seen from leaving New Zealand, the people of this isle received us kindly, we got from them some Sweet Potatoes and fruit, which was of great Service to us, as we were in great want of refreshments, particularly my self who had but just recov[er]ed from a dangerous illness, the most of my people were however pretty healthy. This Island lies in the Latitude of 27°6′S, Longitud of 109° 52′Wt is about 12 leagues in circuit, rather barren and without any wood or good fresh Water or even a safe road consequently my stay was Short, it do not contain many Inhabitants and we saw but few Women in proportion to the Men, they are a Slender people and go almost naked. At this isle are Stone Statues of a vast size, errected along the Sea Coast, we saw some 27 feet high of a proportional thickness and all of one piece, we judged them to be places dedicated to the Dead, their shape was a rude resemblance of a Man and crowned with a great Stone in the shape of a Drum, but vastly larger.

I next visited the Marquases, which lie in 10° South Lat^de^ and inhabited by a friendly and handsome race of people here we got plenty of fruit and some Pork and fresh Water. From the Marquases I steered for Otaheite, where I arrived the latter end of Ap^l^ I now found this isle in the most flourishing state immaginable and was received by the Inhabitants with a Hospitality altogether unknown in Europe. I remained at this and the Society isles till the 4th of June, when I proceeded to the West, touched at Amsterdam and discovered some small isles of little note. After this I fell in with the Land discovered by Quiros and afterwards visited by Bougainville, but explored by neither; I found it to consist of a Group of isles extending from 14 to 20° South Latitude. The Inhabitants of these isles were far less civilized than those more to the East, and composed of three different Nations, one of which was a small race with apish faces and used poisoned arrows; they were all Warlike and obliged us to be continually upon our guard and to work with our arms in hand, they seemed to be very numerous and go almost naked, they are of a very dark Colour, inclining to black and some of them have woolly hair. The isles are fertile and yield fruit and roots; we saw no animals but Hogs and Fowls, they have not so much as a name for Goats, Dogs or Catts, consequently can have no knowlidge of them. Some of them gave us to understand in such a manner as admited of little doubt that they eat human flesh. After leaving these Isles I hauled away to the SW and on the 4th of September, discover'd a large Isl̃and which I called Nova Caledonia, it extends from 19 to 22½ South Latitude: this Country is Inhabited by a friendly race, our landing in their Country gave them not the least apparent uneasiness and they suffered us to go where ever we pleased. They are a Stout well made people of a Dark Colour with long frizled hair and wear little cloathing. The Country is rather barren and very mountainous and rocky, consequently unfit for Cultivation all that can be cultivated is done and planted with yams and other roots and some fruit. This Country produceth fine Timber for Masts and such like purposes which is what I have not found in any other Tropical isle, the Coast is beset with shoals and breakers which, in many places, extend a long way out to Sea, so that we ran not a little risk in exploreing it, and at last was obliged to leave it unfinished. From Caledonia I steered for New Zealand and in the Latitude of 29° discovered a small uninhabited isle, covered with fine Timber.

Octr 19th we anchored the third time in Queen Charlottes Sound in New Zealand, where we remained three weeks. The Inhabitants of this place gave us some account of some Strangers having been killed by them, but we did not understand they were part of our Consorts crew till we arrived at the Cape of Good Hope. That the New Zealanders are Cannibals will no longer be disputed not only from the Melancholy fate of the Adventures people and Captain Morion and his fellow suffer[er]s, but from what I and my whole crew have seen with our eyes. Nevertheless I think them a good sort of people, at least I have always found good treatment amongst them.

After leaving New Zealand I steered directly for Cape Horn, I put in at Terra del Fuego and Staten Land where we met with little worthy of note. On my Passage from the last Mentioned land to the Cape of Good Hope, I fell in with an isle, of about 70 Leagues in Circuit and situated between the Latitude of 54 and 55, which was wholy covered with Snow and ice; again in the Latitude of 59 I met with more land the Southern extent of [which] I did not find, so that I was not able to determine whether it was composed of isles or was a part of a large land, some parts of it shewed a surface composed of lofty Mountains whose summits were lost in the Clouds and every where covered with Snow down to the very wash of the sea, notwithstanding this was the very height of Summer, or rather towards the Autumn when the weather is warmest in the Southern Seas; we also met with a great deal of Ice in the Sea, both Isles and drift ice. After leaving this Land I sought in vain for Cape Circumcision, and on the 22nd of March arrived at the Cape of Good Hope, in great want of both Stores and Provisions, fresh provisions especially, which we had not tasted for a long time, except it was Sea fowl, Seals &c^a^. I left the Cape on the 27th of Ap^l^ touched at St Helena, Ascension and Fayal and arrived at Spithead the 30th of July, having only lost four Men from the time of my leaving England, two was drowned, one killed by a fall and one died of the Dropsy and a complication of other disorders without the least mixture of the S[c]urvy. This Sir is an imperfect outline of my Voyage, which I hope you will excuse, as the multiplicity of business I have now on my hand will not admit of my being more particular or accurate, any thing further you may want to know, you will always find me ready to communicate it.

I did expect and was in hopes that I had put an end to all Voyages of this kind to the Pacific Ocean, as we are now sure that no Southern Continent exists there, unless so near the Pole that the Coast cannot be Navigated for Ice and therefore not worth the discovery; but the Sending home Omiah will occasion another voyage which I expect will soon be undertaken.

Mrs Cook joins me in best respects to you and all your Family and believe me to be with great Esteem

Yours Most Sincerely
JAM^s^ COOK

P.S. My Compliments to Mr Ellerton[1] if he is yet living.

[1] Richard Ellerton was master of Walker's collier *Friendship*, in which Cook sailed as mate, May–November 1753. The muster roll of the vessel is contained in a folio volume in the Whitby Museum, kindly shown me by Miss Dora M. Walker, Curator of the Museum.

17. To Latouche-Tréville

[*Bibliothèque Nationale, Paris, MSS, Nouv.Acq.Fr. 9439, Printed by J. Forsyth in* Mariner's Mirror, *xlv* (*1959*).]

Londres, 10 février 1776

Mon cher Monsieur,

J'aurais répondu sur le champ à votre obligeante lettre du 7 novembre dernier, si je n'avois pas toujours attendu que je pusse vous informer de ma nouvelle entreprise d'un troisième voyage sur l'Océan Pacifique; cette affaire n'a été décidée que d'aujourd'hui et je mettrai à la voile avec deux vaisseaux, vers la fin d'avril. Le premier objet de ce voyage est de reconduire Omaï dans son isle. On n'a point encore déterminé les autres, mais ils se rapporteront certainement aux progrés de la géographie et de la navigation: je serais fort aise de pouvoir vous rencontrer employé ainsi que moi dans une expédition aussi intéressante, d'autant que vous me paroissés avoir quelqu' espérance d'en être chargé et je souhaite que vous réussissiés, puis qu'il y a bien de quoi nous occuper tous deux.

Je vous donnerai, sans aucune réserve, mon avis sur la route à préférer pour achever les découvertes qui restent à faire dans l'hémisphère méridional.

Vos motifs pour continuer ce grand objet ne peuvent pas être contestés. Il est certainement à désirer qu'on visite la partie méridionale de la Nouvelle-Hollande, continent dont je ne doute pas que la Terre de Diemen ne fasse partie, me fondant sur ce que le Capitaine Furneaux en a vu.

Vous ne trouverés ces terres à mon avis qu'autant que vous suivrés la route convenable. Si vous entrés dans l'Océan Pacifique par le cap Horn, je vous conseille de gâgner le 5e degré de latitude méridionale et de traverser une grande partie de l'Océan dans cette latitude; car la partie de cet mer qui se trouve entre le 10e degré de latitude septentrionale et le 10e degré de latitude méridionale est fort peu connue, et il est très probable que cette partie contient plusieurs grandes isles. Le navigateur qui visitera cette mer, en suivant cette route, pourra mouiller aux îles Marquesas où il trouvera de bonnes provisions de toute espéce, et un peuple civil et hospitalier. Je crois qu'il serait à propos d'examiner avec plus d'exactitude la terre qui a été découverte par Mrs. Surville et Bougainville. Je parle des terres qui touchent la Nouvelle Guinée. Il est à présumer qu'elles peuvent produire des épices ou quelque article précieux pour le commerce.

Après avoir pénétré aussi avant, il sera impossible de reconnaître la terre de Diemen, mais il sera peut-être absolument nécessaire de toucher aux Isles de la Sonde.

Si vous entrés dans l'Océan Pacifique par une route de l'Est ou si vous prenés votre point de départ au Cap de Bonne-Espérance ou de l'isle de France, votre premier objet doit être de visiter la côte méridîonale de la Nouvelle-Hollande; ce qu'il faut faire au milieu de l'été, et ce sera l'hiver que vous irés à Otahiti ou aux Marquesas, lorsque les vents d'Ouest régnent le plus, on devrait faire ce passage par la partie de cette mer qui n'a point encor été visitée et qui est située entre les parallèles 30 et 25 Sud, ou même plus bas, si les vents le permettoient, après avoir pris des provisions à Otahiti ou aux Marquesas, mais plus vous irés vers l'Est et mieux ce sera.

La première opération qu'il y aurait à faire ensuite, ce serait de poursuivre la route ci-dessus tracée et de revenir à l'isle de France par les îles de la Sonde.

Les géographes aussi bien que les navigateurs diffèrent d'opinions sur la situation des isles nommées de Salomon. La route que j'ai marquée èclaircira ce point. Si ces idées vous sont de quelque usage pour le voïage que vous avés tant à cœur de faire, je serai charmé de vous les avoir communiquées. Je ne finirai point sans vous exprimer le désir que j'ai de savoir si vos sollicitations auront eu du succés avant que je quitte l'Angleterre.

Je suis, avec autant d'estime que de sincérité, mon cher monsieur,

Votre très humble et très obéissant serviteur,

JAMES COOK

Londres, Mile End, 10 février 1776

P.S. Comme je vois qu'il est trop tard pour profiter de la poste d'aujourd'hui, je vais vous donner une esquisse de mon dernier voyage. Je suis parti du cap de Bonne-Espérance, le 22 novembre 1772. J'ai gouverné au Sud par la latitude de 51 degrés où nous encontrâmes les premiéres glaces. Quand nous fûmes à 55 degrés de latitude et 22 degrés Est de longitude de Greenwich, nous trouvâmes une très grande mer.

Après y avoir été quelque tems je pris le Sud et ensuite je gouvernai vers l'Est jusqu'au méridien du Cap de la Circoncision par la latitude de 59 degrés. Ne voiant aucun signe de terre, je m'en éloignai en prenant le Sud-Est et traversant le cercle antarctique et le méridien de 39 degrés Est par 67 degrés 15 minutes de latitude, où nous sommes arrêtés par un mur de glace que je n'entrepris point de traverser. Je pris du coté du Nord, pour chercher la terre découverte par M. Kerguelen, découverte dont l'on m'avoit informée au Cap de Bonne-Espérance. Je la cherchai en vain entre les 48 et 49 degrés de latitude et entre les 57 et 62 degrés de longitude Est. Je jugeai que je l'avais laissée à l'Ouest de ces méridiens et que les vents très-forts qui venoient de l'Ouest m'en éloignoient. Ici, les deux vaisseaux furent séparés, je continuai ma route avec le vaisseau la Résolution, vers le S.E. à la latitude de 61 et au delà. Je gouvernai toujours à l'Est entre cette latitude et 58 degrés, toujours entre les îles de glace, et sans voir le moindre signe de terre. Après avoir passé le méridien de la Terre de Diemen je pris vers le Nord, et le 26 Mars 1773 je jettai l'ancre dans la Baye de Duskey au Sud-Ouest des côtes de la Nouvelle-Zélande, où je trouvai du bois et de l'eau en abondance, d'excellent poisson et de la volaille sauvage. De là je fis voile pour la rade de la Reine Charlotte, où je rencontrai le capitaine Furneaux.

Après qu'il m'eut quitté, il fit directement route pour la terre de Diemen où il toucha et fit du bois et de l'eau. Ensuite il côtoia les côtes du

Sud et celles de l'Est jusqu'à 40 degrés. Je quittai la rade de la Reine Charlotte avec les deux vaisseaux le 7 juin, et je gouvernai à l'Est par la latitude de 41 et 47 degrés et par la longitude de 134 degrés Ouest de Greenwich. Je tournai alors vers le Nord au 18e degré pour gagner Otahiti, où nous arrivâmes le 18 Aout. Il y a quelques basses isles entre les 17e et 18e degrés et c'est tout ce que nous avons vu de terre dans ce passage. Je passai un mois tant aux isles d'Otahiti qu'à celles de la Société et ensuite je gouvernai pour les isles de Middelbourg et d'Amsterdam, je ne découvris dans cette route qu'une petite isle. Je touchai ensuite à l'une et à l'autre des isles ci-dessus nommées. J'achetai dans l'isle d'Amsterdam des cochons, des volailles et beaucoup de fruit. Ces habitans sont aussi humains que ceux d'Otahiti, mais aussi grands voleurs.

Je partis d'Amsterdam le 7 Octobre et je fis route pour la Nouvelle-Zélande sur les côtes de laquelle nous nous séparâmes tout à fait. Le 3 novembre j'entrai dans la rade de la Reine Charlotte où je restai jusqu'au 26 que je remis en mer. Je gouvernai alors au S.S.E. jusqu'à la latitude de 66 où je m'arrêtai, ne pouvant aller plus loin à cause de la glace. Je tournai après cela vers l'Est entre les 64 et 67 degrés de latitude, les glaces ne nous aiant permis d'arriver que jusques là. Je me fis alors une pointe vers le Nord jusqu'aux 47 degrés, après quoi je revins encore vers le Sud jusqu'à 71 degrés 10 minutes qui est la plus haute latitude à laquelle j'ai été et à laquelle je crois qu'on pût aller.

Nous étions par la longitude de 106 degrés et demi à l'Ouest de Greenwich. Ici nous recontrâmes une muraille de glace et des montagnes de glace dont le sommet se perdoit dans les nues. De là je gouvernai au Nord et je visitai les isles d'Easter (de Pâques) qui sont par la latitude méridionale de 27[d] 16[m] et par la longitude de 110 degrés 10 minutes. Les habitans de ces Isles sont bonnes gens mais grands voleurs, c'est une nation de l'espèce de celle d'Otahiti, ces isles n'ont ni port ni bois ni eau fraîche propre à embarquer. Elles produisent des cannes de sucre, du plantain et des patates. J'y fis peu de séjour et je gouvernai pour les isles Marquesas, où j'arrivai le 7 Avril 1774. Depuis mon dernier départ de la Nouvelle-Zélande jusqu'à mon arrivée dans ces isles, je n'ai découvert absolument aucune terre nouvelle, et je n'en ai pas vu la moindre apparence.

Nous trouvâmes dans les isles Marquesas des fruits en abondance et quelques porcs. De là nous partîmes pour Otahiti et dans notre route nous découvrîmes quelques isles basses. On me reçut très bien à Otahiti, et aux isles de la Société. Je passai six semaines parmi ces peuples. Je fus ensuite à Rotterdam d'où je gouvernai pour les grandes Cyclades que j'appelle les Nouvelles Hébrides. Ce groupe d'isles s'étend depuis le 14 degrés et demi de latitude méridionale jusqu'au 20e. Elles sont habitées par deux ou trois nations différentes qui toutes sont aussi des voleurs. Les productions de ces isles sont à peu près les mêmes qu'à Otahiti. Au sud des Hébrides, je trouvai un grand pays dont les habitans étaient fort humains. Il est situé entre le 19e degré et le 22e et demi et s'étend jusqu'à 80 ou 90 lieues S.S.E. et N.N.O. Sa largeur n'est pas considérable, n'excédant pas 10 à 12 lieues.

Après avoir quitté ces isles, je visitai encore la Nouvelle Zélande d'où je pris directement mon cours pour le Cap Horn. Mais il faut que je finisse ici, n'aiant plus ni de tems ni de place pour continuer.

[*Endorsed:*] Lettre de M. Cook, traduite le 16 Mars
pour la marine.

APPENDIX II

The Controversy over the Resolution

I. Banks to Sandwich

[*Printed from the copy in the Sandwich Papers, Hinchingbrooke, endorsed 'No. 93'. Banks's draft, differing in some respects from this, is in the 'Voluntiers' volume in the Mitchell Library. There are other copies in Sarah Sophia Banks's transcript of Banks's Iceland journal, owned by Sir David Hawley, of Lincoln, and in the Georgian Papers (no. 1322) in the Library of Windsor Castle. The letter has been printed from the Windsor Castle copy by Fortescue*, Correspondence of George III, *II, pp. 343–7; and, with some differences, by H. C. Cameron*, Geographical Journal, *CXVI (1950), pp. 51–3, and in his* Sir Joseph Banks *(1952), pp. 286–90.*]

My Lord

The present Situation of Things regarding the propos'd Expedition to the South Seas, which it was my Intention and Inclination to have taken an active Share in will I trust, render any other Apology to your Lordship for this Intrusion unnecessary.

To avoid the Appearance of Inconsistency, and to justify my Conduct in the Eyes of the Public and your Lordship, I feel it incumbent on me to state the Reasons by which I am influenced to decline the Expedition.

When it was first proposed to me by your Lordship to go to the South Seas again, if His Majesty should think proper to send Ships to perfect the Discoveries that had been begun in the last Voyage, I joyfully embraced a proposal, of all others the best suited to my Disposition and Pursuits, I pledg'd myself then to your Lordship, and have since by the whole Tenor of my conversation and Correspondence, pledged myself to all Europe, not only to go the Voyage, but to take with me as many able Artists, as the Income of my Fortune would allow me to pay; by whose means, the learned World in general might reap as much benefit as possible from those Discoveries, which my good Fortune or Industry might enable me to make.

The Navy Board was in consequence ordered to purchase two Ships, to fit them up in a proper manner for our Reception, that we might be enabled to exert our utmost endeavours to serve the public wheresoever the Course of our Discoveries might induce us to proceed.

Two Ships were accordingly purchas'd; but when I went down to see the principal Ship I immediately gave it as my opinion that she was very improper for the Voyage and went so far as to declare that, if the alterations which I proposed could not be made I would not go in her.

In consequence of this the Surveyor of the Navy was sent to me with a Plan of the Ship; to him I stated my Proposals and laid down upon that Plan, the Quantity of Room that I thought absolutely necessary to be allotted to me and my people, for the carrying on of our respective Employments.

When these Alterations, and those which were judged necessary also for the accomodation of the Captain and the People were made, the Ship, in falling down the River, was found absolutely incapable of pursuing her intended Voyage.

The Navy Board have attributed this Incapacity to the alterations that had been made and are of Opinion that when the Ship is reduced to her original situation, that in which I before refused her, she will be the fittest that can be had for answering the nautical purposes of the Expedition. Without suffering myself to controvert this opinion of the Navy Board that the Ship will be very fit for Sea, although many able Seamen concur with me in doubting it, I must be allowed to say, that the Ship will thus be, if not absolutely incapable, at least exceedingly unfit for the intended Voyage.

We have pledg'd ourselves my Lord to your Lordship and the Nation, to undertake what no Navigator before us has ever suggested to be practicable; we are to attempt at least to pass round the Globe, through Seas, of which we know no Circumstance, but that of their being tempestuous in those very Latitudes, in passing through which, in order to get round one Cape, the whole Squadron commanded by Lord Anson narrowly escaped being destroyed. We have done more; we have undertaken to approach as near the Southern Pole as we possibly can, and how near that may be, no Man living can give the least Guess:

In Expeditions of this Nature the Health and Accomodation of the People are essential to Success; when Sickness and Discontent are once introduced, it will be absolutely impossible to continue the Discovery; by the Alterations made the Accomodations of the people are very much reduc'd; for the Spar Deck being cut away, 30 of the Crew are to be removed under the Gun Deck, before sufficiently crowded which being very low and confined without a free Air, must infallibly in so long a Voyage produce putrid Distempers and Scurvy; and what my Lord, ought more to be dreaded by a Discoverer than such a Calamity, which must soon oblige him to quit his Discovery, and very probably even put it out of his Power to bring Home any Account of what he has done previous to its fatal Influence?

The Accomodations in the Ship are much lessened by the Changes which have been made in the Equipment since the first Plan; the House of Commons have thought the undertaking of so much Importance, as to vote the Sum of £4000 to enable D[r] Lind to accompany us, and assist us with his extensive Knowledge of natural Philosophy and Mechanics, the Board of Longitude have also engaged an Astronomer to proceed in each Ship, and an extraordinary Establishment of Officers was thought necessary, on account of the Difficulties and Dangers, which we were likely to experience in the Course of our Voyage.

Shall I then my Lord, who have ingaged to lėave all that can make Life agreeable in my own Country, and throw on one side all the Pleasures to be reap'd from three of the best Years of my Life, merely to compass this Undertaking, pregnant enough with Dangers and difficulties in its own Nature, after having been promis'd every security and Convenience that the Art of Man could contrive, without which Promise, no Man in my situation would ever have undertaken the Voyage, be sent of at last in a doubtful Ship, with Accomodations rather worse that those which I at first absolutely refus'd; and after spending above £5000 of my own Fortune in the Equipment upon the Credit of those Accomodations which I saw actually built for me? Will the public be so ungenerous as to expect me to go out in a Ship, in which my people have not the Room necessary for performing the different Duties of their Professions; a Ship apparently unhealthy and probably unsafe, merely in conformity to the official Opinion of the Navy Board, who purchas'd her without ever consulting me, and now in no degree consider the Part which I have taken in the Voyage or the Alterations which on my Remonstrance, they concurr'd with me in thinking necessary, but have now taken away, or should I embark, could any thing material be done by People under Circumstances so highly discouraging?

For my own part, my Lord I am able and willing to put up with as small Accomodations as any Man living can be content with; six Feet square is more than sufficient for all my personal Conveniences, nor are any of my people desirous of a larger allotment. Tis our Great Cabbin which is too small and that is in reality the Shop w[h]ere we are all to work, which, if not sufficiently large will deprive the Workmen of a possibillity of following their respective Employments, and prevent me from reaping the Fruit earned by voluntarily exposing myself to Danger and incurring a material Expence:

Neither personal Hazard nor Expence however will I withhold when likely to meet with their proper Encouragement; born with an Attachment to a singular Pursuit, I have already perform'd two Voyages, and in the Course of them have merited, I hope, some Share of the public Regard, and though my Services are upon this Occasion refus'd I shall always hold myself ready to go upon this, or any Undertaking of the same nature, whenever I shall be furnish'd with proper Accomodations for myself and my people to exert their full Abilities.

To explore is my wish; but the Place to which I may be sent almost indifferent to me. Whether the Sources of the Nile or the South Pole are to be visited, I am equally ready to embark in the undertaking whenever the Public will furnish me with the Means of doing it properly, but to undertake so expensive a Pursuit without any Prospect, but distress and disappointment is neither consistent with Prudence or Public Spirit.

As to the position of no other Ship being fit for the Voyage, because no other could take the Ground, I cannot omit putting your Lordship in Mind that within these few Weeks the Emerald one of our sharpest Frigates, lay on shore on the Gunfleet a much longer time, than the Endeavour did upon the Coast of New Holland, after which she was got off. Sir John

Lindsay also hauled up the Stag, another of our Frigates at Trincomaly and shifted her Rudder Irons during the Course of his last Voyage.—What more my Lord, did the Endeavour do, or what more could any Ship have done in that particular Point, on which the opinion of the Navy Board so materially rests?

If these then are capable of taking the Ground, how much more so must the Launceston (the Ship for which we have petitioned your Lordship) be, as all Seamen know that the bottoms of that Class of Ships are flatter than any others employ'd in His Majestys Service? For my own part, I can only say, that was your Lordship to think proper to let us have her for our intended Expedition, I would gladly embark on board a Ship, in which safety and accomodation, both which must be consulted in a Voyage of this kind, are more nearly united than in any other kind of Ship I am acquainted with, and well know that there are many Commanders in His Majestys Service of undoubted Abilities and Experience who would willingly undertake to proceed with her in the intended Expedition, ambitious of shewing the World, that the Success of such an Undertaking depends more upon the Prudence and Perserverance of the Commander than upon any particular built of the Ship that may be employed.

I cannot dismiss this Letter without thanking your Lordship for the many particular Favors, which I have received at your Lordships Hands in the Commencement, and during the prosecution of this my favorite Undertaking, of which I shall ever retain a most grateful Sense. I do not doubt, that was not your Lordship prevented by Forms of Office I should still continue to receive the same Countenance and Assistance, and that if it should be thought proper to alter or enlarge the present Equipment your Lordship would still continue your Protection; as I am not conscious that by any part of my Conduct I have forfieted that Claim to it, which your Lordships great Condescention and Goodness originally conferr'd upon me.

I am with the utmost respect
Your Lordships
most Obliged and most
Obedient humble Servant
JOS: BANKS

May the 30th 1772.

2. NAVY BOARD MEMORANDUM

[*Sandwich Papers, Hinchingbrooke, endorsed 'Observations upon Mr Banks's Letter to the Earl of Sandwich', and 'No. 93'. There is a copy in the Windsor Castle Library, Georgian Papers, no. 1323*. It has been printed by Fortescue,* Correspondence of George III, *II, pp. 350–2; and by Cameron,* Geographical Journal, *CXVI, p. 54, and* Sir Joseph Banks, *pp. 291–2.*]

Mr Banks's first Objection to the Ship respected only the Conveniences for himself and was then no more than this, 'that the forepart of the Cabin

was an Inch or two too low'. As to the proper kind of Ship, and her fitness and sufficiency for the Voyage, his Opinion was never asked, nor could have been asked with any propriety, he being in no degree qualified to form a right Judgement in such a matter; and for the same reason his Opinion now thereon is not to be attended to. As to what concerned himself, as he increased his Suite and his Demands every thing was done to satisfy him, by which it happened that the Properties of the Ship were so much altered that it has been necessary to take away the additional Works that had been done at his request; in doing which it was so contrived that the Difference occasioned thereby to him, was simply this—The great
Feet Ins
Cabin (6 : 6 high between Plank and Plank) was shortned from 22 to 16 feet long, and there was one small Cabin for his Attendants taken away. After this small Reduction, there remained on the whole much better Accomodations than he had in the former Voyage in the Endeavour, and the great Cabin remained in Length and Height though not in breadth equal to those in a 74 Gun Ship[1] for an Admiral, who frequently embarks in such Ships to command His Majesty's Fleets at Sea, whose Cabins are
Feet Ins Feet Ins
only 16 : 2 long, and 6 : 6 high.

Mr Banks seems throughout to consider the Ships as fitted out wholly for his use; the whole undertaking to depend on him and his People; and himself as the Director and Conductor of the whole; for which he is not qualified, and if granted to him, would have been the greatest disgrace that could be put on His Majesty's Naval officers.

His Assertion that the Ship is incommodious to the People, and made worse to them by the late Alterations has a very evil tendency, to raise Discontent amongst the People, and for defeating the Voyage; but it may be averred he is mistaken in the Fact, for the People will be better accomodated, a freer circulation of Air throughout the Ship, and in all respects wholesome and the Men better lodged than they are in any King's-built Ship of the same Dimensions and Burthen.

His Application of the Cases of the Emerald and Stag, and the Conclusion he draws therefrom, discovers him to have less knowledge of Matters relating to Ships than might be expected in one who has associated and conversed so much with His Majesty's Sea Officers. The first was on shore in a smooth Water Channel *at home*, not a *distant strange*, *desolate* or savage Coast at the *Antipodes*. Six Ships instantly anchored by her, hauled alongside, took out her Guns, Provisions &c^{a}, and immediate Assistance of every kind was sent from one of the King's Dock Yards. The Stag, if she was hove up, or hove down, at Trincomaly, it was at a Port where there were conveniences for fitting Ships of burthen, and where undoubtedly they had all the like Conveniences that could be had in the River Thames. Had either of those Ships been in the Endeavours place on the Coast of New Holland, they would never have been heard of again: Even if they

[1] Bellona, Superb, Arrogant &c^{a}. [Marginal note.]

had got off the Rocks, they could not have been hauled up to repair Damages, as was done by the Endeavour.

June 3^{d} 1772.

3. Palliser's 'Thoughts upon the Kind of Ships proper to be employed on Discoveries in distant parts of the Globe'

[*Sandwich Papers, Hinchingbrooke: undated, signed by Palliser. Endorsed 'No. 98'. Hitherto unprinted.*]

Should the advantageous Properties of the Ships be given up or suffered to be in any degree diminished, in order to gain particular Accommodations for Individuals, such a Step may be considered as laying a foundation for rendering the Undertaking abortive at the very time it is set on foot—for undoubtedly the Success of it must principally depend upon that which ought to be the first Consideration, namely, the Safety of the Ships and the Preservation of the Adventurers: Circumstances which will not admit of those Encroachments on the requisite Properties of the Ships:

The greatest Danger to be apprehended in a Voyage on Discoveries to the most distant & unknown Parts of the Globe, is that of running ashore upon desart, uninhabited or perhaps savage Coast[s]:—therefore no consideration in the Choice of a Ship for such a Service should be set in competition with that of a Construction in which a Man may with the least hazard venture upon it: A Ship of that kind must be certainly preferable to any other, and that kind must be one of a large Burthen, and of a small Draught of Water, with a Body that will bear to take the Ground, and of a Size which in case of necessity may be safely and conveniently laid on shore to repair any accidental Damages or Defects.

In such a Vessel an able Sea Officer will be more venturesome and better enabled to fulfill his Instructions than he possibly can (or indeed would be prudent for him to attempt) in one of any other *Sort* or *Size:*—

As to the Position that a three-deckt West India Ship with large Accommodations and being of a finer Body than a Bark, will hold a better Wind, and claw off a Lee Shore when a Bark will not be able so to do—I think it is a mistaken One—for her high built will surely render her as leewardly as the Bark, and prevent her carrying Sail so long, and will moreover greatly increase the Disadvantage of her finer Body in case of taking the Ground, as She would then prove topheavy and overset when the Bark would sit upright.—

I know a Notion has prevailed that when two Ships go on a Service of this Nature, they ought to be of different Constructions, on a Supposition that under any Circumstances of Danger there may be more probability of One of them escaping than if they were both constructed alike, and that the Chance of the Events of the Undertaking being preserved will be thereby doubled, and besides, that in case of the Loss of one of them, her Company may be taken up and preserved by the other: But altho' I readily admit the Propriety of sending out two Vessels in consort upon an

Enterprize of this Sort, yet I cannot by any means see why they should be of different Constructions—for whatever kind is Judged to be the most advantageous for a single Ship, must in my Opinion hold equally so for any greater Number to be employed on the same Service:—This cannot be well denied if it is once admitted that the greatest Dangers and those mostly to be apprehended should be guarded against preferably to any smaller Inconveniencies, and that in this matter the greatest Dangers really are those of going on shore, and the Want of Stores and Provisions necessary to enable the Adventurers to execute the Object of their Mission as already mentioned:—

With regard to the Apprehension of being caught on a Lee Shore in Ships not the best adapted for clawing off—that in my Opinion is not a Matter of sufficient Consideration to outweigh those more important Ones aforementioned, and I am sure that no prudent able *Sea Officer* will with any Kind of Ship whatsoever attempt to run down upon or explore such a Coast as a *Lee Shore*, in parts unknown, but that he will be equally cautious (whatever Kind of Ship he is in) to avoid being caught upon it:—If however, the clawing off a Lee Shore be the principal Object, then the best sailing Frigates ought to be the Ships employed:—

It has likewise been supposed that by the Ships being of different Constructions, an Advantage will accrue that One of them may be sent ahead to find out Channels and lead the other thro', but I believe that Experience will convince any one, that Boats (where small Craft are not to be had) are certainly the best, and perhaps the only Expedients for discovering, and leading Ships thro' unknown dangerous Channels, and that when the Weather is such that Boats cannot be employed in that Service, it will by no means be prudent to trust either of the Ships upon it, therefore the Frame of a small Vessel to be set up on a strange Coast may prove exceeding useful as well for exploring a Coast, as for collecting refreshments upon it, if uninhabited: The frames of two such small Vessels are accordingly put on board the two Ships now going out.—

On the whole, I am firmly of Opinion that Ships of no other Kind are so proper for Discoveries in distant unknown Parts, as the Endeavour (formerly employed) was:—for no Ships of any other Kind can contain Stores & Provisions sufficient (in proportion to their Complements) for the purpose, considering the Length of Time it may be necessary they should last, and if they could contain sufficient Quantities, yet on arriving at the Parts for Discovery, they would still from the Nature of their Construction & Size, be less fit and applicable for the purpose: Hence I conclude it is, that so little Progress has hitherto been made in Discovery in the Southern Hemisphere: for all Ships which attempted the Business before the Endeavour, were unfit for it, altho' those employed did the utmost in their Power: As soon as Mons. Bougainville came in sight of a part of the new discovered dangerous Coast which Cap[t] Cook compleatly explored, he fled from it as fast as possible and durst not approach it with the Ship he was in:—

It was upon these Considerations that the Endeavour Bark was chosen for that Voyage (the first of the Kind so employed) and notwithstanding those on board her who are not proper Judges found fault with her during the whole Voyage, yet it was to these properties in her that they owe their Preservation, and that enabled Cap[t] Cook to stay in those Seas so much longer than any other Ship ever did or could do: and altho' Discovery was not the first Object of his Voyage, it enabled him to traverse far greater Space of Seas, before then unnavigated: to discover great Tracts of Country in high & low South latitudes, and even to explore and survey the extensive Coasts of those new discovered Countries; in short it was those Properties of the Ship, with Cap[t] Cook's great Diligence, Perseverance & Resolution during the Voyage that enabled him to discover so much more, and at greater Distance than any Discoverer performed before during One Voyage, and has very deservedly gained him the Reputation of an able Seaman, an Artist and a good Officer, and a Just Title to the Marks of Favor conferred on him:—

It may be further observed that to embark a great Number of Passengers, claiming great Distinctions and spacious Accommodations with vast Quantities of Baggage, is incompatible with the Idea of a Scheme of Discovery at the Antipodes: If such Passengers do go, they must be content with the Kind of Ship that is fittest:—The Business of Discovery, the Care & Navigation of the Ships and conducting of every thing relative to the Undertaking, must ever depend on the King's Sea Officers only, they being chosen Men, fit for it:—

HUGH PALLISSER

4. SANDWICH TO BANKS

[*Sandwich Papers, Hinchingbrooke. The letter is a draft, with many emendations, in Sandwich's hand throughout. It is endorsed 'Answer to M[r] Banks's letter', and numbered 94. Hitherto unprinted.*]

Sir

As a letter has lately appeared in print addressed from you to the first Commissioner of the Admiralty, giving your reasons for having declined pursuing your original intention of embarking in the proposed Expedition to the South Seas and as it is very possible that his Lordship may not have leisure or inclination to enter into a paper war upon this occasion; having had opportunities of knowing allmost every circumstance that passed relative to the equipment of the Resolution Sloop of War, on board of which you was to have been recieved as a passenger together with several other gentlemen of learning & ingenuity, by whose discoveries as you very properly say the world might reap as much benefit as possible, I cannot refrain from taking the pen in hand, in order to inform the publick of the several facts, which probably occasioned your desisting from an undertaking which you had so much at heart, and from which if it had been executed by you I am perswaded the world would have recieved considerable advantage.

I must begin by desiring you to remember that in your former Voyage in the Endeavour bark you were recieved together with Dr Solander as a passenger on board her, the great Cabbin was in common between the Captain of the ship & yourselves, and all of you in your respective capacities employed your time during the voyage to the illustration of many material points of Navigation, Discovery, & Natural knowledge[;] no complaint whatever was made of want of room or other accommodation, & allmost in your first interview with the noble person at the head of the Admiralty it was agreed that two ships should be prepared instead of one, to compleat the discovery whither there was or was not such a thing as a southern continent, which I must remind you was allways considered as the principal object of the voyage. It was intended that you should embark on board of one of these Ships as before, and there was no idea of enlarging the ship to the quantity of your attendants, but adapting their number to the size of the ship. It was then agreed on all hands, that the opinion of the very great & able Sea officer who lately presided at the Admiralty was well founded; namely that the only ship that was fit for a voyage of this nature was a vessel built for the coal trade, those ships being very roomy in their hold & capable of stowing a very large quantity of provisions, being of a construction that will admit of their going on shore with less danger than ships of war, and because they would work with fewer hands, which in an expedition of this nature is no inconsiderable advantage. in this arrangement you readily acquiesced professing yourself not a competent judge what ship was the fittest for the service, tho' you intimated an opinion of your own that a West Indiaman would be more proper, as being built something sharper & more likely to claw off of a lee shore; but no mention was then made of a Man of War, or the least idea suggested from any one that such a ship was calculated for such a voyage. In consequence of this determination Captain Cooke, of whose knowledge & experience in shipping you yourself had the highest opinion, was directed to go all over the Pool & find out two of the fittest ships for this service, he accordingly executed his orders and the two Vessels that were afterwards named the Resolution & Adventure were purchased in consequence of his testimony in their favour. Hitherto everything went on to the general satisfaction of all parties, but no sooner was the Resolution brought to Deptford to be fitted, than you expressed your discontent: upon your first coming on board her you declared she was not fit for a gentleman to embark in, & that if her cabbin was not heightened and considerable alteration made by building on her to make additional conveniences for yourself and your company, you would not proceed upon the voyage. in consequence of this declaration the great Cabbin was heightened, to 6 feet 6 inches & lengthened to 22 feet, which is the same height with the principal cabbin of many of our ships of 74 guns & six foot longer However that you might not be crouded by the Captain in this *small* Cabbin, he was to have one erected for him above; and that every one of your suite might have ample accommodation a new deck was to be laid over the main deck that they might have seperate cabbins under it. all these alterations were accordingly made, against the express opinion of the principal officers of the Navy; but as Captain Cooke (who had so high an idea of the ship that he thought she could bear all this superstructure) gave it as his opinion that it would not be too much, the weight you had with the noble Lord to whom your letter is addressed occasioned their being over ruled, and the ship was altered and fitted according to your proposal.

We will leave the Resolution at present under the hands of the ship wrights at Deptford who were working upon a plan totally contrary to their opinion, and remind you that during that period several other demands were made by you in which the constant burthen of your song was, that their being complied with or not, should be the decision whither you should or should not proceed on the voyage.

The first demand you made was in a written paper delivered to the first Lord of the Admiralty: it consisted of several articles, the principal tendency of which was, that Captain Cooke should be ordered to follow your directions as to the time of sailing from the several places you should touch at in the course of the Voyage; which was in other words giving you the absolute command of the expedition, & a power of controuling two commanders in his Majesties service; a thing that was never done & I believe never attempted before; but this demand was allso to be a condition of your proceeding or not proceeding on the expedition. However in this point you at last acquiesced on its being suggested to you that it would be fatal to the undertaking that the command should be in the hands of persons not under Military Law, and of course not amenable to the Admiralty, but even then the matter was in a manner compromised not very judiciously in my opinion by his Lordship, who agreed that the Captain should be ordered to consult you about the time of sailing from the different places, but not implicitly to follow your directions, if he thought your ideas were inconsistent with the safety of the ship, and the success of the expedition.

This point being finished another difficulty was started namely the time when it was adviseable the ships should sail from the Cape of Good Hope in order to make Cape Circumsision, the two captains probably two of the best navigators in Europe were clear in the same sentiment that they ought to leave the Cape the latter end of October, but still you adhered so strongly to your own opinion, that it was thought necessary to have a meeting with these two gentlemen, and another Sea officer whose knowledge in his profession as a seamen [*sic*] is as indisputable as in that of an officer, which he has had the good fortune to prove most effectually more than once in the face of the Enemy; yet tho' his opinion was the same you did not alter yours, and you parted from the company leaving it still undecided whither you should or should not undertake the voyage, if this point was not given up.

The next request that was pressed upon the first Lord of the Admiralty in the strongest manner was that the officers in the two ships should recieve promotion thro' your means, and this you urged by suggesting that if they were not to look up to you for preferment you should be considered as nobody, and that it was very hard that you should not be allowed the influence over these gentlemen which such a power would give you. what were the noble Lords reasons for not complying with this request he best can tell, but if a stander by may be allowed to make a conjecture, I should think it very probable that he thought whatever proper influence was to be held over the officers might as well remain in the board of Admiralty as in your hands, and this was another attempt on your part to get possession of the command.

It is now proper to return to the ship at Deptford, where she had been fitted with more conveniences than any ship that ever went to sea, not excepting the Royal Yatchts; I mean conveniences for passengers; for except the Captain Master & first Lieutenant (and there are three Lieutenants belonging to her) none of the sea officers were allowed a place on the upper deck, but were all crouded between decks into that very place, which you now represent in your letter as unwholesome, and as likely to endanger the lives of the common seamen who may be so unfortunate as to undertake the voyage. In this state the Resolution sailed from Deptford, but alas, Captain Cooke was disappointed; whither Mr Banks was or not he best knows, the ship appeared crank or in other words top heavy, & it was agreed on all hands that she could not safely proceed on the voyage till her upper works were taken off, & till she was reduced to the state she was in when she was a merchantman. Here, Sir, was the period in which you exerted yourself to the utmost to obtain another ship in the room of the Resolution. Your letter shews the sort of ship you had pitched upon, and the reasoning which induced you to wish for the change; but as that reasoning appears to me ill funded I must beg leave in a very few words to controvert the point, and to express a distant idea, that you well knew the alteration could not be agreed to, & that you would then be free from the voyage, which it is not a matter of wonder you should begin to be tired of. You mention as an instance of the impropriety of this ship that she was to go thro seas & climates where Lord Anson narrowly escaped, but does that give any reason to conclude that if she had been with L[d] Anson she would not have escaped as well as him; it is a strong presumption that she would, that the Anna Pink a Victualler belonging to that squadron a ship of the same construction as the Resolution did escape those same difficulties, tho' she had only her own complement of men as a Merchantman. the difficulties L[d] Anson had to struggle with in getting round Cape Horn were indisputably owing to his being there at an improper season, but tho' the Pearl and Severn Men of War were obliged to put back, and the Wager Man of War cast away; tho Admiral Pizarro with a squadron of Spanish Ships of the Line failed in the attempt the Anna Pink a collier like the Resolution, did get round & made her way thro these stormy seas, which were so difficult to resist.

As to your attention to the health of the crew, it shews your humanity, but not your experience with regard to the accommodations, that can be given to Seamen in ships of small dimensions; for you may be assured that the men are full as well lodged as in any of our sixth rates, and as well as in many of our fifth rates, especially those taken from the French or built from their dimensions which are most of them as low between decks as the Resolution, tho' their compliment amounts in time of war to 220 men. I perceive that your attention extends only to the common men for when conveniences were made for all your suite the officers were stowed as close as herrings in a barrel, & yet you never took their distress into your humane consideration.

After reciting the many circumstances which make this an improper ship for your purpose you seem to close with that which you think the principal one, namely, that the great Cabbin is too small, & yet that great Cabbin after the necessary reduction has been made is higher and as long, tho perhaps not quite so broad as many of our 74 gun ships which have answered the purpose of the Admirals they were allotted to when they commanded considerable fleets. as to your suggestion that a man of war is as likely to take the ground without recieving damage as a collier, I at once throw down my guantlet in that contest, and will give up all pretensions to the least degree of knowledge on the subject in question, if you can produce one intelligent sea officer, be his connections or party principles what they may, who will join you in that opinion. as to your instancing the case of the Emerald, I own I cannot understand the conclusion you mean to draw from thence, for no one ever said that a man of war never got off a shoal; but every body will say that a man of war that does run upon a shoal has infinitely a worse chance of getting off than a collier which is particularly constructed for taking the ground, but this is a point so universally known that there is no occasion to dwell upon it any longer: I shall therefore only just say that the examples you have cited of the Emerald & Stag are no way applicable to your purpose take them which ever way you please; the former was on shore in a smooth water channel *at home* not in a distant, strange, desolate or savage coast at the Antipodes; six ships immediately anchored by her, hauled along side, took out her guns, provisions, & stores, and immediate assistance was sent from one of the Kings Dock Yards which happened luckily to be at hand; as to the Stag if she was hove up or down at Trincomalé it was in a Port where there were conveniences for fitting ships of burthen, and where undoubtedly they could have as much assistance as in the river Thames. Had either of these ships been in the Endeavour's place on the coast of New Holland they would never have been heard of again: even if they had got off the Rocks they could not have been hauled up to repair their damages as was done by the Endeavour. But before I entirely leave this subject I will beg to reason in your own way, & to cite an example (tho' I own I do not think it a very conclusive one) which must be allowed to be decisive if your case of the Emerald is so. since the reduction of the Resolution to her original state, I have been told that you wished for an old Indiaman, and that such a one had been offered by the India Company. The Wager man of War belonging to Lord Ansons Squadron run ashore & never got off, she was an old Indiaman, Ergo an old Indiaman is an unfit ship for this Voyage.

As to what you say about the Launceston, I shall not scruple to answer that if the board of Admiralty agrees to that proposal they will shew their ignorance, & exceed the limits of their duty: the Launceston is a forty four gun ship which with a proper repair may be rendered very usefull according to her rate in the Navy in time of war. she would take at least half a year and cost £8000 in repairing and after all would be totally unfit for the service; she could not go to sea with less than 180 men, & could not carry provisions for them for half the time they might chance to be out: if she had her proper masts anchors & cables that crew would not be sufficient to work her, if the masts &c were diminished she would sail no better than a collier, and be unable to ride out a gale of wind: if she went ashore she would be in great danger of being cast away; besides which if she was fit for the service, it should seem to me very injudicious in the Admiralty to throw away all the expence that has been allready incurred, to bring a new and unnecessary charge upon the publick, and to deprive the Navy of an usefull ship which is in course of repair, & may be employed very effectually hereafter, in the protection of the trade of his Majesties Subjects, and in the annoyance of his Enemies. I cannot conclude without sincerely expressing my concern that you have changed your intention with regard to this expedition, your publick spirit in undertaking so dangerous a voyage, your inattention to any expence which might contribute to the success of the purpose in which you was engaged, & your extensive knowledge as a naturalist, make it to be lamented that you are no longer one of the crew of the Resolution, but it may not be improper to set you right in one particular which you possibly may have misunderstood, and that is that you suppose the ships to have been wholly fitted out for your use, which I own I by no means apprehend to be the case.

The voyage was undertaken under the direction of the Admiralty, who employed an officer in his Majestys service of known experience, to pursue to the utmost a plan of investigating the Southern Hemisphere, in order to ascertain whither there was such a thing as a Southern Continent and it was supposed that this voyage, in addition to the late discoveries made under his direction, would bring this much controverted point to a final decision. You siezed this opportunity of adding a farther object to this usefull undertaking, and were willing to embark in the expedition in order to make improvements in natural knowledge, you was recieved with open arms by the Admiralty, & it is not their fault that you are not now embarked.

The Royal Society & the board of Longitude were allso desirous to make use of this opportunity for the improvement of Astronomy & to make observations that might possibly lead to a discovery of the Longitude & they have fitted out payed, & instructed an able astronomer for each ship, who they think fully capable to answer these desired ends.

Parlaiment has given their sanction to the expedition by voting a large sum of mony to encourage a person of general knowledge to go with the rest; the person originally intended for this purpose, and who undoubtedly was thoroughly qualified for it, has declined the voyage, but another person has been found who is as well qualified, and more so in one particular, as he carry's his son with him who is a very able designer, and will of course be extremely usefull in that part of the business. Upon the whole I hope that for the advantage of the curious part of Mankind, your zeal for distant voyages will not yet cease, I heartily wish you success in all your undertakings, but I would advise you in order to insure that success to fit out a ship yourself; that & only that can give you the absolute command of the whole Expedition; and as I have a sincere regard for your wellfare & consequently for your preservation, I earnestly entreat that that ship may not be an old Man of War or an old Indiaman but a New Collier.

I am &c

5. Public Information

[*Annual Register, 1772, p. 108.*]

The following particulars have been given as a true state of the proceedings relative to Mr. Banks and Dr. Solander's voyage, and the reason why it is like to be laid aside.—Mr. Banks and Dr. Solander were not consulted on the choice of the ship (the Endeavour) which was bought for them, and on their objecting to her want of accommodation for their draughtsmen, &c. who were necessary for their discoveries, as well as to her want of room to stow the crew; the navy-board undertook to give all these conveniences, and patched the same ship with a round-house and square deck, and, without considering whether the ship could bear it, manned and equipped her for the voyage. Mr. Banks, Dr. Solander, &c. examined her a second time, found her convenient if she could sail, of which they doubted, and reported her top-heavy.—Their observations were disregarded; but a gale of wind arising laid her on her side without her having a single sail unreefed, and she could not for some time recover: they ordered the long-boat to save the crew, when unexpectedly she recovered. Notwithstanding this accident, she was reported good, and fit for the voyage, and was ordered to Plymouth. The pilot obeyed their orders, sending word he could not insure her out of the river. At last it was found the farce could be carried on no longer and the reports on which the navy-board proceeded were found false: expresses were sent along the coast to Deal, &c. to order her into the nearest dock to Sheerness, if they could overtake her: this was no difficult task; for, while the other ships cleared the Downs, she did not make one knot an hour. She was put into dock; they cut off her round-house, and part of her deck, reduced the cabin, and put her in the same unfit situation she was in when first objected to; and then the question was politely put to Mr. Banks, take this or none. Mr. Banks has laid out several thousand pounds for instruments, &c. preparatory for the voyage; Mr.

Zoffani near one thousand for necessaries; and the other gentlemen very considerable sums on that account.

6. Summary by Cook

[*B.M. Add. MS 27888, ff. 5–5v, 6v.*]

To many it will no doubt appear strange that Mr Banks should attempt to over rule the opinions of the two great Boards who have the sole management of the whole Navy of Great Britain and likewise the opinions of the principal sea officers concern'd in the expedition; for a Gentleman of Mr Banks's Fortune and Abilities to engage in these kind of Voyages is as uncommon as it is meritorious and the great additions he made last Voyage to the Systems of Botany and Natural History gain'd him great reputation which was increased by his imbarking in this. This, together with a desire in every one to make things as convenient to him as possible, made him to be consulted on every occasion and his influance was so great that his opinion was generally followed, was it ever so inconsistant, in preference to those who from their long experience in Sea affairs might be supposed better judges, till at length the Sloop was rendered unfit for any service whatever and than she was to be condemn'd altogether, this was carrying the matter so far that even those who favoured Mr Banks most in his other schemes opposed him in this, and when he found he could not carry his point he gave up the Voyage. . . .

Mr Banks unfortunate for himself set out upon too large a Plan a Plan that was incompatible with a Scheme of discovery at the Antipodes; had he confined himself to the same plan as he set out upon last Voyage, attended only to his own persutes and not interfered with the choice, equipmint and even Direction of the Ships things that he was not a competent judge of, he would have found every one concerned in the expedition ever ready to oblige him, for my self I can declare it: instead of finding fault with the Ship he ought to have considered that the Endeavour Bark was just such another, whose good quallities enabled me to remain so much longer in the South Sea then any one had been able to do before, and gave him an oppertunity to acquire that reputation the Publick has so liberally and with great justice bestowed upon him.

APPENDIX III

The Board of Longitude and the Voyage

1. Minutes of the Board

[*The following extracts are printed from the records of the Board of Longitude now in the Royal Greenwich Observatory, Herstmonceux, Vol. V, Confirmed Minutes, 1737–1779.*]

28 November 1771. A letter of the 25th of last month from the Astronomer Royal to the Earl of Sandwich was then read representing that the intended expedition to the South Seas may be rendered more serviceable to the improvement of geography and navigation than it can otherwise be if the ship be furnished with such astronomical instruments as this Board hath the disposal of or can obtain the use of from the Royal Society and also some of the longitude watches and above all if a proper person could be sent out to make use of those instruments and teach the officers on board the ship the method of finding the longitudes: and the Board having taken the same into consideration and concurring in opinion with the Astronomer Royal came to the following resolutions viz.

> That the sending out persons for the above purposes in the two ships intended to make discoveries in remote parts and furnishing them, as well as the officers of those ships with astronomical instruments to make observations will render the said expedition more serviceable to the improvement of geography and navigation;
>
> That one observer be therefor sent out in each ship and the expence attending the same defrayed by this Board;
>
> That the Astronomer Royal and the rest of the professors present be desired to look out for two persons properly qualified and willing to go upon the above service; to know upon what terms they will undertake it; and to report the same at the next meeting; and
>
> That they be further desired to prepare a draft of instructions proper for the said persons and also a list of the necessary instruments; to lay the same before the Royal Society for their approbation; And to bespeak of the proper persons such of the instruments so approved of as this Board are not already possessed of or cannot obtain from the Royal Society;
>
> That the watch made by Mr. Kendall by order of this Board and now in the possession of the Astronomer Royal be sent out for trial in one of the above ships: but that it be previously cleaned by Mr.

Kendall and returned to the Royal Observatory for a months further trial now.[1]

14 December 1771. Mr. William Bayly and Mr. William Wales were proposed by the Astronomer Royal and the other professors as persons well qualified and willing to go out in the ships fitting out for a voyage to remote parts in order to make observations;[2] And the said Mr. Wales who was attending was called in and being asked upon what terms he was willing to engage to perform that service, informed the Board that he expected £350 per annum exclusive of his expences the allowance to be made for which he would submit to their consideration: And the Board understanding from the Astronomer Royal that the above mentioned Mr. Bayly (who could not attend) expects to be paid £300 per annum exclusive of his expences or one guinea a day if his expences are not allowed, which last offer the Board being most inclineable to accept, Mr. Wales was asked if he would go on the same footing, but he declined going for less than £400 per annum if his expences are not allowed him: It was therefore agreed to allow him after the rate of £400 per annum and to make the same allowance to Mr. Bayly to prevent any misunderstanding happening between them on account of the small difference which would otherwise be in their pay; the said allowance to be in full compensation for their trouble and all expences whatever.

The said Mr. Wales then desiring to have an imprest to enable him to fit himself out, And the Board understanding that it would be very convenient for the said Mr. Bayly to have an imprest for that purpose also and Mr. Wales further desiring that his wife may be paid some part of his proposed allowance during his absence, for the subsistence of herself and family

Resolved That the said Messrs. Wales and Bayly have each of them an imprest of £150 to enable them to fit themselves out;

That £150 per annum be paid by ½ yearly payments to Mrs. Wales until her husband's return or, in case he should die during the voyage, til an account of it shall arrive; and that the money which shall be paid to her be deducted from the said Mr. Wales' allowance; And

That a letter be wrote to the Navy Board to desire them to imprest and pay the said sums accordingly.

Mr. Wales then withdrew.

A report from the Astronomer Royal and the other professors[3] was then read containing a list of instruments and heads of instructions which they judge proper for the above mentioned observers with a memorandum annexed signed by Dr. Morton secretary to the Royal Society representing

[1] On the following day these resolutions were reported orally to the Council of the Royal Society by its President, James West; see below, p. 900.

[2] The 'observers' were not nominated by the Royal Society; no names were suggested at its Council meeting of 12 December (see next note).

[3] This report had been approved by the Council of the Royal Society on 12 December (see below, p. 905). A few variants between the list of instruments as enumerated in the Royal Society's draft and in the Board's minutes are indicated in footnotes below.

that the whole thereof had been approved by the council of the said Society who had agreed to lend the following instruments vizt.

1 astronomical quadrant of one foot radius
1 astronomical clock
1 transit instrument
2 common brass Hadley's quadrants.

And it appearing by the said report that the following instruments will also be wanted vizt.

Already in the Board's possession.	1 astronomical quadrant 1 foot radius 1 astronomical clock 1 alarum clock 2 reflecting telescopes Mr. Kendal's watch[1] } now at the Royal Observatory Mr. Arnold's watch[2] } at Greenwich
To be purchased.	2 journeymen clocks 1 alarum clock 2 of Dollond's last improved 3½ feet telescopes with object glass micrometers and moveable wires 2 brass Hadley's sextants with Mr. Maskelyne's improvements 6 variation charts 2 marine barometers[3] 4 common barometers 6 thermometers 2 theodolites 2 wooden frames with glass roofs for observing by reflection[4] 2 large magnetic needles to use at land[5] 2 large magnetic needles of old construction to use at sea 2 magnetic variation compasses 2 Gunter's chains with spare links and rings

Resolved that the secretary do write to Mr. Bradley, mathematical usher at the Royal Academy at Portsmouth for such of the above instruments belonging to this Board as are in his possession
And that the Astronomer Royal be desired to bespeak those necessary to be purchased of the proper instrument makers and get ruby pallets put to the two astronomical clocks by Mr. Arnold as proposed.

[1] R.S. draft adds 'made on Harrison's principle'.
[2] R.S. draft adds 'of new construction'.
[3] R.S. draft adds 'with spiral tubes by Nairne'.
[4] R.S. draft: '2 wooden frames to hold quicksilver, or any other fluid, with ground glass roofs to keep off the air for the purpose of observing altitudes of the sun or stars by reflection with the Hadley's Sextants'. These were artificial horizons.
[5] Instead of this and the next item, the R.S. draft has '2 magnetic dipping needles'.

The heads of instructions being then read and approved;[1]

Resolved that Messrs. Wales and Bayly be directed to attend at the next meeting to hear the same read; and the Astronomer Royal and the rest of the professors were desired to consider and report at the said meeting if anything farther shall appear necessary to be added thereto.

25 January 1772. Messrs. Wales and Bayly attending in consequence of the resolutions of last Board were sent for in, and a draft of their instructions with some additions which the Astronomer Royal had judged proper to make since the last reading was read to them; They then desired that orders may be given for their being supplied with candles and some other necessaries whilst on ship board and that they may be each furnished with a moveable observatory which will be of infinite use to them wherever they may have occasion to make observations on shore and which Mr. Bayly represented he could get made for about £25 each[2]

They were directed to deliver to the secretary a list of the necessaries with which they wish to be supplied; and to furnish themselves with moveable observatories proper for their use; the charge of which should be defrayed by the Board.

They then withdrew.

The Astronomer Royal representing that it will be necessary to provide the undermentioned instruments maps etc for the use of the said Messrs. Wales and Bayly in addition to those which were mentioned at the last Board vizt.

1 journey man clock
2 pair of globes
a pocket watch with a second hand—for Mr. Wales: Mr. Bayly having one
2 of Senex's maps of the Zodiac
2 large magnetic steel bars for touching the variation compasses and dipping needles
12 copies of the Nautical Almanac for 1772, 1773, 1774 and as much as may be printed of 1775.

Resolved. That the same be provided for their use accordingly and the Astronomer Royal was desired to give the necessary directions.

Mr. Bayly then asked for provision to be made for his wife as had been done for Mrs. Wales.

[1] The instructions to the observers formed the second part of the Royal Society's report. Those issued to Wales are printed below, pp. 724–8; the more significant variants between the draft put forward by the Society and the text approved by the Board are shown in footnotes.

[2] 'The Observatory was contrived by my associate Mr. W. Bayly, and is undoubtedly one of the most convenient portable Observatories that has yet been made.'—Wales, *Astronomical Observations*, p. viii. It is shown in pl. II of the book.

7 March 1772. Mr Wales and Mr. Bayly received the stationery they wanted etc.

The instructions for the said Messrs. Wales and Bayly were now signed and copies were ordered to be sent to the Rt. Honorable the Lords Commissioners of the Admiralty with a desire that their Lordships will please to give orders for Mr. Wales with his instruments and necessaries to be received on board the RESOLUTION sloop and Mr. Bayly with his instruments and necessaries on board the ADVENTURE sloop, in order that they may proceed in them on the present intended voyage for the purpose of making the observations which are mentioned in the said instructions; and that their Lordships will please to give the commanders of those sloops directions to assist and support the said persons upon all occasions where they may stand in need of it, to enable them to carry those instructions into execution.

Ordered

That a copy of the said instructions be sent to Mr. Banks who is going out in one of the above sloops for the use of himself and Dr. Solander who accompanies him.

14 May 1772. The Earl of Sandwich having proposed to the consideration of the Board whether it may not be proper to give some directions with respect to the safe custody of the watch machines which are going out under the care of Messrs. Wales and Bayly in the RESOLUTION and ADVENTURE sloops; as well to prevent any improper management or illtreatment of the said watch machines as to obviate any suspicions thereof hereafter; and the Board entirely concurring in opinion with his Lordship that such directions are extremely proper and necessary:

Resolved That such boxes as Messrs. Kendal and Arnold shall judge most proper for the reception of their respective watch machines be immediately provided;

That three good locks of different wards be also provided and affixed to each box;

That the key of one of the locks of each box be kept by the commander of the sloop wherein such box may be; that the key of another of the said locks be kept by the 1st lieutenant of the said sloop or officer next in command to him; and that the key of the third lock be kept by such one of the above mentioned observers (Messrs. Wales and Bayly) as shall be on board: which three persons are daily to be present at the winding up of the said watch machine and comparing them with each other whilst on board and with the astronomical clock whilst on shore and to see that the respective times shown at such comparisons be properly inserted and attested under their hands in the general observation book which the said observers are ordered to keep. But if it shall happen that the commanders, officers or observers or either of them cannot at any time through indisposition or absence upon other necessary duties conveniently attend, their key or keys are in such case to be delivered to such other officer or officers of the sloops as the commanders can best trust therewith, in order that such other officer or officers may attend at the winding up and comparing etc. of the above mentioned watch machines during such indisposition or absence.

Resolved. That the secretary do see to the providing of the said boxes and locks and defray the expence thereof out of any money which may be in his hands.

Resolved. That a copy of the above resolutions be sent to the right honorable the Lords Commissioners of the Admiralty and that their Lordships be desired to give directions to the commanders of each of the above sloops conformable thereto.

2. Instructions to Wales

[*Printed from the Canberra Letter Book.*]

By the Commissioners appointed by Acts of Parliament for the discovery of Longitude at Sea &c.

Whereas you have agreed (on certain Terms) to go on board one of His Majestys Sloops, named in the Margin, which are now fitting out for a Voyage to remote parts, in Order to make Nautical & Astronomical Observations, and to perform other Services tending to the Improvem[t] of Geography & Navigation, you are hereby required and directed to hold yourself in readiness, to Embark on board one of the said Sloops, when the Necessary Orders shall be given for your reception, and then to proceed in her on the above mentioned Voyage accordingly; And whereas we have Order'd you to be supply'd with the Several Instruments, Books, Maps, Charts & other things specified in the Schedule hereunto annexed w[ch] the Astronomer Royal will cause to be deliver'd to you, You are to receive and take into your Charge & Custody the said Instruments, Books, Maps, Charts &c. (Giving our Secretary a Receipt for the Same) and to make use of them for the Several purposes to which they are Respectively adapted, taking all possible care of them during the Voyage and When that shall be finished, returning them to us in the best condition you may be able, And, in the performance of the abovementioned Service you are punctually and faithfully to Observe & Execute the following Instructions.

1.

You are every day if the Weather will admit,[1] to observe Meridian Altitudes of the Sun for finding the Latitude & also other altitudes of the

[1] *every day . . . admit* not in the R.S. draft.

Sun both in the Morning & Afternoon, at a distance from Noon, with the time between measured by a Watch and the Suns bearing by the Azimuth Compass at the 1st Observation[1] in order to determine the Apparent time of the Day and Latitude in case the Sun should be clouded at Noon;[2] You are moreover to Observe distances of the moon from the Sun & fixed Stars with Hadleys Sextants from which you are to compute the Longitude by the Nautical Almanac.

2.

You are to Wind up the Watches Every Day, as soon after the times of Noon as you can conveniently, and compare them together and Set down the respective times, and you are to Note also the times of the Watches when the Suns Morning & Afternoon altitudes, or the Distances of the Moon from the Sun and fixed Stars, are Observed; and to compute the Longitude resulting from the Comparison of the Watches with the Apparent time of the day inferred from the Morning & Afternoon Altitudes of the Sun, and as often as you shall have opportunities, you are to Compare one of the said Watches with one of those which may be under the care of the undermentioned Mr Bayley in the other Sloop, and Note down the respective times Shewn by the said Watches.[3]

3.

You are to Observe, or Assist at the Observations of, the Variation of the compass, and to Observe the Variation of the Magnetic dipping Needle from time to time.

4.

You are to Note the height of one or more Thermometers placed in the Air & in the Shade early in the Morning and about the hottest time of the day, and to Observe also the height of the Thermometer within the Sloop near the Watches; and to make Remarks on the Southern Lights if any should appear; And to make Experiments of the Saltness of the Sea and the degree of Cold by letting down the Thermometer at great Depths, as you may have Opportunity.[4]

5.

You are to keep a Ship Journal with the Log work'd according to the plain dead reckoning (Leeway & Variation only allowed) Noting therein the length of the Log line & times of running, out of the sand Glasses from time to time;[5] And you are to insert therein also another Account corrected by the last cœlestial Observations & a third deduced from the Watches.

[1] *with the time . . . Observation* not in R.S. draft.
[2] *and Latitude . . . Noon* not in R.S. draft.
[3] *and as often . . . Watches* not in R.S. draft.
[4] *and to Observe . . . Opportunity* not in R.S. draft.
[5] *Noting therein . . . time* not in R.S. draft.

6.

You are to teach such of the Officers on board the sloop as may desire it the use of the Astronomical Instruments &[1] the Method of finding the Longitude at sea from the Lunar Observations.

7.

You are to Settle the position of the head Lands, Islands & Harbours in Latitude and Longitude by the cœlestial Observations and also set down what Longitude the Watches give.

8.

Where ever you land you are to make the same observations on shore as you have been directed to make on Ship board, only Observing to take the altitudes with the Astronomical Quadrant instead of the Hadleys Sextants and you are likewise to make the additional observations & to attend to the directions undermention'd.—Viz[t]

Whenever you can land safely (should it be for only two or three days) Set up the Astronomical Clock & fix it very firmly to a Massey peice of wood let deep into the ground and fix the Pendulum at the same exact length as it was of when going at the Royal Observatory at Greenwich before the Voyage and take equal Altitudes of the Sun & fixed stars for determining the rate of its going Noting the arc of Vibration of the Pendulum[2] and the Height of the Thermometer within the clock case[3] at the time; this will not only be usefull with respect to the other Astronomical Observations made on Shore, but also when compared with the going of the Clock at Greenwich, will shew the Difference of gravity from that at Greenwich, which is a very Curious point in Experimental Philosophy.

Compare the Watches with the Astronomical Clock at Noon & also about the times of the Equal Altitudes.

Observe meridian Altitudes of the Sun and also of fixed Stars some to the North & some to the South for finding the Latitude; Observe also differences of right ascension between the Moon & fixed Stars in the Manner explained by the Astronomer Royal (Philos.Trans: Vol 54. p. 348.) in Order to Settle the Moons parallax in right ascension in Various Latitudes.[4]

Make Observations of Eclipses of Jupiters Satellites & Occultations of fixt Stars & Planets by the Moon and any other Observations usefull for settling the Longitude of the place, and you are particularly to exert your best Endeavours to settle the Longitude of the Cape of good Hope with the utmost accuracy, in case you should touch there, by Observations of

[1] *such of the Officers . . . Instruments &:* R.S. draft *the officers on board the ship.*
[2] *Noting the arc . . . Pendulum* not in R.S. draft.
[3] *within the clock case:* R.S. draft *in the House.*
[4] *Observe also differences . . . Latitudes* not in R.S. draft.

occultations of fixed Stars by the Moon and Transits of the Moon & proper stars over the meridian with the transit Instrument; And to send to us, from thence a full & particular Acco[t] of all your proceedings & Observations.[1]

Observe the height of Barometer once at least every day.

Observe the height of the Tides and the time of high & low water, particularly at the full & change of the Moon and Whether there be any difference & What, between the Night & Day tides.[2]

9.

You are to take particular care that all your cœlestial observations, whether made on ship board or on shore, be kept in a clear distinct and regular manner,[3] in a Book wherein the Commander of the Sloop and other Officers may also insert their Observations if they think fit, and that they be written, with all their Circumstances, immediately after they are made or as soon after as they can be conveniently transcribed therein from the loose papers or Memorandum Books in which they may be first Enter'd; which Book is to be always open for the inspection and use of the Commander & other Officers of the Sloop & of Joseph Banks Esq[r] and D[r] Solander who are going the Voyage in one of the sloops: And you are to send to us, by every safe Conveyance which may Offer, the Results of your several Observations and also the Principal Observations themselves.[4]

10.

You are to co-operate with, and assist M[r] W[m] Bayley (who is under engagements with us to go out in the other of the two sloops abovementioned with Instructions similar to these) in whatever may be for the good of the Service wherein you are jointly imployed, we having given him directions to co-operate with and assist you in like manner. And Lastly,

For your care pains & Expences during the time you shall be employed on the above service; you will be allowed after the rate of Four hundred pounds p Annum to Commence from the 25th of January last; And for your further encouragement, we have, at your Request Order[ed] the Sum of One hundred & Fifty pounds to be impress'd to you on Account to enable you to fit yourself out, and One hundred & fifty pounds to be paid Annually during your absence or in case of your Death till such time we shall be apprized of it, by half yearly Payments, to your wife for the

[1] *And to send . . . Observations* not in R.S. draft.

[2] R.S. draft here adds: 'Teach the use of the Astronomical Instruments to such of the Officers of the ship as are desirous of being instructed therein'.

[3] This clause was perhaps prompted by the confusion of Charles Green's records from the *Endeavour*, on which Maskelyne had already animadverted; see I, pp. cxliv–v.

[4] *who are going . . . themselves* not in R.S. draft, which also lacks the two concluding paragraphs that follow.

Subsistance of herself & Family which sums, so to be impressed & paid are to be deducted out of your above mention'd Allowance.

Given under our hands the 7th March 1772

To
Mr Wm Wales

Sandwich
Chas Hardy
J. West
Nevil Maskelyne
Thos Hornsby

John Smith
E. Waring
A. Shepherd
Php Stephens
John Smith

By Order of the Commissioners
Jno Ibbetson

APPENDIX IV

Extracts from Officers' Records

I. Furneaux's Narrative

[*Printed from B.M. Add. MS 27890, ff. 2v–20, with excisions. For the nature of the Ms, see p. cxxxvii above. The text is given as Furneaux wrote it, Cook's alterations being incorporated in the footnotes or otherwise noted.*]

. . . On the 23[d] of November 1772, weigh'd and came to sail in company with the Resolution, directing our Course to the SW but meeting with continual hard gales of wind at West & NW prevented our making any westing, and much damaged our sails and rigging tho' fitted in the best manner, the sea making a continual breach over us, and the decks leaky not only wet the peoples cloaths, but the beds on which they lay, so that they were extreemly fatigued, cold and helpless which they felt more severely by reason of our sudden shift of climate, tossed at the mercy of the waves for near three weeks without one moderate day. We had not reached further than 50° South when we fell in with a very large Island of Ice and was hourly surprized with others, which we at first took frequently for Land, making the signal to the Resolution for that purpose and put us in the greatest consternation for fear of running on them, it being the more dangerous by reason of the thick snow and sleet that fell almost without intermission, which rendered the Horizon extreemly obscure tho' in the midst of summer: from the Latitude of 52°00′ South they became so plenty that we frequently saw Sixteen or more at a time, from a quarter to three quarters of a mile in length and several hundred feet above the surface of the water, that we were often becalmed by them (they are said often to overset when that part that is above the Horizon becomes the heaviest) and at the same time the sea became so covered with the small pieces (we call'd plumpers from the frequent strokes they gave the ship's bows) that it was with the greatest difficulty we could keep clear of the most dangerous ones; thus we went on in the most severe frost, wet and cold, running the gauntlet every day among the Ice accompanied by nothing but whales and a few melancholly birds which differed nothing from those near the Cape of Good Hope, except the Sea Pigeon[1] which are peculiar to those latitudes. We found a strong current setting to SE ever since we left the Cape, that in the Latitude of 54° we were near three degrees to the Eastward of our account. On Monday the 14th of December in Lat[de] 56° South and about four degrees to the Eastward of the Cape we were intirely stopt by the Ice which intirely covered the surface of the water so that there was no part to be seen for half the Compass to the Southward

[1] Probably he means the Snow Petrel, *Pagodroma nivea:* cf. Cook, p. 58 above.

from the Masthead, which in all probability extends to the Pole.[1] The wind being Westerly we kept on the North side of it, saw many Penguins and shot several other Birds: being fine weather, the Resolution hoisted out her Boat and brought onboard her several pieces of Ice, which being melted was excellent water for any use and not in the least breakish: At the back of this field the Ice was extreemly Ragged and mountainous, which afforded a prospect truely severe and winter-like; we kept alongside this field 'till towards the evening, and then hauled off; we soon lost sight of it, but was still surrounded with large and high Islands over which the sea made continual breaches. We continued our Course to the Eastward to the Longitude of Cape Circumsision, then in 60°20′ South, but no land to be found: We began to doubt if there was any such place, or if there was, must be some inconsiderable spot not habitable by reason of the intense cold.

This, together with the extreem danger of Shipwrack among so much Ice, and the favourable opportunity of a strong NW wind was sufficient inducement for quiting our present pursuit of the discovery of Cape Circumcision, and make the best of our way to the Eastward. On the 9th of January 1773 in Latitude 62° South and Longitude 35° East our water growing short, brought to amidst some broken Ice, hoisted out the boats and got onboard Seven or Eight Tons which when melted in the Ship's coppers was very good water; thus recruited in what we most fear the want of at Sea, again encouraged us to proceed on our course to the Southward among the Ice, and try what could be found: 'Twas about this time we had observed the birds had intirely left us and gone (as we supposed) to some Land to breed, for, a few days before there was a great number about the ship tho' now not one to be seen. On the 12th we again brought to hoisted out the boats and got onboard as much Ice as filled all our empty Casks, that we had now as much water onboard as when we left the Cape of Good Hope. We had now several days fair Weather, in which time we got several good Observations of the Sun and Moon, which gave us the Longitude of 39° degrees East; we held on our Course to the Southward till the 18th January when we crossed the Antartic Circle and entered the Frigid Zone, in the evening of the same day in the Latd 67°20′s and Longitude 39°30′ East we were stopt by the Ice which intirely covered the surface of the water, which obliged us to tack and stand again to the Northward, there being at the same time Thirty two Islands of Ice in sight, Tho' I believe had we push'd thro' this archipelago of Ice, tho' it would have been attended with much danger, we might have gone further to the Southward; the Ice in the SW Quarter appearing from the Masthead to be more open, but as this would have answered no end, and in all likelyhood got ourselves hemmed in with Ice, where we should have undoubtedly perished Judged it more prudent to stand to the Northward and beat these seas in such Latitudes where if there is any Land, which might be found habitable and of some use: We accordingly directed our Course to the

[1] Cf. Cook, pp. 59–63.

NNE, 'till the 1st of February, being then in the Latitude of 49°30′ South when we got intirely from among the Ice and seen but a few Islands for these several days past—which is more than we can boast of since we first fell in with it on the 20th of December last. On the 2[d] of February we saw a great quantity of Sea weed and several Divers,[1] then in the Latitude of 48°30′ South and Long. 60° East which gave us some reason to believe we were not far from Land, and believe it was owing to the general opinion being given, together with an Account we had at the Cape of Good Hope of the French having discovered a large Tract of Land near this place about Eighteen months ago, that we again shifted our Course to the Westward and cruized for it several days, had very uncertain weather and hard gales of wind at NNW but no Land to be seen or further signs of any; the Season of the year beginning to advance and a long distance to run to New Zealand (the appointed Rendezvous) together with strong westerly winds, water growing short and no Ice to recruit it, were sufficient motives for us to make the best of our way; and on the 6th bore away and put every man to an allowance of three pints of water a day. On the 7th of Feb[ry] 1773[2] in the morning the Resolution being then about two miles ahead, the wind shifting further to the Westward, brought on a very thick fog, so that we lost sight of her; we soon after heard a Gun, the report of which we imagined to be on the Larboard beam, we then hauled up SE and kept firing a four pounder every half hour but had no answer or further sight of her; tho we kept the course we steered on before the Fog came on, on [*sic*] the evening it began to blow hard and, at intervals more clear, but could see nothing of her, which gave us much uneassiness; we then Tacked and stood to the westward to cruize in the place we last saw her agreeable to agreement in case of separation, but next day came on a very heavy gale of wind and thick weather, that obliged us to bring to and thereby prevented us reaching the intended spot, but on coming more moderate, the fog in some measure clearing away we cruized as Near the place as we could get, for three days when giving over all hopes of joining company again bore away for winter quarters distant fourteen hundred leagues, thro' a sea intirely unknown and reduced the allowance of water to one quart p day. We kept between the Latitude of 52° and 53° South, had much Westerly winds hard gales with squalls, snow and sleet with a long hollow sea from the SW Quarter so that we judge there is no Land in that quarter. After we reached the Longitude of 95° East we found the Variation to decrease very fast, but for a more perfect account I refer you to the Table at the latter end of this book.[3] On the 26th at night we saw a Meteor of an uncom̄on brightness in the NNW, it directed its' course to the SW with a very great light in the southern sky, such as is known to the Northward by the name Aurora Borealis, or Northern Lights: We saw the Lights for several nights running; and what is remarkable we have seen but one

[1] The bird that in his journal he calls 'Dip chicks', 'Divers' being Cook's name for them: *Pelecanoides* spp.

[2] 'of Feb[ry] 1773' inserted by Cook.

[3] No such Table is given.

Island of Ice since we parted company with the Resolution 'till our making the Land, tho' we were most of the time two or three degrees to the Southward of the Latitude we first saw it in. We were daily attended by great numbers of Sea birds, and frequently saw Porpoises curiously spotted white and black.[1] On the first of March we were alarmed with the cry of Land by the man at the Masthead on the Larboard beam, which gave us great joy; we immediately hauled our wind and stood for it, but to our mortification were disappointed in a few hours, for what we took to be land proved no more than Clouds which disappeared as we sailed towards them; we then bore away and directed our course toward the Land laid down in the charts by the name of Van Dieman's land, discovered by Tasman in 1642, and laid down in the Lat^{de} 44° South and Longitude 140° East, and supposed to join to New Holland. On the 9th of March, little wind and pleasent weather, about 9 AM, being then in the Latitude 43°37′ South, Longitude by Lunar Observation 145°36′ East and by Account 143°10′ East a Greenwich, we saw the Land bearing NNE about 8 or 9 Leagues distance; it appeared moderately high, and uneaven near the Sea, the hills further back formed a double Land and much higher, there seemed to be several Islands or broken land to the NW as the shore trenched, but by the reason of Clouds that hung over them could not be certain whether they did not join to the main, we hauled immediately up for it and by noon were within 3 or 4 leagues of it, a point much like the Ramhead off Plymouth, which I take to be the same Tasman calls South Cape,[2] bore North four Leagues of us, the Land from this cape runs directly to the Eastward. About four Leagues alongshore are Three Islands[3] about two miles long and several rocks resembling the Mewstone (particularly one which we so named) about four or five leagues ESE½E off the above Cape which Tasman has not mentioned, nor laid down in his draughts. After you pass these Islands the Land lies EbN and wbs by the compass nearly; it is a bold shore and seems to afford several bays or anchoring places but believe deep water, from the SW Cape which is in the Latitude of 43°39′ South and Longitude 145°50′[4] East to the SE Cape in the Latitude 43°36′[5] s, Longitude 147°00′ East is nearly 16 leag^{s} and Soundings from 48 to 70 fathoms, sand and broken shells three or four leagues off shore: Here the country is hilly and full of trees, the shore rocky and difficult landing, occasioned by the wind blowing here continually from the Westward, which occasions such a surf, that the sand cannot lay on the shore, we saw no inhabitants here. The morning on the 10th of March being calm the ship then about four miles from the shore Sent the great Cutter onshore with the second Lieutenant to find if there was any harbour or good bay, but soon after it came on to blow very hard, made the signal for the boat to return several times but they did not see nor hear any thing of it, the ship then three or four leagues off, that we could not

[1] The description of the porpoises is insufficient to identify them.
[2] South West Cape.
[3] The Maatsuyker islands.
[4] 50′ is altered to 55′ by Cook.
[5] 36′ is altered to 35′ by Cook.

see any thing of the Boat, which gave us great uneasiness, as there was a very great Sea. At ½ past 1 PM to our great satisfaction the boat Returned onboard safe, they landed, but with much difficulty, and saw several places where the Indians had been and one they lately had left, where they had had a fire with a great number of large pearl scollop shells round it, those shells they brought onboard, with some burnt sticks and green boughs: there was a path from this place thro' the woods, which in all probability leads to their habitations, but by the reason of the weather had not time to pursue it. The soil seems to be very rich, the country well cloathed with wood, particularly on the Lee side of the Hills—plenty of water, which falls from the Rocks in beautiful cascades for two or three hundred feet perpendicular into the sea; but did not see the least sign of any place for a ship to anchor in with safety. Hoisted in the Boat and made sail for Frederick Henry Bay. From Noon to 3 PM running along shore EbN at which time we were abreast of the westernmost point of a very deep Bay called by Tasman, Stormy bay. From the West to the East point of this bay there are several small Islands and black rocks we called the Friars; while crossing this bay we had very heavy squalls and thick weather; at times when it cleared up I saw several fires in the bottom of this bay which is near two or three leagues deep and doubt not but good places for anchoring, but the weather being so bad did not think it safe to stand into the bay.—From the Friars, the land trenches away about NbE 4 leagues. We had smooth water and kept in shore and had regular soundings from 20 to 15 fathoms water ½ past 4 we hauled round a high bluff point, the Rocks whereof were like so many fluted pillars,[1] and had ten fath[s] water fine sand within half of a mile of the shore. At 7 being abreast of a fine bay and having little wind, came to with the small bower in 24 fathoms, sandy bottom. Just after we anchored, being a fine clear evening, had a good observation of the Star Antares and the Moon, which gives the Longitude of 147°34′ East, being in the Lat[d] of 43°20′ S. We first took this bay to be that by Tasman called Frederick Henry Bay but find his laid down five leagues to the Northward of this.[2] At Daybreak the next Morning[3] Sent the Master inshore to sound the bay and to find out a watering place; at 8 he returned having found a most excellent harbour clear ground from side to side from 18 to 5 fathom Water all over the Bay gradually decressing [*sic*] as you go inshore. We weigh'd and turned up into the bay, the wind being westerly and very little of it, which baffled us much in getting in. At 7 AM[4] we anchored in 7 fathoms water with the small bower and Moored with the coasting anchor to the Westward the North point of the bay NNE½E (this we take to be Tasman's head,)[5] and the eastermost point we named Penguin Island from a curious one we caught there NEbE½E. The watering place W½N about one Mile from the shore on each side. Maria's Island

[1] Fluted Cape—the name given at this time.

[2] See p. 150, n. 3 above.

[3] 'At . . . Morning' substituted by Cook for Furneaux's 'AM'.

[4] AM is a slip for PM and Cook alters it to 'in the Evening'.

[5] It was not. In any case it was now named, no doubt from its fancied connection with Tasman's Frederick Henry Bay, Cape Frederick Henry; and this it has remained.

which is about 5 or 6 leagues off, shut in with both points that you are quite land-locked in a most spacious harbour. We lay here five days,[1] which time was employed in wooding and watering (which is easily got) and overhauling the Rigging. We found the country very pleasent, the soil of a black rich, tho' thin one; the sides of the hills covered with large trees and very thick, growing to a great height before they branch off: they are all of them of the Ever-green kind of a different sort to any I ever saw; the wood is very brittle and easily split, there is very little variety of sort, having seen but two, the leaves of one is long and Narrow, the seed (of which I got a few) was in the shape of a Button, and has a very agreeable smell: the Leaves of the other are like the bay and has a seed like the white thorn, with an agreeable spicy taste and smell.[2] Out of the trees we cut down for Fire wood there issued some Gum, which the Surgeon called Gum lac. The trees are mostly burnt or scorched near the ground, occasioned by the natives seting fire to the under wood in the most frequented places, and by these means have rendered it easily walking. The Land birds we saw are a bird like a Raven;[3] some of the Crow kind, black, with the tips of the feathers of the Tail and wings, white, their bill long and very sharp[4]—some Paroquets, and several kinds of small Birds. The Sea Fowl, are Duck, Teal, and the Sheldrake.[5] I forgot to mention a large white bird that one of the gentlemen shot, about the size of a large Kite, of the Eagle kind.[6] As for beasts we saw but one which was a Possom but the dung of some which we judge to be of the Deer kind. The Fish in the Bay are very scarce; those we caught were mostly Sharks, Dog fish, and a fish called by the Seamen Nurses, they are like the Dog fish only full of small white spots,[7] and some small fish not unlike spratts.[8] The Lagoons (which are breakish) abounds with trout[9] and several other sort of Fish, of which we caught a few with lines, but being so full of stumps of trees we could not haul the Sein. While we lay here we saw several smokes and large Fires about Eight or ten miles inshore to the Northward, but did not see any of the Natives, tho' they frequently come into this bay as there

[1] According to Furneaux's journal, he worked into the bay on the 11th a.m., and was anchored from 6 p.m. on the 12th (i.e. civil time 11th) to ½ past 9 a.m. on the 15th; so his 'five days' is not highly accurate.

[2] Both these trees were eucalypts, the two commonest about Adventure Bay and its vicinity: the first (its button-shaped 'seed' really the seed-capsule) *Eucalyptus globulus*, the Blue-gum; the second *E. obliqua*, known in Tasmania as the Stringybark.

[3] The raven found in Tasmania is *Corvus coronoides* Vigors and Horsfield.

[4] Perhaps the Clinking Currawong or Bell Magpie, *Strepera arguta* Gould.

[5] The country has more than one sort of duck. The teal would be the Chestnut Teal, *Anas castanea* (Eyton), or perhaps the Grey Teal, *Anas gibberifrons* Müller. The Chestnut-breasted Sheldrake or Mountain Duck is *Casarca tadornoides* Jard.

[6] The White Goshawk, *Accipiter novaehollandiae* Gm.

[7] Seamen were inclined to give the name 'nurse' pretty indiscriminately to sharks and dogfish; from the description of this particular one it was probably the White-spotted Dogfish, *Squalus kirki* Phillips.

[8] This, it seems likely, was *Clupea bassensis* McCulloch, the most common sprat found in Tasmanian waters.

[9] *Galaxias attenuatus* (Jenyns) and *G. truttaceus* (Cuvier) are both found in brackish waters flowing into Adventure Bay at the present time, and it may have been these that were seen.

were several Wigwams or hutts, in which we found some bags and netts made of Grass, which I imagine they carry their provisions and other necessaries in. In one of them there was the stone they strike fire with[1] and Tinder made of Bark, but of what tree could not find out. We found in one of their huts one of their spears, it was sharp at one end done I suppose with a shell or stone: Those things we brought away and left in the room of them, Medals, Gun flints and a few Nails, and an old empty barrel with the Iron hoops on it. They seem to be quite ignorant of every sort of Metal; the boughs of which their Huts are made are either broke or split and tied together with grass in a circular form the largest end stuck in the ground, and the smaller part meeting in a point at the top, and covered with Ferns and bark, so poorly done that they will hardly keep out a showr of rain. In the middle is the fire place surrounded with heaps of Mussel, pearl scollop and Cray Fish shells,[2] which I believe to be their chief food, (tho' we could not find any of them). They lay on the ground on dry grass round their fire, and I believe they have no settled place of habitation, as their houses seem'd to be built but for a few days, but wander about in small parties from place to place in search of Food and are actuated by no other motive. We never found more than three or four huts in a place, capable of containing three or four persons each only; and what is remarkable never saw the least signs of either Canoe or boat, and it is generally thought they have none,[3] and are altogether from what we can judge, a very Ignorant and wretched set of people, tho' natives of a country capable of producing every necessary of life, and a climate the finest in the world. We found not the least sign of any minerals or metals. Having compleated our wood and water, sailed from Adventure bay, intending to coast it up alongshore as high 'till we fell in with the Land seen by Captain Cook and discover whether Van Dieman's Land joins with New Holland. On the 16th passed the Island[s] called Marias, so named by Tasman, they appear to be the same as the main land.[4] On the 17th having passed Schoutens Island, hauled in for the main Land and stood alongshore at the distance of two or three leagues off. The Land here appears to be very thickly inhabited, as there was a continual fire alongshore as we sailed: The Land hereabouts is much pleasenter, low and even, but no sign of a harbour or bay where a ship might anchor with safety. The weather being

[1] Burney, p. 748 below, refers to 'flint and tinder'. It appears that the Tasmanian aborigines made fire both by stone and flint and by friction—and for friction used both the drill and socket, and stick and groove techniques.—H. Ling Roth, *The Aborigines of Tasmania* (London 1890), pp. 96–7.

[2] Mussel: *Mytilus planulatus* Lamarck; Scallop: *Notovola meridionalis* (Tate). Both these molluscs still occur in great numbers at Adventure Bay. One is not sure what Furneaux means by crayfish—perhaps the Spiny Lobster, *Jasus lalandi*, very abundant round the Tasmanian coast (and much appreciated by the *Endeavour's* men on the New Zealand coast); perhaps, though less likely, the small freshwater crayfish *Astacopsis franklinii* (Gray), not uncommon in Tasmanian streams. Burney, p. 748 below, mentions both lobster and crayfish shells.

[3] They used both a primitive sort of a raft, and a very primitive sort of canoe, but they were not habitually waterborne.—Ling Roth, op. cit., pp. 161–4.

[4] Cf. p. 151, n. 2 above.

bad, and blowing hard at SSE, could not send a boat onshore to have any intercourse with the inhabitants. In the Latitude of 40°50′ South the Land trenches away to the westward, which I believe forms a deep bay,[1] as we saw several smokes rising aback of the Island from the deck when we could not see the least sign of Land from the Masthead. From the Latitude of 40°50′ South to the Latitude of 39°50′ S is nothing but Islands and shoals, the Land high, rocky & barran. On the 19th in the Latitude of 40°30′ South, we Observed breakers about half a mile within shore of us. Sounded & had but Eight fathoms; immediately hauled off and deepened our water to 15 fathoms; then bore away and kept alongshore again. From the Latitude of 39°50′ to 39° S we saw no land but had regular soundings from 15 to 30 fathoms. As we stood on to the Northward we made Land again in about 39° and did not stand further to the Northward as we found the ground very uneaven and shoal water some distance off. I think it a very dangerous coast to fall in with. [The Coast][2] from Adventure bay to the place where we stood away for Zealand is S½W and N½E about 75 Leagues, and it is my opinion that there is no Streights between New Holland and Van Dieman's Land, but a very deep bay. I should have stood further to the Northward, but the wind blowing strong at SSE and looking likely to haul round to the Eastward, which would have blown right on the land, I therefore thought it more prudent to leave the Coast and steer for New Zealand. After we left the Coast we had very uncertain weather with rain and very heavy gusts of wind. On the 24th of March we were surprized with a very severe Squall that reduced us from Topgallant sails to reefed Courses in the space of an hour, the sea rising equally quick. We shiped many seas, one of which stove the large Cutter and washed the small one from her lashing into the waist and with much difficulty saved her from being washed overboard: this gale lasted twelve hours. After this we had more moderate weather, intermixed with Calms; we frequently hoisted out the boats to try the Current and in general found a small drift to the WSW; we shot many Birds and had in general good weather, till we came near to the Land, when it came on thick and dirty for several days, till we made the Coast of New Zealand in 40°30′ South having made Twenty four degrees of longitude from Adventure bay (after a passage of fifteen days). We had much southerly winds in this passage, and was under some apprehensions of not being able to fetch the streights, which would have obliged us to steer away for George's Island, so I would advise any that comes to this part to keep to the Southward, particularly in the fall of the year, when the S and SE winds prevails. The Land when we first made it appeared high and formed a confused jumble of Hills and Mountains. We steered alongshore to the Northward, but was much retarded in our Course by reason of the swell from the NE. At noon on the 3d of April, Cape Farewell, which is the South point of the Enterance of the West side of the Streights, EBN½N by the Compass 3 or 4 Leagues. It lays in the

[1] Cf. p. 152, n. 6 above.

[2] These two words are inserted by Cook, no doubt for clarity.

Latitude of 40°30′s and by the Lunar Observations 172°30′ East Longitude from Greenwich, having made 24°51′ from Adventure bay; The Variation is 13 degrees East.[1] About 8 O'Clock we entered the streights and steered NE 'till midnight, then brought to 'till day light and had soundings from 45 to 58 fathoms sand and broken shells. At day light made sail and steered SEbE had light airs. Mount Egmont NNE 11 or 12 Leagues, and Point Stephens SE½E 7 leagues. At Noon Mount Egmont NbE 12 Leagues, Stephen's Island SE 5 leagues. In the Afternoon on the 5th we put the drudge overboard in 65 fathoms, but caught nothing except a few small scollops, two or three Oysters, and broken shells. Standing to the Eastward for Charlotte Sound with a light breeze at NW. In the morning on the 5th of April, Stephen's Island bearing swbw 4 Leagues, was taken aback with a strong Easterly wind, which obliged us to haul our wind to the SE and work to Windward up under Point Jackson. The course from Stephen's Island to Point Jackson is nearly SE by the Compass 11 leagues distant; had from 40 to 32 fathoms sandy ground. As we stood off and on fired several Guns but saw no signs of any inhabitants. In the afternoon at ½ past 2 O'Clock found the Tide set the Ship to the Westward, anchored with the coasting anchor in 39 fathom water, muddy ground; Point Jackson SE½E 3 leagues, the east point of an Inlet about four leagues to the westward of Point Jackson (and appears to be a good harbour)[2] swbw½w. At 8 PM found the Tide to slacken, weighed and made sail (While at anchor caught several fish with hook and Line) found the tide to run to the Westward at the rate of 2½ knots p hour. Standing to the East, found no ground at 70 fathoms. Off Point Jackson NNW 2 Leagues. At 8 had the sound Open, the wind being down the Sound obliged us to work up under the Western shore, as the tide sets up strong there when it runs down in midd Channel. At 10 the Tide being done, was obliged to come to with the best bower in 38 fathoms close to some white rocks Point Jackson bearing NW½N; The Northernmost of the Brothers Ebs, and the middle of Entery Island[3] (which lays on the North side of the streights) NE. We made 15°30′ E variation in the streights. As we sailed up the Sound saw the Tops of high mountains covered with Snow, which remains there all the year. When the Tide slackend we weigh'd and sailed up the Sound, and about 5 OClock on the 7th Anchored in Ship Cove with the best bower in 10 fathom water Muddy ground, and Moored; the best bower to the NNE and small to ssw.[4] In the night we heard the howling of Dogs and People hollowing on the East shore. The two following Days were employed in clearing a place on Motuara Island for erecting our Tents for the Sick (having then several onboard much inflicted with the Scurvy) the Sail-

[1] This sentence, 'It lays . . . East', is deleted by Cook.

[2] The 'east point' was probably Forsyth Island, and the inlet the entrance to Pelorus Sound.

[3] Kapiti.

[4] '. . . this evg was sent to look for watering places, found one where we judge Captain Cook waterd in the Endeavour, the names of several of his people being cut in the Trees'. Burney, Ferguson MS.

makers & Coopers. On the Top of the Island was a post erected by the Endeavour's people with her name and time of Departure on it. On the 9th we were visited by three Canoes with about Sixteen of the Natives, we gave them several things to introduce [*sic*] them to bring us Fish and other things, with which they seemed highly pleased. One of our young Gentlemen seeing some thing wrapt up in a better manner than common, had the curiosity to see, which to his great surprize he found to be a human head lately murdered; they were under the greatest fear of having it forced from them, and particularly the man that seem'd most interested in it, his very flesh crept on his bones for fear of being punished by us, as Captain Cook had expressed his great abhorence to this unnatural act, they used every method to conceal it, by shifting it from one to another, and by signs to signify that there was no such thing amongst them, tho' we had seen it but a few minutes before They then took their leave of us and went onshore. They frequently mentioned the name of Tobia,[1] which was the name of the native of Georges Island (or Otaheite) brought here by the Endeavour, and who died at Batavia. And when we told them he was dead, some of them seemed to be very much concerned, and as well as we could understand them wanted to know whether we kill'd him, or if he died a natural death. By these questions they are the same Tribe Captain Cook saw. In the afternoon they returned again with Fish and Fern roots, which they sold for Nails and other triffles, tho' the nails is what they set the most value on. The Man and woman that had the head did not come off again. We had a catalogue of their words in their language calling several things by name which surprized them much. They wanted it much and offered a great quantity of Fish for it, next morning they returned again to the number of 50 or 60 with their chief at their head (as we supposed) in five double Canoes that is two lashed together by several sticks laid across the two Canoes, at the distance of two feet asunder and seized together with a rope made of grass, which renders them stiff and more convenient. The Single Canoes have an outrigger like the Prows described by Lord Anson.[2] They gave us their implements of War, stone hatchets & cloaths &c[a] for Nails and old bottles, which they put a great value on. A number of their Chiefs, or head men, came onboard us, and 'twas with some difficulty we got them out of the ship by fair means, but on the appearance of a musquet with a fixt baynet, they all then went into their Canoes very quickly: We were daily vis[i]ted by more or less, who brought us Fish in great plenty, for Nails, beads, and other triffles, and behaved very peaceably. I believe they don't stay long in any particular place or have any settled habitation but wander up and down in different Parties, particularly in the summer season, Sometimes laying in the Canoes and sometimes on shore, As there is a number of Hutts in every Cove you

[1] Altered by Cook to 'Tupia'.

[2] The passage 'that is . . . Anson' is deleted by Cook ; and he deletes the whole description of the New Zealanders given below from 'I believe . . .' to p. 740, l. 25, 'their own property'—no doubt as being superfluous. I print it here, however, as some indication of Furneaux's powers of observation.

meet with. Their Huts which at best are but very indifferent, but far superior to those of Van Dieman's Land; they are dry overhead and covered in a most curious manner; but so low you cannot stand upright; the Doors (which generally faces the Northward) are so small that you must crawl in on your hands, and knees. The Fire is near the door, and another in the inside; their bed places are raised about Six Inches above the Ground with dry rushes and Grass, and freathed[1] round of the same height. They are covered with Bark and then thatched with long grass or a kind of Flagg; Their Bread is the Fern root, this they roast and eat it as it is, and some Pound it with a stone on purpose, and form it into little Cakes which they bake on the embers; this, and fish, of which they have great variety, appears to be their chief food as we saw no kind of animals among them but a few Dogs, which they eat and convert the skins into cloathing for their children who adorn their matting at the Corners with tufts of hair. The manner they dress their food, is, they first dig a hole in the ground in which they make a fire and heat a number of stones, which then done are taken out together with the fire that the pit or oven is quite clear, on which they lay their fish or any other food wrapped up in green leaves, and put on the hot stones, and then they rake the coals over them and make more fire if necessary; this method does them quite clean and very good; they never take the guts out, as they prefer them to the Fish, they likewise spit them and place them round the Fire to roast, but this is done only when they are in a hurry. The men are in general stout and nervous,[2] the Women middle sized and round favoured; both Men & Women never stand up right owing to being so much in their Canoes or manner of sitting, they are of a dark copper colour, their hair strong and tied on the top of their head with a Comb or feather stuck in it. All the men that have distinguished themselves in war, are marked with spiral circles which is done by pricking or cuting the skin 'till it bleeds and rubbing the dye on the wounds, this mark continues for life and is called tattowing;[3] they likewise scratch the forehead with a sharp stone for that purpose,[4] after the death of a friend or parent, making a most lamentable noise. They are very fond of red paint and esteem it a great ornament. One of out gentlemen painted upwards of thirty of them one morning with vermilion, they gave him several things and insisted on him taking them. The Ladies go always painted with a dark greasy red of their own making out of Earth mixed with their oil, and have small pieces of it tied up in a piece of cloath round their necks in the manner of a Locket, and often smell to it;[5] their heads decorated with bunches of feathers of different

[1] 'Freath' is a Cornish (and other western county) variant of the dialectal 'frith', to intertwine, twist in and out; 'freathed' might here be rendered 'wattled' or 'woven'. Furneaux, we may remember, was a Cornishman.

[2] 'Nervous' in the eighteenth-century sense of sinewy, muscular.

[3] Tattooing was not a sign of distinction in war, though a distinguished man would generally be heavily tattooed.

[4] This practice and the consequent scars of course had nothing to do with tattooing.

[5] These 'sachets' were scented with gum from the Taramea (spear-grass), *Aciphylla* sp., or the tree called Tarata, *Pittosporum eugenioides*.

colours. Their necklaces of Paroquets' bills, birds bones or other such triffles, at which they hang several ornaments down their breast, they have holes in their ears, at which hangs bunches of human teeth preserved as relicts of a deceased friend, and are in great subjection to the men. Their Cloathing (both Men & women) is a kind of matt or cloth made of silk grass or fine flax, curiously wove and tied about the shoulder that reaches to their knees, it is interwoven with birds feathers of different colours, this they wear next their Skin and call it an *Ahow*,[1] and over it they have one of a coarser sort made of Grass well thrumbed with the same to keep out the wet which they call a Bugy Bugy.[2] They are all of them full of Vermin.[3] Their implements of War are the Hippatoo (or Spear),[4] Battle Ax,[5] patow & Patty patow[6] which is about two feet long and about eight inches wide made either of bone or stone, which they wear by their side and is the last they can use in fighting. They wear it by their side, and contrary to all other Indians they know not the use of Bows and Arrows; they likewise shewd us how they used their implements of war. At the first attack they use the Hippatoo, then to the battle Ax and at last the Patow, keeping all the while a most hideous noise. They shewd us how they disected the bodies as soon as they killed, which is generally by having their Sculls fractured; they cut their head, hands and feet off then open them and throw away their bowells, then cut them up and divide them among them. They are a bold, fearless race of beings, insensible of danger, are great thieves, will steal every thing they can lay their hands on, without being the least confused when caught, and will sometimes even dispute to return it as much as it was their own property. After we had settled the Astronomer with his Instruments and a sufficient guard on a small Island (that is joind to Motuara at low water) call'd the Hippa, where there was an old fortified town, that the Natives had forsaken; their houses served our people to live in, and when sunk about a foot inside made them very comfortable. We then struck our tents on the Motuara and removed the ship further into the Cove on the West shore and moored her for the Winter. We then erected our tents near the River or watering place; and sent ashore all the spars and Lumber off the Decks that they might be caulked and gave her a winter coat to preserve the Hull & Rigging On the 11th of May felt two severe shocks of an Earthquake but received no kind of Damage. On the 17th we were surprized by the People firing Guns on the Hippa, sent the boat, but as soon as she open'd the sound had the pleasure of seeing the Resolution off the

[1] *ahu*.

[2] *pakepake*, often made of undressed flax.

[3] Burney, Ferguson MS: 'many of them Thieves and cursed lousy'. But these qualities were not general, 'some being very cleanly and I believe honest'.

[4] I do not know how the name 'hippatoo' or 'hepatoo', frequently used by the English for a spear, was picked up. *He* (or *e*) *patu* would be a short club. There were various sorts of spear with distinctive names.

[5] The *tewhatewha*, not an axe at all, but a long club, the 'blade' of which was either purely ornamental or designed to give added weight to the blow.

[6] *patu* and *patupatu*.

mouth of the sound. We immediately sent out the boats to her assistance to tow her in it being calm In the evening she anchored about a mile without us, and next morning weighed and warped within us. Both Ships felt an uncommon joy at our meeting after an absence of fourteen Weeks. . . . We left here two Goats a Boar and two Sows. We made a large Garden in the Cove where the watering place was and inclosed it in with a Freath,[1] in which we sowed all sorts of Garden seeds, and cut several good sallads before we came away and left it in a very promising way. We likewise made several Gardens on the Islands and Coves where we transplanted several hundreds of Cabbages. It is remarkable we never saw the least sign of any animal but Rats, of which there is great numbers. On the arrival of the Resolution we prepared the Ship for Sea with all expedition; the Natives visited us after this in great numbers and were much surprized at the sight of another ship larger than they had seen before.

We had the Ship ready for Sea by the first of June, but staid 'till the 7th at which in the morning we sailed in company with the Resolution, directing our Course to the Eastern mouth of the Streights. . . . After we had cleared the Streights we directed our Course to the ESE, but being the winter season had very uncertain weather and were much baffled by the wind and Sea, cold and hard gales from the Eastward; however, we persevered in our Course keeping between the Latitude of 47° and 43° South, till we had made Fifty degrees of Longitude from New Zealand. We found a very hollow Sea from the Eastern quarter, so I believe there is no Land in that quarter before you reach the main Land of America, as we were not 200 Leagues to the Westward of former Voyages. . . .

After a passage of fourteen days from Amsterdam[2] we made the coast of New Zealand near the Table Cape and stood alongshore till we came as far as Cape Turnagain, at which time the wind began to blow strong at West with heavy squalls and rain, which split many of our sails[3] and blew us off the coast for three days in which time we parted company with the Resolution and never saw her afterwards. On the 4th November we again got in shore near Cape Pallisser and was visited by a number of the Natives in their Canoes with a great quantity of Cray fish, which we bought of them for nails and Otaheite Cloath; the next day it blew hard from WNW which again blew us off the Coast and obliged us to bring to for two days, during which time it blew one continual gale of wind with very heavy squalls of sleet, by this time our Decks were very leaky, the peoples beds and bedding wet, several of our people complaining of Colds, that we began to dispair of ever geting into Charlotte's Sound or joining

[1] A wattled fence; cf. p. 739, n. 1 above.

[2] 'from Amsterdam' added by Cook to make the sense clear after a large deletion.

[3] Kemp writes, 3 November, 'N.B. The ship in very bad trim, I imagine from her being so light, as also the rigging and sails in bad order, from the frequent Gales we have had'; and again, 6 November, 'the ship, rigging and sails in bad order, as also short of Water'.

the Resolution,[1] on the 6th of November we being to the North of the Cape, the wind at SW and blowing strong bore away for some bay to compleat our water & wood being in great want of both, having been at the allowance of one quart of water for some days past and not above six or seven days to be come at. We anchored in Tolaga Bay on the 9th in Latitude 38°21′ South, Longitude 178°37′ E It affords good riding with the wind westerly and regular soundings from 11 to five fathoms, stiff muddy ground across the bay for about two miles. It is open from NNE to ESE. It is to be observed Easterly winds seldom blows hard on this shore, but when it does throws in a great sea, that if it was not for a great undertow together with a large River that empties itself in the bottom of the bay a ship would not be able to ride here. Wood and water is easily to be had except when it blows hard easterly, The natives here are the same as those of Charlottes Sound, but more numerous and seemed settled, having regular Plantations of Sweet Potatoes and other roots which are very good; they have plenty of Cray and other Fish which we bought of them for Nails Beads and other triffles at an easy rate.[2] In one of their Canoes we observed the head of a woman Lying in State adorned with Feathers and other ornaments, which had the appearance of being alive, but on examination found it dry and preserved with every feature perfect, and kept as the Relict of some deceased relation. We got about Ten Tons of Water and some wood; and sailed for Charlotte's Sound on 12th. We were no sooner out than the wind began to blow hard dead on the shore that we could not clear the Land on either Tack which obliged us to bear away again for the Bay were we anchored the next morning and rode out a very heavy gale of wind at Ebs which threw in a very great sea, We now began to fear we should never join the Resolution, who we had reason to believe was in Charlotte's Sound and by this time was ready for Sea; we

[1] After losing the *Resolution* finally Burney (Ferguson MS) writes, 'Our Ship in her best trim is not able to keep up, or carry sail with the Resolution, at this time we fall bodily to Leeward being quite Light & so crank that we are obliged to strike to every Squall, and so unmanageable that there is no getting her round either one way or another, on the Morning of the 5th of November being near Cape Pallisser the Wind shifted Suddenly from the NW to the SSW & blew very strong—we had 3 Tryals & were full ¾ of an hour before we could get her head off shore—had she faild the 3d Time we should have cut away our Mizen Mast—the Night of the 5th had a tolerable good chance being to the SE of Cape Pallisser Wind at South, but it being doubtfull whether we should be able to weather the Land (the wind increasing and Night coming on) the Captn did not think it Safe to trust the Ship on a Lee shore. . . . from our being so often baffled in trying to get round Cape Pallisser our Seamen now Christend it, by the significant name of Cape Turn and be damned'. Bayly writes, 7–8 November, 'NB The Wind blew very strong with a mountanious sea with thick hazy weather, the Capt came down off the deck very much terrified to appearance, & said he knew not what to do'. Two lines are drawn through this, whether to score them out as a scandalous aspersion on Furneaux or not is hard to tell.

[2] '. . . were very near having a quarrel with the Natives ashore about a Gallon Cagg of Brandy which they stole—& which I had sent for from the ship for the use of the Wooders & Waterers—Jack Row [*sic*] would fain have had me seizd one or two of the Zealanders & kept them in our Boat till the Liquor was restored—this I thought dangerous as the Zealanders were too numerous—and all our Empty casks ashore—if Sailors won't take care of their Grogg, they deserve to lose it.'—Burney, Ferguson MS.

soon found it was with great difficulty we could get any water, owing to the swell setting in so strong; at last, however, we were able to go onshore and got both wood and water: Whilst we lay here we were employed about the rigging which was much damaged by the constant gales of wind we met with since we made the coast. We got the Booms down on the decks and made the ship as snug as possible and sailed again on the 16th. After this we met with several gales of wind off the mouth of the streights and continued beating backwards and forwards till the 30th of November when we were so fortunate as to get a favourable wind, which we took every advantage of and at last got safe into our desired Port. We saw nothing of the Resolution and began to doubt her safety, but on going onshore we saw the place where she had erected her Tents, and on an old stump of a tree in the garden found the following words cut out 'Look underneath' where we dug and soon found a Bottle corked and waxed down, with a Letter in it from Captain Cook signifying their arrival on the 3[d] Instant and Departure on the 24th, that they intended spending a few days in the enterance of the Streights to see[k] for us; we immediately set about getting the Ship ready for Sea as fast as possible; erected our Tents and Sent the Cooper onshore to repair the Cask, and began to unstow the Hold and to get at the Bread that was in Butts; but on opening them found a great quantity of it intirely spoiled, and most part so damaged that we were obliged to fix our Copper Oven onshore to bake it over again, which undoubtedly delayed us a considerable time; whilst we lay here the inhabitants came onboard as before, and supplied us with fish and other things of their own manufature, which we bought of them for nails &c[a] and appeared very friendly; but they twice in the middle of the night came to the tent with an intention to steal but were discovered before they cou'd get anything in their possession.[1] On the 17th of December, having refitted the ship, compleated our water and wood and got every thing ready for sea, We sent our large Cutter with M[r] Rowe, a midshipman and the Boats crew, to gather wild greens for the Ship's Company with orders to return that evening, as I intended to sail the next morning, but on the Boats not returning the same evening nor the next morning, was under great uneasiness about her, hoisted out the Launch & sent her with the 2[d] Lieu[t2] mann'd with the Boats Crew and Ten Marines in search of

[1] '. . . in the Night some Indians by the Negligence of the Centinel, got to the Tent & took every thing they could lay their hands on to a Canoe which lay among the Rocks—but by being too greedy they were at last discoverd after having made several successful trips & almost compleated their Cargo; they were fired at, but escaped to the woods—one of them must have been wounded as we saw drops of blood along the beach—we found the Canoe well loaded & every thing that was missing except a Shirt & blanket—this is not their first attempt, they came one night last week with 3 Canoes but finding us on our Guard thought proper to retire—we were then so mild as only to fire one Musket over their heads.'—Burney log, 15 December. The same for 17 December: '. . . this forenoon Some Indians came to the Tent & had the impudence to ask for their Canoe, which (as we proposed Sailing next Morning,) we let them have. this forenoon Struck the Tent & got every thing on board'. Bayly's detailed account of these pilfering natives and his own adventures is printed in *Hist.Rec.N.Z.*, II, pp. 214–6.

[2] Cook here inserts 'M[r] Burney'.

her, who returned about 7[1] O'Clock the same night with the melancholy news of her being cut off by the Indians in Grass Cove where they found the Relicks of several and the intrails of five men lying on the beach and in the Canoes they found several baskets of human flesh and five odd shoes new, as our people had been served Shoes a day or two before; they brought onboard several hands, two of which we knew, one belonged to Thomas Hill being marked on the Back T.H. another to Mr Rowe who had a wound on his fore finger not quite whole, and the Head, which was supposed was the head of my servant by the high forhead he being a Negroe, the Launch fired on them where they were assembled in great numbers on the top of a hill making all the signs of joy imaginable. Next morning unmoored & weighed and stood out into the stream and anchored again the wind being unfair; we lay here three days but saw none of the inhabitants; what is very remarkable I have been several times up in the same cove with Captain Cook & never saw the least sign of an inhabitant, tho' there was several old deserted towns which appear'd as if they had not been occupied for several years, and by the report given by the 2d Lieut and boats Crew at their return that there could not be less than 1500 or 2,000 when they came into the bay and I doubt not had they been aprized of our boats coming whether they would not have atacked her, so thought it imprudent to send her up again as we were convinced there was not the least probability of any of them being alive. On the 23d of December weighed and made sail out of the cove[2] and stood to the Eastward to get clear of the streights which we cleared[3] the same evening but were baffled for two or three days with light winds before we could clear the Coast. We then stood to the SSE 'till we got into the Latitude of 56° South without any thing remarkable happening; found a great swell from the Southward: at this time the winds began to Blow strong from the SW and began to be very cold and as the Ship was low and deep loaden the sea made a continual breach over her which kept us always wet and by her straining very few of the people were dry in bed or on deck having no shelter to keep the sea from them. The Birds were the only companions we had in this vast ocean, except now and then we saw a Whale or Porpoise and now and then a seal or two and a few Penguins. In Latitude 58° South, Long. 213° East fell in with some Ice and every day saw more or less, we then standing to the East; we found a very strong current seting to the Eastward for by the time we were abreast of Cape Horn, being in the Latitude of 61° South, the Ship was ahead of our Account eight degrees, we were very little more than a Month from Cape Pallisser (New Zealand) to Cape Horn which is 121 degrees of Longitude, and had continual Westerly winds from SW to NW with a great sea following.[4] On opening some

[1] Altered by Cook to '11'. Burney says 'between 11 and 12'.

[2] Altered by Cook to 'Sound'.

[3] Altered by Cook to 'accomplished'—perhaps because the phrase 'got clear' had already been used a few words earlier, and 'clear' is repeated in the next line.

[4] 'Was very thick & foggy so that we could not see a quarter of a mile ahead—Notwithstanding we stand on at the rate of 5½ Knots tho' the officers are well convinced we

Casks of Pease and Flour that had been stowed on the Coals, found them very much damaged and not eatable so thought it most prudent to stand for the Cape of Good Hope but first to stand into the Latitude and Longitude of Cape Circumscision. After being to the Eastward of Cape Horn found the winds did not blow so strong from the Westward as usual, the wind coming more from the North, which brought on thick ffoggy weather, that for several days together we could not be able to get an observation nor see the least sign of the Sun, this weather last above a month, being then amongst a great many Islands of Ice, which made us be constantly on the look-out for fear of runing foul of them, and being a single Ship made us more attentive. By this time our people began to complain of colds and pains in their limbs[1] which obliged me to haul to the Northward to the Latitude of 54° South, but still the same sort of weather, tho' we had oftener an opportunity of Observations for the Lat^de^ but still if possible to see if there was Land in the place laid down by Bovet, tho' not the least sign of Land as we sailed along yet[2] The Islands of Ice became now more numerous and dangerous, they being much smaller than they used to be, and the nights began to be dark. On the 3^d^ of March being then in the Lat^d^ 54° 04′ South & Longitude 13° East which is the Latitude of the spot[3] & half a degree to the Eastward of it and not seeing the least sign of Land[4] hauled away to the Northward, as our last tract[5] to the Southward was within a few degrees of it, and was in the Longitude of it and about three or four degrees to the Southward; Should there be any Land thereabout it must be a very inconsiderable Island but believe it was nothing but Ice, as we in our first setting out thought we had seen Land several times but proved to [be] high Islands of Ice aback of the large Fields, and as it was thick foggy weather when M Bovet fell in with it, might be very easily taken for Land.

[Furneaux made the land at the Cape on 17 March 1774, and anchored in Table Bay two days later. He stayed there refitting and refreshing until 16 April, when he sailed for England; and anchored at Spithead on 14 July.]

must go to destruction in case any Land should be in our way, as our Ship will not make her course good within 8 Points of the Wind when the Sea is but little agitated.—This has been their method of proceeding ever since we left Zealand, & even when going right before a heavy gale of wind, accompanied with a very mountanious Sea & not knowing how soon we might fall on some Shore.—! *most extraordinary* infatuation.'—Bayly, 26 January.

[1] Cf. Kemp, 16 February: 'The People Continue very healthy, tho' I much fear the continuance of Foggy Wea^r^ and bad Air will cause a change'.—4 March: 'People growing sickly'.

[2] 'but still . . . yet': Cook alters this passage to read, 'but still we continued to have the same sort of weather, though we had oftener an opportunity of geting Observations for the Lat^de^. After geting into the Latitude above mentioned I steered to the East in order, if possible, to find the Land. As we advanced to the East'. . . .

[3] 'the spot' altered by Cook to 'Bouvets discovery'.

[4] Cook inserts here, 'either now or sence we have been in this Parall. I gave over looking for it and'.

[5] i.e. track.

2. Burney's Log

[*P.R.O. Adm 51/4523. Two extracts are here given, the first describing Burney's own landing on the south coast of Tasmania or Van Diemen's Land, and Adventure Bay; the second being his report to Furneaux on the massacre at Grass Cove. The latter has been collated with the copy in his hand in the Alexander Turnbull Library.*]

[VAN DIEMEN'S LAND]

Wednesday March 10th 1773. Little Wind & hazy—at 2 pm hoisted out the Small Cutter and Sent her in Shore—½ an hour after a Fresh Breeze Springing up Fird a gun for her to return—hoisted her in—at 5 & 6 Sounded, 47 fm Coral & Broken Shells, Vartn pr Azth 7..02 E at 8 were abrest the Mewstone it bearing S distance 2 miles. The SW Cape WBN½N had Soundings all the 1st Watch. between 50 & 60 fms fine Brown Sand & broken Shells—at 3 AM it fell Calm—at 4 a Light Breeze Sprung up from the NE with fine clear Weather—at 5 Tackd and Stood in Shore. at 6 The Mewstone W½S 4 or 5 Leagues—Etermost Land in Sight NE. this point we calld the SE Cape—it lays ENE & WSW pr Compass from the Mewstone—Saw a Small Island bearing E¾S distt about 11 Leagues—Variation this Morning pr Ampd 7..13 E—pr Azth 7..01 E at ½ past 6 we passd a fine deep Bay[1] with Several Islands in it—there are 2 pretty high peaks just to the Eastward of it—at 9 The Large Cutter was hoisted out & I was sent in her to see if I could find any fresh water we row'd in Shore a little to the Eastward of the Bay just mention'd. We Observd the Land seemd to part which made me conjecture there was a fresh Water River there—I would gladly have gone to have Seen but it was too far from the Ship—by 11 we got in a Small Bay[2] where we Saw a Sandy Beach but could not Land there for the Surf—however we found a good Landing place on some Rocks. The first thing we Saw when we climbd up was Some Wood Ashes the remains of a Fire which had been kindled there & a great Number of Scollop Shells—We saw none of the Inhabitants—there was a path leading through the Woods which would probably have led us to some of their Huts—but we could not stay to walk up the Wind coming too fresh Obligd us to think of getting on board again—we brought off Several Boughs of Trees—Some Shells & Some of the Burnt Wood—at the Entrance of the Bay on the East Side we saw a fall of Water among the Rocks but did not think it safe for the Boat to go there—at ¾ past 12 we got safe on board—by this time it blew a Fresh gale of Wind from the WSW which had obligd the Ship to Close Reef ye Topsails & hand the Mzn Topsail—The Shore Seems every where to be very Bold—affording plenty of good harbours & Bays all along the Coast. The Land is every Where coverd with Trees making one continued Wood—I allow more Distance this 24 hours than the Log gives for a Swell from the Westward which has set us along shore Latde pr Acct at Noon 43..38 S Longde in 146..56 East—The SE Cape ENE distt about 2 Leagues.

[1] Cox Bight. [2] Louisa Bay.

Thursday March 11th 1773. Fresh Gales and hazy—hoisted the Boat in & Bore away—at ½ past 1 were abrest the SE Cape which makes the SW point of Storm Bay. at 3 Out 3d Reef Main Topsail—[5 p.m.] abrest of Tasman's Head. there are Several Rocks & Small Islds close to it which we nam'd the Fryars—[7 p.m.] Anchord in the Skirts of a fine Bay with the Small Bower in 24 fm—Soft Sand and mud—Many on board Supose this to be Frederick Henry's Bay but from Several Circumstances I am perswaded to the contrary Tasman lays down Frederick Henry's Bay in 43..10 S Latde 9 Leagues Distant in a direct Line from the NE point of Storm Bay & makes it 9 or 10 Leagues deep from the Entrance—The Bay we were in is in 43..20 S only 3 Leagues from Tasmans head & is not quite 3 miles from the Entrance to the bottom of the Bay—Tasman in his Chart has laid down a Small nook or Inlet to the Southward of Frederick Henry's Bay[1] which exactly corresponds with this, & which we calld Adventure Bay. at Day light hoisted out all the Boats & Sent the 2 Cutters in Shore to Sound & look for a watering place at 10 weighd with a light breeze from the WNW & began to Work up the Bay. Little Wind and fair Weather.

Friday March 12th. Light Airs from the Westward with fair Weather—Employd Working into the Bay—at 5 pm Carried out a Kedge Anchor & 3 Hawsers to warp farther in—at 6 Anchord with the Small Bower in 11 fms & Moord with the Coasting Anchor to the Northward—Early in the Morning Sent the Cutter & Launch with a party of Marines to guard them, for Wood & Water to the South Part of the Bay—found the Water very brackish.

Saturday 13th. Modt Breezes from the NW with Cloudy weather & rain in the Night—this Afternoon found another Watering place the Water something better—Started what we got before—Employd wooding & Watering & overhauling the Rigging—carried the Sean ashore & hauld it—caught a few fish, not above 2 Buckets full.

Sunday 14th. The Winds Variable with Cloudy Weather—AM found another Watering Place with excellent Water on the West Side of the Bay—it lays nearly WBS from a Small Island by the South point of the Bay—this Island we calld Penguin Island from our catching one of those Birds there.

Remarks in Adventure Bay

The whole time we Staid here we did not get a Sight of any of the Inhabitants, though they were so near us that we Saw Fires continually on the North Side of the Bay where the Land is lower & not so much overrun with Trees and Underwood as the part we lay in—

We found several of their Huts—& large Old Hollow Trees in which they had liv'd—there were paths which led along the Woods, but almost overgrown with Bushes. The place did not seem to have been inhabited for some months before, so that it was not our coming frightend them

[1] Possibly this 'Small nook or inlet' was the present Marion Bay.

away—it is most likely the Natives never stay long in one place but lead a wandring life, travelling along the Coast from Bay to Bay to catch fish, which by the great quantities of shells we Saw, must make the chief part of their food—Their Huts are very low and ill contrivd, & seem only intended for Temporary habitations: they had left nothing in them but 2 or 3 Old baskets or bags made of a very strong grass—, Some flint & tinder which I believe they make of the bark of a Tree, & a great number of pearl Scollop, Mussel, Lobster & Cray fish Shells which they had roasted.

This Land is situated in a fine temperate & healthy Climate—the Country is exceeding pleasant, but it is almost impossible to penetrate into it on account of the Woods. here are some small snakes, one of which we caught, & a great Number of very large Ants about an Inch & a half long —they bite very sharp & are exceeding troublesome[1]—The Trees are mostly Evergreens, standing very thick and close together—many of the Small ones bore berries of a spicy flavour—the larger ones are in general quite Strait & Shoot up very high before they branch out. they are large enough for Masts for any Ship in the Navy, but are rather brittle and heavy —they have a Soft thick bark which many of them had been strippd of by the Natives—the Wood is of a reddish cast & has a great deal of gum in it—at the back of some of the Sandy beaches are Small Lagoons or Lakes with good Store of Trout, Carp,[2] & other Fish—here is likewise plenty of wild fowl & game but so Shy that I imagine the Natives have some method of catching them— We Shot some Wild Ducks, Crows, Parroquets, a White Eagle & some Small birds. The Eagle was one of the Noblest Birds I ever Saw—we found several tracks of wild Beasts, & the dung of Some which we took to be of the Deer kind—one of our gentlemen Shot a Possown [*sic*], about the Size of a Cat—this was the only Animal we Saw here —from the Tops of the Hills I could see water beyond the Low Land at the North part of the Bay—but whether this has communication with the Sea, or is only a Lagoon we could not determine.[3] if the former it must doubtless be the Bay of Frederick Henry—We Saw the Land again beyond the Water—it seems to be a fine Country to the Northward & by the many fires we saw there, must be well inhabited—we left behind us a small Cask, several Medals tied to the Trees & many other things of little Value—it is very remarkable that no European as we know of, has ever seen an Inhabitant of Van diemen's Land, though it is above 130 Years Since it was first discoverd.[4]

[1] Ferguson MS 'bite most confoundedly'. This formidable ant was probably *Myrmecia forficata* (Fabricius); it is the largest Tasmanian species and stings severely. Specimens over an inch in length are frequently found; and it is common in areas near Adventure Bay. The popular name is 'Inchman'.

[2] This fish seems impossible to identify. The introduced European Carp is found in Tasmania today, but that casts no light on 1773.

[3] The low land was the narrow isthmus that joins the two parts of Bruni Island and separates D'Entrecasteaux Channel from Adventure Bay; the water that Burney saw was Isthmus Bay, on the east side of D'Entrecasteaux Channel.

[4] Marion and his men had seen them, and come into conflict with them, just a year earlier, in March 1772.

The Tide rises here not more than 3 or 4 foot perpendicular the Current or Sett of it is scarcely perceptible, for the Ship always tended to the Wind though ever so little of it—it was 2 days after the full Moon when we came in, so that the Tides were then at the highest. . . .
Monday March 15th 1773. Variable Winds. the Weather Cloudy with Small rain in the first part. Latter fair—PM Compleated our Wood and Water. at Day light hoisted the Launch in, Unmoord & hove in to $\frac{1}{3}$ of the Coasting Cable—at $\frac{1}{2}$ past 9 Weighd with a light breeze from the NW & made Sail out of the Harbour. hoisted the Boats in & Securd the Anchors. Stood away East to go to the Southward of Marias' Islands—had a very good Observation of the ☉ & ☽'s Distce at 11 o'clock—being then 1 mile due North from Penguin Rock At Noon Penguin Rock bore WBS$\frac{3}{4}$S about 5 miles. Tasman's Head SSW & the Southermost of Maria's Islands EBN$\frac{3}{4}$N—Latde Obsd 43..19 S.

[THE MASSACRE AT GRASS COVE]

Saturday December 18th 1773. This morning, I was orderd in the Launch (she being well man'd & armd) to go in quest of the Cutter. My instructions were first to look well into East Bay & then proceed to Grass Cove[1] (the place where Mr Rowe was order'd) & if I heard nothing of the Boat there to go further up the Sound & come down along the West Shore. As Mr Rowe had left the Ship an hour earlier than the time proposed, & in a great hurry, I was strongly perswaded his Curiosity had carried him into East Bay, none in our Ship having ever been there before, or else Some accident had happen'd to the Boat; either gone adrift through the Boatkeepers Negligence, or been stove among the Rocks—this was almost every body's opinion, & on this Suposition the Carpenters Mate was sent with me with some sheets of Tin. I had not the least suspicion of their having receivd any injury from the Natives, our boats having frequently been higher up & worse provided. About 10 we left the Ship—having a light breeze in our favour we soon got round Long Island & within Long Point.[2] I rounded every Cove on the Larboard Hand as we went along, looking well all round with a Spy Glass which I took for that purpose—at $\frac{1}{2}$ past 1 We Stoppd at a beach on the left hand side going up East Bay, to boil some Victuals, as we brought nothing with us but raw meat—while we were cooking I saw an Indian on the Opposite Shore running along a beach up towards the head of the Bay. Our Victuals being drest, we got it in the boat & put off—& in a Short time got to the head of this Reach[3] where we saw an Indian Settlement—as we drew near Some of the Indians came down on the Rocks & waved for us to begone, but seeing we disregarded them, they alterd their Notes—here we found 6 large Canoes

[1] The present Whareunga Bay, outside East Bay and facing between Pickersgill and Blumine islands. Chart XVII will sufficiently illustrate this story.

[2] Another of Cook's names from the first voyage that has not survived; now called Clark Point.

[3] 'Reach' here, I think, in the sense of a distance sailed on one tack: Burney crossed the bay diagonally to a beach farther up on its other side.

hauld up on the Beach—most of them double ones—a great many people but not so many as one might expect from the Number of houses & Size of the Canoes. leaving the Boats Crew to guard the Boat, I stept on shore with the Marines (the Corporal & 5 men) & searchd a good many of their houses, but found nothing to give me any Suspicion—3 or 4 well beaten paths led further into the Woods, where were many more houses—but the people continuing very friendly I thought it unnecessary to continue our search—coming down to the Boat, one of the Indians had brought a bundle of Hepatoos (long Spears) down to the beach—but seeing I lookd very earnestly at him, he put them on the ground & walkd about with seeming unconcern. Some of the people appearing to be frightend I gave a Looking Glass to one & a large Nail to another—from this place the Bay ran as nearly as I could guess NNW a good mile where it Ended in a long sandy beach[1]—I lookd all round with the glass but saw no boat, Canoe or Sign of Inhabitants—I therefore contented myself with firing some Guns which I did in every Cove as I went along. I now kept close to the East Shore & came to another Settlement where the Indians invited us ashore. I enquired of them about the Boat, to which they pretended ignorance—they appeard very friendly here & sold us some fish—within an hour after we left this place, in a small beach adjoining to Grass Cove[2] we saw a very large double canoe just hauld up, with 2 men & a Dog—the men on seeing us left their Canoe & ran up into the woods—this gave me reason to Suspect I should here get some tidings of our Cutter—we went ashore & Searchd the Canoe where we found one of the Rullock ports[3] of the Cutter & some Shoes one of which was known to belong to M[r] Woodhouse, one of our Midshipmen, who went with M[r] Rowe— one of the people at the same time brought me a piece of meat, which he took to be some of the Salt Meat belonging to the Cutter's Crew—on examining this & smelling to it I found it was fresh meat—M[r] Fannin, (the Master) who was with me, supos'd it was Dog's flesh & I was of the same opinion, for I still doubted their being Cannibals: but we were Soon convinced by most horrid & undeniable proofs—a great many baskets (about 20) laying on the beach tied up, we cut them open, some were full of roasted flesh & some of fern root which serves them for bread—on further search we found more shoes & a hand which we immediately knew to have belong'd to Tho[s] Hill one of our Forecastlemen, it being markd T.H. which he had got done at Otaheite with a tattow instrument —I went with some of the people a little way up the woods, but saw nothing else—coming down again was a round spot cover'd with fresh earth, about 4 feet diameter, where Something had been buried:[4] having no

[1] Ruapara Bay.

[2] This beach has no name, but the chart shows it clearly. Burney had now emerged from East Bay, turning the corner, as it were, inside Pickersgill island.

[3] Rowlock ports, ports in the gunwale serving as rowlocks. Burney may have found a length of gunwale including a rowlock port or perhaps the filling piece (today called a poppet) inserted in the port while sailing and attached by a string to the gunwale.

[4] Presumably the *hangi* or *umu*, the 'earth-oven' where the bodies had been cooked.

spade we began to dig with a Cutlass—in the mean time I launchd the Canoe with an intention to destroy her—but seeing a great smoke ascending over the nearest hill, I got all the people in the boat & made what haste I could to be with them before Sunsett—on opening the next bay, which was Grass Cove, we saw 4 Canoes—a Single, & 3 double ones—a great many People on the beach—a large fire was on the top of the High Land beyond the woods, from whence all the way down the Hill the place was throngd like a Fair—those who were near the Shore had retreated to a small hill within a Ships length of the Water side, where they stood talking to us—as we came in I order'd a Musquetoon to be fired through one of the Canoes, as we suspected they might be full of men laying down in the bottom, but nobody was in them—the Savages on the little hill still kept hollowing & making Signs for us to come ashore—however as soon as we had got close in we all fired—the first Volley did not seem to affect them much—but on the 2[d] they began to scramble away as fast as they could, some of them howling—we continued firing as long as we could see the least glimpse of a man through the bushes—amongst the Indians were 2 very stout men who never offer'd to move till they found themselves forsaken by their companions & then they walkd away with great composure & deliberation—their pride not Suffering them to run—one of them however stumbled, & just made Shift to crawl off on all fours—the other got clear without any apparent hurt—I then landed with the Marines & left M[r] Fannin to guard the boat—on the beach were 2 bundles of Cellery which had been gather'd for loading the Cutter—a plain proof that the attack was made here—a broken piece of an Oar was stuck upright in the Ground to which they had tied their Canoes—I then searchd all along at the back of the beach to see if the Cutter was there—we found no boat—but instead of her—Such a shocking scene of Carnage & Barbarity as can never be mentiond or thought of, but with horror.—whilst we remained almost stupified on this spot M[r] Fannin call'd to us that he heard the Savages gathering together in the Valley, on which I returned to the Boat & hauld alongside the Canoes, 3 of which we demolished—whilst this was transacting, the fire on the top of the High Land disappeard & the Indians had gatherd together in the wood, where we heard them at very high words, doubtless quarelling whether or no they should come to attack us & try to save their Canoes—it now grew dark. I therefore just stept out & lookd once more along the back of the beach to see if the Cutter had been hauld up in the bushes—but seeing nothing of her returned & put off—our whole force would have been but barely sufficient to have gone up the Hill, & to have ventured with half (for one half must have been left to guard the Boat) would have been madness—As we open'd the upper part of the Sound we saw a very large fire about 3 or 4 miles higher up—this fire formd a complete Oval, reaching from the top of a hill down to the water Side—the middle space being inclosed all round by the fire, like a hedge—I consulted with M[r] Fannin & we were both of Opinion that we could expect to reap no other advantage than the poor Satisfaction of killing some of the Savages—at leaving Grass Cove we had fired a general Volley towards where we heard the Indians talking—but by going in & out of the boat the Arms had got wet & some 4[1] of the pieces mist fire—what was still worse it began to rain—our ammunition was more than half expended & we left 6 Large Canoes behind us in one place—I therefore did not think it worth while to proceed where nothing could be hoped for but revenge.

Coming between 2 round Islands that lay to the Southward of East Bay[2] we imagined we heard somebody calling—we lay on our Oars & listened but heard no more of it—we hollowd several times but to little purpose the poor Souls were far enough out of hearing—& indeed I think it some comfort to reflect that in all probability every man of them must have been killd on the Spot. We got on board between 11 & 12—

The people lost in the Cutter were Mr Rowe, Mr Woodhouse, Francis Murphy Quartermaster, Wm Facey. Thos Hill. Edwd Jones, Michael Bell, Jno Cavenaugh Thos Milton & James Swilley the Capt^ns^ Man—4 of them belongd to the Forecastle & 2 to the After guard[3]—being 10 in all—most of these were of our very best Seamen—the Stoutest & most healthy people in the Ship—We brought on board 2 Hands—one belonging to Mr Rowe, known by a hurt he had received in it the other to Thomas Hill as beforementiond, & the head of the Capt^ns^ Servant—these with more of the remains were tied in a Hammock & thrown overboard with ballast & Shot sufficient to sink it—we found none of their Arms or Cloaths except part of a pair of Trowsers, a Frock & 6 shoes—no 2 of them being fellows—

I am not inclined to think this was any premeditated plan of these Savages, as the morning Mr Rowe left the Ship he met 2 Canoes who came down & staid all the forenoon in Ship Cove. It might probably happen from Some quarrel,[4] or the fairness of the Opportunity tempted them; our people being so very incautious & thinking themselves to Secure[5]—another thing which encouraged the Zealanders was, they were sensible a Gun was not infallible. that they sometimes mist & that when discharged they must be loaded again,[6] which time they knew how to take advantage of. after their Success I imagine was a general meeting on the East Side of the Sound—the Indians of Shag Cove[7] were there—this we knew by a Cock which was in one of the Canoes, & by a long Single Canoe which I had seen 4 days before in Shag Cove where I had been with Mr Rowe in the Cutter.

[1] In the MS '4' is written interlineally above 'some'.
[2] Pickersgill and Blumine—but neither of them is round.
[3] From the wording in the Turnbull MS we learn that Cavenagh and Milton belonged to the afterguard, the others being the forecastle-men.
[4] The Turnbull MS adds, 'which was decided on the spot'.
[5] 'Mr Rowe had been accustomed to Indians in America for many Years having been in America the greatest part of his time, & put too great confidence in them, for had he been more doubtfull of them he might have Saved his Life & that of his Crew.'—Bayly, 18 December.
[6] 'loaded again': Turnbull MS 'loaded before they could be used again'.
[7] Now Resolution Bay.

3. Clerke's Log

[*P.R.O. Adm 55/103, 'A Log of the Proceedings of, and Occurrences onboard His Majesty's Ship, Resolution Upon a Voyage of discovery towards the South Pole by Cᵗ Clerke'. I print here, first, the statement Clerke prefixes to his journal on his principles of observation and recording; secondly, a selection of his general remarks on places and people; and thirdly, his independent reflections on icebergs and their relation to a southern continent. Headings in square brackets I have supplied; the others are Clerke's own. The 'accounts' come in every case at the close of his daily entries describing incidents at the place visited. I have excised most of the figures he gives so regularly for latitude, longitude and variation; but have been as sparing as possible in altering his punctuation. One or two palpable slips have been silently corrected.*]

[THE EXPLORER'S RATIONALE]

I think its necessary to give some explanation of the contents of this Log to elucidate some matters and give my reasons for introducing others, least they are thought too trivial to have a place in a book of this kind— in the first place every procedure and incident at all relative to the Vessel has been most carefully attended to—the settings of the Sea or Swell I think a very necessary nautical remark as they immediately bespeak a clear Sea for some distance from whatever quarter of the Compass this Sea or Swell proceeds, besides which, an attention to the effect of it must be paid in the correcting of the Course and distance for the day and determining the Ships place, for without this attention, the Log Account wou'd be found much more defective than it is at present.—An account of the various Fowls, Animals &c I think likewise a matter very worthy of observation, particularly those which are suppos'd not to go any great distance from Land—this has ever been said of Penguins—little Divers—Cape Hens and Seals, all of which we've seen at a great distance from any known Land; nor cou'd we find any at all near them—as to the Cape Hens I put totally out of the question, as they doubtlessly are a species of Peterel and of course great aquatic travellers; but in respect to the Penguins, Little Divers and Seals tho' I must confess it a good deal staggers the System, it by no means abolishes it—for tho' we've seen of these Birds and Animals where we cou'd not find Land, and have no reason to conclude there was any; yet we've never discover'd Land but the appearance of these Creatures have intimated our approach to it sometime before we've seen it. The meeting with the White or Snow Peterel is an undoubted sign of being near large quantities of Ice—the Antartick Peterel is only to be seen within, or very near the boundaries of the Polar Circle—these much for the high Latitudes which is the Clime of the Birds and Animals here treated of. When in low Latitudes within or about the Tropics, the Men of War and Egg Birds are the Fowl of intelligence; a few scatter'd ones may be sometimes seen flying at random, but wherever numbers are together, I think its an undoubted sign of being in the neighbourhood of some Isle—wherever you see Land here, there's abundance of these kind of birds and I believe they never travel to any great distance from it, particularly the Egg Bird

—in respect to Seaweed, tho' we meet with it almost throughout the Ocean, I think where large quantities of it makes its appearance, 'tis an Omen not to be wholly neglected— for from the quantities of it and number of Birds above mention'd we fell in with, when cruizing for the Frenchmans Land to the Southward of the Mauritias; I'm firmly of opinion the report they propagated at the Cape of Good Hope is not without some foundation, tho' Monsieur might not chuse to give, or probably has been somewhat mistaken in, the true situation of his new Country.—for these various reasons I think the remarks of the Swell and Fowl are by no means to be neglected as they evidently do give some degree of illustration into matters of discovery.

In the next place this Log Book contains all the Astronomic Observations I've made in the Course of the Voyage. As their Lordships thought proper to signify to us through the Channel of Captain Cook, that they wou'd much approve of our attention to the Longitude by the Lunar System, I took care to equip myself with every essential to act consistently with their Lordships Pleasure, and I flatter myself the result of my endeavours in this particular will prove, that the lands we've met with wou'd have been far from being ill settled, or the Vessels track ill determin'd, had any accident happen'd to our profess'd Astronomer, or in short had there been none onboard her. I've enter'd all my Observations at full length, just as I read them off the Quadrants, to which I've annex'd the errors of those Quadrants—I've taken this method to give a clear and fair Hypothesis, that any Gentleman who may choose to give himself the trouble—having the same foundation for his work as myself, may easily prove if the results of my calculations which I've enter'd with them are fair or defective—by these my Observations I've settled the various Lands this Voyage have brought us acquainted with, and I flatter myself rectified some erroneous settlements of others, all of which are enter'd as they occurr'd in the course of the Log. I've also been very attentive to Azimuths and Amplitudes for the Variation of the Compass, which I've enter'd at large for reasons above asscrib'd—thirdly I've inserted in these books the various qualities of the different Countries we've been conversant with, together with my idea's of the Nature and Genius of its Inhabitants, which I've carefully attended to, whenever the Nature of my Duty wou'd permit and opportunity enable me, to be among them—fourthly and lastly, at the bottom of each days Log after the Columns for Course, Distance and Latitude, is it for the Longitude in by Account—this is the Longitude in by Log beginning its account from the last place sail'd from. I've been particular carefull to settle with all possible exactitude every place we Anchor'd at and from thence took a fresh departure—the next contains the Longitude in by the last Observations, that is, my Account corrected by the last Observations—this is always nearly the true Longitude of the Ship especially in fair Weather when I cou'd make all the Observations I thought necessary—the difference between these two is the error of the Log Account since the last departure which in some places will be found very considerable—in the next Column stands the height of Farenheits Thermometer every day at Noon—this Ther^{m} always stood upon the Quarter Deck in the open Air, and of course shows the temperature of it, thro' the various Climes our business has carried us.

[RUMOUR AT THE CAPE]

The Dutch here gave us to understand, there had lately been a French Ship in the Bay, who had reported that, that Ship with another, had been fitted out at the Mauritias and sail'd thence upon a Voyage of discovery[1] —that due S^{o} from that Isle in the Latitude of 48° they had found Land, which they had coasted to the Eastward 60 Leagues—that they had seen an Opening which they believ'd to afford shelter for their Vessels, in which they propos'd Anchoring; for which purpose they had sent their Boats to sound for the best Ground &c—but that unfortunately during the Time the Boats were employ'd on this service, a Gale of wind sprung up which was so violent as to drive the Ships off the Coast, and that they had left the Boats to make the best shift they cou'd for themselves—The Good People here seem to give the most implicit confidence to this story—not a syllable of it seems to be at all disputed among them—for my own part I think probably there may be something in it, but there certainly is either more or less than what the Dutch give out—for we'll allow that they both found and rang'd Land—that they sent away their Boats and were blown of the Coast—Yet I think its totally improbable that any set of Beings shou'd be so inhumanly unfeeling as not to make the best of their way upon the Coast again, as soon as the Weather wou'd permit, to look after their People, and not leave the poor fellows to perish in wretchedness and want upon a barren Land—unless some very distressing circumstances attended the Ships which we here hear nothing of.

Account of Dusky Bay

I cannot in gratitude take my final leave of this good Bay without doing some justice to its many good qualities— in the first place you Wood and Water here with the utmost facility; the Wood may be cut down close alongside your Ship, and the Water may be fill'd by a fine running Brook about a 100 Yards from the Stern—in the next place it abounds most plentifully in Fish—principally Cold Fish with some Cavally's—Gurnets and Mackarel all large, firm, and exceedingly well tasted:—Here are likewise great abundance of very large and very good Crawfish—A Boat with 6 Hands in a few Hours generally caught enough for the expence of the day—I believe take one day with another our supply of Fish has been about a Hundred Pr Diem and those I'm sure at an average 2 Pounds apeice: so that for near these 7 Weeks past our constant consumption of Fish has [been] 200^{lb} every 24 Hours, and as many Craw Fish besides as we knew what to do with. The Water Fowl here too, I think may justly claim some mention in this Account, of which however I'll say no more, than that I was one of a Party of four that in a days shooting kill'd 41 Ducks and Curlews

[1] The reference is to Kerguelen's voyage.

and did not deem it a very extraordinary days sport—there are many Seals about too which are easily come at, whose Haslets are exceeding good, and some part of the Body properly manag'd make Steaks very little inferior (some of our Gentry sware, far superior) to Beefsteaks, and the Blubber renders very good Oil for Lamps. The frequent and Heavy Rains here Render it very disagreeable at times, however this is my third trip round the World and I suppose somewhere near the Hundred and fiftieth about it, and I cannot recollect any place I ever was at but had some disagreeable quality or other attending it, and I do think that Dusky Bay, for a Set of Hungry fellows after a long passage at Sea is as good as any place I've ever yet met with.

The Tides flow here at full and change days 57′ after 10 O'clock—it flow'd 8 feet at the full Moon, and 5 feet 8 Inches at the Change The Snow was laying on the Tops of some of the highest Hills when we arriv'd here (as I believe it does, the Year round for we observ'd it, when on this Coast in the Endeavour & 'twas then Midsummer) but many days before we left the Bay the Tops of all the Hills were cover'd and it began to grow rather disagreeably Cold.

Latitude of the Cove where we lay by the Mean of several Observations - - - - - - - - - - - -	45°..47′..47″ S
Longitude by the Mean of several Observations of ☽ : ☉ : & * - - - - - - - - - - - - - - -	166..15..30 E
Variation of the Compass here - - - - - - - - -	13..20 E[t]erly

Account of the Isles of Middleburgh and Amsterdam

The Island of Middleburgh is of a moderate heigh[t] to be seen 8 or 9 Leagues from Sea, when you come near it, nothing in Nature can give a more delightfull prospect, particularly when you advance towards the West End—there, the Cocoa Nut Trees intermixt with those of Plantins, Bunanoes and various other Fruits, cover the Ground like a thick Wood close to the Water side—the middle of the Island is the highest—it slopes down gradually to the water—the Trees thin as the Hill rises, but quite to the Top are interspers'd Patches of Cocoa Nut Trees, together with some small Groves or Copses, which variegate the scene with the fine Verdure which covers the rest of the Hills, and adds great Beauty to the Prospect.

At the West End is a good deal of Low Land, where the number of Cocoa Nut and other fruit Trees is totally innumerable—there's an Extent of Ground of 6 or 8 Miles space intirely cover'd with them—Here we Anchor'd about 3 Cables length from the Shore in 25 fathom Water.

The Natives with the happiest confidence imaginable came off to us a mile and half or 2 miles at Sea, they jump'd up the side and into the Ship like old friends and acquaintance—they mostly brought with them a present of Root, which they seem'd exceedingly fond of:—I find it has the same effect upon them as Wines &c. have upon us—they seem'd very desirous of our partaking and becoming a little jolly with them.

We were very sorry to find their Language differ so much from that of the Society Isles; this was really an unfortunate circumstance, as it not only depriv'd us of the pleasure of converse with these good People; but probably of getting some intellegence of Lands or matters within the extent of their Knowledge or Connections which we have no idea of, but this was so much the case that their conversation was nearly as unintelligible to our Indian Adventurers which we brought from those Islands as to Ourselves.

When we went onshore we were reciev'd with every demonstration of Friendship these good people cou'd suggest—the Boats Nose was no sooner landed than a great quantity of Cloath was thrown in as a gift, and in short they seem'd as perfectly solicitous and happy to shew every kind of attention and civility, as any people on Earth, 'be their situation or condition what it wou'd', cou'd be to receive it—this I take to be genuine Benevolence and goodness of Heart, for these People cou'd have no idea of the superiority of our Arms, for they never before our arrival among them had seen but one European Vessel, which was that of Captain Abel Tasman the first discoverer of these Isles in the year 1643—

The regularity of their plantations, and excellency of their Fences here I think is truly admirable—Every Mans or Families private property is divided from his Neighbours by good and strong Fences—in the midst of the Plantation, stands the Houses of the Family, which are of an Oval or Circular form; round about which, is planted a little shrubbery of various flowers, pick'd from the great abundance Nature has given them for their superior scent, and which from the situation of the Climate must be ever green and in blossom—so that when within these houses any Breeze that disturbs the Air, be it from whatever point of the Compass it may, wafts to you the most odouriferous and pleasing Perfumes our olfactory senses can possibly be regal'd with—this Island extends from N to S 13 miles—E & W 6 or 7 miles—Latitude of the West End where we lay 21°..21′ S—Longitude of the West End where we lay 185°..39′ E well detirmin'd by Lunar Observations—which Observations I shall insert just as I read them off my Quadrant at the end of this account.

We staid but one day here, then weigh'd and run down to the Island of *Amsterdam* which we saw was much larger, and consequently more likely to answer our purpose—Amsterdam bears about NW from *Middleburgh* distant 3 or 4 Leagues— We anchor'd off the West End 8 or 9 hours after we left *Middleburgh* in 18 fathom water about 3 Cable's length from the Shore.

The prospect of Amsterdam is very different from that of Middleburgh—here are neither Hills nor Dales, but a fine continued flat surface, and that, totally cover'd with the various Trees adapted by Nature to this Climate; so that the prospect is neither more nor less than one compleat Garden; which in reallity, it absolutely is, and I firmly believe one of the finest in the World; for all the Ground is in a high state of cultivation, and their plantations as regular as any I've ever met with—here are many of the best Tropical Fruits and in such abundance as is scarcely to be describ'd.

The Inhabitants are much the same as at Middleburgh, with whom they keep up a friendly communication—we saw many Canoes passing and repassing during the time we staid among them—the Character of these People in short I think is this—The Men are exceedingly Hospitable and Benevolent, but cannot withstand the temptation of European Toys if there motions are not well attended to—The Women are in general handsome and to the last degree obliging. They have one peculiarity among them which I think is too extraordinary to be omitted—at least ¾ of them have only one; and at least ¼ neither, of their little Fingers: the reason of this strange mutilation we cou'd not fairly ascertain—a very intelligible Lad that attach'd himself to me when I was onshore, gave me and some more of the Officers clearly to understand, 'twas a ceremony at the death of their Father or Mother—We afterwards saw several elderly people with both Sutes of fingers compleat: which in some measure stagger'd this account; however we made a point of getting every information we possibly cou'd into this strange matter; and at last concluded our Young friend had by no means misinform'd us, but that it certainly was a ceremony upon the death of some of their nearest Relations or particular Friends.

The Island of Amsterdam extends N & S 14 miles—E & W 20 miles The circumference is I believe about 16 Leagues—'twas very indifferent anchoring ground where we lay, as will readily be concluded by the rocks cutting one of our Cables intirely, and a good deal chafing the other; however a little to the Northward of us was a very safe & good Harbour, with 2 Channels leading into it—one of which we examin'd and found 3 & ½ fathoms Water through it—the other we did not trouble ourselves about, but 'twas very probably much the best of the two, as 'twas certainly much the widest—so that our Vessel might have been very well secur'd; had we had occasion or inclination to have spent any time among them—the only article I saw wanting among them was fresh water—I cou'd no where see a sufficient quantity of it, to have replenish'd our Water Casks if they had been empty—whether or no, some method might not have been taken to remedy this inconvenience I cannot absolutely say; but think most probably there might.

Latitude of the West End where we lay - - - - - - -	21°..04′ S
Longitude well settled by Lunar Observations which are enter'd on the other side - - - - - - - - - - - - -	185..15 E—
Variation of the Compass - - - - - - - - - - - - - -	11..06 E[t]erly

Account of Easter Island

Easter Island is rather a high Land particularly the N and S Ends of it, which may be seen 15 or 18 Leagues from Sea—as you advance, various other Hills shew themselves which are plentifully interspers'd throughout the Country—when you come near, it affords but a barren Prospect—there are many Plantations of Sugar Canes and Plantin Walks, but they're small. and the general face of the Country appears cover'd with a dry coarse Grass—We first made the SE side and examin'd it for anchorage, but found a strait shore and not the least appearance of any kind of shelter —we then run round the West End (off which lays 2 large rocks, one in a Pyramidical form quite bare the other flat, cover'd with green Shrubs) and examin'd the West side which we likewise found a strait shore and very deficient in Point of Cover for the Vessel—however it being the Lee side of the Island we sounded about the Shore 'till we got good Ground (for by far the major part of it is rocky) and there Anchor'd in 32 fathom—brown sand—the Extremes of the Island bearing from NNE to sthw—distant from the Shore about a mile and half—A little Sandy Beach nearly abreast of us ESE—this is the only sandy spot on this side of the Island—Some Hours before we Anchor'd a couple of the Natives came off and brought us a Bunch of ripe Plantins (a most gratefull Present) then return'd again to the shore seemingly exceedingly pleas'd and happy with a couple of Medals which they got in return. When we landed, the Inhabitants reciev'd us with all the civility they were masters of—they soon understood our business and brought us some sweet Potatoes—Plantins and a few Fowls, which they barter'd very freely for small peices of the White Cloath from the society Isles—this cloath is much esteem'd throughout these Seas—at New Zealand a peice of Cloath which you get for a very moderate size'd nail at the Islands will purchase you there a 100 weight of Fish—Here at Easter Island such a peice of Cloath will purchase 40 or 50 pound of Potatoes—either of which is certainly disposing of a Nail to good advantage. We search'd for Water and a little way from the Seaside found a Well the Water of which the Natives drank very chearfully but it was exceeding brackish and disagreeable—it was situate so near the Sea, that it rose and fell regularly with the Tide—however, bad as it was, we were oblig'd to make the best shift we cou'd with it for we cou'd find no better throughout the Island.

Upon examining the Country we found it a very dry barren soil cover'd with coarse harsh Grass and innumerable large stones—what few things they do cultivate are brought to perfection I believe with great labour from the many disadvantages of the soil they have to work with—the most extraordinary thing among them are the very large Images put over their burying places I imagine to perpetuate the memory of the deceas'd—they are too numerous to ascribe them all to Gentlemen that have sway'd the Sceptre for their number is such in proportion to the Inhabitants as to make it doubtfull whether every Family may not have some pretentions to these Monumental Honours—their number of Figures at one of these places is quite indeterminate and doubtlessly must be govern'd by circumstances; we saw them from one to Ten—these Images are either hue'd out of a black stone or form'd of an exceeding hard Cement and are of a most astonishing size—We measur'd one that was 27 feet by 9 and this was by no means the largest that we met with—We saw one standing which we cou'd not readily come at to measure, but by the best conclusions we cou'd make by standing against it &c &c. we cou'd not suppose it less than 30 feet in height—the Proportion of the Body is not attended to with any extraordinary degree of accuracy but some of the features of the Face are well delineated and strikingly natural—these Images are crown'd with a Stone of an amazing size of a circular form, flat at Top & Bottom, in the middle is made a Hole to fit the Head—several of these Crowns which we met with, I'm sure must weigh many Tons—I firmly believe some of them cou'd not fall short of 12 or 14—now how they cou'd form these Images and afterwards crown them in this manner without any kind of Metal Tool (for they have nothing among them that bears the least affinity to any sort of Metal) or the least knowledge of Mechanic Powers (or the means of using that knowledge supposing they had it, not having a bit of wood that wou'd make a Wedge in the whole Country) is to me the most wonderfull matter my Travels have ever yet brought me acquainted with.

The Natives here are of the middling Stature punctur'd from their Shoulders to their feet with Various figures and stripes—they are of a slim make, totally free from corpulency, remarkably active and swift of foot—The Men in general go naked except a little peice of Cloath about their Middle which is brought up between their Legs I imagine purely for Ornament for it secretes nothing from publick view—the Women wear a Mat about their middle &c &c and frequently a large peice of Cloath about their shoulders—their Cloath here is made of the same materials as the Cloath at the Islands but infinitely worse manufactur'd—these Lasses have tolerable faces—fine form'd Bodies, are very complaisant and perfectly obliging to Strangers—there Auricular Ornaments here are somewhat peculiar and extraordinary—in the bottom of the Ear is a large hole in which, when they dress and mean to look fine they clap in an elastic peice of Matter a good deal resembling a shaving of wood, but I believe 'tis the Bark of some tree work'd very thin for this purpose which extends this Hole to such a degree that I've met with several of them I cou'd very easily have put my fist through—by this mode of dress the Old Peoples Ears hang fairly down upon their Shoulders—the People are by no means numerous, we were throughout the Island and cannot suppose their whole number to exceed 500 Souls—350 of whom I believe to be Men for there seems 2 or 3 of them to 1 Woman—they are very nimble finger'd and will take every opportunity of pilfering but a motion of the Musquet freightens them confoundedly, an idea which I suppose the Spaniards have inculcated, for I must observe this of my friends here, that the dread of the Gun seem'd much more to contribute to their honesty than any innate principle we cou'd observe them to be actuated by—their Houses are low paltry places I believe only intended for sleep & shelter in bad Weather—for they are totally dark and we observ'd that they paid no kind of attention to them in the course of the day—We had an account in England of the Spaniards visiting this place in /69 which is confirm'd to us by some little matters we find among them which must have been left by those Gentlemen—this Island is of a triangular form about miles in circumference—We were there at spring Tides and found them to flow about 27 Inches.

Account of the Marquesas

The Marquesas are 4 Islands discover'd by Alvara Mendana De Neyra's a Spanish Voyager in the Year 1595—he nam'd them La Magdalena—St Pedro—La Dominica and St Christina and gave them altogether the general name of Las Marquesas. We have no account of their ever having been visited, since the first discovery of them to our arrival there in the Resolution—Mendana has given a very good description of their situation in respect of each other in ye account of His Voyage which is translated by Mr Dalrymple in his collection of Voyages, which he publish'd in 1770.

They are a more Hilly and Mountanous kind of Islands than any I've ever yet met with in these Seas—they have a very barren prospect at a distance, 'till you come near enough to discern the breaks in the Hills, or little Vallies, which appear pleasant and fertile—they are totally deficient in that fine salutary Border which is the greatest Beauty, and indeed the greatest blessing (as it produces $\frac{3}{4}$ of their food) of Otahite and the Society Isles—the Hills of the Marquesas in most places break off perpendicular into the Sea—there are very few Vallies near the Water side, and those are small—they have in general strait shores affording very little Cover for Ships. We repair'd to a Roadsted describ'd by Mendana on the Western side of St Christina which we found pretty well shelter'd, and a tolerable safe Place, but generally very bad getting onshore upon account of the Surfe, which laid us under the necessity of landing upon perpendicular Rocks, for the Water is seldom smooth enough to land upon the Beach—at least such was the case during our stay here. The Inhabitants to speak of them in general are the most beautifull race of People I ever beheld—of a great number of Men that fell under my inspection, I did not observe a single one either remarkably thin, or disagreeably Corpulent but they were all in fine Order & exquisitely proportion'd. We saw very few of their Women, but what were seen, were remarkably fair for the situation of their Country and very beautifull—the Men are punctuated (or as they call it tattow'd) from head to foot in the prettyest manner that can be conciev'd—the Women are not tattow'd at all, only 1 or 2 little marks in their Lips, they have very fine long Heads of Hair, which hang down their Backs in a most becoming and gracefull manner—they have the Cloath Plant here, and the same kind of Cloathing as at the Society Isles—the Head dress of the Men has a very pretty appearance—it consists of some twisted Grass, decorated with Mother of pearl shells—Tortoise shells and Cocks Feathers—their Weapons are Clubs—Spears & Slings—I believe they depend a good deal upon their slinging for I've seen them exercise and throw exceedingly well; and go where they will, they always have their slings and stones about them. I was one day a little distance up the Country to one of their Villages, they were exceedingly civil and readily gave me Cocoa Nuts and whatever they had—in examining the Houses I observ'd, that a little net full of smooth, siezable, slinging stones was always a part of the Household furniture—I believe they have frequent Wars and that with very powerfull and consequently very troublesome Enemies—for on the Tops of the high Hills we cou'd percieve Houses and People, and just on the Brink of them Buildings, resembling Fortresses, which they gave us to understand, was their retreat when the Enemy was too strong for them[1] —We cou'd plainly distinguish with our glasses paths to these retreats and People passing and repassing up & down—from all that we cou'd observe of these Islanders we have reason to conclude them a benevolent good people, but a little light finger'd as indeed are all the Indians I ever met with—We were plentifully suppli'd by them with Breadfruit—Bunanoes and Plantins—we likewise got about a 100 Hogs but they were in general very small—the Trade on our part was Beads—Nails and some few Hatchets—We pass'd 5 days very agreeably among these good Folks —got ourselves well refresh'd and our Wants abundantly reliev'd, then took our Leaves and made for Otahite.

Account of Anamocka

Rotterdam, or as the Natives call it Anamocka, to speak of matters in general is a Low and small Island; but in comparison to the many small Isles its environ'd with, is high and large—it is somewhat higher than the generallity of the Low Isles, which are peculiar to these Seas—of a triangular form, and about 9 or at most 10 miles in circuit, with an exceeding pleasant and beautifull appearance—We were reciev'd at our landing with all the civility we cou'd wish—found the Island a charming agreeable spot, with Houses—Gardens—Plantations &c &c in a great measure resembling those at Amsterdam, but by no means in so nice order, nor in so high a state of cultivation—In the heart of the Isle there are 3 large Lakes 2 of salt & one of fresh Water—they all abound in the largest and best Wild Ducks I ever saw or tasted—the quantities of Shaddocks and Yams (both excellent in their kind) which the Island produces is almost incredible—I'm sure we might have loaded the Ship with them, had we set about it—we were also pretty plentifully suppli'd with Bunanoes and Cocoa Nuts—Got some Fowls—Fish and 5 or 6 small Hogs—The Arms of these Islanders are Clubs and Spears—they have Bows and Arrows but I believe they are rather instruments of amusement than Weapons; in short the whole People both Men and Women are much the same in every particular, as those of Amsterdam (which I describ'd last Year) to which place they tell us, they frequently go in their Canoes—the Canoes of Amsterdam—Rotterdam and all this Group of Islands, are by far the best I've met with—they are put together with as much nicety, and their Seams are as fine, as any Cabinet work—they are a strong well proportion'd good Boat—Here are a number of Islands in this neighbourhood; we can reckon 17 from our mast head, all low, pleasant spots, except 2 which lay close together and bear about NWBN they are very high Land. The Canoes run very leisurely throughout the whole and they appear in

[1] The Marquesans built up terraces of masonry, but not for fortresses. They were generally house-platforms, or places for ceremonial use.

a happy state of mutual confidence, and peace with each other. These People have only one bad particle in their whole composition, which is plac'd at their fingers ends, and is eternally itching to be at work upon some matters that's not their own—we staid here but 2 days, during which time they were very industrious in the pilfering scheme—however before we departed, we siez'd 2 of their Canoes and made them return all that their great abilities and strict perseverance had procur'd them—One of the fellows oppos'd this measure so strenuously that we were oblig'd to put a few small shot in him, (however not so as to effect his Life) which had the desir'd effect for they return'd their booty and reciev'd their Canoes.

Account of the People—Country &c &c—of Caledonia

These People are of a dark mahogony Colour—well featur'd—Woolly headed—well form'd bodies, and of the middling Stature—the Features both of the Men and Women are remarkably good, exceeding by far, any woolly Headed Nation we ever met with—their benevolence when they find an opportunity, can be exceeded by nothing but their assiduity in finding it—they're absolutely unhappy unless they can suggest some means of making themselves serviceable and agreeable—when Wooding or Watering—they wou'd either cut or carry—fill the Casks or rowl—and if you interrupted them in this business, they seem'd uneasy that they cou'd not render their best endeavours worthy your acceptance. We have all the reason in the World to suppose ourselves the first Europeans they ever beheld, and that unlimited confidence they immediately plac'd in us, I think speaks greatly in favour of their Honesty and Goodness of Heart—for I'm of opinion, that among any set or Nation of Men, who are accustom'd to catch and maltreat each other; they will naturally suspect all the rest of the World, and I think this argument is particularly applicable to these poor Fellows, whose notions must be so contracted by their situation in Life, that they can form no idea of any kind, but what must immediately have its rise from their mode of deportment to each other—the dress of these our good friends is somewhat singular—when we found them, they were totally naked to the Penis, which was wrapt up in leaves, and whatever you gave them, or they, by any means attain'd; was immediately apply'd there; nor wou'd they care one farthing for any article of dress, that cou'd not in some form, be made to contribute, to the decorating that favourite part. I gave one of them one day a stocking—he very deliberately pull'd it on there—I then gave him a string of Beads, with it he ty'd the stocking up—I then presented him with a medal, which he immediately hung to it—in short let that noble part be well decorated and fine, they're perfectly happy, and totally indifferent about the state of all the rest of the Body. The Womens dress consists of a long string, from which suspends Hemp, work'd into small distinct Ends about 8 inches long—in general dy'd black—this they wrap 4 or 5 times round them, the turns immediately upon each other, just below the Hips; which as perfectly secretes all they want to hide, as all the Petty-Coats &c. &c. I ever saw upon a Woman in my life—the Country about here seems a dry light soil, and I apprehend rather deficient in point of fertility—they have some Yams and Cocoa Nuts among them, and some few Fowls; but I believe their chief subsistance is Fish—for they pay great attention to the ebbing of the Tides—are very busy at low water, and I observe, always get abundance of Shell Fish, with which they frequently regale themselves upon the Beach, as soon as they've caught them.

They have sometimes plenty of large Fish, which they us'd to bring us—We got one that was poisonous among them, of which the Captain and his Mess took a dose—its a confounded ugly looking Animal—Mr Forster calls it a Japan Fish; I think nobody cou'd be twice mistaken in it; however I must leave the description of it to the Naturalists. Their Arms are Spears—Clubs & Slings—they gave us to understand there were People, came from a distant Island sometimes and fought with them, but their Language was so different from any thing we've met with before, that we cou'd get but a very poor account of their Wars, or indeed any other, of their matters—all we know of them is by experience, and they soon convinc'd us by it, that they were a charming benevolent, good People.

They were total strangers to Quadrupeds; we gave them a Male and Female of Hogs and Dogs, which I hope will increase and prove a blessing to them; that they may remember us, with that gratitude and affection, which the knowledge of their Goodness, has implanted in every feeling Heart among'st us, for them. Their Canoes appear rather heavy Vessels, but they navigate them very skilfully:—they have large Mat Sails, with which they work to windward shearly[1] and make very good Weather of it—I believe by the help of these Canoes they get all their large Fish from the reef, which runs here nearly parrellel to the Shore, at 4 or 5 miles distance. Their Houses are built in a Pyramidical form—they are spacious—warm and neat; and really very comfortable Habitations.

All the Astronomic Observations the Weather permitted me to make here, are enter'd as they occur'd in the course of the Log.

The Country hereabouts, Our friends call bellarde, therefore as I know no other name I will distinguish this place by the name of *Bellarde* Harbour. it is in Lat^{de} 20°..16′ s and in Longitude by the Mean of all my calculations upon the Coast - - - - - - - - - - - - - - - - - 164..30 E
Variation by the Mean of 2 sets of Azimuths I took here - - 7..39 E^{t}erly.

Account of Christmas Harbour

These have been 8 such days as I never had the least idea of spending at Terra del Fuego—the Weather fine—Ship safe and abundance of good provision—even the Poor Inhabitants (wretched as they seemingly are) contributed all they cou'd to our enjoyment by their confidence and sociallity.

I avail'd myself of the clearness of the Weather here to make all the observations upon the Country I cou'd from the Hills; and from all I cou'd there observe, or learn from others, who took the same method upon

[1] The word seems here to have the meaning of 'obliquely'.

different parts—this Terra del Fuego is nothing more than a large Cluster of Isles and consequently full of Inlets which run in various directions beyond the reach of our sight and I make no doubt but some of them terminate in the Streights *Magellan*—these Inlets are so numerous upon this Western Coast, that I'm of opinion a Ship may run into very good Shelter upon almost any part of it—there's such an affinity in the appearance of the various Isles, that without the utmost attention any particular place may be easily mistook—the best and indeed the only mark for knowing our Harbour again that fell under my inspection is this—there's a Cluster of small rocky Isles detach'd at a remarkable distance from the Shore (which must be conspicuous if you are at all near the Land) which bears from the SW Point of the Bay S 43° E correct—distant from it 10 Leagues.[1]

The appearance of the Inhabitants here immediately bespeaks your pity —they are a diminitive race—walk exceeding ill, being almost cripple'd from the perpetual attitude of setting upon their heels, and tho' 'twas now midsummer they were continually shaking and shivering as tho' half kill'd with the cold—there cloathing is nothing more than a Seal Skin thrown loosely over their Shoulders every other part of both Sexes is intirely expos'd—their Arms are paltry Bows and Arrows, and long spears pointed with Bones, with which I imagine they kill the Seals—they had a good deal of the flesh of these Animals among them, which they eat raw—bloody—and in short exceedingly nasty—however they were apparen[t]ly a good deal surpriz'd we did not chuse to partake of what they seemingly thought so delicious—their language is very harsh and seems to us scarcely articulate—they make frequent use of the word *Pisheray* which I find Monsr Bougainville has taken notice of—I'm well assur'd its some term of friendship among them, for I observ'd they us'd it most when particularly pleas'd by any little incident and 'twas a very favourite word with the Ladies, which I must do the justice here to observe, that throughout all my transactions and adventures, let what fracas and cabals wou'd, happen; I've ever found *the Indian Lasses* industrious in exerting all their influence upon both parties to bring about reconciliations and introduce friendship. I remember noticing this word Pisheray in both my former Voyages—these People resemble in every respect some I've seen in the Streights of Magellan when I pass'd them in the beginning of /65—We found knives among them so that they've had some traffick with Europeans, most probably upon the borders of the Streights, where I make no doubt but these very people travel, and I think most likely well to the N°ward of y^m^ in the Course of the Winter.

The Isles of direction above mention'd for Christmas Harbour are detach'd 4 Leagues from the Land, and are in Latitude 55°„50′ S°. All the other Islands alongshore are so compact that to all appearance, 'till you come very near them, they form one continued Coast—these Isles may be seen in very Clear Weather just above the Horizon upon Deck when before the Entrance of the Bay. . . .

[1] The Ildefonso Islands.

[ICE ISLES AND SOUTHERN CONTINENT]

In respect to Lands still unexplor'd towards the Southern Extreme of the Globe, I'm of opinion tho' this Voyage has clearly evinc'd there can be no Continent or Isle at all worthy the attention of any People under the Sun, yet that there may be, and is, some extensive Land or a multitude of Isles in that part of the World. I'm induc'd to this way of thinking by the innumerable Ice Isles throughout the Seas in the high Southern Latitudes, which Isles, I make no doubt must be form'd under the Cover of, and contiguous to some Land. Untill this last Southern Campaigne we were very various in our Opinions concerning the formation of an Ice Island, but the sight of those Lands at the bottom of the Atlantic render'd this matter very plain, and gave us a very clear idea of its Origin—increase &c. &c. We there saw Icy Cliffs from which Isles, apparently and evidently had broke off and some Bays only partly full, the rest having separated and floated away to Sea; in short what we there met with, dispel'd all our doubts and clearly convinc'd us, that the Isles are form'd under the Cover of Lands either in Bays or wherever the water is so much shelter'd that the general purterbation of the Sea cannot much effect it, but the surface becoming smooth is of course in a state to be more easily congeal'd which must be soon brought about by the intense Cold that reigns here throughout almost the whole Year—thus Originated, its bulk I suppose to be increas'd to the huge size we found them by the immense quantities of Snow which falls to the share of these happy Climes, which will be found by the account of the Weather in the Log to be almost perpetual even in the height of Summer—this Snow as it falls continues to freeze and embody itself with the Ice, 'till it becomes too enormous to bear its own weight and of course immerges into the Sea; or probably continues till the return of the Vernal Season, which tho' not very mild here, may have influence enough to weaken in some measure a body of Ice, and consequently breaks it adrift and leaves it to cruize at the mercy of the Winds and Seas. Now this being my Hypothesis of an Ice Island I'm led to believe from thence, that the Myriads we've met with, cou'd not have been form'd but by a great deal of shelter and of course large quantities of Land—the Land we fell in with in the Lattitude of 59° was as totally inaccessible to us, as tho' 'twas only a Body of Ice—the shores were form'd of high rocky precipices and the Bays chok'd up with Ice making in high Cliffs, as recorded in the Log—which Cliffs extend themselves in many places beyond the points of Land which form the Bays, so that getting a foot onshore was wholly impracticable—now this was the Midsummer of a Year we had reason to suppose a very mild one, therefore if such was the case in this Latitude, what can be expected when farther advanc'd towards the Pole which we must allow the Center of intense Cold; so what can be expected, supposing there were any Lands comatable which however I believe the Account of this Voyage will put altogether out of the question.

CHA^s CLERKE

4. Pickersgill's Journal

[*Printed from the Enderby MS in the National Maritime Museum, Greenwich, MS 57/038, pp. 91–107, 116–33.*]

We stood off and on all Night, and in the morning [17 August 1773] the People comeing off, with a light wind we stood into a little harbour called *Ohitepeah* in the Map in Dr Hawksworths Voyages to which I must refer; here we Anchor'd and soon after the adventure did the same; here we learnt that the Otahite-Ete Men and the Otahite Nue men had had a War, the latter of which were beat, and our old friend Tutahah and most of his companions were slain—as the King of this part of the Island lived here and had gain'd the Victory we thought to stay here for Hoggs in preferance to the old Bay at Matavie.

The appearance of the Land here was very romantic being high craggy Hill[s], lofty spires and fertile Vallies full of houses and Inhabitants.

After we came to an Anchor, the Natives came on board in such Numbers, that it was with the utmost difficulty we could moor the ship—they brought off fruit but no Hoggs as the King had not yet been down, they durst not sell any, such of the Adventures sick as were able to walk went on Shore in the Day time, the rest were carefully attended on board; whilst the well men were employ'd watering the ships, there being a convenient place for that porpose.

We waited very impatiently for two Days without seeing either King or Hoggs, but on the third he came down, the Captain waited on him with a Present, in return for which he gave two small Piggs, nor would he give leave for any to be sold to us unless the Captain would lett him have our best Boat, for which he offerd Ten Hoggs; This was a mortifying Circumstance to us, and more so as we did not expect it, for its not above Seven years since, there was not a single chief on this Island that would not have walked miles to have given a Hog for an old Nail; this made us quit a place where we could not succeed by fair means to try another, so accordingly we sail'd from Ohitepeah the 25th where I was left with a Boat armed to see if they would trade after the ships were gone, and to follow them to Matavie Bay.

The Ships were no sooner gone then the King with his whole retinue came out of the country to us, but was exceedingly surprized to see so many armed men, and to try what exicution the musketts would do he desired to see on[e] of them fired, which was no sooner done then the whole croud tumbled backward one over another with fear; but as it only made one hole they did not much mind it, so to convince them we could as easily make many I loaded a musket with Small Shot and desireing them to hang up a mark fired at it; when to their utter surprize the mark was torn all to Peices, after this they were so terified that they would see no more; the King by every inducement in his Power wanted me to stay with the Boat which he much wanted bring[ing] down his Women to use their endeavours to allure me not to go any more to the Ship; whilst we staye'd we got 8 hoggs for some Axes.

The King was a tall likely young Man about 18 years of age, with fine flaxen hair, his features regular and his complexion of a Dark Olive, the People strip down to their waists in his Presence and he had a man attending him with a high stool, but as the persons customs and manners &ca of Otahite are so well discribed in Hawksworths Voyages I shall not enter into any pecular detail of them here; as it would be a thing far beyond either my design or abilitys.

Leaveing this place we endeavour'd to stand out to the Ships, but it came on to blow and Rain in such a manner, that we were glad to get near the shore, standing along it, to the westw[d] untell the Evening when we were mett by a Number of Canoes from the Shore, these people came to invite us to their Houses, and strove with each other who should entertain us; one offering food and cloathing another immeadately started up and told me he would not only give me food and cloathes but his Daughter should be my companion whilst I stay'd at his House; this was an offer not to be rejected so he directly came into our Boat and we made for the Shore towards a House where he said his Brother lived who was *Arree* or King of the District his Name *O Rettee* and the same Prince that entertain'd M: de Bougainvelle in 1768 this being the Bay where he lay—as soon as he came into the Boat he striped himself and makeing me do the same, he wraped up my wet cloaths and cloathed me in his dry ones—here Europeans! learn humanity and Cevelity to distressed strangers, from Men who most of you terms Barbarous Nations.

Being landed I was received amidst the acclamations of at least 5000 People who takeing me up in their arms carried me without tutching the ground to their Prince, who gave me a welcome, not to be discribed but imagened; I was led round a numerous Family of reverent old Men a[nd] Presented [to] each of them by the King, they all expressing their utmost Pleasure and satisfaction at my Paying them a Visit, a House was Prepair'd Victuals drest the cocoa Nut trees robbed of their fruit, and all was joy and mirth; we supped together; nor were the men neglected they haveing an other House and every attention shewn them; however for fear I took the precaution to moor the Boat off out of a mans Depth with some of the people armed for fear of this kindness being all Deceat, and when they were angry at my distrust, I appeased them by telling them it was only to keep the Thieves from stealing any thing in the Night, with which they seem'd perfectly satisfied—and after appointing every man his Station in case of an Allarm, for we were but Ten and they 5 or 6000 at least.

The Hymeneal Songs being allready perform'd we retired to rest: untell the Blushing Morn told us it was time to depart—and thus leaveing these friends we took our ways to y[e] Ship my Freind (*Chay oully*) going with us to the ships which we joined off Matavie Bay about 12 OClock that Day, where we received a very agreable Wellcome from what we brought with us.

The 2 Ships Anchor'd in Matavie Bay in the evening and next morning we errected 2 Tents under a guard of the Marines, where the Sick was landed. Many of the Chiefs came on board and promised us plenty of every thing we wanted; bring[ing] fruit but no Hoggs.

On the 29th the Captains waited on the King in his province called *O Parree* about 2 miles from the Ship, he lived in the midst of a number of long sheeds or Houses, and when he received the Captains he placed them by him and treated them with Cocoa Nutts, &c. after the Manner of the country—this visit being over they returnd to the Ships, haveing first obtain'd the Kings Promise to come on board Next Day.

Next morning *Otoo* (The King) came on board but without Hoggs, and indeed many visits were paid without any sign of benifiting so it was resolved to send a boat round to the Back of the Island to a prince called Po-ta-tow, this man tho' under *Otoo* yet is in Power very great and at that time was not upon the best terms with *Otoo*—this made us hope to get some Hoggs from him; accordingly I left the Ship before Day light to get past the Kings house before he could see me which I did and standing along shore with a train of about 100 canoes following; I landed about 1 Oclock in a sandy Bay about six and twenty miles from Matavie, here I left a guard to take care of the Boat and with the rest walkd up about two miles, thro' an agreable country full of Cocoas and wild Roses to his house which consisted of a square yard made by four houses the longest of which was open and situated close to the sea side, here I was receivd by Potatow and seated on Dry'd Grass with his wives and freinds, I opend my Embassy with a Present of a looking Glass to each of the Ladies and a large ax to him. I then asked him to go to the Ships, and to let us have some Hoggs, to which he said I should know presently—desireing me to go with his wives into another house where they loaded me with Cloth, whilst I was here Potatow came again and told me he was affraid to go to the Ships for if he did not give us Hoggs we should shoot him, but if I would stay all Night and bring the Boat to his Door, we should have some in the morning; as this could not be done we parted and was comeing away, with a Promise of some Hoggs in a Day or two, when we missd a horn of Powder which some of those nimble finguerd Gentry had gone off with, which I made Potatow acquainted with, and he addressing the Mob they all run into the woods where he follow'd and soon after return'd with the Horn and Powder all safe, by what means he could so soon procure it I know not, but he certainly carried great command over his teritories and had allways a number of men exerciseing and seemingly kept stricktly to military Duty; he is one of the stoutest men I ever saw, his thigh would measure more round in the Middle then any part of my Body he is very proportionablely made, and his natural Powers are so great that his vast bulk is no impediment to his agility—he and his family attended us to the Boat where we parted and got to the ship thro' rocks sands and many difficultys within the Reefs about 8 o clock being heartily tired.

I must not omit one circumstance; we obs^d down at Potatows a man of the coulour of a Flemmen his Hair Red bad teeth and grey Eyes all which are differant from the Natives of these countries, we at first took him to be a European but on a further examineation we found him to be a Native—how or by what means a white man comes to be born amongst a set of copper coulour'd Indians I leave to the learned to account for.

Whilst we were gone they had not succeeded with *Otoo* who had fled to the woods and trade was run to a stand still upon which I made another essay to the west ward designing to go further if I could not succeed at Potatows. We accordingly set off and called at Potatows about two o clock, where we found no hoggs as he did not expect us, so we told him we would call the Next Day and continued our rout to the West designing to go to the south part of the Island where the old Queen Oberea live'd; in this passage we were followd by vast crouds of people both in Boats and along the shores, about 9 o clock our Indian Pilot could not see to carry us any further, we attempted to land which we did but had scarce got on the Beach in our way to a house before the Chief of the Province met us and told us we must go no further; this was a sad disapointment, however go we must so we got some Musquetts, the Chief seeing them got a Plantain tree and offerd Peace: back went the Muskets, then we must go no farther, up came the Muskets, down came the Plaintain tree and in this manner we continued for three quarters of an hour untell being tired we took our arms and march'd up to a house which we were no sooner in possesion of then they were very good friends with us, this being settled we dress'd our supper and sent for Oberea who lived about two miles off, she came and was very happy to see us but was so poor as not to be able to give us any assistance. She stay'd all Night and inquired about many perticulars but the Otahite people seem not to be bless'd with the most happy memories for I met with few that rememberd Tupia and hardly any who rememberd Oatouro who came a way with M: de Bougainvelle—in the morning the chief was to have let us had a Hogg or two but all at once he got up into the Woods and left orders for us to have none, being thus disapointed in all our hopes we left the Place designing to call on Potatow in our way home.

I think this Part of the Island is more fertile and appears more beautifull then where the ships lay: the sides of the Hills are more Level and the Soil is deep and rich produceing besides the fruit trees plenty of Cotton Indego and wild sugar canes with ginger and various other plants.

We got to Potatows about two o clock; we found him sitting in his long house with a prodegious concourse of people round him, upon the boats landing a lane was made for us and we were seated in the middle and served with Cocoa nutts &c. here we stay'd all Night and were exceedingly well treated and in the morning Potatow offerd to go with us, provided I would promise him on a little bunch of Red feather[s] and calling his God to witness, that he should not be shot: this I did and gave him all the assurance of his being in safty when at the Ship, thus contented he was comeing into the Boat when the beach was lined with people many of them his relations who after attempting in vain to persuade him to stay took an affectinet leave of him, there was not a Dry Eye to be seen so much had these good people the wellfare of their Prince at heart—we got to the Ship by Noon and found them ready for sea, haveing quarrel'd with the Natives which happned thus.

On the Night we went away in the Boat, some of our seamen in company with some of the Adventure's, stragling up in the woods in the Night quarrel'd with some of the Natives and struck them, this being resented by them, it came to an open fight, wherein the Seamen were worsted and forced to call out, this alarmed the ship who sent a Party to take them on board—next morning they were severely punish'd in presence of several of the Natives—this had not the desired effect for instead of satisfieing the people it frightned them, and in a little time the woods who an hour before were full of Inhabitants was now become a Desert. . . .

[7 September] About Noon we were abrest of the S^o^ Point of Uliateah but could not get into the harbour that Night, we stood on our boards all Night and in the morning work'd into a narrow channel between two little sandy Island[s] called in the Maps Oamonenoo; we just got into anchoring Ground and afterward warp'd the two ships within the Reefs near the shore where we moor'd them in comeing in we found a strong currant setting out of the narrow passage, which rendered it very difficult to get in; this currant I fancy is occasion'd by a great southern swell which constantly sets in and breaking upon the Reefs forces a large quantity of water over them, which returns to the Sea thro those small Passages.

We were no sooner in safty then Numbers of the Natives flock'd on board of us from all parts amongst which were many of our old Friends, they seem'd very happy to see us; but few of them either inquired, or I belive thought of Tupia. Amongst the rest that came off was the King named *Oreo*, this man was pecularly fond of Captain Cook; and Insisted on his going on shore that evening to see a Play or Heva, the Principal Parts of which was to be perform'd by his Daughter a young Lady about 15 years of age—and in consequence we all went, and were conducted up to his house amidst a vast concourse of People where we were entertain'd with Cocoa Nuts &ca and Introduced to the young Princess; she was of the middleing stature rather Slender, and Delicate, with good teeth and Eyes and a regular set of features, Black Hair and her complexion so fair that I have seen many Ladies in England much more of a Brunett.

After we had been in this House a little while Miss *Poedoua* for that was her name desired me to go and see her dress; we went to an ajacent House, the front of which was open and opposite it at the distance of about Ten yards between these two Houses was a space neatly cover'd with Matts, on these Matts they acted; in the first house sat the audience and in the second the Musick, one end being inclosed for the actresses to dress in, which was inclosed; into this Place she carried me, where undressing an old woman came in to dress her; her dress consisted of large Pieces of Painted cloths made up in folds and girded tort round her to an amazing thickness, and her head dressed in the Manner of a Turband with fine Platted black hair ornimented with flowers. All the actors being ready they began with a Dance, the Musick consisting of 4 Drums and some Boys to sing, this ending the Men came out and acted their Parts which consisted in rediculeing the Chief People about them so that the whole together made up a kind of a Burletta, indeed the men seem'd to go thro' their Parts exceedingly well but their Danceing consisted of the most ludicrous gestures I ever beheld.

As for the Size Situation &ca. of these Islands I shall refer to Captn Cooks Plan of them as they are laid down in the former Voyages to the South Sea's where a very ample discription is given both of the Islands and their good possesors.

Septr 13th haveing got on Board a great Numb^{r} of Hoggs and nothing to feed them with, our next buissness was to procure food, this we found could not be done in Uliateah but the Natives told us there was plenty in the neghbouring Island of Otaha, to which I was sent the next day with a Party of Soldgers and two Boats, we run down the East side with out being able to procure any thing alltho' we landed at several places whose fertile Vallies seem'd to promise success, the Natives every where gathering round us in Crouds and behaving with the utmost Cevility; about 4 O clock in the Evening we had got to the most Northern Part of the Island, here we found the King named *Otah* he was an old thin Man, he was seated under one of their long houses upon a Stool, with Matts spread before him and the Drums beating for a *heava* or Dance, and had only waited our comeing when they began to perform, this tho' much inferior to what we had seen before yet shew'd their good intentions to entertain us in the most agreable manner they were capable of—as I intended to stay here all Night, we prepair'd for it accordingly by secureing our Boats, roasting a Hog &c. for tho' we could get no greens or fruit yet hoggs were so plenty that we could have had as many as we wanted as likewise Plenty of Wild Ducks and Tame fowles for a glass bead Each. Nothing material happned during the Night exept a Mistake of the Centinal, for we had taken one part of the House to our selves and had a Centinal with a Light, and the King for our greater insurance laid amongst us but as the Devil would have it in the middle of the Night the light went out and a strang[e] man being on Duty, in feeling for the candle which had fallen down caught hold of the old Kings head of hair, and finding it to belong to an Indian immediately concluded he was a Thief who had taken the oppertunity of the Candle's being out to steal some thing and began to lug him by the Hair and beat him about the Head with the Butt end of his musquit, the old man finding himself so roughly handled began to roar out, Both Parties alla[r]med started out of their Sleep in the greatest Confusion, which was increased on both sides untell a light came and set us all to rights, and ended in a hearty laugh at the expence of the Old Man.

When the Morning came, I got up by times for to get a way as early as possible, but enquireing for the people I found most of them absent and on a further examination found them one in one house and one in an other all stragled about the Woods each man with his Mistress.

About 9 Oclock we took our leaves of these good people (the King going with us in our Boat) and began our tour of the west side but found the wind to blow very hard against us—this part of Otaha is mountainous the sides of the Hills being steep and barren, the Bays run in Deep and at the Bottoms is generally a flat Beach and vertile [*sic*] Vallies running far into the Land between the Hills; these Vallies are the most fertile spots in Nature abounding with fine Plantain Walks and groves of Cocoa Nut and bread fruit Trees, under the Shade of which the Natives build their Houses and live generally on the Banks of a revillet which they occasionally turn into their gardens or where the Women sitt and manufacture their Cloth—about one league or three Miles from the Shore there is a flat or border which runs parrellal to the shore and is cover'd with palm and cocoa Nut trees whose ever green appearance on one side and the beauty of the Island on the other, form'd one of the most Pleasant Canals[1] I ever saw; we kept turning to windward untell 3 Oclock when finding the Gale increase and we not likely to get any further, we Landed under a point, and prepair'd for a 2^d^ Night but alass, one missfortune seldom comes alone for as we were dressing our dinner with a croud of people round us, we all at once missed our Trade bag or Treasure; this was at once striking at the root for without that we could do nothing and we had not got half our loading. What steps to take to recover it we knew not, the Peple all fled as fast as they could with their Effects to the Mountains—we divided our forces and leaveing one half with one of the Mates to take care of the Boats, with the other we persued the Inhabitants who by this time had tolerably well cleard the Houses of their Effects and there was hardly a man to be seen, in this manner we follow'd for about 2 Miles where we over took a fat Chief whose Body was so unweildy that he could not move off fast enough, him we took who promise'd to bring back the things stolen from us, provided we would let him go which we did after taking most part of his Effects as a security for his return with which we march'd down to the Boats. Two Objects here struck me much, they were an extream old Man and Woman who thro' age and infirmities could scarce move and not being able to get away with the rest were left in the Woods, and with their utmost exersion crawled to wards us, each with a Dog in their Arms as an offering at the same time with the utmost dejection imploreing their forgiveness—in so pityable a manner, as was truely affecting; we received their Dogs; afterwards letting them loose and gave the Old People each a large Nail with the utmost assurances of their Safty, telling them we did not come to hurt the good people, but to punish the Theivs who had Stole our property, with this they seem'd tolerably satisfied and retired to their Hut. When we got to the boat Mr Bur the Mate that I had left there had dureing our absence, received a large Pigg from the King with assurances of the Things being brought in the morning; thus situated, with so small a party as 23 in all, we did not get much rest that Night, in the first part of it, our Arree or Chief came with half our things and in consequence got half his own back again.

[1] i.e. channels.

In the Morning seeing us prepairing to carry away the rest of the Effects we had seized they produced the rest of our trade and got all their things back, but here a fresh difficulty occur'd for the latter part which consisted principally of looking Glasses were Spoiled for they haveing concealed them in a bush and it comeing on to rain in the Night, they had all got wet, but we were obliged to make the best of a bad bargain and so proceed along the Coast intending to take the first fair oppertunity to return to the Ships, here our luck took a turn for going into a bay from whence we intended to set sail for the Ships, we found such abundance of Fruit that we loaded both boats for little or nothing and that afternoon join'd the Ships.

Here we found the ships allarmd at our long stay as the Uliateah People had left their habitations near the place where they lay without any apparant reason, this occasion'd many Idle storys in the Ships amongst which they did not forget to kill the Officers and make the Men run away with the Boats, &ca; but hearing of our dispute with the Otaha men I believe the Captain and many others laid it to that, and I fancy know no other yet but the true reason was this, after we went away, the Gunner and one of the young Gentlemen being out shooting were follow'd by too numerous a Mob and not being able to keep them back one of them loaded his fowling peice with a little Powder and some Sand and fired amongst the Multitude, who seeing no exicution done exasperated them to a degree of boldness, they advanced and seizeing hold of their Musquits wrench'd them out of their hands bound them Prisners and carried them up to one of their chiefs, who fearing the resentment of the ships orderd them to be unbound their things to be restor'd and a Boat to carry them on Board, telling his own people that Capt[n] Cook would certainly come on Shore and kill them all on his knowing of their behavour—this so effectually frightned them that they immeadately forsook their Houses and fled to the Mountains with their Effects; this never comeing to the Capt[ns] Notice it was laid to the affair of our dispute as they began to come down on our return and in their acc[t] they Pointed to wards the place where it happned which was in a direction towards *Otaha* where we was this seemingly confirmd it.

The Inhabitants of Uliateah told us of many other Islands both to the East and west, but they seem'd to have the greatest knowlidge of those to the NE. One Man said he had been at a large one Called *Miva*, that it was very fertile and spoke much of the largeness of it, and the Cevility, and whiteness of the Inhabitants who, he said were like us but had no fire arms, he set the bearings of it by one of our Compasses NEbE from here—they were ten Day[s] going to it in their Canoes and every Night they slept on an Island; on one of which he said there was a race of Giants whose Bodies were as big as ten of ours, and whose hight he messured out to be about 40 feet; when we laught at him he seem'd very angry and brought many people who all attested to the truth of What he had told us; he further said the Name of the Island was *Oheva* and that he with many others once went to attack three of them, but micarried; and that many of his party was thrown, with much anger half a mile into the Sea; ever since, when they go to Oheva they are very carefull not [to] Offend. On Septr 18th we Sail'd from Uliateah takeing with us a youth about 18 years old who offerd to go, thus we had one in each Ship; in the Night we pass'd two Islands called *Bollobollo* and *Moura*[1] and that Night stood to the SW to avoid two low Islands discoverd by Captn Wallis in 1767. . . .

[1] Maurua; now called Maupiti.

APPENDIX V

Journal of William Wales

[*Mitchell Library MS. Paragraphs consisting entirely of astronomical and other observations are here omitted, except one or two short ones to illustrate Wales's close attention to scientific detail. Also omitted are the astronomical symbols for the names of days. One or two slips have been silently corrected, and a few commas altered.*]

Dusky Sound March–May 1773

MARCH 26*th*. By one o'Clock we began to advance fast into the Bay, which we found to be a large Inlet; but could find no soundings with 50 & 60 fathoms of line. About ½ past One we backed the Main Topsail, hoisted out the Boat, and an Officer went a head of the Ship to sound, and if possible find out a place to anchor in. About Two he made a signal for having found soundings, and by Three we came to an Anchor in fifty fathoms, near a large Island, and moored with an Hawser to the Shore.

In this Inlet there are a prodigeous number of small Islands most of them pretty high; and every one, though ever so small covered with Trees & herbage down to the water's edge; which it will readily be imagined must have a very beautiful appearance to us who had been out at sea between four and five Months, and most of that Time amongst dreary Islands of Ice most of which were larger & higher than those which now surrounded us: but our pleasures were not all merely Ideal; a boat which was sent to fish soon returned with as much fine Fish as the whole Ship's Company could eat. After Dinner I went with one of the Leiut^{s} to examine the Bay and look out for a better Anchoring Place & we were so fortunate as to find one complete as could be wished for. At daylight the boat was sent again to fish and I was entertained in bed with a serenade by the winged Inhabitants of the neighbouring Islands, far superior to any ever enjoyed by a Spainish Lady in the like situation. About 21^{h} we got under way & worked to windward, amongst this Labyrinth of Islands with a fine breeze from the westward, & entered our beautyful Cove by a passage whose breadth was about twice that of the Ship; where we anchored in 25 fath^{m}. In general fine weather, with gentle breezes westerly.

27*th*. At one o'Clock weighed the Anchor again, and warped the Ship opposite to a small cove, at the upper end of which was a Rivulet of fresh Water, where the small Bower was let go, and then the Ship backed into the Cove, where she was secured by Hawsers to both shores: This being done I went with Capt Cook to look out for a proper place for my Observatory & found one at some distance from the Ship which would have been very convenient, had not unforseen Accidents rendered it improper.

In the morning some of the Officers went out to examine the Bay & see what sorts of Game it produced; but had not proceeded far before they discovered some of the Natives on shore, on which they deemed it most prudent to return and acquaint the Capt with a circumstance so material; but they had scarce got on board before a Canoe full of these people came in sight; they stoped not however five minutes before they paddled back again round the point they came from. A sight, so uncommon as our Ship must be to them, would, I suppose, be sufficient to strike terror into the bravest of Mankind! Moderate wind N westerly & heavy Rain.

28*th*. About one o'Clock, the Natives came in sight again, and paddled within about 300 yards of the Ship, where they lay and viewed her with the utmost (seeming) surprize for about half an hour. The Capt ordered all the People to keep below, and then did all he could to entice them to come nearer, but to no purpose: for when they had satisfied their own Curiosity, they put about, and returned the way they came. After Diner I went along with the Capt and some other Officers to the place where they where first discovered: when we landed we found a Canoe drawn up under the bushes, a small Net made of the leaves of a tall sedgy Plant, which grows here in great plenty, and whose fibres are, if possible tougher than those of our hemp or flax, & much finer than the former;[1] several Fishes, some broiled and others raw, and two little Hutts. These Hutts were about 4 or 5 feet high, and nearly of the same breadth, made of bark and the leaves of the same Plant which the Net was; they were round on the top like an arched Vault, and were built in the thickest part of the bushes, I suppose for the sake of more Shelter, so that I could not see their length without creeping amongst the bushes which I did not chuse to do for fear of surprize. The Canoe was composed of two small ones, hollowed out of a tree each, and fastened to one another about a foot asunder by cross pieces, which were lashed to both with bandages made of the hemp Plant, as we called it. The Stems and Stern-Posts rose much higher than the body of the Canoe and the head was attempted to be carved like the upper parts of a man and two limpet shells[2] were put for the Eyes. The workmanship was but rude yet probably were we to see the tools which they have to effect it with we might be rather surprized that we found it no worse. I observed that the Bough of a Tree which lay on the beach appeared to have been cut off with about 4 or 5 strokes of a tool similar to an ax: The bough was as thick as a man's leg. Capt Cook left a hatchet, a looking glass, a medall or two & some other Toys in the Canoe.

In the morning the Capt set the People to work to make a bridge from the ship's Gunnel to the North Shore of the Cove, and as it was now judged improper for me to be so far from the Ship especially on that side where the Natives were, I went on shore there also to see if I could not find a place proper for my Observatory. The remainder of the Day was spent in clearing away the Ground; and I believe that before dinner I had cut down and destroyed more Trees & curious shrubs & Plants, than would in London

[1] *Phormium tenax*. [2] Paua *Halio*

have sold for one hundred Pounds. The former part of the Day heavy Rain the latter Showers & sun-shine alternately: moderate Wind at North-West.

29th. Employed all Day in clearing away the trees and leveling a Place for the Observatory. The Soil, in general seems to be a fine rich black Earth, and very deep; at least 3 or 4 feet. Tolerable fine weather; but frequent Showers: moderate Wind, northerly.

30th. Had two Men from the Ship to assist me in Clearing away, and made much ridance, although many of the Trees which we were obliged to fell would have made fore-Masts for the ship. The greater part of these twenty-four hours Strong Gales Northerly with heavy Rain.

31st. Still employed cutting down Trees, and errecting the Observatory: made a pretty clear opening from WBN to EBN which I judged would be sufficient for my purpose except a vista towards the South for observing Stars South of the zenith. The first part Moderate Wind with Showers; the latter perfectly Clear & fine; which is the first weather of this sort which we have had since we came in.

APRIL *1st.* Set up the Clock, and got a Puncheon filled with stones and gravel as a stand for the Quadrant; but had the mortification to find that neither one nor the other could be fixed with sufficient steadyness to answer any purpose, on account of the loosness of the ground: I was therefore necessitated to look out for another place & pitched on one where two large trees grew almost close together one of which I cut down close to the ground, and the other about 3½ feet above it. The former part fine & clear; the latter cloudy with showers, as usual: Moderate Wind, northwesterly.

2d. Leveled the ground for the observatory round the before-mentioned two Trees put up the Tent, & fixed the Iron frame for the clock on one; and set the Quad[t] on the other; and found them to answer pretty well; although a smart stamp with the foot at 7 or 8 Yards distance would still make the Plumb-line Shake very plainly in the Microscope. Brisk wind, northwesterly, & cloudy with drizzling rain at Times.

3. Fixed up a Thermometer & Barometer, and made a machine for trying the Tydes: It consists of a long square Tube whose internal side is about 3 Inches: A square float is fitted to this Tube & fixed to the end of a long slender Rod which is divided into feet and Inches from the float upwards. I propose to put down this rod into the Tube untill the float just touches the water & then mark the feet & Inches on the Rod which are even with the top of the Tube: As the water is addmited into the Tube only by a small aperture at the bottom the rise and fall of the water occassioned by the surf will be inconsiderable or at least much lessened. Wind northerly & pretty brisk: Cloudy with Rain at Times.

4th. Fixed up my Tyde-Instrument & began to observe; but to my inexpressible surprize found it too short by many feet: It was about 6 feet long & Several People, amongst whom I was one had all along concluded that the Tydes did not rise & fall more than 4 feet or four feet & an half at most; We judged by the Shore; & I mention this circumstance to shew how erroneous estimations of the rise & fall of the Tydes may sometimes be when made in this manner, as I believe they often are. The former part of the Day cloudy with frequent & heavy showers; the latter alternately clear & Cloudy with showers: moderate Wind north-westerly.

5*th*. Set about a new Tyde-measurer, which I now made 11 feet long: Cut down some more Trees which I found would be in my way since I changed my situation. Frequent and heavy showers of Rain & hail: brisk Winds all round the Compass.

6*th*. Finished and fixed up my Tyde Instrument. I placed the bottom of the Tube in the Hollow of a Rock a little below low-water-mark and tyed its top to a Tree which grew out of the bank & hung over the water: Felled the Trees which stood in my south Meridian. The first part of this day mostly cloudy with Showers, the latter constant, heavy Rain: Wind moderate and variable.

7*th*. This afternoon the Cap[t] who had been out surveying of the Bay informed us that he had met with three Natives, a Man and two Women; that the Man called to him as he was going past in the boat, and that they had parted exceeding great friends.—Rain almost without Intermission; Wind moderate & variable.

8*th*. The Cap[t] went again to the Natives & carried with him some things as presents: The whole Family were now assembled to receive him. It consisted of a Man two Women his wives, a young Girl perhaps about 16 or 17, his daughter and 5 smaller children all boys the oldest about 11 or 12 & the youngest under a year. Continued heavy Rain: Wind moderate & Variable in the two western Quarters.

9*th*. Continued heavy Rain: the wind moderate, westerly.

10*th*. The former part Cloudy with Showers, & moderate Winds, northerly: the latter part flying Clouds & almost calm.

11*th*. About Noon the Natives who had been seen by the Cap[t] and Officers as abovementioned were discovered coming towards the Ship in their Canoe. They now came within about 100 yards of the Ship and there went on Shore, hauled up their boat, left it & came over the point & sat down on the Rocks opposite the Ship, and about 20, or 30 yards from it but no perswasion could get them on board. They stayed there all the Afternoon the night & untill noon the next day: they then left us and went we know not whither, for they did not go to the place they came from.

The Man seemed to me to be near 50, was of a midling hight and very broad set; of a pleasing, open Countenance, and not the least ferosity in his looks. His hair was black of a moderate length & curled at the ends. His lips inclining to be thick, his Nose rather flat—it seemed as if the end had been pressed down to his face. His two wives were something younger than himself, and were small sized; their features not disagreeable nor in the least masculine; but one of them was rendered barely not frightfull by a large Wen which grew on her left Cheek & hung down below her Mouth. The Girl's Person was on the whole very agreeable, but rather masculine, exceeding like the old man, and I dare say a very great Pet. She soon singled out a young Fellow, one of the Ship's Company for whom she expressed great fondness & seemed very unhappy whenever he was away from her: but on his offering at some familliarities, to which I suppose he was emboldened by her apparent fondness, she left him, went and sat down between her father & mother, & I never saw her take the least notice of him afterwards except when one of the Officers offered to shoot him for the insult offered to her, and then she seemed much affected and even shed Tears. We afterwards thought she had mistaken him for one of her own sex as his features were rather femnine.

The Man seemed almost continually lost in wonder at the construction of the ship & boats and whenever any of them came near him he examined them in the strictest manner particularly how they were put together and seemed particularly pleased with the motion & effects of the Rudder which he examined & tried over & over.

The Cloathing of the Men and Women, were not that I could perceive in the least different. It consisted of a sort of mat made of the hemp-plant and feathers intermixed: this was hung over their Shoulders, and tied down before; it reached about the middle of their Thighs; below which they had no covering. The hinder part of this Ahou, as they call it, passed between their legs & was made fast to the part before. On very cold days they had over ye Ahou a very thick rug-like Garment, made of Rushes, or the very course parts of the hemp plant, which they called Buggy-Buggy.[1] Every one had a bunch of feathers, Grass &c tied under their Chins by a String which went round their necks, & the Women's hair was tied in a bunch on the Crowns of their heads & adorned with the feathers of Parrots & other birds.

A Corporal of Marines who had learned something of the New-Zeeland language last Voyage asked the Man to let him have his Daughter for a Wife; but was told that it was a matter of too great moment for him to determine on before he had consulted his God. Almost all the Night, and very often in the Day while they stayed near the ship, they Sung and made many strange Gestures, which as far as we could understand, was a conversation which they held with some Being above the Clouds.

To what I have before said of their Boats, I may now add that one is considerably larger than the other, I think that on the starboard side is about ¼th part longer than the larboard one: Those which I have seen being 18 feet & 14 f^t^ respectively. They are fixed so as to approach nearer to each other at the head than at the Stern, which is an useful precaution. The Cross pieces are made fast to the two Canoes with lashings made of the hemp Plant, and they have wash boards above the solid part of the boats fastened in the same manner, so well, that very little water can come

[1] *Pakepake.*

in between them. The Tools which they have to perform this work with are made of a green stone which is very hard and bears working to an indifferent good edge, and are used by them either as Chissells, Axes or Adzes, according as they are without or lashed in different positions to a handle.[1] They had variety of fish-hooks in their Canoes some made all of wood, others all of bone & others again part of wood & part of bone, join'd by tying them together, their lines are made of the hemp Plant some twisted as our Cordage is with two, three & four strands or twists, and others platted like the lash of a whip. The former part of this Day, fine Weather; the latter cloudy with Showers.

12*th*. Early this Evening, our Neighbours the Natives left us and went to a different place from either of those we had before seen them at. Little Wind with Cloudy weather & showers.

13*th*, 14, 15, 16, 17. Almost continual, heavy Rain, with little Wind in the SW & NW Quarters: towards the latter part of Saturday, the wind came Easterly, and the weather cleared up.

18*th*. To day our friends the Natives visited us again, and early on Monday morning the Father & Daughter came round to that side of the Ship where we had the Bridge from the Ship to the Shore, with a premeditated design, I suppose, to go on board the Ship, as they had never come there before although often invited & the way pointed out to them. Before the Man ventured onto the Bridge he stood for at least 6 or 8 minutes talking in the most solemn manner, but whether to himself, the Ship, Us, or some superior Being I dare not even hazard a guess: the Girl stood and seemed all attention. They then went over the Bridge & the Man struck several times against the Ship with a green Bough which he had in his hand before they ventured over the Gunnell. I could not help remarking that they seemed distrustful of every thing which had been our work: A remarkable instance of it was the manner of their passing over the Bridge to the Ship which was made by lying two trees from the shore to the Ship's Gunnel, to which were nailed cross pieces at Convenient Distances, and planks laid over these lengthways to walk on. One of the first mentioned trees grew out of the Bank, horizontally over the water, under which we hauled the Ship's Gunnel; the other was felled, and lay loose Now although they might have walked with the utmost ease as well as safety along the Planks, yet rather than trust to them, they choose to crawl along the single Pole which grew fast to the Shore. Moreover when they got on board the Ship they stamped on the Decks with their feet, as if to try whether or no they were firm nor did they venture into any part of her without using the same precaution.

They brought with them several things, of which we had seemed most fond, as presents to the Capt and others who had been in the boat with him when they first made friends with him. They stayed the whole fore

[1] This seems good evidence for the existence of a Maori axe, as distinct from the adze. Cf. I, p. 285 n.

noon vissited every part of the Ship, with which they seemed much delighted; but most particularly so with a few sheep which we had yet left; and the Cats; the Dogs they seemed much in fear of; nor did they much excite their curiosity from whence I concluded they were no strangers to them.

19*th.* Cloudy at times but very fine Weather. Winds light & variable easterly. The Natives left us.

20*th.* Fine Clear Weather, with gentle Breezes easterly. Capt Cook and others returned from a Cruse towards the head of the Bay where they had met with many more Indians, all of the same friendly disposition with those who left us yesterday.

21*st.* Some Showers, but in general fine weather, all the former Part: the latter Cloudy with Rain. Capt Cook informed me that it was necessary to get my things on board the Ship, as he intended to haul off into a convenient place & go away the first Opportunity.

22*d.* Fine Weather, the wind easterly. Took down the Clock and got it the Iron Work and most other things on board the Ship; but left the Quad^{t} in hopes of getting two or three Equal Altitudes by Mr Kendall's Watch, and the rather as there was to be a visible eclipse of Jupiter's first satellite on the saturday following.

23*d*, 24. Pretty fine weather considering the Place but mostly Cloudy with now & then a shower: Gentle Breezes westerly.

25*th.* Very fine and clear, the wind westerly.

26*th.* Rain most part of the twenty four hours: Wind north easterly. Hove the Ship out of the Cove.

27*th.* Cloudy, with heavy Showers, & moderate winds at North-West.

28*th.* Cloudy with Showers, and light breezes westerly. Got every thing which I had left on shore aboard the Ship.

29*th.* Light breezes westerly with Showers. At 2 oClock we got under sail, and at 5 Anchored in another part of the Bay in 50 fathoms. At 22^{h} hove up the Anchor again and made Sail; and as we passed along one of Nature's most romantic Scenes presented it self to our view; for on the top of a very high mountain, and they are all very high and steep,

> Smooth to the shelving brink a copious flood
> Roll'd fair, and placid; where collected all,
> In one impetuous torrent, down the Steep
> It thundering shot, and shook the country round.
> At first, an azure sheet, it rushed broad;
> Then whitening by degrees, as prone it fell,
> And from the loud resounding Rocks below
> Dash'd in a cloud of foam, it sent aloft
> A hoary mist, in which Sol's lucid beams,

Refracted, form'd a tripple coloured bow.
Nor could the torture'd wave find here repose:
But raging still amidst the shaggy Rocks,
Now flashing o'er the scatter'd fragments, now
Aslant the hollow channel darting swift;
'Till falling oft from graduall slope to slope,
With wild infracted Course, and lessening roar,
It gained a safer bed.

I dare not write *Thomson* at the bottom: I know I have injured him; but it could not be avoided.[1]

30*th*. About 6 oClock anchored near the Shore in 35 fathoms water and made fast to the Shore with a hawser. At 19^{h} weighed & made sail with a gentle breeze at NE. Frequent Showers.

MAY 1*st*. About two o'Clock bore away for a Cove where we Anchored in 30 fathoms and moored with an Hawser to the Shore. Light Breezes, variable, with drizzling Rain at Times.

2*d*. Calm with Showers. About 21^{h} wound up the watches & went up the sound to shoot with some of the Officers. This is the first Days Amusement I have been able to take since I came to this Place.—I might with great Truth have said since I left England.

3*d*. Most part Calm with heavy Rain. About 9 oClock we returned on board the Ship with not a dry thread about us. I am right served for repining in the Morning. We however brought with us great plenty of Ducks, Pidgeons, Curlews, Hens &c &c. Indeed we have never wanted either Wild-Fowl or Fish since we came here. In this Day's excursion we met with a Cove, if possible more beautiful and convenient than that where the Ship lay, & which had escaped the notice of all our surveyors; and a Cascade to which that above mentioned was no more like

—'Than I to Hercules'.

And to which Thomson's description would have suited without the least Alteration; whereas I was obliged to make the *Bow-Lines*[2] entirely new for that, and no man living is less able than I am to bear an expence of that nature. But young Travellers, like young Wits, and young Girls too for that matter, are apt to let their imaginations run riot, and ever think the first that offers a Phoenix; whereas could they but have patience, another infinitely its superior would present it self—Probatum est!

[1] *Summer*, from Thomson's *Seasons*, with some inaccuracies: no doubt Wales was quoting from memory, and he has put Thomson's present tenses into the past. The lines, 'in which Sol's lucid beams,/Refracted, form'd a tripple coloured bow', are his own invention, but in spite of his modesty do not fall noticeably below Thomson's standard.

[2] i.e. the lines about the rainbow. We do not elsewhere find Wales punning, either in his journal or in the reminiscences of his later pupils—some of whom were devoted to puns to the point of aberration. But it is said that 'his ready wit . . . frequently elicited the hearty mirth of his juvenile auditors' (Trollope, *History of Christ's Hospital*, 1834, p. 94); and he may have fallen.

4th. Gentle Breezes variable with frequent Showers. About one o'Clock got under way with a light breeze then at SW which carried us into the mouth of a long narrow Passage or Sound which opened into the Sea; where we anchor'd, it falling Calm, in 30 fathoms Water and moored with a Hawser to the Shore. In the Night we had Thunder & Lightening attended with Hail & in the Morning we saw the Tops of the Hills all round us covered with Snow. We had perceived for a fortnight past, that the Tops of some remote ones which are very high were covered.

5th. Cloudy with Smart Showers, and gentle Breezes chiefly south westerly. At two o'Clock weighed and got under way; and about Eight anchored near a Point which Sheltered us from the Sea in 16 fathoms water and moored with a Hawser to the Shore.

6th. First part Cloudy with showers & moderate Wind at North-west. In the Night we had much Thunder and Lightening with heavy showers of hail & rain & strong Gales of Wind: The latter part strong wind & much Rain.

7th. Strong Gales of Wind at NW and Rainy Weather. The Tops of Hills which are almost perpendicular and whose bottoms are close to the Ship are now covered with Snow; yet none falls with us. We have instead thereof plenty of Rain & cold raw Weather.

8th. Brisk Wind, Variable & mostly Cloudy with Showers. I had frequently to Day an opportunity [of] viewing a Phaenomenon which to me appeared very curious, viz. the descent of the Snow on the Tops of the neighbouring Hills. Very thick whitish Clouds were continually flying over us, and when they approached the Top of any high Hill began to extend themselves towards it in a sort of conical form, as if attracted thereby, & soon after the Top of the Hill was entirely Covered. These Clouds grew visibly less dense by degrees, and in a little were entirely dispersed by the wind; and it then appeared that all that part of the Hill which had been hidden by the Cloud was covered with Snow.

9th. The former Part tolerable fine weather; the latter strong Gales from the NE with rain.

10th. First part and Night moderate wind with Showers of Hail and Rain: The latter gentle Breezes with flying Clouds. At 21^h got under way with a fine Breeze at SE and at Noon the Northermost Entrance into Dusky Bay (out of which we came) bore ESE dist. by estimation 5 Miles. The outermost Island which lies off the said Entrance SEBS about one Mile. The most southerly land in sight bore S 28°W and the most Northerly N 8°E. The meridian Altitude of the Sun was 26°21¼′ and consequently the Latitude 45°34½′S.

We are now (thank God) leaving this dirty, and, on that Account, disagreeable Place;[1] after a stay of near Six Weeks, during the greater part

[1] Cf. Clerke on 'this good Bay', pp. 755–6 above.

of which I was continually troubled with severe Colds, attended with a fever owing to my being almost always wet, and sometimes so bad that it was with the utmost difficulty that I attended my bussiness. But before I quit it entirely it may not be amiss to give the best Account that I can of it; and what future voyagers may expect to find there.

And amongst the most material, he may be certain of meeting with an almost continued series of rainy weather, at least at this time of the year; owing, I suppose to the number, and prodigeous height of the Hills, which not only surround, but are also scattered up and down in the Bay: For every Island, of which there are almost an infinite number, is a mountain; and the Country a heap of Mountains piled one upon another, untill you lose their Tops in the Clouds. There were some whose Tops I scarce ever saw while I was there. Their sides are almost perpendicular and covered with tall Trees almost down to the waters edge. The Mold is black and very deep; evidently composed of decayed Vegetables, and so loose that I could make the plumb line of my Astronomical Quadrant shake when placed on the Stump of a large tree by jumping on the Ground at 10 or 12 Yards distance; and this I conceive to be the reason why we meet with such great numbers of large trees, as we do, blown down by the Wind even in the thickest parts of the Woods. All the Ground amongst the Trees is covered with Moss and Ferns, of both which there is a wonderful variety; but very little herbage of any other sort, and none that was eatable that we found, except about a handful of water-cresses, which Mr Pattin, the Surgeon found just before we came away. The Trees are of various kinds but all new to me. Some, of a kind somewhat between the Spruce & Ceader large enough to make main Masts for Ships of 500 Tun's Burthen,[1] and others, which I dare say would make excellent Timber for the use of Cabinet-makers, &c; one in particular whose wood is almost as hard as Lignum Vitae and as beautiful as Cedar.[2] The Number, and Variety of aromatic Trees and shrubs are very great, most of the myrtle kind amongst which the pimento[3] is very plentiful. But amidst all this great variety we met with none which bore fruit fit to eat. I saw not one of the Apple or Nut Tribe, & but one of the Plumb. This much resembled a small Olive and was very full of an oil of a yellowish Colour, which smelt & tasted exactly like Turpentine.[4] The seeds of all the rest were of the berry kind; full of seeds and of a disagreeable tast. In most parts the woods are so over run with supple-Jacks,[5] that it is impossible to force one's way amongst

[1] The Rimu, *Dacrydium cupressinum*.

[2] Hardness suggests first the Southern Rata (sometimes called Ironwood), *Metrosideros umbellata;* but mention of the cedar suggests also the straight-grained Matai or Black Pine, *Podocarpus spicata*—hard, though not so hard as the Southern Rata. Wales would find them both.

[3] Probably the myrtle Rohutu, *Myrtus pedunculata*, a large-leaved form of which is abundant throughout the southern fiord district of New Zealand.

[4] This must be the unripe fruit of the Miro, *Podocarpus ferrugineus;* the fruit ripens in the winter and then takes on a bright red colour. It has, as Wales notes, the smell and taste of turpentine.

[5] *Rhipogonum scandens*, still a marked and sometimes maddening feature of the New Zealand bush.

them: several which I have seen are at least 50 & 60 fathoms long. Some species of the Ferns have stems 18 & 20 feet high and as thick as a man's thigh. The leaves, or rather branches, all shoot out horizontally at the Top and form a Circle at least 3 or 4 Yards in diameter.[1] These Fern-Trees as we called them contradict part of the note p. 139 of Mr Lee's Introduct. to Bot.[2] in as much as the stem here spoken of, has the very characteristic which he mentions.

Of Fowl we had great plenty, amongst which we enumerate large and very beautiful Wood-Pidgeons;[3] Ducks of a variety of sorts, all exceeding good; one, which on account of its varigated plumage, we called the *painted Duck* was the most beautiful bird I ever saw.[4] Besides these we had Teal, Curlews, Water hens, Parrots, Parakeets[5] & innumerable birds of a lesser size: amongst these I must not omitt to particularize two or three, on account of their singularity.

First the Wattle-Bird, so called because of its having two Wattles under its beak as large as those of a small dunghill Cock, is considerably larger, particularly in length, than an English Blackbird. Its Bill is short & thick, and its feathers of a dark lead-colour; the colour of its Wattles is a dull yellow; almost an Orange-colour.[6]

Another remarkable one was by the Gentlemen in the Endeavour's Voyage, called the poy-Bird.[7] This also is larger than a Black-Bird; but less than the Wattle-Bird. The feathers are of a fine Mazarine Blue except those of its neck, which are of a most beautiful silver Grey; and two or three short white ones which are on the pinion-joint of the wing. Under its Throat hang two little tufts of curled, snow-white feathers, called its *poys*, which is an Otahitee word for Ear-rings.[8] On the whole, whatever Idea this description may convey, the plumage of this bird is exceeding remarkable and beautiful.

The last I shal mention is the Fan-Tail. Of these there are different sorts, but the body of the most remarkable one is scarce larger than a good Filbert, yet spreads a tail of most beautiful plumage full ¾ of a semi-circle, of, at least, 4 or 5 Inches radius.[9]

[1] Wales may have been thinking in particular of the Tree Fern *Cyathea smithii*.

[2] James Lee (1715–95), a well-known Hammersmith nurseryman, was a correspondent of Linnaeus, and translated some of his work into English, under the title of *An Introduction to the Science of Botany* (1760 and later eds.). In the 1765 edition, a footnote on p. 139 describes '*Filices, Ferns*', otherwise called '*Acaules*, without Stems; for in these Plants, what rises out of the Ground is plainly a Leaf only: One of the Characters of a Stem or Trunk is to be alike on every Side; but in the Stalks of Ferns, there is manifestly a Front and back . . . which shews them to be Leaves'.

[3] The Kereru, *Hemiphaga novaeseelandiae*.

[4] The Paradise Duck, *Casarca variegata*.

[5] The Red-fronted Parrakeet or Kakariki, *Cyanoramphus novaezelandiae*, was collected in Dusky Sound by both Sparrman and Forster, and first described by Sparrman. The other birds in this list are identified in the notes to Cook; the 'Water hen' being with Cook simply another name for the Woodhen or Weka.

[6] The South Island Crow or Kokako, *Callaeas cinerea*.

[7] The Tui or Parson Bird, *Prosthemadera novaeseelandiae*.

[8] *Poe*, a pearl.

[9] The New Zealand Fantail, *Rhipidura fuliginosa* Sparrman, is a dimorphic species. A specimen was taken by Forster the day after the *Resolution* entered Dusky Sound, and this is probably the bird to which Wales refers.

It appeared odd enough, at least to me, to see the Birds here so very familiar with us, as if they had not the least Idea of our being their Enemies. It was not uncommon for them to perch on the barrel of the Gun in our hands, already loaded for their destruction. This makes either for or against the Doctrine of Inate Ideas: for either they were possessed of none, and so perched there indifferent or else they were, & knew there was less danger to be apprehended whilst there, than when at a few yards from the muzzle.

The Hens, as we called them were a sort of *Rail*, which would stand & stare at us untill we knocked them down with a stick, so that at length it was accounted rather a descredit to have shot one.[1]

But our principle, and indeed an inexhaustable Store was the Fishery. A boat with a petty Officer and Six Men constantly supplied the whole Ship's Company with as much as they could eat, and yet used nothing to catch them with but hooks and lines. Nor was the plenty greater than the variety, of which most are, I believe, peculiar to this place; but there are not wanting Several Sorts that are well known; such as Mullet, Cavallas, Guard-Fish, Horse-Mackeral &c. Amongst the crustacous Tribe we found Craw-Fish, Muscles, Cockles, Scollops Whelks Periwinkles, and many others whose Names I am not acquainted with.

I met with no minerals, or fossills, except a few inconsiderable pieces of Talk, but was informed that some of the Gentlemen met with a specimen of silver Ore.[2]

With respect to Nautical and Geographical Remarks, I have little to say. My Bussiness confined me entirely to the Ship, and had it been otherwise, boats would have been wanting; but I regreted it the less, as Cap[t] Cook, whose Skill & experience in these Matters, is perhaps inferior to none, made them his particular Bussiness: But it may, I believe with great truth be said that no place affords a greater variety of safe and convenient Coves for a Ship to lie in; better shelter from the Winds, or greater plenty of good Water & wood.

Queen Charlotte Sound May–June 1773

18*th*. Very little wind & fine weather. Towed up the Sound. About 2[h] the Adventure's boat came on board with two officers who informed us they were all well, and had been in Charlotte Sound about six weeks. That they had made the South point of New Holland, where they wood[ed], watered, and stoped 4 or 5 Days, after which they traced the Coast within a few leagues of the Place where Cap[t] Cook fell in with it in his last Voyage. About 3[h] came to an Anchor in 15 fath[ms]. In the morning weighed, and towed nearer the Shore, where we anchored in 11 fathoms and moor'd with a Hawser to the Shore. As soon as this was done I desired Cap[t] Cook to set me on Shore to make observations; but he informed me that we should not stop here, and that he had already desired Cap[t] Furneaux to order M[r] Bayley on board without delay.

[1] The Weka, *Gallirallus australis*.
[2] No other gentleman has ever met with one.

19*th.* Little wind south-westerly and pleasant Weather. This morning early two Boats were sent to fish, and a party of Men to haul the Sean; but all returned without success. Capt Cook was more successfull, who went to look for Greens, for he returned with the Pinnace loaded with wild Cellery, Lambs-quarter, &c, which it may be supposed were very acceptable to us after so long an absence from every thing of that nature. The Adventure's People also on their first arrival here had sown great quantities of seeds such as Mustard, Cresses, Radishes &c. and they were no churls of what they had. At noon I returned from a visit to Mr Bayley with a large handkerchief full of these last; which were not less welcome than the former.

20*th.* Moderate Wind Northerly, and Cloudy Weather. Having now reasons to suppose it would be at least 3 or 4 days before we were ready to sail, I got my astronomical Quadrant on shore at a Beach near the ship, and set up a Cask filled with water for a Stand, in order to get a few equal Altitudes, & if possible see what Rates the Watches now had: but the place was very inconvenient as the hills to the westward were so high that I could not get the sun later than about 20 minutes past two o'Clock.

21*st.* Wind moderate, & variable almost all round the Compass: mostly Cloudy.

22*d.* Moderate Wind northerly, and Cloudy weather. Several of the Natives came on board us without any ceremony. I had conceived vast things from report of the New-Zeelanders to the Northward of Dusky Bay But must confess my self much disappointed.

23*d.* Light Breezes south-westerly, and fine Weather for the most Part: More of the Natives on board: I cannot help again making a comparison between these and our late friends at Dusky Bay. These are importunate for every thing they see, and are as great thieves as the Eskimaux; but want much of their ingenuity in concealing it: whereas those at dusky Bay scarce ever asked for any thing, or ever received any considerable Present without making one in return, and that in Articles which to them must be very valuable. As to stealing, for aught that I saw to the contrary, their Creator had utterly deprived them of the Idea.

24*th.* Brisk Wind, Westerly and tolerable fine Weather, all the first part; afterwards Cloudy with Rain.

25*th*, 26, 27, 28, 29. Mostly cloudy with showers; the Wind generally pretty brisk, and chiefly south-westerly. The Natives, more or less of them on board almost every Day, to try what they could either beg or steal; and nothing came amiss. One of them ventured up to our Top-Gallt Mast head; and, if we did not misunderstand him told us he could wish to go with us. He and three others refused to go away with the rest, and were left on board: In the Evening they had something given them to eat and had a clean dry sail spread for them under one of the Gang-ways where they lay down and slept 'till about 10 oClock when two old men came alongside in a Canoe to enquire for them. The Officer then on deck shewed them where they were & waked them: Two were preswaded by the Seniors to go with them, but the others absolutely refused, and lay themselves down & slept untill Morning seemingly without the least dread; notwithstanding it was afterwards discovered that one of them was in possession of a Vol. of Tom Jones, which he had stole out of an Officers Cabbin, who had done every thing he could to entertain them; and the other of a hand lead which he had *found* on the Quarter Deck.

29*th*. When we came to wind up the Watches at Noon, it was found that the middle Lock to Mr Arnold's Watch was damaged, and could not be opened, I suppose by its being opened yesterday with a wrong Key through mistake. It was proposed to open the Box by sawing of the Staples in to which the Bolts of the lock shoot; but being apprehensive that the action of the saw might shake the watch too much, I proposed that the screws which fast[n] these Staples to the cover of the box might be wrenched out, by introducing the blade of a screw Driver, & turning it round; and which was accordingly put in execution. As some damage was done to the Lock by this Accident, the Lock was taken off and the Watch trusted under the other two untill it was repaired.

30*th*. Moderate Breezes westerly and fine Weather. Many Natives on Board who stole the Centry's Lamp & 4 hour Glass, but had not address enough to get off with them undiscovered.

31*st*, JUNE 1*st*, 2*d*. Mostly Cloudy with Showers. The Natives continue to come and go.

3*d*. Fine Clear Weather with Moderate Wind at SW. Several Cannoes of Natives whom we had not seen before came along side: these seemed to make a little more Conscience, or at least were more afraid of stealing from us, than what those we had seen before were.

⁂One of our Boats which had been out on duty was chased by two Canoes of strange Natives.—Put the middle Lock on M[r] Arnold's Watch again.

4*th*. Moderate Wind southerly, and Cloudy Weather. Many Natives whome we had never seen before came along-side of us. Before they ventured to come very near us two of the Men who seemed to be Chiefs amongst them pronounced very loud and long Orations, at the same time holding in their hands a green bough, all the others observing much attention. Our old Neighbours who were now also on board us were much terifyed at the sight of them. The Men trembled the women made loud Lamentations; both joined in assuring us that these New-comers were their Enemies & would Murder them, if we did not shoot them with our Guns. We assured them in the strongest manner we could they should not be hurt; but it was to no purpose, for as soon as ever they saw them along side, they all sliped into their own Canoe, which happened to be on the other side of the Ship, and crept away close along shore for fear of being discovered. We afterwards found that there were seven large Cannoes of these New-comers, and that they came from somewere towards, if not actually from the Northern Island. They were much better Clad, and provided with Arms than any we had seen before, so that the other poor Wretches had Cause enough to be alarmed; but before we had done with them we brought them nearer on a par by purchasing all their weapons that we could, either offensive or defensive. Neither party came on board us any more; but we had reasons to suppose they had settled matters amicably as we frequently saw Canoes go from one place to another.

5*th*. Strong Wind at SSE with rain. Computed the Rates of the Two Watches from the Equal Altitudes that I had taken here & found that M[r] Kendall's was gaining 9″.05 P. Day & M[r] Arnold's losing 94.158 P. Day on mean Time.

6*th*. The former part of this Day strong Gales at SSE & Cloudy with rain: the latter Moderate Wind, south-westerly and tolerable fine Weather. At 16[h] the Ship was unmoored, & about 19[h] under way: At Noon the Two Brothers bore WBN dist. about a Mile, & were in a line with Cape Koamaroo. The Latitude observed was 41°08⅓′S. The Adventure, once more, in Company.

Being going to leave this land of Canibals, as it is now generally thought to be, it may be expected that I should record what bloody Massacres I have been a witness of; how many human Carcases I have seen roasted and eaten; or at least relate such Facts as have fallen within the Compass of my Observation tending to confirm the Opinion, now almost universally believed, that the New Zeelanders are guilty of this most detestable Practice. Truth, notwithstanding, obliges me to declare, however unpopular it may be, that I have not seen the least signs of any such custom being amongst them, either in Dusky Bay or Charlotte sound; although the latter place is that where the only Instance of it was *seen* in the Endeavour's Voyage. I know it is urged as a proof positive against them, that in the representation of their War-Exercise, which they were very fond of shewing us, they confessed the Fact. The real state of the Case is this. They first began with shewing us how they handled their Weapons, how they defyed the Enemy to Battle, how they killed him: they then proceeded to cut of his head, legs & arms; they afterwards took out his Bowels & threw them away, and lastly shewed us that they went to eating. But it ought by all means to be remarked that all this was shewn by signs which every one will allow are easily misunderstood, and for any thing that I know to the contrary they might mean they Eat the Man they had just killed; but is it not as likely that after the Engagement they refreshed themselves with some other Victuals which they might have with them? It ought farther to be remarked that I did not see one out of the many who went through those Massacres, who did not stop before he made the sign of eating; or that did it before some of us made the sign, as if to remind him that he had forgot that part of the Ceremony. This circumstance is brought as a proof both that they are, and that they are not Caniballs. One says, it is plain they Eat their Enemy after they have killed him, but are ashamed to acknowledge it, because they know we disapprove of it. The others say no; it is plain they looked on the Action as complete & stoped, untill you reminded them that it was necessary to take some refreshment after their Labour.

No stronger proofs, than the above have been seen by any person on board the Resolution this Voyage: but more substantial ones are said to have been seen on board the Adventure. One of the Gentlemen found amongst the Baggage in a Canoe, a raw human head, cut off close to the shoulders. This discovery is said to have produced much consternation amongst the People in the Canoe, who put it out of sight again with all possible expedition, nor could it be found afterwards. But hard as this circumstance is made to bear against them, it does by no means follow with certainty that this Head was preserved to be eaten: Saul, had he been a stranger to the Affair, might with equal justice have concluded that David was a Caniball when he was brought before him with the Head of Goliath in his hand. On the other side it must be admitted that after what is reported to have been seen here in the Endeavour's Voyage it was most natural to conclude that this head was intended for a very different purpose than that which David carried his up to Jerusalem for.

I cannot help relating a circumstance or two before I quit the subject entirely, as they tend to shew how far we are liable to be misled by Signs, report, & prejudice. Two Canoes of Natives came alongside one of the Ships & after they had traded such little matters as they had, went away out of the Sound. Sometime after One Canoe only returned & the people of the ship enquired ernestly what was become of the other. They made the same sign they do at the conclusion of their Exercise and it was immediately concluded that they had met with Enemies who had killed & eaten them; and it would certainly have passed so, had not the other Canoe returned a day or two after with every soul in it alive & well. Another circumstance is the following. A person on board the Adventure not only asserted that he saw one Indian killed by the others, but also related the particulars and manner in which it was done: nay it had gone so far on board our Ship with some as to suppose that a fire which we saw on shore, had been kindled to dress him at, & it was expected that Cap[t] Cook who was gone on shore at the place would surprize them in the very fact & probably bring on board some part of the unhappy Victim, to silence all unbelievers of this Custom for the future. The Cap[t] notwithstanding returned without having seen any thing of the sort; & it was afterwards certainly known that the man was not only un-roasted, but even alive and well.

Tahiti and the Society Islands August–September 1773

AUGUST 17*th*. Enquired of Cap[t] Cook about carrying on Shore my Observatory, and Instruments, who told me he should not Stop long here, and that it would not suit him to have a Guard on shore, without which I did not think it would be prudent to go my self, having already seen too much to think I was capable of guarding against such expert Thieves;—

I therefore set my self to make the best Observations which I could on board the Ship. Light Breezes, chiefly from the Land and fine Weather.

18*th.* To Day Isaac Taylor, a Marine, died and was buried. I find little time is left for a Man to come to life again. There is however one comfort attending burials at Sea, if they give no time for them to come to themselves before they are buried, there is no danger of their doing it afterwards; and I know not of a more dreadfull Idea which can come across a man's mind, than that of being deposited in a Vault, merely on this Account. But to recur once more to Isaac Taylor whose disorder was a Dropsy.— He was the first Person who has died on board the Resolution since we left England.— The Natives still continued to bring us off plenty of Breadfruit, Cocoa-Nuts Bananas Apples Nectrines &c which we purchased at a very moderate rate, viz. 3 or 4 cocoa Nuts for a Glass Bead and others in proportion; but notwithstanding all that has been said of Hogs & Poultry by former Voyagers, I have not yet seen one of either sort which they would part from.—Very fine Weather, with light, Variable Winds but chiefly from the Sea in the Day-time & from the Land in the Night.

19*th.* The Weather pretty much the same as yesterday. Vast Numbers of the Natives on board the Ship some to trade and others to see what they can steal: but I believe the value of those Articles which they have hitherto got by traffic bears but a very small proportion to that of those which they have stolen. . . .

20*th.* Very little wind all day from the South East and very fine Weather: the Heat being more moderate than on the former days which we have lain here. The Natives again on board following both their Occupations as unconcerned as ever.

21*st.* The former part little wind and fine Weather. Having Completed watering the ship, Unmoored her at 5 & rode with the best Bower, and a whole Cable, intending to sail in the Morning for another Part of the Island; but instead of that we had a very strong Wind from the NW which brought in a heavy swell. The Natives still continue to bring us plenty of several sorts of fruits, also Yams & another very agreeable Root which they call *Tarra.* It is not found any where, I believe, except here and in the neighbouring Islands; but we have not got one Hog yet.

22*d.* Calm, and the Air extreamly hot. The Capt[t] went in search of the *Aree*, or King of this part of the Island, whose Name it seems is *Owhyadoa* to see if he could not procure some Hogs, for this Article, as far as we can gather from those Natives who Visited us is entirely under his direction, and they dare not part with one without permission from him.—Several of our People being on shore to Day, told us on their return that they had seen an European who ran directly from them into the Woods, and that by his appearance they judged him to be a Frenchman:[1] some Gentlemen who were then on shore endeavoured to enquire of the Natives concerning him and understood that a French Ship had been late here whose Cap[t] had told them he would return in 5 Months and that the Person who had been seen was left behind untill his return.

23*d*. Light breezes from various points of the Compass, and Cloudy with Showers. The Cap[t] returned from his Visit to the King, Owhyadoa, having with much difficulty, and expince in presents &c procured three Hogs. He found him a very young Man, who had but newly arrived at his present dignity, on the death of his Father. He seemed, I am told much frightened, and was surrounded with a vast number of the inferior *Arees*, who had been on board the Ship, and who it was supposed had contributed a good deal to increase his fears in order to keep him from us. To day a more strict enquiry has been made into the Affair of the Frenchman by some who pretend to understand the language best, and they bring back a very different Story. The ship is now spanish; and the Cap[t], whilst here, hanged three or four of his People,[2] and this escaped from him. I for my part, after examining the two persons who pretend to have seen him, think there is not the least reason to imagine that the Man they saw was an European. His Dress was not in the least it seems different from the others, only he was whiter than they, and ran away into the Woods as soon as he saw them. On the whole that there may have been a French or spanish Ship here since the Endeavour is very probable; but, in my opinion, all the rest of the story is a mere Fiction.

About 18[h] we weighed, and were towed out of the Harbour by the Boats; but the Cutter was left behind under the Command of an Officer to try if he could not purchase a few Hogs, after they saw the Ship gone, and no hopes remaining of getting our Axes any way else. At Noon the Point of Land which forms the eastern side of the Bay bore SW about 2 Leagues distant, and the most northerly land in sight NW$\frac{3}{4}$W. The Latitude Observed was 17°42′S. In general, the wind has blown off the Land from about 5 or 6 o'Clock in the Evening untill 9 or 10 in the Morning about which time a light breeze came in from the sea; but this was by no means regular, and indeed we had very little wind all the time we lay here. The Bay which we lay in here is called Oaiti-peha, and takes its name from the neighbouring districts.

24*th*. At 6 o'Clock the northermost land in sight bore W$\frac{1}{2}$N and the most southerly SBE. We stood West & west $\frac{1}{2}$ North about 10 Miles untill 12 o'Clock, when it fell calm and continued so untill 4 in the Morning, when

[1] According to Burney, Ferguson MS (following 18 August), 'one of the men spoke to him in broken french, "parly vou francee Mons[r]" the supposed frenchman made no answer, but on the question being repeated ran away laughing—I won't pretend to determine whether or not this was a frenchman but I am very much inclined to think our people were mistaken, however M[r] Forster wrote a Letter in french which he gave to one of the Natives, but we never heard the fate of it.'

[2] According to Forster, I, p. 308, this story, quite untrue, came from Vehiatua. It is rather curious that Cook ignores the whole matter in his journal.

a small breeze sprung up at east, but which soon veered round to the south-west & from thence WBN & we then steered SBW and at Noon Point Venus bore WSW about 3 Miles.

25*th*. About 2 oClock Mr Pickersgill joined us in the Cutter having picked up 8 Hogs at divers places as he came along shore & which was to us an almost invaluable Acquisition. About 4 oClock stood into Matavi Bay through the Passage which lies between the Larboard Reef & Dolphin Bank, and at 5 came to an Anchor in 7 fathoms Water and Moored with the stream Anchor. The wind beginning to slacken our boats & Men were sent to assist the Adventure, and about 7 oClock she also came safe to an Anchor.—In the Morning a Party of Marines being sent on Shore as a Guard, I landed my Observatory and Instruments and begun to put them up on the Spot where Mr Green Observed the Transit of Venus in 1769, which has every advantage which could be wished for such a purpose.—Light, variable Winds with flying Clouds.

26*th*. Employed in putting up the Observatories & Instruments, & in making Observations. The former part Cloudy, the latter quite clear; Weather Very hot & little Wind.

27*th*, 28*th*, 29*th*, 30*th*. Employed making various sorts of Observations on shore (Vide Observ^n^ Book) During all which time we had little Wind and exceeding Hot Weather. It was generally Cloudy in the Afternoons and exceeding Clear all the forenoons. The Clouds began to Gather about the high Peak of Otahitee about Noon & soon after spread themselves towards the North untill the whole Hemisphere was covered by them. I scarce ever in my life passed four more agreeable Days than these were; for the few spare Hours which I had I never wanted amusement, as we had seldom less than four or five hundred of the Natives of All Ranks & sexes round our little Encampment, and I did not fail to profit by the Opportunity of trying and studying their Tempers & disposition with the Utmost Attention. It may surprize some to be told that an extent of 60 Yards in front, and near 30 in depth, was guarded from such a body of People by only 4 Centinals, with no other lines to assist them, but a rope stretched from Post to Post, & that often so slack as to lay on the ground; but it is nevertheless true, and that so effectually that none of us ever received the least insult or incivillity from any of them, nor did any of them come within our lines without leave: so terrible did Capt Wallace make the sight of a Gun to the Inhabitants of Otahitee!

31*st*. A little after 9 oClock in the Morning we began to take down the Observatories Clocks Instruments &c and by ½ past 11 they were all packed up and ready to put into the Boat, and by Noon they were all safe on board the Ship again.

Although so many Visits have now been made to this celebrated Island, and so much said of it by Europeans that it may be supposed nothing material can be added on the Subject; yet, since it appears to me that some particulars have either been misrepresented, or Misunderstood, and others omitted which I know will by many Persons be deemed Curious, I hope I may be excused in adding a word or two on the Subject & representing matters as they appeared to Me.

As to its Geography, little is left to be said. My Latitude of Point Venus does not differ two seconds from that which Mr Green & Capt Cook had before found it, and its Longitude, for anything that I yet know to the Contrary is as exact. But the Occultation of β Capricorni which we observed here will determine that point to great precission if the Moon's place shall have been observed at Greenwich, on the same day. The Bay of Oaiti-peha, where we first anchored lies in Latitude 17°46′28″ s and Longit. 0°21′25½″ E from Point Venus, that is in 210°46′36″ E from Greenwich. The Latitude results from taking a Mean of 6 Observations of the Sun's Meridian Altitude and the Longitude is that shewn by Mr Kendall's Watch, allowing its dayly gain on Mean time to be 8″.863 a day, which is what I have found it to be, when on shore at this place.

I looked in vain for its situation in M. Bougainville's Voyage, although the Article *Geographical* situation stands in the Margin. He seems industriously to have concealed his Latitudes and longitudes during his whole run across this vast Ocean: the reasons for which are difficult to assign; since he has given Maps, which if any thing near the truth will be sufficient to defeat any purpose which he could have in concealing them. His Map of this place errs about 1°¼ in the Longitude of the north point of the Island; and, which is a much more unpardonable Error, about ⅓ of a Degree in its Latitude. It is very possible these errors may not belong to Mr Bougainville, as I have only the English Edition, where the Maps are expressly said to be altered and Corrected, the Method of doing which by persons who have never seen the place, I must confess, I do not understand.—It appears very strange to me how the Observations which were made here by *Mr Veron*[1] could differ 7 or 8 degrees from one another, unless there was some very great defect in the Instrument, or want of Care in the Observer. I should imagine, Observations of the kind which he mentions when made on the same day ought not to differ more than as many minutes.

The face of the Country, making some allowance for a warm imagination, is not badly described by Mr Bougainville; but some allowances must be made by every Person, who has not seen the Place, and would not be deceived. That Gentleman seems to have been almost lost in admiration of its Beauties, and those of its Inhabitants all the time he was here. His colouring is indeed so high, that one cannot help suspecting a false glace;[2] for his description suits much better with Mahomet's Paradise, than any terrestial Region: It must notwithstanding be allowed to be a very beautiful Island, and appears, no doubt, to great advantage after a long Voyage. I remember well that England does so, and run no risk in asserting that Otahitee would make but an indifferent appearance if placed beside it.

The Lands here do not seem to be considered as private property, any

[1] Properly Verron—the astronomer with Bougainville.
[2] i.e. gloze.

farther than as they are planted with fruit Trees, Yams, &c all which are manifestly so: and it appeared to me that the property of the land was rather determined by the Trees which were Planted on it than that of the Trees by the Land whereon they were planted, as in England.[1] I conceive that it is lawfull for any person to raise a Plantation on Ground not already occupied by another.

With regard to the Personal Beauties of the Otahitean Ladies, I believe it would be most prudent to remain entirely silent; since by a contrary preceedure I must expose in the grossest manner my own want of tast, or that of those Gentlemen who have asserted that 'they may vie with the greatest beauties of Europe', and that 'the English Women appeared Verry ordinery on their first arrival there' from this celebrated Cythera: but it is no new thing for the itch of writing to get the better of prudence; it will not therefore be wondered at if I run all risks of this kind to have the pleasure of describing their persons; at least, so far as there appears to be any national characteristic in it. In the first place then their stature is very small, and their features although rather regular have a masculine turn. Their Complexion is a light Olive, or rather a deadish Yellow; their hair is of a glossy black and cut short in the bowl-dish fashion of the Country People in England; but had here, I think, a pretty effect, as it corresponded more with the simplicity of their Dress than any other form would. Their Eyes are exceeding black and lively but rather too prominent for my liking. Their noses are flat especially towards the lower end and their nostrils in consequence wide, as are also their mouths. Their lips are rather thick than otherwise; but their teeth are remarkable close, white, and even. The Breasts of the young ones before they have had Children are very round and beautifull, but those of the old ones hang down to their Navals. I have no occasion to call in the Aids of Imagination to describe every part of them, down to their very toes, as there were plenty of them who were not solicitous to hide any of their beauties from our Eyes; but it may be best to stop here, and proceed to say a little in defence of their Characters, which have, in my opinion, been as much depreciated as their beauties have been Magnifyed.

All our Voyagers both French and English have represented them without exception as ready to grant the last favor to any man who will pay for it. But this is by no means the Case; the favours of Maried Women are not to be purchased, except of their Husbands, to whose commands they seem to pay implicit obediance, and therefore it is possible a thing of this kind may sometimes be done, where a woman happens to be married to a man who is mean enough to do it; but these instances are undoubtedly very rare, & cannot be charged to the woman's Account. Neither can the Charge be understood indescriminately of the unMarried ones. I have

[1] It is clear that all land on Tahiti was held by someone or other as personal property, irrespective of what trees were planted on it. But Wales may have been right about separate ownership of trees.—See Williamson, *Social and Political Systems of Central Polynesia*, III, pp. 270–87.

great reason to believe that much the greater part of these admit of no such familiarities, or at least are very carefull to whom they grant them. That there are Prostitutes here as well as in London is true, perhaps more in proportion, and such no doubt were those who came on board the ship to our People. These seem not less skilfull in their profession than Ladies of the same stamp in England, nor does a person run less risk of injuring his health and Constitution in their Embraces. On the whole I am firmly of opinion that a stranger who visits England might with equal justice draw the Characters of the Ladies there, from those which he might meet with on board the Ships in Plymouth Sound, at Spithead, or in the Thames; on the Point at Portsmouth, or in the Purlieus of Wapping.—I am not altogether of opinion that the Natives of Otahitee are indebted to any of our *late* Voyagers either French or English for the Disorder above hinted at: there is not the least doubt but that they can cure it; and it seems difficult to conceive how they should so soon find out a remedy for a disease, which baffled the most skilful Physitions of Europe for so many Years. But be this as it may, the English have certainly got the credit of it, as the natives have no other name for it, that we know of, than Opay[1]-no-Britannia so that if the French had realy the honour of introducing it, as some suspect, they are now even with us for calling it the French-Disease.

Their notions of Religeon, like those of every other People whom we visit but for a short Time and whose language is but imperfectly understood by us are difficult to come at nor do I believe that any thing on this head is yet known with certainty, except that they believe there is one Supreme Being; but whether they think it Necessary to pay him any sort of Adoration I could not discover. I am told that they sometimes sacrifice Hogs which if true I suppose must be to him, though this does not absolutly follow. It is likewise said that they believe their servants, or inferior People, do not go to the same place of abode after death, which their Principals do, and if so, they must believe in a future state although their notions concerning it are directly repugnant to ours. It is now pretty certain that those who have asserted that they are Idolaters are mistaken: The Images which have been mentioned being merely [men?] and considered by them in the same light as we do the Statue of a deceased friend, or the figures on his Monument. It was almost impossible to travill half a mile without meeting one of them, which they always told us distinguished a *Mari* or burying Place:[2] and at the Burying places of some of their Chiefs, there are not only great numbers of these Images errected but also a very large Pile of Stones.[3] I saw one in the Province of Oati-peha which contained more stones than would load both our Ships. Round these *Maris* they plant a sort of Trees, which at first I mistook for Cypress,[4] and I am not yet clear, they are not something of that kind; on these they hang great

[1] 'a rotten sore'—marginal note by Wales.

[2] Wales here refers to *ti'i*, symbolical effigies of the dead or of ancestral deities, set up to protect sacred sites or to mark boundaries. Cf. I, p 108.

[3] Presumably this is the *ahu*, the principal feature of the *morai*.

[4] *Casuarina equisetifolia*.

quantities of fruits of every sort, which we understood were for the use of the departed; but it is very possible we might herein mistake their meaning as we often did in other matters. They do not bury their dead when they die, but erect a sort of shed not far from the House, and place the body under it on a kind of Bier, wraped up in some of their whitest Cloth: The Shed also is sometimes covered over & hung round with Cloth, and here the Body lies untill the flesh is mouldered away, & the Bones are then buried.

Their Government and Policy seem as little understood as their Religeon. I had no opportunity of forming the least Idea of it; and those who had, or pretended to have, differ so widely in their accounts, that I dare not depend on any. It seemed the opinion of most that the Whole Island is divided between two principal Arees, or Kings, Viz. Owhyadoa who governs the lesser, and Otow, who governs the greater Peninsula; to whom all the other Arees, of which there are great Numbers, are subordinate. When the Endeavour was here *Toutaha* (mentioned by M. Bougainville) governed this latter; but on the Accession of the present Owhyadoa, some disputes arose between the two Kings,[1] which involved the whole Island in a War, wherein Toutaha and several of his Chiefs were killed about 5 Months before our arrival. As all European Ships before us had anchored in Toutaha's Dominion, and of course were supposed to be his friends; it might cause, or at least increase the fears of Owhyadoa whilst we lay at that part of the Island.[2]

Some are of opinion that they are governed by a body of Laws, whereby those who offend against them are punished; but this does not seem absolutly certain. There is no doubt but that certain Crimes are punished amongst them; but I am rather inclined to think their punishment lies in the breast of the Chief. Murderers, for example, are put to death, and a Post set up in some conspicuous place to represent them, at which all those who pass by throw stones.

They sometimes, instead of eating their fruits as they grow, make a sort of Bread, composed of different kinds, broken & mixed well together; this they leaven & keep for a considerable time: it seemed very disagreeably sour to most of us; but some eat of it and declared that it was very good after they became used to it. They also make a very strong beverage from the roots of a plant of the pepper kind, which will intoxicate—they also eat the Root it self very greedily.[3]

Next to their Plantations, which are their chief care, the manufacturing of their Cloth requires their greatest attention. It is a very laborious & teadious piece of Work, and falls entirely to the Women's share; but they employ none but the Old and ugly in works of so laborious a nature.[4] It is made from the Bark of a Plant, which they cultivate with great Care,

[1] Wales's history is here wrong; see p. 202, n. 3 above.

[2] Cf. I, p. clxxxv.

[3] Eating the root was unusual; Wales had probably seen them chewing it, like a quid of tobacco.

[4] This is quite wrong: the young and fair also beat *tapa*.

by beating the bark on a Plank with a piece of heavy wood made four-sided; the four sides are all fluted, but one finer than another, and they begin to beat it with the widest Side first and end with the finest. The Cloth is kept moist with water all the Time they are beating it. When it is finished to their mind, they sometimes dye it red or yellow with the Juice of two Berries which grow pretty common here. Since Europeans have come amongst them they sometimes print it in diverse figures by diping the End of a Bambo, cut properly, into the juice, in imitation of our Handkerchiefs; but they seldom ever wear it thus printed themselves, at least I never saw them do it.

On my first going on shore I was much charmed with the friendliness & seeming hospitality of these People: every one almost invited me to his house to eat Fruit &c. I could not resist their kind Invitations and had no sooner sat down amongst them but one beged Beads another nails, a third a Knife & a fourth My Handkerchief, Neckcloth, Coat, Shirt &c. I had stocked my self pretty well with some of the former Articles and thought it incumbent on me to give to every one of my kind Entertainers whilst they lasted, but was not well pleased to find many things gone which I had not the satisfaction of giving; but my chagrin was much greater on finding that I quitted no house without leaving more Persons unsatisfied than otherwise with what I thought generosity. I pursued this Plan the two or three first days: at the end of which I found my stock in Trade considerably decreased, & scarce any thing in return for it but Tyo! Tyo! As this way of proceeding seemed to give so little satisfaction to either Party, I resolved to alter my conduct for the future, and neither give or receive any thing by way of Friendship; but proceed by the less noble & generous, though perhaps more just and equitable way of Barter & Trade, and have the utmost reason to be satisfied with having done so; as none left me without being pleased with his bargain, and I was generally pleased with mine, I walked where ever my bussiness or pleasure called me in company or alone, armed or otherwise as it might happen, and never had the least quarrel with, or received incivillity from one of them, whilst very few of those who acted on the score of friendship escaped without.

Could I have prevailed on my self to have again altered My Conduct, and make choice of a Tyo, or Friend, as is the Custom here, it should have been Ereti the Friend of *M. Bougainville*; not that he was less importunate & craving than others; but because he was much more sensible and inteligent. He was also much more inquisitive & had a stronger desire to learn the Affairs & Customs of the Country we came from than any other that I met with; and this desire of learning made him, I conceive take more pains to communicate than any others were. It was the Day after our going a shore on Point Venus, that this good natured & sensible Man paid us a Visit at our little Encampment, and his name was a sufficient Introduction. We scarce ever after Breakfasted or dined without Ereti making one at our Table; and as he had but little of that prejeduce which hindered the rest of his Countrymen from even tasting our Victualls, they soon became palatable too him, but especially Tea, Biscuit, and butter, though it may be supposed the last was none of the Best. Nor would he refuse to take his Glass of Port, & drink to King George: It is true he made strange faces at the first, and some wryish ones even at the 3[d] & 4th Glasse; but before we parted, Ereti could drink it with almost as good a grace as ourselves. Thus our correspondence continued to our coming away; we every day got from him some intelegence which we thought useful; he, I suppose, did the same, and we were pleased with each other; yet were not Tyo's or Friends, in their sense of the word. That I chiefly admired in him was the readiness wherewith he comprehended our meanings, and enabled us to understand his own; and it is to him that I am indebted for many of the foregoing Hints.

No Animals besides Hogs, Dogs and Rats have yet been seen on this Island and it is highly probable that they are acquainted with no other, since they call every strange Animal they see by the Name of one of these. It may appear strange that we should get so very few Hogs at this place where all former Voyagers met with such plenty. Perhaps the Island has been drained by them & is not yet got replenished; Our Axes may not now be so valuable to them; or lastly, as they knew that it was Hogs we most wanted, it is probable they might Keep them up, as we did our Axes to increase the price.

We found Fowls almost as scarce as Hogs notwithstanding they were so very plentiful formerly. The Wild-Fowl are Ducks, Pidgeons, very beautiful green Doves,[1] and a great variety of the Parrot-kind; one very small one was of the most beautiful Mazarine-blue that I ever saw.[2] Besides these there were great variety of other small Birds which I did not Attend to.

The Fruits I have enumerated before, and a more particular Account seems unnecessary, as they are all very Common in every Tropical Country except the Bread-Fruit, and that is exceedingly well described both by Dampier and Lord Anson.

With regard to minerals I can say nothing. A few specimens of Iron Ore was found, I am told in Cap[t] Wallace's Voyage; possibly there may be great variety of others since People who Visit Countries for such short times, as voyagers generally do, have little opportunities of examining its subterraneous parts. Some pretend to know that the Whole Island of Otahitee has been produced by a Volcano. Islands may be formed so, and this amongst the rest for any thing that I know to the Contrary; but I saw no signs of its having been a Volcano, unless, it be the dark colour of the sand on the Beaches, and a few pieces of pumice stone which I met with at Oaiti-peha. And as to the Rocks being chiefly Lava, I can only say that I saw none which had the least appearance of being so, any more than the rocks in other Countries.

Such are the Hints which my short stay, and leasure from more impor-

[1] Fruit Doves, *Ptilinopus* sp.

[2] The Blue Lory, *Vini peruviana*. Sparrman called it *Psittacus cyaneus*, but owing to the law of priority his name did not obtain currency.

tant Bussiness have enabled me to give of this Island, and its Inhabitants; in all which I have endeavoured to come at truth, and can safely say that if I deceive, I am deceived, which in deed is very possible, where a person lies under the disadvantages of want of Time, and knowledge of the People's language he has to speak of. . . .

SEPTEMBER y[e] *1st.* At 4[h] the Cutter returned from a Cruse round the Island in search of Hogs & brought two. At 5[h] weighed, & made Sail out of the Bay, and as soon as we were Clear of the Reef Brought too and Hoisted in the Boats. At half past 6 o'Clock, Point Venus bore ESE dist. about 3 or 4 miles. We then steered NWBW & WNW and at Noon, *Eimeo*, or York Island bore SE and the Island of Huaheine WBN and the Latitude Observed was 16°51½'S.—The former part of the Day Brisk Wind at North West; the latter a moderate Gale S Easterly, and flying Clouds.

2d. We now steered West, & WBN½ N untill 5 oClock, at which time the Northern Point of Huaheine bore WNW and the Southern Point SWBW & then hauld up SSW under the Topsail. At 6 o'Clock brought too on the Starboard Tack Main-topsail to the Mast. At 12 Wore Ship & brought too on the other Tack untill 15[h] when we made sail & ranged close along the Reef which surrounds the Island in order to be as much to windward as possible when we came off the Harbour's mouth, where we had to work in through a gap in the Reef scarce more than a Cable's length wide, which we happily effected without touching on either hand: But the Adventure attempting to follow us when we were about half through unfortunately missed stays the first time and droped on the Larboard Reef. Cap[t] Cooke immediately Ordered the Resolution's Lanch, with Hands, to her Assistance although it may be well supposed that we could but ill spare them in so perilous a situation as we then were, which by carrying an Anchor out for them on which they hove presently got them off; but as they were going to carry out another, the first came home, and she fell again on the Reef where she lay untill we got to an Anchor, when the Master was sent with Hands to assist them farther, and by Noon they were clear of the Reef, & soon after safe at an Anchor.

3d. The former part light Airs, and sultry Weather; the latter brisk Wind with flying Clouds. Many of the Natives on board trading for Hogs Fowls & Fruits: The two former Articles seeming to be much more plentifull here than at Otahitee. 47 Hogs & about twice the Number of Fowls being purchased already on board the Resolution.

4th. Moderate Wind and Pleasant Weather. In the Morning I went on shore and walked quite a cross the Island which is not broad here. M[r] Bayley only was with me and our Road lay along one of the pleasantest Vallies that I ever saw. It is a perfect Orchard from one end to the Other, interspersed with the Houses of the Inhabitants who nowhere offered us the least incivillity unless picking our Pockets, unknown to us, may be thought so. They every where met us with Hogs and Cocks intreating us to purchase them; but I observed not one Hen was offered to us, nor did I see any about their Houses: a circumstance which I am at a loss how to Account for. Neither the Country or its Inhabitants that I could perceive differed in any respect from those we have left except that they seem to have a greater plenty of Hogs, and Fowls; & fewer Fruits.

5*th*. The Winds & Weather much the same as yesterday. As this Island is deemed remarkable for the largest and best constructed Canoes of any in this part of the South seas, I was very desirous of seeing some of them, and accordingly went this After noon to view one which belongs to the Principal Aree of the Island. It was a double one; that is, consists of two Canoes, joined together by Cross-Beams in the manner that I have described those of New Zeeland to be. The Cross-Beams extended beyond the outer Gunnels of the Canoes both ways, and are again crossed by three longitudinal Poles on each side the Canoes & by one between them, there by forming eight squares in breadth, viz 3 on each side & two between; and as there are 19 of the Cross-Beams they form 18 of those squares in length. In each of these squares sits a Rower: the Cross Beams, which are neatly squared serve[g] for their seats, so that there is room for 144 Rowers besides those who sit in the Canoes themselves to steer. This rowing Stage, as we may call it, is 66 feet in length by 24 in breadth. Towards the Midships rise four Pillars each 4 feet 8 Inches high, two from the outer Gunnel of each Canoe & support a stage 24 feet long by 10 broad. These Pillars are round, about a foot diameter, and ornamented with a sort of rustic Carving, not inellegant. This last mentioned Stage is for the fighting Men, for those large Canoes are never used but in their Wars. The Length of the Canoe from Head to stern is 87½ feet & breadth from the outer edge of one Gunnel to that of the other is 3 feet & 2 Inches. Both Head and stern of each Canoe is ornamented with a Human Figure carved in their taste, that is a large head & Body with two Hand[s] & two feet but neither Arms, Legs or Thighs. The hight of the Head, above the Keel is 4[f].. 10[in] & of the Stern 15½ feet. A transverse section of the body of the Canoe is in the Margin. The Parts as well of the frame-work as body, or hull are all fastened together with Cordage made of the outer rind of Cocoa-Nuts and they contrive by tying and cross tying to make their Joinings exceeding firm and tight.

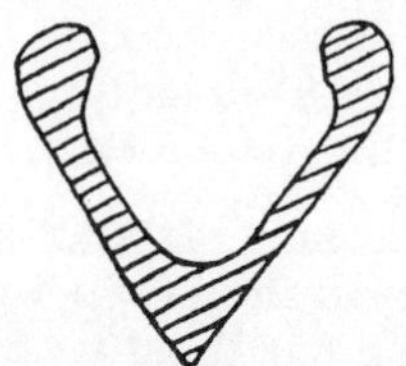

We went from hence to the Kings House. He is a thin elderly man, very grave & seems to be much reverenced by his Subjects. Cap[t] Cook gave him, when here in the Endeavour a Copper Coin of some kind, and a piece of lead with His & the Ship's Name &c and told him that if any ships like the Endeavour visited his Island to shew them that & they would be friends with him: accordingly the first time Capt Cook saw him he pulled the Coin & bit of lead out of a small Bag & presented them to him, Capt Cook returned them to him along with some Medalls & a piece of Copper on which were the Names of the present ships & the Year &c, with the same advice which he gave him before, which there is no doubt will be treasured up by his family for many Generations if no ships Visit this Island sooner.

6th. Moderate & very pleasant Weather. Having long had a great desire of examining the Reefs with which all these Islands are surrounded I took the opportunity of this Afternoon's Low Water, & being landed on it, I walked for about the space of half a Mile that being as far as I could get without going above the Middle in Water. It seems to be one continued firm Rock of very hard, white Stone, not much unlike Limestone except in hardness, and almost every where covered with large Bunches of Coral, mostly white, here & there a Branch only of a pale dullish brown. The Rock is every where full of small holes, which are larger underneath the surface & every one contains a Shell with a live fish in it; the greater part of which are too large to be got out, so that it appears either that the Shell is much grown since it got into the Hole, or that the Rock has grown over it: which of these is the Case more expert Naturalists must determine.—I suspect both.

In the Morning, unmoored and made sail, Having Purchased upwards of 400 Hogs at this small, but plentiful Island. I have but one remark to make of its Inhabitants, which is that they seem much less dependant on their Arees than those of Otahitee.

The Name of the Bay which we lay in is called Owharre; and I found the Latitude of the Ship when at Anchor to be 16°44¾'S by a mean of 4 Meridian Altitudes of the Sun. Its Longit from Point Venus as shewn by Mr Kendall's Watch 1°32'32½"W that is 208°52'38"E from Greenwich. The Variation of the Compass I found to be 4°50¾'E.

At Noon the Northermost point of Huaheine bore NEBE and the Eastermost point of Uliateah WBS. The Latitude Observed was 16°50⅔'S.

7th. The Weather very fine, with moderate Winds South Easterly, which is the point it b[l]ew from all the time we lay at Huaheine. At 6 o'Clock the East end of Uliateah bore SSE½E and Ohamaneno Harbour, which is that we are bound for NNE dist 4 or 5 Miles.—but Night coming on, we were obliged to tack and stand off and on untill morning when we attempted to work in; but finding it impracticable, the Anchor was let go off the point of the starboard Reef, and warps carried out a head to warp the ship through the Passage into the Harbour. This Passage is an opening in the Reef, like that at Huaheine, and something wider than that; but so great a surf sets in here on the Reef, that great quantities of Water washes over it into the space which is between the Reef and Island and this

Water having no way out again but by these small openings, causes a strong Current to set out at them continually, unless perhaps for a small space of time when the Tide of Flood runs strongest. At Noon the Resolution's Launch and Hands were sent to Assist the Adventure.

8*th*. Went on Shore with Mr Pickersgill to look out for a proper place to erect the Observatory on, as Capt Cook talked of having a Tent & Guard on Shore, & found one Convenient enough: indeed the principal thing to be considered was the End of the Solar Eclipse which will happen on the 16th Inst which I had some notion might possibly be seen here. We afterwards walked a considerable way up the country, along the banks of a small River which runs into the Bay where the ships lie, and found it not inferior to either of the Islands which we have left in any respect whatever. Brisk Wind at south-East & very hot on shore but pleasant enough on board the Ships.

9, 10. Moderate Wind South-Easterly with Showers.

11*th*. The former Part Moderate Wind; the latter more brisk, at South and SE, with Showers.—This Afternoon went with some of the Officers to the House of the Aree of the district where the Ships lay, and who is Brother to the Principal King, or Aree of the Whole Island; where we were entertained with what they call a *Heava*; that is an entertainment of Music and Dancing. The Music was performed on three Drums of different Tones, arrising from their different magnitudes & form. The Base, or deepest toned one, was about 12 or 14 Inches high, and perhaps as much in diameter: The Middle one was about 2½ feet high and about 10 Inches diameter; and that which had the highest tone, might be near 3½ feet high and about 7 or 8 Inches Diameter. Their Heads were made of Shark's Skin and braced much in the same Manner as ours are, only without the slides which ours have for bracing and unbracing; and they beat them with their fingers. The Dancing, as we called it, was performed by two Girls, one of whom is the daughter of the Aree, and accounted a capital Performer, under the direction of an old Man, who travills from place to place for that purpose, and is said to have made great improvement to this divirsion, on which account he is held in great Esteem. The Dress of the Performers is extraordinary and very grand on these Occasions. It consists of a great quantity of their cloth of different Colours bound very tight around the Waist with Cords, and disposed so as to stand off sideways from the Hips in a vast number of plaits or folds, to the extent of a fine Lady's Hoop-Peticoat when in a full Dress. To this is attached a parcel of Coats below, and a sort of Waist coat without sleeves above. Round the Head is wound a great quantity of plaited Hair in such Manner as to stand up like a Coronet, and this is stuck full of small floures of various colours which renders the Head-Dress, in My opinion, truly elegant. The Dexterity of the Performers does not lie in the Motion of the feet; but in that of the Hips, Arms, Fingers and Mouth: all which they keep in motion together, and ye principal skill of the performer seems to lie in contriving to have these several motions as opposite & contrary to one another as possible. These Motions they perform in all attitudes viz standing sitting kneeling Lying, as also with their face in all directions as East, west &c. all which is directed by the above mentioned old Man who not only gives the word, but sets the example also. In this part of the *Heava*, although the principal with them, there is little very entertaining to an European Eye. The wriggling of their Hips, especially as set off with such a quantity of Furbeloes, is too Ludicrous to be pleasing, and the distortion of their mouths is realy disagreeable, although it is for this the young Princess is chiefly admired. Her face is naturally one of the most beautiful on the Island; but in these performances she twists it in such a manner that a stranger would some times realy question whether her right Eye, Mouth & left Ear did not form one great Gash passing in an oblique direction across her face.

It may be supposed this Exercise is too violent to last long at a time, especially in this climate and under such a load of dress: accordingly the dancing seldom lasts longer than about 5 or 6 Minutes at a time, and in the intervals we were entertained with the performances of 5 or 6 men which sometimes consisted in a sort of figure Dance, wherein they were very carefull that their feet kept exact time to the Drums; at others in the action of short Interludes, which were in my opinion by far the best parts of the Performance, and realy diverting. The subjects of these were sometimes tricks which they are supposed to put on one another either through cunning, or under cover of a dark night; but oftener turn on intimaces between the Sexes, which at times they carry great lengths. These Parts were performed exceeding well, the command which they have over their Features and Countinance is extraordinary, and I am not certain that I ever saw Mr Garrick perform with more propriety than one Man did most of his parts. Their Stage, if I may be allowed the Expression, is under a Shed, open in the Front, and at one end is their dressing Room; into, and out of which they make their *exits*, and enterances as occasion requires; & the floor is spread with very curious Mats: In short, it may be said without exaggeration, that the Drama is advanced in these Islands, very far beyond the Age of Thespis.

12*th.* Finding it not possible to observe the Sun's Meridian Altitude on board the Ship, on Account of the Island of Otaha which intercepted the Horizon I took the Astronomical Quad^t on shore to a point of Land which I had previously determined to lie due East from the ship by means of the Azimath Compass, and Allowing the Variation to be as at Huaheine the distance between the two places is about a Mile & Quarter, and found the Latitude to be 16°45′20″s by taking a mean between both Arches. Out of Curiosity several of us dined to day on shore off a Hog, dressed by the Natives in their own Manner. . . .

13*th.* Brisk South-Easterly Winds and Pleasant Weather. The Launch was sent under the Command of an Officer to Otaha to purchase Fruits for a

Sea Stock. One of the Natives being caught with two shirts which he had stole from a person who was washing, the Cap[t] ordered him to be tyed up to the shrouds & punished with two dozen Lashes. He had served one so before, and it is remarkable that none of the Natives who were round the Ship in their Canoes would let either of them come into them; but they were both obliged to swim to the Shore. I observed the Latitude again to day & found it 16°45′26″: the mean of this and the former 16°45′23″s.

14th. Strong Gales with Showers. Dined with y[e] Aree at his house, along with the two Cap[ts] & Officers of both Ship[s], off a Hog dressed in their way, which has been described before; after Dinner we were entertained with another *Heava*; and parted in the strictest friendship at Night when we came on board; the King embracing every one severally. In the morning we were very much surprized to find that not one Canoe came off to the ships, which they never failed to do before as soon as it was light. On inquiry, it was found that two of the Adventure's People had been left on shore all Night, & it was immediately concluded that they had had some quarrel with the Natives & were murdered. A boat went on shore directly, and found them at the place where they had been left the night before by the Person who ought to have brought them off. They had been kindly treated by the Natives & taken care of all night; but not one of them was now to be found any where on this part of the Island; and their Houses were striped of every thing valuable. Cap[t] Cook afterwards went on Shore and after much search found the Chief, who sometimes said that we had murdered some of his People, near where the Ships lay, and at other times that it was our boats people who had done it at Otaha; but nothing certain could be made out; and Cap[t] Cook endeavoured to preswade him that no such thing had happened, which he seemingly believed & promised to return to his House.

15th. Strong Wind with Rain. None of the Natives came near us all the former part of this day. The wind blowing very strong, at 6 oClock hove on the larboard Hawser, & let go the small Bower Anchor, being moored before on[l]y with the Stream & a Kedge Anchor, and veered out to half a Cable. In the Morning the Natives returned as usual.

16th. Strong Gales at SE and showery weather. This evening the Launch returned from Otaha, having been detained there by the blowing Weather, which was directly against them. The Natives just as familliar as before, nor have we been able by any means to discover the Cause of their late fright. At 18′ past 6 o'Clock in the Morning the Sun rose over the land; the Eclipse being entirely over. At 7 AM weighed and sailed out of the Harbour; and at Noon it bore ENE and the Latitude observed was 16°..51⅓′s.

Tonga October 1773

OCTR *1st* Made sail and passed between the south point of the large Island which we now found to be Tasman's Middleburg, and the small one above mentioned. The passage between them is about 2 Miles wide.— We ranged the SW side of Middleburge about ¾ of a mile from y[e] shore, and at 20[h] the SW Point bore NBE½E dist about 2 Miles, & the north point was then opening. As soon as we got the length of the Point we hauld the Wind & at ½ past 21[h] anchored about half a Mile from the Shore in 25 fathoms, and a sandy bottom: the north Point bearing NNE½E, the South-West point S½W and the highest part of the Land ESE. The south point of Amsterdam Island W¾N, its north-east point NNW½W & a small Island which lies of that point NBW. We saw no signs of any inhabitants untill we had got near the South West point, probably on account of its being early in the Morning. We than saw one or two standing on a sandy Beach, and soon after several hundred who ran along the Beach as we sailed along. Soon after we had doubled the point we saw several Canoes coming off to us, on which we shortened sail for them to come up, and one Canoe in which was an elderly man and two young ones was presently along side. We made signs for them to come on board & hove them a rope to tow their Canoe by and the old man hesitated not a moment but was up the side before the Canoe was well up with us and sat himself down on the quarter deck in the midst of us without the least concern; and the others instead of holding longer by the rope and waiting for him, let it go and paddled away with as much seeming indifference as if they had left him amongst the best known friends in the World. He had plenty of Nails and beads given to him, with the former of which he seemed much pleased but made no account of the latter. Every thing that was given him he put on the Crown of his head, before he put it away. He brought in his hands a root of the Pepper Plant which grows at Otahitee, and of which they make there their favorite Drink, and gave it to the first man he met on the gang-way, and seemed by the manner in which he presented it to think it of great Value. Soon after several others came on board with the same freedom and unconcern, amongst whom was one, who by the bustle they were in at his appearance, we judged to be of some consequence amongst them. He happened a small misfortune when about 200 Yards from the ship, in his Canoe being overset; but that in itself was of small consequence he left it to the care of his people and swam to the Ship without difficulty or ceremony. The greatest misfortune was we did not at first know his Majesty again in this trim, and his Attendants, Cloaths & pepper-Plants which should have announced him were lost & left behind with the Canoe. But he was a sharp man and soon found up the Mistake & also a remedy; he began to order such of his Country men as was on board before him with so much Authority and was obeyed so implicitly that we knew who he was and waited not for his presents which he had sent for before we shewed him proper respect. As he was naked and seemed very Cold the Cap[t] made him a present of a large Piece of red Cloth to cover him which pleased him much & others gave him Nails and other things equally agreeable. His presents which he had sent for were not long a coming; they consisted of a sort of glazed Otahitee Cloth, fine Mats & roots of pepper-plants, and he soon distributed them about him. It is remarkable that every one who came off to us brought with them roots of the Plant above mentioned, which they presented to us, taking at the same time much pains to let us know its virtues and value, and seemed much surprised that we set none by it, which they attributed no doubt to our extreme ignorance.

As soon as the Ship was at an Anchor, the Pinnace was hoisted out and the Capt went on Shore. The Chief went with him and they were met on the rocks by many hundreds of the Inhabitants who seemed to welcome them on shore with Huzzas. The Chief took him to his house where he was regaled with a Cup of their Liquour which is the same & made from the same Plant as that at Otahitee. I mean the pepper-tree. The Cup was a large leaf having its sides folded up in a very curious Manner so as to hold the Liquour. But this hospitable King did not stop here but gave him fruits to bring off & shewed him every other mark of respect & friendship that seemed in his power; and when the boat came off it was almost loaded with Cloth, Mats & other things which were hove in by the People.

2d. Immediately after dinner I went on shore with several of the Officers; the two Cap^ts were gone before us. We found them at the house of the Chief where a great number of the Inhabitants were assembled, and singing in a manner which was very agreeable, accompanying the Music with clapping their Hands so as to keep exact time to it. Not their voices only but their music also was very harmonious & they have a considerable compass in their Notes. There were some also who played on very large Flutes, which they fill with their noses as at Otahitee; but these have 4 holes or stops, whereas those of Otahitee have but two. They had also an Instrument which they blow into with their mouths composed of 10 small reeds of unequal lengths, bound together side by side, as the Doric Pipe of the Ancients is described to have been done.

After I had stayed some time here I left the house and walked up into the Country with intent to have seen the farther side of the Island but was obliged to return before I had gained the highest ground for fear of being left on shore by the boats. I had notwithstanding an opportunity of seeing a considerable extent of the Island, which every where seemed fruitful and pleasant, and the roads as good as in England. When I got back I found the Capt^ts still with the Chief, who had ordered great quantities of fruit & Yams to be dressed for them to take on board. About 7 oClock we took our leaves of this friendly Man, who with all his family attended us down to the boat and about 8 o'Clock the next Morning weighed & sailed from this beautifull and agreeable Island.

Our knowledge of the place and people must were it only on account of our short Stay, be very imperfect; but I endeavoured to see as much and make as many Observations as possible. The Men seem in general strong and raw boned, pretty tall, and well proportioned, of a complexion some what between the Inhabitants of Otahitee & those of America, that is of a very light copper Colour. The women also are rather tall, well formed, and have very regular and soft features, but are rather to[o] fat to be esteemed beauties any where but in Holland; and this fault seems general. They are certainly the most lively laughing creatures I ever saw, and will run dancing & chattering by ones side without the least invitation, or consideration whether or no they are understood or any Answer returned to what they say provide one does but seem pleased with them. They appeared to me strictly modest, I mean in general; for there were here, as well as in every other place that I have been at, some of a different Stamp. The hair of the women was all black; that of the men was of different colours & sometimes on the same Head, caused, I conceive, by something which they put on it; and both sexes wear it very short and combed upwards. Many of the Boys had it cut quite close except a single lock on the top of the Head, and a small quantity on each side which was quite long. Their Eyes are of a dark hazel, and beautifull enough, but their teeth are not in general either so white or even as those of some other Indian Nations. Their Dress is very simple, consisting only of a piece of cloth which is wraped round their waist & hangs down below their knees; & both men and women go naked from the Waist upwards except some ornaments of Shells & beads of mother of pearl, Tortoise shell &c which they tye round their necks & Arms, and are very pretty so that it is no wonder that they dispised ours, trumpery glass ones.

Their Cloth is of the same texture and made from the same materials as that of Otahitee, but stronger & not so fine, and they have a method of glazing it so as to turn Wet for a considerable time. From the unsuspicious manner in which they first came on board, we had entertained a notion that the Idea of an Enemy was unknown to them, but on going ashore we found that they had several sorts of very formidable Weapons, such as Clubs and spears made of very hard wood; also very good bows, but their Arrows were but indifferent being made only of light reeds tiped with a bit of hard wood: Had our first conjecture been right it should seem that they would have had no need for those Weapons of offence. We could not help remarking one very singular circumstance amongst them, which was this: the greater part of them both Men and Women had lost the little finger of one hand; some had lost both; and others one, and a joint or two joints of the other. I endeavoured much, but in vain to find out the reason of this custom. It was neither peculiar to Age or sex; nor, that I could discover a mark either of rank or infamy, none seemed ashamed to have it known whether they had lost them or not but were equally ready to shew us the state which their Hands were in: moreover, notwithstanding I expressed great surprize at the circumstance none of them seemed to take any pains to remove it.

We saw no Animals here except Hogs, and of these not many. They have exceeding fine Poultry of the large white dunghill kind, and some ducks both tame and wild; besides these they have exceeding fine, large blue wood-pidgeons,[1] and great variety of Doves, some very beautifull green

[1] There are no large blue wood pigeons in Tonga to-day

ones, with a patch of scarlet feathers on the top of the head;[1] besides these I saw several other sorts both large & small birds that seem peculiar to this Island.

Their Fruits are Cocoa Nuts, Plantains & Bananas, of each of which there are great plenty and all very good. There are some Bread-Fruit, but it is not so plentifull here as at Otahitee & the society Islands. We found here also, a fruit not much unlike a Lemon, except in size: this being as large as a Cocoa-Nut. It is known both in the East and West Indies, and called there a Pumplenose; & sometimes in the latter Place, a Chaddock from the Name of the Person who first carried them there. I saw also a few Nectrines but they were not yet ripe. These are the same sort which we had at Otahitee &c, and are, I am told, called in some places the fever Fruit, being sometimes reccommended in that distemper on account of their fine cooling qualities. I saw no Roots except Yams, which are excellent, but were not plentiful no[w as] it was a wrong season. There were prodigeous large patches of them newly pla[nted and] fenced in.

I found, by a single observation for each, that the Latitude of the Ship at Anch[or was] 21°20½'s. and the Longit. by Mr Kendall's Watch 184°55¾'E. I had not opportunities of making more Observations but these were very good, and May be depended on.

This Island is called *Eaoowe* by the Natives, is of a Moderate hight, or rather what may be called high towards the south End, and rises gradually up from the sea, by a gentle Ascent to the highest part of the Island, and thence descends in like manner, on the other side, and that so regularly, that a furrow might be run with a Plough from one end of the Island to the other.[2] For the space of half a mile or more from the shore it is one continued grove or Orchard of fruit Trees, not planted at random as in Otahitee but in Enclosures, neatly fenced in with a sort of Lattice work made of reeds. The Doors to these Enclosures hang in a frame, and are sometimes made of thin boards, and at others of a Mat stretched on a light frame of wood; and every ones House is in the Midst of his little Plantation. Their Houses have not so good an Appearance on the Out side as those of Otahitee, but they are infinitely more so on the Inside being entirely lined both Top sides & floor with very fine Mats. Between the Enclosures belonging to different Persons, are Lanes, or Roads to go inland, or from one Plantation to another.

The Inland parts, are but very thinly inhabited; but it is not over run with Wood as in most other uncultivated Countries, but appears from the Offing like a very large Park, laid out by design, having here and there large Clumps of spreading Trees, in others very large single ones, and here and there long ranges of high Cocoa Nut Trees planted in rows on either side of the roads.—Most of The young Plantations of Yams which I saw were amongst the large Clumps of Trees just Mentioned the trees in the

[1] The Crimson-crowned Fruit Dove, *Ptilinopus porphyraceus*.

[2] This, anyone will agree who has walked or ridden over Eua, is an overstatement. But from the sea, the rise and fall of the island certainly appears very regular.

Middle of the Clumps being cleared away for that purpose; but all the outside ones are left standing, as if by disign, I suppose probably to afford shade & shelter to the Plants. The Yams are planted in rows at equal intervals each way so that each plant is in the Corner of a square. Every part of the Island, which is not planted is covered with long grass, seemingly of a very good Nature, and the soil is a very deep red Earth.

We saw not a drop of fresh water on the Island, but make no doubt of some being there, and I ground my opinion on the height of the land, which must afford Springs. Moreover the Inhabitants brought off to us great quantities of sugar-Cane which those Gentlemen who have been in the West Indies said was in every respect as good as any there and yet we saw none growing; and I have been told these Canes will not thrive without great plenty of water.—It has moreover been ever held impossible for an Island which is inhabited to be without water; but I do not build much on that head here, the Natives being so well supplied with the milk of Cocoa Nuts as to render this invaluable Article to other countries of less use to them: moreover their whole diet being fruits renders them less liable to thirst.

We steered WNW from the Place where we lay, and when we had run about 7 Miles the North point of Middleburg bore EBN & the south Point SE. The south point of Amsterdam WBS and the North East point N½W. The two extreme points of Middleburg subtended an angle of 57°8′ by Hadleys Quad[t] & I had intended to have veryfied all the other Angles in like Manner had not a misfortune rendered one unable untill it was to[o] late. We now steered WSW and were abreast of the south point of Amsterdam when we had run 5 Miles. We now set every point as it opened & carefully measured the run from point to point by the Log & my Watch; and we set the most remarkable ones again as they shut in, from whence the annexed Map of the Two Islands is drawn.

3*d*. About 4 oClock we came to an Anchor under the West side of the Island, in 18 fath[ms] water, foul rocky Ground, and full of Coral. About ⅜ of a Cable's length from the Shore; and having veered out two Cables, let go the Coasting Anchor in 40 fathoms. When moored, the point South of us bore S 17°W and that north of us N 40°E the dist. between these points is about 4 Miles. There is a reef of rocks which is bare at Low-water, about 2½ Miles without us bearing WNW.

The Island of Amsterdam, called by the Natives *Tongatabo* is low land except towards the South End where it may be said to be of a moderate height: It has not by much so beautifull an Appearance as Middleburg, when sailing along it purely I conceive on this Account. These two Island[s], like all those of Otahitee Huahine, &c. are encompassed with reefs of Coral Rock, only with this difference that they are here close to & form the Shore, whereas they are there at a considerable distance from it with deep water between. It appears highly probable to me that the shores of those Islands may in time extend themselves to the reefs also, as these now do.—But this by the bye.

As soon as we got near the shore, the Natives of this Island came off to us in the same familliar manner as those of Middleburg did: they all likewise brought with them by way of present, or I now rather think sign of Peace, the same root, and were equally surprized that we held it not in more estimation. In the Morning they began to bring off to us plenty of Fruits, Yams, Pigs, & Fowls which we purchased for nails. It is very remarkable that Knives and Hatchets were very little esteemed either here or at Middleburg; probably for want of being acquainted with their use: Nails either large or small, were very good Articles at both places, I suppose because they were acquainted with their use as we saw several at Middleburg which must have been left here by Tasman, as we know of no other person who has visited these Islands before us.

4th. This Afternoon went on Shore, and walked a-cross the Island to Maria's Bay, to get a sketch of that side of the Island. An odd Circumstance happened at my landing. At least 4 or 500 of the Natives were assembled at the landing place, and as the boat could not come near the shore for want of Water sufficiently deep, I pulled of my Shoes &c to walk through, and when I got on dry ground put them down betwixt my legs to put on again, but they were instantly snatched away by a Person behind me. I turned round & just saw him mixing with the Crowd but it was in vain for me to attempt following him bare-footed over such sharp coral rocks as the shores are here composed off; and my situation and Attitude may be supposed ludicrous enough. The Boat had put back to the Ship & my Companions had each made his own way thro' the Croud, and I was left in this Condition alone, and not able to stir from the place without having my feet cut to pieces with the Coral. Luckily I saw Capt Cook coming along with one of their Chiefs, to whom I made my complaint he went into the Croud found out the thief and brought my shoes back in a little Time. I rewarded his Trouble & honesty with a large nail, and both parties were well pleased.

This Island seems to be in the highest state of Cultivation; there being scarce a foot of land which is not enclosed and planted, except the public roads, one of which runs between every Plantation, and as they are nearly square the roads generally intersect each other at right angles. At several of these intersections there are square areas of perhaps 50 to 100 yards left unenclosed, and planted round with large spreading Trees. Towards the upper end there is raised a small mount, whose top is enclosed with a sort of low parapet of square flat hewn Stones, set on edge in the ground, and the mount is ascended in the front by a flight of steps of the same stone. All the Top of the Mount within the Parapet is covered with gravel, or very small pebbles, and in the midst is a Building, which I took the liberty to enter, and found in one of them two, and in another one small wooden Image, and in both they were placed on the left hand as I went in. On the Middle of the floor lay a heap of black small pebbles (those which covered the floor of the building & top of the mount were of the common brown Gravel) disposed into an Oval form, which took up about ⅜ of the breadth & length of the whole Building. The building might be about 4 Yards long & near 3 Yards wide. The Gravel both within and without was kept very neat & clear from weeds, and the Area before the Mount was a level patch of short green Grass. The Trees which are planted round these places were of three sorts: the largest not much unlike a Beech-Tree;[1] the other two, were a sort of Palm-Tree,[2] and the Cypress which I have remarked to be planted near the burying places of Otahitee and the Society Islands.—

I returned on board in the evening, after making a considerable circuit in the Island, without meeting with the least insult or incivillity from any one of the Natives, after that which happened at my landing. Although I met with many hundreds in the roads I travelled & that frequently in large bodies, and we no more than three without any Arms except my Gun, of the effects of which they seemed totally Ignorant.—In the Morning, a petty officer going on shore in the Pinnace to trade for fruits &c they seized the boat, unhung the Rudder, & took away some of the Implements belonging to her by force, on which the Officer of Marines was ordered on Shore, with his Party, to protect the Boat while trading.

5*th*. This afternoon I stayed on board to have got altitudes of the Sun for finding the Time & Longitude by the watch; but was hindered from doing anything by the Cloudyness of the Weather. In the Morning I went on shore to try the height and time of the Tides & found that the Water rose 3 feet 11⅛ Inches, and that it was high water about half past 11 oClock AM. When I was coming off again & had just got into the Boat I observed a Jacket which belonged to one of the boats Crew go over the boats side: I saw no visible Agent; but looking over the boats side after it I saw one of the Natives runing away with it under water. I immediately alarmed the people in the Boat & several shot was fired after him by the Midshipman & Coxswain but in too much hurry & Confusion to take place, and the rogue would certainly have gone clean off with it, had it not been for an Officer who was on shore that fired a load of small shot into him, after calling to him repeatedly to quit it without effect; but he droped it instantly on being hit with the shot, and walked off. It is remarkable that although there were several hundreds of the natives about us when this happened, yet not one of them seemed concerned or alarmed at our firing. I must confess I should not have been sorry to have seen this Man drop, for an example to the rest, for their Audacity and our lenity had been Carried now to such lengths that they had several times attempted to take the Cloaths of our Back: one thing is very remarkable, that those things were done nowhere but at the landing Place; our people being never offered the least incivillity when walking inland, although they frequently did it alone & un-armed. I had scarce got on board the ship but one of them was

[1] Probably the Miro or Milo, *Thespesia populnea*. This, like the other trees mentioned, had sacred associations in more than one part of Polynesia.

[2] Ti, *Cordyline terminalis*.

discovered coming out at the scuttle of the Masters Cabbin, out of which he had taken his and the Ship's Log books, his Daily assistant, Nautical Almanack & some other Books, there were two or three more in the Canoe & though they were called to repeatedly & threatened with being fired at if they did not bring them back, they paid not y[e] least regard, but made off as fast as they could untill a Musquet Ball was fired through their boat, when they threw the books overboard & all jumped after them. The Books were all picked up, & the Canoe filled & sunk along side.

6*th*. Went again on shore to look after the Tyde and found that it was low-water, a little before 6 o'Clock in the Evening; and that the fall was nearly the same as the rise. The shore being flat, and the water in consequence thereof ebbing out a long way; I could think of no other Method of finding the rise & fall but by setting up a Pole at the low water mark and my level at the high water Mark, and after adjusting it very car[e]fully taking the difference of the Altitudes of the Center of the Telescope & the part of the pole which was cut by the horizontall wire. As I was very particular not only in adjusting the Instrument but also in placing the pole to agree with the Vertical wire of the Telescope & in measuring the difference of the Altitudes afterw[d] I am willing to flatter myself that I am not much wrong, notwithstanding its disagreement with Tasman's relation. It should also be observed that Tasman was here about two days after the Change, & the ☽ was now almost three-quarters old. Our Times of high-water differ also Considerably: For Tasman says that a sw Moon makes high-water; from whence I cannot suppose that the time of high-water preceeded the Moon's southing more than 3 hours, whereas mine preceeds it about 4½ hours; and I am certain I cannot have erred more than a quarter of an hour, or 20 minutes, and I hope not so much. I have said so much on this head, because I have found Tasman's relation so very accurate in every other respect both here and at New-Zeeland. He is perfectly right in what he says concerning the direction of the flood & Ebb; and the reason seems to be that this is the direction of the Coast in this part of the Island. I cannot help remarking that Tasman says not a word of the Reef which lay without. Can it bee that so accurate an observer neglected this? It is impossible to miss seeing it. Or can it be that this Reef has increased so as to become visible since he was here? I beg Tasman's pardon, I had not seen his Map when I wrote the Above, in which it is accurately laid down as it appears at present.[1]

We had pleased ourselves, since coming to this Island, with thinking that we had found out the reason why they cut·off their little Fingers here, viz. that they cut off a joint on the death of any near Relation; but this Evening I met with an exceeding old man who had both hands quite perfect: yet so old a man must have lost many relations, his Parents in particular. Another thing about which much dispute has arrisen is the design & use of those neat little buildings which I have mentioned to be

[1] This last sentence is a later addition, interlinear.

situate at the intersections of the Roads; some asserting that they are Temples & the Images Idols, and others that they are Burying Places & the Images merely Ornamentall. If the former opinion be true they pay little regard to their Gods for one of the Natives set one of them up for us to shoot at: For my part I believe they are approp[r]iated to both, here as well as in Europe & that the Images, are put there in memory of ye persons interred.

Queen Charlotte Sound November 1773

NOVEMR 2*d*. About one o'Clock came to an Anchor in 12 fathoms between Cape Terrewitte and Cape Pallisser in a fine sandy Bay; going into which we found the Soundings remarkably regular. This Bay is pretty deep, and there was the appearance of a very good Harbour beyond some Islands which form the bottom of the Bay. We had scarce got to an Anchor before several Canoes full of the Natives Came along side, and the people came on board without any ceremony from whence I concluded that they had been on board some of our Ships before, probably in Q. Charlotte's Sound; we got a few fish of them which were acceptable enough. That this Bay may not be mistaken, it is necessary to observe that there is the appearance of another deep Bay between a point of Land which forms the East side of this, and Cape Pallisser, that being close under Cape Pallisser, as this is under Terrewitte, and the point which separates them does not come out by much so far as either of the two Capes. It seems highly probable to me that this point is only an Island & that the two Bays may join beyond it.[1] The Entrance into what we conceived to be an Harbour is at the NE Corner of the Bay we anchored in, and there are several Rocks which stretch across it;[2] but notwithstanding this the Passage did not seem either difficult or dangerous, and it would certainly have been examined, if a fine Breeze had not sprung up at SE about 3 o'Clock, in consequence whereof we got under way, and made all the sail possible in hopes of reaching Q. Charlotte's Sound before dark. The Breeze freshened, and we ran 7½, 8 & 8½ Knots; yet at 7 oClock the Brothers were 3 Miles to the westward of us. At ½ past seven hauled the wind & stood for the sound; it now began to blow exceeding strong, and soon became very dark and rainey moreover so strong, and contrary a Tide ran here that the ship frequently would not steer, and to add to the Misfortune our rigging was become so very bad with long beating of the straight's mouth that some part or other of it went away almost every minute. In this trim we were running directly on a lee-shore for the Wind had pinched on us, so about 8 oClock tacked, & stood across the sound, judging ourselves too near the shore to bring up. At ½ past 8, endeavoured to Tack again; but the ship missed stays twice, & was obliged to be wore at last, by which means she was very near driving out again into the straights; and to prevent it, the

[1] Not a good guess. See Cook, p. 285, n. 3 above.

[2] The rocks hardly 'stretch across' the entrance to Port Nicholson; they are on its western side.

Anchor was let go in 18 or 20 fathoms. It proved strong Clayey Ground, & having veered out a great length of Cable, we rode safely untill Morning. About 17^h weighed and made sail; but it falling Calm, came too again, and about 21^h weighed a second time, and about Noon moored in Ship Cove with a Cable each way. The former part brisk Wind and Cloudy, the Middle strong Gales, with rain, & the latter part Little Wind & fine weather.

3d. The former Part little Wind and fine Weather, the latter some showers. In the Afternoon I went with Capt Cook to see if we could not find a place which would be tolerably convenient for my Observatory, and also for the People who were to be employed on various points of Duty on Shore, as we should thereby be a mutual protection to each other, and pitched on the Beach at the bottom of the Cove, where I observed before. In the Morning I got the Observatory &c on Shore and began to put it up. We had not anchored before great numbers of the Natives came along side in their Boats, amongst whom we soon recognized several of those who came into the sound a day or two before we left it in June last: Capt Cook also remembered one old Man who was chief at this place, and resident in it all the time that the Endeavour lay here but there was not one of the family amongst them who was here all the time the Resolution lay in this place in June last, and were so much frightened at the arrival of the new-comers. Our People soon learned *with certainty* that they had all been killed and eaten.

4th. Variable Wind and Cloudy, the latter part Rain. Finished the Observatory & set up the Astronomical and Assistant Clocks: fixed up a stand for the Quad^t and Adjusted it ready for Observation.

5th. The former part strong Wind with Rain, and very cold disagreeable Weather for living in Tents: the latter part flying Clouds, and more Moderate. It having been discovered on board that most of [the bread] which we had in Butts was damp and Mouldy; to day a Copper Oven was brought on Shore and fixed up by the Tent to rebake it.

6th. The former part Cloudy, the latter fine and clear, with brisk Wind, variable. This Morning it was discovered that a surtout Coat, and a Bag of foul Linen which had been brought on shore to be washed were stolen out of the Tent in which we lay. They had been seen by some of the people after sun-rising; three or four of us had been in, or near the Tent all the morning; and we had never suffered any of the Natives hitherto to land near us for fear they should discover our weakness. There therefore remained no other way for them to go but for some of the Natives to have come through the woods at the back of the Tent, creep under its side, take them out and return the way they Came: but this was an enterprize so difficult and dangerous to those who must have done it; and at the same time so alarming to ourselves that we were neither able or willing to believe it possible to have been done. It nevertheless proved true; for Capt Cook going on shore at the place where they resided, found the very things amongst them and learned that some of them had crossed over the point of Land which seperates the Cove where they were from that where we were, & is about a Mile broad, full of Wood, & very high, had watched 'till we were all out of the tent and then sliped in & taken them away. We now agreed to watch by turns, two hours at a time, which as we had but 6 persons on Shore came to one watch P. night apiece.

7th. Mostly cloudy with Rain, and brisk Wind northerly. Got on Shore a Chest of Arms, &c. & more People coming on shore, on various points of Duty, we began now to muster strong. We were but 5 persons on shore the first Night, & those divided in two tents; for I did not dare to leave the Instruments, but especially the Time-Keeper, without any one in the place with them, & it would not hold all, neither had we any arms, except one pair of Pistols, and my Gun; so that I should have been very unhappy had I then suspected that these people were capable of yesterday's enterprize.

8*th.* The former part cloudy with Rain, and very cold Weather: the latter flying Clouds & variable Winds.

9*th.* The former part very fine with moderate Wind southerly: the latter part Heavy Rain.

10*th.* The former part mostly cloudy with Showers: the latter much rain & very disagreeable weather.

11*th.* The first part cloudy: the latter pretty clear with moderate Winds, chiefly southerly.

12*th*, 13*th*, 14*th*, 15*th*, 16*th.* Moderate Wind at South-East; South, & South-West and very fine Weather. In the course of these five Days The Man and his family who were here in May & June last made their appearance amongst us, having had (I suppose) a joyful Resurrection from the Bowels of their Brother Cannibals; for nothing, it seems, could be more certain than our Information that they were eaten! This is the third time, however, that I have been witness to our intellegence of this nature being false, or misunderstood.

17*th.* The former part brisk Winds northerly, with Rain; the latter frequent Showers. I expected this change all yesterday & the latter part of Monday, since then about the tops of the Mountains in the Northwest Quarter, being the highest hereabouts, began to be covered with thick white Clouds which would frequently extend themselves half way down the sides nearest to us, and again contract themselves in-to a very small space, and hang only about their sumits: But yesterday about Noon half-way-down did not serve their turn, for a strong gust of wind brought them quite down, with great violence & overspread the whole sound in a little time.

18*th.* The former part flying Clouds; the latter heavy Rain & Hail: Strong North-westerly Winds.

19*th.* Most part Cloudy with Rain, and moderate Wind, north-westerly.

20th. The former part mostly Cloudy; the latter heavy Rain: Wind southerly, and moderate.

21st. The former part cloudy with moderate Wind North-westerly: the latter fine pleasant Weather. Received Orders to get my Observatory & Instruments on board the Ship.

22d. Fine pleasant Weather with Moderate Winds at North-West. After geting the Corresponding Altitudes Took down the Observatory Clocks & Instruments packed them up and put them on board the Ship.

23d. I have this day been convinced beyond the possibility of a doubt that the New-Zeelanders are Cannibals; but as it is possible others may be as unbelieving, as I have been in this matter, I will, to give all the satisfaction I possibly can, relate the whole affair just as it happened. After dinner some of the Officers went on shore at a place where many of the Natives generally dwelt to purchase Curiosities, and found them just risen from feasting on the Carcase of one of their own species. It was not immediately perceived what they had been about; but one of the Boats Crew happening to see the head of a Man lying near one of their Canoes, they began to look round them more narrowly, and in another place found the Intestines Liver Lungs &c lying on the ground, as fresh as if but just taken out of the Body, and the Heart stuck on the points of a two pronged spear & tied to the Head of their largest Canoe. One of the Natives with great gayety struck his spear into one lobe of the Lungs, and holding it close to the Mouth of one of the Officers made signs for him to eat it; but he beged to be excused, at the same time taking up ye Head & making signs that he would Accept of that which was given to him, and he presented them with two Nails in return. These Gentlemen saw no part of the Carcase nor even any of the Bones; but understood that the unhappy Victim had been brought from Admiralty Bay, where these natives had lately been on a *hunting Party*; and one of them took great pains to inform them that he was the person who killed him.

When the Head was brought on board, there happened to be there several of the Natives who resided in another part of the sound, and who although in friendship with were not of the Party of whom the Head was purchased. These were, it seems very desirous of it; but that could not be granted: However one of them who was a great favorite was indulged with a piece of the flesh, which was cut off carried forward to the Gally, broiled and eaten, by him before all the Officers & ship's Company then on board. Thus far I speak from report: the Witnesses are however too credible & numerous to be disputed if I had had no better authority; but coming just now on board with the Capt and Mr Forster, to convince us also, another Steake was cut off from the lower part of the head, behind, which *I saw* carried forward, broiled, and eaten by one of them with an avidity which amazed me, licking his lips and fingers after it as if affraid to lose the least part, either grease or gravy, of so delicious a morsel.

The Head as well as I could judge had been that of a Youth under twenty, and he appeared to have been killed by two blows on the Temple, with one of their *Pattoos*, one crossing the other; but some were of opinion that the whole might have been done at one blow, and that what appeared to have been caused by the other, was only a cross fracture of the Scull arrising from the first.

My Account of this matter would be very defective, was I to omitt taking notice of the Behavior of the young Man whom we brought with us from Uliateah & who came on board with the Captain, &c. in the Pinnace. Terror took possession of him the moment he saw the Head standing on the Tafferal of the Ship; but when he saw the piece cut off, and the Man eat it, he became perfectly motionless, and seemed as if Metamorphosed into the Statue of Horror: it is, I believe, utterly impossible for Art to depict that passion with half the force that it appeared in his Countenance. He continued in this situation untill some of us roused him out of it by talking to him, and then burst into Tears nor could refrain himself the whole Evening afterwards.

From this Transaction the following Corollaries are evidently deducible, viz—1st) They do not, as I supposed might be the Case, eat them only on the spot whilst under the Impulse of that wild Frenzy into which they have shewn us they can & do work themselves in their Engagements; but in cool Blood: For it was now many Days since the Battle could have happened.

2d) That it is not their Enemies only whom they may chance to kill in War; but even any whom they meet with who are not known Friends: since those who eat the part of the head on board, could not know whether it belonged to a friend or Enemy.

3d) It cannot be through want of Annimal food; because they every day caught as much Fish as served both themselves and us: they have moreover plenty of fine Dogs which they were at the same time selling us for mere trifles; nor is there any want of various sorts of fowl, which they can readily kill if they please.

4th) It seems therefore to follow of course, that their practice of this horrid Action is from Choice, and the liking which they have for this kind of Food; and this was but too visibly shewn in their eagerness for, and the satisfaction which they testified in eating, those inconsiderable scrapts, of the worst part on board the Ship: It is farther evident what esteem they have for it by the risks which they run to obtain it; for although our neighbours feasted so luxuriously, we had abundant reasons to conclude that they came off no gainers in the Action, since almost all of them had their foreheads & Arms scarrified, which is, it seems, their usual custom, when they lose any near Relation in War.

To Day unmoor'd and hove short to half a Cable. Fine pleasant Weather: Winds moderate and Variable.

24th. Winds and Weather Variable. Went on shore with some of the

Officers to the Indian Village where I saw the Man's Heart sticking on the spear, and tied to the Head of the Canoe as described above; the Intestines also were lying in the same place; but were now, all parched by the heat of the sun, which is a manifest proof that they had been taken out of the Body only the Day before; but the Liver & Lungs were now wanting; I suppose they had now found an appetite for these also, the Carcase being all done.

At ½ past 15^h weighed, and sailed out of Ship Cove; but about 19^h falling little wind, Anchored under the End of Long-Island. About 20^h weighed again and came to sail with a fine Breeze at North-West. At Noon the Two-Brothers bore SE dist. about 2 Miles. Set studding sails & directed our Course for the Northern shore of the straights in search of the Adventure, on whose Account we are under some uneasiness; more especially as we had while in the Sound, near a whole week running of very favourable Winds and Weather for her coming in.

Easter Island March 1774

MARCH ye 13*th*. Moderate wind south-easterly, and flying Clouds. About 3 o'Clock the Cutter was hoisted out & the Master sent in her to examine a small Bay which is on the west side of the Island. He returned about five and brought with him one of the Natives who had swom off to the Boat. This man was of a middle height, rather slender and seemed to be about 50 years of Age. His Complexion was of a dark Copper-Colour, his Eyes a dark brown & his hair black and cut short. His beard was black short and bushy, and his Features did not seem to differ materially from those of Europeans. He appeared very brisk and Active, and to take much notice of what was round him, at least more than is usual for other Natives of the Southern Islands to do. The pendant parts of his Ears had long slits in them, and were extended to at least 2 Inches in length; when he saw us taking notice of them, he turned the slits over the upper parts, so that at first look it might have been conjectured the small flap had been cut away. At a little past 6 oClock the Ship anchored off the Above mentioned Bay in 36 fathoms water with the small bower.

About three oClock in the morning it was discovered that the ship was driving, on which the Anchor was hove up, and sail made to windward in order to gain the bank again. At 8 oClock the Pinnace and Cutter were hoisted out and the Capt & some other Gentlemen went on shore to see what might be expected from the Island and particularly if any water could be had: as I had nothing material in hand I made one of the Company; and the Ship stood on and off in the interim. The Native, who without the least concern had staid on board all night went in the [Pinnace]. Several hundreds of the Natives were gathered together on the Shore to receive us; and many swom off to meet the boats some of which we took up, but the boats would not carry the tenth part of them who swom off. As we approached the Shore, we discovered a sort of breast work of very neat hewn stone which we conceived had been the work of some European, more especially as there was the appearance of an Embrasure on that side which faced us; but on going on shore we found it to be entirely the work of the Natives, and that there had formerly stood on it two of those Colossean Statues which are mentioned above; but that they were now fallen down, and broken to pieces: What we took for an Embrasure was a Place where a very large stone had fallen out of the wall. The workmanship was not inferior to the best plain piece of Masonry that I have seen in England. The side Walls were not perpendicular but inclining a little inwards, in the manner that the Breast works and forts in Europe are; but there was no sort of Cement in the Joints. We landed without the least ceremony, for we saw not a weapon of any sort in the hands of any of the Natives; and as soon as we had done so they crow[d]ed round us & brought us roasted Potatoes, & sugar-cane, both of which were very acceptable; but the latter did not contain much juice. We presented them with some Nails and Trinkets in return; but I observed that when any one gave to us, I observed that there were at least half a dozen others ready to beg it of us again, and I had one snatched out of my hands: from whence I concluded that property is not quite equally divided here any more than in England. They were exceeding loving, and desirous of walking arm-in-arm with us; but we were not long in discovering their drift in doing so: my handkerchief was gone in an Instant, and one of our people detected another of them taking away a small brass achromatic spy-glass which I had in my Pocket. After much fruitless search and Enquiry by signs, I was at last lucky enough to find out a well, pretty convenient for watering at but the water was neither fresh nor sweet: it however determined the Cap[t] to come to an Anchor & stay a day or two. All round the beach where we landed the Island seemed very barren, and entirely covered with stones. There were Notwithstanding some plantations of Potatoes, and we saw a few Fowls, but not many and they would part with none. We saw, I think, at least 500 Men; but not more than 6 or 8 women a disproportion which surprized us much. There can be no doubt but that some European Ships have been here since Roggewein's time, as we saw one man who had a pretty good European hat on: it had a very broad brim, like those usually worn by the Portuguese or Spaniards. Another had one of those Jackets on, usually known by the name of *Grekos,* and it was in no bad plight. I saw one who had got the handle of an English pewter spoon hung by a string round his Neck; I call it English because it had on the back part an X with a crown over it: this last might have been left by Roggewein; but the others, I think, could not.

A little before Noon we returned on board and the Ship anchored in 32 fathoms, the bottom a dark sand. . . .

14*th.* Moderate breezes Easterly and flying Clouds. Went on Shore to Examine the Tide by a mark which I had made in the morning, and found that it rose about 2 feet; but this could not be determined with any great nicety on account of the great surf which sets in; and I think it was highest ab[t] 3 oClock; but this is even much more uncertain than the other, for the same reason; to which must be added the small rise and fall of the Water.

After having determined this point in the best Manner I was able M[r] Hodge [*sic*], the Draughtsman, & myself set out to Cross the Island; but had not proceeded far before the Natives became too troublesome to venture farther, so we turned again for a Musquet, which those People have by some persons or other been taught to pay a great deal of difference[1] to, and we now walked untill we saw the other side without much molestation, all leaving us but one Man, who would be very kind, and very officious offering frequently to carry the Musquet for us, which we on our part declined with proper Acknowledgements, to his great grief. He ever and anon called to such of his Countrymen as he saw near the road we passed, and when they came to him they droped behind and seemed to consult together concerning us; but as none of them had any weapons we walked on without the least regard to him or them, and they soon left him & he picked up others. We continued our Course untill we could see the greatest part of the South East[2] side of the Island, and then sat down to take a sketch of it and rest ourselves. After we had done what we were about I got up to return & took up the Musquet, when the Man walked past Mr Hodge snatched his hat off from his head & ran away with it. I cocked and pointed the Musquet without thought of any thing but firing at him; but when I saw a fellow Creature within 20 Yards of its muzzle I began to think his life worth more than a hat, *and as to the Insult*, rot it! let him who next offends on the presumption of haveing gone clear this time punish it. As to the Owner of it

> He sat like Patience on a Monument
> Smiling at Grief.—

We varied our road in our return, for

> The Land was all before us where to chuse

and nothing to hinder us; but wherever we came whether Cultivated or not the Ground was covered with large rough stones, not much unlike the Matter which is thrown out of an iron furnace.

We saw no sort of wood on the Island but one, the leaf and seed of which are not much unlike those of the common Vetch, only the Pod resembles perhaps more that of a Tamrind in its size & shape. The seeds have a most disagreeable bitter tast and the Natives when they saw us chew them made signs for us to spit them out, from whence we concluded that they think it poysonous. The Wood is pretty hard, of a redish colour & rather heavy; but very crook'd and small: we saw none above 6 or 7 feet high. The Natives call it Torromedo.[3] We passed through many Plantations of sweet-Potatoes; but most of them poor and small, and one or two Plantain-Walks;

[1] i.e. deference.
[2] MS *sic*; but I think he must mean south-west.
[3] Toro-miro, *Sophora toromiro*.

but saw no fruit on any of the Trees. We met not with one drop of water in all this circuit, and on the whole the Island seemed to us scarce sufficient for the sustenance of Human Nature.

We visited several of their Houses which are miserable enough. They are formed by setting sticks upright in the Ground at 4 or 5 feet distance and bending them towards each other and tying them together at the top, forming thereby a sort of Gothic Arch; the longest sticks are in the Middle, and they place shorter & shorter each way, and at a less distance asunder by which means the Building is highest & broadest in the Middle & lower & narrower towards each end. To these, which serve as Raftors are tyed others horizontally, and the whole is thatched over with the leaves of sugar Canes, or some such like Plant. The Door way is in the Middle of one side and is formed like a sort of Porch, and may be about as high & large as the mouth of a common Oven, so that a man can barely crawl in on his hands and knees. They are exceeding dark holes, without any kind of Utensils, seemingly calculated for no other purpose but to creep into when it rains.

The Capt having ordered a Party to go round the Island & see what it produced, I took that Opportunity of doing the same, as also to enable myself to give a better sketch of the Coast, as this may be done with much more exactness from an Eminence within the land than it can from the ship; by this means too I could in some measure add to the certainty of its dimensions by observing car[e]fully the Time we were walking from point to point. We set out about 9 oClock in the Morning, and crossed directly from the little Bay where the ship was at Anchor to the south west side of the Island followed by a great Croud of the Natives who pressed much upon us: but we had no[t] proceeded far before a middle aged Man punctured all over from head to foot and painted, or rather daubed with a sort of white earth on his face appeared with a spear in his hand and walked along side of us, making signs to his Countrymen to keep at a distance and suffer us to walk unmolested and when he had pretty well effected this he hoisted a piece of white cloth on his spear and carried it before us stopping when we stopped, and when he saw us preparing to set forward he placed himself in the front & led the way with his Ensign of Peace, as we interpreted it to be. For the greater part of the distance across the ground was every where covered with stones as hath been described above; but notwithstanding this there were amongst them many large tracks of land planted with sweet Potatoes and here and there a Plantain walk; but I saw no fruit on any of the Trees. Towards the highest part of this end of the Island the soil seemed to be much better than any I had seen before, being of a fine red earth and not covered with stones as in the other parts; but here there were neither houses nor Plantations; for which no doubt a Reason is to be assigned although I did not see any.

On the other side near the sea, we met with three Platforms of Stonework, or rather the ruins of them equal[ly] neat and curious with that already described. On each of these had stood four of those large Statues but they were all fallen down from two of them, and also one from the third, every one except one were broken with the fall and otherways defaced; but I measured the whole one and found it 15 feet in length & 6 feet broad over the shoulders. Each Statue had on its head a large Cylindric Stone of a red Colour and worked so truly round that some insisted that they must have been turned into that form; but I suppose the size will be a sufficient refutation of that opinion, as one, and that apparently not by far the largest was 52 Inches high and 66 in diameter. In some the upper corner of the Cylinder was taken off in a sort of concave quarter-round; but in others the Cylinder was entire. The Statues themselves are of a soft greyish stone very different from any other which I saw on the Island, and had in my opinion much the Appearance of being factitious. The Walls of one of the Platforms had on it a Coping of the red stone rounded on the upper side, and in the under one were deep Mortices into which [words illegible] formed on the upper stones of the Wall in a very neat & artful manner; yet has not [words illegible], Pains and sagacity been able to preserve these curious structures from the ravages of all [word illegible] Time.[1]

We went from hence North eastward according to the direction of the Coast, and presently crossed a place where the earth had been taken away for some purpose or other to the bare Rock which seemed to be a very poor sort of Iron Ore. As we continued our March we discovered that this was by far the more fertile part of the Island. It being frequently interspersed with large Plantations of Potatoes, sugar-Canes and Plantain Trees, and those not so much cumbered with stones as those which we had seen heretofore. On this side also the Natives twice or thrice brought us water, which although brackish, (I might say salt) and intolerably stinking, our excessive thirst made very acceptable. We also passed four or five Huts, the Owners of which came running out to us with roasted Potatoes & Sugar Canes & having placed themselves ahead of the foremost of us, for we all wa[l]ked in a line, on account of the Path-way) gave to each as he passed by one. They observed the same method in distributing the water which they brought us, and were very careful that the foremost by drinking more than his share should not leave none for the Hindmost. At the last day, when the Widow's two Mites are remembered, may this hospitallity of the poor Easter Islanders not be forgot!—It was relieving the thirsty & hungry indeed! and what reccompence was in our power to bestow was small enough, it seemed however acceptable; and if it did but do them the good they deserve it will do them much indeed. But at the same time impartiallity obliges me to confess that there were not wanting, especially amongst those who followed us several who endeavoured to steal from us at every Opportunity, and sometimes carried it so far as to snatch from us the very things which had been given us by others. Nay at last, to prevent worse Consequences, we were obliged to fire a load of small shot at one,

[1] The curious reader may easily restore the ravages Time has made on this last statement from Cook, pp 357–8 above.

who was so audacious as to snatch a bag which contained every thing we had brought with us from the Man who Carried it. The shot hit him in the back, on which he droped the Bag, ran a little way & then droped; but he afterwards got up & walked, and what became of him afterwards I know not, some of the others led him off. As this affair stoped us some little time the Natives gathered together & presently we saw the Man who had led the way hitherto & one or two more come runing towards us when they came up to us they did not stop but run round us repeating in a kind [of] recitative manner a few words, and they continued to do so untill we set forwards again when our old friend hoisted again his Cloth & led the way as before, & none ever attempted to steal from us the whole day afterwards.

About the Mid-way, on this side, on a small eminence we met with several of the Natives amongst which was one whom we soon discovered to be a Chief amongst them: to him our friend, after some ceremony, delivered his white flag, & he gave it to another who carried it before us the remainder of the day: some presents of Nails, Otahitee Cloth, &c. were made to the Chief, by the Officer who commanded the Party, after which we took our leave, & proceeded on our way.

Towards the eastern end of the Island we met with a Well whose water was perfectly fresh; being considerable above the level of the sea; but it stunk much, owing to the filthyness, or cleanliness (call it which you will) of the Natives who never go to drink without washing themselves all over as soon as they have done, and if ever so many of them are together, the first leaps right into the middle of the hole drinks & washes himself without the least ceremony, after which another takes his place and does the same. This water however, as being perfectly fresh, was highly acceptable to us, notwithstanding, at least twenty of them had drunk & washed themselves in it immediately before we came up.

This side of the Island is full of those Colossean Statues which I have mentioned so often, some placed in Groups on platforms of Masonry others single and without any being fixed only in the Earth, and that not deep; these latter are in general much larger than the others. I measured one which was fallen down & found it very near 27 feet long & upwards of 8 feet over the breast, or shoulders and yet this appeared considerably short of the size of one which we dined near: its shade at a little past 2 oClock being sufficient to shelter all our party, consisting of near 30 persons from the Rays of the sun.

The Workmanship of these stupendous Figures, although rude is not bad, nor the features of the Face ill formed: their Noses and Chins, in particular, are exceeding well executed. They are as near as I guess about half length ending in a sort of Stump at the Bottom on Which they stand. In the Accounts which we have of Roggewein's Voyage, they are said to be Idols and that the Natives were seen paying adoration to them at sunrise: How these Gentlemen could see this I must confess I cannot tell, it is certain they were not then on Shore, & I am confident few People would venture to anchor within less than a Mile & half from any of the shores of this Island.—a long distance to speak so positively of what these people were doing! But be this as it may it is very certain They have now gotten much the better of those Idolatrous Practises seeing that not one Person amongst them was observed to pay them the least reverence or respect whatever. Was I to hazard a conjecture I should rather think they have been errected to the Memory of some of their Ancient Chiefs & possibly may mark the places where they were buried: It is certain that we found pieces of Human bones amongst the ruins of some of them and this circumstance has already been brought to prove that human Sacrifices have formerly at least been made to them.[1] They give different Names to them, such as Marahate, Hadarego, Arrahoa &c &c to which they always prefix the word *Moi*, and sometimes annex *Areki*: the former, as near as we could gather signifies a burying place, and the other a Chief although some say they understood it to Mean Sleep.[2]

It appears very surprizing to me how they could bring and raise those prodigeous Masses of Stone, and still more how they could place the large Cylindric Stones which has been mentioned on the Heads of them afterwards: if indeed the former are factitious they might have been put together on the place and in the position they now stand, and I know not or have heard of any probable Means which could have been used to effect the latter unless a sort of Mount or scaffolding of Stones or Earth has been raised in shelving form equal to the hight of the Statue up which they may have rolled the Cylinder, and even then it would have been found no easy matter to have placed it on its head without throwing it down: This it must be owned must have been a work of immense Time Labour and Patience, and therefore no wonder it seems now to have been long discontinued for not one that we saw has the least appearance of being modern; however if it be a reason for discontinnuing the errecting of them it could be none to the taking care of those which were already set up, in which point there seems to be as great a difficiency amongst the present Natives as in the former, and there is some reason to believe that in a few years there will be few or none standing.

15*th*. At dinner we could get no fresh Water except two Bottle[s] which we had brought with us from the last mentiond Well. What was brought us here by the Natives being rank salt Water; but I observed that some of them drank pretty plentifully even of this; so far will necessity and Custom get the better of Nature! On this account we were obliged to return to the Well, where having drunk round we directed our rout right across the Island towards the Ship, as it was now four o'Clock, and in this walk which for about 5 Miles was all up-hill we suffered exceedingly through thirst. In a small Hollow On the highest part of the Island we met with several of y[e] Cylinders which I have observed were placed on the Heads of the Statues, some of which appeared larger than any which we had seen before

[1] Death from natural causes is much more likely. See p. 344, n. 2 above.

[2] *ariki*, of course, a chief; *moe*, as a noun, sleep; as a verb, to sleep or to die.

but it was now too late to stop to measure them. Is it not possible this might have been a quarey where those stones might formerly have been dug, from whence it would have been no difficult matter to rol them down after they were formed.

On the declivity of the Mountain towards the west, we met with another Well; but the water was a very strong Mineral, had a thick green scum on the Top and stunk worse than that of Harrogate in Yorkshire:[1] necessity however made it go down, and I drank a pretty large draught of it; but had not gone One hundred Yards before I got eased of it the same way it went down: in short it made me so sick that I could not proceed for some time, and I did not join the Party again before I got to the Beach off which the Ship lay.

In all this long Excursion, or in that I took yesterday I saw no tree or indeed wood of any sort except that I have mentioned above; we saw indeed in several places the Otahitee Cloth Plant; but very poor and weak never more than two or at most 2½ feet high. There was indeed in one place at y[e] South west corner of the Island a small shrub whose leaf was not much unlike that of an Ash. The wood of it was white & brittle in some measure resembling that of the Ash.[2]

We saw not one Animal of any sort, or bird, except a few tame fowls, and a Noddy or two, which also were kept tame by the Natives, and of which they seemed very fond and [? Careful][3] or, on the whole, any thing which can induce ships that are not in the utmost distress to touch at this Island. The Tide, as I was informed by one of the Masters Mates[4] who was on shore filling water, and whom I desired to look after it, for this day, rose 2 feet and 3 or 4 Inches and was highest between 3 and 4 oClock.

In the Morning a Man came along side in a Canoe with a single Fowl, and wanted some very particular thing for it; but what we could never find out: it was at last purchased for a Cocoa-Nut-shell; and I believe it was that he wanted. In this Canoe there were two planks more than 12 Inches broad; whence they had been got puzzled not only me but others much. It is certain no trees which will make Planks of half their breadth or even ⅓ of it grow on this Island: Can it be possible they have been made out of drift wood which has been drove on the Shore of this Island from America or [page torn] other Islands in the Neighbourhood from whence they have been got. It is certain we saw [page torn] nor were we able to get the least information on this head from any of the Natives although [page torn] and every Method we could think off to Obtain it. We Have been equally unfortunate in our enquiries concerning the native Name of

[1] Harrogate had risen to great popularity as a spa at this time, particularly among the northerners of England. Wales, a Yorkshireman, had probably some direct experience of it.

[2] Marikuru, *Sapindus saponaria*. Cook (p. 347 above) turns Ash into Asp.

[3] One may guess that this was part of the bird-cult of Easter Island; the 'noddy' was probably the Sooty Tern, the centre of this cult. See Buck, *Vikings*, pp. 229–30.

[4] 'Mates Mates', the second word interlinear. 'Master's mates' seems the natural emendation.

the Island; for on comparing Notes I find we have got three several Names for it, viz. *Tamareki*, *Whyhu*, and *Tuapij:* They have but few words common with those of Otahitee, and did not appear expert at conversing by signs.

About 9 oClock in the Morning the Wind came from the seaward with heavy Rain on which the ship was got under way, and stood to and from whilst the Boats went on shore to purchase what Potatoes might be brought down to the landing Place by the Natives.

The Latitude of the Place where the Ship lay, and which is about 3 Miles from the South west corner of the Island, is 27°07′¾ s and in Longit. 249°03′ East of Greenwich by Mr Kendall's Watch.

The Marquesas April 1774

APRIL *7th.* About Noon we began to enter the Straits mentioned by Mendana, as seperating the Islands of St Christina and La Dominica which we found to answer very well to the description which is given of them in the Account of his Voyage as translated by Mr Dalrymple. When we were about half way through we saw a Bay in Christina which appeared so nearly to answer the description which is given of *La Greaciosa* in that Voyage except in the circumstance of being on the North side of the Island, instead of the West that Capt Cook was in some doubt whether or no that might not be a mistake in some transcript or other, and this the Identical Bay in which Mendana Anchored; but at last he considered to proceed, and having passed the straights and turned a little towards the South we met with another which was thought to Answer much better: but here the Wind blew almost right out and came down a deep Vally which is at the bottom of the Bay in such sudden and violent Gusts, as I do not remember to have seen else where. One of them took the Ship whilst in stays, and was very near driving her on the Large perpendicular Cliff which forms the South west point of the Bay, and she had scarce got clear of that danger before another laid her flat down on her beam-Ends, and as she was now very light, and is naturally a little tender sided, I verily believe a few Minutes would have filled & sent her down if the Topsails &c had not been let go. Through these two Misfortunes we drove a considerable way to leeward of the Harbour's Mouth; but as the Water was very smooth without she soon fetched to windard again, and about 5 oClock the small Bower was let go, Just within the Mouth of the Bay in 30 fathoms, and a sandy bottom & two thirds of a Cable Veered out.

We had soon great Numbers of the Natives round us in their Canoes, but they were very cautious, and did not chuse to come very near the Ship. At length I enticed one of them to come so near as to take a sheet of writing paper from me, and when he had got it he made signs to me to send him down a rope to which he tyed a sort of Weapon which he had in his hand made not much unlike an Oar, only it is straight. After this several came near and began to barter for bread fruit which they sold us for small nails &c. when it was almost dark one of them brought us a small Pig which was bought for a broken knif.—How much I wished to see another in its Throat! may be guessed by those who have not tasted fresh meat for four or 5 Months. We observed that every Canoe had a heap of stones in its bow & every Man had a sling tied round his head.

All the Night we had Violent squalls of Wind attended with frequent and heavy showers, and early in the Morning the Natives came off again with Bread fruit which we purchased at the same rate as before viz 4 bread fruit for a sixpenny Nail, and they were by much the finest and largest fruit that I have ever seen. One of them who I suppose had got a little of the Pickeroon[1] in him when he had got the nail refused to send up his fruit, on which the Capt after taking exceeding good Aim not to hit him fired a musket ball close by his head the report wind and whistle of which frightened him so that he run to the other end of his boat for the fruit and sent them up Instantly.

About 7 oClock the Pinnace was Manned and I went with Capt Cook to see whether or no the shores were accessible what the Country was likely to furnish and if there was any convenient place for Errecting My Observatory. Just as we had got into the Boat one of the Natives who was on the Opposite Gang-way catched up one of the Iron stantions to which the Man-ropes are fixed & leaped with it into the Canoe on which a Musquet was fired over him by one of the Officers, but it had no effect, another was called for, and Capt Cook called out not to kill him but the Natives about the ship made too much noise for him to be heard. He then ordered the Pinnace to pull round as fast as possible but before it could be done two more Musquets were fired the latter of which hit him and he droped down dead in the Boat just as we got in sight. Another Man who was in the Canoe with him instantly hove the Stantion over board, and when we got along side of the Canoe sat baling out the blood, in a kind of Hysteric Laugh.

Leaving a Spectacle so dissagreable, we rowed round the Bay and sounded in several places, in which we found as near an Agreement with those Mentioned by Mendana as could well be expected, after so long an interval. We saw several fine streams of fresh water; but no great promisses of any thing else, as not a fruit Tree of any kind was to be seen, and so great a surf set every where on the shore that we could not see a place where it seemed possible to land with safety to the Boat. On this the Capt concluded it would be best not to stop here longer than was necessary to get off a few Casks of Water, & if possible, a little fruit, and then make the best of our way to a More favourable Port. When we returned to the Ship we found that every one of the Natives had quitted her; but in two hours time they returned and trafficked as before. After Breakfast a Party of Marines were ordered on Shore to protect the Watering, and as the Horizon was Land locked both to the North & south from the Ship, I took my Sextant & a Bason of Quicksilver & went on shore with them to observe the Sun's Meridian Altitude but was disappointed. We now found it tolerable Landing amongst some Rock[s] which we had not seen before; but even here, it is not to be done without great Care, especially towards High-Water.

[1] i.e. picaroon, from Spanish *picaron*, a thief, knave.

8th. About One oClock, or perhaps a little later, for there was no determining to any nicety on account of the surf which is the greatest here that I ever saw, it was high Water; and I took marks at three different places which appeared to me most convenient for the purpose, in order to Measure how much it fell. After winding up the Watch & Observing some Altitudes for the Time, I went again on shore with the Guard, and walked a considerable way up the Country but saw neither Person, House or Plantation of [any] sort, nor even a single Fruit Tree. Their Houses being it should seem a long way up the Country, at least in this part of the Island. There are many which we can see from the Ship on the Ridge of a very high Range of Mountains; or rather Cliffs for they are in most places almost perpendicular. These Houses seem all Pallasaded round; but whether this be by way of fortification against an Enemy, or only as a fence to prevent Accidents by tumbling down the Precipiece may be doubted.—A little before 7 oClock we went on board, at which time, according to the best measurements I could Make the Water had fallen 3½ feet from two of the Marks; but near 4 feet by the other. I could not be certain, but believe it was pretty near if not quite low-water, as I could not perceive that it fell any for sometime before.

In the Morning when the Party went on shore, I took My Sextant & Quicksilver; as also the Diping Needle, and found by a mean of 12 tryals, in which the face of the Instrument was turned East and west Alternately, that the Needle's South End dipped 18°20′ below the Horizon. At Noon I found that the Supplement of twice the Sun's Altitude (for I was obliged to use the back Observation) was 35°18′, and that the Index of the Quad[t] stood 1⅜′ off the Arch of the Quadrant; and hence that the Latitude of the Place is 9°55′¼s. This forenoon the Natives brought down to us several small Hogs, a few Chickens, and a considerable quantity of Plantains and Bread-fruit; but no Cocoa Nuts, except two, and these were both old and good for little. Strong Gust[s] of Wind with Showers.

9th. The Party coming off before the time of High-Water I could not get it to day, and as I knew it would be dark before the time of Low-Water I went not on shore this Afternoon but took the Opportunity of Observing some Azimuth's of the sun, and doing some other things which could not be done so well as on board the ship. We had all the Afternoon great numbers of the Natives trading with fruit & now & then a Hog, which they have always done with the utmost Honesty & fairness since the first day. In the Morning I got on shore Early enough to observe the low water which happened at or near 9 oClock, and there was less surf now than heretofore, yet far too much to determine any thing with precision. After changeing the Poles of the Needle, the Mean of twelve trials, made with the face of the needle turned alternately East and West as before, gave the dip of the Needle's south End 17°56¼′. The supplement of twice the sun's Altitude on the Meridian was 36°03′, and the Index stood off the Quadrantal Arch 1′50″; and hence I compute the Latitude 9°55¾′s.

We trafficked while on shore for a Boat Load of fruit, some small Hogs and a few fowls. The Weather these last 24 Hours has been somewhat more regular than on the two preceeding days.

Hitherto we had not been indulged with the sight of one Woman since we came to these Islands: but this forenoon a party of several Hundreds of the Natives came down with one of their Chiefs at their Head in great pomp and form, and amongst them one Woman. She certainly was, or appeared to be considerably on the wrong side of thirty; but notwithstanding that was in the opinion of Most who saw her one of the most beautiful women that has been seen at any of the Islands in these seas. She was clad from head to foot pretty much in the same Manner, and with the same sort of Cloth as the Women of Otahitee are. She was remarkably fair; but had some freckles on her Nose and Cheeks, and her Feature[s] were extreamly regular, soft, and agreeable, and her whole deportment meek affable, and apparently, modest in the Utmost Degree so that if this was a just sample their women must be exceedingly desirable. There was along with her a Man who carried in his Arms an exceeding beautiful Girl about 6 Years old which they gave us to understand was hers, from this circumstance & the attention which seemed paid to her by those which were About her I concluded that she was of some Rank amongst them & that Curiosity had brought her down, rather on this day than any other, as thinking probably it might be done with more safety: but some of our Gentlemen, who it must be owned are much quicker sighted, in matters of this sort, than Me, were *positive* she was brought down for a *certain purpose*, and I was near getting my self into danger by doubting it. All that can be said to the Matter is, *that if it was so* either the Women of this Island are ill qualified for, or the Men who brought her down were bitter bad judges in the Choice of a Whore seeing that there did not appear to be the least spark of Concupiscence in any one feature or Action; on the contrary her whole Person and demeanour bespoke her one of that sort of Women which a Man of any tolerable degree of Modesty could never think of Attempting with success.

10*th*. I found the time of High water this After noon to be about half past three o'Clock: it was certainly after three and before four. It had risen 4 feet, or nearly so, by two of My Marks and something more than 3½ feet by the other. These Marks are on different and pretty distant parts of the Shore. This Afternoon I changed the Poles of the dipping Needle again and it then gave me the four following dips of its south End, viz. 11°30′; 11°20′; 11°40′; 11°45′; the difference between which and the first I am much at a loss to account for, unless I made a mistake yesterday, and did not actually change the Poles as I intended, which is very possible, and in that Case the difference is not to be wondered at, seeing that the construction of this Instrument is such as to require two seperate and very tedious adjustments, as often as the Dip Changes, and on this Account this Needle however Accurate in other particulars it may be is not convenient for a Voyage of this kind where we are continually moving from place to place & thereby changing the Dip very considerably & at every Place have many things to do, often in a little Time and under many inconveniencies.

In the Morning I went on shore again & found that the Tide Ebbed out about 4 feet from the last nights High-water Mark, and that it was low-water about 10 oClock;—certainly not sooner; but my chief Errand was to try if I could not get the dipping Needle properly Adjusted; but had not time to effect it. This Circumstance is the more vexatious as I shall probably never have another Opportunity of landing so near the Equator: Clouds dissappo[int]ed me also of the Sun's Meridian Altitude. The Weather Yet Squally with Showers; but rather more Uniform than it was the first Day or two.

11*th*. About 3 o'Clock weighed and stood along shore to the southward, and at half past 4 tacked and stood over towards the Island *Ohevahoa* (Mendana's La Dominica) to look, as I suppose, for a Harbour in it; but after standing along the west end & finding none we stood southward again. . . . These Islands were first discovered by Mendana in his last Voyage when he went to settle the Salomon Islands which he had discovered in a former one and called by him *Les Marquesas de Mendosa*. There are five of them although neither he nor we have seen more than four; for it is plain from his Account that we have not yet seen that which he Calls *La Magdalena*, nor did he see that which we first fell in with which is the most northerly of them all. . . . The Account which is given in Mendana's Voyage of the Harbour is not more minute than Accurate, unless that most persons perhaps would expect to have found its Enterance narrower in proportion to its breadth than it realy is; but we know not how Horse-shoes were made at that time in South America. The Gaps which he speaks of in the trees are, I presume Ridges of the Hills on which no Trees grow here; but these things are too subject to Mutabillity for much stress to be laid on them at almost 200 Years distance. Even his Town is fled away the Lord knows whither; but there yet remain many stones which appear to have been its foundation, & his Brooke & 'spring of water pouring out of the Rock at the hight of a fathom as thick as a mans Arm', and they are as pure water as I ever tasted. The Bay is about a Mile and half Deep, and about the same breadth where broadest and it may be about a Mile wide at its Enterance. On the whole, the Account (which was written by Quiros) does, in my humble judgement great honour to his Accuracy and integrity; and if he was a small matter out in the situation it is not to be wondered at considering the Early times in which this Voyage was made.

The Natives of these Islands taken Collectively, are undoubtedly the finest Race of People that I or perhaps any Person Else has ever seen. They are not like the Otahiteans One a great fat Overgrown, unweildy fellow and the next perhaps you meet a poor meagre half starved Wretch, over run with Scabs and blotches, but are, almost without exception all fine tall stout-limbed, and well made People, neither lean enough for scare-Crows, nor yet so fat as in the least to impede their Activity. Their Features are also very regular, and not that sameness in them which is so frequently Observed to obtain throughout a whole Race or Nation of Indians. In the Articles of Teeth and Eyes indeed the People of Otahitee, as well as the Natives of North America have greatly the Advantage; for many of these have very bad Teeth, and their Eyes are neither so full or lively as those of the others besides many are grey; but in general they are of a lightish brown. Their Hair, which in colour is as various as in England, except that I saw none which had red, they were[1] short except a bunch on each side of the Crown which they tye on a knot. Some of them also part their Beards, which are very long & tye them in two Bunches under their Chins, others Plat them, some were them loose and others quite short.— In this respect it seems to be *Chacun a son Gout*, as his Majesty of Prussia is reported to have said on a very different Occasion.[2]

They are punctured from head to foot in various figures and the Men in general go entirely naked, except a slip of Cloth which they pass round their Waist and then bringing the two Ends forwards betwixt their legs turn them up and stick them in the part which goes round them: this indeed is the dress of the Common People at Otahitee and the Society Isles;[3] and simple as it is it answers every purpose which modesty can require as completely as our own. As to the Women both here and at the society Isles they go cloathed from the Neck downwards in a manner which is both simple and elegant.—Some of the Men wore a small piece of Cloth round their Heads; others again had nothing but their slings; but many wore a sort of broad fillet platted in a very neat Manner of the fibrous parts of the Husk of Cocoa Nuts: in the front is placed a large Mother of Pearl Shell worked round; and before that another less of Tortoise Shell; also before that one still less of Mother of Pearl. These are so large as wholy to cover the forehead of him that Wears it and all round the Fillet are fixed long feathers of Cocks and Tropic Birds which when the Fillet is tied on stand upright so that the whole together forms not only a complete piece of Armour for their foreheads against the stones which may be thrown by an Enemy but also an excellent shelter from the sun and a very sightly Ornament at the same time.

Besides the Weapon mentioned at the beginning of these remarks they have slings with which they throw stones to an Amazing Distance and with great Velocity but it did not appear to me that they did it with much Aim. Their Canoes are composed of pieces joined to gether with a bandage made chiefly of the Bark of a soft wood which grows here in great plenty, and is very tough:[4] the workmanship is very rude, & they are from 15 to

[1] i.e. wear.

[2] What this occasion was is not very clear. The reference is possibly to the remark of Frederick the Great, when in 1740 the education, Catholic or Protestant, of the children of his Guards was under discussion, that in his kingdom everybody was at liberty to get to heaven in his own way.

[3] The *maro*.

[4] Marquesan canoes were 'built-up' on a basic hull of a single hollowed tree-trunk; the best were made of Tamanu, *Callophyllum inophyllum*. What soft wood bark Wales had seen

20 feet long, and about 14 or 15 Inches broad, some may be an Inch or two more and they end in two solid pieces fore and aft. That at the stern rises up in an irregular direction and ends in a point. The Head projects straight out in an horizontal direction and at the end is carved into some faint resemblance of an human face; but this is not spoken with intent to depreciate their workmanship in this Art, which in some other Instances which I have seen exceeds that of most other Islands in these seas. They use a paddle as is done by all other Indians which I have seen except the Exkimaux. I saw none of their houses except 3 or four small Huts in which nobody now lived and were miserable beyond description; but those whose Leasure permitted them to make more frequent, & longer Excursions into the Country give a Much better Account of them, as indeed those which we see on the ridge of Mountains seem to deserve.

These Islands are all very high land, vastly irregular and Cliffy, the higher parts being mostly covered with Clouds, at least it was so whilst we were there; but the Land, especially in the Vallies, seems to be exceeding rich and fertile mostly covered with wood; but it is almost all of that soft kind mentioned above; very pithy and good for nothing except to burn and scarcely that: On the sides of the Hills indeed grow a pretty many Etoe Trees as they are called almost all over the south seas which is exceeding hard and heavy but brittle: it is of this wood that they make all their weapons, and from thence it has its Name. It is the Cypress which I formerly mentioned to be planted round their *Maris* or burying Places at Otahitee.

We got here in all near 100 small Pigs, perhaps half that Number of Chickens; and a prodigeous quantity of Bread fruit and Plantains which were without exception the largest and finest that I have ever seen and allowed to be so likewise by those who had seen much more of these Fruits than I have done and in point of goodness and flavour exceeded by none.

We saw no Animals here beside Pigs, nor any tame Fowls except Chickens; nor did the Woods seem to afford much Game; but they abounded with small Birds of very beautiful Notes and Plumage but the fear of Alarming the Natives hindered Us from shooting so many of them as might otherwise have been done.

Tahiti and the Society Islands April–June 1774

APRIL 22*d*. Having represented to Cap[t] Cook that it would be of considerable use to get the rate of the Watches going at this Place, and the longitude shewn by it; as it would tend greatly to corroborate the Longitudes of Many Places which we have lately passed more especially as this is now so well determined; I got every thing ready for going on Shore by Noon, & soon after a Guard being Appointed, I got on Shore the Clock Astronomical Quad[t] and Reflecting Tellescope: the two former I proposed

converted into 'bandages' or lashings it is hard to say—perhaps hibiscus; they were usually of broad three-plait coconut-fibre cord.—See Ralph Linton, *Material Culture of the Marquesas Islands* (B. P. Bishop Mus. Memoirs, VIII, no. 5, Honolulu 1923), pp. 298–319.

to set up in the Enterance of the Ship's Tent as Capt Cook told me he could not Allow above two or three Days for this bussiness.

I got the Tent up and my Clock jogging before it was dark in doing of which I was the more Earnest as I found there would be an Occultation, or at least a near Appulse of both C & r Leonis to the ☽ that Night; but when I came to open my Tellescope I found it utterly spoiled, at least so far that not the least use could be made of it untill the Metalls are re-polished, and I could not then get on board for another; nor indeed was there then Time to put it together if I could. Hence we may see one great advantage which refracting Telescopes have over reflecting ones in long Voyages, more especially where no provision is made of a proper place to stow them in; but where a Person is glad to put them away in any hole or Corner that he himself can find. In the Morning however I got on shore Mr Dollonds Refracter, put up a Barometer, Thermometers &c as usual, and Observed Altitudes for the Time. The weather very variable; but in general the Wind was moderate with flying Clouds and sometimes showers.

23*d* to ye 28*th*. I continued my Observations in the Ship's Tent; but finding then that Capt Cook's stay at this place was likely to be considerably longer than was at first expected; and that it was not only inconvenient but that my Instruments without great Care were liable to be disturbed I sent for my own Tent on Shore; and having first removed the Great one errected it over the Clock & Quadrant as they Stood. During these 6 Days the Winds & Weather were very variable sometimes moderate pretty fine at others Strong squals of wind atended with thick Clouds and heavy showers of Rain, Thunder and Lightening, especially when the wind came Westerly.

APRIL 28 to MAY ye 10*th*. I continued my Astronomical Observations with all the Attention possible, especially those which tended to settle the Longitude of the Place, and am willing to flatter my self that I have contributed something towards it both this time and last, although the weather was very unfavourable for the first three or four Days when most might have been done. On the tenth I took down every thing by Capt Cook's direction and Carried them on board the Ship.

The Attention which I found necessary to my Astronomical Observations did not allow me time to keep a regular Journal while on shore; but as several circumstances occurred to me which I am willing to think worthy notice I shall put them down here, and flatter my self they will not be thought the worse of for wanting that regularity and order, usually kept up in a Work of this kind. . . .

MAY 10*th* to the 13*th*. What I have to offer concerning the Place and Inhabitants consists chiefly of little Circumstances, which in themselves, are not of the least moment; but, in my humble opinion, contribute more towards giving a tolerable Idea of the Genius and disposition of the People than a thousand Volumes of private Opinions written concerning them, unsupported by such like Facts, especially as we have every day repeated proofs that not one amongst us knows so much of their Language as to understand them always, even in the Common Transactions of buying and selling; much more in things of so intricate a nature, that they can scarcely be known with tolerable certainty of our next-Door Neighbours.

The first I shall mention happened one evening while I had gone on Board to supper. We were alarmed with the report of a Musquet at the Tent; a Boat was sent & I got on shore immediately where I found it had been discharged by one of the Centinals at a Native, who had found Means to steal a Water Butt almost from under his Nose, and was swiming it off down the River which runs at the back of the Tent. The man quitted his prize and ran on shore immediately, where he was found hid in a bush, and carried on board the Ship. In the Morning *Otoo*, the Aree or Chief Man of all the greater Peninsula of Otahitee, and who indeed claims Dominion over the lesser also, as we do over France,[1] happened to go on board the Ship with several of his Nobles (as we called them) and amongst the rest one who is a near Relation & called *Toowha*. Cap[t] Cook shewed the Man, and represented the Case to Otoo, at the same time insisted on the Man's being punished to deter others from the like practices in future: Otoo petitioned much for him but finding it to little purpose gave his consent, and the Man was brought on shore tied up before at least a thousand of them and had two dozen lashes given him, which almost flayed his back, after which he was set at liberty. The Natives were all going away seemingly very Much displeased; Otoo hung his head and seemed much frightened; but Toowha, stepping forward onto a little Eminence, called them back, and spoke for a full half hour, or more: If his language was as elegant as his Action was gracefull he must be a very great Orator. The substance of it, as near as we could gather, was to the following Effect 'How can you act in so shamefull a Manner as to steal from your friends, who bring you every thing that is good & usefull? do not they bring you Axes, Knives, Nails, Red Feathers, Beads, &c., and give them to you for Hogs, Breadfruit Cocoa-Nuts, &c. things that you can spare; and could they not, if they were not your friends, easily kill you, and take them for nothing? but they do not so.—They are your friends! Why then do you rob them? If you will steal, Steal from the Tiarabo-Men, and the Men of Eimeo, who are your Enemies, & fight with you; but steal not from them.—Go, and bring Cocoa Nuts and bread-fruit to them as usual.'

Otoo and his friends having been frequently very solicitous to see our Exercise, and the Great Guns fired Cap[t] Cook at last Consented; and the Party of Marines were drawn out and exercised before him and his Chiefs, and as the time had been Appointed two or three days before I believe almost half the Island had been informed of it for the Point was full of People from one End to the Other: They went very well through all their Manouvres, and fired many Vollies with Ball: It is impossible (and therefore it would be Nonsense to Attempt it) to describe the Amazement they

[1] This is an excellent instance of Wales's perceptiveness; unlike the majority of his countrymen, he obviously did not accept Tu's claims at their face value.

were under the whole time; but especially at the distance which the Balls fell at in the Water, and the Expedition with which they repeated their firing, and for which I thought the Marines had great Credit as it must convince them how inadequate their weapons are to ours: On the whole I verily believe that Otoo and his Gentry went away scarcely more pleased than frightened: he notwithstanding forgot not to insist on the Great Guns; and Sunday Evening was appointed for that purpose; but an Accident happened on Saturday night which put it by to a future Day.

The accident hinted at was this. One of the Centinals happening to nod a little in the Middle Watch, as some much greater Men are said to have done before him, one of the Natives, who no doubt was, as I believe some of them always were, on the look-out for what they could steal made free enough to take his Musquet; and was fortunate enough to get clear of with it without any others seeing him. By sun-rise there was scarce one Person of any Account left on the part of the Island where we were, and their Houses were all striped quite naked. A while afterwards four or 5 large Canoes appeared Coming round the Point on which Cap[t] Cook maned the Boats, and went to Intercept them in hopes that Otoo or some principal Person might be there whom he might detain Prisoner untill the Piece and some other things of Value which had been stolen were brought back; but found none who he Judged of consequence enough to Answer his purpose. There were however none who would not the Day before have been very much offended at our barely supposing they were not very considerable Arees, yet now absolutely denied their being so; nay assured the Cap[t] they were such inconsiderable persons that should they even presume to speak to Otoo he would beat them very severely, and probably they spoke no more than truth for their Arees are not very ceremonious on these Occasions but were it otherwise there are but few I believe who on a similar Occasion might not have done the Like.

Otoo, however, before he fled had dispatched one of his principal People in search of the Musquet; and he was lucky enough to hear of it; and brought it back to the Tent in the Afternoon for which Cap[t] Cook made him a very hansome Present, and went with him next day to Otoo where all was made up again, I believe, to our Mutual satisfaction. It is realy strange that People who are so well acquainted with the effects of fire Arms as these are should be guilty of such desperate Actions; nay a more extraordinary one than either of these above recited happened for one of them in the Night got into the Tent amongst us notwithstanding there were 3 Centinals no doubt with intent to carry off the first thing he could lay his hands on and would certainly have succeeded had he not unfortunately tumbled over one of our People who had that night spread his bed on the ground that he might enjoy to more advantage the fruits of a bargain he had made the Evening before: Nay it is certain that several instances of this sort happened for we lost many very Bulky things out of the Tent which could not have been carried away in the Day time unperceived; and this was one very great reason why I moved my Instruments out of the Ship's tent.

But not withstanding all these *fracas*, Otoo would not give up the Great Guns, and another day was appointed to which they were very punctual, and two or three rounds were fired some with round and others with Grape which terrified them if possible more than the small Arms; but they were much better pleased in the Evening, when several pieces of fire-works, such as sky Rockets Serpents Air Balloons &c &c. were played off, which diverted without Alarming them.

Otoo is a Young Man, very tall but slender, and stoops much: He has the appearance of a very stupid Man but His Actions and Government seem to bespeak him a wise active & great Prince; or if not, he must have very able Counsellors: He seems very fond of Millitary Matters: War Canoes are building in every part of his Kingdom; & they had whilst we were here Reviews of one sort or other almost every day, especially Naval ones of which Matters we understand that *Toowha* has the Management. . . .

After the Marine Review was ended we went on shore where we saw a number of Men drawn up with spears, and soon after discovered others which were (pretendedly) hid amongst the Grass & shrubs under the Cover of which (as was to be supposed) they advanced to attack the others: They began by throwing their spears at a distance, whilst their Opponents stood with the points of theirs rested on the ground before them; that is in a right line between themselves & the Assailants, with the other ends up as high, and right before their Eyes so that when they saw their Enemy's spear come at them, by a swing of their Arms this way or that as was most convenient they put it past them with a dexterity that was realy admirable. As they advanced the Attack was made by pushing and striking; the former they parryed somewhat in the same manner as is done with a foil in fencing, and avoided the blow by turning half round on one heel. During this Mock-Engagement, Otoo, very good-naturedly, frequently desired us not to be afraid, for that the People would not hurt us; a piece of politeness which I much fear none of us ever thought of paying him, when he attended our exhibitions of this kind; although we are, I suppose, willing enough to believe much more necessary.

I must not forget to remark the Attention which was paid here to the Youth who went with us from Uliateah by every one and by Otoo in particular who spared nothing which he thought would entice him to stay behind. He got him married to one of the finest young Creatures on the Island, the daughter of a principal Aree, and a great favourite of Otoos; offered him lands, honours in short, every thing that a king could offer; & *Oediddee* would certainly have been wise enough to accept of them, if Capt Cook had not insisted on his returning to Uliateah: in which he was the More particular, as none yet who had gone from any of these Islands had returned to their native Place. I believe he had the fate of a traveller amongst many; who seemed not to credit much his storys of seeing the New-Zeeland[er]s eating one another, of the White Land (as he called the Ice Islands) the perpetual Day, and some other things of that Nature; but this is no wonder some of them will no doubt want believers even in

England. I have always thought the situation of a Traveller singularly hard: If he tells nothing which is uncommon, he must be a stupid fellow to have gone so far, and brought home so little; and if he does, why—it is hum,—aye—a toss up of the Chin; and,—'He's a Traveller'!

I have had abundant reason this time to be convinced of the injustice which is done the Women of this place by those who represent them as ready to prostitute them selves to any who come up to their price, as I have seen very many Instances where things have been rejected with disdain which in their Estimation must be almost invaluable, and I was once witness to a piece of delicacy which even I did not expect to have met with here: it was a Relation, or at least one who claimed to be such to Oedidde who was with much difficulty hindered from thrashing another Woman for complaining before me and some others of the backwardness of her Bedfellow the night before; but though we prevented the Beating, we could not hinder her from belabouring her with her Tongue; and amongst other things she told her that such as she would make us spit at them, and say when we got home that the Otahitee Women stunk; for that we should think all like those who did as she did. Another Circumstance which confirms me in this opinion is that not one Woman we know of who has had any connections with the English are yet Married: the greater part are now in appearance little better than Vagabonds; and the few who have fared better, are only in keeping by a sort of Men who either by their Profession or otherwise, are forbid the Use of Women;[1] but who like many others in the same situation, hold no short Dalliance with them in private. One of the Most agreeable Women that I have seen here is in this situation, and scrupled not to acknowledge that she had murdered a Child or two because the Father dared not be known to have had any Commerce of that kind. And this is a thing which we have some reasons to believe is not very uncommon amongst them. . . .

MAY y[e] 14*th*. About 3 PM Weighed and got under [sail] soon after which one of the seamen slid down the ship's side with intention to leave her and swim on Shore and would certainly have Escaped had not the Lieut. of Marines been Accidentally looking out of the Gun-Room Ports & seen him drop astern; on which a boat was hoisted out, and he was taken up and Confined. . . .

15*th*. At 2 PM the North Point of Huaheine bore SWBW½W dist. some 5 Miles or so. And at ½ past 3 came too at the mouth of the Northern Enterance into Owharre Harbour, and carried out Warps; by the Means of which we came to an Anchor about 7 with the small Bower; and in the Morning the Stream Anchor was Carried out to steady the Ship. We lie here about a Mile and half to the Northward of where we did last Year: It had not long been Daylight before the Old Chief of whom I spoke when here last came on board with his Medall and Copper 'Graving; and soon

[1] Presumably this refers to the *arioi*, and it is of course a misconception. See I, pp. clxxxviii–ix. Women as well as men belonged to the order.

After great Numbers of the People came off with Hogs Fowls and Fruit. Moderate Breezes Easterly & flying Clouds.

16*th*. Mostly Cloudy with Showers. In the Morning M[r] Forsters going on Shore their Servant was attacked, and an Attempt made to strip him by some of the Natives.

17*th*. Mostly Cloudy with showers. I found that the Tide flowed very near two feet at the Harbour's Mouth to Day, and I have some reasons to believe I did not see it untill some time after it had been low Water. In the Evening I went, amongst others to see one of their Dramatic Entertainments and soon recognized my old Friend the Uliatean Garrick amongst the Performers; who entertained us with two or three little Pieces which appeared to be Extempore: They were certainly *Pro-Tempore*, and his Part of them was most Excellently well performed; It was that of a Girl, and the Piece represented her as runing away in the Ship from Otahitee with the English, and concluded with the Reception which she was supposed to Meet with from her friends at her return, which was not represented to be of a very indulgent Nature. Now this was Actually a piece of true History, and the Girl was present at the Representation of her own Adventures, which if they knew, as I make no doubt they did, was a very Cruel; although they perhaps might think a very wholsome, and even Necessary piece of Satire. It was with the utmost difficulty she kept her seat, and she stood in need of all the Comfort & support her new friends could give her to keep from Tears. It is not foreign to the Purpose to add that two *Ladies*, Natives of this place, who had been previously engaged to sleep on board the Ship, but went on shore to see the *Heavah* (as they call it) broke their Engagements, and could not by any Means be prevailed on to return on board the Ship.

18*th*. Light breezes Easterly with showers. Three of the Petty Officers who were out on a shooting Party were Robbed of a Bag wherein were some Hatchets Nails &c. One of their Guns (they had but two) missing fire, the Natives coaxed the other to fire at a Mark; think them, I suppose they might play their intended Prank with safety; but it missing fire Also, 'tis possible they might think themselves equally safe, for they seized the Bag immediately, and set out with such speed that the others thought it useless to follow them; but stood snaping their Guns to no Purpose.—The Audacity of these People is so great that I cannot go on shore even Close to the Ship to observe the Meridian Altitude without a Guard.

19*th*. First part flying Clouds; the latter frequent Showers: Wind Moderate, easterly.

20*th*. Moderate Wind easterly, and fine Weather. This After noon we heard from some of the Natives that two of the Lieut[s] and one of the Master's Mates who were out on a Shooting party had been Attacked, and their Arms and Cloaths taken from them; on which the Cap[t] Went on shore to Enquire into the Affair; and soon after they all three Came on board having got their things again through the interposition of some of the Chiefs of the Island: We were all eager to learn the story; which I could not help observing could scarcely be said to *run on all four*, as the Critical Gentry express it.—In the Morning, 'The Capt with several of his Officers and Seamen, and the Officer of Marines and his Party, armed, went into the Country, in search of the People that were Guilty of this Robbery'; to which Party were super-added some 'Gentlemen Volenteers', as they were pleased to denominate themselves; one of whom having lost the Bayonet belonging to his own Piece, had one of the ship's Bayonets tyed on the Muzzle of it.

21st. About 4 PM the Armed Party returned; having, according to the strict, literal meaning of some Poet or other; who, I have utterly forgot,

March'd up the Hill, and then—March'd down again.[1]

The weather very fine, with loose, flying Clouds, and Moderate Wind, easterly....

23d. Flying Clouds; the Wind Moderate and Variable towards the East: Stood on & off all night under the Lee of the Island, and in the Morning worked to Windward in order to Gain the Harbour's Mouth.

24. The former part Moderate Wind ESE with flying Clouds; the latter light Airs with Rain. About 2 PM came too off the Harbour's Mouth with the small Bower and carried out Warps ahead to warp the ship into the Harbour. At 7 Came too again with the Small Bower for the Night, and in the Morning it was weighed and the ship Warped into the Cove which is about ¾ of a Mile to the Eastward of where we lay last Year. Here she was moored with the stream Anchor to leeward; and we had soon the pleasure of seeing all our old friends at this place in good Health, and very happy to see us once more.

25th. Brisk winds south-Easterly and Cloudy with Rain. It was High-water to Day at 11 AM perhaps, a little later for there is no determining those things to great nicety here on account of the small & slow rise of the water.

26th. The former Part Moderate Wind at ESE & Cloudy with rain; the latter, brisk wind Easterly, and flying Clouds. It was high-water to day about Noon and the rise of the Water was 8¼ Inches: this last point may be determined with the utmost Accuracy here, as the water has not the least Motion; I find it by taking the Altitude of the Water above a flat stone, which is the foundation of one of their *Maris* or burying Places, with a two foot Rule & it may be very well determined to the ⅛ of an Inch, so that an Error of a ¼ Inch can scarcely happen at both high & low-water even if the Errors should both tend the same way.

27th. Brisk winds easterly, and cloudy weather. This Afternoon, amongst

[1] No doubt he is thinking of the classic lines—anonymous, alas!—on the noble Duke of York, who had ten thousand men: 'He marched them up to the top of the hill And he marched them down again'.

several others, I walked a considerable way up the Country, and came at last to one of the most beautiful Vallies I have ever seen: a little way up the Ascent on one side stood a small Hut and in the bottom ran a stream of water, which, poetry appart, might be justly called chrystaline, and said to tinkle as it fell from Rock to Rock, and Murmur along the Pebbles. We walked up towards the Cottage: they seemed to be poor indeed; and had little to give us either to eat or drink except the water which ran below: he however did what he could, and if he had not wherewithall to allay our hunger he attemp[t]ed to charm it, for without speaking five words he placed himself on his back-side and in an instant called forth more Music out of two pieces of dryed sticks laid hollow, than I had before heard at these Islands. After he had finished his Solo, Sonata Overture, or whatever else you may please to call it, for I am no dab at your Musical Matters, we distributed our C[r]umbs of Comfort amongst his Women & Children, and set off homeward. He accompanied us a little way, till finding a favourable Opportunity, he snatched two Chissells, which one of the Lieutennants (in a very tempting manner it is true) carried under his Arm, and flew with them through the woods like an Arrow. When we got back I found that the Princess *Poydoa* performed that Evening for the Entertainment of the strangers, as these were my favorite amusements, I made scarce more than a hop skip & Jump to the Play-house where I found she could twist & distort a set of very delicate features with as much dexterity as ever. 'Tis true this did not divert me much; but sufficient Amends were made by some of the Interludes to me, whose tast is not over-&-above delicate. The Concluding Piece, they called *Mydiddee Arramy*. Which I know not how to translate better than *The Child-Coming*. The part of the Woman in Labour was performed by a large brawny Man with a great black bushy beard, which was ludicrous enough. He sat on the ground with his legs straight out, between the legs of another who sat behind him and held the *labouring man's* back hard against his own breast. A large white Cloth was spread over both which was carefully kept close down to the Ground on every side by others who kneeled round them. The farce was carried on for a considerable time with a great many wrigglings and twistings of the body, and Exclamations of *Away! Away! Away to perea!*[1] (which I dare not translate) untill at length, after a more violent than ordinary struggle out crawled a great lubberly fellow from under the Cloth, and ran across the place between the Audience and Actors, and the *he-Mother* stradling after, squeezing his breasts between his fingers and dabing them across the youngsters Chaps, & every now & then to heighten the relish of the entertainment mistooke and stroaked them up his backside. On the whole it was conducted with decency enough for a Male Audience, had not Mididdee dragged a great wisp of straw after him which hung by a long string from his Middle. The Women did not however retire even from this part of the Entertainment, or even turn their faces but sat with

[1] '*Aue! Aue! Aue to piria!*'—*Aue*, alas!—here no doubt a shout of mock grief; *to*, to push; *piria*, from *piri*, to be pressed; the general effect being that the midwives were hard at work.

as demure a Gravity as Judges are said to do when hearing baudy Causes. I asked some who sat round me why they also did not laugh as I did & one of them replied '*Mididdee tooatooy*', the aptitude of which expression pleased me as much as the Entertainment itself, because the latter word has exactly the same meaning and is applied in the same manner as the word *Impotent* is with us.[1]

After the Entertainment Capt Cook desired the Company of Poydoa her Mother Brother &c &c to dinner the next day, and they came to breakfast. I was much diverted with the polite and Easy behaviour of the Lady we had brought with us from Otahitee on this occasion, for when they arrived she ran to the Gang-way received every woman as she came up the side in her Arms and kissed them with as much easy cordiallity (and perhaps hypocrisy) as ever a fine Lady in Great Britain could have done: but she was in truth a cute Girl and deficient in no one point, that I know of, unless it was Chastity, and as to that it was not seemingly considered as one of the Cardinal Virtues at our house. It was Low-water this morning about 7 AM.

28*th*. Moderate Wind easterly and fine Weather. It was high water about One o'Clock, and the rise of the Water $7\frac{3}{4}$ Inches. I dined along with Orehow[2] the Aree of Uliateah and father of Poydoa in the Cabbin; His Wife, Daughter, and some other Females who Came with them being not allowed by their Customs to eat with their Lords and Masters the Males, eat their Victuals in another Room. I believe the Old Gentleman drank a full Bottle of wine to his own share which at length made him Noisy, and he insisted on our going on shore with him where Poydoa should Entertain us with another *heavah*. Much about the time that the Entertainment began, we lost the old Gentleman and did not see him again untill after it was over, so concluded his wine had put him to sleep, and were going away without enquiring for him and had just got to the boat, when he came running through the Croud, caught hold of the Cap[t] & lead him back, where we found two or three Hogs, and a heap of Cocoa Nuts and bread fruit almost sufficient to load the Boat which he told the Cap[t] he must take on board with him; so that notwithstanding his being drunk we found he had been employing his time to Much better purpose than sleeping. The *Heavah* was as usual; but I shall describe one Interlude which I had not seen before, as I think it may perhaps tend to throw some light on an order of Men here which we are but little Acquainted with I mean those who are forbid the use of Women but whom we discovered a little before we left Otahitee have a considerable share in the Management of their Millitary Affairs, and are called *Aree-Owhee's*.[3]

The principal Actors were 4 Men and a Boy, and after some parade which I did not understand, One of the Men took of a piece of Cloth which he shewed to those round him, and then dancing up to the drums, in doing

[1] *Tuatuai*, 'straight-laced', modest. What the lady seems to have told Wales was that a modest woman did not laugh at such things.
[2] Cook always gives the name of this chief as 'Oreo'; 'How' =*fau*, principal chief?
[3] i.e. *arioi*. Wales gives us a good rendering of the pronunciation of the word.

which he kept exact time to the music, shewed his Cloth spoke some words and then came and threw it with an Air of defiance on the Ground. Another Man did the same in every respect; and after him the Boy also; only the latter instead of throwing down his Cloth with that menacing Air which the others did he hid it under a Mat which Covered the Floor, and stood on one side while the two Men stood each by his Cloth with their Arms folded in a sort of sullen posture. Another Man then pulled a very small bit from his Garment, and in immitation of the former, danced up to the Music, with a great Many Ludicrous Gesticulations, and shewed his shred of Cloth with much Pomp and many Airs of defiance, spoke the same words which they did, and then came in the face of the two Men and blew it away with his Mouth; when folding his arms as they did and affecting their Gravity, he asked them if they were *Aree-Owhees* to which they Answered in the Affirmative; and he replied (literally) *Sweet Aree Owhees!* and instantly prepared to attack them on which they took up their Cloth & tied round them in manner of a sash and one of 'em engaged him but was soon beaten, his Cloth taken from him and he turned away in disgrace; he then Attacked the other but was now beat in his turn on which the Victor was Crowned with green boughs &c by his Companions who afterwards danced round him & the Piece concluded.

It was low-water about ½ past 8 AM. . . .

30th. The Weather yet very fine, and the Wind Easterly. . . . This forenoon one of the Natives came on board who measured 6 feet 4 Inches & ⅜; he was slender and exceeding upright, & had a sister along with him almost as tall as himself.

31st. Wind & Weather as above. High water between 3 and 4 o'Clock and the rise of the Water was 7½ Inches.

JUNE *1st.* Wind and Weather still the same. To Day one of the Natives arrived in a Canoe from Huaheine, and told us there were two ships come to that place: that one was Capt Furneaux, and the other Mr Banks; that he had been on board them, and that in one they made him drunk. In short he told his story in as clear and particular a Manner as I could have done it, and added that Capt Furneaux' Ship was less and Mr Banks' Greater than the Resolution.

2d. The Wind and weather yet the same. Many Rockets, Balloons, and other fire-works were this Evening played off for the Amusement of the Natives; but they had been so long on board the Ship that very few were good for any thing. Many of the Natives still insist on Mr Banks, and Capt Furneaux being at Huaheine. In the Morning Orehow, and his whole Family came on board, amongst whom was a Young Woman, who when we were here last accompanied Poydoa in her Theatrical Exhibitions; but now declined it on account of being with Child. She made not the least scruple of telling us that she should strangle it as soon as born, because the father was an *Aree-Owhee.* We should have got more Intelligence from her, I believe, on this head, had it not been for Oediddee, who stopped her short with great earnestness, and told her that such things were not done in Britannia, and that we thought them bad. After this we might as well have hoped to extract Oil out of Tinder, as another word from her on this subject; and tho' I was very angry with the Boy for disappointing me, yet could I not help being pleased with him on the whole as I was convinced that he was actuated by a fear of his Country's suffering in our opinion: therefore though he must be damned to all Eternity as a Philosopher; yet as a Patriot, a good natured Man, & a lover of humanity; I think he must certainly be saved! Indeed every Action of his life shewed him possessed of one of the most humane hearts that ever Man was.—May he live long, and enjoy that happiness which such a heart only can give!—The Maxim that a Prophet has no honour in his own Country was never more fully Verified than in this Youth—he was not the least notice taken of here, so that I believe every one without exception were now sorry he was not left at Otahitee, although all joined then in thinking it expedient that we should bring him hither.

3d. The Wind and weather yet continues the same. In the Morning the ship was unmoored and by ten oClock, under-way. Orehow, and his whole Family had been on board all the Morning, and frequently in Tears at the thoughts of our Departure; and more especially as Cap[t] Cook had told them he did not expect ever to come again. The utmost minute being now come, for we were without the harbour's Mouth, the old man and his whole family without exception went over the side into their Canoe which waited for them bathed in tears: But if this was the Case with those whose Acquaintance with us had been so short; what must have been the Conflict in poor Oediddee's breast whose Accquaintance had been so long & whose heart was certainly made of Nature's softest Materials. His legs seemed scarce Able to support him over the side into the Canoe which waited for him, and when it droped a stern of the ship he gave a look up at her of unutterable anguish, burst into tears and droped down in the stern of it. Nothing I believe could have torn him from us would Cap[t] Cook have given him the least hopes of his being ever able to return.—The Affection which the Natives of this Island in particular have taken to the English has something remarkable in it. Those off Otahitee are certainly not inferior to them in the goodness of their dispositions, and have had a longer Acquaintance with us, yet although a look of silent sorrow is always visible in their Countinance at our departure yet they always manage so as to keep it within very decent bounds, whereas these are able to preserve none. The Natives of Huaheine, although situate between the two, seem of a much less gentle disposition than either, nor are they much liked by them, which appears to me a little odd. At Noon Ohamoneno Harbour bore East, distant about 5 Miles, and the Latitude observed was 16°44½′ s.

On computing the Observations made in this Harbour, I find the Watch gives 208°25′8″ E which is only 1⅗″ in time different from what it gave last Year. . . .

Tonga June 1774

26*th*. . . . at 5 oClock we came to an Anchor under the North side off great Annamocka in fathoms Water after sailing NNW 3¾ Miles, NNE 3¾ and ENE 1¾ the wind being SE the whole Afternoon. When brought up the Extreams of the Island bore N88¾ E & S34½ W.

Ever since 9 or 10 oClock in the Morning we have had Natives round the ship in their Canoes from the different Islands as we came along, and who came without hesitation on board the Ship as often as asked to do it. They brought off with them the Yauva, or pepper-Root, Cocoa-Nuts Plantains Chaddocks Yams & fowls. As soon as we had Anchored the sea was almost covered with Boats bringing Roots & fruit which we purchased for Nails; that Article of Commerce being as valuable here as at any place we have seen before.

In the Morning the Cap[t] and Officers went on shore to look for water, and found three large Ponds or Lakes; but two were perfectly salt-water, and that in the third was very brackish, full of Insects, and stunk intolerably; so that Either they did not meet with Tasman's Pond (which I suspect) a great Alteration has happened in it (which is possible) or he has much misrepresented Matters, which we have not known of him before. In the Morning we saw to the Northward a great Multitude of Islands, all of which were small and low; and two to the North-West which were high. The Extreams of the larger of these bore N40⅓°W & N33¾°W and the Middle of the Other N29½W. A large Cluster of y[e] low ones bore N½E and four which were nearest us N31°E, N19°E, N15°E & N12°E.

27*th*. This Afternoon I went on shore, and when we landed met the surgeon, who had been left behind in the forenoon. The Natives had by surprize snatched and wrested his Gun from him, and it was with some difficulty he kept them from Striping him by presenting a tooth-pick Case which they Mistook for a Pistol; but as soon as we appeared they left him and shifted for themselves. We walked a Considerable way in the Island & found the Houses and Plantations to be exactly like those of *Tongatabu* and *Eaoowe*, but not near so Elegant nor was the Island by much so well Cultivated, as the former of those, although from the Accounts of Tasman I expected to have found it more so. The Persons, Manners, and Dress of the People are also perfectly corrispondent to those of Tongatabu; and I cannot again forbear expressing My Admiration of the sweetness, softness & Melody of their singing and playing on their flutes & ten reed pipe, and as to the address & behaviour of their women it has a delicacy and softness in it utterly unknown to any other Indian Women whatever; I must however acknowledge that on a second review of both that in point of. . . .[1] The Island as far as I could perceive does not differ in any respect from other low Reef Islands, except that the Lakes or Lagoon in the Middle of

[1] This is the end of a page, and some words are missing. The next page goes on immediately, as in the printed text; possibly Wales had to break off his writing, and on resuming forgot that he had not finished a sentence.

it seems almost filled, or grown up, probably owing to the luxuriance of the Vegetation which is evidently much greater than the Consumption, as we saw vast quantities of fruit lying roting under the Trees for want of Gathering, and this I suppose must greatly increase the soil. Two salt springs were seen here, one of them which I saw appeared to me considerably above the surface of the sea & I am told the other was so likewise, a circumstance which [I] think rather extroardinary, unless they proceed from some of the Inland Lakes, which perhaps by their being filled up may raise the water, above that in the sea, and so feed those springs. To us the Natives behaved with great Civillity owing probably to the Number of our Party.

In the Morning the Boats went again on shore to get Water, and trade for fruits, Roots &c, an Officer who went to superintend the Work had his piece seized, and several others were Robbed of divers Articles, On which several Guns loaded with Shot were fired from the Ship into that part of the Island, & the Capt went on shore with a party of Marines; seized two of their large sailing Canoes; and one Man who attempted to defend them was Much hurt in his wrist & thigh by a load of small shot; those proceedings terrified them so much that they immediately brought down both Guns & every other thing of any vallue which they had stoln & restored them, in return the Canoes were given up and Mr Pattin went on shore & dressed the Man's Wounds, and found them not very dangerous. They appeared it seems vastly pleased at the attention paid to the Man's hurt and both sides parted, seemingly with great good friendship to one another, and our trade went on as before; but without any Thievery.

28. The Capt and Mr Cooper being both on shore, and not coming off untill late in the Afternoon I could not wind the Watch up at the usual Time, and by some fatallity or other I forgot afterwards untill it was down;[1] I have, two or three times before, been near let it go down on the same Account but luckily recollected before it was down. I took several Altitudes this Morning from whence I find it is $2^h10'41''$ slower than it was before; and as I had got several at this place before it was let go down no inconvenience can possibly Arrise from this Accident; however as I had now kept it going two years I had begun to flatter my self with the hopes of carrying it home without any thing of this sort happening.

Having Got a large Cargo of Yams, which I think the best root in the World, and Fruit, a few Fowls and two or three small Pigs, we weighed about 7 oClock, and after sailing NNW 4¾, tacked, & stood SWBS 3½ Miles then tacked & stood NNW 3 Miles to Noon, when we were close to a small sandy Island which lies NBW from the place where we lay at Anchor, and I observed the Latitude 20°05′50″ S.

[1] During the later exchange of pleasantries between Wales and Forster, Forster took some credit for not mentioning this lapse in his book; to which virtuous claim Wales made reply, 'P.S. As to the watch being forgot at Anamoka, you know your father told every officer on board the ship that he would publish it; and so he undoubtedly would, if he had not thought it would have tended only to shew his malevolent heart'.—*Remarks*, p. 47.

The People of these Island[s] resemble so much those of Tongatabu that it would be only repeating the same words were I to say any thing concerning those. Their Canoes also are exactly the same as those; but as I cannot find that I have there said any thing concerning them, it may not be amiss to do it now. They are from about 16 to 20 feet long & about 20 or perhaps 22 Inches broad in the Middle, and taper off gradually in breadth towards each end: One way they carry their whole depth, or at least nearly so to the very extermity but the other way they come off to nearly a point, the Keel or under part being taken away.[1] They are Covered for about ¼ part of their whole length at ea. end, and in the Middle are open. They are formed of several pieces joined together with bandage in so neat a Manner that on the outside it is difficult to see the Joints, all the fastenings being on the inside & pass through ridges left, or rather worked on the several boards which compose the vessell at their edges & ends, for that purpose. No Canoes that we have seen in these seas can bear the least Comparison with these in point of neatness & workmanship. Besides these, of which every Man seems to have one, they have others, which are formed by fixing two very large ones, exactly resembling these in shape, together by Cross pieces: these have a Mast & yard & Carry very large sails of Matts, which Jibes round when they want to Tack in a very convenient Manner; but how the Manoeuvre is performed I could not see. In rigging these Vessells they employ Ropes near as thick as our 5 In Hawsers, which are laid in the same Manner with ours but, I think neater than any I ever saw before, the strands having so very regular and sharp a twist: I know not of what Materials they are made.[2] Two or three of these Vessells & a vast Number of the small ones which also Occasionally carry a small Latine sail Accompanied us all this Day, and tacked when we did so that it is possible that some who have seen more of working various kinds of Vessells than I have may be able to describe in what manner those do it.

The Longit. of this Place as shewn by the Watch is 184°59′36″ E; but by a Mean of 27 Lunar Observations, 15 of which were Made before we came there, 3 at the Place, and 9 after leaving it, the Longitude comes out 185°29′01″ E. Those Observations which were not made at the Place were reduced to it by the Watch as usual. The Latitude by a Mean of 4 good Meridian Altitudes with two Hadley's Quad^{ts} was 20°15′ S. And the Variation by a mean of 4 Azimuths and 2 Amplitudes was 9°47′ E but this is considerably less than any we had taken for some time before at sea, possibly owing to the ship's head being a different way. I had no opportunity of determining anything concerning the Tides except that it was low Water about 20′ past 4 o'Clock on Monday ye 27th which was the only time I had any opportunity of being on shore: By the Marks on the shore it should seem as if it rose about 5 feet but I know by repeated Experience how very fallacious this way of Judging is.

[1] The Tongan canoe is still built to this pattern.
[2] Coconut husk; see Mariner, II, p. 201.

The New Hebrides July–August 1774

JULY ye 21*st.* The Shores of the Island, laid down by M. Bougainville, to the South-West of Whitsuntide Island,[1] are on the North-West side exactly like those of the former three, bold, and without Inlets; but on the south west side they are flat. The land is very high and to wards the North Point is a very high Hill which I am convinced is a Volcano, as it continually vomits up vast Columns of black Smoke; but I heard no noise: Some say flames were seen in the Night. The Whole Is well covered with Wood, but I saw no Plantations or Inhabitants; however Smokes were seen in many Places. Its south side was flat & more regular, and seemed indeed very beautifull; but we passed at too great a distance to distinguish any thing Particular.

Soon after we had Tacked at Noon we discovered the Appearance of two very good harbours in the land to the Westward;[2] on which the Boats were hoisted out & sent to Examine that to Leward. There were several Hundreds of the Natives on the Shores viewing us, and several Canoes which ventured off a little way. They were all armed with Bows & Arrows & small Clubs, which they slung across their shoulders. They seemed to look at us & our Boats with Admiration but did not attempt to come near or meddle with them. After due Examination the Boats made the signal of there being a good Harbour and safe Enterance, on which we bore away for it and about 5 oClock Anchored in 20 fathoms, bottom sand and Rocks; being sheltered on all sides by the Land & reefs except about 5 or 6 Points to the Northward & that might be shut up by going farther in. We had not been long at Anchor before many of the Natives came round the Ship seemingly in a very friendly manner, but would sell nothing except now and then an Arrow, and I observed that every man had his Bow lying in the Canoe, ready bent and several Arrows beside it. Towards the Evening two or three came on board the Ship; but I was then bussy below & did not see them: they stayed about the ship till near 8 oClock & then went on Shore.

In the Morning several Canoes were round the Ship by Day light; but still refused to barter any thing whatever; and soon after several hundreds swom off to her and came on Board, so that in a little Time the Decks & rigging were full from the topmast head to the Chains; but none had any Arms who came on board that I saw except one, who had a small neat Club slung at his back. They are universally a small and ordinary race of People, not quite but very near as dark as the Negros, and do something resemble them in their Countenances, although neither their Noses are remarkably flat or their Lips Thick. Their Hair also is quite short & curled like theirs, but not so soft and woolly. They go entirely Naked except the Penis for which they have a very fine Case, fringed; & a String to the end of it by which they tye it up to a sort of Belt or String that goes round their

[1] Presumably he means Ambrim, and by 'the land to the westward', in the next paragraph, Malekula; but in Bougainville's map both are south-west of Pentecost.

[2] Sasun Bay and Port Sandwich.

wast so very tight that the shape of their Bodies is not much unlike that of an over-grown Pismire; but their limbs are well shaped & Clean made enough.

Most of them had a wild Boars Tooth, or some such like thing bent circular round their right wrist, and a round piece of wood with a hole through it on their left: the hole was so small that it would barely come over their hand. Some had very large Scabs or blotches on their Arms & Legs; but this was far from being general.

The People who kept the Boats along side had orders not to let any of the Natives come into them for fear of their stealing any thing: but one, more positive than the rest insisted on doing so, and when the Man pushed his Canoe of with the Boat hook, pushed a long Bamboo at him, and the Man, then, pushed the Boat hook at him; on which he very deliberately laid down the Bamboo, took up his Bow, and picking, very carefully an Arrow out of his Quiver applied it drew it up to the head & was taking Aime at the Man, and would, I make no doubt, have shot him dead if Cap[t] Cook had not at that Instant discharged a load of small Shot into his face & shoulders, on which he droped his Bow a little, just wiped his hand across his face, and then took it up pointed it at the Cap[t] but before he could get Aime to his mind one of the Officers fired another load into his Breast & Shoulders, on which he disisted & rowed off. Several Arrows were now shot over the Ship, and all the Natives who were on board her leaped into the sea & swom on shore: and a Great Gun being fired amongst the Trees, which reechoing from all the Adjacent Woods & Mountains made a most terrible Report and frightened them Much; however no farther Mischief was done, and so ended Affair the first. The Man had shot his Arrow long before Cap[t] Cook was ready with his Musquet had it not been for the Motion of his Canoe which hindered his taking Aime, and he several times turned round with much Anger in his looks to scold the Man who Managed her for not keeping her steady, by which time some of those in the ship had leaped overboard swom to him, & catched hold of his Bow with intent to stop him; but he seemed resolute, shook them off & would, I beli[e]ve certainly have executed his purpose had he not been fired at.

Their Canoes are hollowed out of one Tree, have no side-boards, and may be from 10 to 15 feet long & perhaps 15, 18 to 20 Inches wide: They are fitted with an out-rigger, as is usual in all the other Islands in the South Sea, and rise a little towards ea. end; but not so much forward as aft.

After Breakfast the Cap[t], Lieu[t] and the Lieu[t] of Marines with his Party went on shore With People to Cut wood: It was then about Low-Water, so that the Boats could not come near the Shore. The Cap[t] leaped into the Water & walked towards the shore without Gun where several Hundreds of the Natives were Standing with Bows Arrows and other Weapons: but when they saw him advance alone without Arms, one who seemed to be a Principal Man amongst them gave his Bow & Arrows to another & came into the Water to Meet him, and spread[g] his Arms open as if to receive him; and when they met took the Cap[t] by the hand & led him on shore. The

Officers and Marines followed him armed and were drawn up on the Beach, and the Natives stood with their Bows & Arrows as a Counter-guard, all the time they were on Shore. The Capt made the Chief understand he wanted Wood, and he made signs for them to cut down what they had occasion for. At Noon they came on board again without having had the least squabble; but the Natives would not suffer any of our People to go of the Beach; but always stopped them when they offered it and pointed to them to go back to their Company.

22d. This Afternoon we had no Natives Came near the Ship: The Capt and some others went up the Sound & found the Ground & soundings every where good: in short that it was a most excellent Harbour. The Shores were in many places Swampy and covered with Mangroves; but they did not meet with any fresh Water. A Plan of it taken as well as I could from on board the ship is Annexed.—In the morning Weighed & got under-way but it falling Calm we were scarce clear of the Harbour's Mouth at Noon.

As soon as they saw us get under way they became much freer & seemed willing to part from any thing even their Bows, of which they had hitherto been very Carefull. They seemed most pleased with Marbled Paper & some of them immediately converted it, before our Eyes into a Covering for the only part which is covered about them. In this traffac they exhibited remarkable proofs of their honesty & Integrity for the ship at first had good way through the Water, by which means several of them droped a stern after they had received what they had agreed for & before they had time to deliver their part of the Bargain in return, and it is almost incredible to conceive what efforts they made to Come up with us again & deliver it. One in particular did not get up before it was Calm & the thing had been forgot; he came up however a long side & held it up, several offered to buy it which he absolutely refused untill he saw the Person he had before sold it to to whome he gave it & when he offered to give him something else he refused to take it & shewed him the thing he had before received....

There were seen here Cocoa-Nuts Bread fruit & one or two Oranges: We saw and heard plenty of Fowls & got one Pig which the chief made a Present off to the Capt. Several others were seen; but they would part with no more. I believe it to be a very plentiful Country could we have seen it. The Shores, as far as we have yet seen are flat for a considerable way inland, after which the Country rises gradually to a considerable height, and has a very beautiful appearance. The Natives told us they called it *Mallicola*, and that the Name of that Island on which the Volcano is is *Ambrym*, and the large Island which first opened off its south west End is Called *Ahpe*....

AUGUST ye *5th.* After dinner the Capt and Officer of Marines landed with the Party. There were vast Numbers of the Natives on the Beach all Armed with Spears, Bows & Arrows & Clubs, who drew close to our people as soon as they got on shore; and it appeared to me, for we saw every thing from the Ship as plain as if we had been with them, that they were irresolute & knew not whether to Attack them or not. They shewed the Capt a Pond of Water close to where they landed at which they filled three or four small Casks, and then Came on board. They carried no more Casks with them as this was intended only as a *Coup d'Essai*, and the Water Casks served as an Excuse. When our People reimbarked, the Natives gathered Close round the Boat & we then fully expected an Attack, and everything was ready for it on board; but they yet were too irresolute & seemed as though they had not had time to pre-concert a Scheme for so that this time the Boats all got safe on Board without a skirmish.

All night the flames from the Volcano were very visible over the hills. The Mouth seems not to be above 4 or 5 Miles from the Harbour, about West from it. In the Morning Many of the Natives Came again round the Ship in their Canoes. Amongst the rest one old Man who had the day before made many trips for Cocoa Nuts Plantains and Yams, continued to do the same now untill he was interrupted by the following Accident. A Man who had been very Insolent in brandishing his Club, striking the Ship & Committing other Acts of defiance, at length Offered it to the Capt for a Medall, or some such thing, but on receiving it refused to give his Club, and rowed away with it; and after repeatedly Calling & Making signs to him to bring it back the Capt fired a Charge of Small Shot at him which hit his face & breast; but notwithstanding this he still Continued to paddle away as fast as he Could & being now at a great Distance the Capt ordered One of the Wall-Pieces[1] to be fired at him, which was done with such good Aime, although he was a quarter of a Mile from the ship, that the Ball struck not a Yard from him. Several others were fired at him untill he got on Shore & though none hit him yet every ball fell very near him even when near ¾ of a Mile of, and caused so great a consternation and Astonishment in all the Rest that in an hour Afterwards the Abovementioned old Man, was despatched off to us with Green boughs & other Ensigns of Peace, and a present of a large Bundle of Sugar Canes, which was accepted, and a very Considerable present Made to him in return. The Capt at the same time endeavouring to make him understand why the Man was fired at, and that we wished they would throw away their Spears & Bows &c &c & be friends with us, in which Case we would hurt none of them. When he got on Shore they all gathered round him & he seemed in very earnest discourse for some time but to what purport or effect was impossible to know.

Soon after the Capt gave Orders for another trial to land, which now seemed a serious Affair, as I believe some thousands were on the Beach on each side of the Watering Place all Armed. The Ship was brought broadside too by means of a Spring, and all the 4 Pounders which could be mounted on that side were loaded & brought to bear on the Place where

[1] Cook calls them swivel-guns; a wall-piece was a heavy musket mounted on a swivel, on top of a wall (here no doubt the bulwarks) for defence. See below, p. 915, 25 February.

the Landing was intended to be made. When the Boats drew near the shore, the Capt[t] made signs to them to draw back. The Old Man, our friend also was there & two others who endeavoured to make them do so but [to] no purpose, on which a Musquet was fired over them which made some run; but one more Audacious than the rest set up his backside at them & claped his hand on it—this was not to be put up with a Musquet was fired at him & some others amongst the Croud who yet staid & the Officer on board thinking the battle general, gave orders to fire also; 5 four-pounders, some loaded with round, and others with Grape Shot, four or five Wall pieces, and two or three Swivils were fired from the Ship, which cleared the beach so that not a Man was to be seen in two Minutes time except the three old Men who had endeavoured to make them retire, & these never stirred, so confident were they that we would not hurt those who we thought our Friends. But what is most remarkable we had no reason to suppose that any Person was much hurt by all this firing, notwithstanding there were so many: and was a very happy Circumstance as it Answered our Purpose without. The People then landed, filled a Boat Load of Water & then returned on board.

6*th*. This Afternoon I went on shore with the Boats which went for Water, which happened as near as I could determine at 4^{h} 48′ and to look at the Place which was said to be Absolutely improper to establish a Post on; I did not see any reasons to be affraid of trusting my self on shore there with a proper Guard; but as I cannot be supposed a proper Judge of these Matters, It was my duty to submit to better Judgments & Contrive some means of getting at least the Rate of the Watch without staying on shore All Night. I did not Judge it safe to Carry the Watch backward & forwards every day for fear of Accidents, as we had to land in a surf on a flat shore, and, since the Misfortune which happened to my Pocket Watch[1] it did not seem easy to do it without. There was no way but by Signals; & those must go through three hands beside my own, which must render the Method Precarious, but it was better than none, and I resolved to make use of it only with this precaution to venture the Watch on Shore the first & last Day, & be as carefull as possible in the others; being certain of one steady hand to assist me always in it.

When we got on Shore there was not one Native to be seen; but in about an hours time they began to make their Appearance on the Beach & by degrees drew nearer; but there was not one who brought a Weapon of any sort; but all left them stuck up at a distance, and we endeavoured all in our power to convince them how happy we were at it & how little occasions they had for them on our Account; and before we went on board a sort of Intimacy & dependance on each other began to come on. Besides filling a Boat Load of Water, the Sean was hauled with great good luck several times & we encouraged them to run amongst & help us and at y[e]

[1] A meddlesome midshipman, on the previous 27 January, had invaded his cabin while he was at breakfast, and in examining the watch, dropped and broken it.

same time gave them some fish which pleased them much but at the same time the Guard was not remitted in the least; We brought on board about 20 dozen of fine fish, mostly Mullet, which furnished the Whole ship's Company with a fresh Meal.

The Water is taken out of a Pond, at the back of the Beach; it is very high Coloured but exceeding frish and sweet. The Country round the Harbour is covered with Cocoa-Nut Trees full of fruit, of which the Natives seemed to make no Account for if we only pointed to them one of them would run up like a squirrel, and clear the tree in an Instant whilst others would gather & throw them to us, without expecting any thing for them for they seem not to have the least notion of Buying & selling neither were they fond of, or indeed willing to touch any thing we had.

All beyond the Beach, which in some places might be about 40, in others not more than Ten Yards broad the Country seems one entire forrest of low Trees and Bushes over-grown with a sort of vine which makes it almost impenetrable except by some narrow tracks, or Avenues, made by the Natives. I went up one of those about a ¼ of a Mile & saw in two or three Places patches of Plantain Trees which seemed to grow wild but not one House or Native. However as the Path was very narrow & crooked I did not chuse to go far for fear of surprize.

In the Morning I took the Watch & Astron. Quad[t] on shore & got Altitudes: I moreover made many trials of the Dip of the Needle & found that its south end dipped 44°51′. I changed the Poles of the Needle between every 4 or 6 trials.—By taking equal Altitudes I found that the Low-Water was at $11^h42'$ and the Latitude by the dble Alt of the Sun, taken with Hadley's Quad[t] from a Quicksilver Horizon was 19°32′18″ s. . . .

7th. . . . We had many of the Natives round us all day, some with Arms, others without; but they were in general very quiet and good natured, giving us any thing they had except their Arms, which they refused to part with but for ours, which I thought but reasonable.—In the Evening the Sean was again hauled but with very indifferent fortune as we did not catch above 5 Dozen of Fish & most of them small. All the Morning it was Cloudy so that I got no Altitudes nor the Meridian Altitude at Noon.

8. This Evening the Sean was hauled again; but with less Success than Yesterday. In the Morning it was very fine & Clear and I got Altitude[s] for the Time by the Watch and also the double Alt. of the Sun on the Meridian which gave the Latitude 19°32′33″ s.

Yesterday and to day the Volcano has ceased to make that horid noise it used to do; but yet vomits forth vast quantities of black Smoke, and in the Night flames of Fire are sometimes seen. Many pieces of Pumice stone have been found in different parts of y[e] harbour; but none have been seen to fall since we came in; nor have we been able to see any thing of the kind come out of it with the smoke. One of the Natives came off with us, and dined on board the Ship.

9th. This Afternoon I got but two wires of the Corresponding Altitudes & those were rendered useless by some Mistake Committed on board the Ship in the Times by the Watch, so that this Day's Labour, and it is not a little, is entirely thrown away. In the Evening hauled the Sean three times and caught three sea Spiders,[1] a small Bream & a little sting-Ray. Some who went to get Ballast to day scalded their fingers in a stream of Water which bubbled up amongst the stones they were gathering to carry on board the Ship.

In the Morning the Sean was hauled again and they caught about a dozen fine Mullets; but this & some other things hindered me from getting on shore till near half past ten oClock, and of course the Observations of to day cannot be much depended on. This way of going to work is very inconvenient as my whole time is taken up in trying to get a few Equal Altitudes since there is no getting on board again for several hours after I have done, & have no way of spending my time but in sauntering too & from on the Beach for I dare not go inland on account of the Natives.— It has also another bad tendency, for having nothing else to do, I write down all the Nonsense that comes in my head & thereby swell my Journal, as Falstaff did his Belly, out of all reasonable Compass.

10th. It came on Cloudy at Noon, so that I got no more than three Wires of the corresponding Altitudes & those gave the Gain of the Watch 10".81. After I had done Observing, as I could not get on board, and having long had a great desire to make a short Excursion inland, I prevailed on two of the Officers to accompany me, so taking our Guns we struck into a Path which seemed to lead right across the point of the Island, and had not gone a quarter of a Mile before we came to some of their Plantations, through which we walked near half a Mile before we came to any of their Houses. These Plantations consisted of Yams & Tarro (an excellent Root met with at Otahitee & all the Society Islands) and several other sorts of Vegetables which we were utter strangers to. There were also great numbers of Plantain Trees almost all of which had fruit on in one state or other: There were also Cocoa Nut, Fig & Nectrine Trees all with fruit on, & many others with which we were not acquainted. The Ground appropriated to the Roots was formed into Beds as is usual in England & the Mold was very rich & fine as if it had been sifted through a sive. The Yams were planted in a large, high, round heap of very fine Earth, at one End of the rectangular Bed which appertained to them along each side of which were reeds stuck up and others laid across from those for the Plants which are of the Viny kind to run along and Cling to. At the End of this range of Plantation we came to a Place, where there was no bramble or under-wood; but many very high spreading Trees under which was a sort of Village Consisting of about 20 houses in which there were a prodigious number of Inhabitants, both men & women. The Houses are

[1] Any spider-like marine creature was called a sea-spider; what precisely these were it is impossible to say.

about 10 Yards long & three broad & mostly built in form of a semi Cylinder, by setting the Ends of sticks in the Ground & bending them together & tying them at the Top; but there were some built like the roof of an English house without any Walls: both sorts are thatchd with Palm-tree Leaves. We saw many exceeding fine Hogs & plenty of Fowls feeding about the Houses so that those People seem to abound in every thing that is needfull for life. They seemed a little alarmed at our first Coming on them so suddenly; but when they saw we were so few, made signs of friendship & were car[e]full not to meddle or come near any thing, they seemed much pleased & were extreamly civil & obliging. We told them we wanted to go to the farther side of the Island & look out for more Land, and an old man stepping out from amongst the rest made signs for us to follow him & led us the way quite across the Island, several others followed us but not one brought a weapon of any sort along with him. When we got to the farther side we saw two Islands but I believe there are four because they gave us four Names & pointed different Ways they called the two I saw *Irroname* & *Amatum* the other two Names were *Etonga* & *Fotona.*[1] *Irroname* is, I think, the same which we saw to the Eastward the Morning we came into the Harbour, but I could not be certain as I had no Compass; if it be not, that we saw then is called *Fotona.* Having satisfied our Curiosity here, we returned with our Guides, the Old Man still leading the Way, and answering such questions as we put to him in the best manner he could. Indeed they were all very civil & obliging Answer[g] and shewing us every thing they could, and were very ready to get us specimens of any Plant, Tree or fruit we passed by untill we came back to the Village, where our old Gentleman stoped and a young one came on with us and shewed us a much shorter track down to the Beach than that we went by, and I returned exceedingly delighted with my Afternoon's Excursion.

In the Morning I got on shore something earlier than usual & took two sets of equal Altitudes. While I was observing some of the Guard Called out the Volcano! The Volcano; and turning round I saw a prodigeous Column of black smoke, Earth & large Stones rising up into the Air to an amazing height, and presently after heard an Explosion greater, I think than any Clap of Thunder I can remember. There were several Explosions after this, but none so large; nor did I afterwards see it emitt any thing but smoke.

11*th*. Got Corresponding Altitudes at 10 Wires; but on computing them found they made the Watch's Gain since Yesterday, almost 20″, whereas yesterday's with the first made not quite 11″ and of Course there must be a great error in some of them, as the Watch never yet varied half that quantity from one day to another. Indeed I begin to despair of doing any thing to the Purpose here, and yet am so great a slave to it that I have scarce time to eat.

[1] Erronan was an alternative name for Futuna: possibly 'Etonga' was an alternative likewise for Aneityum. Or it may have been a name for one part of the island, possibly a sign of Tongan settlement. Forster speculates upon it, II, p. 310.

In the Morning it was Cloudy till near 10 o'Clock so that I could get no Altitudes before that time and soon after came on a Shower of Mire, I can call it nothing Else, as it was Compounded of Water Sand Earth, and some other matter like small particles of Asbestos. I make little doubt but it came from the Volcano although [the] Wind blew now directly from the Opposite Quarter & from the Sea; Moreover I dare say these Sort of Showers are not unfrequent here as all the Trees, Bushes Plants &c are covered with the same Matter.

12*th*. The same dissagreeable kind of Shower continued almost without intermission the Whole Afternoon; only the Matter fell dry. I collected a quantity of it which fell into My Quad^{t} Case & on the head of the Cask which I used for a Quad^{t} Stand & find by comparing it therewith that it is the same Matter which Composed the Beach all round the Harbour. It was with the utmost Pain & difficulty that I got 3 wires of the Equal Altitudes on this Account, and thought I had entirely lost my Eyes in the Evening with attempting to get the Dist. of the ☽ & Antares because the Star was so near the Zenith. The Sean was hauld this Evening & we caught a considerable quantity of Fish.

In the Morning it was Cloudy, yet I made a shift to get 10 Wires, out of two or three sets of Altits. By conversing with some of the Natives on the Beach I learned that the name of the small Island which lies of the Harbour's Mouth is *Immer*,[1] and that of the Island where we Anchored a day or two before we came in here is *Irramango*.[2] I believe that I forgot to mention that the Name of this we are now at is *Tanna*.

13. Cloudy all the Afternoon so that nothing could be done. And as I could neither leave the Beach were my Instruments were nor get on board the time was wearysome enough, for Amusement, I got some of the Natives to throw their spears at two stakes which had been driven down to fasten the Boats too. One of them hit a Stake which was about 6 Inches broad & 20 high several times. This Stake was of soft rotten wood about 3 Inches thick and the Spears went quite through it several times; he stood at 11 & 12 Yards from it; beyond which none of them choose to stand; nor could they throw with any great aime at much longer distances; although when they throw only for distance they can throw them 50 or 60 Yards with great force. The abovementioned Person threw with much the best Aime; others threw several times (one 7 or 8) and hit the Stake but once. However, at the distance of 8 or 12 Yards they seemed all of them Certain of hitting a Man's Body. The other stake was of white Pine: It was a piece of a Studding sail Boom & perfectly sound: those spears which struck it full went into it about an Inch. I got one man to shoot Arrows at a Cocoa nut which I set up on a stick at about 8 Yards distance: he shot four or 5 times but never hit it and came but once within the Compass of a Moderate sized Man. It is probable he might be a bad shooter, since one of them, I am told, shot a small fish swiming in the Water, or possibly this last might

[1] Aniwa. [2] Eromanga.

be mere Chance. I have been more particular on this head as we may hereby form some estimation what Execution they can do with their Weapons. I measured all the distances, so that there can be no deception on that head.

In throwing their Spears they use a short stiff String platted of Rushes, or some such thing, which at one end has a large Knot, and at the other a small Noose which goes onto the fore finger. They take a turn round that part of the Spear where it is nearly on an Equipoise, bringing the noose End over the Knot, which when drawn tight by the finger jambs the Knot against the Spear, and thereby holds it fast. They hold the Spear between the Thumb and the remaining fingers, which serve only to give it direction the Velocity or force being communicated to it by the string & fore-finger, the former, on account of its stiffness, imjambing & flying off from the Spear as it becomes slack, which will be the instant there is no more occasion for it, viz. when the velocity of the Spear becomes greater than that of the hand. This Evening the Volcano flamed out more than usual.

In the Morning it was cloudy with drizzling rain so that no Observations could be got, and having long had a desire & probably might never have another opportunity I embraced this of going up the Mountain towards the Volcano, in Company with several Others, all imagining it not to be above 4 Miles off; but after we had climbed Hill after Hill, and gone near that distance from the Ship, we did not find ourselves in a jot better situation for viewing it, but were to appearance as far off as at first setting out. Not above half a Mile from the Shore, on the side of the hill next y[e] Bay are several places where smoke issues from Cracks & Fissures in the Earth, and which we had hitherto taken for fires made by the Natives. These must, I am now convinced, be at least 6 or 7 Miles from the Place where the Principal Appearance is, and there are vast tracks of Plantations, and Many Villages between them. The Ground where these Smoking Places are rised up like a Mole-Hill of two or three Yards diameter. The Earth is a bluish Clay, soft & wet, as if with the steam of boiling water, and crusted over on the outside with a Substance in tast like Allum, and in many places are little heaps of real Sulphur, of which those places smell very strong to a considerable distance. The Trees Shrubs & herbage are exceeding fresh, green & flourishing close to the place where the Smoke rises, and some low fig-trees, loaded with green fruit hung directly over one of them yet seemed exceeding fine and healthy. I dug a hole in one of those Places in which I put a Thermometer of Fahrenheits construction made by M[r] Ramsden & Covered the Bulb for some depth with the Earth that I dug out, and in one Minute it rose to 210°. It remained in 2½′ but did not rise higher; and I could have wished it might have stood longer; but as the Thermometer was the property of another Person who did not chuse it should,[1] & having none of my own which go high enough I was obliged to be content with this Experiment, which I do not think quite satisfactory, because I know by experience, that a Thermometer carried

[1] This seems to point to the elder Forster.

into a greater degree of heat will rise at first higher than its natural State and after some time fall to it, and it may be, that in such extream degrees of Heat as this was, the Aberration I am speaking of may be considerable. Below this place, and close to the Shore I am told there is a spring so hot as to boil Perriwinkles, which I intend to try with a Thermometer the first Opportunity I have of landing there for there is no going to it by land.

We found the Natives here far less friendly than on the other side of the Harbour, where I made my former Excursion. Here they opposed our proceeding farther with their spears, Bows & slings, all ready Charged; and although we got past them on[c]e or twice yet they slipped through bye-ways and formed a-head of us again, and we found at last that we must either desist or come to blows with them, which we thought no-ways Justifiable as our Errand was little more than shere Curiosity. It is but justice to add that when they found we had given up the Point, and were returning in earnest they called to us to stop & brought us Sugar Canes and Cocoa-nuts; and a bunch or two of Plantains, and then made signs to us to go away, which we did.

But the greatest satisfaction this Ramble gave me was in an irrefragable Proof of the fallacy of a Notion some had taken into their heads that the Natives of this Island were sodomites. This opinion they grounded on one of the Natives endeavouring to entice certain of our People into the Woods for a purpose I need not mention. I had at first presumed to undertake their defence, and argued that they might possibly mistake those Persons for Women, as had been the Case with some of our Own People, and particularly one at Otahitee where we are much better acquainted than those people can be supposed to be with us: but there are People who, either through Custom, Education, or something worse, are not capable of defending the Whims they Adopt otherwise than by *It is so.—I know it.* and falling into a violent passion because their word is not taken in Cases where no man can give his word with certainty: and some of this Cast have asserted, and I make no doubt *written down* as *Dogberry* says that most of the People we have lately been among are Sodomites, or Canibals, or both, in which last predicament stand the poor Souls we are now with. It hapened moreover unfortunately for the retailers of those Opinions that no person had been attempted who had not either a softness in his features, or whose employment it was to Carry bundles of one kind or other which is the Office of their own Women, and of this sort was the Instance I am going to relate. The Man who carried Mr Forsters Plant Bag had, I was told, been two or three times attemp[t]ed, and he happening to go into the Bushes on some occasion or other whilst we were set down drinking our Cocoa-nuts &c. I pointed it out to the Natives who sat round us, with a sort of sly look & *significant action* at the same time, on which two of them Jump'd up and were following him with great glee; but some of our Party bursting out into a laugh, those who were by (suspecting it I suppose) called out *Erramange! Erramange!*[1] (Its a Man! Its a Man!) on which the

[1] From *eruman* or *yeruman*, a man. Is the name of the island also derived from this?

others returned, very much abashed on the Occasion, and the mistake was so palpable that every one present, and there were some of the most positive on y[e] other side of the question, were obliged to acknowledge that they had taken him for a woman, and had not the least notion of executing their purpose, after they found it otherwise.

14*th*. Cap[t] Cook being desirous of seeing the Place where the Natives dwell who are so friendly I went with him to the Village, where I began now to have some little Acquaintance. Some of my old Friends met us at the Enterance & seemed much pleased at our Coming. They shewed us all round their little Village which is a perfect Paradise in the rural tast, and at every house almost we were desired to sit down, and Victualls of several sorts brought us to Eat & Cocoa-Nuts to drink, and when we had staid with them as long as we thought proper, two or three were sent along with us down to the Beach to carry some fruit they had pulled for us, a Yam or two & some sugar Cane. In the Morning it was Cloudy; but I got a few Wires of the Equal Altitudes & afterwards employed my self in taking a draught of the Harbour; in doing of which I found at one Corner, under the Hill where the Smoking Spots are a stream of Water running out of the Rock which seemed to me nearly as hot as boiling Water; but having with me no thermometer I could not then determine its Absolute heat.

15*th*. This Afternoon it came pretty Clear, so that I was Employed the whole Afternoon and Evening about my Observations. In the Morning I borrowed a Thermometer of Cap[t] Cook as I had none Graduated high enough intending after I had got the morning Altitudes, to try the heat of the Spring I saw yesterday; but got it broke so strangely in carrying out of the boat that I was not less surprized at the Manner, than vexed at the Matter of the Misfortune.—This Morning the Chief of the Island, came down to see us. He was a very old Man of the most open Countenance that I have seen amongst them, unless we except that of the old Man who so early became our friend and benefactor; but then his was a merry open Countenance, which seemed as it could laugh at all the Pomps and Vanities of this World, whereas this Man's was rather solemn & beneign. He was not distinguished from the rest by any thing that I saw unless it was a broad red & white Checkered Belt that he wore round his Wast. The material & manufacture of which seemed the same as those of the Otahitee Cloth. His name was *Geogy*, and his Title *Areki*.

16*th*. The Afternoon & Evening were very Cloudy and so hot that the Thermometer stood at 83 a little after sun-set. The Morning also was very cloudy untill near 9 oClock, when it began to clear up & Continued fine untill Noon.

17*th*. This Afternoon Cap[t] Cook tried with a Fahrenheits' Thermometer the heat of the Spring which rises on the Shore opposite the Ship and found that the Thermometer rose to 191. I could not now go with him; but his Account of the Matter was so distinct that I have no doubt of the experiment.

In the Morning while I was observing the Altitudes Capt Cook tried the Hot-Spring, which rises opposite the Ship again; but the Thermometer rose no higher than 187°. These Experiments were made by digging a small [hole] into which the water ran, and immersing the Thermometer in it; but it occurred to me that this method is exceptionable, for the water at the Bottom of the Hole where the Bulb of the Thermometer lies will grow Cold, and the hot water as it comes out of the Spring only run over the Top of it. I therefore proposed that in trying that we were then going to at the corner of the Beach, the Thermometer might be laid along in the Stream, with but a small Elevation above the Plane of the horizon, with its bulb close to the hole in the Rock where the Water Issues & but just below the surface of the stream: It was necessary the Stem of the Instrument should be a little elevated to be sure the Mercury did not run along it by means of its gravity. This method was now used & the Thermometer had not been in quite 2 Minutes before it rose to 202½. It staid in 6 or 7 Minutes & fell only half a degree. I think it is not possible to have a fairer Trial than this was.

I estimated the time of Low-Water this Morning at three quarters past Eight o'Clock.

18*th.* The time of high Water this Afternoon was at $2^h55'$, as determined by equal Altitudes of the Water, and it rose 3 feet & one Inch, which is higher by an Inch than on the Day of the Change. By estimation the Time of low-water in the morning was at half past 9 o'Clock, after getting of which, and the Altitudes, an Opportunity offering I went on board the Ship to make some Calculations and presently after one of the Natives was Shot by a Centinal for drawing his bow at him. he had drawn it, it seems once before; but not liking the Arrow he put it bye & chose another & as he was drawing it the Man fired & shot him through the left Elbow Joint into that side, among the Ribs, and the Ball broke one of them in its Passage. He walked a little way, and then Staggering Side-ways fell into the Water, whence he was drawn by some of his Country men & carried off a little way. The Surgeon was sent for Instantly, but the Man was dead before he could well examine him. The Circumstances relating to the Wound I had from Mr Pattin on his return; the rest from Mr Whitehouse, one of the Mates who was present at the time it happened.

19*th.* By equal altitudes the Time of High water was at $3^h50'$, and it flowed 3 feet 5 Inches. This Evening I met with a young Fellow (It was he who dined on board the Ship) who could throw a Spear with exceeding good Aime & great velocity 20 Yards. I believe he could be morally certain of hitting a Man at that distance, and miss him but very seldom at 30 Yards, but it did not appear to me that any great danger was to be apprehended by us who are cloathed in the latter Case, unless it happened to be attended with some accidental Circumstances. He could throw it 60 or 70 Yards when he attempted to throw as far as possible, and once threw it over a Cocoa nut Tree which could not I think be less than 15 or

16 Yards high, and at last threw it so far into one of the Nuts which were on the top of that tree that it hung there. It was a very light spear that he used on this Occasion. I saw no other who could throw a Spear so well as this. He found fault with me, in Shooting with a Bow & Arrow for drawing the Bow too much, and I observe they draw it but little when they shoot at a Mark; but they throw their Spears with all their Might, let the dist. be what it will.

I must confess I have been often lead to think the Feats which Homer represents his heros as performing with their Spears A little too much of the Marvelous to be admitted into an Heroic Poem, I mean when confined within the straight Stays of Aristotle; nay even so great an Advocate for him as M[r] Pope acknowledges them to be *surprizing*. But since I have seen what these People can do with their wooden ones; and them badly pointed and not of a very hard nature either, I have not the least exception to any one Passage in that Great Poet on this Account. But if I can see fewer exceptions I can find an infinite number more beauties in him as he has I think scarce an Action circumstance or discription of any kind whatever relating to a Spear, which I have not seen & recognized amongst these People as their whirling motion & whistling noise as they fly. Their quivering motion as they Stick in the Ground when they fall. Their meditating their aim when they are going to throw & their shaking them in their Hand as they go along &c &c.

As to the Persons of these People they are in general pretty well made, but I think rather low, very brisk & Active as indeed most Indians are, probably from the Joints not being Cramped, or their bodies cumbered with Cloaths.

Their hair is chiefly brown, and curled but not short, and they seperate it into small locks & bind, or wold them round with the rind of a long slender plant or Shrub down to within about an Inch of its end, and as the hair grows they continue the binding so that it appears like a parcel of small Strings hanging down from the Crowns of their heads: They have brown Eyes, are very dark Complexioned; but cannot be called black nor have they the least characteristic of the Negro about them. The men go entirely naked except the Penis which they wrap up in a bundle of leaves or Grass and stick the End of this Covering, which they sometimes make half a yard, or two feet long into a String or belt that goes round them. The Women wear their hair Cut short, which is an universal fashion with that Sex throughout all the South Seas, except at the Islands of Tonga Tabu, Annamocka &c, and have all a kind of Pettycoat made of flags or some such thing that reaches below their knees, except such as are not arrived at the Age of puberty, and who have many of them only a few flags hanging down before like an Apron.

I have described their habitations already; but to what I have said of their plantations may be added that their whole time is employed about them, or at least between that labour & the Exercise of their Arms in which they are exceeding dexterous: Every Man is a Warrior, and after we became acquainted, seemed to take great pleasure in shewing us their skill in that Art; but more especially in the use of their spears in which they seem to place their principal dependance. They have some Canoes large enough, perhaps 30 feet long, two broad and three deep: they carry a sort of latine sail like the smaller sort at Tongatabu &c & have out riggers like them; but the Workmanship is very rude when compared with those of that truly ingenious People. The Bottoms of them are mostly of one Piece, and the boards which compose their sides are sewed on with bandage as they are done at Otahitee &c; but the Joint is covered on the outside by a thin battan, champhered off at the edges, over which Strings pass.

The fruits of this Island are Cocoa Nuts, Plantains, Breadfruit, Oranges,[1] Figs, Nectrines, Wild nutmegs and many others whos[e] Names I know not. Their Roots are Yams, the largest by far that I ever saw, Tarra Root & a sort of Potato, and they have great Plenty of large Sugar Canes. Fowls & Hogs are in abundance; but they would part with none. Indeed we had nothing which they seemed to place any Value on, and they were even afraid to touch any thing that belonged to us, so that there was no great danger of their thieving. In the morning we weighed & sailed out of the Harbour without any Accident happening, although the Passage in & out is I believe very intricate & dangerous full of Rocks and Shoals, and has an ugly bar across which causes a great swell and in bad weather is in some places near breaking. As soon as we were out the Ship was brought too the Boats Hoisted in and at 11 AM made Sail when the Extreams of Tanna bore N 50 W. 6 Lea. and S33°E. . . .

New Caledonia September 1774

SEPTR. y[e] *4th.* About 8 oClock came off an Opening in the reef about 1½ Miles wide which seemed to promise a Good Harbour within. The Boats were therefore hoisted out and sent to examine it. About 9 they returned & reported that the passage was clear, and the Soundings within regular from 14 fathoms downward: the Bottom sand with Coral intermixed. There were a great number of the Natives in their Canoes, which carry a fore sail & Mizen, m[a]de of Mats, who seemed to be fishing on the Reef; but seeing our Boats go towards the Opening they drew up both ways & lay on the two Points of the Reef, admiring them all the Time they were employed sounding; but never attempted to meddle with, or come near them. One indeed that came from the Shore & had it seems one of their Chiefs on board went up to the Boats without ceremony & in the most friendly manner took several fish out of their own Boat & hove into ours; & the Officer who was in her presented them with some Medalls, & such other Trinkets as he happened to have with him with which they seemed Pleased & went off.

On hearing this Report, the Cap[t] Sent a Boat to lie on the point of the southern reef & hauled the ship close round because the Tide of Ebb set very Strong to the northward. These precautions were no more than

[1] We must here have again the fruit that Cook calls Barreeco, *Citrus macroptera.*

necessary for we did but just go clear of the Northern Reef, the point of which lies somewhat within the other. All this time the Natives to the number of 10 or 12 Canoes lay on the two Points of the Reef seemingly wraped in astonishment at the address with which so large a body was turned & twisted about, and as soon as we were past them, they all up with their sails & followed us so that (to illustrate small things by large ones) we seemed like a Man-of-War, with a large fleet of Merchantmen under Convoy. We sailed thus between three & four Miles; the soundings being from 12 to 14 fathoms Clean Ground, and then came to the point of another Reef which extended South Eastward & seemed to Join the other about 5 or 6 Miles higher up. Over the end of this we passed in 5 & 6 fathoms, having all the Way a Boat a head sounding & Making signals. Within this reef lies a small sandy Island, under the Lee of which the Cap[t] proposed to Anchor, and for that purpose made two or three boards to windward, the Natives following us all the time, tacking when we did, and making signs of friendship, & satisfaction at our arrival.

5*th*. Between 12 & 1 o'Clock we anchored in 5 fathoms; the small Sandy Island, mentioned above & on which I now proposed to Observe the Ensuing Solar Eclipse bearing S 88°E dist. about a Mile; The most easterly point of y[e] Main in sight S 68′E. The Point of the Inner Reef N 11½E and the Opining in the outer one N 4 or 5 W for it could not be set with Certainty. The most Northerly point of the Main in sight N 76 W. The Extreams of the large Island to the Northward N 69½W, and N 61W, and a small one between it & the Main N 70½°W.

We had not been long at Anchor before the Natives ventured so near as to take from us pieces of Otahitee Cloth which were lowered down to them by a String, and before night many of them Came on board the Ship with a Confidence surpassed by nothing but the Behaviour of the People of Tonga-tabu, Annamocka, on the like occasion. They appeared perfectly good natured, friendly & honest which is more than can be said of any others in these seas on our first Acquaintance with them. They are quite naked except for a bit of Cloth or a leaf which they tye round the Penis, and which sometimes does not cover above half of that. Some of them fasten the end of this covering up to a string which goes round their waist but in General they let it hang down. Some few have a bit of Cloth tied round the forehead but not many. In short those People approach nearer to the Dress of Adam before he sewed the fig leaves together, than any we have seen before. They are an hansome well-made People enough, and like all other naked people very Active and nimble. Their Complexion is a very dark Copper, with Jet-black Hair & Beards. Their hair is very much frizzled, and most of them keep it cut quite short so that at first sight it looks very much like that of Negros, but on examination I found it as strong & coarse, if not more so than ours. I think the Hair of the Mallicola People is not so strong & hard as that of those, in other respects they are exactly Alike. Their Weapons are short Clubs, Slings, and Spears which they throw in the same Manner, as the Tanna People do but these are much more neatly made & more desperate Weapons.

Their Canoes, are all double, with a very heavy Platform over both, on which they have a fire hearth, & generally a fire burning. The whole Boat is very clumsey & heavy, which enables them to carry so much sail as they do; but they move very slowly without. They do not Paddle, as all the other Nations in these seas do, but work them with large Oars, which pass through holes in the Platform, in the same manner that small Boats are sometimes done in England by a single Person with an Oar over its Stern; which I believe is generally termed sculling it along.

In the Morning I landed on the above mentioned Small Island, and got Altitudes for the Time by Mr Kendall's Watch, and also of the Water for determining the time of low Water. Seeing us land here, a great number of the Natives came over to us in two Canoes & landed on the Island; but thinking them too Many, and that some of them might take away things which I could but Ill spare, I made signs to them to go away, and they all Instantly retired to their Canoes which lay half hauled up on the Beach, and there sat and observed our Operations.

About Noon it was Low-water, and nearly dry between the Island & the Main. When 40 or 50 of the Natives Chiefly women & Children walked over to us; but these were no great trouble to us for we needed but look toward them and they would all run into the Water: 'tis true they grew bolder by degrees, and in a little time some of the most Audacious would stand & look at us untill we came within half a score Yards of them, before they ran.

The dress of the women is a sort of fringe, made of a Substance not much unlike hemp twisted into strings, and passed at least 20 or thirty times round their wast; it is cut very even at the bottom & reaches not more than half way down the Thighs. This is all their dress except that some very few wear a small piece of Cloth like the Men tied round their forehead but this is not common, and may probably be some mark of distinction.

6th. The unfavourableness of the Weather hindered me from seeing the beginning of the Eclipse, and it continued so untill near the Middle, when it became pretty Clear and continued so to the End, which I got with great Precision at $3^{h}28'49\frac{1}{4}''$ Apparent Time. . . .

The time of Low water, as appeared by Equal Altitudes was at $00^{h}18'$, and I made the Latitude of the Island by the Sun's Meridian Altitude $20^{\circ}17'$ S.

In the Morning as early as possible I went on Shore at the Watering Place, which is a small Brook SW of the Ship to have got the time of High Water, but found that at $18^{h}50'$ it was past the water having then fallen about $2\frac{1}{2}$ Inches as appeared by a stick which was set up last night. It was easy to see how high it had been by the Wet part of the Stick as there was not the least surf.

7th. At Noon I went to look after the Low-water but found the Natives had taken away my mark, so that I could determine nothing relative to the quantity the Water fell, but the time of Low Water was at 58′ past Noon. I set up another Mark in another Place; but when I went again in the Evening it also was gone.

This Afternoon I took an Opportunity which Cap[t] Cook offered me of going with him a few Miles down the Coast in the Boat. We landed opposite one of their Villages, which consisted of 6 or 7 Houses: But there were very few Natives about them I suppose they were up at the Watering Place & on board the Ship. The Houses were all circular; about 6 or 7 Yards diameter as I judged by steping across them. The Upright sides may be about 5 feet after which the roof begins and runs up to a pretty sharp point and so high as to make two stories of about 7 or 8 feet each into which they are divided by a flooring of Sticks laid Cross-wise. The upper one seems appropriated to a sort of Store house for their Arms Utensils &c &c. The Walls are made by setting pretty strong Posts in the Ground, to which are fastened Rails, or Cross-pieces all round at different heights. Against those rails on the outside Reeds are placed upright, which are fastened by putting long slender Rods all round on the out side directly opposite to the Rails or cross pieces which are within & the two are tyed tight together by strings which pass between the Reeds at short distances from one another, and there by keep the Reeds in their Place. These Walls may be about 3 or 4 Inches thick & the Reeds are laid in very close. The Roof is thatched in the same Manner, and is at least 6 or 8 Inches thick so that it readily appears that their houses are not only neat & convenient but also very warm; but notwithstanding this and the temperate Climate they are in, there are none of them without a fire Hearth; but they have no Window nor so much as a hole to let the Smoke out on which account they must be dark, and very disagreeable. The Door-way is about 2 feet or 2½ feet wide, and the same height with the upright part of the Wall. Instead of a Door, there hang down a great many Flags like a Curtain, which they put aside each way when they want to go in or out. The Door posts are in general two Terms,[1] the Faces on which are not badly Executed; and all the difference between them & those we meet with in English Architecture is, that the Sheath or Stem, is here a semi-Cylinder, carved into Shells &c whereas those of the latter are I think usually square & plain. Round some of the Houses were Plantations of Yams, Tarro Roots, &c but these were rare & the Plantations small. There were Cocoa-Nut-Trees round most of them—but not many, and they were all small and low. Indeed the Soil of the whole Country seems sterile, being a dry Sandy mold, that produces no underwood, but is every where covered with a long dry Grass. The Trees, are chiefly of one sort, whose bark is very white & hangs in rags, the leaves also, which are long, narrow & few in number, are of a very pale dead Green, so that at a

[1] 'Term' in the architectural sense: a pillar out of which rose a carved figure—the traditional form in which the Roman god Terminus was represented.

distance they look only like dead Trees[1] & the Country quite bare. This is to be understood of the Country in general, for there are exceptions, where the Ground is low & swampy, and all these parts are covered with Mangrove trees which are of a very lively Green & look beautifull enough at a distance; but when you come amongst them it is much the worst part of the Country, unless we except again the tops of the Mountains which are bare Rocks, very full of Mundic. I should have mentioned that the White Tree above Mentioned is an exceeding hard wood & a very fine aromatic.

The Inhabitants boil their Victuals in a large long Earthen Pot which they set over a fire on three stones with its mout[h] inclined side-ways, I suppose for handiness in getting things in and out. These Pots are very neatly made of a fine red clay, and they seem tolerably Cleanly about them. Their Principal food seems to be fish which they catch on the Reefs, and the Bark of a certain tree which they roast, and are almost continually chewing; it is of a very insipid tast; but some of our people who chewed a good deal of it said it began to be very agreeable.[2] In short this Country seems to be no Land of Canaan. However if little can be said in Praise of the Country, much may of the goodness of its Inhabitants. Their honesty is the greatest I ever saw; and it is certainly from principle, for they are as fond of our things as any other People whatever: that of the Tanna People was supposed to proceed from their contempt, or rather dread of touching any thing we had, even when it was given to them for few would take it otherwise than in a leaf, or some such thing.[3] Nor is the Good-nature, Friendship, or hospitallity of these People a jot inferior to their Integrity: and Ill befall the Person who ever gives them Cause to act otherwise. To what I have before said relating to the Manner in which those People wear their Hair, may be added that many of the men have a lock on each Temple left long, which they dress up into two such Wings as our Jemmy Mercurys[4] at home did a little while ago; but in point of cleanliness our present neighbours have much the preference; since I have not seen any of their wings clogged with a pound-weight of greasy Past[e], as was generally the Case with the others.

In the Morning Equal Altitudes of the Water were taken by two Marks, and the top of high Water marked on each. The High-Water was at $19^h29'$. The Marks now made Use off were two Trees which had been blown down and now lay fast in the sand with their branches standing up, one is in the Mouth of y^e^ Brook & the other a good way out to seaward, for the shore is very flat & the Water Ebbs out in some places near half a Mile. I made choice of these because I think it not Easy for the Natives to remove them.

I have learned from some of the Natives that the Name of the large Island we see to the Northward is *Ballabea*, & that the small one on which I observed the Eclipse is *Pudyoua*; but I cannot find out that they have any

[1] One of the eucalypts. [2] An hibiscus; see p. 542, n. 4 above.
[3] For fear of the effect, by contact, of some personal 'magic'.
[4] A contemporary nickname for a dandy.

General Name for the Main land. It is divided into many districts over each of which there is a Chief whom they entitle *Areki*. The Name of that District off which the Ship lies is *Ballade*, and its Areki is called *Teabooma*, who has been on board. The little Island Pudyoua also belongs to him. The Areki of Ballabea is called *Teaby*, and besides it, he is Areki of a province on the Main, or the little Isle which lies between Ballabea & the Main, I could not tell which, but believe it is the latter; however be it which it will, it is called *Caddy*,[1] and I shall therefore distinguish that little Isle by this Name. I got the Names of 12 or 14 Districts or Islands with their Arekis, but as I was neither certain of the Extent, or even order of them it is to no purpose to Enumerate them.

8th. It was low-water, at least as near as I could Estimate, at 5′ or 10′ past 2 o'Clock, at which time I fixed a Rod up at the Place, and by means of the Astronomical Quad^t^ found the difference of height between the two high-water Marks of this Morning, and the Low-water mark at this time, which were 2 feet 11 Inches & a $\frac{1}{4}$, and 3 feet no Inches & $\frac{7}{8}$ of an Inch. I then removed the Rod to a Place where the low-water had been marked on a Rock the Day before & found the difference between that & the two high water-Marks, and found them 3 feet one Inch & a quarter, and three feet: It is obvious that the two former & two latter ought to have been the same; I know not why they are otherwise,—perhaps the differences are pardonable. . . . To Day the Launch & Cutter were sent with ye 3d Lieut. & Master to examine & survey ye Western Part of the Land.

9th to the *11th.* We had strong Wind & Cloudy weather with Rain at times, on which Acount and the scarcity of Boats I had no opportunity of getting once on Shore at either the Times of high or Low Water. . . .

Norfolk Island October 1774

OCTOBER *10th.* The Boats being hoisted out I took the opportunity of seeing our new Discovery, and found the Shores exceeding Steep and Rocky, and in most places inaccessible on that Account. In one Place we found a short beach composed of very large Pebbles; but here there would have been no landing on Account of the surf, had it not been for some high Cliffy Rocks which stand at a little distance from the shore and break off the Sea in some Places, making it thereby tolerable landing, especially towards low-water, which as near as I could Judge would happen to Day between 5 & 6 oClock.

Near the shores the Ground is covered so thick with the New-Zeeland flax-Plant that it is scarce possible to get through it. This Plant was now nearly in its greatest perfection, the flowers being just opening, and as might naturally be expected from the Climate vastly more exuberant than at New Zeeland; but a little way in-land the woods were perfectly clear and easy to walk in. The Soil seemed to be exceeding Rich and deep

[1] Ile Pam.

resembling that of New Zeeland, and like it probably formed chiefly by ye decay of its Vegetable Production. The Pines mentioned above[1] are something, but not very different in their Foliage from those we saw at the last Islands; but the wood is of a very different Texture having a red coarse Grain; whereas the other is close white and fine, and the Wood it seems, very tough. I saw many trees which were as thick, breast high, as two Men could fathom and at the same time exceeding straight and high: I believe much larger Ships than the Resolution might on Occasion supply themselves with Main-Masts.

I took on shore with me a Bag which I soon filled with Wood sorrel[2] Sow-Thistle,[3] and samphire,[4] with which the shores in some places abound; but the greatest rarity we met with here was the Cabbage Tree,[5] of which there are many, and we brought the Cabbages of several on board. Those Trees are of the same Genus with the Cocoa nut Tree & not readily distinguished from them at first sight; but they bear no Nuts at least none that are fit for use. What they call the Cabbage is properly speaking the Bud of the Tree, of which as the Tree has but a Stem without Branches Each tree produces but one Cabbage, which is situate at the Crown, where the leaves spring out, and is enclosed in their Stems. This Vegetable is not only wholesome but extreamly palatable also, and proved the most agreeable repast whe had had for some Time. Variat. by Azim. at $18\frac{1}{2}^{h}$ hours $11°28\frac{1}{6}'$, $11°25\frac{2}{3}'$, & $10°15\frac{1}{3}'$ E.

OCTOBER y^e 11*th*. The Island we have Just left the Capt Calls Norfolk Island after the Dutchess of Norfolk. It abounds with Rails,[6] Parrots, and Pidgeons; the latter are exactly like those of New-Zeeland, and are perhaps the largest in the World, and as fine flavoured, when young.[7] The Parrots are I think rather smaller than the Parrots there but their Plumage is more beautiful.[8] Besides these there were many sea Birds such as Gulls, Gannets, Divers &c.

We saw no Inhabitants nor the least reason to believe it had ever been trod by Human feet before.

[1] The Norfolk Island Pine, *Araucaria excelsa*.
[2] *Oxalis* sp.
[3] *Sonchus oleraceus*.
[4] The plant that would look most like samphire to Wales's English eyes would probably be *Apium prostratum*, the 'wild celery' of New Zealand.
[5] *Rhopalostylis sapida*, the New Zealand Nikau.
[6] The Banded Rail, *Rallus philippinensis* Linn.
[7] The extinct Norfolk Island Pigeon, *Hemiphaga novaeseelandiae spadicea* (Latham).
[8] Probably he refers to the Norfolk Island Parrot, *Cyanoramphus novaezelandiae cookii*.

APPENDIX VI

The Antarctic Muse

[*Dixson Library, 'Captain James Cook Relics and MSS'. A note appended to the MS by Miss Louisa Jane Mackrell, the great-niece of Admiral Isaac Smith, reads, 'This song composed by Thomas Perry one of the Sea Men that went round the world with Captain Cook and was very much valued by the Captain. Mrs Cook kept it with the Gold Medal till her death'. The 'Gold Medal' was presumably either the Copley medal or the medal struck by the Royal Society to commemorate Cook after his death.*]

It is now my brave boys we are clear of the Sea
And keep a good heart if you'll take my advice
We are out of the cold my brave Boys do not fear
For the Cape of good Hope with good hearts we do steer

Thank God we have ranged the Globe all around
And we have likewise the south Continent found
But it being too late in the year as they say
We could stay there no longer the land to survey

So we leave it alone for we give a good reason
For the next ship that comes to survey in right season
The great fields of Ice among them we were bothered
We were forced to alter our course to the Northward

So we have done our utmost as any men born
To discover a land so far South of Cape Horn
So now my brave Boys we no longer will stay
For we leave it alone for the next Ship to survey

It was when we got into the cold frosty air
We was obliged our Mittens and Magdalen Caps to wear
We are out of the cold my brave Boys and perhaps
We will pull off our Mittens and Magdalen Caps

We are hearty and well and of good constitution
And have ranged the Globe round in the brave Resolution
Brave Captain Cook he was our Commander
Has conducted the Ship from all eminent danger

We were all hearty seamen no cold did we fear
And we have from all sickness entirely kept clear
Thanks be to the Captain he has proved so good
Amongst all the Islands to give us fresh food

And when to old England my Brave Boys we arrive
We will tip off a Bottle to make us alive
We will toast Captain Cook with a loud song all round
Because that he has the South Continent found

Blessed be to his wife and his Family too
God prosper them all and well for to do
Bless'd be unto them so long as they shall live
And that is the wish to them I do give.

APPENDIX VII

The Ships' Companies

THE muster-books of the two ships, from which this list is principally compiled,[1] are preserved in the Public Record Office (*Resolution*, Adm 36/7672; *Adventure*, Adm 36/7550). As in Volume I, Appendix V, the order and numbering of the names follow those of the muster-books, and an alphabetical index has been added. Places of origin and ages on joining, when known, are given immediately after the names. For the fourteen men who had been in the *Endeavour* with Cook and now served under him again, reference should also be made to the biographical notes in Volume I, pp. 589–601. The letter 'E', preceding certain comments, signifies a quotation from a list given in the memoirs of John Elliott (see p. cxxxvi above). Elliott's memory seems to have been fairly accurate, except about ages: he was probably right in noting William Dawson (*Resolution*, no. 25), clerk in the muster-book, as 'Acting Purser', because a purser's work Cook would naturally depute to his clerk; and his description of Daniel Clark (*Resolution*, no. 133), ship's corporal, as 'Cap^ns^ Clerk' is borne out by Mitchel's note that this man was 'Writer'. Elliott lists as many as fourteen midshipmen.

The captain's responsibility for keeping muster-books, as the authority for pay and victualling of his ship's company, has been described in relation to the *Endeavour* (I, 588–9). The muster-books and 'dead tickets' of the *Adventure* were delivered by Furneaux to the Admiralty on 8 August 1774; those of the *Resolution* by Cook on 30 July 1775.

On 27 November 1771 the Admiralty approved complements of 110 for the *Drake* (afterwards *Resolution*) and 80 for the *Raleigh* (afterwards *Adventure*). These were, on 28 February 1772, increased to 112 and 81 by the authorisation of additional carpenter's mates. Two widows' men were carried on the books of the *Resolution*, one on those of the *Adventure*. On 25 December 1771, when the ships' names were changed, new commissions and warrants were issued for all the officers already posted.

The manning of the ships did not go forward smoothly. By the end of February 1772 thirty-six men (including the armourer, a warrant-officer) had 'run', i.e. deserted, from the *Resolution*, and twenty-two more ran before she sailed from Plymouth on 13 July; twenty-nine had been discharged and one drowned. It is hardly surprising that, calling at Madeira at the end of July 1772, Cook ordered boatmen to be hired 'to attend on the ship, no man being suffered on shore in case of running'.[2] Of the

[1] There is also a list in B.M. Add. MS 27958.
[2] Adm 36/7550, 29 July 1772.

Adventure's crew, thirty-seven ran before sailing, and eleven were discharged. All these men, who are omitted from our list, were replaced, and both ships sailed with a full complement.[1]

To clarify the resultant confusion in the muster-books, Cook was on 4 May 1772 ordered to bear any 'overplus' men as supernumeraries for wages and victuals as far as Plymouth; and on 2 June Furneaux was instructed to bear one supernumerary to Plymouth.

Losses from the *Resolution* during her voyage were made good by taking on A.B.s at the Cape in November 1772 (1) and in April 1775 (4); those from the *Adventure* by transfer from the *Resolution* (2) and entering A.B.s at the Cape in November 1772 (1) and in March 1774 (7). As usual, the muster-books present some puzzles. Where and when did Cook take on board the *Resolution* the two men (nos. 197 and 198) first entered on 1 August 1773, when he was in the open sea near Pitcairn Island, or the other man (no. 200) entered on 23 December 1774, when the ship lay in Christmas Sound, Tierra del Fuego? And how did Cook account for the pay and victuals of John Keplin, Richard Lee and John Leverick, punished at various times for various misdeeds, but never entered in the muster-books?

The *Resolution* carried a lieutenant and eighteen marines, the *Adventure* a second lieutenant and eleven marines. On 25 January 1772 the Plymouth division was ordered to find, for the *Resolution*, a recruit capable of playing the bagpipes and a drummer who could also play the violin; and on 9 May the Nore division was required to produce two men to play the bagpipes. This search was apparently successful, for in Dusky Sound, on 11 April 1773, Cook 'caused the Bagpipes and fife to be played and the Drum to be beat'—the first of a number of musical performances which fell on the Pacific.

Of Banks's 'people', nine were carried on the *Resolution*'s books, as supernumeraries for victuals only, from 8 May to 5 June 1772, two on those of the *Adventure* from 1 May to 18 June; their names are included in this list. The supernumeraries (for victuals only) who sailed from Plymouth were, in the *Resolution*, William Wales the astronomer and George Gilpin his assistant, the painter William Hodges, Francis Masson 'the King's gardener', who was to be carried to the Cape, and the two Forsters with a servant; and in the *Adventure*, the astronomer William Bayly and his servant. It will be noted that, while the Raiatean 'Oedidee' and his 'servant' were carried by Cook as supernumeraries from August 1773 to June 1774, Furneaux took Omai on his books at Huahine in December 1773 as an A.B. Other supernumeraries (omitted from this list) included the yard artificers who worked on the ships in the Thames, pilots, boatmen and customs officers, caulkers and riggers employed at Cape Town, and the seven East India Company soldiers (of the St Helena garrison) brought home by Cook from the Cape.

[1] In fact, at the first muster (15 July) after leaving Plymouth, Cook found himself one man over strength 'owing to a mistake in the Clerk' (above, p. 18).

The *Adventure* was paid off on 16 July 1774, the *Resolution* on 28 August 1775.

The only previously published list of those who sailed in the ships is Kitson's (1907, pp. 513–5); it is neither complete nor accurate.

RESOLUTION

1. COOK, James (1728–79). Commander, per commissions 28 November (from *Scorpion*) and 25 December 1771. Joined 30 November. Appointed post-captain *Kent*, 9 August 1775. Appointed captain in Greenwich Hospital, 12 August 1775, with permission to resign if called to more active service. E 'An Exelent Seaman and Officer—Sober—Brave, Humane'.

2. ELLIOTT, John. Walton, Yorks, 15. A.B. Joined 30 November 1771. Born 1759; in 1770 entered in the navy by his uncle John Wilkinson, but first went on merchant voyages to St Kitts and the Mediterranean and had some schooling in navigation. Taken into *Resolution* through his uncle's influence with Palliser. East India Company voyage to India, December 1775–7; and then in *Colebrook*, wrecked in Simon's Bay, 24 August 1778. Resumed naval service, 4th lieutenant *Ajax* 1779, West Indies service under Rodney; 1st lieutenant 1780; badly wounded by an explosion of powder at 'The Great and Glorious Action of the 12th April 1782', i.e. the Battle of the Saints. After this seems to have retired from navy. Only wrong advice and the death of his uncle, he thought, kept him from being a post captain at the age of 20 and an admiral at 32 or 33.—*Memoirs*, B.M., Add. MS 42714.

4. MANLEY, Isaac George. London, 18. Midshipman. Joined 3 December 1771; discharged per Admiralty order 8 April 1772. Midshipman *Endeavour*, first voyage (I, 593).

5. WALLIS, James. Carpenter, per warrants 28 November and 25 December 1771. Joined 3 December. Had served in North America; compared Norfolk Island pines to 'the Quebeck Pines'. Appointed carpenter *Firm*, 6 October 1775.

6. COOPER, Robert Palliser (–1805). First lieutenant, per commissions 28 November and 25 December 1771. Joined 4 December. Had served in Newfoundland (2nd lieutenant *Niger* 1766) and West Indies. A kinsman of Sir Hugh Palliser. E 'sober, steady good officer'. Appointed commander *Hawk* sloop, 10 August 1775. Posted captain, 1778; superannuated rear-admiral, 1796.

7. PIRIE, John. Aberdeen, 33. A.B. Joined 6 December 1771.

8. RAMSAY, John. Cook, per warrant 6 December 1771 (from *Scorpion*). Joined 6 December. A.B. *Endeavour*, first voyage (I, 590). Gunner's mate *Resolution*, third voyage.

9. REYNOLDS, Peter. Deptford, 22. Carpenter's mate. Joined 9 December 1771. Carpenter *Discovery*, third voyage.

11.} 181.} CHAPMAN, William. Gravesend, 39. A.B. Joined 10 December 1771. Discharged 23 July 1773 to *Adventure* as cook, although 'aged', and without the use of two of his fingers.

13. PICKERSGILL, Richard (1749–79). Third lieutenant and lieutenant at arms, per commissions 29 November (from *Scorpion*) and 25 December 1771. Joined 11 December. Master's mate *Endeavour*, first voyage (I, 592). Much used by Cook in small boat work; romantic, enthusiastic; E 'a good officer and astronomer, but liking ye Grog'.

15. SEAMER or SEYMOUR, John. Thame, Oxon, 22. Carpenter's crew. Joined 11 December 1771. Entered as A.B. in *Resolution*, third voyage, but ran before sailing.

19. ANDERSON, William (1750–78). Surgeon's mate, per warrant 3 December 1771 (from *Barfleur*). Joined 12 December. An enthusiastic and able self-taught naturalist. Valuable to Cook for his ability in native languages and for his ethnological observations. Made botanical and zoological collections, which he bequeathed to Banks. Surgeon *Resolution*, third voyage; died at sea 3 August 1778. E 'a Steady clever Man'.

20. PATTEN, James. Surgeon, per warrant 11 December 1771 (from *Senegal*). Joined 12 December. Skilful professionally, and spoken highly of by the Forsters. E 'a Steady clever Man'.

21. ROBERTS, Henry (c. 1757–96). Shoreham, Sussex, 15. A.B. Joined 13 December 1771 (from *Mary* yacht). A skilful cartographer and draughtsman. E 'very clever young man'. Master's mate *Resolution*, third voyage. Second lieutenant *Dragon*, 1780. Employed 1781–4 in drawing charts of third voyage for engraving. In 1789 appointed to command the sloop *Discovery* (not Cook's ship) on an expedition either to examine sites for colonies in West Africa or to survey the north-west coast of America; the expedition being delayed, the *Discovery* was paid off in December 1790, Roberts went on half-pay, and Vancouver was appointed to command this expedition. Captain *Undaunted*, 1795–6; took part in capture of Essequibo and Demerara; died in West Indies 25 August 1796.

24. SMITH, Isaac (1752–1831). London, 18. Master's mate. Joined 17 December 1771 (from *Scorpion*). Master's mate *Endeavour*, first voyage (I, 590). E 'Clever and steady'; a useful surveyor and draughtsman. Appointed lieutenant *Weazle* sloop, 19 August 1775.

25. DAWSON, William. Deptford, 22. Clerk. Joined 17 December 1771. Elliott says he was 'Acting Purser' and, 'a Steady clever Man in his Situation'. A.B. *Endeavour*, first voyage (I, 590). Appointed purser

Spy, 17 April 1776; later *Crescent* and *Phaeton*. Wrote to Banks from Port Royal, Jamaica, 2 July 1788, stressing his unblemished character and misfortunes (shipwreck, capture by the French), and consequent loss 'of almost every farthing I had acquired during twenty six years servitude in the Navy'; his health was now impaired and he sought Banks's interest in securing some small office.—Mitchell Library, Banks Papers, 2, f. 24. See also I, p. 590.

26. COLLETT, William. High Wycombe, 22. A.B. Joined 17 December 1771. A.B. *Endeavour*, first voyage (I, 592). Master-at-arms *Resolution*, third voyage.

27. COLNETT, James (1752?–1806). Plymouth, 19. Midshipman. Joined 17 December 1771 (from *Scorpion*). E 'Clever & Sober'. First to sight New Caledonia. Subsequently served as gunner *Juno*, master *Adventure* store-ship, and lieutenant *Bienfaisant* and *Pégase*. Between 1786 and 1791 made two trading voyages in furs to north-west America, China and Japan; employed 1793–6 surveying for Admiralty on coasts of South America and England. Promoted captain 1796. In 1802–3 commanded *Glatton*, taking convicts to Sydney.

29. EWIN, William. Pennsylvania, 28. Boatswain's mate. Joined 17 December 1771. Boatswain *Resolution*, 13 September 1775; and on third voyage.

30. MARRA, John. Cork, 25. Gunner's mate. Joined 17 December 1771. A.B. *Endeavour*, first voyage (I, 596–7). Punished for mutiny and desertion before leaving England, and for insolence at Tahiti, April 1773. Attempted to desert at Tahiti, 14 May 1774, and put in irons for it; again (but query whether desertion really intended) in Queen Charlotte's Sound, New Zealand, November 1774, and flogged for it. 'An Irishman by birth, a good Seaman and had Saild both in the English and Dutch Service' (Cook). Wrote a surreptitious journal published by Francis Newbery in 1775. Noted by Banks at some later date, post-1800, as at Port Jackson.—Mitchell Library, Banks Papers, 9, f. 23.

31. COLLETT, Richard. High Wycombe, 18. A.B. Joined 17 December 1771. Master-at-arms, *Discovery* and *Resolution*, third voyage.

32. GOULDING, Robert. Birmingham, 24. Carpenter's crew. Joined 17 December 1771.

33. HARVEY, William. London, 20. Midshipman. Joined 17 December 1771. Midshipman *Endeavour*, first voyage (I, 592). E 'steady officer'. Master's mate and third lieutenant *Resolution*, third voyage. Promoted commander, 1790.

34., 142. SHAW, Thomas. London, 19. A.B. Joined 17 December 1771.

35. WYBROW, John. Edinburgh, 19. A.B. Joined 17 December 1771 (from *Scorpion*).

38. CAVE, John. Durham, 25. Quartermaster's mate. Joined 17 December 1771.

41. PRICE, Joseph. Westminster, 20. Midshipman. Joined 17 December 1771. E 'Unsteady and drink[g]'.

45. WHITEHOUSE, John. London, 31. Master's mate. Joined 17 December 1771. E 'Jesuitical, sensible but an insinuating litigious mischief making fellow'. Promoted lieutenant in August 1775; superannuated commander, 1811.

46. ANDERSON, Robert. Inverness, 30. Gunner, per warrants 12 and 25 December 1771; requested by Cook. A man of character, who brought home to Marra the authorship of the surreptitious journal published by Francis Newbery in 1775. Quartermaster *Endeavour*, first voyage, but more than once in trouble (I, 592). Gunner *Resolution*, third voyage.

50. BURNEY, James (1750–1821). London, 21. A.B. Joined 17 December 1771. Son of Dr Charles Burney, the musician and musical historian, and brother of Fanny Burney. Went to sea at age of 10 as captain's servant, *Princess Amelia* and *Magnanime*, serving in fleet off Brest, 1760–2; captain's servant *Niger* frigate 1763–5, and *Aquilon* frigate 1766–9; for last six months A.B. 1770–1 voyage to Bombay in *Greenwich* Indiaman as ordinary seaman. Appointed to *Resolution* through Burney-Sandwich connection; passing certificate for lieutenant January 1772; discharged to *Adventure* as 2nd lieutenant at Cape, 17 November 1772. December 1774–5 2nd, then 1st, lieutenant, *Cerberus* frigate, on American service. 1776 1st lieutenant *Discovery* on Cook's third voyage; after Clerke's death 1st lieutenant *Resolution*. For a few months in 1781–2 temporary captain *Latona* frigate, North Sea; May 1782 captain *Bristol*, 50 guns, took out convoy to Madras, served under Sir Edward Hughes against Suffren, was then employed in coastal service till invalided home at end of 1784. No further command, though he repeatedly offered his services. His great literary work the *Chronological History of the Discoveries in the South Sea or Pacific Ocean*, 5 vols., 1803–17, and *Chronological History of North-Eastern Voyages of Discovery* . . . , 1819; author also of pamphlets on defence, scientific and geographical papers, and *An Essay by way of Lecture, on the Game of Whist*, 1821. Elected F.R.S., 1809. Promoted superannuated rear-admiral 1821. Highly regarded by a circle of friends ranging from Dr Johnson and Sir Joseph Banks to Charles Lamb.

51., 143. STALKER, John. Ayrshire, 31. A.B. Joined 17 December 1771.

54. HORN, Andrew. Co. Kildare, 21. A.B. Joined 17 December 1771.

55. SIMMS, James. London, 20. A.B. Joined 17 December 1771.

62. READING, Solomon. London, 25. Boatswain's mate. Joined 23 December 1771. Saved Thomas Fenton from going overboard, 10 March 1773. Wounded by a spear at Eromanga. There are three letters in three different hands from this man in Mitchell Library, Banks Papers, 2, ff. 20–22 (if Soloman Redden of f. 20 is the same, as Banks evidently thought he was)—all asking for help. The second, dated *Colossus*, Spithead, 30 October 1787, humbly takes leave etc., 'Having the Honor to go round the Wold in the Endeavour with You'—which was not true. He wants Banks to get a boatswain's warrant for him; he has had 30 years in the service, and has a wife and family. The third letter, with no date but 'June 24th', relates that 'I have Been Grievously Afflicted with the Gravel in My Kidneys, But Being Now Much Better I am about shipping My self For the East Indias'; and requests the loan of 'a Trifle to Fit Me for the Voyage . . .'. There is the draft of a testimonial from Banks, 10 January 1791, certifying (apparently without deep enquiry) that Solomon Redding behaved himself in the *Endeavour* with diligence and activity (Banks Papers, 2, f. 19); and a later note that he was living at 11, Ratcliff Highway (ibid. 9, f. 23).

63. BLACKBURN, John. London, 26. A.B. Joined 23 December 1771. Mitchel says he was the cook.

65. CLERKE, Charles (1743–79). Second lieutenant, per commissions 28 November and 25 December 1771. Joined 23 December 1771. Third lieutenant *Endeavour*, first voyage (I, 593). E 'a Brave and good officer, and a genal favorite'. Appointed commander *Favourite* sloop, 26 August 1775. Commander *Discovery*, third voyage; died at sea, 22 August 1779.

66. WHITE, Thomas. Scotland, 26. A.B. Joined 23 December 1771.

68. BURR, John Daval. London, 27. Master's mate. Joined 24 December 1771. E 'steady good officer'. Lieutenant, 10 August 1775, in *Hawke* under Cooper (no. 6).

71. INNELL, John. London, 18. A.B. Joined 26 December 1771. Punished for drunkenness 13 February 1774, for insolence 6 April 1774.

72. BEE, William. Barton, Yorks, 25. Quartermaster's mate. Joined 26 December 1771.

79. WILLIS, Thomas. Holywell, 17. Midshipman. Joined 3 January 1772. First to sight Willis Island, South Georgia, January 1775. E 'Wild & drinking'. Promoted lieutenant, 1778.

81. GRAY, James. Leith, 27. Boatswain, per warrants 12 December (from *Cruizer*) and 25 December 1771; requested by Cook. Joined 3 January 1772. Quartermaster *Endeavour*, first voyage (I, 592). Appointed boatswain *Essex*, 13 September 1775.

82. PETTERSON, Emmanuel. Bombay, 21. A.B. Joined 3 January 1772. Punished for riotous behaviour at Tahiti, 31 August 1773.

87. SCARNELL, Francis. Portsmouth, 22. Quartermaster. Joined 3 January 1772. A.B., 10 July 1772. 'Purser's steward' (Mitchel).

88. GILBERT, Joseph (1733?–1824?). Boston, Lincs. Master, per warrant 3 January 1772 (from *Asia*). Joined 7 January. Had been master of *Guernsey*, surveying coasts of Newfoundland and Labrador (with Michael Lane), 1764–9; then master of *Pearl* (surveyed Plymouth Sound, 1769) and of *Asia*. Wounded at Eromanga, 4 August 1774. Responsible for surveying and chartwork in *Resolution*. E 'a steady good officer'; and Cook had a high opinion of his judgment. Master Attendant at Portsmouth Dockyard, 1776–91, with rank of lieutenant, and duty of 'teaching the young gentlemen at the Academy the practical part of seamanship . . . and shewing them the nature of fitting rigging,' at £13 per annum; Master Attendant at Deptford Dockyard, 1791–1802. Said to have died at Fareham at age of 91.

89. DRAWWATER, Benjamin (1748?–1815). Surgeon's 2nd mate, per warrant 7 January 1772. Joined 7 January. E 'a Steady clever Man'.

91. WHEILON or WHELAN, Patrick. London, 30. Quartermaster. Joined 7 January 1772. Quartermaster *Resolution*, third voyage.

93. DAWSON, Edward. Scotland, 30. A.B. Joined 7 January 1772. Carpenter's mate, 10 July 1772.

96. DAY, James. Scotland, 27. A.B. Joined 7 January 1772.

98. DRIVER, Thomas. Orkney, 31. A.B. Joined 7 January 1772.

101. GRINDALL, Richard (1750–1820). London, 22. A.B. Joined 7 January 1772. E 'Steady Clever young Man'. Sixth lieutenant *Barfleur*, 1781. Commanded *Prince* at Trafalgar. Vice-Admiral 1810; created K.C.B. 1815.

102. LOGGIE, Charles. Plymouth, 17. A.B. Joined 7 January 1772 (from *Nautilus*). '. . . M[r] Charles Loggie, a Midshipman, and the Son of a very old Post Capt[n] in the Navy, had for some time taken to drinking, a thing that he, of all young Men, should not have done, as he had when a Child, most unfortunately cut his head, and had been trapan'd, consequently when he got Liquor he was a Mad Man, at other times, as good a temperd young Man as any in the Ship'. —Elliott *Mem.*, f. 42. Sent before the mast for bad behaviour, 6 January 1773; flogged for assaulting Maxwell, 2 January 1774; threatened to stab cook, 18 March 1775; killed in a duel 1782.

111. ANDERSON, David. Dalkeith, 24. Boatswain's mate. Joined 21 January 1772.

112. ROLLETT, Richard. Lynn, Norfolk, 22. Sailmaker; requested by Cook. Joined 22 January 1772. Kept a journal 'Interlin'd in his

bible'. He seems to have had some objection to sailing with Cook, and writes to Banks, 9 June 1772, asking for 'the Honour of a birth in your Service, in the Capacity of Mas^tr^ Sail maker . . . I am very desirous to proceed on the Voyage, but in the ship with Which you & Dr Solander goes, I should have gone with the Adventure, if you had not been going in the Resolution when I first shipd my self. . . . It is the Desire of my friends, I should go this voyage, which If I Do not, the Disadvantage will be very great to me As it Lyes in there power to do very genteel for me at My Return, Which I must & will suffer Reather than go in this Ship, altho I am so Desirous of Proceeding the Voyage. . . . I hope youll please to let me know your pleasure Which I Impatiently wait for & hope it will be a profound Secret to Cap^tn^ Cook For if it Dont sute you, & he heres of it my time will be Very Miserible to me'.—Alexander Turnbull Library, *Miscellaneous material relating to Cook's Voyages, 1768–84*. He died in 1814.

114. MITCHEL or MITCHELL, Bowles. Deptford, 20. A.B. Joined 22 January 1772. Midshipman, 12 June 1772; A.B. 1 July 1773. E 'Steady young Man'. Promoted lieutenant, 1777; superannuated commander, 1810.

117. VANCOUVER, George (1757–98). Son of John Jasper Vancouver, collector of customs, of King's Lynn. London, 15. A.B. Joined 22 January 1772. E 'a Quiet inoffensive young Man'. Midshipman *Discovery*, third voyage. Lieutenant *Martin* sloop 1780, and served in West Indies 1781–9. In 1789 appointed to proposed expedition under Captain Henry Roberts (no. 21), on recommendation of Commodore Sir Alan Gardner, and superintended fitting out of *Discovery*. Served under Gardner in *Courageux* in 1790. Succeeded Roberts in command of *Discovery* in December 1790, and surveyed north-west coasts of America, returning in 1795. Post-captain 1794.

118. BEVAN, William. Glamorgan, 25. Carpenter's crew. Joined 22 January 1772.

119. BRISCOE, William. Scarborough, 21. A.B. Joined 30 January 1772. Ship's tailor; punished for theft, 15 February 1773.

122. JACKSON, George. London, 41. Carpenter's mate. Joined 4 February 1772.

123. PECKOVER, William. London, 21. Gunner's mate. Joined 4 February 1772. (Perhaps to be identified with the man of this name who was A.B. in *Endeavour*, first voyage; see I, 595–6.) Gunner *Discovery*, third voyage. A man of thwarted ambition, he writes to Banks (n.d.), '. . . as you was so good to me During your last Voyage & so generous sinc your Return I Am Determind to haxard my Life Again with you in the Same Vessil from Motives of Gratitude & Ragard I ham now Emboldend to solicit your Goodness to have me appointed Supernumery Midshipman in one of the Ships

newly Commissiond for the South Seas. . . .'—Mitchell Library, Banks Papers, 'Voluntiers', p. 553.

124. WHITE, Stephen. London, 32. A.B. Joined 4 February 1772.

133. CLARK, Daniel. Essex, 32. Corporal. Joined 10 February 1772. Master-at-arms, 1 July 1772. E 'Cap[ns] Clerk Clever but liking Grog'. Mitchel calls him 'Writer'.

138. FREEZLAND, Samuel. Holland, 23. A.B. Joined 13 February 1772. Sighted 'Freezland Peak', 31 January 1775.

140. ATKIN, Anthony. Fife, 30. Quartermaster. Joined 13 February 1772.

141. BORDALL, Samuel. Topsham. 21. Quartermaster. Joined 19 February 1772. A.B., 10 July; quartermaster, 30 July 1772.

145. WILLIAMS, Charles. Wapping, 20. A.B. Joined 28 February 1772. Punished for losing his tools (as cooper's mate) at Raiatea, 28 May 1774.

146. TERRELL, Edward. London, 21. A.B.; requested by Cook. Joined 2 March 1772. A.B. *Endeavour*, first voyage (I, 590).

147. SMALLY, John. Deal, 26. A.B. Joined 2 March 1772.

148. MONK, Simon. Brentford, 30. A.B. and ship's butcher. Joined 5 March 1772. Died at sea 'by a fall down the hatchway', 6 September 1774; 'a man much esteemed in the ship' (Cook). For other tributes, see p. 533, n. 3 above.

149. HOOD, Alexander (1758–98). London, 14. Son of Samuel Hood, of Kingsland, Dorset, purser R.N. and first cousin of Admirals Lord Hood and Lord Bridport. A.B. Joined 5 March 1772. Nearly crushed by an arms-chest in a storm, 25 October 1773. First to sight land in the Marquesas (Hood Island), 6 April 1774. Discharged to *Marlborough*, 5 August 1775. Subsequently served in West Indies and North America; promoted captain in 1781. From 1790 employed in Channel; and while commanding *Mars* (74 guns) he was killed in a desperate action against the French ship *Hercule*, April 1798.

152. BARRETT, Edward. London, 15. Cook's mate. Joined 10 March 1772.

153. FENTON, Thomas. London, 18. A.B. Joined 10 March 1772. One of the armourer's assistants. Fell from the catharpings, 10 March 1773.

154. SMOCK, Henry. Portsmouth, 30. Carpenter's mate. Joined 18 March 1772. A.B. 20 August 1772. Drowned at sea, 'at work over the side fitting in one of the Scuttles', 29 October 1772. 'His good-natured character, and a kind of serious turn of mind caused him to be regretted *even* among his shipmates' (George Forster).

156. Ellwell, John. London, 45. Quartermaster. Joined 20 March 1772.

158. Whattman or Watman, William. Reigate, 25. A.B. Joined 20 March 1772. A.B., *Resolution*, third voyage; died at Hawaii 1 February 1779.

163. Drew, William. London, 21. Armourer's mate, per warrant 20 March 1772. Joined 24 March.

164. Brown, Matthew. York, 26. Armourer, per warrant 27 March 1772 (in succession to Edward Ireland, run). Joined 27 March.

165. Mills, John. Banff, 24. A.B. Joined 2 April 1772.

175. Corbett, Richard. Limehouse, 26. A.B. Joined 20 April 1772. Mitchel says he was the barber.

177. Maxwell, James. London, 21. A.B. Joined 28 April 1772 (from *Rose*, at his request). One of the 'young gentlemen'; E 'an Hypocritical canting fellow'. Ordered before the mast for damaging a sail, 6 February 1774; confined for threatening to stab the cook, 18 March 1775.

178. Hayes, James. Bridgwater, 25. A.B. Joined 13 June 1772.

179.
195. Coghlan, John. Glamorgan, 15. A.B. Joined 21 June 1772. E 'Wild and drinking'. Discharged to Supernumerary List at Cape 30 October 1772, 'having one man more than the complement'. While midshipman, sent before the mast for quarrelling, 1 February 1773.

180. Frazer, John. London, 41. Ship's corporal. Joined 1 July 1772 (from *Reasonable*, in lieu). Claimed to have been taken on as an experienced diver (see also Sparrman, p. 60), and to have 'invented an instrument for taking up things out of the sea'. In December 1775, being unable to go to sea 'on account of pains in his body, caused by frequent diving', he petitioned Sandwich for 'a boats warrant'; Cook thought him unqualified for preferment calling for seamanship, but suitable as master-at-arms.

190. Lockton, John. Bristol, 43. Quartermaster. Joined 10 July 1772 (from *Somerset*, in lieu).

191. Snowden, Thomas. Whitby, 22. Sailmaker's mate. Joined 10 July 1772 (from *Dublin*, in lieu).

192. Harrison, John. North Shields, 21. A.B. Joined 10 July 1772 (from *Torbay*, in lieu).

193. Perry, Thomas. London, 39. A.B. Joined 10 July 1772 (from *Solebay*, in lieu). Wrote a song about the voyage (Appendix VI).

194. Atkinson, William. Westmoreland, 30. A.B. Joined 10 July 1772 (from *Kent*, in lieu). Punished for theft, 15 February 1773.

196. Gilbert, Richard. Boston, Lincs. A.B. Entered 27 November 1772 (from Cape Town?). Perhaps a relative of Joseph Gilbert, master, also of Boston (no. 88). Discharged at Cape Town 30 April 1775, by request.

197. Cook, James. London. A.B. Entered 1 August 1773. Discharged at Cape Town 30 April 1775, by request. (Perhaps the same man who was an officer's servant in *Endeavour*, first voyage; I, 596.)

198. Cook, Nathaniel. London. A.B. Entered 1 August 1773. Discharged at Cape Town 30 April 1775, by request. A.B. *Endeavour*, first voyage (I, 596). A.B. *Resolution*, third voyage.

199. Hodges, William. (See Supernumeraries, no. 21).

200. Edes, Abraham. Warwickshire, 20. A.B. Entered 23 December 1774.

201. Smith, John. Bristol, 33. A.B. Entered at Cape 1 May 1775.

202. Adams, Francis. Cork, 35. A.B. Entered at Cape 1 May 1775.

203. Elmes, James. Suffolk, 19. A.B. Entered at Cape 1 May 1775.

204. Hendrick, John. Hanover, 25. A.B. Entered at Cape 1 May 1775.

MARINES

(Nos. 1–20 joined at Sheerness, 29 May 1772; nos. 21 and 22 at Plymouth, 9 July 1772. All from Chatham division except nos. 1, 20–22.)

1. Edgcumbe, John. Second lieutenant, per Admiralty order 25 January 1772 (from *Royal Oak*). Portsmouth division. Sergeant *Endeavour*, first voyage (I, 598). E 'a Steady Man, and a good officer'. Promoted 1st lieutenant 1775; captain 1779; placed on half-pay list 1781.

2. Hamilton, John. Sergeant.

4. Beard, Robert. Corporal.

5. Brotherson, Philip. Drummer. Punished for theft, 15 February 1773.

6. Scott, James. Private. Described in muster-table, Add. MS 27958, as 'Gentleman Caditt', and discharged 12 June 1772 to *Adventure* as second lieutenant. See also under *Adventure*, Marines, no. 13.

7. Commena, —. Private.

8. Baldy, Richard. Private. Punished for his inefficiency as a sentry at Tahiti, 8 May 1774.

9. Phillips, John. Private.

10. Carpenter, Richard. Private.

11. Tow, William. Private.

12. Harper, John. Private.

13. Wedgeborough, William. Private. Punished for drunkenness and nastiness, 19 March 1774; fell overboard off Eromanga, 1 August 1774; killed a native of Tana, 19 August 1774, and confined for two months for it. Drowned, probably when drunk, in Christmas Sound, Tierra del Fuego, 22 December 1774: 'it was supposed that he had fallen over board out of the head where he was last seen'.

14. Waterfield, Richard. Private.

15. Woodward, George. Private. Punished for riotous behaviour at Tahiti, 31 August 1773.

16. Twitty, Charles. Private.

17. Taylor, Francis. Private. Punished for theft, 15 February 1773.

18. Buttall, John. Private. Punished for theft, 15 February 1773; and for riotous behaviour at Tahiti, 31 August 1773.

19. Monk, William. Private.

20. McVicar, Archibald. Private. Portsmouth division. Presumably the 'Highland Scotsman' engaged to play the bagpipes, 'to the great distress' of Mr Sparrman's ears and to the delight of the Tahitian ladies.

21. Gibson, Samuel. Corporal. Plymouth division. Private, *Endeavour*, first voyage (I, 598). Sergeant, *Resolution*, third voyage. Of some use as an interpreter: 'He it was among our people who possessed the best knowledge of the [Tahitian] language' (Sparrman, who also suggests that Gibson, deserting at Tahiti in 1769, had 'aspired to no less than the throne of Otaheite itself').

22. Taylor, Isaac. Private. Plymouth division. Unwell from the time of leaving England; died at Tahiti 18 August 1773 of consumption, or 'a complication of disorders without the least touch of the Scurvy', culminating in a dropsy.

SUPERNUMERARIES

(Nos. 2–10 were members of Banks's 'retinue', borne on the ship's books 8 April–5 June 1772 for victuals only, per Admiralty order 24 June 1772.)

2. Miller, Joseph [James]. Draughtsman; accompanied Banks to Iceland.

3. Miller, Benjamin [John Frederick]. Draughtsman; accompanied Banks to Iceland.

4. Wilson [Walden?], John.

5. Briscoe, Peter.
6. Roberts, James.
} Banks's Lincolnshire servants. Sailed in *Endeavour*, first voyage.

7. Sidsaft [Sidserf?], Peter. Servant.

8. ASQUITH, John. Servant.

9. ALEXANDER [Sander], John. The Eurasian servant engaged by Banks at Batavia on the first voyage.

10. YOUNG, Nicholas. Sailed in *Endeavour*, first voyage (I, 600).

11. WALES, William (1734?–98). Astronomer; joined 29 June 1775, per Admiralty order of 25 June. A Yorkshireman, born near Wakefield 'of parents of humble circumstances'; is said to have 'walked to London with a Mr Holroyd . . . Plumber to George 3rd'. Married the sister of Charles Green, astronomer in the *Endeavour*. An able man in his profession, who had in 1769–70 observed the transit of Venus for the Royal Society at Hudson's Bay. After his return with Cook in 1775, he edited the record of his and Bayly's observations (published 1777), engaged in controversy with George Forster, and was elected F.R.S. (1776). Edited the *Astronomical Observations* of the Byron-Wallis-Carteret-*Endeavour* voyages (1788). Secretary of the Board of Longitude, 1795–8. In 1775 appointed master of the Mathematical School at Christ's Hospital. Characterised by Charles Lamb in his 'Recollections of Christ's Hospital' as 'that hardy sailor, as well as excellent mathematician, and co-navigator with Captain Cook', and as a severe but genial man with 'a perpetual fund of humour, a constant glee about him, which, heightened by an inveterate provincialism of north-country dialect, absolutely took away the sting from his severities'. Leigh Hunt's *Autobiography* describes Wales as 'a good man, of plain simple manners, with a heavy large person and benign countenance. When he was at Otaheite, the natives played him a trick while bathing and stole his small-clothes; which we used to think a liberty scarcely credible'. According to William Trollope, his grandson, 'by his energies the Royal Mathematical School of Christ's Hospital was first seen to realise the objects of its foundation, and gave the promise of becoming one of the first naval seminaries in the world' (*History of Christ's Hospital*, p. 95). Buried in the cloisters of Christ's Hospital.

12. GILPIN, George. Wales's 'servant'; joined with him. E 'A Quiet y[oun]g Man'. Assistant at Royal Observatory 1776–81; Clerk of Royal Society 1785–1809; Secretary of Board of Longitude 1801–1809. Died 1810.

21. HODGES, William (1744–97). 'Landskip painter'. Joined per Admiralty order 30 June 1772; taken on strength as A.B. 7 September 1774; discharged to supernumerary list 30 April 1775. E 'Clever good Man'. Born in London; a pupil of Richard Wilson; appointed official artist in the *Resolution* by interest of Lord Palmerston. Energetic in drawing and painting landscapes and portraits of South Sea islanders. On his return, employed by the Admiralty to work up oil paintings from his sketches and to supervise engraving. In India

from 1778 to 1784, painting picturesque views under patronage of Warren Hastings. Exhibited at Royal Academy 1776–94; A.R.A. 1786, R.A. 1789. In 1795 gave up painting and opened an unsuccessful bank at Dartmouth. Died by his own hand at Brixham, Devon.

33. MASSON, Francis (1741–1805). 'The King's gardener'. Taken on board per Admiralty order of 5 May 1772 for passage to the Cape, and discharged there 22 November 1772. The first of the plant collectors sent out from the Royal Botanical Gardens at Kew, he made expeditions to the Cape in 1772–4, the West Indies in 1776–1781, and the Cape again in 1786–91, bringing back many plants 'unknown at that time to the Botanical Gardens of Europe' (Banks). F.L.S. 1796.

37. FORSTER, Johann Reinhold. (1729–98.) 'Gentleman' and naturalist. Joined per Admiralty order 25 June 1772. E 'a clever, but a litigious quarelsom fellow'. Of Scottish-Prussian descent, and very wide interests in learning; a Lutheran minister near Danzig 1753–1765, during which time he turned to natural history; in 1765, under Russian patronage, investigated conditions in the Saratov colony on the lower Volga; in 1766 went to England, where he was an unsuccessful school-teacher and hack-writer. F.R.S. February 1772; D.C.L.(Oxon) November 1775. After the voyage spent some years in poverty, sponging and back-biting; in 1779 appointed to a chair at Halle university, where he remained till his death, a more prominent than useful member of academic society, never escaping the necessity of constant translation and miscellaneous low-powered scientific writing.

38. FORSTER, Johann George Adam (1754–94). 'Gentleman' and naturalist. Joined per Admiralty order 25 June 1772. E 'a Clever, good young man'. The eldest son of J. R. Forster. Educated mainly by his father, but with a strong original bent towards botany and a gift for languages. From an early age helped J. R. Forster with hackwork for the maintenance of the family, and sailed in the *Resolution* as his assistant and natural history draughtsman. After return to England engaged in literary and scientific work arising from the voyage, and then, visiting Paris and Germany, at last through his own fame and amiability managed to get his father the chair at Halle. F.R.S. January 1777. Was appointed professor of natural history at the Carolinum (officers' school) at Cassel; where, with only light academic duties, he wasted a great deal of time; he wrote a little, joined the Rosicrucians for a few years, and was always in money difficulties. In 1784 accepted the chair of natural history at Vilna; here, in a coarse and unlearned society, he was bored and disappointed; in 1788 became an easy-going librarian at Mainz; in 1790 visited England again, with Alexander von Humboldt. Married 1785; his wife left him in 1793, by which time, though in

poor health, he was deeply implicated in the revolutionary movement, a cosmopolitan seeking French annexation of the Rhineland. He went to Paris as a deputy of the Rhenish-German National Convention in March 1793, stayed on suffering some moral discomfort under the Terror, caught pneumonia in December, and died on 10 January 1794. After leaving Vilna he wrote a great deal to make ends meet, work which was generally superficial and uneven; he nevertheless became a very respectable figure in German literature, and, through Humboldt, a great influence on German scientific thought.

39. SCHOLIENT, Ernest. 'Servant to Mr Forster'. Joined per Admiralty order 25 June 1772. 'A feeble man . . . set upon [in Huahine] by five or six fellows who would have strip'd him' (Cook, 16 May 1774).

40. SPARRMAN, Andreas [Anders] (1748–1820). 'Servant to Mr Forster'. Studied at the University of Uppsala under Linnaeus, and made his first voyage at the age of 17 to India and China as surgeon in a Swedish East Indiaman. In 1768 joined the Swedish Chirurgical Society as student; 1770 qualified as a physician. In January 1772 sent by the Swedish government, on the nomination of Linnaeus, to the Cape for botanical exploration. E 'Clever steady Man'; certainly a rather proper young man, but interested in food and drink. The victim of assault at Huahine, 6 September 1773. Left the *Resolution* at Cape Town on her homeward passage, for further botanical and ethnological exploration, returning to Sweden in July 1776. Published a narrative of his travels in 1783, 1802, 1818; the first part appeared in an English translation in 1785. In 1787 went to Senegal to study the possibility of founding a Swedish colony there, visiting Paris and London on the way home. From 1778 to 1798 he presided over the 'Cabinet' of the Royal Academy of Sciences, to which he had presented the greater part of his ethnological collections. Apart from his travel volumes, he wrote a number of scientific papers.

42. OEDIDDY.
43. POETATA, his servant.
} 'Natives of Otaheite'. Entered at Raiatea 17 August 1773 [*sic*]. Discharged at Raiatea, by request, 4 June 1774.

ADVENTURE

1. FURNEAUX, Tobias (1735–81). Commander, per commissions 28 November and 25 December 1771. Joined 30 November. Fourth son of William Furneaux, of Swilly House, Stoke Damerel, Devon. Served in various ships, 1755–66, in West Indies, on coast of Africa and in Channel. Second lieutenant in *Dolphin* under Wallis (his cousin by marriage) 1766–8; described by George Robertson as 'a Gentele Agreable well behaved Good man and very humain to all

the Ships company'. Appointed Captain *Syren*, 10 August 1775, and served in North America. Died at Swilly 18 September 1781.

2. SWILLEY, James Tobias. A.B. Joined 30 November 1771. Furneaux's servant, 'a negroe', and presumably named by him. Killed by Maoris 17 December 1773.

3. WOODHOUSE, Thomas. Midshipman. Joined 1 December 1771. A.B. 1 January 1773. Killed by Maoris 17 December 1773.

4. MOODY, Robert. Dundee, 27. Quartermaster. Joined 3 December 1771.

7. SHANK, Joseph. First lieutenant, per commissions 28 November and 25 December 1771. Joined 28 November. Subject to gout, and discharged sick at the Cape of Good Hope, 19 November 1772, per order of Captain Cook.

11. FREEMAN, Thomas. Plymouth, 22. A.B. Joined 7 December 1771.

12. CONSTABLE, Love. Midshipman. Joined 7 December 1771. A.B. 1 January 1773; midshipman 19 December 1773.

13. FANNIN, Peter. Master, per warrants 3 December 1771 and 6 January 1772. Joined 9 December 1771 (from *Flora*). Retired from the navy in 1775 and settled in Douglas, Isle of Man, where he set up a school of navigation. In 1789 he published a valuable map of the Isle of Man.

15. JOHNS, Edward. Boatswain, per warrants 3 and 25 December 1771. Joined 12 December.

17., 122. HART, Edward. London, 18. A.B. Joined 16 December 1771.

18. HERGEST, Richard. A.B. Joined 16 December 1771 (from *Marlborough*). Midshipman 2 January 1773. Midshipman, *Resolution*, third voyage. Lieutenant commanding *Daedalus* storeship, sent to Pacific in 1792 to supply Vancouver's expedition. Killed at Oahu by Hawaiians, 11 May 1792. 'For many years . . . my most intimate friend'—Vancouver.

19. ROWE, John. Master's mate, 26 or 27. Joined 17 December 1771 (from *Torbay*). A.B. 1 November 1773; master's mate 2 December 1773. Related to Furneaux by marriage.[1] Had served most of his time in America and West Indies. Killed by Maoris 17 December 1773.

23. BARBER, Robert. Kilkenny, 23. Quartermaster. Joined 17 December 1771. A.B. 1 January 1773.

[1] The families of Furneaux (of Swilly) and Rowe (of Landrake, five miles away across the Tamar) were closely connected by marriage. John Rowe's first cousin, Elizabeth Rowe, married James Furneaux, elder brother of Tobias. Her sister Anne married John Wallis, elder brother of Samuel the circumnavigator; and their uncle, Samuel, married Anne Furneaux, aunt of James and Tobias Furneaux.

24. GLOAG, Andrew. Gunner, per warrants 13 and 25 December 1771. Joined 18 December 1771.

26. MURPHY, Francis. Dublin, 31. Quartermaster. Joined 18 December 1771. Killed by Maoris 17 December 1773.

27. GIBBS, James. Perth, 29. Boatswain's mate. Joined 21 December 1771.

28. BAZIL, Antony. 'East India', 22. A.B. Joined 21 December 1771.

29., 120. THOMAS, William. London 21. A.B. Joined 21 December 1771.

30. DEWAR, Alexander. Clerk. Joined 1 January 1772 (from *Torbay*). Clerk, *Resolution*, third voyage.

32. ANDREWS, Thomas. Surgeon, per warrants 13 December 1771 and 3 January 1772. Joined 25 December 1771 (from *Somerset*).

35. HAWKEY, William. Master's mate. Joined 8 January 1772. A.B. 1 April 1773.

39. BELL, Michael. Deptford, 21. A.B. Joined 8 January 1772. Killed by Maoris 17 December 1773.

40. MOOREY, George. A.B. Joined 13 January 1772. Midshipman 2 January 1773. Though 'a very sober young man' (Bayly) had a vision of his father, 4 March 1773.

41. KEMP, Samuel. Midshipman. Joined 10 January 1772. Died at sea 9 September 1772, 'by the same unlucky means as M[r] Lambrecht' (see no. 51).

42. HALEY, John. Cork, 27. Boatswain's mate. Joined 20 January 1772.

45. LANGFORD, John. Shepton Mallet, 20. A.B. Joined 25 January 1772.

47. LIGHTFOOT, Henry. Midshipman. Joined 28 January 1772.

49. HILL, Thomas. Portsmouth, 27. A.B. Joined 29 January 1772. Punished for insolence 12 December 1773; killed by Maoris 17 December 1773.

51. LAMBRECHT, John. 18. A.B. or midshipman. Joined 1 February 1772. Died at sea 24 August 1772, 'of a Fever he caught at S[t] Jago by bathing and making too free with the water in the heat of the day'.

52. KEMPE, Arthur (–1823). Second lieutenant, per commission 3 January 1772. Joined 1 February. First lieutenant, per commission 18 November 1772. Had served at the siege of Quebec, 1758. Post captain 1780; rear-admiral 1799; vice-admiral 1804; Admiral of the Red 1821.

53. MEDBERRY, William. London, 19. Carpenter's crew. Joined 5 February 1772.

55. FALCONER, John Richard. A.B. Joined 5 February 1772 (from *Somerset*). Master's mate 1 April 1773.

59. OFFORD, William. Carpenter, per warrant 7 February 1772. Joined 11 February.

61. ARROWSMITH, Noble. London, 23. A.B. Joined 11 February 1772.

62. WEAVER, Robert. London, 24. A.B. Joined 11 February 1772.

64. HILL, Andrew. Sailmaker, per warrant 12 February 1772. Joined 12 February (from *Tweed*).

65. SANDERSON, William. Hull, 29. Gunner's mate. Joined 13 February 1772 (from *Torbay*). Punished at Raiatea, 17 September 1773, for insolence and 'uttering prophane Oaths'.

69. FISH, John. Epping, 22. A.B. Joined 23 February 1772.

71. PRYOR, Henry. Alton, 36. A.B. Joined 23 February 1772.

73. FITZGERALD, Thomas. Ireland, 20. A.B. Joined 25 February 1772.

75. CARLO, Thomas. London, 32. A.B. Joined 25 February 1772.

77. GAMESON, James. Armourer, per warrant 25 February 1772. Joined 25 February.

78. LANYON, William. A.B. Joined 26 February 1772 (from *Terrible*). Midshipman 10 September 1772; master's mate 19 December 1773. Master's mate *Resolution*, third voyage. Lieutenant 1779; superannuated commander 1814; died 1817.

80. KENT, John. Surgeon's first mate, per warrant 3 March 1772. Joined 3 March (from *Torbay*).

81. YOUNG, John. Surgeon's second mate, per warrant 6 March 1772. Joined 14 March.

84. WHITE, George. Chichester, 24. A.B. Joined 7 March 1772. Carried as supernumerary for wages and victuals from 2 May 1772.

88. WILBY, John. A.B. Joined 14 March 1772. Midshipman 1 February 1774. Lieutenant 1776; became a Knight of Windsor; died 1803.

90. CAVANAGH, John. Kilkenny, 30. A.B. Joined 14 March 1772. Killed by Maoris 17 December 1773.

92. UPTON, John. Deptford, 26. Gunner's mate. Joined 14 March 1772.

93. CRAVAN, James. Dublin, 22. A.B. Joined 14 March 1772.

94. FAGAN, John. Woolwich, 20. A.B. Joined 14 March 1772. Carpenter's crew 15 July 1772.

95. VOWELL, Cornelius. Cork, 35. A.B. Joined 22 March 1772. Carried as supernumerary for wages and victuals from 23 June 1772.

96. TRENEER, Francis. Falmouth, 25. Quartermaster. Joined 22 March 1772 (from *Torbay*).

97. MOLLOY, Richard. Dublin, 39. A.B. Joined 22 March 1772.

98. BROWN, Robert. A.B. Joined 22 March 1772 (from *Nautilus*).

101. MAHONY, Mortimer. Cook, per warrant 23 March 1772. Joined 26 March. Died of scurvy at sea 23 July 1773. A naturally dirty and indolent man.

103. HARRISON, Robert. Prestonpans, 24. A.B. Joined 10 April 1772.

104. FINLEY, John. Fife, 26. A.B. Joined 10 April 1772. Quartermaster 19 December 1773.

106. WILLARD, Nathaniel. Maidstone, 45. Carpenter's crew. Joined 12 April 1772. Carpenter's mate 15 July 1772.

107. LEWIS, David. N. Wales, 25. A.B. Joined 12 April 1772. Carpenter's crew 16 July 1772.

108. JONES, James. Gosport, 25. A.B. Joined 12 April 1772. Killed by Maoris 17 December 1773.

109. SOWREY, William. Lancaster, 24. A.B. Joined 12 April 1772. Quartermaster 2 January 1773.

112. DYKE, Thomas. A.B. Joined 4 June 1772 (from *Torbay*). Master's mate 30 July 1772; A.B. 1 December 1773.

113. FACEY, William. Lancaster, 25. A.B. Joined 4 June 1772. Killed by Maoris 17 December 1773.

114. ROBERTS, William. Beaumaris, 29. A.B. Joined June 1772. Sail-maker's mate 30 July 1772, per order of Captain Cook.

115. MILTON, William. Fayal, Azores, 19. A.B. Joined 19 June 1772. Killed by Maoris 17 December 1773.

116. CRISPIN, William. Carpenter's mate. Joined 24 June 1772.

118. CRONEAN, John. Limerick, 23. A.B. Joined 25 June 1772.

119. CARR, William. A.B. Joined 2 July 1772. Master-at-arms 30 July 1772, per order of Captain Cook.

121. MCALLISTER, Dugal. A.B. Joined 4 July 1772 (from *Dublin*).

122. HART, Edward. A.B. Entered 11 July 1772 (from Supernumerary List).

123. RAYSIDE, John. A.B. A stowaway from a Portuguese ship at Funchal, Madeira. Entered 25 August 1772 (from Supernumerary List where he had been entered on discovery 2 August, per order of Captain Cook).

124. WIGHT, Henry. A.B. Joined 1 November 1772, at Cape.

125. BURNEY, James. Second lieutenant, per warrant 20 November 1772. (See muster-book of *Resolution*, no. 50.)

126. CHAPMAN, William. Cook. Entered 24 July 1773, from *Resolution*, per order of Captain Cook.

127. TETUBY HOMY [Omai]. Huahine, Society Islands. 22. A.B. Entered 19 December 1773 (from Supernumerary List, where he had been entered 9 September 1773).

[The seven men following were entered at the Cape of Good Hope on 21 March 1774.]

128. HUTCHINSON, Alexander. A.B., from *Seahorse*.

129. GARDNER, James. A.B., from *Seahorse*.

130. NICHOLLS, —. A.B.

131. GARRET, Abraham. A.B.

132. RYAN, William. A.B.

133. WILSON, Thomas. A.B.

134. ANDERSON, William. A.B.

MARINES

(Nos. 1–12, all of Chatham division, joined 29 March 1772.)

1. MOLLINEUX (Mollonex), John. Sergeant.
2. MILLS, Alexander. Corporal.
3. LANE, John. Drummer.
4. LEAR, Daniel. Private.
5. STEWART, Donald. Private. Punished for fighting, 29 August 1772.
6. ALLDEN, William. Private.
7. REED, Richard. Private.
8. THOMAS, John. Private.
9. KEARNEY, William. Private.
10. SOMMERFIELD, Bonaventure. Private.

12. ROSS, Alexander. Private. Punished for riotous behaviour at Tahiti, 31 August 1773.

13. SCOTT, James. Second lieutenant, per commission 11 June 1772. Joined 7 July (from *Resolution*). A man of unbalanced mind, suspicious and quarrelsome; 'a great stikler for *Honour*' (Bayly). Promoted 1st lieutenant 1776; placed on half-pay list 1779.

SUPERNUMERARIES

(for victuals only)

18. BAYLY, William (1737–1810). Astronomer. Entered 1 May 1772 per Admiralty order of 25 June. Born at Bishop's Cannings, Wilts., the son of a farmer. A self-taught mathematician and astronomer; in household of 3rd Duke of Richmond at Goodwood, 1769–70,

and subsequently assistant at the Royal Observatory; in 1769 observed the transit of Venus at the North Cape for the Royal Society. Astronomer in the *Discovery*, third voyage; his astronomical observations were published in 1777 (Wales and Bayly) and 1782 (Cook, King and Bayly). Headmaster of the Royal Naval Academy at Portsmouth, 1785–1807. He does not seem to have got on very well with Furneaux.

19. MACKY, Robert. Bayly's servant. Joined 1 May 1772, per Admiralty order.

20. BACSTROM, Sigismund (*fl.* 1770–99). 'Secretary to Mr Banks'. (Nos. 20 and 21 were carried on the books 1 May to 18 June 1772, per Admiralty order 24 June.)

21. CLEVELEY, John. 'Draughtsman to Mr Banks.' Went to Iceland with Banks.

NOMINAL INDEX

(References are to the muster-book numbers. Numbers preceded by 'M' refer to Marines by 'S' to Supernumeraries)

Resolution

Hendrick, John, 204
Hodges, William, S 21
Hood, Alexander, 149
Horn, Andrew, 54
Innell, John, 71
Jackson, George, 122
Lockton, John, 190
Loggie, Charles, 102
McVicar, Archibald, M 20
Manley, Isaac George, 4
Marra, John, 30
Masson, Francis, S 33
Maxwell, James, 177
Miller, 'Benjamin' [John Frederick], S 3
Miller, 'Joseph' [James], S 2
Mills, John, 165
Mitchel or Mitchell, Bowles, 114
Monk, Simon, 148
Monk, William, M 19
Oediddy, S 42
Patten, James, 20
Peckover, William, 123
Perry, Thomas, 193
Petterson, Emmanuel, 82
Phillips, John, M 9
Pickersgill, Richard, 13
Pirie, John, 7
Poetata, S 43
Price, Joseph, 41
Ramsay, John, 8
Reading, Solomon, 62
Reynolds, Peter, 9
Roberts, Henry, 21
Roberts, James, S 6
Rollett, Richard, 112
Scarnell, Francis, 87
Scholient, Ernest, S 39
Scott, James, M 6
Seamer or Seymour, John, 15
Shaw, Thomas, 34, 142
Sidsaft [Sidserf?], Peter, S 7
Simms, James, 55
Smally, John, 147
Smith, Isaac, 24
Smith, John, 201
Smock, Henry, 154
Snowden, Thomas, 191
Sparrman, Andreas, S 40
Stalker, John, 51, 143
Taylor, Francis, M 17
Taylor, Isaac, M 22
Terrell, Edward, 146
Tow, William, M 11
Twitty, Charles, M 16
Vancouver, George, 117
Wales, William, S 11
Wallis, James, 5
Waterfield, Richard, M 14
Wedgeborough, William, M 13
Whattman or Watman, William, 158
Wheilon or Whelan, Patrick, 91
White, Stephen, 124
White, Thomas, 66
Whitehouse, John, 45
Williams, Charles, 145
Willis, Thomas, 79
Wilson [Walden?], John, S 4
Woodward, George, M 15
Wybrow, John, 35
Young, Nicholas, S 10

Adventure

Allden, William, M 6
Anderson, William, 134
Andrews, Thomas, 32
Arrowsmith, Noble, 61
Bacstrom, Sigismund, S 20
Barber, Robert, 23
Bayly, William, S 18
Bazil, Antony, 28
Bell, Michael, 39
Brown, Robert, 98
Burney, James, 125
Carlo, Thomas, 75
Carr, William, 119
Cavanagh, John, 90
Chapman, William, 126
Cleveley, John, S 21
Constable, Love, 12
Cravan, James, 93
Crispin, William, 116
Cronean, John, 118
Dewar, Alexander, 30
Dyke, Thomas, 112
Facey, William, 113
Fagan, John, 94
Falconer, John Richard, 55
Fannin, Peter, 13
Finley, John, 104
Fish, John, 69
Fitzgerald, Thomas, 73
Freeman, Thomas, 11
Furneaux, Tobias, 1
Gameson, James, 77
Gardner, James, 129
Garret, Abraham, 131
Gibbs, James, 27
Gloag, Andrew, 24
Haley, John, 42
Harrison, Robert, 103
Hart, Edward, 17, 122
Hawkey, William, 35
Hergest, Richard, 18
Hill, Ambrose, 64
Hill, Thomas, 49
Hutchinson, Alexander, 128
Johns, Edward, 15
Jones, James, 108
Kearney, William, M 9
Kemp, Samuel, 41
Kempe, Arthur, 52
Kent, John, 80

Lambrecht, John, 51
Lane, John, M 3
Langford, John, 45
Lanyon, William, 78
Lear, Daniel, M 4
Lewis, David, 107
Lightfoot, Henry, 47
McAllister, Dugal, 121
Macky, Robert, S 19
Mahony, Mortimer, 101
Medberry, William, 53
Mills, Alexander, M 2
Milton, William, 115
Mollineux, John, M 1
Molloy, Richard, 97
Moody, Robert, 4
Moorey, George, 40
Murphy, Francis, 26
Nicholls, —, 130
Offord, William, 59
Pryor, Henry, 71
Rayside, John, 123
Reed, Richard, M 7
Roberts, William, 114
Ross, Alexander, M 12
Rowe, John, 19
Ryan, William, 132
Sanderson, William, 65
Scott, James, M 13
Shank, Joseph, 7
Sommerfield, Bonaventure, M 10
Sowrey, William, 109
Stewart, Donald, M 5
Swilley, James Tobias, 2
Tetuby Homy [Omai], 127
Thomas, John, M 8
Thomas, William, 29, 120
Treneer, Francis, 96
Upton, John, 92
Vowell, Cornelius, 95
Weaver, Robert, 62
White, George, 84
Wight, Henry, 124
Wilby, John, 88
Willard, Nathaniel, 106
Wilson, Thomas, 133
Woodhouse, Thomas, 3
Young, John, 87

APPENDIX VIII

Calendar of Documents

THE documentation of this voyage is full and complicated, and much that could have been legitimately included in the following list—particularly on the unofficial side—has been deliberately omitted in the struggle against distension. Thus almost the whole bulk of the papers bearing on the voyage accumulated by Banks, and now in the Mitchell Library, has been ignored, although a few are so valuable as to demand printing in full. On the official side commissions and warrants of appointment (P.R.O. Adm 6/20, Adm 106/2898–9; National Maritime Museum ADM/A/2649–50) have also been ignored; as have been certain entries (e.g. in minutes) which merely show one step in an administrative process which is already clear enough. In some cases, however, every step has been documented, mainly to show how immediately Cook's requests were met. The In Letters of the Victualling Board for this period have been dispersed, but a number have come to rest in collections outside England, and have been listed when possible. Some are in the volume in the Dixson Library, entitled *Captain James Cook Relics and MSS*; this I have referred to as Dixson R. Many letters exist in several copies, and Cook had his own correspondence entered in the volume I have called the Canberra Letter Book (CLB) from its existence now in the Commonwealth National Library, Canberra. (This is a separate volume from the Canberra Letter Book of the first voyage, and covers the years 1771–8.) It is another useful source for Victualling Board transactions. Where more than one source is given for letters from Cook, the original always comes first; similarly for letters with minutes or endorsements. Cook's holograph letters, whether given in full or not, are denoted by an asterisk *; documents printed in the *Historical Records of New South Wales*, Vol. I, Part 1 (1893), by a dagger †. Other principles adopted are as described in the introduction to the calendar in the first volume of this edition, Appendix VI.

The following table indicates the classes of official documents that have been drawn on.

Public Record Office

Adm 1/1609	In Letters: Captains' Letters 1741–71
„ 1/1610	„ „ „ „ 1772–75
„ 2/97	Admiralty Secretary, Out Letters: Orders and Instructions 8 May 1771–June 1772.
„ 2/546	„ „ Out Letters to Public Offices and Admirals July 1771–May 1772.

Adm 2/547 Admiralty Secretary Out Letters to Public Offices and Admirals June 1772–May 1773.

„ 2/549 „ „ Out Letters to Public Offices and Admirals August 1774–July 1775.

„ 2/550 „ „ Out Letters to Public Offices and Admirals August 1775–January 1776.

„ 2/731 „ „ Common Out Letters, 20 May 1771–September 1772.

„ 2/733 „ „ Common Out Letters, 15 September 1774–13 December 1775.

„ 2/745 „ „ Correspondence General 1759–72.

„ 2/1135 „ „ Letters to Greenwich Hospital 1767–May 1780.

„ 2/1166 „ „ Out Letters.

„ 2/1167 „ „ „ „

„ 2/1332 Secret Orders and Instructions 1762–78.

„ 3/78 „ Minutes of the Board November 1770–August 1771.

„ 3/79 „ Minutes of the Board September 1771–February 1773.

„ 3/80 „ Minutes of the Board March 1773–January 1775.

„ 3/81 „ Minutes of the Board February 1775–December 1775.

„ 18/116–7 Accountant General, Bill Book.

„ 97/86 Medical Department [Sick and Hurt Board] In Letters: Letters from Officers in Command 1766–75.

„ 98/10 „ „ Out Letters to the Admiralty 1764–1774.

„ 98/11 „ „ Out Letters to the Admiralty 1775–1779.

„ 99/47 „ „ Minutes of the Board.

„ 106/1208 Navy Board In Letters: Admiralty to Navy Board, Miscellaneous C 1772.

„ 106/1227 „ „ In Letters: Admiralty to Navy Board, Miscellaneous C–D 1775.

„ 106/2201 „ „ Out Letters to Admiralty 1771–2.

Adm 106/2203 Navy Board Out Letters to Admiralty 1775–6.
„ 106/2204 „ „ Out Letters to Admiralty 1776–7.
„ 106/2585 „ „ Minutes of the Board 1771.
„ 106/2586–7 „ „ Minutes of the Board 1772.
„ 106/3316 „ „ Deptford Yard Letter Book Series 1, 1768–1772.
„ 106/3317 „ „ Deptford Yard Letter Book Series 1, 1772–75.
„ 110/25 Victualling Board Letter Book 1771–3.
„ 110/26 „ „ Letter Book 1773–5.
„ 111/68 „ „ Minutes, Board and Committees 1771.
„ 111/69 „ „ Minutes, Board and Committees 1772.

The relevant Admiralty indexes are Adm 12/4806, Digest of In Letters, and Adm 10704/17, Abstract of letters from Admiralty to Navy Board, Series 1, from January 1768.

National Maritime Museum

ADM/A/2647 Admiralty Letters to Navy Board September 1771.
ADM/A/2651–2 Admiralty Letters to Navy Board January–February 1772.
ADM/A/2654–6 Admiralty Letters to Navy Board April–June 1772.
ADM/A/2694 Admiralty Letters to Navy Board August 1775.
ADM/A/2696 Admiralty Letters to Navy Board October 1775.
ADM/B/185–6 Navy Board Letters to Admiralty April 1771–September 1772.
ADM/C/604–6 Admiralty Letters to Victualling Board October 1771–June 1772.
ADM/DP/104 Victualling Board Letters to Admiralty 1772.
ADM/E/41–2 Admiralty Letters to Sick and Hurt Board 1770–80.
ADM/FP/18 Sick and Hurt Board Letters to Admiralty 1775.

The Board of Longitude's orders for payments on the Treasurer, sealed and signed, are bound up with the Admiralty Letters to the Navy Board.

1771

29 August. *Admiralty to Victualling Board.* The Board is to allow on account of Lieut. Cook, late commander of *Endeavour*, some wheat and barley which was expended during his late voyage.—Adm 2/97.

29 August. *Admiralty Minutes.* Cook appointed to *Scorpion*, to be fitted out at Deptford for Channel service. Complement 120 men; 14 carriage guns and 14 swivels.—Adm 3/78.

29 August. *Admiralty to Cook.* To fit out at Deptford for foreign [*sic*] service. —Adm 2/97.

29 August. *Admiralty Secretary to Cook.* To hasten to the Nore with his ships, agreeable to their Lordships' orders of 9 January last.—Adm 2/731.

25 September. *Admiralty to Navy Board.* Instructions to purchase two proper vessels of about 400 tons for service in remote parts.—ADM/A/2647.

1 October. *Admiralty to Victualling Board.* To allow of some particular charges in account of Lieut. Cook, late of *Endeavour*, for employment of purchaser to procure necessary provisions at Rio de Janeiro at 5% commission and 5% discount off bills of exchange; onions at Madeira; vegetables at Batavia (an extraordinary quantity because of sickly state of crew's health).—Adm 2/97. Cf. vol. I, p. 640.

9 October. *Admiralty Secretary to Mr Charles Irving.* To attend Navy Board with his ship's hearth.—Adm 2/731.

9 October. *Admiralty Secretary to Navy Board.* To examine and report on Mr Charles Irving's new hearth, and if thought advisable to suggest which ship it might be tried on.—Adm 2/546.

30 October. *Admiralty Secretary to Victualling Board.* A letter has been received signed Marinus about inspissated juice of malt and it is requested that a report may be made on it. Enclosure: London, 14 October, 14 page letter about scurvy and the preparation of inspissated juice of malt and two extracts from Glauber. Suggests use of gum senega also.—ADM/C/604; Adm 2/546.

15 November. *Victualling Board to Admiralty.* Cook having informed the Board that salted cabbage keeps at sea and is as effective as sour krout in preventing scurvy, has asked for 4 tons of casks to be filled with it for present intended voyage to southern parts of globe. Approval from Admiralty is sought. Minuted '29th Nov[r] To approve the quantity proposed.'—ADM/DP/103.

15 November. *Navy Board to Admiralty.* In accordance with order of 25 September, two barks have been purchased: *Marquis of Granby* 450 tons, *Marquis of Rockingham* 336 tons. Orders have been given for fitting them and proposals will be made for numbers, guns and complements.—ADM/B/185.

19 November. *Navy Board to Admiralty.* Report upon Mr Charles Irving's new constructed ship's hearth. Navy Board has ordered two to be made by Messrs Crowley & Co. under Irving's inspection, one for ship of 74 guns and one for frigate of 20 guns. Will propose ships proper for experiment when hearths are completed.—ADM/B/185.

25 November. *Admiralty Minutes.* Victualling Board to prepare quantity of Baron Storsch's carrot marmalade for trial.—Adm 3/79.

25 November. *Admiralty to Victualling Board.* The Society for the Encouragement of Arts, Manufactures, and Commerce have forwarded a receipt thay have received from Baron Storsch at Berlin for making a marmalade of yellow carrots as one of the best remedies against scurvy.

A proper quantity is to be prepared in the manner specified and experiments made thereof in such ships as shall be thought fit by their Lordships. Enclosure: Copy of Storsch's letter, dated Berlin 12 February.—ADM/C/604; Adm 2/97.

25 November. *Admiralty Secretary to Secretary of Society for Encouragement of Arts, Manufactures, and Commerce.* Informing him that Victualling Board has been directed to provide carrot marmalade from Baron Storsch's recipe.—Adm 2/731.

27 November. *Navy Board to Admiralty.* Further to their letter of 15th inst. Complements are proposed as follows: *Marquis of Granby*, carriage guns 12, 6 pounders; swivels 12; no. of men 110. *Marquis of Rockingham*, carriage guns 10, 4 pounders; swivels 8, no. of men 80. Instructions are required for fitting the ships, sheathing and filling their bottoms and information of the names to be used for registration. Minuted '28th November. To be registered as sloops, former as *Drake*, latter as *Raleigh* and to be with the number and nature of guns and complement of men as they have proposed.'—ADM/B/185.

27 November. *Admiralty Minutes.* The two barks bought by Navy Board for service in remote parts to be entered as *Drake* and *Raleigh. Drake* to have 12 guns, 110 men; *Raleigh* to have 10 guns, 80 men. James Wallace to be carpenter of *Drake*, Jas. Adcock of *Raleigh.* Cook to command *Drake*, Lieuts. Robert Pallisser Cooper and Chas. Clerke 1st and 2nd Lieuts. Furneaux to command *Raleigh.* Lieut. Jos. Shank 1st Lieut. —Adm 3/79.

28 November. *Board of Longitude Minutes.* Resolving that two astronomical observers be sent in Cook's ships and that the Royal Society approve their instructions and the list of instruments to be provided. Royal Greenwich Observatory. Printed above, p. 719.

29 November. *Royal Society, Minutes of Council.* 'The President [James West] acquainted the Council, that yesterday he had attended a Board of Longitude;[1] when the Commissioners agreed to appoint two of the best observers that could be found for an expedition into remote parts with liberal appointments; and the Astronomer Royal, and the professors were desired to draw up a Plan, forthwith, with full directions to the observers in the respective ships to be sent, and also jointly as occasion may happen; together with lists of proper instruments adjoined to the said Plan: and that the same is ordered to be laid before the Royal Society for any alterations or additions they shall think proper: And the whole report of the Astronomer, Professors &c &c is to be laid before the board of Longitude at their next meeting, which is to be on the 14th Decr next.'—R.S., Council Minutes, vol. VI, p. 119.

[1] The minutes of this meeting of the Board are printed in Appendix III, pp. 719–20 above.

29 November. *Admiralty to Navy Board. Drake* and *Raleigh* to be sheathed, filled and fitted out for voyage to remote parts, established with complements according to the scheme, and victualled to 12 months of all provisions.—ADM/A/2651.

29 November. *Admiralty Minutes.* Lieut. Pickersgill to be 3rd Lieut. of *Drake.*—Adm 3/79.

30 November. *Admiralty to Cook.* 'Having appointed you Commander of his Majesty's Sloop Drake at Deptford, which we have ordered to be Sheathed, filled, fitted, and Stored at that Place for a Voyage to remote parts, Manned with one Hundred & Ten Men, agreable to the Scheme here unto annexed,[1] & Victualled for twelve Months for the said Complement with all Species of Provisions except Beer of which she is to have as much as she can conveniently Stow; You are hereby required & directed to use the utmost dispatch in getting her ready for the Sea accordingly, & then falling down to Galleons Reach take in her Guns & Gunners Stores at that place & thence proceed to the Nore for further order.'—CLB.

30 November. *Navy Board to Victualling Board.* Instructions to victual *Drake* and *Raleigh* for voyage to remote parts for 12 months of all allowances except beer, of which 1 month, and brandy in lieu of remainder. Attached: Scheme of Officers and men to be established.—ADM/C/604.

30 November. *Admiralty Minutes.* Orders to be given for about 4 tons salted cabbage to be sent on board *Drake.*—Adm 3/79.

30 November. *Admiralty to Victualling Board.* Whereas by Victualling Board letter of 15th inst. information was sent that Cook had acquainted the Commissioners that it was found in course of his late voyage that cabbage simply salted will keep any length of time at sea, and that he thought it would be equal value to sour krout in preventing scurvy, and asked for about 4 tons of casks to be filled with it for present voyage, it is approved for his request to be granted and the required amount of salted cabbage is to be provided as soon as possibly may be.—ADM/C/604; Adm 2/97.

[?] December. *Solander to Lind.*[2] 'My Dear Doctor/ This Letter is wrote when I am in such raptures of wishing it may be attended with success, that I am afraid it will hardly be intelligible—our mutual friend Mr Cummins has promisd that he will back the proposition.

'Government have resolved to send out two Ships upon Discoveries into the South Seas. Mr Banks and My self have got leave to go in one of them. No expense whatsoever is to be spared. Every thing is to

[1] This 'Scheme' is not here printed, being almost identical with that given by Cook, pp. 11–12 above; Cook has 112 men in all.

[2] This letter, in Solander's hand, is obviously to Lind, but it lacks its final page and signature. There is no date, apart from 'December 1771' pencilled at the top of the first page in a different hand. It must have been written some time in the first week of the month.

be made as agreable as possible to them that go. Capt[n] Cook (who commanded the Endeavour) is to have the command of the Drake which is the Ship we propose to go in & Capt[n] Furneaux to command the Raleigh. Most all the Officers that were upon the former expedition go again; and many of the common Men—a sign that our fatigues were well paid with the pleasure we had in making acquaintance with the generous people we met with, and from the many new things we saw. From not knowing how to properly equip ourselves we were not half so well provided last voyage as we now shall be; We did notwithstanding Discover a prodigious deal in all Branches of Natural History, Geography, astronomy &c, &c. Now it is the Desire of the King, of all great Men in power, particularly the Admiralty People, &c that this next Expedition shall be as compleat as possible. The Board of Longitude have resolved to send out two Astronomers and wish very much, that one of them at least, should be a Philosopher at the same time; They are willing to be very liberal in their reward. Great many want to go—but most all of them are mere Observers—M[r] Banks, whose character, I dare say you have heard; and who deserves all possible praise for his Spirit in promoting real Knowledge, is by the Admiralty Board, the Board of Longitude, and all them that have any thing to do with the Equipment of this Expedition, continually consulted and very much attended to. He and myself have been Desird by the Board of Longitude to think of, and propose to them proper Persons fit for these undertakings.

'Now I come to the great point which I utter with the greatest overflow of wishes to succeed. Will You my Dear Doctor give us leave to propose You, to the Board of Longitude, as willing to go out as an Astronomer. Your well known character makes us all, beg, pray & long for your affirmative answer. What great thing could you not do, preferable to any body else in the creation. Don't think I flatter, I write from sincere conviction. All them that know You, say the same. Now figure to yourself what real pleasure you would find, in being so useful to Mankind. I don't propose this, thinking a reward of a few hundred a year would prevail upon you—but as an undertaking suitable to your Inclination, that has allways been tending to increase Science and to do good. A field of very great extent is now open to You. All the world will be glad, if you will take a walk in it. Every man will be benafited by it.

'M[r] Banks, who has not the pleasure of being personally known to you has desired me, to acquaint you with his warmest wishes of having You, My Dear Sir, as a fellow Traveller. He has it so much at heart, that he has resolved to send this, by Post-express, to you—& begs that you will be so good and return to him or me, an answer by the same conveyance as soon as possible. The expenses of which he will most thankfully repay. The Reason for this haste is: the Meeting of the Board of Longitude, Saturday Dec[r] the 14th, when proper

Persons are to be proposed.[1] We are afraid no Letters by the common Post could be recieved time enough; We ought to have the answer by friday afternoon or as much sooner as possible. I am just now informed that an express may go between London and Edinburgh in something less than three days, hope therefore to have your answer if possible by friday Morning. We are then to meet the astronomical People i.e. the Different Professors from Oxford, Cambridge & Greenwich to consult about what is to be said to the board, the Day following

'How we all have been so thoughtless & not before this, apply'd to you, is a thing we will talke over, when we walk the quarter-deck together.

'Both Mr Banks & Myself, and I likewise can answer for Capt. Cook, shall do our utmost to make life agreable during the Voyage which will probably be a three years one. I hope we shall be a very comfortable Society.

'Mr Cummins who has so much friendship for Mr Banks & myself, that he interests himself very much in our behalf, gives his best Compliments to You—has not time to write with the express but will send You a letter with this nights post.

'It is proposed that we shall leave England in March next—touch at Madeira—go to the Cape of good Hope, stay there a Month or more—from thence proceed to the Southward of New Holland and stop for a short time at some place in New Zeland—afterwards set out upon Discoveries farther to the South than any European Navigator has been. In those high Latitudes spend two or three Summers & every Winter go up within the Tropics to compleat our former discoveries. Good God, we shall do wonders if you only will come and assist us.'—Dixson Library MSS.

2 December. *Victualling Board to Cook.* Orders received to supply *Drake* with twelve months' provisions except beer; what quantities did he require? —CLB.

2 December. **Cook to Admiralty Secretary.* Sends list of petty officers and foremast men belonging to *Scorpion*. Asks that they may be discharged into *Drake*.—Adm 1/1609.

2 December. **Cook to Admiralty Secretary.* 'Mr James Grey, who was with me in the Endeavour Bark and at Present Boatswain of the Cruizer Sloop, has signified his desire to go out again with me. I pray you will be pleased to move my Lords Commissioners of the Admiralty to appoint him Boatswain of His Majestys Sloop Drake.—Permit me Sir to recommend to their Lordships Thos Hardman who has Saild with me sence the beginning of the year 1767, in the Stations of Boatswain Mate & Sail-maker—he is well quallified to be Boatswain

[1] This was the date when Wales and Bayly were proposed by Maskelyne, following the meeting of the Council of the Royal Society on 12 December; p. 720 above.

of any of His Majestys Sloops in ordinary or Home Service his constitution at present is not Sufficient to stand such a Voyage as I am going otherwise I should have applied for him to have been appointed my Boatswain.—P.S. I shall recommend Rob[t] Anderson, who was also with me in the Endeavour, to be appointed gunner of the Drake provide he quallifies himself for that Station.'—Adm 1/1609.

2 December. *Victualling Board Minutes.* Navy Board 30th past. *Drake* at Deptford *Raleigh* at Woolwich to be victualled for voyage to remote parts to 12 months. Write to Captains as usual.—Adm 111/68.

2 December. *Admiralty Minutes. Drake* to be supplied with such additional stores and provisions as she can conveniently stow; also camp forges, copper ovens, apparatus for making stinking and salt water fresh and sweet. Ed. Johns to be boatswain of *Raleigh.*—Adm 3/79.

3 December. **Cook to Admiralty Secretary.* Prays to be paid for *Scorpion* without passing an account.—Adm 1/1609.

3 December. *Admiralty Secretary to Navy Board.* Refers application from Cook to be paid wages for *Scorpion* without passing any account for her.—Adm 2/546.

5 December. *Admiralty Secretary to Cook.* To apply to Victualling Board for supply of portable soup to be issued when fresh provisions cannot be obtained.—Adm 2/731; CLB.

5 December. *Admiralty Secretary to Furneaux.* Letter identical with foregoing. —Adm 2/731.

5 December. *Admiralty Secretary to Sick and Hurt Board. Resolution* and *Adventure* are to be issued with additional quantity of portable soup and instructions for its issue to well men will be given to their commanders.—ADM/E/41.

5 December. *Admiralty to Navy Board.* Order to supply *Drake* and *Raleigh* with stores and provisions proper for the service for which they are intended. Camp forge and copper oven to be supplied and coppers to be fitted with Irving's apparatus for rendering salt water fresh, and with Lieut. Osbridge's[1] machines for rendering stinking water sweet. —ADM/A/2650.

5 December. **Cook to Admiralty Secretary.* Acknowledges receipt of order of 30 November.—Adm 1/1609.

6 December. *Navy Board Minutes.* To be proposed to Admiralty to furnish *Drake* and *Raleigh* with frames of two vessels of 20 and 17 tons, to be set up here and afterwards taken asunder when wanted.—Adm 106/2585.

6 December. *Navy Board to Admiralty.* Propose that *Drake* and *Raleigh* may be furnished with the frames of 2 vessels of 20 and 17 tons, for ex-

[1] 'Orsbridge's' in original.

ploring and surveying any coasts where they may touch.—ADM/B/185; Adm 106/2201.

6 December. *Navy Board to Victualling Board.* Additional quantities of provisions to be issued to *Drake* and *Raleigh.* Minuted: '6th—Write the Captains and desire to know what additional quantities will be wanted.' —ADM/C/604.

6 December. *Victualling Board Minutes.* Captain Cook 5th December. Ordered that the following good new tight tanks be seasoned and prepared for *Drake.* Butts 200; puncheons 220; hogsheads 60; barrels 80; half hogsheads 60; 20 gal. casks 20; barricoes[1] 20. The Master Cooper to take care that they be made of very best materials, and that they be in all respects suitable for a voyage to remote parts. Acquaint Cook. Navy Board 6th December. *Drake* and *Raleigh* to be supplied with such additional provisions as they can conveniently stow. Write Captains to know what additional provisions they will want.—Adm 111/68.

6 December. *Victualling Board to Cook.* An order had been received to supply an additional quantity of provisions. What quantities does he require? —CLB.

6 December. *Navy Board Minutes.* Officers at Deptford and Woolwich yards to appoint a ship in ordinary at each port for reception of such seamen as may enter for *Drake* and *Raleigh.*—Amd 106/2585.

6 December. *Admiralty Secretary to Victualling Board.* Refers an application from Furneaux that he may be allowed for extra allowance of wheat, oatmeal and spirits issued under Cook's orders.—Adm 2/549.

11 December. *Admiralty Minutes.* Lieut. Robert Parker to be 2nd Lieut. of *Raleigh.* Jas. Gray of *Cruizer* to be boatswain of *Drake.*—Adm 3/79.

11 December. *Victualling Board Minutes.* Furneaux 9th. Ordered the following good new tight casks to be seasoned etc: Butts 160; puncheons 160; hogsheads 60; barrels 20; half hogsheads 60; 20 gal. flasks 20; barricoes 20; Master Cooper to take particular care that they be made of very best materials, and that they be in all respects suitable for a voyage to remote parts.—Adm 111/68.

12 December. *Royal Society, Minutes of Council.* The draft report for the Board of Longitude read to the Council by Maskelyne; some additions made; the report approved and signed. It includes (i) 'a list of the Instruments, proper to be sent', noting those already in the possession of the Board, those to be lent by the Royal Society, and those to be ordered from the instrument-makers; and (ii) 'instructions for the direction of the observers'.[2]—R.S., Council Minutes, vol. VI, pp. 123–30.

12 December. *Admiralty to Navy Board.* The Navy Board's proposal that

[1] Kegs.

[2] The Royal Society's report was presented to the Board at its meeting on 14 December (above, pp. 720–2). The list of instruments and instructions to the observers, as approved by the Board are printed above, pp. 721–2, 724–8.

two decked vessels of 20 and 17 tons might be useful to *Drake* and *Raleigh* for exploring and surveying is agreed to and frames of such dimensions are to be set up and then packed in cases for the purpose. Minuted: 'Give orders to the Officers of each yard to cause 2 vessels according to the draught herewith sent and to be put on board the sloops accordingly.'—ADM/A/2650.

13 December. *Admiralty Minutes.* Two decked vessels of 20 tons to be sent out to *Raleigh* and *Drake* for surveying coasts etc. Andrew Gloag to be gunner of *Raleigh.*—Adm 3/79.

13 December. *Navy Board Minutes.* Deptford and Woolwich officers to fit *Drake* and *Raleigh* with same number of blocks cooked and pinned[1] as is established to ships of 28 guns.—Adm 106/2585.

14 December. **Cook to Admiralty Secretary.*† 'Having some business to transact down in Yorkshire as well as to see an Aged Father, please to move my Lords Commissioners of the Admiralty to grant me three Weeks leave of absaance for that purpose.'—Adm 1/1609.

14 December. *Board of Longitude Minutes.* Wales and Bayly appointed and their terms of employment approved. The Royal Society's report considered and the provision of instruments agreed.—Royal Greenwich Observatory. Printed above, pp. 720–2.

15 December. *Furneaux to Sick and Hurt Board.* Asking that *Raleigh* be supplied with portable soup in the same proportion as supplied to *Drake. Raleigh*'s complement is 80.—Adm 97/86.

16 December. *Cook to Victualling Board.* 'Agreable to yours of the 6th inst I here send you an account of the quantitys of each species of Provisions, which I judge the Drake will stow, including those already orderd, the sugar which the Endeavour Bark was supply'd with on her late Voyage was bad in the very utmost sence of the word, I hope care will be taken, that what the Drake & Raleigh Sloops are Supply'd with will be of a better sort.

'Provisions for the Drake Sloop

Bread in Butts	26880 Pounds
ditto in Baggs	26880 ,,
Flour as Bread	15000 in barrls & half Hhds
Beef in Puncheons	6000 } Pieces
Pork.. ditto	12000 } Pieces
Flour as Beef	1980 Pounds
Beer	60 Puncheons
Spirits	1500 Gallons
Port Wine	600 ,,

[1] i.e. coaked and pinned, fitted with coaks and pins. Coaks are the small metal bushes inserted in the sheave of the block, to prevent wear by the pin on which it turns.

Pease in Butts	300 bush[ls]
Suet	1500 Pounds
Raisins	3300 d[o]
Oatm[l] in Small Casks	150 } Gall[s]
Wheat in d[o]	1200 }
Butter	1500 Pounds
Cheese	1500 ,,
Oyl	200 Gall[s]
Sug[r]	2000 Pounds.'—CLB.

16 December. *Cook to Sick and Hurt Board.* Applies for portable soup for 120 persons.—Adm 97/86.

16 December. *Cook to Sick and Hurt Board.* 'The Secretary of the Admiralty having acquainted me by Letter date 5 Inst[t] that my Lords Commissioners of the Admiralty had order'd you to cause His Majesty's Sloop Drake under my command, to be supplyed with some Portable soup to issue to her Crew, as you should direct, when fresh Provision cannot be got, I take the liberty to acquaint you that her Crew will not consist of less than 120 persons, & that the Voyage will (very probably) be upwards of three Years, during which time I cannot fore see that more then two Months Provisions can be got. I hope that proper Attention will be paid to the quality of this most valuable Article. . . .'—CLB.

17 December. *Admiralty Secretary to Cook.* Grants him leave for private affairs as asked by letter of 15th inst.—Adm 2/731.

17 December. *Admiralty Minutes. Drake* and *Raleigh* to be furnished with particular letters of recommendation to governor of Rio de Janeiro on account of previous treatment to H.M.'s ships.—Adm 3/79.

17 December. *Navy Board Minutes.* Captain King of *Asia* to be acquainted that we have removed his master to *Drake*. *Drake* to try Irving's hearth while in dock. Acquaint Cook.—Adm 106/2585.

17 December. *Navy Board to Cook.* He is to try Irving's hearth, and report thereon—CLB.

20 December. *Victualling Board Minutes.* Captain Cook 16th. Let provisions mentioned therein be sent to *Drake* except sour krout and salted cabbage. Acquaint Cook that we do not think proper to give positive orders about these yet. Acquaint him that we have in store c. 31,009 lb. sour krout packed in 98 barrels; salted cabbage c. 7137 lb. in 13 hogsheads. Said quantity will at rate of 2 lb. per man per week serve the 190 men of *Drake* and *Raleigh* c. 100 weeks. Ask him to acquaint us whether Sloops can take aboard whole of this amount—if so we shall order same to be sent aboard in proportion to their complements.—Captain Furneaux 15th. Let provisions therein mentioned be sent to *Raleigh* except sour krout and cabbage.—Ordered that the respective officers be particularly careful that provisions for *Drake* and *Raleigh* be

the best and newest in store, that water casks be new, that casks with provisions in them be in every respect good and fit for foreign voyage and the provisions be packed in tight casks. Ordered purchase of 40 quarters of newest and best wheat, to be kiln dried at Red House, packed in tight casks. Also 700 lb. newest and best mustard seed, unground, packed in tight casks.—Adm 111/68.

20 December. *Victualling Board to Cook.* Giving directions for the provisions to be brought on board when the ship is ready to receive them; quoting 2 lb per man per week (for 100 weeks) for sour krout and salted cabbage.—CLB.

20 December. *Lord Rochford to Lord Sandwich.* 'My dear Lord / I, as well as many others, have been struck with your naming the two ships that are going out the *Raleigh* and the *Drake*; for be assured, though a mere trifle, it will give great offence to the Spaniards. They hold in detestation those two names, and will believe we do it on purpose to insult them. I had some conversation with the King upon this subject to-day, and he wished I would write you a private letter upon it that you might consider it. What do you think of the Aurora and the Hisperus which two names are just come into my head? But after all, you will do just as you please, but I thought it right to give you this hint.'—Sandwich Papers, Hinchingbrooke.

23 December. *Victualling Board Minutes.* Ordered purchase of 140 quarters newest and best wheat, to be kiln dried at Red House, then sent to mills at Rotherhithe and ground and dressed into flour (through the same sort of cloth as fine households) and packed into tight barrels and half hogsheads for *Drake* and *Raleigh.*—Adm 111/68.

25 December. *Admiralty Minutes.* Names *Drake* and *Raleigh* to be changed to *Resolution* and *Adventure.*—Adm 3/79.

25 December. *Admiralty to Navy Board.* The two barks lately bought are to be registered under names of *Resolution* and *Adventure* and not as formerly stated *Drake* and *Raleigh.*—ADM/A/2650.

26 December. *Admiralty Secretary to Cook.* Authorising change of name of ship from *Drake* to *Resolution*, and corresponding change of commissions and warrants.—CLB.

27 December. *Navy Board Minutes.* Orders according to Admiralty instructions of 25th inst., for registration of *Resolution* and *Adventure.*—Adm 106/2585.

30 December. *Deptford Yard Officers to Navy Board.* Giving a list of materials and their prices used on construction of round house and captain's cabin.—Adm 106/3316.

36 December. *Victualling Board Minutes.* 5 coopers to be entered on piece work to assist in raising casks for *Drake* and *Raleigh.*—Adm 111/68.

31 December. *Navy Board to Victualling Board.* Their Lordships have

directed that *Drake* and *Raleigh* shall be registered by names of *Resolution* and *Adventure*. Minuted: '1st January Read—Let notice be given to proper officer.'—ADM/C/605.

1772

1 January. *Victualling Board Minutes*. Write Cook that present contractor for fresh beef has been ordered to supply *Resolution* with what may be wanted.—Adm 111/69.

1 January. *Victualling Board to Cook*. Stating that Mr William Preddy is authorised to supply fresh beef to the ship.—CLB.

1 January. *Admiralty Secretary to Furneaux*. 3 weeks' leave granted for private affairs.—Adm 2/731.

3 January. *Admiralty Minutes*. Lieut. Arthur Kempe to be 2nd Lieut. of *Adventure*.—Adm 3/79.

3 January. *Cook to Captain William Hammond, Hull*. 'Ayton . . . / I am sorry to acquaint you that it is now out of my power to meet you at Whitby nor will it be convenient to return by way of Hull as I had resolved upon but three days ago M[rs] Cook being but a bad traveler I was prevailed upon to lay that rout aside on account of the reported badness of the roads and therefore took horse on Tuesday Morn[g] and road over to Whitby and returned yesterday. Your friends at that place expect to see you every day. I have only my self to blame for not having the pleasure of meeting you there. I am inform'd by letter from Lieut[t] Cooper that the Admiralty have altered the names of the Ships from Drake to Resolution and Raleigh to Adventurer [*sic*] which, in my opinion are much properer than the former. I set out for London to morrow morning, shall only stop a day or two at York'. Endorsed: 'from my freind Capt Cook the great Navigator'. Whitby Museum.[1]

8 January. *Victualling Board to Admiralty*. Mr Henry Pelham sends details of method of making beer at sea from the inspissated juice of malt, and his own experiments. He refers to the letter he addressed to the Admiralty under the signature of 'Marinus'.—ADM/DP/104.

8 January. *Victualling Board to Admiralty*. Samples of inspissated juice of malt have been received and Commissioners recommend preparation of a quantity for trial. Letter signed 'Marinus' is returned. Minuted: '15th January. To make a quantity of each for 200 men for 6 weeks, Lordships intending to have trial of it on Resolution and Adventure.' —ADM/DP/104; Adm 110/25.

13 January. *Admiralty Minutes*. No servants to be borne. Officers to be paid sums equal to wages of servants allowed them.—Adm 3/79.

13 January. *Admiralty to Cook and Furneaux*. Orders according to foregoing minute.—Adm 2/975; CLB.

[1] Presented to the Museum in 1951 by Mr R. Lionel Foster.

13 January. *Victualling Board Minutes.* To write Admiralty Secretary that Board had made some carrot marmalade, and send sample. Storsch writes that one spoonful mixed with water taken now and then will prevent scurvy, and even cure it if taken constantly; one tablespoonful usually taken to be ½oz, so that marmalade for 3 months for 200 men would amount to c. 90 gals.; 5 bushels carrots will produce gallon marmalade. Carrots are 4/6d bushel picked. How much of said marmalade are we to make?—Adm 111/69.

13 January. *Victualling Board to Admiralty.* A sample of marmalade of yellow carrots prepared in accordance with proposals of Baron Storsch is forwarded. Minuted: '17th January—Send copy of Storsch's letter and of this report to Commissioners for Sick and Hurt and desire them to have a proper quantity made for 200 men for 6 weeks to end that experiment may be made of its efficacy. Mr Marsh suggests to Stephens that it would be easier for S & H to prepare the quantity as they have suitable pans for making it in—the pans used for making Portable Soup.'—ADM/DP/104.

13 January. *Cook to Victualling Board.* The ships would take in the whole of the sour krout and salted cabbage prepared for them.—Dixson R.

14 January. **Cook to Sandwich.* Asking Sandwich's favour on behalf of Richard Hutchins.—Adm 1/1610.

14 January. *Admiralty to Navy Board.* Directing that officers of *Resolution* and *Adventure* be paid by bill allowances equal to the wages of the number of servants allowed them.—ADM/A/2651.

15 January. *Navy Board Minutes.* Orders to Clerk of Cheque at Woolwich and Deptford for allowance to officers of *Resolution* and *Adventure* to be paid by bill equal to wages of number of servants allowed them; able seamen to be entered in their room.—Adm 106/2586.

15 January. *Victualling Board Minutes.* Cook 13th desiring the cabbage and sour krout may be sent to *Resolution* and *Adventure* with Young's report thereon. Write Cook a mistake in ours of 20th past—sour krout in store being 89 barrels instead of 90: we have ordered 55 to be sent to *Resolution*, 34 to *Adventure*.—Adm/111/69.

15 January. *Victualling Board to Cook.* Letter in terms of foregoing minute. —CLB.

16 January. **Cook to Admiralty Secretary.* Acknowledges order of 13th inst., not to bear servants, able seamen to be entered in their room.—Adm 1/1610; CLB.

16 January. *Admiralty to Victualling Board.* To cause quantity of inspissated juice of malt, as recommended by Pelham, to be prepared for trial on *Resolution* and *Adventure*—sufficient for 200 men for 6 weeks, of the two kinds of juice, i.e. 1. Juice impregnated with the virtue of hops. 2. Juice impregnated with virtue of hops and fermented, in

order to avoid inconvenience of sending hops to sea and difficulty of always having yeast.—ADM/C/605; Adm 2/97.

20 January. **Cook to Navy Board.* 'Inclosed is an Account of the Additional Stores which I judge will or may be wanting for His Majestys Sloop the Resolution under my command in the Course of her intended Voyage, which I humbly submit to the consideration of your Board, and if approv'd, beg you will be pleased to give Orders for her to be supply'd therewith.—I earnestly request that the Seins may be both larger and of a superior quallity to those usualy supply'd the Navy, they being made of soft loose twine soon decay and have not Strength to hold large fish, which we too Sencibly experienced in my last Voyage; in short too great Attention cannot be had to the goodness of all the Fishing Geer as being Articles that may be of the utmost utillity to us.'—Adm 106/1208; CLB.

20 January. *Admiralty Minutes.* Baron Storsch's marmalade for 200 men for 6 weeks to be prepared. To be tried by *Resolution* and *Adventure.*—Adm 3/79.

20 January. *Admiralty to Sick and Hurt Board.* The Board is to make enough carrot marmalade for experiment by the *Resolution* and *Adventure.*—ADM/E/41.

20 January. *Victualling Board Minutes.* Admiralty order 16th January directs Victualling Board to have sufficient hopped and unhopped juice of malt to be made for 200 men for 6 weeks. The Board itself having no means of preparing this quantity, orders Mr. Jackson, an eminent chemist, to undertake it. Mr. Raymond, the Master Brewer, ordered to supply him wort and beer.—Adm 111/69.

22 January. **Cook to Navy Board.* Recommending Richard Rollett as sailmaker.—Adm 106/1208.

22 January. *Navy Board Minutes.* Rollett to be appointed sailmaker of *Resolution.* Acquaint Cook.—Adm 106/2586.

22 January. *Navy Board to Cook.* Appointing Richard Rollett as master-sailmaker.—CLB.

22 January. *Admiralty Secretary to Navy Board.* Forwarding for their advice Cook's letter requesting to be paid his wages for *Scorpion* sloop without passing any account. Cook's letter to be returned.—ADM/A/2650.

22 January. *Navy Board to Admiralty.* Have no objection to pay Cook's wages for *Scorpion* sloop, without passing an account.—ADM/B/186; Adm 106/2201.

23 January. *Admiralty Minutes.* Cook to be paid his wages for *Scorpion* without passing any account.—Adm 3/79.

23 January. *Admiralty to Navy Board.* Directing Navy Board to dispense with Cook's not passing an account for *Scorpion* and to cause him to be paid his wages for her.—ADM/A/2651.

24 January. *Navy Board to Cook.* Additional stores asked for would be supplied, with a few exceptions, specified.—CLB.

25 January. *Admiralty Secretary to Colonel Boisrond, Portsmouth.* To put Lieut. Edgcumbe of *Royal Oak* in orders for *Resolution.*—Adm 2/1166.

25 January. *Admiralty Secretary to Colonel Bell, Plymouth.* To order a recruit who plays bagpipes to hold himself in readiness to embark on one of ships fitting out for making discoveries.—Adm 2/1166.

25 January. *Admiralty Secretary to Colonel Bell, Plymouth.* To order a drummer who plays violin to hold himself in readiness to embark on one of ships fitting out for making discoveries.—Adm 2/1166.

25 January. *Board of Longitude Minutes.* Instructions read out to Wales and Bayly. Further instruments to be provided.—Royal Greenwich Observatory. Printed above, p. 722.

27 January. **Cook to Admiralty Secretary.*† 'The Complement of men to His Majestys Sloop Resolution being compleat, and more are coming daily to enter, some of whom, may be better then those already born; and as it will be necessary to have choise pick'd men, which I am of opinion may easy be got, was I impower'd to discharge such men, as upon trial are found any ways defective, and to enter others in their room.—If this method is approved of please to move my Lords Commissioners of the Admiralty to give orders accordingly; But if their Lordships are pleased to detain in the service, all the men I may, or can enter; an order to bear them on the Supernumerary List for Wages and Victuals untill they are turn'd over to some other of His Majestys Ships will answer every purpose.'—Adm 1/1610.

27 January. *Victualling Board Minutes.* The Board finds that *Resolution* and *Adventure* will want 2,700 gals. brandy in lieu of some of their beer; propose to Stephens obtaining it from Guernsey as amount in store is insufficient.—Adm 111/69.

27 January. *Victualling Board to Admiralty Secretary.* Proposing arrangements for purchase of 2,800 gals. French brandy from Guernsey.—Adm 111/25.

28 January. *Sick and Hurt Board to Admiralty Secretary.* In obedience to Admiralty order 20th inst. had prepared small quantity carrot marmalade (herewith send sample) and as it seems to be very well done would cause the quantity ordered for *Resolution* and *Adventure* to be prepared in like manner without loss of time.—Adm 98/10.

29 January. *Board of Longitude to Navy Board.* Board of Longitude appoint Mr William Wales and Mr William Baillie to go out in *Resolution* and *Adventure* to make nautical and astronomical observations, each to be allowed £400 per annum. Minuted: 'Imprest to be granted accordingly. Imprest 29th Jan. to Mr. Wales £150—To Baillie £150.'—ADM/A/2651.

29 January. *Cook to Ordnance Board.* Recommending Edmund Ireland as armourer, *Resolution.*—CLB.

30 January. *Admiralty Minutes.* Victualling Board to be allowed to send to Guernsey for 20 pipes of French brandy for *Resolution* and *Adventure.*—Adm 3/79.

31 January. *Admiralty to Victualling Board.* Gives approval to proposal that French brandy should be bought from Guernsey.—ADM/C/605.

31 January. *Admiralty Secretary to Cook.* Gives leave to discharge defective men.—CLB.

5 February. *Admiralty Secretary to Furneaux.* To recommend a carpenter in room of James Adcock who has obtained leave to resign.—Adm 2/731.

6 February. *Cook to Navy Board.* Reporting that Irving's ship's hearth was inferior to those in use in H.M. ships.—CLB.

6 February. **Cook to Sandwich.* 'My Lord / I beg leave to lay before your Lordship a Map of the Southern Hemisphere S[h]ewing the Discoveries that have been made up to 1770, to which is subjoined my opinion respecting the rout to be pursued by the Resolution and Adventure All which are humbly submited to Your Lordships consideration, by / My Lord / Your Lordships Most Obedient Humble Serv[t] / Jam[s] Cook'.—Mitchell Library, Safe PH 17/11. Map reproduced in *Charts and Views*, Chart XXV; subjoined opinion printed in I, cxiii–iv, and pp. xx–xxi above.

7 February. *Navy Board to Admiralty Secretary.* Report on trial of Irving's hearth, not equal to those in use. Enclosures: copies of letters from Officers of Deptford Yard and Cook.—ADM/B/186; Adm 106/2201.

7 February. *Admiralty Minutes.* Wm. Offord to be carpenter of *Adventure*; former resigning.—Adm 3/79. Warrant for Offord, ADM/A/2652.

8 February. *Royal Society, Minutes of Council.* Dr James Lind recommended to the Board of Longitude 'as a person who will be extreamly useful in the intended voyage for discoveries in remote parts; on account of his skill and experience in his profession, and from his great Knowledge in Mineralogy, Chemistry, Mechanics, and various branches of Natural Philosophy; and also from his having spent several years in different climates, in the Indies'.—R.S., Council Minutes, vol. VI, p. 131.

10 February. **Cook to Victualling Board.* Asks for water casks, i.e. 30 butts, 20 hogsheads, 10 puncheons. Minuted: '10th Let the Casks be sent and acquaint the Captain'.—Dixson R.

11 February. *Cook to Navy Board.* 'D[r] Knights Azimuth Compasses now in use are (I beleive) universally allowed to be defective at Sea, on acc[t] of their very quick Motion when the Ship is the least agitated, this

has caused Mr Gregory Compass maker in Leaden Hall Street, to add some very engenious contrivence to the Drs Compasses, which in my opinion will in part, if not Wholy, remedy the defect, & which I have heard asserted by Several Capt^ns of India Men, who have used them, as the assertaining the variation of the Compass in remote Parts of the world must be of use to Navigation, I pray you will be pleased to order His Majestys Sloop Resolution under my Command to be Supplyed with one of Mr Gregorys Azimuth Compass's of an improved construction.'—CLB.

11 February. *Navy Board Minutes. Adventure* and *Resolution* to be supplied with one of Mr Gregory's improved azimuth compasses. Acquaint Cook.—Adm 106/2586.

11 February. *Navy Board to Cook.* Authorising the supply of Gregory's improved azimuth compass.—CLB.

11 February. *Furneaux to Navy Board.* Recommending sailmaker. Minuted: 'appointed and Furneaux told.'—Adm 106/1208.

14 February. *Victualling Board to Cook.* No wine in store locally and not enough spirits to meet sloops' demands (wine 1000 gallons; brandy 2700 gallons). Will he take what is now available, or ship the whole quantity at Portsmouth?—CLB.

15 February. **Cook to Admiralty Secretary.*† 'Edward Terrel Seaman who Saild with me in the Endeavour Bark and now belongs to His Majistys Ship Barfleur, hath apply'd by letter to Sail with me again and his friends have likewise made application in his behalf, and as he is a young man on whose conduct I can rely I pray you will be pleased to move my Lords Commissioners of the Admiralty to order him to be discharged from the Ship in [*sic*] now belongs into His Majestys Sloop Resolution.'—Adm 1/1610; CLB, dated 14th.

19 February. **Cook to Victualling Board.* Thinks it advisable to take in the whole of the spirits and wine demanded at Portsmouth.—Nan Kivell coll.

20 February. *Admiralty to Cook.* He is to enter and bear two properly qualified carpenters in addition to present complement until further orders. —Adm 2/97.

20 February. *Admiralty to Furneaux.* To bear one carpenter.—Adm 2/97.

21 February. *Admiralty Secretary to Charles Irving.* Navy Board is of opinion that his fire hearth is not equal to those already in use.—Adm 2/731.

21 February. *Cook to Victualling Board.* Applies for beef, pork, suet, pease, wheat, sour krout, salted cabbage, common salt, oil.—CLB.

21 February. *Cook to Victualling Board.* Applies for twenty bushels of Bay salt.—CLB.

21 February. *_Cook to Victualling Board._ Asks for cooper's tools, and encloses a list in a clerk's hand headed 'Coopers Tools Necessary to be taken on a Long Voyage'.—Dixson R; CLB.

21 February. _Victualling Board to Admiralty Secretary._ No French brandy at Guernsey. Agent has sent samples of Spanish which seems good. Is Spanish to be bought, or wine supplied to _Resolution_ and _Adventure_ in lieu thereof?—Adm 110/25.

21 February. _Victualling Board to Cook._ Authorising the supply of more salt, also cooper's tools.—CLB.

24 February. _Admiralty Secretary to Victualling Board._ With reference to Victualling Board's letter of 21st inst., directions are sent to purchase the Spanish brandy for _Resolution_ and _Adventure._—ADM/C/605.

25 February. *_Cook to Admiralty Secretary._† 'Long Musquettoons, Swive[l]'d,[1] will be of infinate use on many occasions to His Majestys Sloops the Resolution and Adventure in the Course of their present intended Voyage, I beg you will be pleased to move my Lords Comiss^rs of the Admiralty to order the former to be Supply'd with Twelve and the latter with Eight and the Resolution to be supply'd the Armourers Tools mentioned in the Inclosed list—in addition to those already order'd.'—Adm 1/1610; CLB.

25 February. *_Cook to Navy Board._ 'I beg you will be pleased to order the great Cabbins of His Majestys Sloop Resolution under my Command to be fitted with Brass Furniture in stead of Iron, that she may be supply'd with a Top Lanthorn and Green Base in stead of Red.' Minuted: 'The Capt^ns Cabbin to be fitted with Brass Locks . . .'—Adm 106/1208.

25 February. _Navy Board to Cook._ Informing him of foregoing decision.—CLB.

27 February .*_Cook to Admiralty Secretary._† 'Men that are Masters of the two Professions of Ship-wright and Caulker, will be Very much wanting to His Majestys Sloops the Resolution and Adventure in the Course of their present intended Voyage, and as I find these men are not to be got without more than common incouragement, I beg you will be pleased to move my Lords Commissioners of the Admiralty to order two additional Carpenters Mates to the Resolution, and one to the Adventure, the pay of this Station will induce these Men to enter.'—Adm 1/1610; CLB.

27 February. _Admiralty Minutes._ According to Cook's request _Resolution_ to be supplied with 12 musquetoons, swivelled, _Adventure_ with 8 and also armourer's tools given in his list.—Adm 3/79.

[1] No doubt it was one of these that is referred to by Wales as fired at Tana, p. 852 above.

28 February. *Admiralty Minutes.* Two more carpenters' mates to be allowed to *Resolution*, one more to *Adventure.*—Adm 3/79.

28 February. *Admiralty Secretary to Navy Board.* Informs Navy Board of foregoing.—ADM/A/2652.

28 February. *Admiralty Secretary to Cook.* In answer to his request of 25th inst., *Resolution* and *Adventure* are to be supplied with 12 and 8 musquettoons respectively, and former with some armourer's tools.—Adm 2/731.

29 February. *Navy Board to Victualling Board.* Transmits orders about carpenters' mates. Minuted: '4th—Let notice be given to proper officers.' —ADM/C/605.

2 March. **Cook to Victualling Board.* Wants the remaining part of provisions demanded except beer, butter, cheese and spirit.—Dixson R.

2 March. **Cook to Navy Board.* Applies for two years' surgeon's necessaries. Minuted: 'Write to contractor to order the supply. Acquaint him.'—Adm 106/1208.

2 March. **Cook to Navy Board.* 'I am sorry I was not more explicit when I applyed for Brass Furniture to the Great Cabbins of His Majestys Sloop Resolution under my Command, for by your Answer I find you have been pleased to order Brass Locks to the Doors of the Great Cabbin only, whereas I meant to apply, not only for Locks, but Hinges, Turnbuckles and every other article that is usualy fitted with Iron, to be of Brass both to the Great Cabbin & Round House, in which manner I beg you will be pleased to order them to be fitted.' Minuted: 'Acq^{t} him we cannot comply with his request.'—Adm 106/1208.

3 March. *Cook to Navy Board.* Sending five pay lists.—Adm 106/1208.

3 March. *Navy Board to Cook.* Surgeon's necessaries will be hastened on board.—CLB.

3 March. *Navy Board to Cook.* Acquaints him that *Resolution* cannot be supplied with brass furniture he requested.—CLB.

4 March. *Victualling Board to Cook.* Four barrels of experimentally cured beef sent; to be reported on.—CLB.

7 March. *Board of Longitude Minutes.* Instructions for Wales and Bayly signed. Admiralty to be requested that the astronomers be received on board the ships.—Royal Greenwich Observatory. Printed above, p. 723; with the Instructions, pp. 724–8, from CLB.

9 March. **Cook to Victualling Board.* 'I think it will be necessary to examine every Cask of Beef and Pork after it is stow'd in its place, on board the Resolution under my Command, and to fill such up with Pickle as are found the least diff[i]cient and this to be repeated as often as the Casks can conveniently be come at, for which purpose I beg you will be pleased to ord[er] her to be Supply'd with Two Hogsheads of Strong Pickle.' Minuted: '9 Let the Pickle be sent and Acq^{t} him'.—Dixson R.

9 March. *_Cook to Victualling Board._ Wants bread in bags that had been demanded, and 80 puncheons additional of Sea Beer. Appends list of bread, beef, pork, pease, wheat flour needed. Minuted: '9 Let the Provisions &c[a] be sent.'—Dixson R.

[9 March].[1] *_Cook to Banks._ 'I received a Note from M[r] Marsh of the Victualing Office wherein he desires that we will call upon him on Friday Morn as he is obliged to Attend at the Admiralty on Thursday. I left a line at your House yesterday desireing to know your Sentiments concearning a Stove for the Cabbin, it being necessary the officers of Deptford Yard shou'd know how to act. If you approve of a Green Base floor Cloth for the great Cabbin I will demand as much Cloth from y[e] Yard as will make one. As you mean to furnish the Cabbin well I think you should have Brass Locks & Hinges to the Doors &c[a]: this however will be a private affair of your own as nothing of this kind is allow'd, the Round House will be fitted in this manner at my Expence.

'Thus far I had got with this letter when your note arrived, I think it a good thought to take M[r] Buzagios Stove with you as it may be very usefull on many Occasions. I shall go to Deptford to morrow to give directions about the other. Whenever it is certain that D[r] Lynd goes with us I beg you will let me know by the Penny Post. My Respects to the D[r] and am / Dear Sir / Your very humble Serv[t] / Jam[s] Cook. Monday Eving 6 o'Clock.'—Mitchell Library, _Banks Papers_, 'Voluntiers', pp. 331–2.

10 March. *_Cook to Admiralty Secretary._† 'When the Endeavour was fited out to go on her late Voyage, she was supply'd from the Sick and Hurt Office with a quantity of Rob of Oranges and Lemons, which we found of great use in preventing the Scurvey for laying hold of her crew. I therefore pray you will be pleased to move my Lords Commissioners of the Admiralty to order His Majestys Sloops the Resolution and Adventure to be supply'd with a quantity in proportion to what the Endeavour had.'—Adm 1/1610.

10 March. *_Cook to Navy Board._ 'The Surgeon of His Majestys Sloop Resolution under my command, having represented to me that the Currants and Almonds supplyed in his Necessarys are perishable articles and of little use to the Sick, and desires he may be supply'd with Sugar to the Value, in lieu thereof, I beg you will be pleased to order the Contractor to comply with his request.'—Adm 106/1208; CLB.

10 March. *_Cook to Navy Board._ 'Machines for Warping Ships in unfathomable depths, may be of great use to His Majestys Sloops Resolution and Adventure in the Course of their present intended Voyage; I beg you will be pleased to order each of them to be supply'd with two.

[1] The sole indication Cook gives of the date of this letter is his 'Monday evening'. It seems reasonable to date it 9 March, the first Monday after the Navy Board's letter of 3 March denying the brass furniture for the cabin.

The construction of these machines are very simple and known to Mr Cosway Master Atendant of Deptford Yard—Also Ice Anchors and Hatchets, such as used by Greenland Ships, may possibly be wanting on some Occasion, I think it would not be a miss for each of them to have two of each of these Articles.'—Adm 106/1208; CLB.

10 March. *Sick and Hurt Board to Admiralty.* In accordance with orders 20 January a quantity of marmalade of carrots has been prepared for 200 men for 6 months and it is ready to be disposed of. Minuted: '11th March. To be sent on Board R & A. Their Capt^s^ to issue it & report on efficacy.'—ADM/FP/15; Adm 99/47.

10 March. *Joseph Yorke to Lord* [*Rochford*].[1] He had been negotiating at the Hague for recommendatory orders for the *Resolution* and *Adventure* from the Dutch East India Company: as Lord Sandwich had signified that the ships would be ready to sail by the middle of the month, it would be idle to wait for the deliberations of the Chamber of Seventeen, and the Prince of Orange, as Governor and Director-General of the Company, had signed 'Ostensible Recommendations', and answered for the Chamber's acquiescence in renewal of orders of 1761. Document sent in duplicate, one for each ship.—CLB.

10 March. *William Prince of Orange and Nassau to all Governors and Ministers of the Dutch East India Company.* Order referred to in foregoing .—CLB.

11 March. *Navy Board Minutes.* Ask Cook to give description of warping machines. Write to contractor to supply *Resolution* with sugar instead of currants and almonds. Acquaint Cook.—Adm 106/2586.

11 March. *Navy Board to Cook.* Desires further information regarding machines for warping ships, and ice anchors and hatchets.—CLB.

11 March. *Admiralty Secretary to Sick and Hurt Board.* Cook has requested a supply of rob of oranges and lemons for *Resolution* and *Adventure.* Information is to be forwarded stating what supply of said rob is in store. —ADM/E/41.

11 March. *Navy Board to Cook.* Authorizing the supply of sugar in lieu of currants and almonds.—CLB.

11 March. *Victualling Board to Cook.* Authorizing the supply of Saloup.—CLB.

12 March. *Furneaux to Navy Board.* Asks for a supply of paper.—Adm 106/1208.

12 March. *Furneaux to Navy Board.* Desiring sugar in lieu of currants and almonds. Minuted: 'Write to contractor to supply sugar.' —Adm 106/1208.

[1] Sir Joseph Yorke was British ambassador at The Hague, 1761–80. There is no indication in the Letter Book of the person addressed, apart from 'My Lord'; but I presume it was Rochford, as secretary of state for the southern department.

12 March. *Admiralty Secretary to Cook.* A supply of Baron Storsch's marmalade of carrots will be sent to the ship; Cook to report at the end of the voyage as to its efficacy in the prevention of scurvy. Encloses a copy of Storsch's letter.—Adm 2/731; CLB.

12 March. *Admiralty Secretary to Furneaux.* Letter identical with foregoing.—Adm 2/731.

13 March. *Admiralty Secretary to Sick and Hurt Board.* Directions have been given for experiment with carrot marmalade in *Resolutiou* and *Adventure.*—ADM/E/41.

13 March. **Cook to Victualling Board.* 'Out of 240 Baggs of Bread sent on board the Resolution under my command we have only been able to take into the Bread room 201, the remaining 39 (which are return'd back to store) please to order to be Packed in Butts and sent on board again.' Minuted: 'NB Mr Collier had orders to do it the 12th . . .'—Dixson R.

13 March. **Cook to Navy Board.* 'I have been informed that, by your order, the Resolution under my Command was to have been supplyed with three Saines made of the same sort of twine as Salmon Netts usualy are, but that they could not be got in proper time. I beg leave to acquaint you that Saines of any length made of three threed twine (not inferior to salmon twine) can be got at the Shortest notice of James Davidson N° 27, Fish Street Hill.—I therefore humbly pray. you will be pleased to reconsider the great utillity these Saines will be of to us in the Course of the Voyage and order the Resolution to be Supplyed therewith.' Minuted: 'Mr Slade the Purveyor to purchase three Sein Netts for the Resolution one of 80 one of 70 & one of 60 fathom of the sort Capt Cook describes, and also two for the Adventure of 60 fathom each . . . Acq^t^ the Capt.'—Adm 106/1208.

13 March. *Navy Board Minutes.* Directions as to purchase of nets for *Resolution* and *Adventure.*—Adm 106/2586.

13 March. *Navy Board to Cook.* Authorising the supply of nets as requested.—CLB.

13 March. *Sick and Hurt Board to Admiralty Secretary.* In reply to letter of 11th inst., no robs of oranges and lemons in store; as *Endeavour*'s surgeon died on voyage received no information about the robs on *Endeavour* and no mention made of efficacy of robs in journal of surgeon's mate, but learnt in conversing with him and several others from *Endeavour* that the robs were useful. Quantity of same proportion cannot be supplied for *Resolution* and *Adventure* in less than fortnight.—Adm 98/10; Adm 99/47.

17 March. *Furneaux to Navy Board.* His cook has absented himself; desires another.—Adm 106/1208.

17 March. *Navy Board Minutes.* Write to contractor to supply sugar in lieu of currants and almonds to *Adventure.*—Adm 106/2586.

17 March. *Navy Board Minutes.* Cook's letter of this day. Orders to Deptford officers to cause machines, ice anchors and hatchets he mentions to be made under his inspection. Acquaint Cook and ask him to let us know upon what occasion the machine for warping is intended to be useful, in what instance he has seen it applied and with what success. —Adm 106/2586.

18 March. **Cook to Victualling Board.* 'Please to order .... Six firkings of Butter in addition to what she has been supply'd with .... P.S. Please to order me the usual compliment of Tongues'. Minuted: '18 Let the Butter, and Tongues, if Due, be sent, and acq^t him.'—'Tongues due D.'—Dixson R.

18 March. **Cook to Navy Board.* 'Mr Banks informs me that Dr Lynd goes out in His Majestys Sloop Resolution under my command, and at the same time desired me to apply to your Board to have another Standing Cabbin built for the D^r or one of his people, I therefore pray you will be pleased to order a Cabbin to be built on the lower Deck on the Starboard side abaft the Pump Deal.' Minuted: 'To be complied with give orders to Deptf^d Officers accordingly.'—Adm 106/1208.

19 March. *Royal Society, Minutes of Council.* Such astronomical instruments 'as are come back from the late expedition to the south'[1] to be sold by auction, except those lent to the Board of Longitude.—R.S., Council Minutes, vol. VI, p. 147.

19 March. *Admiralty to Sick and Hurt Board.* Instructions are given for rob of oranges and lemons to be put on *Resolution* and *Adventure* for trials of its efficacy. Report to be made on return of said sloops.—ADM/E/41; Adm 2/97.

19 March. *Admiralty Secretary to Cook.* In answer to his request 10th inst., Victualling Board to supply proper quantity of rob of oranges and lemons.—Adm 2/731; CLB.

20 March. *Sick and Hurt Board to Cook.* 3000 lb portable soup had been sent on board *Resolution* for use of the well men as well as the sick, to be issued when fresh provision could not be had; also quantity of marmalade of carrots.—Adm 99/47; CLB.

20 March. *Sick and Hurt Board to Furneaux.* Letter similar to foregoing; 2000 lb portable soup sent.—Adm 99/47.

20 March. *Victualling Board to Cook.* Directions had been given to agent in Portsmouth to issue 441 gallons of brandy and 600 gallons of wine, which with the 1059 gallons of spirits already drawn, made up the quantity requisitioned. Further supplies would be forthcoming if thought necessary.—CLB.

[1] i.e. the *Endeavour*'s expedition.

23 March. *Cook to Sick and Hurt Board.* Acknowledging letter of 20 March on supply of portable soup, etc.—Adm 97/86.

23 March. *Cook to Sick and Hurt Board.* Asking for order for *Resolution* to be supplied with elixir of vitriol, Dr James's powders,[1] copper pots, saucepans etc.—Adm 97/86.

23 March. *Admiralty Minutes.* Cook to be allowed £101 2s 0d for some extraordinary expenses in *Endeavour.*—Adm 3/79.

24 March. *Navy Board Minutes.* Furneaux's letter of 17th inst. Let another cook be supplied to *Adventure.* Acquaint Furneaux.—Adm 106/2586.

25 March. **Cook to Navy Board.* 'As His Majestys Sloop Adventure does not take out the yawl that was built for her at Woolwich, I beg you will be pleased to order His Majestys Sloop the Resolution under my command, to be supply'd with it in the room of the one intended for her at Deptford, as I think she will answer much better.' Minuted: 'To be complied with, give orders to each yard accordingly.'—Adm 106/1208.

25 March. *Cook to Navy Board.* Applies for an additional number of spare copper forelocks for pump chains. Minuted, Deptford Officers to supply him with as many as he should ask for.—Adm 106/1208.

25 March. *Admiralty Secretary to Cook.* Usual order to make remarks on coasts, etc.—Adm 2/731.

25 March. *Admiralty Secretary to Furneaux.* Similar letter to foregoing.—Adm 2/731.

30 March. *Furneaux to Sick and Hurt Board.* Requesting that *Adventure* may be supplied with Dr James's fever powders and elixir of vitriol.—Adm 97/86.

30 March. *Furneaux to Sick and Hurt Board.* Acknowledging theirs of 20th inst. on portable soup and marmalade of carrots, which directions he will comply with. Will keep carrot marmalade in his own charge.—Adm 97/86.

31 March. *Admiralty Secretary to Cook.* Is he willing to take Mr James Maxwell, midshipman H.M.S. *Rose,* who wishes to be transferred to the *Resolution*?—CLB.

[1] 'Dr James's Fever Powder' was exactly the sort of universal remedy a seaman would pick on. Dr Robert James (1705–76) made a great name, and an appropriate income, for himself by the invention of this powder, a mixture of antimony and phosphate of lime; certainly no other medicine before aspirin was ever swallowed so universally by the British, and none other was ever the subject of such hymns of praise from men generally rational. An up-to-date publicity after Cook's return would undoubtedly have capitalized on its use by him. The rights of sale were held by Newbery the bookseller, who comes otherwise into the Cook history (see pp. 961–2 below). There is a reproduction of one of Newbery's ornamental advertisements in *Johnson's England* (ed. A. S. Turberville, Oxford 1933), II, p. 144; and an amusing article by Bruce Dickins in *Life and Letters,* II (1929), pp. 36–47. See also the index to L. F. Powell's edition of Boswell's *Johnson* (1950) under 'James'.

31 March. *Furneaux to Navy Board.* Requests surgeon's necessaries for two years.—Adm 106/1208.

1 April. *Admiralty Secretary to President of College of Physicians.* Refers to him Priestley's proposal for rendering salt water fresh, by introduction of fixed air,[1] procured from chalk by means of diluted oil of vitriol.—Adm 2/546.

1 April. *Admiralty Secretary to Dr Priestley.* Asks him to attend the College of Physicians that they may examine the water distilled by his method from sea water.—Adm 2/731.

3 April. **Cook to Admiralty Secretary.* Is willing to receive James Maxwell as midshipman.—Adm 1/1610; CLB.

6 April. *Secretary of College of Physicians to Admiralty Secretary.* The College had examined Priestley's method of impregnating water with fixed air, was satisfied with the experiments, and would allow the method to be tried on His Majesty's ships.—CLB.

9 April. **Cook to Navy Board.* 'His Majestys Sloop Resolution under my command is so very full of Provisions & Stores that it will be impossible for me to allow any one Man, or set of Men, a single Chest to keep the few necessary Cloathing &c[a] they may have; I pray you will be pleased to order for this purpose, canvas bags to be made for each man, about a yard in length, and the Resolution to be supply'd therewith.' Minuted: 'To be supplied as desired'.—Adm 106/1208.

10 April. *Navy Board Minute. Resolution* to be supplied with canvas bags Cook requested. Acquaint him.—Adm 106/2586.

10 April. **Cook to Admiralty Secretary.* 'Agreeable to their Lordships order, I have purchased all the Articles intended to be sent out in the Resolution and Adventure (and which are now on board) amounting to Three hundred and Nine pounds One Shilling and Four pence, as will appear by the inclosed papers, which I pray you will be pleased to lay before their Lord Ships and move them to order me to be repaid.

'Accompt of Sundrys purchased by order of the Right Hon[ble] the Lords Commissioners of the Admiralty and put on Board the Resolution and Adventure—

			£		
To Shott of Dan[l] Gow as p[r] Bill			10..	3..	—
— Caps & Hatts of	Hen. Dekor	D[o]	6..	0..	—
— Ribbans	Jos. Vaux	D[o]	4..	17..	9
— Sundrys	Jn[o] Baker	D[o]	155..	19..	6
— Beads	Jn[o] Howard	D[o]	26..	5..	—
— Kettles & Wire	Geo. Pengree	D[o]	22..	15..	7
— Sundrys	W[m] Wilson		31..	10..	—

[1] 'Fixed air' was the gas now known as carbon dioxide, discovered by Joseph Black (1728–99), professor of chemistry at Glasgow and Edinburgh. Priestley's process was in principle the same as that which gives us soda-water.

		£		
— D° ———— Eliz. Batts ——— D° ———		43..	6..	—
— Steel ———— Jn° Berdoe ——— D° ———		3..	6..	—
— Grindstones &c^{a}—Coulson & Co.—D° ———		3..	5..	—
— Waterman for puting the Above on board —		1..	11..	6
		£309..	1..	4'

—Adm 1/1610.

10 April. *Sick and Hurt Board to Cook.* Surgeon of *Resolution* had been supplied with proper proportions of elixir of vitriol and Dr James's fever powders; also 24 pint bottles each of robs of oranges and lemons.—Adm 99/47; CLB.

10 April. *Sick and Hurt Board to Furneaux.* Similar letter to foregoing; 16 pint bottles each of robs.—Adm 99/47.

11 April. *Admiralty Minutes.* A list to be sent to Cook of hardware to be supplied by Mr Boulton of Birmingham as presents with which to win natives' friendship etc. Iron utensils, shot; Cook to supply jackets, trousers, ribbons, beads and other articles.—Adm 3/79.

11 April. *Admiralty Secretary to Cook.* 'It being judged necessary that the several things mentioned in the enclosed Account, should be provided & Sent on board the Resolution & Adventure in the proportions therein Mention'd, in order to be exchanged for Refreshments with the Natives of such New discovered or unfrequented Countries as they may touch at, or to be destributed to them in presents towards obtaining their friendship, & winning them over to our Interest, And their Lordships having directed Mr Boulton of Birmingham to pack up in proper Cases, & send to the Storekeeper at Deptford to be put on board the said Sloops the Several Articles Mark'd B in the said Account, I am commanded to acquaint you therewith, & it is their Lordships directions, that you provide the other Articles, and transmit me an account of the Cost thereof, that their Lordships may order the same to be paid.

			For the Resolution &	Adventure
B	Adzes	⎫	12	8
B	Axes	⎪ with Helves........	200	140
B	Broad Axes	⎪ in Bundles	24	16
B	Hatchets	⎭	300	200
B	Spike Nails		500 Weight	300 Weight
B	Nails 40 pence & upward		500 w^{t}	300 w^{t}
B	Chizzles		24	16
B	Saws		12 N	8
B	Coopers Augers		50	30
	Knives		20 Dozen	14 Dozen
	Scissars		6 Dozen	4 Dozen

B	Tweezors—broad	6 Dozen	4 Dozen
	Combs Small tooth	10 Dozen	6 Dozen
	D° Large	6 Dozen	4 Dozen
	Looking Glasses, wood frames	20 Dozen	14 Dozen
	Beads in Sorts	£15 worth	£10 worth
	Old Shirts not Patch'd	3 Dozen	2 Dozen
	Red Baize	200 Yards	140 Yards
	Old Cloaths	£5 worth	£3 worth
	Hatts	£6 worth	£4 worth
	Fine Old Sheets	20	12
	Kettles or Potts	24	16
B	Hammers NB with Helves	24	16
	Grindstones	12	8
	Whetstones	6 Dozen	4 Dozen
	Steel	100 wt	60 wt
Wyer, Brass & Iron		100 wt	60 wt

One thousand Pound weight of small Shot & 30 dozen Yards of Ribbond to be destributed between the two Sloops Jackets & Trousers of fearnought made up one for Each Man

Obs. The Articles Mark'd B in the Margin Mr Boulton of Birmingham will Supply, & send in Proper package to the Storekeeper of Deptford Yard to be put on board the Resolution & Adventure.'
—Adm 2/731; CLB.

13 April. **Cook to Admiralty Secretary.*† 'The Commissioners of the Victualing were pleased to inform me some time ago, that His Majestys Sloops Resolution and Adventure were to call at Spithead to compleat their proportion of Spirit and Wine.—I beg leave to acquaint you that they are already so full of Provisions, Stores &ca that it will be next to impossible for them to take in any more Spirit, and that they have Sufficient of this article to last untill oppertunity offers to take in more when they will have room to stow it away; and as they can be supply'd with Port Wine at Plymouth, I am humbly of opinion that the touching at spithead will be attended with Loss of time, and that it will be more adviseable, and attended with less delay, for them to call at Plymouth, to take in their Wine, Party of Marines and to be paid two Months Pay advance.'—Adm 1/1610.

13 April. **Cook to Admiralty Secretary.* Requesting to be paid £309 1s 4d for articles he had purchased for *Resolution* and *Adventure.*—Adm 1/1610.

13 April. *Admiralty to Navy Board.* Cook to be repaid £309 1s 4d mentioned in foregoing. ADM/A/2654.

13 April. *Admiralty Secretary to Cook.* Is ordered to be repaid £309 1s 4d.—Adm 2/731.

13 April. *Admiralty Secretary to Cook.* A supply of instruments had been sent for Mr Wales's use; to be stowed in a proper manner and place.—CLB.

15 April. *Admiralty Secretary to Cook.* Covering note enclosing inventory of goods sent by Mr Boulton, Birmingham, for exchange with native peoples.—Adm 2/731; CLB.

16 April. *Admiralty to Navy Board.* Messrs Boulton and Fothergill of Birmingham to be paid £80 14s 3d for articles provided for *Resolution* and *Adventure*, and further £50 for making a die and striking off 2,000 medals to be distributed to natives of such new discovered countries as the sloops may touch at.—ADM/A/2654.

20 April. *Victualling Board Minutes.* 140 butts and 20 puncheons of water, which will be wanted for *Resolution*, to be got ready to ship when captain may demand.—Adm 111/69.

21 April. **Cook to Navy Board.* 'Having examined the Carpenters Crew of His Majestys Sloop Resolution under my command and find them in a manner wholy without caulking Tools, and as there will be a great deal of Caulking on board the Sloop which must be perform'd wholy by her crew, I pray you will be pleased to order her to be supply'd with the under mentioned Tools'. List of nine different sorts of tools appended. Minuted: 'Woolwich Officers to supply them.'—Adm 106/1208.

21 April. *Navy Board Minutes. Resolution* to be supplied with caulking tools requested by Cook. Acquaint him.—Adm 106/2586.

22 April. **Cook to Admiralty Secretary.*† 'Please to acquaint my Lords Commissioners of the Admiralty with the arrival of His Majestys Sloop Resolution under my command at Long Reach, in order to take in her Guns and other Ordnance Stores, which could not be done in Gallions Reach, there not being there a sufficient depth of Water for the Sloop to lay with safety'.—Adm 1/1610.

22 April. *Admiralty Secretary to Cook.* Admiralty had been notified of ship's arrival at Longreach in order to take in her ordnance stores.—CLB.

23 April. *Admiralty Secretary to Cook.* Ordering the master and lieutenants of *Resolution* to include a current number of the *Nautical Almanac* and *Astronomical Ephemeris* with their books of navigation, and to continue taking succeeding numbers.—Adm 2/97; CLB.

23 April. *Admiralty Secretary to Furneaux.* Similar letter to foregoing.—Adm 2/97.

23 April. *Admiralty Minutes.* College of Physicians having reported that no noxious qualities are communicated to water by Dr Priestley's method, captains of *Resolution* and *Adventure* are to give it trial.—Adm 3/79.

23 April. *Admiralty to Cook.* Order to experiment with water impregnated

with fixed air on Priestley's method, and to report on it as an antiscorbutic.—Adm 2/97; CLB.

23 April. *Admiralty to Furneaux.* Similar order to foregoing.—Adm 2/97.

24 April. *Admiralty Secretary to Furneaux.* To fall down to Longreach.—Adm 2/731.

24 April. *Admiralty Secretary to Marine Officer Commanding Portsmouth.* To order Edgcumbe not to fail to embark in *Resolution* at Longreach by Wednesday next.—Adm 2/1166.

27 April. **Cook to Admiralty Secretary.*† 'The party of Marines, which I understand are ordered immediately on Board his Majestys Sloop Resolution under my command, will increase the number of her crew above the established Complement, which is already nearly compleat; to discharge seamen in the River may be the means, not only of the Sloop leaving England Short of Complement, but not being man'd with such able Seamen as might be wished: I therefore pray you will be pleased to move my Lords Commissioners of the Admiralty to order the overplus men to be born on the Supernumerary List untill th[e]re is an oppertunity to discharge them into some of His Majestys Ships at one of the out Ports, after first compleating the two Sloops complements therefrom.'—Adm 1/1610.

27 April. **Cook to Admiralty Secretary.* Acknowledges orders of 23 April on *Nautical Almanacs* and Priestley's method of impregnating water with fixed air.—Adm 1/1610; CLB.

28 April. *Admiralty Secretary to Priestley.* Desires him to communicate his method of improving water used at sea to commanders of *Resolution* and *Adventure*, and to furnish their surgeons with instructions, especially the process of impregnating sea water with fixed air.—Adm 2/731.

30 April. **Cook to Admiralty Secretary.*† 'Before I sail'd from England in the year 1768 on my late Voyage, my Lords Commissioners of the Admiralty were pleased to allow me a Set of Mathematical Instruments in order to make Surveys, Observations &c[a]: the same Instruments being much in use in the course of that Voyage, received considerable damage, which I have caused to be repaired and put on board the Resolution; I have likewise provided my self with a proper quantity of Stationary, which with the Instruments amounts to Thirty nine pounds Seven Shillings & four pence as will appear by the inclosed Vouchers, which I pray you will be pleased to lay before their Lordships & move them to order me to be repaid.'—Adm 1/1610.

2 May. *Admiralty Secretary to Victualling Board.* The inspissated juice of malt, prepared in accordance with instructions of 16 January last, to be sent on board *Resolution* and *Adventure*, $\frac{3}{5}$ to former, $\frac{2}{5}$ to latter, with instructions to commanders for making proper experiments of its

efficacy. 'P.S. These sloops will have their sailing orders on Monday or Tuesday next'.—ADM/C/606; Adm 2/546.

2 May. *Admiralty Secretary to Cook and to Furneaux.* To make experiments of the inspissated juice of malt and to report thereon.—Adm 2/731.

4 May. *Victualling Board Minutes.* Write Stephens on inspissated juices of malt; appears that by being evaporated in coppers that were much deeper than they would have been had they been made expressly for purpose they have by their long continuance over the fire acquired a deep colour and taste somewhat empyreaumatick or burnt; but upon being mixed with water they ferment very well, yield good small beer differing only in colour, tastes rather like beer made with treacle. As no time to prepare juice more perfectly in proper shallow vessels, have ordered the barrels to be sent on *Resolution* and *Adventure*, and have sent instructions to captains, and have observed that if because of their colour and taste they are too disliked to be used, at least it will be possible to see how they keep in different climates. Write Furneaux and Cook accordingly.—Adm 111/69.

4 May. *Victualling Board to Cook.* Inspissated juice of malt sent, and Dr Hales's recipe for making fresh yeast; Cook to report on both at end of voyage.—CLB.

4 May. *Admiralty to Furneaux.* To proceed to Downs and there await further orders.—Adm 2/97.

4 May. *Admiralty Order to Cook.* In reply to Cook's letter of 27th April about marines: Cook is to bear his overplus men on a supernumerary list for wages and victuals till his arrival at Plymouth, there dispose of them as Rear-admiral Spry shall direct.—Adm 2/97; CLB.

4 May. *Admiralty Secretary to Cook.* As Cook wishes to be absent a few days longer, he is to order his 1st lieutenant to proceed to Downs with sloop, there to remain till further orders.—Adm 2/97; CLB.

5 May. *Admiralty Secretary to Cook.* To give Francis Mason, a gardener sent out by the king, a passage to Cape of Good Hope.[1]—Adm 2/97; CLB.

6 May. *Victualling Board Minutes.* Write Stephens that barrels of inspissated juice of malt contained but little more than one quarter of quantity which Admiralty ordered to be prepared 16th January. Also submit that beer made thereof should be issued accordingly to discretion of the commanders without any abatement being made in men's usual allowance of beer, wine or spirits.—Adm 111/69.

6 May. *Victualling Board to Admiralty Secretary.* Letter in terms of foregoing minute.—Adm 110/25.

[1] Francis Masson (1741–1805), rather inadequately described as 'a gardener', was one of the great botanical collectors of the eighteenth century, and the first sent out from Kew. He returned after three years greatly successful. He made two other botanical journeys from the Cape into the interior, the last again of great scientific importance.

6 May. **Cook to Admiralty Secretary.* Acknowledges order 4th May, lieutenant to proceed with *Resolution* to Downs.—Adm 1/1610.

7 May. **Cook to Navy Board.* 'Judgeing that His Majestys Sloop Resolution under my command was too deep in the Water, I caused 20 Tons of Iron Ballast to be taken out of her sence she arrived at Long reach; if upon tryal it should be found necessary to replace it, I pray you will be pleased to lodge an order at Plymouth for her to be supply'd therewith.' Minuted: 'Give orders to Plymouth to supply what Iron Ballast the Captain may demand'.—Adm 106/1208.

8 May. *Admiralty Minutes.* Navy Board to pay £39 7s 4d for repair of Cook's mathematical instruments used in *Endeavour*, and for stationery for intended voyage.—Adm 3/79.

8 May. *Victualling Board Minutes.* Cook's letter of 7th that *Resolution* and *Adventure* are to go to Plymouth immediately; and request that there they may be supplied with as much wine as they can conveniently stow, and fresh meat every meat day during their stay there. Write him that Agent has been so instructed. Write Agent accordingly.—Adm 111/69.

8 May. *Victualling Board to Cook.* Authorising a supply of wine and fresh meat whilst ship is at Plymouth.—CLB.

8 May. *Navy Board Minutes.* Plymouth officers to supply what iron ballast Captain requires. Acquaint Cook.—Adm 106/2586.

8 May. *Navy Board to Cook.* Authorising a supply of ballast at Plymouth.—CLB.

9 May. *Admiralty to Navy Board.* Payment to be made to officers and men of *Resolution* and *Adventure* in advance, 6 months' wages, so that they can make provision for their families.—ADM/A/2655; CLB.

9 May. *Admiralty Secretary to Cook.* To apply to Captain Collier, Nore, for and embark two marines with bagpipes on board *Resolution* and *Adventure* and to discharge to headquarters at Chatham two marines to make room for them.—Adm 2/1166; CLB.

9 May. *Admiralty Secretary to Cook.* To make out paylists for six months for his company that they may be paid at Plymouth. Two months' advance are ordered to his men.—Adm 2/731; CLB.

9 May. *Admiralty Secretary to Furneaux.* Similar letter to foregoing.—Adm 2/731.

9 May. *H. Pelham, Secretary to Victualling Board, to Cook.* Detailed letter on experiments in making beer at sea.—CLB.

11 May. *Furneaux to Navy Board.* Monthly books sent.—Adm 106/1208.

11 May. *Admiralty to Furneaux.* To proceed to Plymouth Sound. Await there further orders.—Adm 2/97.

11 May. *Admiralty Secretary to Victualling Board.* It is agreed that beer made

from juice of malt may be issued on the orders of commanders without any abatement being made in the men's allowances of beer, wine or spirits.—ADM/C/606; Adm 2/546.

11 May. *Admiralty Secretary to Cook.* Beer made from inspissated juice of malt to be issued without any abatement in men's issue of wine, spirits and beer.—Adm 2/731.

11 May. *Admiralty Secretary to Furneaux.* Similar letter to foregoing.—Adm 2/731.

12 May. *Cook to Navy Board.* Paybooks sent.—Adm 106/1208.

12 May. *Admiralty Minutes.* Furneaux is unable to procure two carpenter's mates. Commissioners at Plymouth to be ordered to let him have any two shipwrights out of the yard who are willing to go and if none offer to discharge two from the guardships into the sloop.—Adm 3/79.

12 May. *Navy Board Minutes.* Orders for payment to companies of *Resolution* and *Adventure* of six months' wages at Plymouth, also two months' wages in advance. Officers not to pass accounts at present, but accounts for whole time are to be passed before they receive any further pay. Pay books will be sent away to-night.—Adm 106/2586.

13 May. *Admiralty Secretary to Cook.* Enclosing letters from Priestley explaining directions for his process.—Adm 2/731; CLB.

13 May. *Admiralty Secretary to Furneaux.* Similar letter to foregoing.—Adm 2/731.

13 May. *Admiralty Secretary to Priestley.* His account of process for improving water used at sea has been sent to the commanders of *Resolution* and *Adventure*.—Adm 2/731.

14 May. *Board of Longitude to Navy Board.* Board of Longitude assigns rewards as follows: To Mr Larcum Kendall of Furnival's Inn Court, watchmaker, for a new watch machine constructed by him in consequence of Board's orders, wherein some of the expensive parts of that made by Mr John Harrison for the discovery of longitude at sea have been left out, and other alterations made in order to reduce the price and so bring such watch machines within general use—£200. Mr Wales and Mr Bayly £100, to fit themselves for their voyage, by way of imprest.—ADM/A/2655.

14 May. *Admiralty Secretary to Navy Board.* Captain Cook has forwarded a letter from his first lieutenant and written himself about the unsafe state of the *Resolution*. Suggests improvements.—ADM/A/2655.

Enclosures (1) *Cooper to Cook.* 'Resolution in Hole Reach Wednesday afternoon 13th May, 1772. / I take this opportunity of informing you of our leaving Gravesend this morning with a moderate breeze with the wind from ENE to ESE and in working down the River, find the ship so exceedingly crank that though the light colliers working down the river, some with top gallant sails and *all* their whole topsails and staysails when we could not with safety (though the wind was steady and without flurries) carry our single Reeft Topsails with the Jib and main topmast staysails: the two latter we was obliged to haul down, the ship frequently fell down within 3 streaks of the port cills, at the same time the ship not at all under command, with great difficulty and attention able to get her about. The Pilot desires me to inform you that he cannot think of taking her further than the Nore with security to the ship or without hazarding his reputation in the attempt, unless with a fair wind. I thought it my duty to give you the earliest notice of our situation. I beg leave to offer you my own private opinion and to assure you that I think her an exceeding dangerous and unsafe ship. However, in the morning we shall proceed in our way for the Nore when I shall write to you again and enclose you a letter to the Admiralty for your perusal with my further sentiments as to the qualification of the ship. At present being in great haste'.

(2) *Cook to Stephens.* '14th May 1772 / This morning I received the enclosed letter from Lieut. Cooper informing me that the ship is so exceeding crank that he thinks it unsafe to proceed with her any further than the Nore.—I beg leave to offer it as my opinion that she is too deep in the water to carry sail, being loaded below her bearings, and that by cutting down part of her upper works, shorting her masts and exchanging her guns from 6 to 4 pounders would lighten her to a proper depth of water and make her very fit to proceed on the voyage'. Minuted: '14th May—Send them to Navy Board and direct them to take the same into their most serious consideration and to report to their Lords as soon as possible what they consider may be proper to be done to her at Sheerness to enable her to prosecute her present intended voyage.'—ADM/A/2655.

14 May. *Admiralty Minutes. Resolution* to proceed to Sheerness, to remain there till further orders.—Adm 3/79.

14 May. *Admiralty to Cook.* Notwithstanding former orders, to go to Sheerness and remain till further orders.—Adm 2/97; CLB.

14 May. *Board of Longitude Minutes.* Instructions for the safe custody of the chronometers.—Royal Greenwich Observatory. Printed above, pp. 723–4.

15 May. *Clerke to Banks.*† 'Resolution in Sea Reach / Sir / The Interest you must necessarily have in matters I now trouble you with, flatter myself will render any kind of apology unnecessary so will proceed without farther preface. We weigh'd anchor at Graves-End this morning about 10 O'clock, with a fine Breeze from the Eastward, the wind from that quarter, laid us under the necessity of working down the Reaches which work, I'm sorry to tell you, we found the Resolution very unequal to; for whilst several light Colliers were working down with

their whole Topsails, Staysails &c. one small Brig in particular with her Top Gallant Sails; these Light Vessels so upright, that a Marble wou'd hardly rowl from Windward to Leeward, the Resolution I give you my honour, under her reeft Topsails, Jibb & Main Top Mast Staysail, heel'd within three Streaks of her Gun Ports. She is so very bad, that the Pilot declares, he will not run the risk of his Character so far, as to take charge of her, farther than the Nore without a fair Wind, that he cannot with safety to himself attempt working her to the Downs. Hope you know me too well, to impute my giving this intelligence to any ridiculous apprehensions for myself, by God I'll go to Sea in a Grog Tub if desir'd, or in the Resolution as soon as you please; but must say, I do think her by far the most unsafe Ship, I ever saw or heard of: however, if you think proper to embark for the South Pole in a Ship, which a Pilot, (who I think is, by no means a timorous man) will not undertake to carry down the River; all I can say, is, that you shall be most chearfully attended, so long as we can keep her above Water by / Sir / Your Much Oblig'd & H'ble Serv[t] / Cha[s] Clerke'.—Mitchell Library, *Banks Papers*, 2, f. 1.

15 May. *Navy Board to Admiralty.* There is much concern at news of *Raleigh* proving so crank, as she has a very promising body and good dimensions and did well as a merchant ship. The trouble must be attributed to the accommodation for passengers and the quantity of heavy stowage. It is proposed that she should be ordered to Sheerness and alterations made in her and the guns altered from 6 pounders to 4 pounders. Minuted: '15th May—Direct them to do as they have proposed and to consider whether the shortening of the masts may not also be an advantage to her.'—ADM/B/186; Adm 106/2201.

15 May. *Admiralty to Navy Board.* In reply to Navy Board's letter of 15th May, it has been decided that the alterations proposed should be undertaken with all dispatch. The shortening of her masts will also be considered.—ADM/A/2655.

15 May *Admiralty Minutes. Resolution* to proceed to Sheerness to have her round house removed and alterations made to decks in order to correct excessive crankness.—Adm 3/79.

15 May. *Navy Board to Cook.* Ordering the pilot employed in carrying *Resolution* from Longreach to the Nore to report to Navy Office.—CLB.

16 May. *Admiralty Secretary to Navy Board.* Information being received from the Nore List that the *Resolution* is sailed from thence, their Lordships have sent orders to the Downs to her commander to proceed either to Sheerness or Portsmouth for the alterations which are proposed.—ADM/1/2655.

16 May. *Admiralty Secretary to Cook or Commanding Officer of Resolution.* To proceed either to Sheerness or Portsmouth for alterations to ship.—

In margin: 'Returned and cancelled the ship having put back to the Nore'.—Adm 2/731.

16 May. *Admiralty Secretary to Furneaux.* He is to give an account of behaviour of ship in passage from Longreach to Downs and thence to Plymouth.—Adm 2/731.

16 May. *Admiralty Secretary to Navy Board.* Orders the fitting of Irving's apparatus for rendering salt water fresh to be fitted in *Resolution* and *Adventure* and spare tubes for apparatus to be supplied. Minuted: 'Write to Stephens the Brazier immediately to provide spare tubes for these sloops and to send them to Deptford Direct Deptford Officers to send them to Sheerness and Sheerness Officers to put them all on board Resolution that those for Adventure may be delivered on board her when they meet.'—ADM/A/2655; Adm 2/546.

19 May. **Cook to Admiralty Secretary.*† 'In concequence of Lieut[t] Cooper representing to me that the Resolution Sloop under my command was found, upon tryal, to be so Crank that she would not bear proper sail to be set upon her; I gave it as my opinion that it was owing to the additional works that have been built upon her in order to make large accomodations for the Several Gentlemen Passengers intended to embark in her, and proposed that she might be cut down to her original state, which proposeal I laid before you in my letter of the 14th Inst and likewise attended the Navy Board who were pleased to inform me of the alteration they proposed to make—which alteration, I am of opinion will render her as fit to perform the Voyage as any Ship whatever. I understand that it has been suggested, that I never thought her, or these kind of Vessels proper for the service she is going upon: I beg you will acquaint their Lordships that I do now, and ever did think her the most proper Ship for this service I ever saw, and that from the knowlidge and experience I have had of these sort of Vessels I shall always be of opinion that only such are proper to be sent on Discoveries to very distant parts.'—Adm 1/1610; CLB.

19 May. *Navy Board Memorandum.* 'Navy Office . . . / William Appleby Pilot of the Resolution Sloop attending was call'd in and discours'd on the qualities of the said Sloop. He acquainted the Board that he took charge of her at Deptford and Piloted her to the Warp below Sheerness. That she is very crank owing to her being over built with the additional Works raised on her. That he is well acquainted with these kind of Ships having served his time in them, and been Mate and Master of several of them, and that they are of a built for burthen and stowage. That he is of opinion if the additions were taken away, she will be as good as any Ship of that kind. That he never heard of her being esteemed Crank when a Merchant Ship or could say any thing to that effect having never seen or known the Ship before.' Copy in Windsor Castle Library, Georgian Papers No.; 1316 attached to Cook's letter of same date. Not in the Navy Board Minutes in P.R.O.

19 May. *Navy Board Minutes.* Deptford Officers to let us know tomorrow by messenger whether both the coppers of the *Resolution* and *Adventure* are completely fitted with Irving's apparatus. If not, what has prevented it? Cook representing that part of bread on *Resolution* is very mouldy, Sheerness Officers are to examine into state of bread and report thereon. Direct Master Shipwright at Deptford to attend us to-morrow to tell us in what manner and with what stuff the bread was laid.—Adm 106/2586.

20 May. *Admiralty Secretary to Cook.* Admiralty had received notification of the arrival of *Resolution* at Sheerness.—CLB.

20 May. *Navy Board to Admiralty.* In return to letter of 16th ordering the fitting of Irving's apparatus to *Resolution* and *Adventure.* Said apparatus was ordered 5 November last, and sent to store at Deptford, but not fixed for want of someone to do so. Irving had been asked to instruct how to do this in *Adventure,* and there would be the same trouble with *Resolution.* Spare tubes would be ordered as requested. Minuted: '27th May—Send copy to Irving and desire him to give the necessary instructions for fitting his apparatus.'—ADM/B/186; Adm 106/2201.

20 May. *Admiralty to Navy Board.* Directions that such accommodation is to be made on *Resolution* for the captain, officers and passengers as may be proper, and is consistent with the alterations ordered on 15th inst. —ADM/A/2655.

21 May. **Cook to Admiralty Secretary.*† 'Please to acquaint their Lordships with my repairing to His Majestys Sloop Resolution under my Command yesterday, that the intended alterations go on with great alertness, and that I shall not only forward them but take every other step to put the Ship in a condition to put [to] Sea with all Possible expadition—I beg leave also to acquaint you, that sence the Ship came along side the Jetty, a stranger came into the yard who knew her in the Merchant Service, he with great confidence, and some warmth, asserted that at that time she, not only was a stiff Ship, but had as many other good quallities as any Ship ever built in Whitby, this tends to refute some false suggestions that have been thrown out against her. I can only assure you that there does not remain the least doubt but what she will a[n]swer every wish'd for purpose & am' etc.—Adm 1/1610; CLB.

21 May. **Cook to Navy Board.* 'Having with the officers of this yard, considered the dimentions of the Masts and yards of His Majestys Sloop Resolution under my Command, am of opinion that the lower Masts will bear to be shortend about two feet, but think it will not be necessary to reduce them in thickness, the yards will have sufficient strength if they are reduced to the same thickness her origional yards were, I pray you will take the same into consideration and give orders accordingly. It may not at this time be amiss to inform you that a Man

has been in this yard sence the Ship was here, who knew her in the Merchant service, he confidently asserted that she was a Stiff Ship before we got her, and seem'd much displeased at the report that had been raised against her, this was before I came down so that I had no opertunity to see him.' Minuted: 'Send a Copy to the Admiralty . . . Give orders accordingly.'—Adm 106/1208; CLB.

21 May. *Admiralty Secretary to Cook.* Acknowledging Cook's of 19 May.—Adm 2/731; CLB.

21 May. *Admiralty Secretary to Cook.* Acknowledging Cook's of 21 May.—Adm 2/731.

21 May. *Cook to Victualling Board.* Reporting bread supply to be found damp and mouldy due to the greenness of the wood lining of the bread store. Suggests a new supply of fresh bread to be issued in lieu.—CLB.

22 May. *Navy Board to Admiralty.* Further to their Lordships' of 15th inst., asking for a report on the shortening of masts in *Resolution*, a copy of letter from Cook is forwarded. Officers at Sheerness have been instructed accordingly. It is hoped that this will be approved. Copy of letter from Cook, Sheerness 21 May enclosed.—ADM/B/186; Adm 106/2201.

22 May. *Navy Board to Admiralty.* In accordance with directions in order of 20th inst., a plan has been prepared of *Resolution* with the best accommodation that can be contrived for captain, officers and passengers. The accommodation on *Endeavour* when she was fitted for like voyage is shown in red. Minuted: '28th May—Mr Banks does not go in her and that therefore only to make accommodation for Captain and Officers and astronomer. Plan is enclosed.'—ADM/B/186; Adm 106/2201.

22 May. *Navy Board to Cook.* Authorising the shortening of the lower masts and the reduction of the yards on the *Resolution* by two feet.—CLB.

22 May. *Victualling Board Minute.* Captain Cook 21st. Let 130 empty bisket bags be forthwith sent to sloop to bring up her bread. Write Cook that we shall send him other bread in lieu when he acquaints us that sloop is ready to receive it.—Adm 111/69.

23 May. *Admiralty Secretary to Cook.* Telling him that information in his letter of 21 May had been passed to Lords of Admiralty.—CLB.

24 May. *Cook to Navy Board.* 'As it will be necessary to take out of His Majesty's Sloop Resolution, under my Command, such Boatswain, & Carpenters Stores, as we can best spare I pray you will give orders that they may be received into Store at this Place, & also that She may be supply'd with about fifteen tons of Iron ballast, some Hammacoes, Boats oars, & some other trifling Articles I find we are Short of'. Minuted: 'Give orders accordingly'.—Adm 106/1208; CLB.

24 May. *Cook to Ordnance Officer, Sheerness.* Requesting him to receive surplus ordnance stores.—CLB.

24 May. **Cook to Admiralty Secretary.*† 'Sence I have been down here, I have been inform'd that a report prevails in Town that the Crew of His Majestys Sloop Resolution under my command, are so terrified with her former cranckness that they are afraid to stay in her; I pray you will be pleased to acquaint their Lordships that I do not find this report has any foundation in truth, and that altho the Sloop has been along side the Jetty head sence she put in here, where the people can go on Shore at pleasure not one man has left her.'—Adm 1/1610.

26 May. **Cook to Navy Board.* 'You have been pleased to order the Masts of His Majestys Sloop Resolution under my command to be Shorten'd, please to order her Sails to be made agreeable thereto.' Minuted: 'Give orders accordingly'.—Adm 106/1208; CLB.

26 May. *Navy Board Minutes.* Orders to Sheerness Officers to supply iron ballast and other stores to Cook.—Adm 106/2586.

26 May. *Navy Board to Cook.* Ordnance Officers, Sheerness, had been instructed to receive surplus boatswain's and carpenter's stores and authorised to supply fifteen tons of iron ballast.—CLB.

26 May. **Cook to Victualling Board.* Bread room would be ready in two days; please to order down 21,280 pounds to replace what had been taken out. Minuted: '. . . And care is to be taken in Shiping and sending the same down that no wet or damp may come thereto.'—Dixson R; CLB.

27 May. *Admiralty Secretary to Navy Board.* Having received Navy Board letter of 22nd inst., with enclosure from Cook proposing the lower masts of *Resolution* should be shortened 2 feet and the yards to be reduced to same thickness her original yards were, their Lordships direct this to be done.—ADM/A/2655; Adm 2/546.

27 May. *Navy Board Minutes.* Orders to Sheerness Officers to shorten masts and make sails agreeable to Cook's letter of 26 May.—Adm 106/2586.

27 May. *Navy Board to Cook.* Authorising the alteration of the sails, as requested.—CLB.

27 May. *Victualling Board to Cook.* Reporting that a fresh supply of bread was being sent to the *Resolution* forthwith.—CLB.

27 May. *Admiralty Secretary to Irving.* Desires him to instruct in the fitting of his apparatus for rendering sea water fresh on board *Resolution* and *Adventure*.—Adm 2/731.

28 May. *Admiralty Secretary to Navy Board.* With reference to letter from Navy Board with plan of *Resolution* of 22nd inst., Banks has this day informed their Lordships that he does not intend to proceed in *Resolution* on her present voyage, accommodation therefore has to be prepared only for captain, officers and the astronomer who is to proceed at request of Board of Longitude.—ADM/A/2655; Adm 2/546.

28 May. **Cook to Navy Board.* 'Inclosed is an account of all the Stores I can think of that are wanting for His Majestys Sloop Resolution under my command, Iron Ballast excepted.—The smallest anchors we have on board are much too heavy for the Boat in frame, and as here are several small old ones in Store, I will, with your approbation, take two on board. The Masts are shorten'd and we wait for orders to fit the sails thereto.' List appended of boatswain's and carpenter's stores: brooms, boat sail, small anchors, oars, log and deep sea lines, boats' mast and yards. Minuted: 'Direct Sheerness Officers to supply these particulars . . .'—Adm 106/1208.

The copy of this letter in CLB has some marked differences, the principal of which is the absence of the final sentence and the substitution of the following:

'The Transome Cabbin you have ordered to be fitted up will not be taken in Hand, untill M[r] Bankes determination is known, for if he does not go there are already two Cabbins more on that deck then will be want'd, & which must come down, likewise the two foremast Cabbins on the Gun Deck, provided D[r] Linde also declines going.'

29 May. *Navy Board Minutes. Resolution* to be supplied with stores requested. Acquaint Cook.—Adm 106/2586.

29 May. *Navy Board to Cook.* Letter in terms of foregoing.—CLB.

29 May. *Admiralty Secretary to Cook.* His letter of 24 May had been read to their Lordships.—CLB.

30 May. *Cook to Victualling Board.* Reporting the receipt of the fresh supply of bread and the return of the mouldy.—CLB.

30 May. *Banks to Sandwich.* Protesting against latest alterations in *Resolution.*—Sandwich Papers, Hinchingbrooke. Printed above, pp. 704–7.

31 May. *Clerke to Banks.*† 'Resolution at Sheerness / Sir / I yesterday receiv'd your favour, and indeed am very sorry, I'm not to have the honour of attending you the other bout: Am exceedingly oblig'd to you, my good Sir, for your kind concern on my account: but have stood too far on this tack to think of putting about with any kind of credit, so must have recourse to my old Maxim, "if I can't do as well as I wou'd, I'll do as well as I can" and fear not, but I shall weather all,—Thank you very heartily for the trouble you have taken in calling upon Lord Rochford; your civilities to me have been such, that go where I will, do me the justice to believe Sir, I shall ever carry a most gratefull sense of them, and joyfully embrace any opportunity to convince you how ready I shou'd be to express it. Captain Cooke never explain'd his scheme of Stowage to any of us. We were all very desirous of knowing, for it must have been upon a new plan intirely: know he kept whatever scheme he had quite a secret: for Cooper ask'd my opinion, and repeatedly declar'd he cou'd form no idea how it was possible to bring it about.

Mr Pallisser was here yesterday, spent some time in looking about and examining her; they're going to stow the major part of the Cables in the Hold, to make room for the People even now: I ask'd Gilbert, if such was the present case, what the divil shou'd we have done, if we had all gone: Oh by God that was impossible; was his answer— Won't say farewell now, for if you'll give me leave, will tell you from Plymouth how we're likely to start, and how matters are dispos'd of. Wish you'd send a Venture by me, of one of your small Cags of large Nails, for by what I hear, they are much better than any of my freight; give me leave to trouble you with my best Respects to Doctor Solander & believe me / Sir / Y^r Highly Oblig'd & Humble Servant / Chas Clerke'.—Mitchell Library, *Banks Papers*, 2, f. 2.

1 June. **Cook to Navy Board*. 'Mr Hunt, Master Builder of this Yard, being desireous that tryal may be made, in the Resolution, of the composition he has invented to prevent Worms from eating into Ships Bottoms &c^a I pray you will be pleased to order two of her Boats bottoms to be paid therewith to be supply'd with two or three hundred weight for such other tryals as may offer in the Course of the Voyage, or you are pleased to direct, all which is humbly subm[i]tted to your consideration by' etc. Minuted: 'Give orders accordingly . . .'—Adm/1208; CLB.

1 June. *Victualling Board Minute*. Captain Cook 30th May. That he has received on board 21,280 lb bread in 190 bags, and returned by the vessel 18,922 lb in 173 bags, also 183 empty bags.—Adm 111/69.

2 June. *Navy Board Minutes*. Authorising the supply of Hunt's composition, and the painting of two of the ship's boats with the same.—Adm 106/2586.

2 June. *Navy Board to Cook*. Letter in terms of foregoing.—CLB.

2 June. *Admiralty to Furneaux*. To bear one supernumerary till he arrives at Plymouth then turn him over to one of the guardships.—Adm 2/79.

2 June. *Sandwich to Banks*. Comments on letter of 30 May on *Resolution*, and advises Banks not to make it public: '. . . I am sure if you will give yourself time to think coolly, you will at once see the impropriety of publishing to the world an opinion of your own, that one of the King's ships is unfit for a voyage she is going to be employed in, and that her crew will be in danger of losing their lives if they go to sea in her . . .' —Sandwich Papers, Hinchingbrooke. (A modern copy.)

2 June. **Cook to Banks*.† 'Sir / I receiv'd your letter by one of your People acquainting me that you had order'd every thing belonging to you to be removed out of the Ship and desireing my assistance therein.

'I hope Sir you will find this done to your satisfaction, and with that care the present hurry and confused state of the Ship required— some few articles which were for the Mess I have kept, for which together with the Money I have remaining in my hands I shall account with you for when I come to Town.

'Taught by experience not to trust to the knowlidge of Servants the whole of every necessary article wanting in such a voyage, I had, indipendent of what I purchased for the Mess, layd in a stock of most articles which will be now quite sufficient for me, and is the reason why I have not kept more of yours.

'The Cook & two French Horn men are at liberty to go when ever they please. Several of the Casks your things are in belong to the King, are charged to me and for which I must be accountable I shall be much obliged to you to send them to the Victualing Office when they are emptied but desire that you will by no means put your self to any ilconveniency on this head as I shall not be call'd upon to account for them untill my return.

'If it should not be convenient to send down for what may be still remaining in the Ship of yours they shall be sent you by / Sir / Your Most Ob^t^ & very humble Servant / Jam^s^ Cook

'I Pray my best respects to the D^r^ & sence I am not to have your Company in the Resolution I most sin[c]erely wish you success in all your exploring undertakens.'—Mitchell Library MSS.

3 June. *Navy Board to Sandwich, memorandum.* 'Observations upon Mr Banks's letter to the Earl of Sandwich.'—Sandwich Papers, Hinchingbrooke. Printed above, pp. 708–9.

—June. *Palliser to Sandwich, memorandum.* 'Thoughts upon the Kind of Ships proper to be employed on Discoveries in distant parts of the Globe.' —Sandwich Papers, Hinchingbrooke. Printed above, pp. 709–11.

3 June.[1] **Cook to Admiralty Secretary.* 'Several applycations hath been made to me by John Dodsworth of His Majestys Ship Barfleur to go out in the Resolution Sloop under my command previous to my receiving the Inclosed; as he is known to some of my officers to be a good man and the great desire he seems to have to go the voyage induceth me to pray that you will move my Lords commissioners of the Admiralty to grant his request.' *Enclosure:* 'His Majesties Ships Barfleur Spithead May 30th 1772.—Honnoured S^r^ / I have made bold to trouble your Honnour once more hopeing your Honnour will be so Good as to Make Intrest for to Get me ALong with you. I Wrote to Edward Turrell before but not haveing an Answer I had Given all Expectation Over till hearing from him this Preasant Instant and he desires me to Apply to Your Honnour a Gain which News Gives me a Great Satisfaction and hopes to Gain my point So far as to have the pleasure to Sail with Your Honnour, but not hearing for So Long time had Given all hopes over and I Endeavourd, very hard to Gett out in the prudent to the East Indies but Could not have that Liberty and had been Since Made a Quarter Master but if they was to Make me

[1] Dated by Cook 3 May, an obvious slip.

ten times better it would not be So A Greeable to me as to proceed with Your Honnour which if Your Honnour will be so Good as for to Gett that Grant from the Board for with out that I Am very Certain that I shall not have the Liberty to Leave this Ship on any Consideration so S[r] Your Honnours Complience in this will Always Oblidge me to think my Self in Duty Bound to pray for Your Honnours Health and well fair and all belonging their to but pray S[r] if this is not Granted be So Good as not to mention it farther or other ways possible I May Gain displeasure So S[r] Subscribe my Self S[r] Your Most humble Servant to Command / John Dodsworth'.[1]—Adm 1/1610.

5 June. *Navy Board to Cook.* Asking the reason for keeping the pilot on board during her stay at Longreach from 7 April to 11 May.—CLB.

— June[n.d.] *Cook to Navy Board.* Giving reasons for the keeping of the pilot on board for period stated.—CLB.

5 June. *Cook to Navy Board.* Sending a pay ticket for Wm. Bilby.—Adm 106/1208.

7 June. **Cook to Admiralty Secretary.*† 'All the alteration that have been made in His Majestys Sloop Resolution under my command, are now in a fair way of being finished in a few Days, painting excepted, I pray you will be pleased to move my Lords Commissioners of the Admiralty to grant me a Weeks leave of absence from the Sloop in order to come to town to settle some private affairs of my own before I take my final departure.'—Adm 1/1610.

8 June. *Sandwich to Lord North.* Advises North not to consider the possibility that Banks might change his mind again.—Sandwich Papers, Hinchingbrooke.

8 June. *Admiralty Secretary to Captain Suckling, Senior Officer, Chatham.* Cook to have week's leave for private affairs.—Adm 2/547.

8 June. **Cook to Navy Board.* 'There being only one apperatus for Distillation on Board His Majestys Sloop Resolution under my command and as I understand that there are some at Deptford which were intended for her, I pray you be pleased to order them down, and to be fitted to her Coppers—The Adventure Sloop is likewise in want of some'. Minuted: 'Acq[t] him Deptford Officers are directed to send them as soon as they can get them from the Contractor.'—Adm 106/1208.

10 June. *Admiralty Secretary to Furneaux.* To receive on board and to bear John Dodsworth as supernumerary till he joins *Resolution.*—Adm 2/731; CLB.

10 June. *Navy Board Minutes.* Cook's 8th inst. Acquaint him that Deptford Officers are to send Irving's apparatus to Sheerness as soon as they get it from brazier.—Adm 106/2586.

[1] He did not go the voyage, in spite of the letter to Furneaux, 10 June below

11 June. *Admiralty Secretary to Suckling.* To discharge Mr James Scott of the Marines from *Resolution*, being appointed 2nd lieutenant.—Adm 2/1167.

11 June. *Admiralty Secretary to Rear-admiral Spry, Commanding Officer, Plymouth.* To embark Scott in *Adventure*, discharging one of marines for that purpose.—Adm 2/1167.

12 June. *Suckling to Cook.* To discharge Scott.—CLB.

12 June. *Admiralty Secretary to Navy Board.* It being His Majesty's pleasure that John Reinhold Forster and George Forster, gentlemen skilled in natural history and drawing should proceed in one of the vessels, their Lordships direct that accommodation should be made in *Resolution.* 'P.S. Orders will be sent this being to save time.'—ADM/A 2656; Adm 2/547.

13 June. *Victualling Board to Admiralty Secretary.* Baron Storsch's carrot marmalade: sample sent, instructions asked for as to quantity to be prepared.—Adm 110/25.

13 June. *Board of Longitude to Navy Board.* Following payments to be made: To Dr Stephens, Messrs Wright etc., and to Messrs Peter and John Dollond, for instruments supplied to Messrs Wales and Bayly £168 10s 0d; to Mr Nairne for instruments for said observers £119 3s 6d; to Mr Burton for same reason £79 13s 0d; and to Mr George Adams £27 9s 0d.—ADM/A/2656.

15 June. **Cook to Navy Board.* 'Understanding from Mr Stephens that two Botanists will be sent out by the King in His Majestys Sloop Resolution under my command, I pray you will be pleased to order the two fore mast Cabbins under the Quarter Deck to be rebuilt for their reception, with all possible dispatch.'—Adm 106/1208.

15 June. *Admiralty Minutes. Resolution* to proceed to Plymouth.—Adm 3/79.

15 June. **Cook to Victualling Board.* Wants 1000 lb stockfish, if any in store at Sheerness or Plymouth. Minuted: 15th, to supply 1066½ lb in store to Plymouth by first vessel from Portsmouth.—Dixson R.

15 June. *Admiralty Secretary to Furneaux.* To send names of Banks's draughtsman and secretary, whom he desires an order to victual, and discharge.—Adm 2/731.

16 June. *Admiralty to Cook.* To proceed to Plymouth.—Adm 2/97; CLB.

16 June. *Navy Board Minutes.* Acquaint Cook that Sheerness officers have been directed to rebuild the cabins he desires.—Adm 106/2586.

16 June. *Navy Board to Cook.* Letter in terms of foregoing.—CLB.

17 June. **Cook to Navy Board.* Pilot wanted. Minuted: Write for a pilot. Acquaint him.—Adm 106/1208.

17 June. *Navy Board to Cook.* 'Mr Irving's tubes' would be sent to Sheerness as soon as received.—CLB.

17 June. *Clerke to Banks.*† 'Resolution at Sheerness / Sir / I receiv'd yours by your servant and am very much oblig'd for the Cagg of Nails—think I now set out compleatly freighted for the South Sea Marts, hope to make a good trading Voyage of it, go matters how they will, and stow away in a curious Cabinet of *Miti*[1] curiosities at my return.—flatter myself with the hopes of making an addition to the Burlington Street collection, will certainly make some increase, and I hope a good one; for shall be happy my actions shou'd bespeak my sense of your civilities and friendship.—Must again express my unhappiness that I cannot have the pleasure of attending you, but can't help it, two or three Years will blow all over, and replace me again in Old London and its Purlieu's, Captain of at least my own Carcass, to dispose of it as I please: when I assure you, you shall never want a Sailors attendance to run any where on this side of H— so long as remains above Water / Your Much Oblig'd / & Devoted Servant Chas Clerke

'Believe our stay here will be 12 or 14 days longer—the Gentlemen of the Gunroom intreat your acceptance of their respects & Compliments'.—Mitchell Library, *Banks Papers*, 2, f. 4.

18 June. *Admiralty Secretary to Victualling Board.* The naturalists who are going out in *Resolution* have stated that it would be of great use if they were provided with 4 puncheons of double proof spirits of 80 gals. each for preserving specimens, their Lordships direct that these are to be provided without a moments loss of time, as sloop is under sailing orders. An order will be sent in form, this being to save time. Minuted: 'Received ¾ past 2 and Mr Frankland immediately ordered to enquire after the spirits.—19th Read and Mr Frankland and Dixon ordered to purchase it.'—ADM/C/606; Adm 2/547.

18 June. *Admiralty to Victualling Board.* Order in form as preceding.—ADM/C/606; Adm 2/97.

18 June. *Admiralty Secretary to Hon. Daines Barrington.* Informed that Victualling Board are directed to furnish 4 puncheons of 80 gals. each to *Resolution* as he proposed, for preservation of such animals as naturalists might collect.—Adm 2/731.

18 June. *Admiralty to Cook.* To cause 4 puncheons double proof spirits to be put on *Resolution* for use by naturalists to preserve such animals as they may happen to collect.—Adm 2/97.

19 June. *Victualling Board Minutes.* Frankland and Dixon to buy 320 gals. of double proof spirits to preserve animals from putrefaction: same to be packed in 4 iron bound puncheons which are to be properly seasoned, and to be sent on *Resolution* at Sheerness without moment's loss of time. Write to Excise and Customs to allow *Caesar* to carry it to Plymouth if *Resolution* should have sailed.—Barbe and Dixon to buy 1,000 lb best and newest stock fish. To be sent on *Resolution* at Sheerness or Plymouth.—Adm 111/69.

[1] He seems to be using the Tahitian word *maitai*, good, beautiful.

19 June. **Cook to Admiralty Secretary.* Applying for order to victual nine persons belonging to Banks's party from 8 April to 5 June. List given. —Adm 1/1610; CLB.

20 June. **Cook to Admiralty Secretary.* Asks for duplicate of order to victual Banks's men to be sent to Clerk of Cheque at Woolwich.—Adm 1/1610.

20 June. *Hunt to Cook.* Giving directions for application of his composition. —CLB.

20 June. *Sandwich to George III.* Sends the king 'a sketch of a letter in answer to that written to him by Mr Banks, which may possibly be proper to be printed in case the other is made publick. Your Majesty will observe that it is under a fictitious name, which for many reasons is most adviseable'.—Georgian Papers, No. 1342, Windsor Castle Library. The enclosure does not appear in this collection.

— June. *Sandwich to Banks.* Draft of unsent and unpublished letter referred to in foregoing.—Sandwich Papers, Hinchingbrooke. Printed above, pp. 711–7.

22 June. *Cook to Navy Board.* 'The Quarter Deck and Poop awning of His Majestys Sloop Resolution, under my Command, are made of old Canvas, as such as may be fit for home service, Yet far from being of Sufficient Goodness to last even, one half of her intended Voyage, I therefore pray you will be pleas'd to order her to be supply'd with others at plymouth, either made of New Canvas, or of Canvas not above one third worn.' Minuted accordingly.—Adm 106/1208.

24 June. *Navy Board Minutes.* Cook's of 22nd past. Give orders to Plymouth officers to supply *Resolution* with awnings either of new canvas or $\frac{1}{3}$ work. Acquaint Cook.—Adm 106/2586.

24 June. *Admiralty Secretary to Cook.* To bear persons belonging to Banks for victuals 8 April–5 June, during which time they were on board on supernumerary list. Names: Joseph Miller, Benj. Miller, John Wilson, Peter Briscoe, James Roberts, Peter Sidsaft, John Asquith, John Alexander, Nich. Young.—Adm 2/97; CLB.

24 June. *Admiralty to Furneaux.* To bear some persons belonging to Banks and Board of Longitude for victuals for time they have been or may be on board.—Adm 2/97.

25 June. *Admiralty Minutes.* Messrs Forster (*Resolution*), Wales (*Resolution*), and Bayly (*Adventure*) to be received on board ships. Captains to give them every assistance. Captain of *Adventure* to put himself under command of Cook.—Adm 3/79; CLB.

25 June. *Admiralty to Cook.* He is to give the naturalists, John Reinhold Forster and Geo. Forster, and observers, Wm. Wales and Wm. Bayley, who are to go out in the sloop he commands (with exception of Bayley who will be in *Adventure*) all convenient accommodation, facilities to land when opportunity arises. Also very particular instructions about

the watch machines which are going out for trial under the observers. To make use of recommendation of Prince of Orange in case of touching at any of ports or settlements of Dutch East India Company. —Adm 2/97; CLB.

25 June. *Admiralty to Cook.* Secret instructions.—Adm 2/1332; CLB. Printed pp. clxvii–clxx above.

25 June. *Admiralty to flag officers, captains and commanders of H.M. ships and vessels.* They are not to demand of Captain Cook, *Resolution*, or of Captain Furneaux, *Adventure*, to see the secret instructions received by them from the Admiralty, nor to detain the ships, but to render all assistance to both captains to enable them to put the instructions into execution.—Adm 2/1332; CLB.

25 June. *Admiralty to Furneaux.* To be under command of Cook.—Adm 2/97

26 June. *Admiralty Secretary to Cook.* Sends the East India Company's private signals for his and Furneaux's guidance.—Adm 2/731; Adm 2/1332.

26 June. *John Ibbetson, Secretary of Board of Longitude, to Cook.* Entrusting to his care the deal case containing three mahogany boxes and keys and the clock machines to be used on the voyage.—CLB.

26 June. *Cook to Furneaux.*† Passing on orders received regarding Bayly's appointment to the *Adventure.* Also instructions given on care of the watch machines.—CLB.

27 June. *Admiralty Minutes.* William Hodges is to be received on *Resolution* and victualled as one of her company.—Adm 3/79.

30 June. *Admiralty to Cook.* Order for the appointment of Mr William Hodges to the *Resolution* as artist and painter, and instructing Cook to include him on the ship's strength.—CLB.

30 June. *Admiralty Secretary to Cook.* To receive on board William Hodges, landscape painter, and see that he does diligently employ himself.—Adm 2/97; Adm 2/731; CLB.

3 July. *Cook to Admiralty Secretary.* 'Resolution in Plymouth Sound . . . Please to acquaint my Lords Commissioners of the Admiralty with the arrival of His Majesty's Sloop Resolution Under my Command at this place, and that the fault She formerly had in being Crank is now intirely removed, a doubt of a contrary Nature does not, I am persuaded, remain in the breast of any one person on board; In turning into the downs with a fresh of wind at sw in company with several vessels, not one of which but what was oblig'd to take in their Top Gallant Sails, and one ship, Reef'd her Fore topsail, Yet at this time we carried Top Gallant Sails with ease. In coming down channell we had an oppertunity to find that she will hold her side up to as much sail as can be set without endangering the Masts. With Respect to her other qualities, we have not had sufficient tryal to Report with

certainty, but upon the whole I believe she will be found to steer and Work well and to sail as fast as most deep Laden Ships of her con-[s]truction.'—Adm 1/1610; CLB.

3 July. *Captain Edward Hughes, H.M.S. Somerset, Senior Officer Plymouth, to Cook.* Instructing him to receive a marine to fill a vacancy in the ship's company.—CLB.

3 July. *Cook to Furneaux.*† Directing Furneaux to serve under his command. Adm 1/1610; CLB.

3 July. *Cook to Furneaux.* Instructions on reception of Bayly, and his duties. —CLB.

4 July. *Cook to Admiralty Secretary.* Acknowledges his of 25th June with enclosed orders and instructions, and his of same date with private signals.—Adm 1/1610.

4 July. **Cook to Navy Board.*[1] 'You will no doubt be desirous to know how the Resolution answers after the alterations that have lately been made, I beg leave to inform you that the fault she formerly had in being crank is now entirely removed and that from the little tryal we have had of her sailing and working she promises to answer very well in these respects.'—B.M., Add. MS 37425, f. 134.

5 July. *Cook to Admiralty Secretary.* Acknowledges order of 30 June on Hodges. —Adm 1/1610; CLB.

7 July. *Admiralty Secretary to Cook.* Acknowleges Cook's letter of 3rd inst., with account of his arrival at Plymouth, and the advantage in ship's sailing due to the late alterations.—Adm 2/731.

8 July. *Navy Board Minutes.* Acknowledges receipt of Cook's letter of 4th inst. Acquaint him we are very glad crankness removed, and that there is so good a prospect of ship's sailing and working well.—Adm 106/2587.

9 July. *Captain Hughes to Cook.* To discharge five men into other ships as specified.—CLB.

11 July. *Cook to Robert Palliser Cooper, 1st lieutenant Resolution.*† Passing on the orders received regarding Wales's appointment to *Resolution*, and care of chronometers.—CLB.

11 July. **Cook to George Perry, Victualling Office.* 'I thank you for your care in looking over my Charts and am pleased to find there are so few Errors, or rather none but what has been corrected. Lagoon Island &c^{a} will not be engraved or any other but what you have, I think some of these Islands were seen by Quiros but not by Schouten, his rout was farther to the northward.—As I have declined every applycation that has been made to me for taking on board Madeira Wine, I will

[1] The lower part of the sheet on which this letter is written has been torn away, the lost portion carrying with it the name of the body addressed and most of a minute, but the form of the subscription leaves no doubt that Cook was writing to the Navy Board, on his arrival at Plymouth.

not promise you. perhaps I may find room in some corner of the Ship for a Hħd which is all you must expect from him who is with great truth. . . Jam[s] Cook.—P.S. I intend Sailing tomorrow'.—Nan Kivell coll.

13 *July. Admiralty Secretary to Captain Hughes, Senior Officer, Plymouth.* Approves of diving machine being bought and put on *Resolution.*—Adm 2/547.

15 July. *Cook to Furneaux.* Passing on Prince of Orange's recommendatory letter together with a translation in French sent previously to Cook.—Adm 1/1610; CLB.

15 July. *Cook to Furneaux.* Copy of secret instructions: copy of order to flag Officer.—Adm 1/1610; CLB.

15 July. *Cook to Furneaux.* Giving first, second and third rendezvous. Further instructions and procedure should *Resolution* become parted from *Adventure.*—Adm 1/1610; CLB. Printed above, pp. 683–4.

29 July. *Cook (Funchal Road, Madeira) to Furneaux.* Instructing him to order wine for *Adventure.*—Adm 1/1610; CLB.

30 July. *Furneaux to Cook.* Reporting shortage of beef and asking for permission to record shortages on the list attached to the head of each cask.—CLB.

30 July. *Cook to master and master's mates, Adventure.* Ordering an examination to be made of the contents of casks of beef, at the time of opening, and a record of shortages to be made.—CLB.

30 July. *Furneaux to Cook.* Requesting the appointment to *Adventure* of Mr William Roberts as sailmaker's mate.—CLB.

30 July. *Cook to William Roberts.* Appointing him sailmaker's mate *Adventure.*—CLB.

1 August. *Furneaux to Cook.*† Requesting permission to allow William Carr to act as master at arms.—Adm 1/1610; CLB.

1 August. *Cook to W. Carr.*† Appointing him master at arms *Adventure.*—Adm 1/1610; CLB.

1 August. *Cook to Daniel Clark.*† Appointing him master at arms, *Resolution.*—CLB.

1 August. *Cook to Admiralty Secretary.* Reporting arrival at Madeira.—Adm 1/1610; CLB. Printed above, pp. 684–5.

1 August. **Cook to* . On voyage to date; and on Mrs Burnett.—Windsor Castle Library, Georgian Papers, no. 1359. Printed above, p. 685.

1 August. *Cook to Victualling Board.* Informing Board of the drawing of supplies of fresh beef and onions for both ships.—CLB.

1 August. *Cook to Navy Board.* Had drawn money for the replacement of ship's bell on *Resolution,* in favour of Mrs Elizabeth Cook.—CLB.

2 August. *Furneaux to Cook.*† Reporting that an Englishman, John Rayside, seaman on a Portuguese vessel at Madeira, came aboard *Adventure* unperceived and secreted himself overnight: asking for instructions as to his disposal.—Adm 1/1610; CLB.

2 August. *Cook to Furneaux.*† Ordering John Rayside to be taken on the supernumerary list for victuals and wages until further orders.—Adm 1/1610; CLB.

11 November. *Furneaux to Cook.* Reporting mouldy bread, and asking for a survey.—CLB.

11 November. *Cook to master and one mate of Resolution and Adventure.* Ordering a survey of the mouldy bread and the disposal of that condemned.—CLB.

13 November. *J. Gilbert, P. Fannin, James Whitehouse to Cook.* Report on survey of bread.—CLB.

16 November. *Joseph Shank to Cook.*† Requesting permission to return home on grounds of ill health.—Adm 1/1610; CLB.

16 November. *Cook to Surgeons Resolution and Adventure.*† Requesting a medical report on Shank.—Adm 1/1610; CLB.

16 November. *Surgeons Resolution and Adventure to Cook.*† Reporting the medical examination of Shank and recommending that he be allowed to return home, this being absolutely necessary on account of his health.—Adm 1/1610; CLB.

16 November. *Cook to Shank.*† Giving permission to return home.—Adm 1/1610; CLB.

16 November. *Cook to Admiralty Secretary.* Reporting on inspissated malt and beer making.—Adm 1/1610; CLB. Printed above, p. 686.

18 November. *Cook to Kempe.*† Appointing him 1st lieutenant *Adventure.*—Adm 1/1610; CLB.

18 November. *Cook to Burney.*† Appointing him 2nd lieutenant *Adventure.*—Adm 1/1610; CLB.

18 November. *Cook to Admiralty Secretary.* Reporting on voyage up to date, and enclosing copies of orders consequent on Shank's illness.—Adm 1/1610; CLB. Letter printed above, pp. 686–7.

18 November. **Cook to Banks.*† Reporting on the voyage to date.—Mitchell Library MSS. Printed above, p. 688.

18 November. *Cook to Admiralty Secretary.* Enclosing 'State and Condition of H.M. Sloops *Resolution* and *Adventure*', Cape of Good Hope, 18 November 1772.

18 November. *Cook to Navy Board.* Advising the drawing of money to purchase medical supplies and stores for caulking etc. on *Resolution* and *Adventure.*—CLB.

18 November. *Cook to Victualling Board.* Reporting the drawing of money for the purchase of provisions at Cape of Good Hope.—CLB.

19 November. *Cook to Admiralty.* Reporting on the voyage.—*General Evening Post,* 19 April 1773. Printed above, p. 689.

20 November. **Cook to John Walker.* A brief leave-taking.—General Assembly Library, Wellington. Printed above, p. 689.

23 November. *Cook to Furneaux.*† Advising procedure should *Adventure* become separated from *Resolution.*—Adm 1/1610; CLB.

6 December. *Cook to Furneaux.*† Authorising an extra half allowance of spirit and wine on such days as thought necessary, and an issue of boiled wheat or oatmeal for breakfast each Monday, and requesting that an exact account of same be kept.—Adm 1/1610; CLB.

14 December. *Cook to Furneaux.*† Second letter advising procedure should *Adventure* be separated from *Resolution.*—Adm 1/1610; CLB.

1773

28 March. *Cook to Furneaux.*[1]† Owing to scorbutic complaints being contracted by ship's company, gives orders to purchase and boil any vegetables obtainable, with wheat or oatmeal, and portable broth, and to serve every morning for breakfast. Orders the continuance of the boiled wheat or oatmeal for breakfast, but the cancellation of the issue of half allowance of spirit mentioned in the order of December 6.—Adm 1/1610; CLB.

30 April. *Victualling Board to Admiralty Secretary.* Advice of bills drawn by Cook at Cape of Good Hope: 12,864 rix dollars 47 stivers.—Adm 110/25.

6 May. *Admiralty Minutes.* Victualling Board to accept and pay bills of exchange Cook has drawn on them at Cape of Good Hope for 12,864 rix dollars and 47 stivers, at 48 stivers per rix dollar.—Adm 3/80.

4 June. *Cook to Furneaux.*† Advising procedure of *Adventure* after departure from Queen Charlotte Sound, should ships become separated.—Adm 1/1610; CLB.

17 July. *Cook to Furneaux.*† Cancelling the breakfast issue of boiled wheat or oatmeal on Mondays.—Adm 1/1610; CLB.

24 July. *Cook to William Chapman.* Appointing him cook *Adventure.*—CLB.

25 October. *Admiralty Minutes.* Shank to be paid his wages for time he was 1st lieutenant of *Adventure.*—Adm 3/80.

5 November. *Cook to Master, Boatswain and Mate, Resolution.* Ordering an examination of all bread remaining in casks and the throwing over-

[1] There is a minor problem here. The order is 'Given under my hand . . . in Dusky Bay this 28th day of March 1773'. Furneaux was not, and never was, at Dusky Bay, having parted company with Cook seven weeks before. On this date he was in the Tasman Sea, six days' sail from New Zealand. 'Purchase' is used in the sense of 'procure'.

board of any found to be unfit for consumption, and the reporting of the proceedings.—CLB.

18 November. *J. Gilbert, James Gray and Isaac Smith to Cook.* Reporting proceedings at examination of bread, stating deterioration due to bread being packed in new casks made of unseasoned wood.—CLB.

4 December. *Cook to James Gray, Boatswain Resolution.* Directing that the decayed rigging on the main and fore topsails and sheets, main and fore lifts, & stoppers to anchors be made into oakum for the immediate caulking of the sides, decks, etc. of *Resolution.*—CLB.

1774

10 April. *Cook to James Gray.* Further order for all decayed rigging to be converted into oakum for the purpose of caulking sides, decks etc. of *Resolution.*—CLB.

14 April. *Furneaux to Sick and Hurt Board.* He had that day drawn on Board three bills of exchange for 123 rix dollars 6 stivers at 48 stivers each rix dollar with exchange of 8% payable to Messrs Dijkes and Mulder, merchants Amsterdam or their order, value received of Mr Christoffel Brand the same being for payment of board and lodging of sick men sent on shore.—Adm 97/86.

28 April. *Cook to master, boatswain and mate, Resolution.* Ordering casks of bread to be taken ashore for further examination, and all bread unfit for consumption to be thrown into the sea, and a report of the proceedings to be made.—CLB.

1 May. *Cook to James Wallis, carpenter Resolution.* Order to make two iron grapnels for the ship's boats.—CLB.

10 May. *J. Gilbert, James Gray and Isaac Smith to Cook.* Reporting further examination of bread, stating that the deterioration was due to the sudden extreme changes of temperature.—CLB.

14 July. *Admiralty to Furneaux.* To proceed to Nore immediately, and there await orders.—Adm 2/99.

15 July. *Navy Board to Admiralty.* Recommending that *Adventure* should be paid off and laid up at Deptford.—Adm 106/2203.

16 July. *Admiralty to Furneaux. Adventure* to be paid off.—Adm 2/99.

5 August. *Adventure*: To dispense with officers and petty officers not delivering or producing journals or log books.—Index 10704/17.

10 August. *Admiralty Minutes.* Furneaux and officers to be paid allowance equal to the number of servants deficient, no servants being entered on books.—Adm 3/80.

[— August.] *Accountant-General, Bill Book.* To Captain Tobias Furneaux, *Adventure*, allowance for deficiency of servant's wages from 28 November 1771 to 8 August 1774 at 19s per man, £133 13s 8d.—Adm 18/116, no. 4368.

[— August.] *Accountant-General, Bill Book.* To Lieut. James Burney, *Adventure*, allowance for deficiency of servant's wages from 20 November 1771 to 8 August 1774, £21 5s 6d.—Adm 18/116, no. 4343.

18 August. *Deptford Yard Officers to Navy Board.* Sending carpenter's account of defects of *Adventure*.—Adm 106/3317.

19 August. *Solander to* [*Lind?*][1] 'Hertford / Dear Sir / In my last letter, wherein I gave You a compleat Account of what has been done by Capt. Furneaux, during the last South Sea Expedition, I mention'd that he has brought with him a Native of one of the Society Isles. I will now give You an Account of him.

'His Name is *Omai*. He is borne in Ulaietea, where his father was a Man of considerable landed property, but about 12 years ago the King of Bola-bola conquer'd that part of Ulaietea where Omais father had his estates, which still are possessed by the Conquerors friends. Omai's father was killed in one of the Battles and the Boy obliged to leave the country with a few servants—Omai then retired to Otaheite, where he was, when Capt. Wallis arrived thither. *Omai* was wounded with a Musket bullet in his side, the famous day, when Capt Wallis fired upon the Otaheiteans on *One tree hill:* The Wound is still very visible. He has also been wounded in his arm with a Spear in one of his arms, in one of their civil wars. After Capt. Wallis's departure Omai bound himself prentice to a Priest or Wise Man of Otaheite, in this Capacity we found him, at our arrival in the Endeavour. He still was a Boy and not so remarkable as to make us remember him, but he perfectly well remember'd all of us, who had been there. A Short time after our departure from Otaheite he retired to Huaheine, where he lived as a private Gentleman of a small fortune when Capt. Cook & Furneaux last year came there. He soon became a favorite of the Surgeon and the Armourer and resolved to go with them to Europe. He had 4 Servants, who all endeavoured to perswade [him] from going, so did also the King of Ulaietea, but Omai was resolute, and parted from his own country in high Spirits after he had formally taken leave of the king and all his friends. The king of Ulaietea recommended him to Capt. Furneaux's attention. He is not above 21 or 22 years old. He has grown a little during the time he was on board of the Ship. He is very brown, allmost a[s] brown as a Mulatto. Not at all hansome, but well made. His nose is a little broadish, and I believe we have to thank his wide Nostrills for the Visit he has paid us—for he says, that the people of his own country laughed at him

[1] There are two persons to whom this letter could have been addressed, to judge from its first paragraph: Lind, and John Ellis the naturalist. Solander gave them both 'a complete Account' of Furneaux's voyage: Lind, in a letter of 27 July 1774, now in the Dixson Library; Ellis, in one dated 22 July, printed in J. E. Smith's *Correspondence of Linnaeus and other Naturalists* (1821), II, pp. 14–18. The reference to Miss Burnet in the last paragraph, however, inclines me in favour of Lind, who mentions her in correspondence with Banks as an Edinburgh friend.

upon the account of his flatish Nose and dark hue, but he hopes when he returns and has so many fine things to talk of, that he shall be much respected. When he Saw M[r] Banks who happen'd to have no powdre in his hair he knew him instantly; The first intercourse with me was droll enough; I came into Capt. Furneaux room and began to converse with him, which Omai heard who was in the next room, and came running in calling out—I hear Tolano's voice (obs. Tolano = Solander) but coming into the room he recollected not my figure, so he walked quite round me, constantly looking at me, but at last thought himself mistaken. He then desired Capt Furneaux to make me speake, which I had not sooner done than he cried out, he was sure I was Tolano, but much encreased in bulk. We soon made ourselves known by conversing pretty freely with one another in his Language. It has been very pleasing to us, to him and many others, that both M[r] Banks, myself, & M[r] Banks's servant James have not forgot our South Sea Language.—So we all can well keep up a Conversation with him. He first of all lived at M[r] Banks's house, and afterwards removed to Hertford, where he has been inoculated by Baron Dimsdale. He is now quite recovered, and to morrow we propose to go up for good to town. M[r] Banks & Myself have almost Constantly been with him here at Hertford, and M[r] Banks Serv[t] James Roberts and the Surgeon of the Ship he came home in (Mr. Andrews) have lived in the Inoculation house with him during the whole time. Omai is [a] sensible communicative Man, so he is a valuable acquisition. He has pleased every body, and is quite contented and pleased with his reception here. We *think* that the King has promised to send him back; It is a thing so much wish'd for, by us, I mean that an other S.S. Expedition should take place, that I have onely said we *think* so— I am sure the king said so—but .L[d] Sandwich and M[r] Banks are now quite cordial again—we are soon to go down to Hinchinbrook. I suppose You are tired by this time of reading so much upon a subject which can't be much interesting to You. But I can hardly get any thing else now in my head to write about. Especially as my friend Omai sits by my side, quite elevated by having been informed that he to morrow is to leave this place of confinement. If it had not luckely for us happend that the blue Horse Guards were quartered here at Hertford, I believe we as well as Omai should have been tired of the place; But we have lived in a very agreable Society of the Officers of that Corps, among them is Capt. Arch[d] Stewart, an old Acquaintance of mine. M[r] John Stewart has twice been down to pay his brother and us a visit. The other day L[d] Elibank Gov[r] Geo Jonstone and Capt Blair spent a day with us. Poor Omai was then in his worst Prickle, so they did not see him to great advantage. Omai don't yet speak any english, but I think he will soon learn it, as he has got several words and begins to pronounce S tolerably well; as yet he cannot pronounce K, but I am sure he will even conquere that, as he is desirous of learning to speak English. He is well behaved, easy in his Manners, and remarkably complaisant to the Ladies. I will onely mention one thing as a proof of his good breeding. We dined with him at the Duke of Gloucesters, at going away the Dutchess gave him her pocket handkerchief, which he properly recieved with thanks, and observing her Name marked upon it, he took an oportunity when she looked at him to Kiss it. Many more instances of his own Gallantry could I mention If I had not already dwelled to[o] long upon this subject.

'My best complts to Miss Burnet and all other friends. Banks presents his Complts and I am for ever / My Dear Sir / Your most obedt servant & sincere friend / Dan. Solander.'—Alexander Turnbull Library, *Holograph Letters and Documents* . . . , no. 24.

1 September. *Cook to J. Ramsay, cook Resolution.* Ordering 400 lb of cooking fat to be made into tallow.—CLB.

16 September. *Victualling Board to Admiralty Secretary.* On acceptance of bills of exchange drawn by Furneaux at Cape of Good Hope 14 April last.—Adm 110/26.

24 November. *Navy Board to Admiralty.* William Offord, late carpenter of *Adventure*: on dispensing with some deficiency of stores. Navy Board is of opinion that dispensing with the deficiency of stores alleged by Captain Furneaux may prove very prejudicial to His Majesty's service if drawn into a precedent, as the same reasons may be pleaded in other cases where the like deficiencies may happen, whether it should arise from negligence, waste or embezzlement. Nevertheless submit to their Lordships whether his request may not be granted on account of the particular voyage he has made.—Adm 106/2203.

29 November. *Admiralty Minutes.* At Furneaux's request orders are to be given to dispense with W. Offord, late his carpenter, passing an account for some stores charged against him for not being regularly expended.—Adm 3/80.

1775

24 January. *Admiralty Minutes.* Curiosities brought back by Furneaux to be sent to trustees of British Museum.—Adm 3/80.

19 March. **Cook to Admiralty Secretary.* Within two days' sail of Cape. Promises full report when he arrives there.—Adm 1/1610. Printed above, p. 690.

22 March. *Cook to Admiralty Secretary.* Reporting on voyage.—Adm 1/1610; CLB. Printed above, pp. 691–3.

31 March. *Victualling Board to Admiralty Secretary.* In return, on allowing Furneaux for sundries issued to *Adventure* by order of Cook.—Adm 110/26.

3 April. *Victualling Board to Admiralty Secretary.* In return, on allowing Fur-

neaux for sundries condemned by survey after time of warranty.—Adm 110/26.

4 April. *Admiralty Minutes.* Furneaux to be allowed the extra wheat, oatmeal and spirits issued to his men.—Adm 3/81.

[10?][1] April. *Cook to Admiralty Secretary.* Advising the sending of journal, charts, paintings, etc. of the voyage, by Captain Newte, *Ceres*, and the sending of two journals or log-books by Captain Clements, *Royal Charlotte*.—CLB. Printed above. p. 693.

10 April. *Cook to Victualling Board.* Had drawn on Board in favour of Mr Jacob Speer at the Cape, £100 sterling.—CLB.

10 April. *Cook to Navy Board.* Had drawn on Board in favour of Mr Jacob Speer, for repairs and stores, £100 sterling.—CLB.

12 April. *Admiralty Minute.* Victualling Board to allow Furneaux credit on his accounts for the provisions condemned by survey, and for rum and brandy stored and lost in bad weather on his making affidavit to the truth of what he has set forth.—Adm 3/81.

24 April. *Cook to Navy Board.* Had drawn on Board, in favour of Mr Christoffel Brand, for 730 rix dollars and 22 stivers, for stores and caulking.—CLB.

25 April. *Cook to Victualling Board.* Had drawn on Board in favour of Mr Gabriel Bourcourt at Amsterdam, for 1600 rix dollars, for purchase of provisions.—CLB.

25 April. *Cook to Victualling Board.* Had drawn on Board, in favour of Mr Pieter Johannis Dewit, for 800 rix dollars, for purchase of provisions.—CLB.

26 April. *Cook to Victualling Board.* Had drawn on Board, in favour of Mr Christoffel Brand, for 513 rix dollars, for purchase of provisions.—CLB.

27 April. *Cook to Victualling Board.* Had drawn on Board, in favour of Mr Christoffel Brand, for 1056 rix dollars and 21 stivers, for purchase of provisions.—CLB.

24 May. *Cook to Admiralty Secretary.* Further journals and charts sent.—Adm 1/1610; CLB. Printed above, p. 694.

28 June. *Solander to Banks.* '. . . As a Copy of Capt Cooks Letter was sent down to Ld Sandwich, I take it for granted you know all concerning his Voyage. I[t] does not appear from any thing Capt Cook has wrote if Oridi is on board or not. I should rather think that he is; as they mustered the day they came into the Cape of good hope as many men as when they left the Cape—and I think one man fell over board of[f] New Zealand. If he should arrive before your return, shall it be mention'd to him, that Omai wishes he would live in the same house

[1] The letter is not given a precise date; but the *Royal Charlotte* sailed on the 10th, and Cook writes, 'I thought proper herewith to transmit to you, by the Royal Charlotte', etc.

with him? It seems Mr Omai has desired Mr Vigniol to take him in, in case he should come.—In all the Letters that are come from the Gentlemen on board the Resolution, they speak much in praise of our friends and all other Sth Sea Inhabitants that they have met with; and Nova Caledonia is described as a paradise without thorns or thistles. Mr Penneck [?] has seen Mr Forsters Letter to Mr D. Barrington and made the following abstract: 260 new Plants, 200 new animals —71°10′ farthest Sth—no continent—Many Islands, some 80 Leagues long—The Bola Bola savage incorrigible Blockhead—Glorious Voyage —No man lost by sickness.'—Mitchell Library, *Banks Papers*, J, 1–2.

30 July. *Cook to Admiralty Secretary.* Transmitting copies of orders (26) given in writing on proceedings of *Resolution* and *Adventure*, 1772–3, including further copies of those already sent from Cape, 18 November 1772.—Adm 1/1610. All enclosures have been entered chronologically above.

30 July. *Cook to Navy Board.* Enclosing muster books and dead tickets of *Resolution.*—CLB.

30 July. *Clerke to Banks.*† 'Resolution Sunday Morn: 5 o'clock / Dear Sir / We're now past Portland with a fine fresh NW Gale and a young flood Tide, so that in a very few Hours we shall anchor at Spithead from our Continent hunting expedition. I will not now set about relating any of the particulars of our Voyage, as I hope very soon to have the Honour and happiness of paying my personal respects, when I can give you a much clearer idea of any matters you think worth inquiring after, than its possible to do at this distance.

'I hope I need not assure you that its utterly out of the power of length of time, or distance of space, to eradicate or in the least alleviate the gratitude your friendly offices to me has created—I assure you I've devoted some days to your service in very distant parts of the Globe; the result of which I hope will give you some satisfaction; at least it will convince you of my intentions and endeavours in that particular. I shall send this away by our civil Gentry, who will fly to Town with all the sail they can possibly make. God bless you send me one Line just to tell me you're alive and well, if that is the case, for I'm as great a stranger to all matters in England as tho' I had been these 3 Years underground—so if I receive no intelligence from you I shall draw bad conclusions and clap on my suit of black; but you know I never despair, but always look for the best, therefore hope and flatter myself this will find you alive and happy, which that it may, is the sincerest Hope and Wish of / Dear Sir / Your Gratefully Oblig'd & most H:ble Servt / Chas Clerke.—Excuse the Paper, its gilt I assure you, but the Cockroaches have piss'd upon it.—We're terrible busy—you know a Man of War—my respects & every social wish to the good Doctor—I'll write him as soon as possible—here's too much damning of Eyes & Limbs to do any thing now.'—Mitchell Library, *Banks Papers*, 2, f. 4.

[1 August?] *Cook to Admiralty Secretary.* Reporting arrival at Spithead and giving further details of voyage.—CLB. Printed above, pp. 694–5.

[1 August?] *Cook to Admiralty Secretary.* Reports on provisioning and health of the ship. '. . . We were happy in having few or no opportunitys in giving a full & fair Tryall, to either ye Marmalade of Carots or Water Imprignated with Fixed Air, my opinion is not very favourable to either & that the Surgeons worse, but this ought not to Discourage further experiments. I must beg leave to mention Some further Articles which their Lordships caused to be put on board the Efficacy whereof had been before tryed.

'Wort made of Malt, is without doubt one of ye best Antiscorbutic Sea Medecines yet found out and if given in time will, with proper attention to other things prevent ye Scurvy from making any progress, but I am afraid it will seldom be found to cure it, we have been a long time without any, without feeling ye Want of it, which might be owing to other Articles.

'Sour Krout can never be enough recommend[ed], it is not only a Wholesome Vegitable diat but highly Antiscorbutic & spoils not by keeping.

'Portable Broth is a very nourishing & valuable Article & that which we had was Excellent & kept good to ye last.

'The Rob of Lemon & Orange was Wholy under ye Surgeons care, I must refer to his Journal for its Efficacy and use.

'We were supplyed with sugar in ye room of Oyle & Wheat in ye room of Oatmeal & were certainly gainers by ye Exchange.

'Sugar I apprehend helps to prevent ye Scurvey & Oyle to promote it, I am of opinion it would contribute to ye health of Seamen if Oyle was totaly banished out of ye Navy, & likewise Butter & cheese in Sea Victualing & Sugar Introduced in their room ye Ships would be clear of that disagreeable Smell, caused by rotten cheese, and I can make it appear it would be a saving to ye Crown.

'Wheat keeps better than Oatm^l^ and makes a far more wholesome diet & what Seamen like much better, indeed I no [*sic*] nothing that can equal it for a breakfast when sweetned with sugar. But ye Introduction of ye most Salutary Provisions or Medecines will sometimes lose their Effects unless suported by some well regulated rules. I hope it will not be taken amiss my Mentioning these which I caused to be observed during ye Whole Voyage, as they are founded on many Years experience & some information I had from Sr Hugh Pallisser, Capt: Campbell, Captain Wallis & other experienced Officers & which certainly contributed not a little to that good State of health we, I may say, constantly enjoyed. The Crew were at three Watches, except on some extraordinary occasions, by this Means they were never broke of their rest & were seldom Wet, consequently had always dry cloaths to shift themselves. There persons as also their Hammacoes, Bedding

& cloaths were kept constantly clean & frequently examined into, especially after Wet rainy Weather; when they were spread on deck to air, the Ship was kept clean betwixt decks & aird with fires or Smoakd with gunpowder mix'd with Water, or Vinegar so long as we had any to spare, this was done once or twice a week, as well in hot as in cold Weather, it is equally Necessary in both; to this & Cleanliness among ye people too great attention cannot be paid, ye Consequence of ye least Neglect, is a putrified Air and a disagreeable Smell below which nothing but fire & smoak will purify.

'Proper methods was taken to keep ye Ships Coppers constantly clean & ye Beef & pork fat was never given to ye people as there can be no Doubt but it promotes the Scurvy.

'I took care to take in water when ever it was to be got, even tho' we did not want it, because I look upon Water from ye shore to be more wholesome than that which has been kept in Casks, some time on board a Ship, of this Assential Article we were never at all at allowance, but had always plenty for every Necessary purpose.

'We came to few places w[h]ere either ye art of Man or Nature had not provided some sort of refreshments or other, either in ye Animal or Vegitable way, & it was first care to procure them by every Means in my power & Oblig'd ye people to make use of them, both by example & authority. It is from these kinds of refreshments I can only Account for the Resolution having few or no Scorbutic people on board on our passage from New Zealand to Otahiete the first time, when at the same time ye Adventure had many of her best men far gorne [*sic*] in that disease; for except Fish they had hardly any refreshments from ye time we left ye Cape till I join'd them in Queen Charlotte's Sound, which was about Six Months; they were unacquainted with the method of making Spruce Beer & Strangers to many of ye Vegitables with which that place abounds, consequently not benefited by them, whereas ye Crew of ye Resolution had been living on Fish, Spruce beer & Vegitables for upwards of two Months, which eradicated every seed of ye Scurvy, & this was not ye only time we received this Benefit during the Voyage.'—CLB.

1 August. *Cook to Victualling Board.* Reports on experimentally cured beef, inspissated juice of wort and beer, and proceeds: 'Since I am upon the Subject of Victualling, it may not be a Miss to inform you that the Bread which we had in Casks and the pease were but indifferent and the Mustard seed (if it was such) was so bad that not an Animal on board would eat it, the pease were never good not even at first, But this was not the case with the Bread, better could not been made than it was at first and I cannot yet well Account for its being damaged as I am well Satisfied that no care was wanting either in baking or packing of it in any respect whatever, we at first thought it was owing to

the casks being New and the Bread being pack'd in Winter and perhaps in Wet Weather, and this was probably the cause, for in most of them, the bread which lay neer and in Contact with the wood, was rotten while that in the Middle of the cask was good. The first Opportunity we had after making this discovery, we had it all well pick'd aird and some baked, the cask were cleaned and the best bread repacked in them and the other put into the Bread room for first Expence, this lasted between two & three months and then we began to use of that in Casks and found it neer as bad as ever & to grow daily worse. We now thought that the damage was Occasioned by the cold & Dampness of the hold, when we were in the Icy sea & oblig'd frequently to take on board Ice to Serve in stead of Fresh water, returning in a short time from Extreme cold Weather to that of hot, the bread in the Cask, for want of fresh air, began to heat, mould and rot and before we had an Opportunity to give it a Second overhauling it was irrecoverably Spoild, this convinced me that after bread is once damaged it cannot be recovered on board a Ship. In putting bread on board Ships for long Voyages, or packing it in casks for the same purpose, too great attention cannot be paid, and it ought never to be done in Wet Weather if it can be possible avoided, for tho it may be done under Cover the air will nevertheless, be full of moist particles which the bread will imbibe sufficient to spoil it, if it is kept any time in a close place and excluded from fresh air, this the Bakers at the Cape of Good Hope are so sensible of that they never will pack their bread in casks in Rainy Weather, the Casks ought to be made of the best seasoned Wood and made very dry before the bread is pack'd in them. The Board may think me a little tedious about the bread, especially as I can charge none with any neglect, but every hint of this Kind must tend to some information and this was my sole Motive for mentioning of it. All our other Provisions turned out exceeding good the Beef & Pork would have been thought excellent to the very last had we not lived so long upon it. Before I conclude I beg leave to acquaint you, that among some remarks, I have sent to their Lordships, I have taken the liberty to recommend Sugar to be issued in the Navy in the room of Oyle, Butter & Chesse and Wheat in the room of Oatmeal, the Experience gained in two long Voyages, has Convinced me that the Introductions of these two Articles in the room of the Others would be conducive to ye health of Seamen, that of Sugar especially, as it is highly Antiscorbutic, which Oyle, Butter & Cheese cannot,[1] were these Articles abolished we should be free from that disagreeable Stench caused by rotten Stinking Cheese which we always have in a greater or less degree so long as any remains on board, besides Sugar I apprehend would be cheaper in the end if not at first, for if the Navy was provided with a good dry sort it would never decay, whereas there is hardly an article of Provisions w[h]ere there

[1] *sic*, probably for 'are not'. The text of this copy seems rather corrupt.

are more Surveys upon than Butter & cheese and not without good reason, Oyle is what very few Seamen like, but boil'd Wheat sweetned with Sugar, I have not met with one who did not like it nor can there be a better breakfast for a seaman.

'The Sour Krout which you caused to be made and put on board kept good to the very last, the Introducing of this Article in the Navy would be of great use but Saloup might very well be omitted in any future Voyage.'—CLB.

[1 August]. *Solander to Banks*. 'Two oClock Monday / This moment Capt Cook is arrived. I have not yet had an oportunity of conversing with him, as he is still in the board-room—giving an account of himself & Co. He looks as well as ever. By and by, I shall be able to say a little more.

'Give my Compl[ts] to Miss Ray and tell her I have made a visitation to her Birds and found them all well.

———————————————[1]

'Capt[n] Cook desires his best Compl[ts] to You, he expressed himself in the most friendly manner towards you, that could be, he said: nothing could have added to the satisfaction he has had, in making this tour, but having had your company. He has some Birds, in Sp. V.[2] for you &c &c that he would have wrote to you himself, about, if he had not been kept too long at the Admiralty and at the same time wishing to see his wife. He rather looks better than when he left England. M[r] Hodges came up in his chaise, I saw him and his Drawings. He has great many portraits—some very good. He has two of my friend Tayoa. Otu is well looking man—Orithi whom they call Ohieriri was really a handsome man according to his pictures.

'Foster Sen[r] and Jun[r] are also come up, but I have not seen them, they did not call at the Admiralty.

'Hodges says the Ladies of Otaheite & Society Isl[ds] are the more hansomer they have seen. But the Man of the Marquesas seem to carry the prize. Hodges seems to be a very well-behaved young Man. All our friends are well.

'Inclosed You will find a Letter from Ch' Clark / Compl[ts] to all / I am for ever / Your sincere friend / Dan. Solander

'I have seen Cooks maps; the tract you have is not much erroneous

'The Groupe of Islands near Amsterdam Cook calls the *Friendly Islands*, because the People behaved very friendly

'Terra del Sp. *Scto* he calls *Hebrides*—there the People were not so friendly, he there was obliged to kill some

'Nova Caledonia is a narrow slip of an Island, as he could see from Mountains—People rather well behaved than otherwise.'—Mitchell Library. *Banks Papers*, L 1–3.

[1] Here Solander draws a line across the page—apparently to denote the lapse of time.
[2] i.e. Spirits of Vinum, alcohol.

3 August. *Admiralty Minutes. Resolution* at Portsmouth to be ordered up to Galleons Reach.—Adm 3/81.

9 August. *Admiralty to Cook.* To proceed to Deptford to be paid off.—Adm 2/100.

9 August. *Admiralty Secretary to Navy Board.* Directing Navy Board to solicit Treasury for money to pay off sloop *Resolution* and to cause her to be paid off and laid up at Deptford.—ADM/A/2694.

9 August. *Admiralty Minutes.* Mr James Cook to be appointed captain of *Kent.*[1] *Resolution* to be paid off and laid up at Deptford.—Adm 3/81.

10 August. *Admiralty Minutes.* At his request Cook to fill up vacancy in Greenwich Hospital and to be permitted to resign it again if called to more active service. *Kent* to be paid off and laid up at Plymouth.—Adm 3/81.

11 August. **Cook to Admiralty Secretary.*† 'Last night I received a letter from Mr Cooper acquainting me with the Arrival of His Majestys Sloop Resolution at the lower end of Long-reach and that he expected to be at Gallions to day. . . . Mile end Friday Morn^g^ 7 oClock.'—Adm 1/1610.

12[2] August. **Cook to Admiralty Secretary.*† 'The death of Captain Clements one of the Captains in the Royal Hospital at Greenwich, making a Vacancy there, I humbly offer my self to my Lords Commiss^rs^ of the Admiralty as a Candidate for it, presuming if I am fortunate enough to merit their Lordships approbation, they will allow me to quit it when either the call of my Country for more active Service, or that my endeavours in any shape can be essential to the publick; as I would on no account be understood to withdraw from that line of service which their Lordships goodness has raised me to, knowing myself Capable of ingaging in any duty which they may be pleased to commit to my charge'.—Adm 1/1610; Adm 12/4806.

12 August. *Admiralty Secretary to Cook.* Is appointed Fourth Captain in Greenwich hospital, and according to his wish he will be allowed to quit it again when there is service for him.—Adm 2/733; Adm 2/1135.

14 August. *Solander to Banks.* 'Our Expedition down to the Resolution, made yesterday quite a feast to all who were concerned. We set out early from the Tower, reviewd some of the Transports; Visited Deptford yard; went on board the Experiment, afterwards to Wolwich, where we took on board Miss Ray & Co and then proceeded to the Galleon's where we were wellcomed in board of the Resolution—and Lord Sandwich made many of them quite happy.

[1] The *Kent* was a 74-gun ship, built in 1762.

[2] The date of this letter as Cook gives it is 12 August; but as the Admiralty minute on the matter is dated 10 August, and the letter of appointment and the commission 12 August, Cook may have made a slip. Alternatively, he may have first asked for, or been offered, the post in conversation, and written his letter later (it was written at the Admiralty Office), to give Stephens something to answer on paper and thus regularise the matter.

'Providentially old Captn Clements died 2 or 3 days ago, by which a Captains place of Greenwich was made Vacant—This was given to Capt Cook—and a promise of Employ whenever he should ask for it. Mr Cooper was made Master and Commander—Mr Clerke was promised the command of the Resolution to carry Mr Omai home; Mr Pickersgill to be his 1st Lieutenant. 3 Midshipmen were made Lieutenants viz Smith, Burr & ....[1] The Master Mr Gilbert is made Master Attendant at Sheerness.

'All our friends look as well as if they had been all the while in clover. All inquired after You. In fact we had a glorious day and longd for nothing but You and Mr Omai. Mr Edgcomb & his Marines made a fine appearance.

'Ld Sandwich asked the Officers afterwards to dine with us at Woolwich.

'Most of our time, yesterday on board, was taken up in ceremonies, so I had not much time to see their curious collections. Mr Clerke shew'd me some drawings of Birds, made by a Midshipman, not bad, which I believe he intends for You. I was told that Mr Anderson one of the Surgeons Mates, has made a good Botanical Collection, but I did not see him. There were on board 3 live Otaheite Dogs, the ugliest most stupid of all the Canine tribe. Forster had on board the following Live Stock: a Springe Bock from the Cape, a Surikate, two Eagles, & several small Birds all from the Cape. I believe he intends these for the Queen. If I except Cooper & 2 of the new made Lieutenants I believe the whole Ship's Company will go out again. Pickersgill made the Ladies sick by shewing them the New Zealand head of which 2 or 3 slices were broiled and eat on board of the Ship. It is preserved in Spirit and I propose to get it for Hunter, who goes down with me to morrow on purpose, when we expect the Ship will be at Deptford....' —Mitchell Library, *Banks Papers*, M, 1–3.

15 August. *Cook to Navy Board.* Transmitting pay books, slop book and alphabet.[2]—Adm 106/1227.

16 August. *Admiralty Secretary to Navy Board.* Instructions to dispense with journals and log books.—ADM/A/2694.

17 August. *Admiralty Secretary to Navy Board. Resolution* not to be dismantled further than may be necessary to her being taken into a dock to be refitted for foreign service.—ADM/A/2656; Adm 2/550.

17 [August]. **Cook to Admiralty Secretary.* 'Mr Isaac Smith, whom my Lords Commissioners of the Admiralty have been pleased to promote to the Rank of Lieutenant, acquaints me that he has pass'd his examination touching his abilities to serve as such, but cannot get the necessary certificate from the examiners untill they have an order to dispence

[1] The third was Whitehouse.

[2] Alphabetical list of all persons in the pay books, which were set out in numerical order (cf. Appendix VII above).

with his not producing any Journals of the Ships in which he has served, and this he cannot do as they are lodged in the Admiralty agreeable to their Lordships Instructions to me; as several more of my Petty officers will want to qualify themselves for promotion and none of them have Journals of the Resolution to produce, I beg you will move their Lordships to give such orders as may be necessary on this head.'—Adm 1/1610.

18 August. *Victualling Board to Admiralty Secretary.* Bills of exchange drawn up by Cook at Cape of Good Hope: for 1,600 rix dollars; for 800 rix dollars; and for 1,050 rix dollars 48 stivers. To be accepted?—Adm 110/26.

19 August. **Cook to John Walker.* 'Dear Sir / As I have not now time to draw up an account of such occurrences of the Voyage as I wish to communicate to you, I can only thank you for your obliging letter[1] and kind enquiryes after me during my absence; I must however tell you that the Resolution was found to answer, on all occasions even beyond my expectation and is so little injured by the Voyage that she will soon be sent out again, but I shall not command her, my fate drives me from one extream to a nother a fews [*sic*] Months ago the whole Southern hemisphere was hardly big enough for me and now I am going to be confined within the limits of Greenwich Hospital, which are far too small for an active mind like mine, I must however confess it is a fine retreat and a pretty income, but whether I can bring my self to like ease and retirement, time will shew. Mrs Cook joins with me in best respects to you and all your family and believe me to be with great esteem / D^r^ S^r^ / Your Most affectionate friend and Humble Servt / Jam^s^ Cook.'—Phillips coll., Salem, Mass.

22 August. *Solander to Banks.* '... Several of the Resolutions Men have called at Your house, to offer you their curiosities:—Tyrrell was here this Morning. Poor Clarke, as I hear, has been in a sad scrape. Upon going out, he gave a joint Bond with his Brother, for paying Sir John Clarke's debts. I've wondered much why I had not seen Mr Clarke since the Ship came up to Deptford, but I this day learnt, that he has been obliged to live among Lawyers &c 'till he could quiet the Creditors, which I hope he has now done, at least I was told so. Sr John Clarke has sent some Money home from India but not enough—and now I

[1] Cook evidently refers here to a letter of 2 August 1775, which (or part of which) is copied on the back of Cook's own letter to Walker from the Cape, 20 November 1772 (p. 689 above), as follows: 'I was pleas'd to read in the publick Papers of thy arrival at Portsmouth in the Resolution and I hope in good Health after so long an Absence from the land of thy Nativity which no doubt would be matter of great Joy to thy father, thy wife was so kind as to give a few lines in June last Advising thy safe Arrival at the Cape of good Hope the 22^d^ of March which was very Acceptable, also thine of the 20 of Novr 1772 from the said place which gave me pleasure to hear of thy being so well Satisfy'd with the Ship after so much Stir talk & bustle before your Sayling, I shall be glad to hear at thy leisure, such Occurrinces as thou may Judge necessary [?] that have Happen'd during the Voyage.'

have been told Ch Clark is to pay them 100£ immediately and part of his pay quarterly. However I don't know if it is so.

'Capt Cook has sent all his curiosities to my apartments at the Museum. All his Shells is to go to Lord Bristol—4 Casks have your name on them and I understand they contain Birds & fish &c. the Box D° with Plants from the Cape. . . .'—Webster coll.

28 August. *Navy Board to Admiralty. Resolution* sloop paid off at Deptford.—Adm 106/2204, loose letter.

6 September. *Cook to Latouche-Tréville.* In French. Informing Latouche of the results of the voyage.—Bibliothèque Nationale, MSS, Nouv. Acq. Fr. 9439. Printed above, pp. 695–6.

13 September. *Cook to Sick and Hurt Board.* Reporting favourably on portable soup.—Adm 97/86.

13 September. *Admiralty Minutes. Resolution* to be put into condition for voyage to remote parts, and to report when she will be ready to receive men.—Adm 3/81.

14 September. **Cook to John Walker.* Giving an account of the voyage.—Dixson Library MSS. Printed above, pp. 696–9.

18 September. **Cook to Admiralty Secretary.*† 'Last Saturday Morning I examined Mr Anderson the gunner about the Publication of my late Voyage, said to be in the press, and told him that he was Susspected of being the Author; he afirm'd that he had no knowlidge, or hand in it, and would use his Endeavours to find out the Author, and yesterday made me the Inclosed report, to day Marra Called upon me and confirmed what is therein set forth, and further added that Bordel, my Coxswain and Reardon the Boatswain mate, each kept a Journal which they had offered to the Booksellers but they were so badly written that no one could read them. I have no reason to suspect this story, but will however, call on the Printer and endeavour to get a Sight of the Manuscript, as I know most of their hand writings. This Marra was one of the gunners Mates, the same as wanted to remain at Otahiete. If this is the only account of the Voyage that is printing, I do not think it worth regarding; I have taken some measures to find out if there are any more and such information as I may get shall be communicated to you by' etc.

Enclosure: 'Sir—According to your derection I overhauld Every Booksellers Shop in S^t^ pauls till at Last I Came to m^r^ fran^s^ Newburrys. I fairly Caught his Shopman, who answer'd me, (when I demanded the Resolutions voyage) that they had not time to print it yet. I then ask'd him if it was the Captains Journal they had, on which he Looked at me and said they had no Journal at all yet, but stood as fair a Chance to publish the voyage as others, by this tim[e] he understood I was pumping of him So went & brought me one of the Shop bills & bid me a good day, telling me that befor the voyage was publish'd it would be advertis'd. I then drove to marra & peckovers Lodging found the former at home I told him I had a mesuage from you S^r^ to deliver to peckover, on wch marra went & found him I told him that there would be nothing Ever don for him or me, unless we Could find out who it was that was publishing the voyag, this made all present very sorry. ther was present some of your Late Crew. Some told me reading wrote a Journal which Enell produc'd I deposited five guineas if he would Let me show you the acc^t^ he Consentd others told me Rollet Keept a Journal Interlin'd in his bible. I wrote down all these Informations for your Satisfaction. at Last marra pulld the paper from befor me, wrote at the angel, angel Court in the bourgh southwark [please to turn over] Send that to Captain Cook, if he pleases to send a Line for or to me, Ill Clear Every man that is Suspected, adding Im the man that is publishing the voyage. I wants no preferm^t^ and God forbid I should hinder those whose bread depends on the Navey. and m^r^ anderson as you have allways been my frend Com with me I^ll^ Convince you further that the name of anderson was never Intended to be perfixt to the voyage. he order'd the Coach to Drive to newburrys Carried me into a back parlor, Informd m^r^ newburry his frends was keept out of bread. therfor he had discoverd all now says he what name is my Journal of the voyage to Come out in, in no nam at all says the Book seller then say the other Let it Come out in the name of Jno Marra at Length. adding if Captain Cook pleases to Call here m^r^ newburry give him all the Satisfaction in your power. m^r^ newburry said he would, after which Mr Newburry Invited us both to dener.

'I should S^r^ have waited on you Last night but Im so Lame I Could not Come up. if you will be pleas'd to Let me know when you will Send for marra I^ll^ wait on you at the same tim[e] to Confront him. but there is too many wittness for him to Retract.

'Honour'd sir you'l please to observe that this is twice I Inocently fell under your displeasure which god has been please to Clear me off—I am S^r^ with the greatest Respect / your most obedient and most Humble / Servant / R. Anderson'.—Adm 1/1610.

8 September. **Cook to Admiralty Secretary.*† 'I found it necessary, while we were in the high Southern Latitudes, to order an additional half Allowance of Spirit to be served to each man per day, and an allowance of Wheat to be boiled every Monday for Breakfast, besides the usual Allowance for dinner, in order the better to inable them, to endure the Cold and hardships they there under went; I also caused Wheat with Portable Soup and Vegetables to be boiled every Morning for Breakfast, whenever the latter was to be got, as will more fully appear by the Inclosed Vouchers, which I beg you will be pleased to lay before their Lordships, and move them to order these over Issues to be allowed me on My Victualling Account.'—Adm 1/1610.

20 September. *Admiralty Secretary to Victualling Board.* Referring to Board foregoing letter and accounts from Cook for its opinion on Cook's application to be allowed the over issue on his victualling account for extra half allowance of spirit, and extra wheat between 6 December 1772 and 22 March 1775.—Adm 2/550.

3 October. *Sick and Hurt Board to Admiralty.* Surgeons for *Resolution* and *Endeavour* [*sic*] have reported their observations on marmalade of carrots and rob of oranges and lemons as preventatives for scurvy, also on malt for making wort and on portable soup. Marmalade was unsuccessful but this might be because it was administered in very small doses. Wort was very successful with assistance of portable soup, sour krout and usual surgeon's necessaries and a proper attention to cleanliness. Cook states that with portable soup they were able to make many wholesome and nourishing messes of wild vegetables. Minuted: 'Read 18th November—To be entered in minutes and reference to be had thereto when any more ships are sent on voyage to remote parts.—ADM/FP/18; Adm 98 11.

28 October. *Board of Longitude to Navy Board.* Orders that William Wales be paid allowance at rate £400 p.a. from 25 January 1772 to 25 August last; also £50 extra for some extraordinary trouble since in completing such of the computations and drawings as his daily business on the voyage did not allow him time for; also £25 12s 5d, being bill for carriage of instruments at different places—deducting £250 which has already been imprested to him, and sum advanced to his wife during his absence.—ADM/A/2696.

7 November. *Sick and Hurt Board to Admiralty Secretary.* Report upon application by Patten to be allowed his extra expenses on account of men attended by him at Cape of Good Hope. Recommends that he be reimbursed £5 10s, the amount spent on medicines; and £8 10s, being five shillings a day for 34 days, the expense he was at while attending the sick at that place, upon his verifying truth of disbursements by affidavit, especially as there appears to have been great economy used respecting sick from *Resolution*, no other charge than that of £8 14s 7d, paid for sick quarters at Cape, having been incurred during the whole voyage.—Adm 98/11.

15 November. *Admiralty Minutes.* Cook to be allowed credit on his accounts for 709 gallons of spirits, and wheat, issued in high southern latitudes. Patten, late surgeon, allowed £5 10s for medicine bought at Cape of Good Hope and £8 10s for attending the sick men 34 days while on shore there.—Adm 3/81.

15 November. *Admiralty to Victualling Board.* Conveying decision on Cook's application, as noted in foregoing entry.—Adm 2/100.

18 November. *Admiralty Minutes.* Report of Sick and Hurt Board on carrot

marmalade etc. to be entered in the books of this office—regard to be had thereto whenever a ship is sent to remote parts.—Adm 3/81.

[— November]. *Accountant-General, Bill Book.* To Captain James Cook, *Resolution*, allowance equal to wages of 5 servants 30 November 1771 to 28 August 1775 at 19s per man, £232 1s 3d.—Adm 18/117, no. 4586.

— December. *John Frazer, petition to Sandwich.* Had gone in the *Resolution*, 'as the properest Person to dive; having acted in that Capacity, with good Success, in taking up His Majesty's Naval Stores.—That your Petitioner has been informed, by Dr Solander, that Captain Cook, upon his Arrival, recommended your Petitioner to the Board of Admiralty, as a Person that had been singularly useful in the Voyage. —And that your Petitioner has, by a studious Application and long Experience, invented an Instrument for taking up Things out of the Sea...'. He therefore solicits a boatswain's warrant, on board a ship in ordinary, 'not being able to go again to Sea, on Account of the Pains in his Body, caused by frequent diving, from the Pressure and Coldness of the Water.... would then be ready at Hand, to seek after any Thing very particular of His Majesty's that may be lost'. Minuted: '20th December. Send petition to Captain Cook and desire him to inform me whether the man is deserving the preferment he prays for'.—Adm 1/1610.

26 December. **Cook to Admiralty Secretary.*† 'In Answer to your letter of the 20th Inst. respecting the Petition of Jno Frazer, I am to acquaint you, that I do not think him Qualified for the Preferment he prays for, or any other in which Seamanship is necessary. He has lately applyed to me to Solicit their Lordships to appoint him Master at Arms; as he is a Steady Sober Man and served several years as a Soldier in the East India Companies Service I believe he may be well enough qualified for that station.'—Adm 1/1610.

1776

10 February. *Cook to Latouche-Tréville.* (In French) Advising on the route to be taken in exploring the Southern Hemisphere and giving an account of the last voyage.—Bibliothèque Nationale, MSS, Nouv. Acq. Fr. 9439. Printed above, pp. 700–03.

5 March. **Cook to Sir John Pringle.*[1] 'As many Gentlemen have expressed some surprise, at the uncommon good state of Health, which the Crew of the *Resolution*, under my Command, experienced during her late long voyage; I take the liberty to communicate to you the methods that were taken to obtain that end....' Abstract follows of

[1] Sir John Pringle (1707–82) was the President of the Royal Society. A most eminent physician with notable army experience, he was the great reformer of military medicine and sanitation in his day, and so had a particular interest in Cook's procedure. It was this letter which, as a paper presented to the Society, gained for Cook the award of the Copley medal.

methods used.—Royal Society *Letters and Papers*, Decade VI, No. 163. Printed in Pringle's *Discourse upon some late improvements of the Means for Preserving the Health of Mariners* (1776) and *Phil. Trans.* LXVI (1776), pp. 402–6. There is a MS copy in B.M., Add. MS 8945, ff. 58–9 v.

23 April. *William Anderson to Pringle.* 'An Account of Some Poisonous Fish in the South Seas.'—Royal Society *Letters and Papers*, Decade VI, No. 185. Printed in *Phil. Trans.* LXVI (1776), pp. 544–52. Refers to the sickness suffered from the fish eaten at Malekula (pp. 469–70 above). 'I must observe, that it may well be doubted, whether this species is always poisonous, as our men ate another of the same sort about a month after, without being affected by it.'

3 May. **Cook to Sick and Hurt Board.* 'I have Receivd your letter of the 30th of last Month, Respecting the Attendance, which Mr Patten late Surgeon of His Majestys Sloop the Resolution, gave to the Invalids that were on Shore in Tents at the Cape of Good Hope. It appears by my Log Book that the Tents were set up on the 24th of March, and taken down on the 22nd of Apl following. To the best of my recollection, there were some Invalids at them the whole of this time, for except the Cooper and Sail-maker, the party on shore was mostly composed of these sort of Men. . . .'—Adm 97/87.

ADDENDUM

1775

22 March. *Cook to Sandwich.*[1] '*Resolution* Cape Good Hope / My Lord, / Permit me to acquaint you of my arrival here this day and to assure your Lordship that it gives me the highest pleasure to find you still preside over that high department I have the honour through your Lordship's favour to be a member of. Being conscious of having exerted my utmost to fulfill every intention of the voyage your Lordship trusted to my care, will give me but little satisfaction if it meets not with your Lordship's approbation and give me hopes for a continuation of your Lordship's favours on / My Lord / your Lordship's most devoted humble servant / James Cook.'

[1] This letter is printed from a copy inserted in an interleaved and grangerized copy of G. W. Anderson, *A . . . Collection of Voyages round the World*, 2 vols., London, A. Hogg, [1784], now in the National Maritime Museum, MS 58/112, and in the 1880's the property of Robert Edward Barker. A MS footnote (p. 193) reads, 'The letter sent on this occasion [i.e. accompanying the copy of the journal sent home from the Cape in the *Ceres*] was in the possession of Frederick Barker March 1882. It was all in Captain Cook's autograph and addressed to the Earl of Sandwich'. This reference seems to be to the letter inserted. Frederick Barker was a well-known collector of autographs. The original of the letter is not now known; it is not specified in the sale catalogues of Barker's collection, 1906. The phraseology of the first sentence is not at all characteristic of Cook, but one cannot pronounce dogmatically against the authenticity of the document.

INDEX

The proper names and titles heading main entries are those of Cook's time, with the variant spellings used in the sloops in brackets. Information editorially supplied is in square brackets. Cross-reference from modern geographical names is given. Names of ships, titles of books, foreign words and systematic biological names are in italics. The form 'xli*n*' or '233n' indicates a note only, but 'xli, n' or '233, n' indicates a note and a reference on the page specified. In so close a text, a particular person or thing may be mentioned more than once on the page; or may be mentioned indirectly. A native dignitary known to Cook by name, for instance, may sometimes be mentioned as 'the chief' or 'the old man'. In alphabetical order, New Zealand comes before Newbery; St (for Saint) Bartholomew before Ste (for Sainte) Barbe.

ADDENDA AND CORRIGENDA

p. xxv, l. 10: *for* sloops-of-war *read* ships

p. xxxiv, l. 20: 'rather late, at the age of 20, in 1755, as a midshipman'. The date of Furneaux's entry into the navy is unknown, but he did become a midshipman in 1755.

p. xli, ll. 18–26: 'He was not . . . Hodges.' There is confusion here, between Cook's second and third voyages: Jones told Hodges his story in August 1775. See Bernard Smith, *European Vision and the South Pacific* (Oxford, 1960), p. 92.

p. liv, l. 1: 'may have been a libel'. The story was hardly a libel: see John Dunmore, *French Explorers in the Pacific*, I (Oxford, 1965), pp. 209–10.

l. 2 from bottom: 'Marc Macé'. Marion du Fresne's Christian names are sometimes given thus in the documents, but were properly Marc Joseph. See Dunmore, *French Explorers*, p. 168, n. 2.

p. lv, l. 1 of notes: *for* J.D. *read* John

p. lix, l. 27: *for* probability *read* probabillity

p. lxvii, l. 24: *for* Dusky *read* Doubtful

p. lxxv, l. 5 from bottom: *for* son of the *read* grandson of Mumui, the 12th

p. lxxxviii, l. 11 from bottom: *for* superter- *read* suprater-

p. xcii, l. 10: *for* Towha *read* 'Towha' or To'ofa

p. cii, n. 2, l. 5: *for* 1752 *read* 1757

p. cvi, l. 20: *for* wth *read* with

p. cix, n. 3: James and Nathaniel Cook were Cook's sons. See Vol. III, Part Two, of the present work, pp. 1458–9. In the *Addenda and Corrigenda* to Vol. I the last sentence of the entry relating to p. 589 should be deleted.

p. cxv, l. 4 from bottom: *for* three *read* four; *and see next entry.*

p. cxxix. To the list of MS copies of Cook's journal must now be added one in the National Library of Ireland, Dublin, Joly Collection, MS 7–8. It appears to be a late copy running from 9 April 1772 to the end of the voyage, and most closely resembles the Greenwich MS, G; it includes twelve engraved charts. It seems to be in the hand of Cook's third voyage clerk, the hand of P.R.O. Adm 55/111–113. These are the conclusions of Mr J. L. Cleland, of the National Library of Australia, who has very kindly acquainted the editor with the facts, and made a detailed examination of the two-volume manuscript.

p. cxl. To the list of 'Other Logs and Journals' should be added the journal of Peter Fannin, master of the *Adventure*, now in the Admiralty Library.

p. clix, l. 2, on Roberts's age: he seems more likely to have been 25 than 15. See Vol. III, Part Two, p. 1462.

p. clxii, *Ferguson Collection: for* H. *read* A. The reference is to the present Sir John Ferguson.

p. 3, l. 11: *for* sould *read* s[h]ould

p. 13, l. 2 from bottom: *for* Provisinos *read* Provisions

p. 91, l. 25: *for* our *read* [h]our

p. 106, l. 14: *for* 86° 40′ *read* 86° 40′ [E]

p. 113, Wednesday 31*st*. The little bluff used by Wales for his observations was, we learn from the charts (e.g. Chart XXIX) called Astronomers Point.

p. 199, n. 1, l. 1: *for* wha *read* what

p. 242, l. 1 of notes: *for* possibly Niau . . . long. 145° 20′ W *read* probably Tauere, in approximately lat. 17° 22′ S, long. 141° 30′ W.

l. 4 of notes: *delete* Niau

p. 249, n. 5, l. 3: *for* son *read* grandson

p. 263, n. 4, l. 5: *for* Brongniart *read* Brogniart

p. 309, n. 5: *add to last line* perhaps a male elephant seal.

p. 331, n. 2: *delete last sentence*

p. 377, n. 2, l. 1: *for* Tehavaroa passage *read* Tehavaroa passage of Takaroa

p. 378, n. 3, l. 5: *for* two or three *read* five or six

ll. 5–6: *for* two fine canoes *read* a double canoe

p. 409, n. 3: This note is rather too dogmatic. The situation is not absolutely plain.

p. 420, n. 3: *for* afterbirth *read* afterbirth or umbilical cord

p. 433, n., l. 2: *for* probably Makatea . . . 148° 14′ W *read* probably but not certainly Rekareka, in latitude 16° 48′ S, longitude 141° 35′ W.

l. 3: *for* The two . . . apart *read* Dalrymple identified La Sagitaria with Tahiti.

p. 463, n. 8, second sentence: This should be deleted. Neither Cook nor the present editor was necessarily wrong in identifying Manicolo with Malekula; Vanikoro must certainly be ruled out, as not answering the description a 'great land' which Quiros picked up. G. S. Parsonson, in Celsus Kelly (ed.), *La Austrialia del Espíritu Santo* (Hakluyt Society, Cambridge, 1966), II, p. 378, argues in favour of the Fijian island of Vanua Levu.

p. 504, n. 2, l. 3: The 'particular plant' referred to by Forster was *Canarium commune*.

p. 508, n. 1, l. 1: *for* was *read* had become

l. 2: *for* seems likely . . . action *read* was raised by the great earthquake of 1878.

p. 512, n. 3: *for* Sakau *read* Sakau or Ladhi (Lathi-hi)

p. 542, n. 1, l. 2: *for* '*viridiflora*' *read* '*leucadendron*'

p. 551, l. 9: There should be a note on Cook's Cape Coronation. The name has disappeared from the map: the cape is now not Coronation but Puareti.

p. 552, l. 7 from bottom of notes: *for* that *read* than

p. 556, l. 16: *for* we *read* we[re]

p. 559, l. 3 from bottom: *for* one *read* [n]one

l. 2 from bottom: *for* state *read* s[t]ate

p. 562, n., ll. 2–3: 'but so far . . . Scotland' is a slip. Cook had seen the coast of Scotland while serving as master of the *Solebay* in 1757.

p. 594, n. 3, l. 1: *for* '*Apium graveolens*' *read* '*Apium australe* Thouars'

p. 596, n. 3: *substitute for first sentence* They were Alacáluf, a different 'nation' from those Cook had seen in Success Bay, who were Aush or Eastern Onas, and did not use canoes.

p. 597, n. 1, l. 11: *for* Dr *read* The Rev.

p. 599, n. 3: *add* There are two species of mussel, the cholga, *Aulacomya ater* Molina and the smaller mejillon, *Mytilis edulis platensis* (d'Orbigny); both are 'well tasted'.

n. 4: *for* Magellanic Steamer *read* Magellanic Steamer or Flapping Loggerhead

p. 610, nn. 1 and 2: Mrs T. D. Goodall of Estancia Harberton, Ushuaia, Tierra del Fuego, writes to the editor, 'The west end of Staten Island is the flattest! The mountains soon go up, but the most jagged are in the middle-west—in fact it is nothing but mountains. Only that one beach long enough for a plane to land, and the south side has absolutely no beaches at all, just mountains down into the sea. I agree it very seldom has snow, although most books say it is continually covered. Cook was right about the vegetation—it is like a jungle.'

p. 612, n. 2: *add* Or they may have been *Empetrum rubrum* Vahl, thinks Mrs Goodall.

p. 614, n. 1: *for* Magellanic Steamer *read* Magellanic Steamer or Flapping Loggerhead

p. 657, ll. 1–4 of notes: Perhaps a better identification for 'Daybreak Island' is Tafahi (Dunmore, *French Explorers*, p. 192), in approximately lat. 15° 53′ S, long. 173° 50′ W. It is about 2000 feet high.

n. 2, l. 7: *for* 'Land of Assassins' *read* 'after the Arsacides commonly called Assassins'.

p. 707, l. 6 from bottom: *for* 93 *read* 95.

p. 777, n. 2: *for* '*Halio*' *read* '*Haliotis* sp.'

p. 795, n. 1: *for* Properly Verron *read* Pierre Antoine Véron

p. 873, para. 3: The question about the two men (nos. 197 and 198) is answered by the fact that they were Cook's sons (cf. entry above for p. cix, n. 3). The question about Keplin, Lee and Leverick is happily answered by Commander W. E. May, who found in the Public Record Office a Supernumerary List of men entered in the crew. They should appear in the *Resolution* ship's company as follows:

185. LEVERICK, John. London, 21. A.B. Joined, Supernumerary List 29 May 1772, transferred to muster book 30 June 1772.

188. KEPPLIN, John. London, 20. A.B. Joined, Supernumerary List 29 May 1772, transferred to muster book 30 June 1772.

189. LEE, Richard. London, 20. A.B. Joined, Supernumerary List 29 May 1772, transferred to muster book 30 June 1772.

p. 880, No. 114, MITCHELL: *Add* There is extant a formal testimonial to his character signed by Cook, very likely connected with his 'passing certificate', granted after success in his lieutenant's examination: 'These are to Certify the Right Hon[ble] the Lords Commissioners of the Admiralty, that M[r] Bowles Mitchell served as Midshipman under my Command, Onboard His Majesty's Sloop Resolution, from the 22nd January 1772, to the date hereof, during which time he behaved with diligence & Sobriety and was always obedient to Command.—Given under my hand Onboard His Majesty's said Sloop this 28th August, 1775. Jam[s] Cook'.—Phillips coll., Salem, Mass.

p. 880–81, No. 123, PECKOVER: *Add* He served as gunner in the *Bounty*, and was in the boat voyage with Bligh.

p. 882, No. 158, WHATTMAN or WATMAN: The age of 25 here given must be wrong. He appears in the *Resolution*'s muster book, third voyage, as 44, but King refers to him as an old man.

p. 882, No. 179, Coghlan: The age of 15 is probably wrong. He appears in the Supplementary List referred to above as aged 45, entered as A.B. 29 May 1772, transferred to muster book 30 October 1772; so there is a good deal of confusion.

p. 883, Nos. 197, 198, Cook, James and Nathaniel: Cook's sons, as noted above.

p. 887, No. 1, Furneaux: *Substitute*

1. Furneaux, Tobias (1735–81). Commander, per commissions 28 November and 25 December 1771. Joined 30 November. Second son of William Furneaux, of Swilly House, Stoke Damerel, Devon. Served in various ships, 1755–63, in West Indies, the Channel, on coast of Africa and West Indies again. Half-pay July 1763–July 1766; second lieutenant *Dolphin* (16 July 1766) under Wallis (his cousin by marriage) 1766–8; described by George Robertson as 'a Gentele Agreable well behaved Good man and very humain to all the Ships company'. Appointed captain *Syren*, 10 August 1775, and served in North America 1775–7, when his ship was driven ashore and he was made prisoner. Returned to England in autumn 1778; half-pay 1 January 1779. Died at Swilly 18 September 1781.

p. 888, No. 12, Constable: *Add* First lieutenant *Queen*, 98, in 1793; 'an excellent sailor and an indefatigable first lieutenant. The devil on board, but an angel on shore'.—*Recollections of James Anthony Gardner* (Navy Records Society, 1906), p. 124.

p. 889, No. 52, Kempe: *Add after 1758* Midshipman with Byron, 1764–6.

pp. 892–3, No. 18, Bayly: *Add* Bayly published 'Astronomical Observations made at the North Cape, for the Royal Society', in *Phil. Trans.*, 1769, pp. 262–72; and with Jeremiah Dixon produced 'A Chart of the Sea Coast and Islands near the North Cape of Europe'. See also Vol. III, p. 1477.

p. 904, 5 December. *Admiralty to Navy Board*, l. 5: *for* Osbridge's *read* Orsbridge's

p. 908, l. 3 from bottom: *for* 36 *read* 30

ADDENDUM TO THE CALENDAR OF DOCUMENTS

1772

28 May. *Cook to Captain William Hammond.* Sheerness. 'Dear Sir/ As you cannot be Ignornant [*sic*] of what is said in Town for and againest the Resolution, I beg you will sit down and give me a full detail thereof, and if you suspect her to be, or ever thought her a tender ship let me find so much friendship from you as to trust me with the secret, as I can now Load and trim her accordingly; for my own part I am in no doubt of her Answering now she is str[i]ped of her Superfluous top hamper—Believe me to be/ Dr Sir/ Your Most Affectio[n]ate friend/ & Humble Servt/ Jam^s Cook'.—Dixson Library.